Water-Soluble Vitamins							Minerals						
Vitamin C (mg)	Thiamin (mg)	Riboflavin (mg)	Niacin (mg NE)‖	Vitamin B_6 (mg)	Folacin¶ (μg)	Vitamin B_{12} (μg)	Calcium (mg)	Phosphorus (mg)	Magnesium (mg)	Iron (mg)	Zinc (mg)	Iodine (μg)
35	0.3	0.4	6	0.3	30	0.5**	360	240	50	10	3	40
35	0.5	0.6	8	0.6	45	1.5	540	360	70	15	5	50
45	0.7	0.8	9	0.9	100	2.0	800	800	150	15	10	70
45	0.9	1.0	11	1.3	200	2.5	800	800	200	10	10	90
45	1.2	1.4	16	1.6	300	3.0	800	800	250	10	10	120
50	1.4	1.6	18	1.8	400	3.0	1200	1200	350	18	15	150
60	1.4	1.7	18	2.0	400	3.0	1200	1200	400	18	15	150
60	1.5	1.7	19	2.2	400	3.0	800	800	350	10	15	150
60	1.4	1.6	18	2.2	400	3.0	800	800	350	10	15	150
60	1.2	1.4	16	2.2	400	3.0	800	800	350	10	15	150
50	1.1	1.3	15	1.8	400	3.0	1200	1200	300	18	15	150
60	1.1	1.3	14	2.0	400	3.0	1200	1200	300	18	15	150
60	1.1	1.3	14	2.0	400	3.0	800	800	300	18	15	150
60	1.0	1.2	13	2.0	400	3.0	800	800	300	18	15	150
60	1.0	1.2	13	2.0	400	3.0	800	800	300	10	15	150
+20	+0.4	+0.3	+2	+0.6	+400	+1.0	+400	+400	+150	††	+5	+25
+40	+0.5	+0.5	+5	+0.5	+100	+1.0	+400	+400	+150	††	+10	+50

United States under usual environmental stresses. Diets should be based on a variety of common foods in order to provide other nutrients for which human requirements

activity of diets as retinol equivalents.

vitamin E activity of the diet as α-tocopherol equivalents.

enzymes ("conjugases") to make polyglutamyl forms of the vitamin available to the test organism.
ances after weaning are based on energy intake (as recommended by the American Academy of Pediatrics) and consideration of other factors such as intestinal absorption;

by the existing iron stores of many women; therefore the use of 30-60 mg of supplemental iron is recommended. Iron needs during lactation are not substantially different advisable in order to replenish stores depleted by pregnancy.

Trace Elements†						Electrolytes		
Copper (mg)	Manganese (mg)	Fluoride (mg)	Chromium (mg)	Selenium (mg)	Molybdenum (mg)	Sodium (mg)	Potassium (mg)	Chloride (mg)
0.5-0.7	0.5-0.7	0.1-0.5	0.01-0.04	0.01-0.04	0.03-0.06	115-350	350-925	275-700
0.7-1.0	0.7-1.0	0.2-1.0	0.02-0.06	0.02-0.06	0.04-0.08	250-750	425-1275	400-1200
1.0-1.5	1.0-1.5	0.5-1.5	0.02-0.08	0.02-0.08	0.05-0.1	325-975	550-1650	500-1500
1.5-2.0	1.5-2.0	1.0-2.5	0.03-0.12	0.03-0.12	0.06-0.15	450-1350	775-2325	700-2100
2.0-2.5	2.0-3.0	1.5-2.5	0.05-0.2	0.05-0.2	0.1-0.3	[illegible]-1800	1000-3000	925-2775
2.0-3.0	2.5-5.0	1.5-2.5	0.05-0.2	0.05-0.2	0.15-0.5	[illegible]	[illegible]-4575	1400-4200
2.0-3.0	2.5-5.0	1.5-4.0	0.05-0.2	0.05-0.2	0.15-0.5	[illegible]	[illegible]	1700-5100

National Research Council, Washington, D.C.
RDA and are provided here in the form of ranges of recommended intakes.
trace elements given in this table should not be habitually exceeded.

de back cover.

Introductory Nutrition

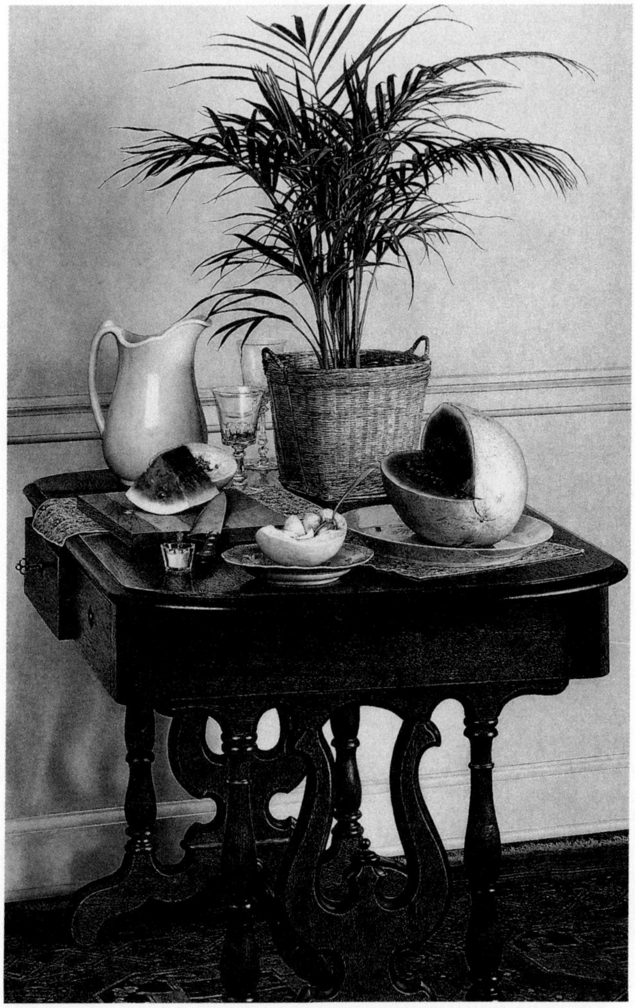

STILL LIFE WITH WATERMELON AND PALM
1984
John Stuart Ingle

Courtesy Tatistcheff Gallery, New York

Introductory Nutrition

HELEN A. GUTHRIE, Ph.D., D.Sc., R.D.,
Professor and Head, Nutrition Department,
The Pennsylvania State University,
University Park, Pennsylvania

Revised with the assistance of
Robin S. Bagby, M.Ed., R.D.,
Instructor, Nutrition,
The Pennsylvania State University,
University Park, Pennsylvania

SEVENTH EDITION

with 449 illustrations
Illustrations by Cathelia C. Maxin

Times Mirror/Mosby College Publishing

ST. LOUIS • TORONTO • BOSTON • LOS ALTOS 1989

Publisher: Nancy K. Roberson
Editor: Ann Trump
Developmental editor: Kathy Sedovic
Project manager: Kathleen L. Teal
Production editor: Teresa Breckwoldt
Designer: Susan E. Lane
Manuscript editor: Emma Dankoski
Production: Ginny Douglas, Susan Trail

SEVENTH EDITION

A division of The C.V. Mosby Company
11830 Westline Industrial Drive
St. Louis, Missouri 63146

Printed in the United States of America

Library of Congress Cataloging in Publication Data

Guthrie, Helen Andrews.
Introductory nutrition / Helen A. Guthrie ; illustrations by Cathelia C. Maxin.—7th ed. / revised with the assistance of Robin S. Bagby.
p. cm.
Includes bibliographies and index.
ISBN 0-8016-2201-8
1. Nutrition. I. Bagby, Robin S. II. Title.
TX354.G8 1989 88-25910
613.2—dc19 CIP

GW/VH/VH 9 8 7 6 5 4 3 2 1

Preface

A comparison of the first edition of this text published a mere 22 years ago with this new seventh edition provides a vivid demonstration of the rapid transition that has occurred in college publishing. Whether it is a cause of or a result of the rising expectations of professors and their students is not clear. Pedagogical features a few years ago consisted of several essential tables, an occasional graph, and an even more occasional photograph to demonstrate deficiency conditions. Today authors depend on graphic artists to illustrate and thus reinforce the meaning of their words and on designers and production editors to create the most visual appeal from the arrangement of the text on a page. They draw on a well-developed science, which dictates the number of lines on a page, the width of the lines, the amount of "white space," and the type face. Chapter openers, usually with a strong visual impact, are reminders to the readers that they are making a transition to a new issue or topic. Color is chosen and used with great care, as is the size of the page and the quality of the paper.

As an author I am grateful that Times Mirror/Mosby College Publishing has recognized that this attention to the smallest detail affects acceptance of the book, almost even before the content of the pages has been judged. In spite of the changes in all these physical features that lead the professor and his or her students to choose the book and then read it, my purpose and philosophy in writing the seventh edition are virtually unchanged from the first edition. This book remains an attempt to respond to the inquisitiveness of students, their families, and their friends about the quality of the food supply and its impact on the health of their and future generations. It is my hope that in studying nutrition in a systematic way, students will acquire sufficient sophistication about the principles of nutrition. This knowledge will enable them to evaluate the dietary advice with which the whole population is constantly confronted, not only from health professionals but also on TV and in almost every form of printed material and every advertising medium.

The growth and evolution of this text over the years reflect not only the careful and extensive market research by the publisher but peer review by competent professionals who themselves are current or potential users of the text and the frank but thoughtful and astute comments of their students. It is these contributions that have shaped this text to most closely meet the needs of both instructors and students of the introductory nutrition course.

MAJOR CHANGES

What are the ways in which this edition reflects a fresh editorial approach? Most important among the many changes are the following features.

Readability

Robin Bagby, who has provided invaluable assistance with this revision, has contributed not only with her insights and enthusiasm, but with her infinite attention to detail. Her experience in teaching several approaches to introductory nutrition courses at The Pennsylvania State University is reflected in the student perspective, which she continually kept in the forefront. With the help of reviewers, editors, and Robin, I have tried to keep the style refreshing without sacrificing the basic scientific style that has characterized previous editions.

Reorganization

Reorganization of the sequence of chapters is the result of recommendations from current and potential users of the book. Although there will always be instructors who will choose to meet the needs of their course and their personal teaching style in a different format, there was a clear mandate to move the chapter on the Selection of an Adequate Diet (Chapter 3) to the beginning. This should now help stimulate interest in the application of the principles of nutrition to making appropriate food choices. Similarly, the majority of the instructors responding wished to have the principles of digestion, absorption, and metabolism (Chapter 2) presented before a discussion of the major energy yielding nutrients. These changes have been made and the rest of the text modified to accommodate this innovation.

Updating

In the 3 years since the preparation of the sixth edition there have been many advances in the science of nutrition that now warrant the attention of professors and their students. Examples of these updates or additions are many, including but not limited to the following topics which have been included in this new edition.

The synthetic fats made from glucose and egg whites are discussed in Chapter 4, as are the essentials of the information explosion regarding fatty acids in fish oils and related metabolites. New uses for vitamin A-related compounds are covered in Chapter 12 and newly recognized roles for trace elements, boron and aluminum, are discussed in Chapter 11.

In the applied sections, discussions of pregnancy-induced hypertension, eating disorders, and drug-nutrient interactions of special significance for older citizens are highlighted in Chapters 15, 17, and 18 respectively. Chapter 17 features recently available data on the unique composition of human milk in comparison with cow's milk. The chapter on Nutrition and Physical Fitness (Chapter 19) contains new theories on carbohydrate loading and a discussion of the effects of dehydration on performance.

Pedagogical Features

Awareness Checks. The "Have You Ever Wondered" feature of the last edition has been replaced by *Awareness Checks*, a group of four to six statements reflecting the content of the upcoming chapter about which students may have some knowledge or interest but about which they need more information if they are to be confident of their answers. The students are asked to make their best judgment as to whether the statement reflects truth or fiction. At the end of the text, students are provided with the page number on which they will find the information needed to support the correct answer. These statements are designed to motivate students to seek the answers as they read the chapter and to stimulate their interest in the material to follow.

Marginals. The marginal material has been carefully evaluated to ensure that each carries a message that reinforces and/or reviews the information in the chapter. Extensive use of margins includes definitions of key terms, cross-references, notes, and *new consumer tips*. We have taken great care to see that concepts and terms are adequately defined the first time they are used. Marginal illustrations have been designed to emphasize or draw attention to the textual material.

Consumer Tips. *New* "tips for the consumer" focus on the application of information provided in the chapter to improve dietary and food selection practices. These tips are identified by their appearance in color in the margin, and they contribute to our goal to personalize the presentation of basic principles of nutrition.

Chapter Summaries. These "By now you should know" features are a series of succinct statements that highlight the most salient points of the chapter, emphasizing those that are related to the issues and questions which most frequently arise in applying the principles of the topics discussed. They serve to further sensitize the student to the timeliness of the topic.

Applying What You've Learned. This *new* section is a series of activities or projects that direct the student to further address their new knowledge to some practical issues. These activities encourage them to use the resources of the text or sensitize them to nutrition information readily available to them in their environment.

Suggested Readings. This feature of previous editions has been retained and expanded to include short summaries of the content of journal articles that can lead the instructor and often the motivated student to a more thorough discussion of aspects of the topic which are attracting scientific interest. Although there are often very fine items that could have been used, we have selected only those that should be readily available in most libraries in schools teaching nutrition. We have all experienced the frustration of being tantalized by being directed to a resource that is hidden in a remote publication that does not find its way into library holdings or is printed in a restricted or inaccessible source. Our philosophy has been if it's not accessible, it does little good to know of its existence.

Additional Readings. It was with great personal restraint that I was able to suppress my intrigue and respect for the history of nutrition and the sophistication of the earlier contributors to follow the wisdom of publishers that users of introductory texts are more focused on advances in a field than on the historical perspective. Thus references in this section are drawn predominantly from the 1980s, focusing on current research and review articles.

Focus. Focus sections dealing with a current issue relating to the topic of each chapter added in the sixth edition have evoked most favorable responses. The most successful of these have been retained, often slightly modified to update or clarify them. Several new focus topics have been introduced in the seventh edition to reflect emerging issues in nutrition (like RDAs and U.S. RDAs in Chapter 2, Sweetness Mania in Chapter 4, Fish Oils and Health in Chapter 5, and Osteoporosis in Chapter 10). They remain more informal extensions of the chapter, some speculative, some provocative, and others merely topics of related importance that were not appropriate to the chapter content.

Glossary. The glossary has been expanded to include all terms that may be new to the student. A *pronunciation guide* has been added to the glossary to aid the student in the pronunciation of difficult terms.

Appendices. Most of the appendices from previous editions have been retained in a thoroughly updated and expanded form. Data on nutritive content of fast foods, a compelling interest of many college students, have been changed to reflect the changing menu emphasis in these restaurants. In addition, a *new* appendix on Nutrient Analysis (E) has been added. This appendix assists students in assessing their own nutrient intake by applying concepts presented in the text.

Illustrations. Once again we have been fortunate to draw on the skills and creative competence of Cathelia Maxin to produce new and modified graphic illustrations. In addition we have had the resources of our colleagues willing to share their photos to illustrate the relevant techniques, symptoms, and marketing approaches.

Use of the Metric System

Since this text is widely used both in the United States, which has not converted to the metric system, and in countries such as Canada, where the metric system is almost universally used, we have indicated units of measurement in both systems. In a few cases in which the metric system is routinely used, such as in setting some dietary standards or measuring blood amounts, measurements are in the metric system only.

Findings from Dietary Surveys

Data from the two major surveys, the NFCS (Nationwide Food Consumption Survey), conducted by the U.S. Department of Agriculture, and the NHANES (National Health and Nutrition Examination Surveys), conducted by the Department of Health and Human Services, along with the Total Diet Study and the more recent Continuing Survey of Food Intakes of Individuals (CSFII), are used throughout the text to provide information on the adequacy of nutrient intake and nutritional status in various segments of the population.

Endpapers

Two resources to which students frequently refer have again been placed as endpapers inside the front and back covers.

Recommended Dietary Allowances. Although revised RDAs had not been released at the time of publication, the text includes a discussion of the rationale for these allowances, some of which would have changed appreciably. The most up-to-date data available, the 1980 RDAs, are presented inside the front and back covers.

Metropolitan Height/Weight Tables. The most current for height and weight, published in 1983, have been included in this edition. They can be found inside the back cover of the book.

SUPPLEMENTARY MATERIALS

Instructor's Manual and Testbank

Prepared by Robin S. Bagby, M.Ed., R.D., of The Pennsylvania State University, this comprehensive, unique Instructor's Manual has been revised to reflect the changes made in this edition of the text. It includes the following practical features:

- Chapter objectives
- What is different in this edition
- Chapter outlines with corresponding notes and transparency masters
- Nutrient analysis exercises that can be photocopied and given to students as assignments
- Teaching suggestions to stimulate ideas for clarifying difficult concepts for students
- Related issues, including topics for class discussion such as fiber and cancer; relevant suggested references are included
- Student activities (group and individual activities)
- Media resources, including information on video and audio cassettes, films, slides, and computer software
- A Testbank of approximately 1000 examination questions, including multiple choice, true/false, matching, and essay questions
- Transparency masters of the most important and useful illustrations found in the text, as well as some new masters not found in the text

Nutrient Analysis Software

A *new* nutrient analysis software program is available to adopters of the seventh edition of this text. It enables students to analyze their own food intake with interactive disks that contain a data base of food items. In addition, it includes a calorie expenditure analysis based on the specific activity level of the student.

ACKNOWLEDGMENTS

Even more than in previous editions, this seventh edition represents the input of a great many people. The constant feedback from students, including both favorable and critically constructive comments, has alerted me to their reactions and opinions as some of the most sensitive barometers of impact. Very early in the revision process, Stacy Tessaro spent many hours painstakingly checking consistency, as well as accuracy, of content.

The critical element in the success of this revision, as it reflects the needs of the book's current or potential users throughout the country, were the thoughtful, explicit, and stimulating comments of the following reviewers, who offered invaluable suggestions for revisions:

Lyndon Carew
University of Vermont

Susan Crockett
North Dakota State University

Jean Freeland-Graves
University of Texas–Austin

Michael Jenkins
Kent State University

Louise Little
University of Delaware

Pat Munyon
San Diego Mesa College

Janice Peach
Western Washington University

G.G. Robinson
University of South Florida

Susan Saffel-Shrier
University of Utah

G. Rickey Welch
University of New Orleans

I can only hope that at least some of these dedicated individuals gained something as they provided me with a breadth of perspective on the uses and needs for an introductory level text.

Facilitating the efforts of all of us was Kathy Sedovic who developed the project and coordinated the review process. Ann Trump carried the responsibility for almost all major decisions, while Susan Lane masterminded the design of the book. Teresa Breckwoldt served nobly as manuscript editor, offering many suggestions to enhance the readability of the manuscript and anticipating the need to clarify many points for the student. My neighbor, Cathelia C. Maxin, takes credit for almost all of the illustrations, graphs, flow-charts, and marginal illustrations. Her patience knew no bounds as she applied her infinite ability to grasp the message and reduce it to a few well-chosen lines—as only a talented artist can—to produce the finished artwork.

Most important has been the dedication of Robin Bagby as we pooled our time and perspectives to produce what we are confident will continue to be a scientifically relevant and widely accepted text introducing the current generation of college students to the challenge of nutrition as a health science.

In earlier editions, I recognized the help of three children and a very supportive husband. The three children, Barbara, Jane, and Jim, are now established in their own professions but continue to offer moral support. My husband, George, has once again provided endless encouragement throughout the ups and downs of a revision.

Helen A. Guthrie

Contents in Brief

Contents

PART I

Basic Principles of Nutrition

PART II

Applied Nutrition

Appendixes

Introductory Nutrition

PART I

Basic Principles of Nutrition

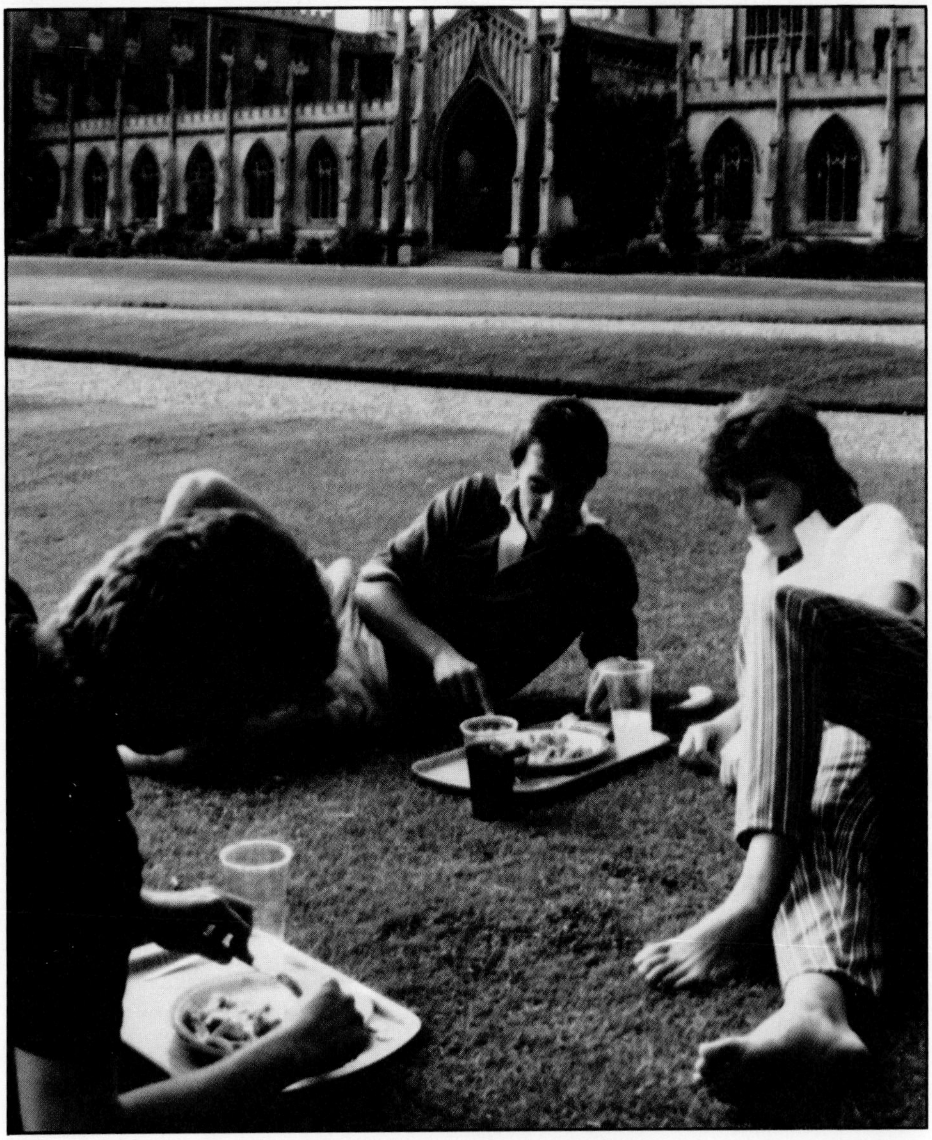

AWARENESS CHECK

Truth or Fiction?

- A person hospitalized is at risk for developing malnutrition.
- The diet of a pregnant woman has little impact on the infant's physical condition at birth.
- Weightlessness changes an astronaut's nutritional status.
- Development of new foods such as low-cholesterol cheese can have only a positive effect on degenerative diseases.
- To reduce the incidence of heart disease, cancer, bone diseases, and diabetes everyone should follow dietary modifications.
- Nutrients needed in small quantities have less important functions in the body than nutrients needed in larger quantities.
- Today is described as the naturalistic era of nutrition.
- A dietitian is limited to working in a hospital or institutional setting where emphasis is on diet therapy, menu planning, and food service.

CHAPTER 1

Overview of Nutrition

Although nutrition has been recognized as a science for at least half a century, it has only been in the past two decades that it has captured the imagination and interest of the public and policymakers. Today we are surrounded by evidence of a heightened awareness and concern about nutrition—health food stores and magazines are flourishing; nutrition is discussed on television talk shows; the public is seeking out nutritionists for counsel and advice; the federal government is supporting nutrition intervention programs, as well as research and training; private industry is "selling" nutrition; and nutritionists are finding many new career opportunities. Accompanying this increased awareness of nutrition, however, is an increased opportunity for the promotion of unfounded and unscientific theories. This book is designed to provide you, the college student, with basic nutrition information for making informed food choices in the face of an ever-changing food supply promoted with sophisticated marketing strategies.

As you begin your study of nutrition, perhaps the first step should be to understand how the discipline or field is defined. Nutrition, as a science, has been defined in many ways. Most simply it has been identified either as the science of nourishing the body properly or as the analysis of the effect of food on the living organism. It has also been defined as the relationship between man and his food with psychological and social, as well as physiological and biochemical, implications. More specifically it has been identified as the science of food, the nutrients and other substances therein, their action, interaction, and balance in relation to health and disease and the processes by which the organism ingests, digests, absorbs, transports, utilizes, and excretes food substances.

Regardless of definition, there is general agreement that nutrition is concerned with the way food is produced, with any changes that occur in it before it is eaten, and with the way the body uses food until it is either built into body tissues or excreted. This includes the study of digestion, absorption, and transportation of nutrients to and from cells and the way in which nutrients are used within the many types of body cells. In addition, nutritionists are becoming increasingly concerned with the factors that determine what food is available; what a person chooses to eat; and how these choices affect the nutritive quality of the diet and, as a result, the health of the individual.

As more is learned about the role of nutrients in maintaining health, there has been rising interest in the role of nutrition in the immune system, its interaction with genetics, and the ways in which nutrition can influence development and the aging process and the quality of life. It is ironic that one of the challenges for today's nutritionist is to persuade many people that their diets are adequate, that their use of nutrient supplements is unnecessary, and that some nutrient and food excess can lead to other illnesses.

In the late 1960s, interest in nutrition escalated in the United States when a shocked and outraged American public began to realize that hunger and malnutrition existed in the midst of plenty. As a result of a notable television documentary, the first White House Conference on Food, Nutrition, and Health was convened in 1969. This conference represented a commitment by the federal government to identify problems of hunger and malnutrition and to take steps to alleviate them. A follow-up conference in 1974 to assess what progress had been made resulted in the initiation of a number of federally supported nutrition activities. These included nutrition programs for the elderly; Women, Infants, and Children (WIC), a program for high-risk women, infants, and children; standards for nutrient labeling of processed food products; and nutrition education in elementary schools. Other established programs such as school feeding and food stamps were expanded. Along with these developments, our nutrition-conscious nation has shown its concern with nutrition by spending increased amounts on health foods, relying more and more on alternate food patterns, and preoccupying itself with the relationship between nutrition and health.

Dietary Goals for the United States, a statement issued by the Senate Select Committee on Nutrition and Human Needs early in 1977 and revised in 1978, provided further evidence of increasing government interest in the nutritional health of the country. Subsequently, a joint **Department of Health and Human Services** (DHHS) and **United States Department of Agriculture** (USDA) publication, *Dietary Guidelines for Americans,* was released early in 1981. A National Academy of Sciences (NAS) publication, *Diet, Nutrition, and Cancer,* and the first joint report on nutrition to Congress from the USDA and DHHS in 1985 further highlighted the relationship of nutrition to health problems and provided background material for the second report in 1989.

DHHS
Department of Health and Human Services

USDA
United States Department of Agriculture

Some Agencies Internationally Concerned about Nutrition

- United Nations
  - Food and Agricultural Organization (FAO)
  - World Health Organization (WHO)
- United States Agency for International Development (USAID)
- League for International Food Education (LIFE)
- Peace Corps
- Agency for Overseas Blind (AOB)

On an international level the first authorized agency within the United Nations was the Food and Agricultural Organization, commonly known as the FAO. In 1944 it was charged with the responsibility of devising ways to improve the nutritional status of the world's population as a major pathway to peace. Another UN agency, the World Health Organization (or WHO), allocates resources for the solution of nutrition problems. U.S. groups such as the Agency for International Development, or USAID, have similar goals.

In spite of these efforts, malnutrition and undernutrition, existing along with a rapidly expanding population and inadequate medical care, remain dominant health problems in the world today. The worldwide distribution of nutritional deficiency diseases (Figure 1-1) shows that they are concentrated in tropical countries with high population density.

IMPORTANCE OF GOOD NUTRITION

Before beginning an intensive study of individual nutrients, the student of nutrition may legitimately ask, "What evidence is there that nutrition makes a difference?" The USDA suggests that appropriate nutrition intervention activities can reduce morbidity and mortality from heart disease by 25%, from respiratory and infectious diseases by 20%, from cancer by 20%, and from diabetes by 50%. The Senate Committee on Nutrition and Human Needs cited anemia, obesity, alcoholism, allergies, dental decay, arthritis, and osteoporosis among the many conditions for

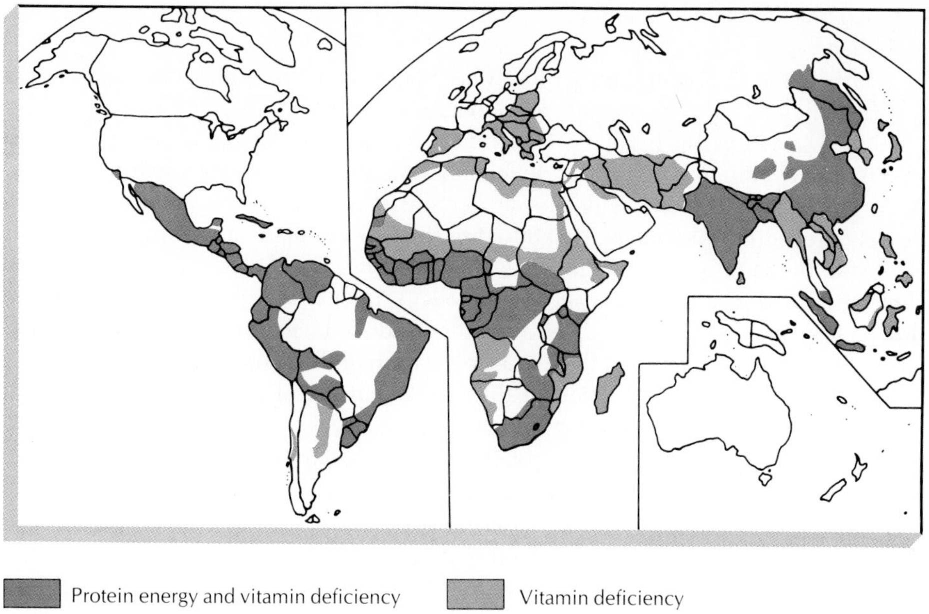

Figure 1-1 Distribution of protein-energy and vitamin-deficiency diseases in the world.

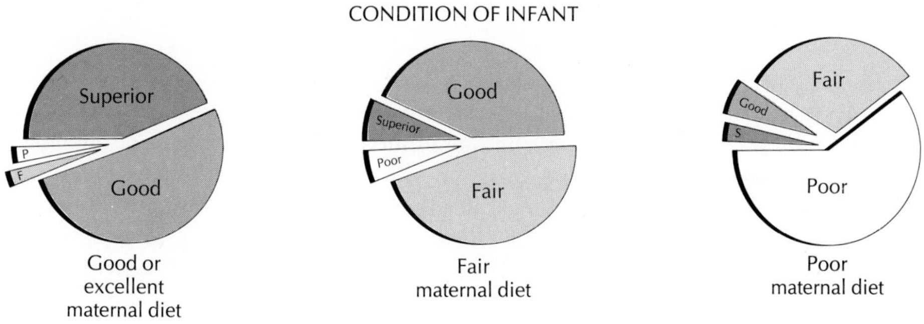

Figure 1-2 Relationship between quality of mother's diet and condition of infant at birth.
Modified from Burke BS: Journal of Nutrition 38:453, 1949.

which improved diet would result in substantial savings and relief of human misery. The preventable costs attributable to such conditions are estimated at billions of dollars annually. Thus it appears that good nutrition may indeed be one of our most valuable and underutilized resources.

In one of the earliest systematic studies of the relationship of diet to health, Burke worked in 1946 with pregnant women at the Boston Lying-In Hospital at Harvard. Of the infants born to mothers whose diet was rated good or excellent, 94% were judged to be in superior or good physical condition at the time of birth, and only 6% were rated in fair or poor condition. When the mothers' diet was assessed as poor, however, only 8% of the infants received a superior or good rating; 92% were judged in fair or poor condition. These observations are illustrated in Figure 1-2. Because people change food habits slowly, even when highly motivated by a condition such as pregnancy, these dietary ratings undoubtedly reflected long-standing patterns of eating rather than those prevailing only during pregnancy.

The increase in the height of American children in the past few decades is partly attributable to improved nutrition. In 1951, Philadelphia schoolchildren in first through fifth grades in all socioeconomic groups were, on the average, 3 inches (5 cm) taller and 3 pounds (1.35 kg) heavier than their counterparts in 1925. In 1880, only 5% of male college freshmen were over 6 feet (1.8 m) tall, whereas in 1955, 30% reached this stature. Before giving too much credit to nutrition, however, we should also keep in mind that advances in other areas of health care have

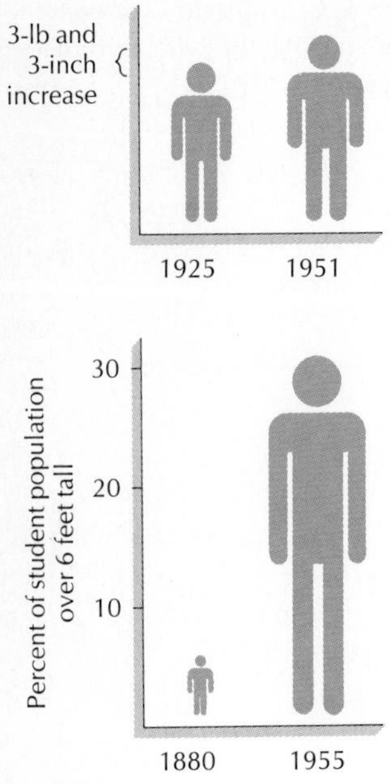

Increase in size of American children between 1925 and 1951 and American college students between 1880 and 1955

reduced the incidence of infection and other deterrents to optimal growth at an early age.

Early in the history of nutrition, we were mainly concerned about diet preventing severe deficiency diseases such as pellagra (niacin), beriberi (thiamin), scurvy (vitamin C), and goiter (iodine). These diseases are now rare, and iron-deficiency anemia is the only major nutrient deficiency remaining as a public health concern. As we have accumulated evidence of the role of diet in health maintenance and disease prevention, the focus has shifted to the role of nutrition in the major causes of death. Perhaps most convincing is the data showing that levels of total blood cholesterol and of a special type of low-density lipoprotein cholesterol, which are risk factors in coronary heart disease, can be reduced when the total fat, saturated fat, and cholesterol content of the diet is lower and/or the content of polyunsaturated fat is higher. Each 1% reduction in the blood cholesterol level is associated with a 2% reduction in coronary heart disease. Similarly, there is a growing conviction that adequate, but not excessive, fiber in the diet may reduce the risk of colon cancer, and, as reported in popular literature, that excessive fat intake is a risk factor for obesity and hence diabetes, atherosclerosis, and some types of cancer.

Still further evidence that the health authorities in the United States consider that nutrition does make a difference is the inclusion of eight specific nutrition objectives in the Surgeon General's health objectives for 1990 to promote health and prevent disease. Those listed in Table 1-1 are the result of a midcourse review in 1985 of the objectives developed originally in 1980.

HISTORICAL BACKGROUND

Nutrition is a relatively new science, recognized as a distinct discipline only since 1934 with the founding of the professional organization, the American Institute of Nutrition. As a science relying on the techniques and basic findings of chemistry and biology, nutrition emerged only after development of these other branches of science. Nutrition, like other sciences, does not stand alone. It not only draws on, but also contributes to, advances in biochemistry, microbiology, physiology, cellular biology, medicine, and food science. One of the more recent technological breakthroughs, genetic engineering, offers both a tool and a challenge for nutritionists.

Although most of the organized study of nutrition has occurred in the twentieth century, there has been a long-standing curiosity about the subject. A few well-conceived nutritional experiments were performed earlier than the 1900s, but these stimulated only vague interest. The history of nutrition can be aptly divided into four eras:

- **Naturalistic era** (400 BC to AD 1750)
- **Chemical-analytical era** (1750 to 1900)
- **Biological era** (1900 to 1955)
- **Cellular or molecular era** (1955 to the present)

No attempt will be made to discuss all the findings of each era. However, a few important discoveries will be highlighted to give a picture of the extent of nutrition knowledge at each stage. It is also important to recognize that chemical, analytical, and biological investigations continue to contribute to our knowledge.

Among the Contributors to Nutrition in the Naturalistic Era

Hippocrates	Father of Medicine
Sanctorius	Insensible perspiration
Harvey	Circulation
Spallanzani	Digestion
Lind	Scurvy cure

Naturalistic Era (400 BC to AD 1750)

The naturalistic era was characterized by many vague ideas about taboos, magical powers, or medicinal value of food. Just as millions do today, early men and women recognized that food was essential for survival. In Biblical times, Daniel observed that men who ate **pulses** and drank water thrived better than did those who ate the king's food and drank wine. As the Father of Medicine, Hippocrates considered food one universal nutrient when he discussed food, health, and disease in 400 B.C.

pulses
Legumes (vegetables), usually peas and beans

Table 1-1 ◆ Nutrition objectives for 1990

Category	Objective ("By 1990 . . .")	Baseline Data*
High Priority		
Improved health status	Eliminate growth retardation of infants and children caused by inadequate diets	Estimated 10% to 15% of infants and children among migratory mothers and some poor rural populations (1972–1973)
Reduced risk factors	Decrease prevalence of significant overweight (120% or more of "desired" weight) to 10% of men and 17% of women, without nutritional impairment	14% of adult men and 24% of adult women (1971–1974)
	Reduce mean serum cholesterol in adults 18–74 years old to ≤200 mg/dl	Mean cholesterol = 223 mg/dl (1971–1974)
	Reduce average daily sodium ingestion by adults to the 3–6 gram range	Estimated averages of 4–10 grams (1979)
	Increase the proportion of women who breastfeed their babies to 75% at hospital discharge and 35% at 6 months of age	45% at hospital discharge, 21% at 6 months (1978)
Increased public-professional awareness	More than 75% of population can correctly associate suspected diet-disease links for heart disease, high blood pressure, dental caries, and cancer	—
	70% of adults can identify the major foods which are low in fat, low in sodium, high in calories, high in sugars, or good sources of fiber	—
	90% of adults should understand that to lose weight people must either consume fewer calories or increase physical activity—or both	—
Improved services-protection	Virtually all routine health contacts with health professionals should include some element of nutrition education and nutrition counseling	—
	All states should include nutrition education as part of required comprehensive school health education at elementary and secondary levels	Only 10 states mandated nutrition as a core content area in school health education (1979)
Improved surveillance-evaluation system	A comprehensive national nutrition status monitoring system should have capability for detecting nutrition problems in special groups and as baseline data for national policy decisions	—
Medium Priority		
Improved health status	Proportion of pregnant women with iron deficiency anemia should be reduced to 3.5%	7.7% (1978)
Reduced risk factors	50% of the overweight population should have adopted weight-loss regimens, combining an appropriate balance of diet and physical activity	—
Improved services-protection	Labels of all packaged foods should contain useful caloric and nutrient information to enable consumers to select healthy diets; similar information should be displayed along with nonpackaged foods	—
	More than 50% of employee and school cafeteria managers should be aware of and actively promoting the USDA/DHHS Dietary Guidelines	—

Adapted from Glanz K, and Damberg CL: Meeting over nation's health objectives in nutrition, Journal of Nutrition Education 19:211, 1987.
*A dash (—) indicates that baseline data are not available.

In the early seventeenth century the Italian physician Sanctorius weighed himself before and after each meal. His only explanation for his failure to gain weight in keeping with the amount of food taken in was that there must be weight loss, resulting from **insensible perspiration.** It was during this period that such men as Harvey and Spallanzani, interested in circulation and digestion, made observations that eventually facilitated the study of nutrition. In 1747, at the end of the naturalistic era, the first controlled nutrition experiment was carried out by a British physician, Lind. He attempted to find a cure for scurvy (now known to result from vitamin C deficiency) by treating 12 sailors ill with the disease with six different substances. He determined that either lemon or lime juice cured scurvy; the other five substances—oil of vitriol, cider, nutmeg, seawater, and vinegar—did not.

insensible perspiration
Loss of water through the skin that is so slow that it goes unnoticed

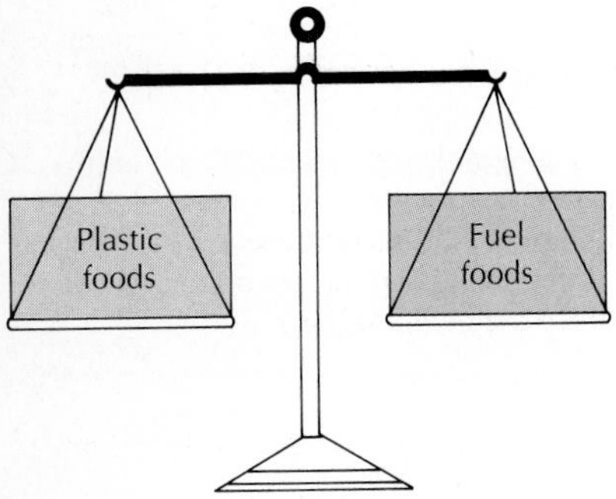

Liebig's original theory of a balanced diet

Chemical-Analytical Era (1750 to 1900)

In the eighteenth century the chemical-analytical era was initiated by Lavoisier, who became known as the Father of Nutrition. He studied the way we use food energy (calories) and was the first to study the relationship between heat production and oxygen use in the body.

Early in the nineteenth century, methods were developed for determining the elements carbon, hydrogen, and nitrogen in organic compounds. Analyzing foods to find amounts of each of these led Liebig to suggest that the nutritive value of food was a function of its nitrogen content. He also proposed that an adequate diet must provide what he then called plastic foods (protein) and fuel foods (carbohydrate and fat). In 1871 Dumas, a French chemist, tried to produce a synthetic milk of carbohydrate, fat, and protein in the proportions found in cow's milk. When the infants to whom he fed it died, Dumas logically concluded that milk must contain some unknown nutritive substance.

A similar conclusion was reached in 1881 by Lunin. He found that mice died when fed a diet of purified casein (a protein in milk), milk sugar (a carbohydrate), milk fat, and the minerals from milk, whereas those fed milk thrived. Between 1881 and 1906 the use of similar diets in other animal experiments led to essentially the same conclusion: the addition of "astonishingly" small amounts of natural foods was necessary to promote growth and to maintain health in animals. Food obviously contained other substances besides carbohydrate, fat, protein, and minerals; just what they were remained a mystery.

Among the Contributors to Nutrition in the Chemical-Analytical Era

Lavoisier	Father of Nutrition
Priestley	Study of oxygen
Liebig	Balanced diet
Dumas	Synthetic milk
Lunin	Synthetic diet for rats

Biological Era (1900 to 1955)

By 1912 it had been well established that there was another dietary essential besides carbohydrate, fat, protein, and minerals. Casimir Funk, recognizing that this elusive dietary component was essential to life (*vita* in Latin) and believing it to be *amine*, or nitrogen-containing, introduced the term *vitamine* to describe it. Soon after, two independent studies showed that there were at least two vitamins—fat-soluble vitamin A and water-soluble vitamin B. One study showed that some fats such as butter contained an essential growth factor, whereas others such as lard did not. From another we learned that a water-soluble substance in rice bran prevented beriberi, a disease common in the Orient. By 1920, when it was established that all vitamins did not contain nitrogen, the final "e" was dropped to obtain the term **vitamin,** which is now a household word.

The concept that the classical deficiency diseases such as beriberi, scurvy, rickets, and pellagra were the result of an absence of nutrients needed in very small amounts did much to stimulate attempts to identify the nature of these dietary essentials. It soon became clear that there were several components of both fat-soluble A and water-soluble B. By 1940, four fat-soluble and eight water-soluble vitamins had been identified as essential elements in the human diet; several others had been identified as essential for various species of animals. The chemical

Among the Contributors to Nutrition in the Biological Era

McCollum	Vitamin A
Davis	Vitamin A
Sebrell	Weight control
Stearns	Vitamin D
Elvejehm	Niacin
Gyorgy	Vitamin B_6
King	Vitamin C
Macy	Milk composition
Rose	Amino acids

vitamin
An organic substance needed in very small amounts that is, nevertheless, essential for life and must be provided in the diet

structure of each vitamin had been established, many had been synthesized, and knowledge of their biological roles was accumulating rapidly. Since 1940 only two essential vitamins (folacin and vitamin B_{12}) have been identified.

During this same period minerals in the diet were studied. Minerals, like vitamins, proved to be a complex mixture, with 20 elements having been established as dietary essentials for humans. The essentiality of several others is still uncertain.

Cellular or Molecular Era (1955 to the Present)

Since 1955 many technological developments, such as the electron microscope and the ultracentrifuge, have made it possible to study the nutrient needs of the individual cells and even the subcellular components, or organelles, of the cell. As a result, an understanding of the intricacies of cell structure and the complex and vital role that nutrients play in the growth, development, and maintenance of the cell is accumulating rapidly. Nourishment of cells is essential for the nourishment of tissues; in turn, nourishment of tissues is basic to the nourishment of organs and ultimately of the whole body. Failure to form an essential enzyme or other cellular components results in the malfunction or death of a cell. This process eventually results in a specific physical symptom of ill health.

After 1960 emphasis in nutrition research changed from a search for essential dietary components to a study of the interrelationships among nutrients, their precise biological roles, the determination of human dietary requirements, and the effect of processing on the nutrient quality of foods. More recently, to help narrow the gap between our theoretical knowledge of nutrition and its practical application in the improvement of nutritional status, nutritionists are seeking the help of educators, communicators, and anthropologists.

It is important to remember that, although we depend on studies at the molecular level to enhance our understanding of nutrition, food is the ultimate source of nourishment. Thus food is the only source of the many nutrients on which cell growth and function depend. It is only through an understanding of how our food habits are formed that we will be able to influence food intake.

Sophisticated Tools in Nutrition Research

Electron microscope (cell structure)
Ultracentrifuge (separate cell fraction)
Radioactive isotopes (trace element metabolism)
Stable isotopes (trace element metabolism)
Radioimmunoassays (hormone analysis)
Atomic absorption spectrophotometry (trace element analysis)

Among the Contributors to Nutrition in the Cellular/Molecular Era

DeLuca	Vitamin D
Mertz	Trace elements
Hegsted	Calcium
Young	Protein
Goodman	Vitamin A
Munro	Protein
Sandstead	Zinc
Harper	Amino acids
Horwitt	Vitamin E

PRESENT STATUS

It has been a mere hundred years since we learned that carbohydrate, fat, and protein were not the only food components needed for normal growth and development. Today we have a vast, complex, and rapidly expanding knowledge of over 45 nutrients that must be supplied in the diet. The absence of any one of these nutrients, whether it is needed in small or large amounts, can have a profound effect on health.

Although the last vitamin was discovered over 30 years ago, we are still identifying essential mineral elements. In addition, the discovery of the many complex interactions among vitamins, minerals, and macronutrients presents a scientific challenge. Translating our knowledge of nutrient needs into meaningful dietary advice for a public concerned about the impact of dietary practices on health, longevity, and behavior is an even greater challenge for the nutrition educator.

The fact that nutritional deficiency diseases are still occasionally found in affluent and developing countries alike is stark evidence of our failure to apply all the nutrition information that we have. These diseases, in addition to problems of overnutrition that occur primarily where people are affluent enough to overeat, have led nutritionists to seek help from social scientists in encouraging behavioral changes to improve nutritional health.

Many new approaches to the study of nutrition are emerging. Variation in individual needs has stimulated interest in the effect of genetics on nutritional needs. Knowledge of the role of genetics in human development has led to cures for some metabolic defects. The effect of nutrition on brain development and behavior and on resistance to infection, stress, environmental factors such as pollution, and drug use are only a few of the new concepts being studied.

Some Reputable Nutrition Journals
- Journal of Nutrition
- Journal of the American Dietetic Association
- The American Journal of Clinical Nutrition
- Journal of Nutrition Education
- Nutrition Research
- Ecology of Food and Nutrition
- Lipid Research
- Proceedings of the Nutrition Society
- Nutrition Reviews
- Journal of the Canadian Dietetics Association

Recognition that nutrition plays a part in the development or treatment of cardiovascular disease, hypertension, diabetes, and cancer, commonly known as "killer diseases," has led to extensive study of its role. Many premature claims have been made about the effectiveness of specific foods or nutrients in preventing or curing degenerative diseases. As a result, the nutritionist is now as concerned with combating misinformation as with delivering sound nutrition information.

The number of recent scientific publications in the field of nutrition indicates how much nutrition research has increased since the concept of vitamins was first presented. In 1913 there were four nutrition articles, all by Casimir Funk. The number has risen constantly until in 1988 reviews on single nutrients routinely list from 200 to 500 references, and over 4000 papers with implications for nutrition are presented at a single scientific meeting. Research papers relating to vitamin E alone are appearing at the rate of over 700 per year.

The number of investigators who consider nutrition their major interest is obvious from membership in scientific organizations devoted to nutrition. The American Institute of Nutrition, whose members have made significant contributions to the field, has over 2200 members. The Society for Nutrition Education, formed in 1971 to provide a forum for professionals concerned with the application of nutrition knowledge, has over 5000 members. The American Dietetic Association, with 57,000 members, is the largest and oldest established professional organization devoted to both practice and research in dietetics.

The U.S. government provides grants in support of human nutrition research, training, and education. In addition, federal support fosters many nutrition intervention programs. When the support from private industry and foundations is added in, we see a growing commitment on the part of both public and private sectors to further nutrition knowledge and to promote the dissemination of that knowledge.

CONTEMPORARY TOPICS IN NUTRITION

Interest in nutrition has escalated partly because many people recognize that nutrition is one of the few determinants of health status over which they can exert some control. So while physiologists, food scientists, and nutrition scientists are attempting to unravel the complexities that determine what goes on within the body, its cells, and its subcellular components, there is also a growing interest from the general public about the relationship of our changing food supply to dietary practices and health. The following overview includes some of the issues of current concern.

Iatrogenic Malnutrition

iatrogenic
Arising from the practice of medicine

total parenteral nutrition (TPN)
Feeding a person totally by infusing nutrients directly into the blood

The increasing use of drugs and surgery to treat many physical ailments has led to unexpected complications relating to nutritional needs, known as **iatrogenic** malnutrition. For instance, oral contraceptives now used by many young women are associated with increased needs for several nutrients. Not only do they have an effect on the immediate needs of the young women, but they also influence their needs during subsequent pregnancies and lactation. Another example is the use of antibiotics, which interferes with the synthesis of some vitamins in the gastrointestinal tract and results in an increased need for a dietary source of these vitamins. Anticonvulsant drugs have a marked effect on the need for vitamin D, and bypass operations to shorten the intestinal tract of very obese people reduce their ability to absorb many nutrients in addition to the calories they hope to limit. The use of **total parenteral nutrition (TPN),** in which patients who have trouble eating or absorbing nutrients are fed entirely through their veins, has led to many nutritional problems as scientists struggle to formulate a TPN solution capable of meeting all

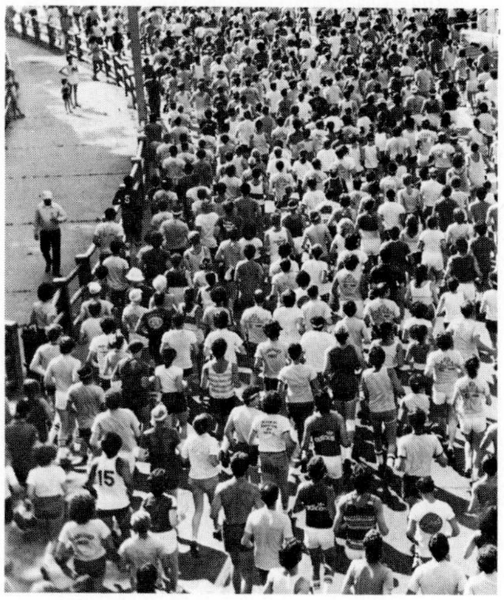

The current fitness craze has stimulated many athletes, both professional and amateur, to turn to nutrition to help improve their performance. For more information on nutrition and physical fitness, see Chapter 19.

nutritional needs. Physicians are constantly on the lookout for unsuspected nutritional complications resulting from the use of modern medical practices.

Athletic Performance

A relationship between nutrition and fitness has been recognized only recently. Athletes are now turning to nutrition, as well as psychology, to try to gain a competitive edge. The result has been the emergence of a whole new focus in nutrition called sports nutrition, which emphasizes the positive effect of nutrition and eating patterns on athletic performance. Sports nutrition research attempts to either document or refute much of the anecdotal information that has become the basis of a very lucrative "sports health" business and a source of at least some false hope for aspiring athletes.

Behavior

Interest in the relationship between nutrition and behavior usually falls into one of two distinct areas: (1) a concern with the effect of severe malnutrition, especially during early life, on the development of the brain and on other parts of the central nervous system and with long-term consequences of this on learning ability and performance, and (2) interest in the effect on behavior of certain essential nutrients, food additives, normal dietary constituents such as sucrose, and contaminants such as lead. There has been long-standing interest in diet and hyperactivity in young children. Nutritionists and behaviorists are now investigating the role of diet in the treatment of other mental problems such as autism and Down syndrome. There is also continuing study of the effect of hunger on learning and behavior.

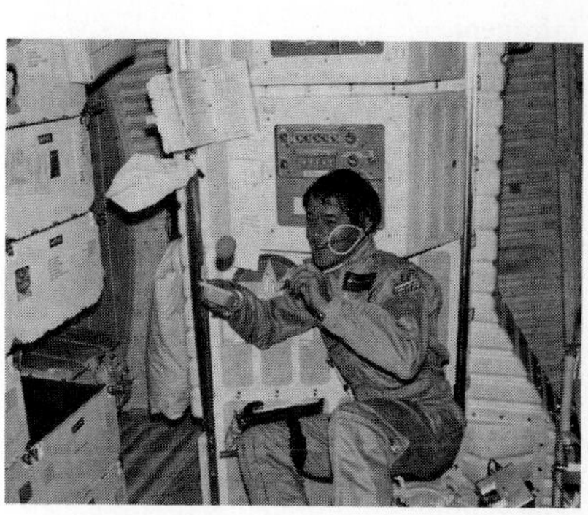

An astronaut eating in space

Space Exploration

Prolonged travel in space is raising many questions about special dietary requirements, not only regarding the form in which food must be fed but also the way the body uses nutrients under conditions of weightlessness. Of special interest are questions about changes in taste perception: the effect of dehydration; loss of appetite; distribution of blood throughout the body; and changes in calcium and nitrogen needs. Although the number of us who will have firsthand experience with space flight is probably small, the application of what is learned about the way the body uses food in space will have much wider implications and may affect all of us.

Safety of Our Food Supply

The **Food and Drug Administration (FDA)** and the USDA are responsible for seeing that our food supply is safe and wholesome. The almost universal use of herbicides and pesticides on plants and frequent use of antibiotics in animal feed that ensures quality food can be produced at a reasonable cost but elicits a high level of concern about the impact of these substances on health. The use of a growing list of additives to enhance the keeping qualities, flavor, texture, and palatability of our food is also a focus of questions. Nutritionists and food scientists share these concerns and are constantly assessing the effect that substances may have on the use of and need for nutrients. Both groups are careful to balance the risks of using particular substances against the benefits. In addition to studying the effect of additives, scientists are becoming increasingly sensitive to unintentional or incidental additives, which include a number of naturally occurring toxins and those that may either develop during storage or enter food during processing.

Food and Drug Administration (FDA) A federal agency responsible for the enforcement of regulations regarding the manufacturing and distribution of food, drugs, and cosmetics

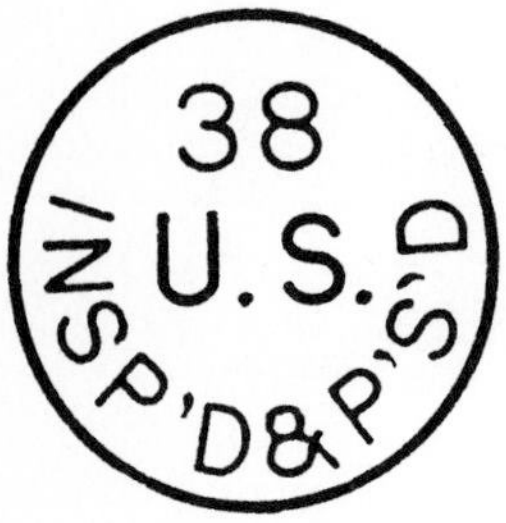

Stamp indicating meat has been inspected for wholesomeness

Health, Organic, and Natural Foods

Health, *organic*, and *natural* are terms that have crept into advertising, labels of food products, and many popular articles about foods and nutrition. In reality none of them has any legal or even generally accepted definition. As a result, they are used very loosely and with widely varying interpretations, many of them more emotional than scientific. All foods are in fact organic, most are natural in the sense that they are produced in nature, and the vast majority of foods make a positive contribution toward health. (If they don't, it is usually because they are overused rather than because of anything inherently unhealthy about them.) These three terms are usually used to connote *absence* of something rather than *presence*. For example, they are used to describe foods raised without the use of inorganic fertilizers, pesticides, or herbicides; foods sold without any processing or minimal processing; or those with nothing added, such as sugar, preservatives, or coloring, and nothing taken away, such as outer skin or fibrous parts.

Supplementation

Concern about nutrition and its relationship to health has led a great many people to begin prescribing supplements for themselves. The multibillion dollar supplement business is testimony to the fact that American people have lost faith in the ability of the food supply to meet their nutrient needs. The public has also become overconfident in its ability to diagnose problems and make appropriate prescriptions. In most cases the results are relatively harmless although economically unsound. In some cases, however, they are potentially lethal. The term "megavitamin therapy" is often used to describe this practice, but in reality it involves minerals and many nonnutritive substances, as well as vitamins.

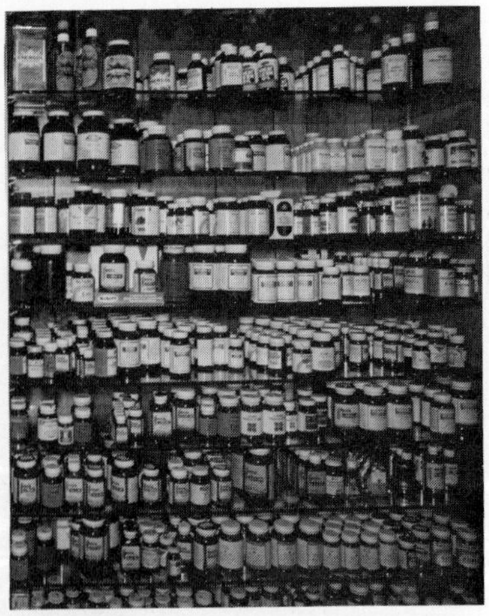

The public is presented with a confusing array of nutrient supplements

Immunity

In little more than the past decade, we have accumulated enough information to know that adequate nutrition is important in allowing our immune system to function to protect us against infection and to help us recover from infectious diseases once they do occur. There is great interest in learning which nutrients are specifically involved, but until these are determined the best advice is to maintain good nutritional status. A possible role for nutrition in modifying the course of acquired immune deficiency syndrome (AIDS) is attracting much attention.

Biotechnology

As a result of rapid advance in genetic engineering of bacterial cells, it has been possible to develop bacteria that can change the nutrients in our food supply. Because the foods that are produced in this way are not "natural" foods, they have been termed "novel" foods. Although these foods may have some of the nutritional qualities we are seeking, for instance low-cholesterol cheese, the FDA is concerned that we do not know enough about the long-term effects of their use. It is therefore reluctant to approve them for sale to the public.

biotechnology
Using modern technology to modify living systems, including changing the structure of plant, animal, and bacteria genes

Education

Although nutrition has long been taught in school as part of health and sometimes home economics classes, nutritional concepts are also now being taught within many subjects such as reading, science, and mathematics. In addition, many industries are recognizing that well-nourished workers lose fewer days due to sickness and may also live longer, and are thus emphasizing nutrition as part of a health promotion disease prevention program at the worksite. Nutrition is being offered on television and in community health programs, and many people are seeking private consultation to learn the components of an adequate diet. Nutrition is also the focus of required or elective classes for students in medical school.

Changing Life-styles

With an increasing number of single-parent homes and many more families with both parents employed outside the home, there have been changes in eating patterns that have implications for dietary adequacy. The three main concerns are the number of children who are responsible for their own food preparation without adequate adult supervision; the perceived reliance on "fast food" or "convenience food" chains; and the number of adults who "eat on the run" or "graze" on food throughout the day. The nutritional implications of these practices, either good or bad, can be judged only by their influence on the total diet.

Degenerative Diseases

The possible relationship between nutrition and the so-called degenerative diseases—cancer, coronary heart disease, hypertension, arthritis, diabetes, and osteoporosis—has led to growing interest in nutrition in the past decade. The publication of several state-of-the-art papers on these topics has heightened the public's interest. More importantly, these reports have focused the attention of Congress on the need to support investigations to study these relationships so that sound nutritional guidance can be provided to the public. Dietary modification undoubtedly benefits groups of people whose heredity makes them susceptible to a particular condition; it may also benefit people who are not predisposed to the condition. There is debate, however, about the appropriateness of suggesting a dietary change to everyone if it is helpful to a small group but probably unnecessary for others.

Degenerative Diseases
- Cancer
- Coronary heart disease
- Hypertension
- Arthritis
- Diabetes
- Osteoporosis

Public Policy

Because the nutritional status of a population is ultimately determined by the availability of an appropriate food supply, it is critical that policymakers be aware of the nutritional implications of policies relating to agricultural subsidies, import/export tariffs, public works, and credit. The development of a national nutrition policy directed toward ensuring that all people have access to a nutritionally adequate diet is essential. Nutritionists who have traditionally not become involved in political activities are now recognizing that they have a responsibility to support programs designed to promote a high level of nutritional health.

THE FOOD/NUTRIENT LINK

Food fulfills many roles for the individual. Its psychological value, its social significance, and its satiety value are more likely to be determinants of when, how much, and what foods are consumed than are nutritional considerations. Although all of these are of great importance, the role of food that we are primarily interested in is that of nourishing the body. If we emphasize "variety" and "moderation" in choosing food, we will very likely be provided with all the nutrients essential for the normal functioning of the body. If food is not properly chosen, we will risk experiencing a deficiency in one or more of the essential nutrients.

essential nutrient
A nutrient that must be provided by food because it cannot be synthesized by the body at a rate sufficient to meet bodily needs

An **essential nutrient** is defined as one that must be provided by food because the body cannot synthesize it at a rate sufficient to meet our needs. Nutrients essential for one species may not be essential for another. For example, vitamin C is an essential nutrient for humans and guinea pigs but not for rats. The essential nutrients function in the body to:

- **Supply energy**
- **Promote growth and repair of body tissues**
- **Regulate body processes**

The nutrients that perform these functions can be divided into six main categories:

- **Carbohydrates**
- **Lipid**
- **Protein**
- **Minerals**
- **Vitamins**
- **Water**

It is clear from Figure 1-3, which classifies nutrients according to functions, that lipid and protein perform all three functions, whereas certain minerals and water are involved in only two, and vitamins and carbohydrate are directly involved in only one. Nonetheless, a nutrient that performs only one function is just as essential as one that is involved in all three functions.

A listing of the essential nutrients in each of these main categories is shown in Table 1-2. The nutrients listed are absolutely essential for human growth and the maintenance of life. Some nutrients are present in a wide variety of foods, so that there is little likelihood of a deficiency occurring. On the other hand, some are distributed in a limited number of foods and will be present in less-than-optimal amounts if the variety in the diet is limited. There are, however, an infinite number of ways in which foods can be combined to provide an adequate amount of these nutrients.

A comparison of the nutrient composition of five representative foods is listed in Table 1-3. From this table it is evident that water, carbohydrate, lipid, and protein constitute over 98% of the weight of food, and that vitamins and minerals

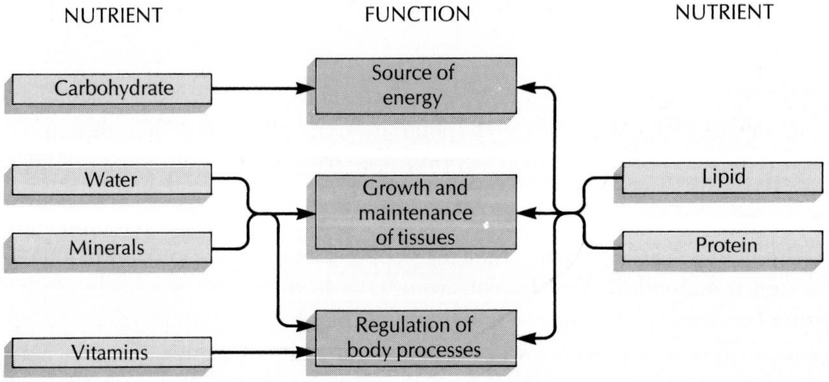

Figure 1-3 Relationship among major nutrient groups and functions of nutrients. Vitamins and minerals are indirectly involved in supplying energy and in growth and maintenance. They are necessary to facilitate the biochemical changes involved in these processes.

constitute an extremely small portion. However, these small amounts are enough to make the difference between a healthy, well-functioning body and one with nutritional inadequacies. Nutrients that have been identified as "problem nutrients," or those most likely to be consumed in less than recommended amounts, in the United States are indicated in Table 1-2.

Although each of the essential nutrients is needed for normal body functions, the amount needed bears no relationship to that nutrient's importance. For instance, the nutritional needs of an adult man vary from 2 μg (1/14,000,000 oz) of cobalamin (vitamin B_{12}) to 56 grams (2 oz) of protein. A deficiency of a nutrient needed in extremely small amounts may cause more severe symptoms more rapidly than a deficiency of one needed in much larger amounts. For instance, iron deficiency is much more common than calcium deficiency, yet the requirement for calcium is 80 times the requirement for iron. Besides being the result of inadequate intake,

Table 1-2 ◇ Essential nutrients as classified in 1988

Carbohydrate	**Minerals**	**Vitamins**
Glucose	Macronutrient elements	Fat-soluble
	*Calcium	*A (retinol)
Fat or **Lipid**	Phosphorus	D (cholecalciferol)
Linoleic acid	†Sodium	E (tocopherol)
Linolenic acid	Potassium	K
Arachidonic acid	Sulfur	Water-soluble
	Chlorine	‡Thiamin
Protein	†Magnesium	Riboflavin
Amino acids	Micronutrient elements	‡Niacin
Leucine	*Iron	Biotin
Isoleucine	Selenium	†Folacin
Lysine	†Zinc	*Vitamin B_6 (pyridoxine)
Methionine	Manganese	Vitamin B_{12} (cobalamin)
Phenylalanine	Copper	Pantothenic acid
Threonine	Cobalt	Vitamin C (ascorbic acid)
Tryptophan	Molybdenum	
Valine	‡Iodine	**Water**
Histidine	Chromium	
Nonessential nitrogen	Vanadium	
	Tin	
	Nickel	
	Silicon	
	Boron	
	Arsenic	
	Fluorine	

*Most likely to be a problem in the United States (based on Nationwide Food Consumption Survey, 1977-1978).
†Potential problems.
‡Previous problems; they have now been corrected.

Table 1-3 ◇ Approximate composition of some representative foods

	Whole Milk (%)	Bread (%)	Carrots (%)	Chicken (%)	Bananas (%)
Water	87.0	35.8	88.2	69	74
Carbohydrate	5.0	50.4	8.4	0	24
Lipid	3.5	3.2	0.2	8	0.9
Protein	3.7	8.7	1.1	19	0.9
Minerals	0.7	1.1	1.9	1	1
Vitamins	0.1	0.1	0.1	0.1	0.1

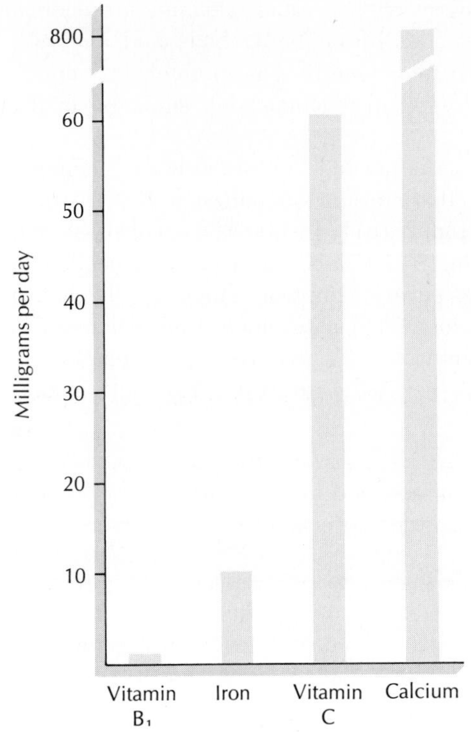

Relative amounts of essential nutrients needed; those needed in smallest amounts just as important as those needed in much larger quantities.

nutrient deficiencies can result from increased needs, decreased absorption, or depressed utilization of a nutrient.

One important factor in the development of deficiencies is how quickly body reserves are depleted in times of dietary deficiency. The marginal shows that this time varies from a few hours in the case of **labile** amino acids, which the body has virtually no capacity to store, to about 60 days for many water-soluble vitamins, to 7 years for calcium. The major site of storage differs with the nutrient—the liver stores iron, vitamin A, and carbohydrate; the adrenal gland stores vitamin C; and bone stores calcium. For some nutrients there is no storage site. In these cases, deficiency symptoms will become evident as soon as individual cells have become depleted of the nutrient.

From this point on we will be learning about the way the body uses certain nutrients and the consequences of getting either too much or too little of any of the essential and nonessential nutrients in food. Most of the information will be well established, but in a constantly changing field such as nutrition, some of the information will of necessity be speculative. To fail to include some of this would deprive the student of the excitement of the discipline—a cost too high compared with risking retraction of statements in later editions.

labile
Easily broken down or destroyed

Extent of Body Reserves of Nutrients and Time Required to Deplete Reserves

Amino acids	Few hours
Carbohydrate	13 hours
Sodium	2-3 days
Water	4 days
Fat	20-40 days
Thiamin	30-60 days
Ascorbic acid	60-120 days
Niacin	60-180 days
Riboflavin	60-180 days
Vitamin A	90-365 days
Iron	125 days (women) 750 days (men)
Iodine	1000 days
Calcium	2500 days

BY NOW YOU SHOULD KNOW

- At this time over 45 nutrients have been identified as essential to human nutrition.
- Essential nutrients must be provided by food.
- Nutrients function in the body to supply energy, promote growth, repair body tissues, and regulate body processes.
- Nutrients fall into six major categories: carbohydrate, lipid, protein, minerals, vitamins, and water.
- Although some nutrients are needed by the body in greater amounts than others, all nutrients are important, working either alone or together to maintain health.
- Nutrition as a discipline has only existed since 1934.
- Evidence of nutrition knowledge dates back to biblical times.
- Interest in nutrition is at an all-time high, ranging from concerns about the relationship between nutrition and degenerative diseases to nutrition for athletes and astronauts.
- This text is designed to provide the fundamentals of nutrition for those planning to pursue a career in a nutrition-related field and for those who wish to obtain enough information to allow them to be informed consumers.

STUDY QUESTIONS

1. Make a time line of events that were legendary in nutrition. Divide the time line into the appropriate eras of nutrition.
2. List the six major categories of essential nutrients. Which three provide energy? Which one only regulates body functions?
3. When vitamins were first discovered they were spelled "vitamine." Soon after the spelling changed and the "e" was dropped. Why?
4. Define "essential nutrient" and explain how they are available to the body for energy, growth, and maintenance of body tissue and for regulatory processes.
5. You have recently read an advertisement claiming that eating oat bran is a more cost effective means of lowering blood-cholesterol levels than cholesterol-lowering drugs. List three steps you can take to find if this is true and a safe practice.
6. How are degenerative diseases approached in the Nutrition-Related Goals for the Nation for the Year 1990?

Applying What You've Learned

1. **Starting a Nutrition File for Current Issues**

   One of the best ways to get familiar with current issues in nutrition is to review the popular press. By keeping up with the popular press, you will begin to understand how the basic principles can be applied. Look through a recent issue of a women's or men's magazine, a weekly magazine such as *Time* or *Newsweek*, a Sunday newspaper magazine, and your local newspaper. Note the range and number of articles relating to nutrition. When you can, clip or photocopy the articles to start a nutrition file system. Some of the possible file categories include nutrition and athletics, alcohol, cancer, heart disease, osteoporosis, and vitamin/mineral supplementation. Popular issues in nutrition are constantly changing, so over time you may need to change your file categories.

2. **Notions about Nutrition**

   Many people have beliefs about nutrition that may be correct or incorrect. Listen to conversations among your friends about food or nutrition. Make a list of the beliefs or statements you hear. As we read the chapters in which these beliefs are related to basic principles, try to decide if each statement was based on fact. When you are not sure, ask your instructor. Discussing beliefs and myths that surround nutrition will enhance the classroom experience.

3. **Labeling and Advertising as a Source of Nutrition Information**

   We often acquire nutrition beliefs from food advertising and labeling. Begin to note the nutrition claims. Try to judge whether they are factual or misleading. Bring labels and advertisements to class to share with your instructor; these will enhance the classroom experience.

4. **Creating a Time Capsule**

   Write down 10 nutrition-related questions you have now. Put these into an envelope. At the end of the course, open the envelope and see how many you can then answer.

5. **Investigate Career Opportunities in Nutrition**

   Write to the American Dietetic Association for a brochure on careers in dietetics: American Dietetic Association, 216 W. Jackson Blvd., Chicago, IL 60604-1003.

SUGGESTED READINGS

Califano JA: America's health care revolution: Health promotion and disease prevention, Journal of the American Dietetic Association 87:437, 1987.

Califano writes a commentary on the revolutionary way of health in the United States. This article provides a short overview of heart disease, cancer, substance abuse, injuries, and teenage pregnancy and the importance of teaching disease prevention in medical schools, to the poor, and to those who overindulge.

Glanz K, and Damberg CL: Meeting our nation's health objectives in nutrition, Journal of Nutrition Education 19:211, 1987.

This article recaps the role of nutrition in preventive health services, health protection, and health promotion for the nation. The 17 health promotion objectives that focus on nutrition in the Nation's Health Objectives for 1990 are addressed. It reports on the 1985 midcourse review that measured the progress toward achieving these 17 health objectives.

Sorenson AW, Kavet J, and Stephenson MG: Health objectives for the nation: Moving toward the 1990s, Journal of the American Dietetic Association 87:920, 1987.

This article provides a historical perspective to the development of the Nation's Health Objectives for 1990. Likewise, it summarizes the 1985 midcourse review and suggests the development of objectives for the year 2000.

ADDITIONAL READINGS

Food Technologists Expert Panel on Food Safety and Nutrition: Effects of food processing on nutritive values, Food Technology 40:109, 1986.

Food Technologists Expert Panel on Food Safety and Nutrition: Food biotechnology, Food Technology 42:133, 1988.

Gussow J, and Clancy KL: Dietary guidelines for sustainability, Journal of Nutrition Education 18:1, 1986.

Harper AE: Nutrition: from myth and magic to science. Nutrition Today 23:8, 1988.

Haughton B, Gussow JD, and Dodd JM: An historical study of the underlying assumptions for United States Food Guides from 1917 through the basic four food group guide, Journal of Nutrition Education 19:169, 1987.

Hayes JR, and Borzelleca JF: Nutrient interaction with drugs and other xenobiotics, Journal of the American Dietetic Association 85:335, 1985.

Herbert VH: Unproven (questionable) dietary and nutritional methods in cancer prevention and treatment, Cancer 58:1930, 1986.

Kris-Etherton PM, Dreon DM, and Wood PD: Diet and coronary heart disease: the challenge before us, Journal of Nutrition Education 19:242, 1987.

McCollum EV: A history of nutrition, Boston, 1957, Houghton Mifflin Co.

Nair PP: Diet, nutrition intake and metabolism in populations at high and low risk for colon cancer, American Journal of Clinical Nutrition 40:879-963, 1984.

Pao E: Changes in American food consumption patterns and their nutritional significance, Food Technology 31:43, 1981.

Ryan AS, Foltz MB, and Finn SC: The role of the clinical dietician. I. Present professional image and recent image changes. II. Staffing patterns and job functions, Journal of the American Dietetic Association 88:671, 684, 1988.

Schneider H: What has happened to nutrition? In Ingle, DJ, editor: Life and disease, New York, 1963, Basic Books, Inc., Publishers.

Simoupolis A: Diet and health, scientific concepts and principles. American Journal of Clinical Nutrition 45:5, 1987.

Stephenson MG: The 1990 national objectives for improved nutrition, Journal of Nutrition Education 19:155, 1987.

Willett WC, and McMahon B: Diet and cancer—an overview, New England Journal of Medicine 310:633 and 697, 1984.

FOCUS Careers in Nutrition

Some of you who are using this text as an introduction to nutrition have undoubtedly already made a decision to seek a career in nutrition. On the other hand, most of you have probably selected the course as an elective to explore and use nutrition information for your personal benefit. Among this second group will be some who may want to consider nutrition as a career.

For those of you who decide to continue the study of nutrition there are many and diverse career opportunities, ranging from dietetics to research. The starting point for everyone is the study of the fundamentals of nutrition. Most students have not had any prior study of biochemistry and physiology, but both of these will be necessary before the in-depth knowledge of nutrition needed for professional competence is possible. The end point of nutrition study is the acquisition of a unique set of skills for a specific position to complement fundamental nutrition know-how.

If you are confused about the distinction between a "dietitian" and a "nutritionist," you are not alone. In general, a *dietitian* is someone who has completed an undergraduate program that meets the academic requirements of the American Dietetic Association and has then obtained the necessary experience to meet the requirements to qualify for professional registration. Successful completion of these academic and experience requirements and a qualifying "registration" examination permit the use of the designation "Registered Dietitian" (R.D.). The academic requirements consist of a core of courses in the basic sciences, nutrition, and foods and an introduction to related subjects such as economics, educational psychology, and management. Beyond that a student may choose to emphasize one of four options—community, management, clinical, or general, each with its own academic requirements. In addition to meeting the requirements for many positions, the registered dietitian has the credentials to justify third-party payments from the many insurance companies that consider nutrition counseling a reimbursable medical expense.

A *nutritionist*, on the other hand, is someone who has completed undergraduate and/or graduate training in the discipline of nutrition without necessarily meeting the academic and experience requirements to qualify for the R.D. This person, who in most cases has the same or more advanced training in nutrition than the dietitian, may not have the required supporting courses. Whereas almost all dietitians have had some experience in counseling people on therapeutic diets for conditions such as diabetes or kidney problems, nutritionists are more likely to have competence in dealing with the concerns of normal nutrition. Unfortunately, there is no restriction on the use of the term—the result is that many untrained and unqualified persons call themselves nutritionists.

Up until the past 10 or 20 years, career opportunities for a person trained in nutrition or dietetics were confined to hospital or institutional settings. In these settings it was expected that nutrition professionals would be concerned with the day-to-day operation of the hospital's or institution's foodservice, including menu planning, food purchasing, kitchen layout, and personnel management. In addition they were expected to provide nutritional counseling to inpatients, as well as those referred for dietary help on an outpatient basis. With the recognition of the complexities of both the management and counseling aspects of the dietitian's role, an individual is now frequently prepared for a position either as a clinical nutritionist/dietitian or as an administrative dietitian. Many, however, are still qualified as generalists to meet the needs of situations in which one dietitian must still assume full responsibility for the dietary or nutritional care program.

Within a hospital setting clinical dietitians are responsible for the nutritional quality of the meals served, but most of their time is devoted to patient education. This involves instructing the patient about the basis for a prescribed diet to provide an understanding of the limitations on food selection. This instruction often includes an analysis of the patient's usual food habits and consultation with other family members to plan a diet that will ensure maximum compliance after discharge from the hospital. To succeed in this role, the dietitian must have effective counseling skills. In many situations the dietitian's responsibilities include providing similar counseling services to groups or individuals as outpatients. In an institutional setting, such as a nursing home for the elderly, a residential center for the mentally or physically handicapped, or a prison, there inevitably will be those who have special dietary problems requiring a clinical dietitian to play a similar counseling role. Many hospitals have recently begun to contract nutritional care services to large national organizations. These organizations are now becoming major employers of dietitians.

In recent years there have been increased opportunities for the clinical dietitian or nutritionist to function outside an institutional setting. Most notable of these opportunities is the establishment of private practices, which offer nutritional counseling to the general public on a fee-for-service basis similar to that of the psychological counseling offered by many clinical psychologists in private practice. Additionally many physicians, especially those in group practice, are including nutritionists as part of their health-care team. To succeed in these roles it is almost essential to be an R.D. and to have had several years' experience in a clinical setting.

Many dietitians have responded to the need that many small nursing homes and child-care facilities have for at least part-time consultation in nutrition; they have set up consultation services that meet the needs of a group of such facilities. Dietitians also serve as consultants to volunteer organizations such as the March of Dimes, American Heart Association affiliates, Easter Seals, and the many other volunteer agencies that deal with specific health problems and nutritional needs. Summer camps for children with diabetes or weight problems, both requiring the expertise of nutritionists, are becoming more popular, as are year-round facilities for the obese. The role of nutrition in athletics has been highlighted by the inclusion of a nutritionist as a member of the Olympic support team and as consultant to several major football teams; this opens the door for similar activities in a wide variety of sports and athletic programs. Already many fitness programs are operating with a staff of nutritionists and exercise physiologists. Similarly, executive health programs and health-in-the-worksite programs are incorporating nutrition education as an integral part of their activities.

With the growing recognition that the success of nutrition education programs depends largely on the communication skills of the professional, persons with skills in written, oral, or video communication have a unique opportunity to contribute to the many corporate, government, and education programs for public education in nutrition. Those who have primary skills in the communication field but who acquire some training in nutrition concepts and issues can also function as nutrition educators.

The area of public health nutrition is primarily concerned with state and local government programs and also with some at the federal level. The responsibilities of these nutritionists are largely administrative, but they also involve coordination of programs in which many nutritionists are employed as community nutritionists. These programs include Meals on Wheels and Congregate Feeding Programs for the elderly; WIC (Women, Infants, and Children), directed to nutritionally vulnerable people; and the Food Stamp Program for low-income families. While the administrative positions require advanced work in public health nutrition, those at the local level represent very viable opportunities to start on a career ladder in either dietetics or nutrition.

New career opportunities are springing up in the corporate setting. Management is recognizing that employees are the most valuable company asset and that a healthy employee who comes to work regularly is an asset worth preserving. As a result, many nutritionists are functioning in a worksite setting, providing group classes and individual counseling and planning programs to enhance the nutrient adequacy of the diets of the employees. Many combine their nutritional skills with skills in exercise science.

For those with a strong physical or behavioral science orientation, nutrition offers many opportunities in research, ranging from solving practical problems addressed largely by food and pharmaceutical industries, to basic research supported largely by federal government agencies and industry, to research to be carried out in a research organization or academic setting. A career in research usually requires an advanced graduate degree. This same academic preparation qualifies you for admission to professional schools of medicine, dentistry, osteopathic medicine, and veterinary medicine.

Perhaps one of the major challenges to nutritionists today is finding effective ways to combat the misinformation that is being spread by health food stores and the media. This requires diplomacy, communication skills, and a strong scientific base in nutrition. It also requires an in-depth understanding of the principles of nutrition and a constant effort to remain informed about new advances. For those interested in the health or helping professions, careers in nutrition provide an excellent opportunity to develop those interests in a discipline that is evolving and emerging at an increasingly fast pace. There is little doubt that nutrition, a discipline that is at the heart of preventive medicine and that affects a person from conception until death, is here to stay. A key question to ask when making a nutrition career choice is which direction to choose, among the many now established or on the horizon. Obviously there is overlap—the important thing is to enter the field with an in-depth appreciation of the scientific base and social applications of nutrition.

For more information on careers related to nutrition, see:

Caldwell, Carol C: Opportunities in nutrition careers, VGM Career Horizons, Lincolnwood, Ill., 1986, National Textbook Co.

Kane J: Exploring careers in dietetics and nutrition, New York, 1987, Rosen Publishing Group.

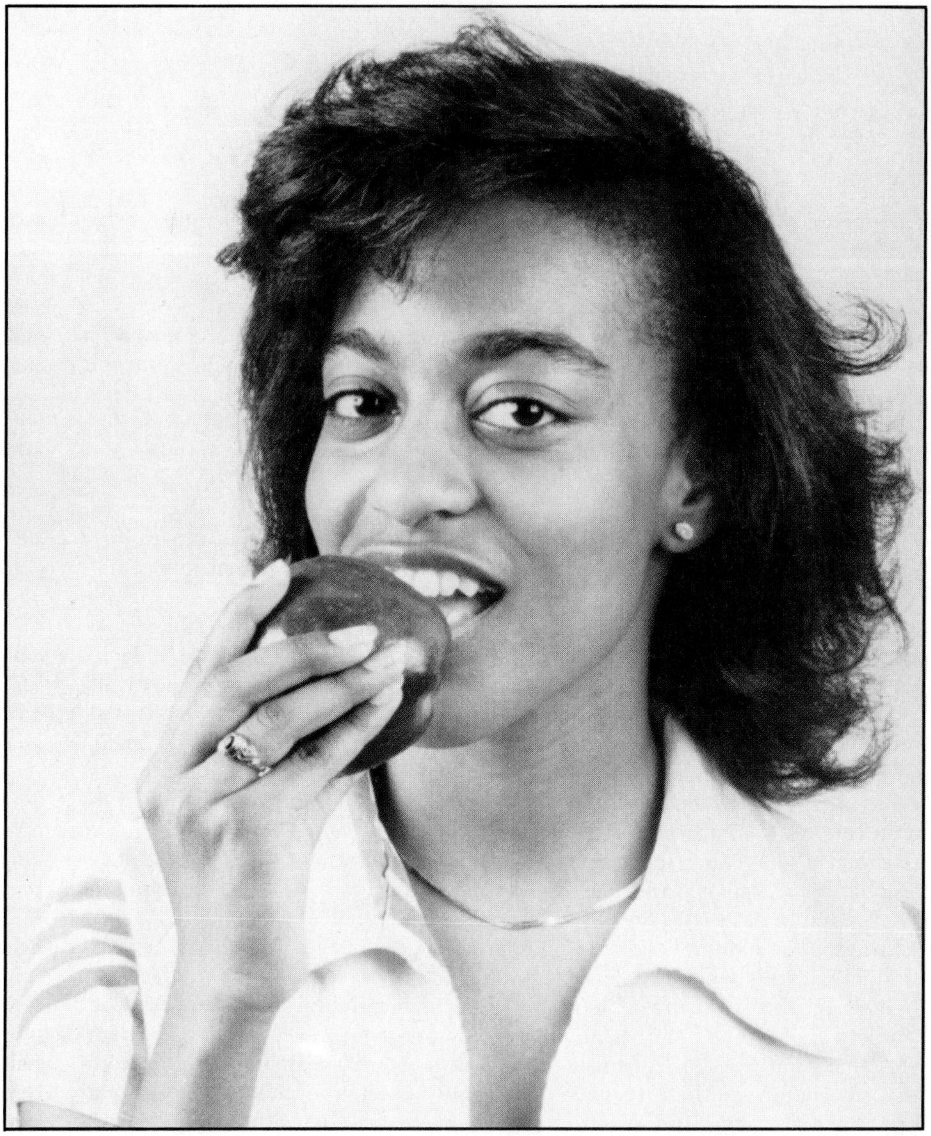

AWARENESS CHECK

Truth or Fiction?

- The stomach is the main organ of digestion.
- External cues such as seeing or smelling food will trigger your appetite whether you are hungry or not.
- The muscular tube of the small intestine is smooth to aid in the movement of nutrients in, out, and down the gastrointestinal tract.
- The acid level of the stomach and small intestines influences digestion.
- Water passes freely across membranes by osmosis whereas solids cross by passive diffusion or active transport.

CHAPTER 2

Fundamentals of Digestion, Absorption, and Metabolism

Although it is quite possible to have a good understanding of nutrition without any appreciable knowledge of physiology, biochemistry, or cell biology, it is helpful to be familiar with a few fundamentals of these sciences. If you are going to be able to appreciate the complexities of releasing the nutrients from the food that supplies them, it is important to start with an understanding of the human digestive system.

While the intricate details of digestion, absorption, and metabolism may be beyond the interests of students of introductory nutrition, it is not unusual for students to develop curiosity about how the various processes work together. Many others will already have studied these processes in high school. For them this chapter serves as a review. This chapter discusses how the body deals with the wide variety of food that is taken in as the body uses it to nourish the millions of cells. Details of digestion and metabolism of major nutrients will be discussed in the appropriate chapters.

The initial step in nourishing the body is the eating, or *ingestion*, of food. Ingestion is regulated by hunger and appetite, which respond to both internal and external stimuli. The internal stimulus is the sensation of hunger that accompanies either a drop in blood glucose levels or the contraction of the stomach in the absence of food. When food is in the stomach again, hunger gives way to feelings of satiety as the blood glucose level rises, and hunger pangs subside.

For information on the basics of biochemistry and cell biology as related to nutrition, see Appendix A.

The external stimuli, or external cues for eating, are as complex and varied as the internal. For many individuals, the sight or aroma of food will trigger the appetite. Others respond to social and environmental cues, eating (1) in social situations whenever food is available; (2) at a prescribed time of day or in a prescribed place; (3) as a defense mechanism against times when no food is available; (4) as a response to frustration, anxiety, or unhappiness; or (5) as a reward. External cues turn off the desire to eat as readily as they turn it on. Some people respond only to internal cues, but for most, eating is triggered by both physiological internal cues and environmental external cues.

DIGESTION

digestion
The process by which food is prepared for absorption

digestive tract
The tube that passes from the mouth to the anus and includes the esophagus, the stomach, the small intestine, and the large intestine

Before food can be used, it must undergo many changes to reduce it to a simple enough form so that it can pass through the intestinal wall to be absorbed into the blood, which in turn transports it to the cells for use. The process of changing food into these simple components is called **digestion,** and the changes occur primarily in the digestive tract (Figure 2-1).

The **digestive tract** is essentially a tube about 30 feet (9 m) long that passes through the center of the body from the mouth to the anus. Food travels through this muscular tube from the time it is swallowed until any undigested residue is excreted in the feces. Until food is absorbed through the walls of the digestive tract and into the blood, it cannot be used by the cells. Technically it is still outside the body. The cells lining the digestive tract control not only the form in which nutrients enter the body but also, in many cases, the amounts of nutrients that enter. These "walls" also have the ability to keep substances out of the body that are of no value or are potentially dangerous.

The Mouth

The first physiological response to either the anticipation or presence of food is the flow of saliva into the mouth. As a thin, mucuslike fluid coming from the four sets of salivary glands in the mouth, saliva performs two major roles. Its first function is to mix with food, lubricating dry foods and diluting thicker foods. Its second function is to provide starch-splitting enzymes.

For details of how enzymes work, see Appendix A

An enzyme is a protein that acts on a particular class of nutrients and makes very specific changes, usually converting complex substances to less complex forms.

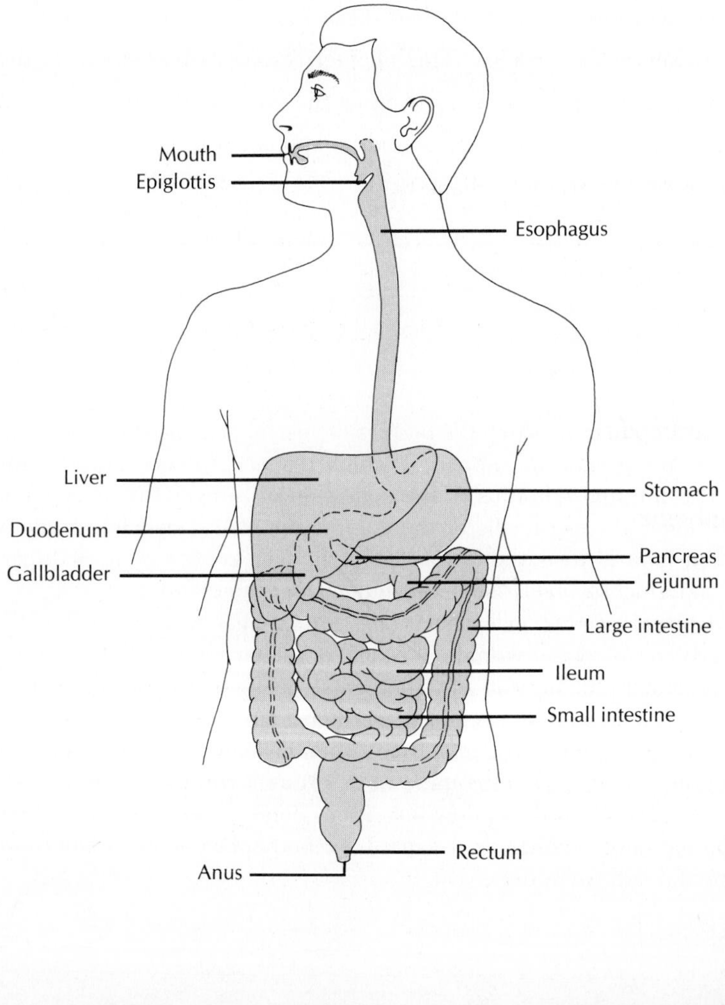

Figure 2-1 The human digestive system passes from the mouth through the esophagus to the stomach, where acids facilitate some chemical changes. From the stomach, food passes to the small intestine, where some nutrients are further broken down to very simple molecules to be absorbed into the bloodstream, and then to the large intestine or colon, where water is resorbed and the residual material is compacted. Exit is through the rectum and out the anus. Above the stomach is the liver, which plays many important roles in digestion; under the liver is the gallbladder; and nested below the stomach is the pancreas, which secretes many of the digestive enzymes into the small intestine.

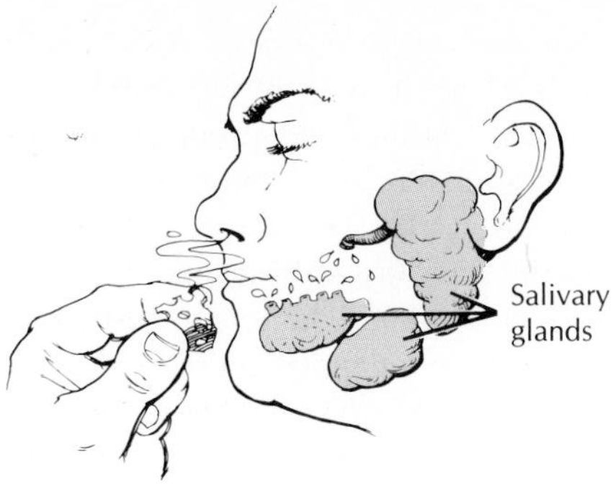

Ingested food is lubricated and mixed with fluid secreted by salivary glands in response to the aroma and taste of food.

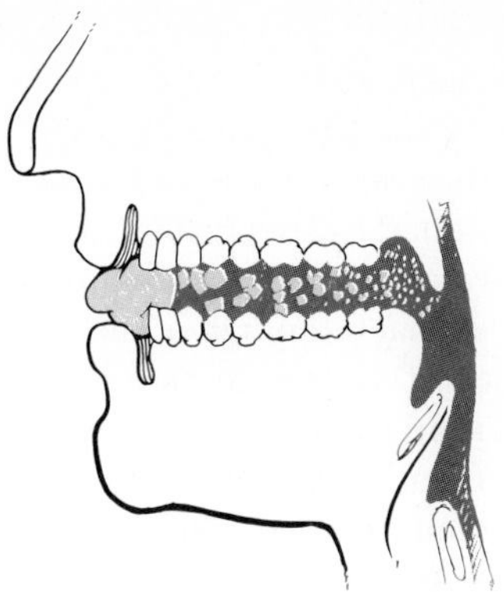

Food is broken into small pieces by the action of chewing.

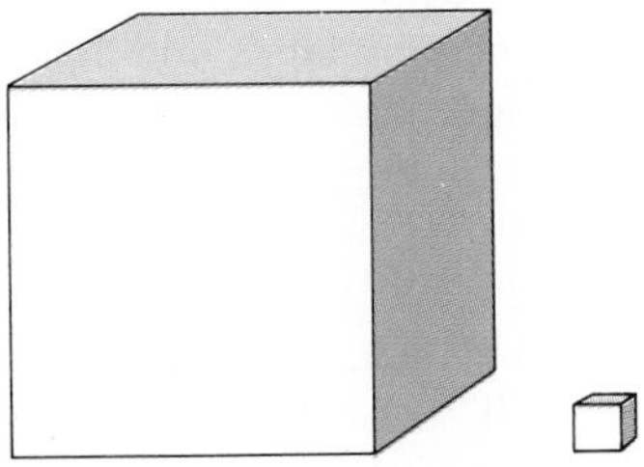

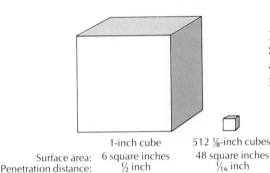

Effect of chewing on a food particle: Smaller units have a larger surface area and a shorter distance for enzymes to penetrate.

The character of ingested food is chemically changed by the action of enzymes. All enzymes have names that end in "-ase" and a prefix that tells what substance it changes; for example, a lipase is an enzyme that acts on fat, while a protease acts on protein. Salivary enzymes act best at the neutral pH of saliva. Saliva contains no enzymes that act on lipid or proteins, only amylases which acts on the carbohydrate, starch. However, there is an enzyme released at the base of the tongue that changes lipids.

The action of chewing in the mouth mechanically divides the food into small particles. This breaking up serves two purposes: the enzymes have a larger surface area on which to act, and the distance through which the enzymes have to penetrate is greatly reduced.

The Esophagus

The esophagus is a muscular tube about 10 inches long that connects the mouth to the stomach. Once food has been lubricated with saliva and broken into small pieces by chewing, the tongue can roll it into a small ball, or **bolus,** and thrust or toss it to the back of the mouth. From there it can be placed at the top of the esophagus. Simultaneously, a small flap called the epiglottis slips over the top of the trachea, or windpipe, to prevent food from entering the respiratory tract and lung; thus, food is directed into the esophagus.

bolus
A portion of food rolled into a small ball by the tongue and swallowed

Once the bolus is in the esophagus, it is propelled to the stomach by **peristalsis.** Peristalsis is the churning, wavelike action resulting from the contraction and relaxation of the muscles of the digestive tract. Peristalsis reduces the size of food particles still further and mixes them thoroughly with digestive secretions.

peristalsis
Successive wavelike contraction and relaxation of the walls of the intestinal tract to mix and move ingested food

chyme
Homogenous mixture of saliva and food that enters the stomach from the esophagus

cardiac sphincter
The muscle between the esophagus and the stomach that controls the entrance of the digestive mass into the stomach; referred to as *cardiac* because of its proximity to the heart

hormone
A messenger released in response to a condition (such as food in the stomach) that will affect the function of metabolic activity of one or more tissues. For more details on how hormones work, see Appendix A

gastrin
A hormone secreted from the wall of the stomach in response to the presence of food in the stomach; gastric juices are in turn released that aid in digestion

mucosa
The inner lining of the digestive tract

The Stomach

Although we often think of the stomach as the major organ or site of digestion, in reality it plays a minor part. The stomach, located at the end of the esophagus, consists of three sets of muscles surrounding a cavity that can extend to hold up to 2 quarts of food and fluid. Food reaches the stomach after being mixed with saliva into a slightly alkaline homogenous mass called **chyme.** Chyme passes into the stomach through a muscular opening called the **cardiac sphincter.** The presences of chyme in the stomach triggers the release of the hormone gastrin. A **hormone** is a messenger that is released in response to a condition that will affect the function or metabolic activity of one or more tissues. Once chyme enters the stomach, **gastrin** responds and stimulates the release of hydrochloric acid from the lining of the stomach. This hydrochloric acid changes the pH of the stomach to approximately 2.0, which is strongly acidic, and makes it possible for other enzymes to function to aid in the digestion of food. The wall of the stomach is protected by mucus secreted at the same time as the hydrochloric acid; it coats the stomach lining, or **mucosa,** and protects it from damage from the action of the acid. The enzymes secreted in the stomach function in the acid environment, but the starch-splitting enzymes from the saliva are inactivated. The chyme churns in the stomach for approximately 6 to 8 hours. During this time peristalsis and digestive secretions continue to prepare the nutrients for absorption.

pylorus
The muscle between the stomach and the small intestine that controls the entrance of the digestive mass into the small intestine

lumen
The inside of the digestive tube

bile
Substance that is made in the liver, stored in the gallbladder, and released to aid in the digestion of lipids

secretin
Hormone secreted from the intestinal wall in response to food in the intestine, triggering the release of pancreatic juices to aid in digestion

The Small Intestine

The small intestine is the major organ of digestion. It is 20 feet in length, the longest organ in the body. It is called "small" only because its diameter is less than that of the large intestine. By the time chyme leaves the stomach, it is almost completely liquefied. This liquid then passes slowly in regulated amounts through the **pylorus,** a muscular opening that separates the stomach from the small intestine, into the **lumen** (or center) of the intestinal tract. The enzymes needed to complete the reduction of complex nutrients to units that are simple enough to pass into or through the intestinal wall are available in the small intestine. **Bile** is made up of acids manufactured in the liver from cholesterol. Bile is stored in the gallbladder, and from there it is released into the small intestine to aid lipid digestion by breaking fat into small particles. Once the chyme enters the small intestine, a hormone, **secretin,** is released. This hormone stimulates the pancreas to release its digestive juices. The pancreas also secretes sodium bicarbonate, an alkali, which acts to neutralize the acid chyme. This, in turn, activates the enzymes in the pancreatic juice.

The final stage of digestion, known as membrane digestion, takes place in the intestinal wall. This reduces nutrients to sufficiently simple components that can be absorbed into the blood to be transported to nourish the cells. The sites and nature of the changes in digestion are summarized in Table 2-1.

portal vein
The vein that carries blood and absorbed nutrients from the intestinal wall to the liver

ABSORPTION

Absorption is the process by which the simple nutrient components which are the result of digestion pass out of the digestive tract, into the cells lining it, and from there into the bloodstream or the lymphatic system, which carry nutrients to the body cells. Most nutrients are absorbed directly into the blood and are taken in the **portal vein** first to the liver. However, some go first to the lymphatic system, a secondary circulating system that collects lipids and excess fluids; from there they go to the general circulation, or bloodstream (Figure 2-2). From this point, they are distributed to the liver and body cells in the same way as nutrients that first entered through the portal vein. All nutrients pass from the blood into the extracellular fluids between the cells; from these fluids the cell obtains the nutrients

Table 2-1 ◆ Summary of sites and nature of digestion

Site	Type of Action	How Accomplished
Mouth	Mechanical	Chewing
	Chemical	Salivary enzymes
		Lingual enzymes
Stomach	Mechanical	Peristalsis
	Chemical	Action of hydrochloric acid
		Gastric enzymes
Small intestine	Mechanical	Peristalsis
		Bile
	Chemical	Pancreatic enzymes
		Intestinal enzymes
Intestinal membrane	Chemical	Intestinal enzymes

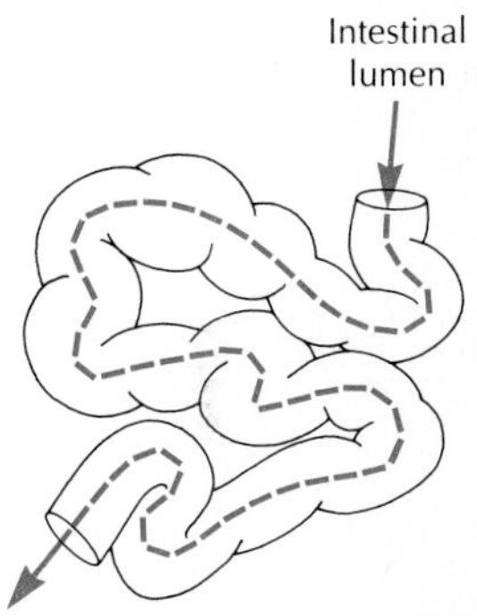

The interior of the intestinal tract through which food passes during digestion is called the lumen.

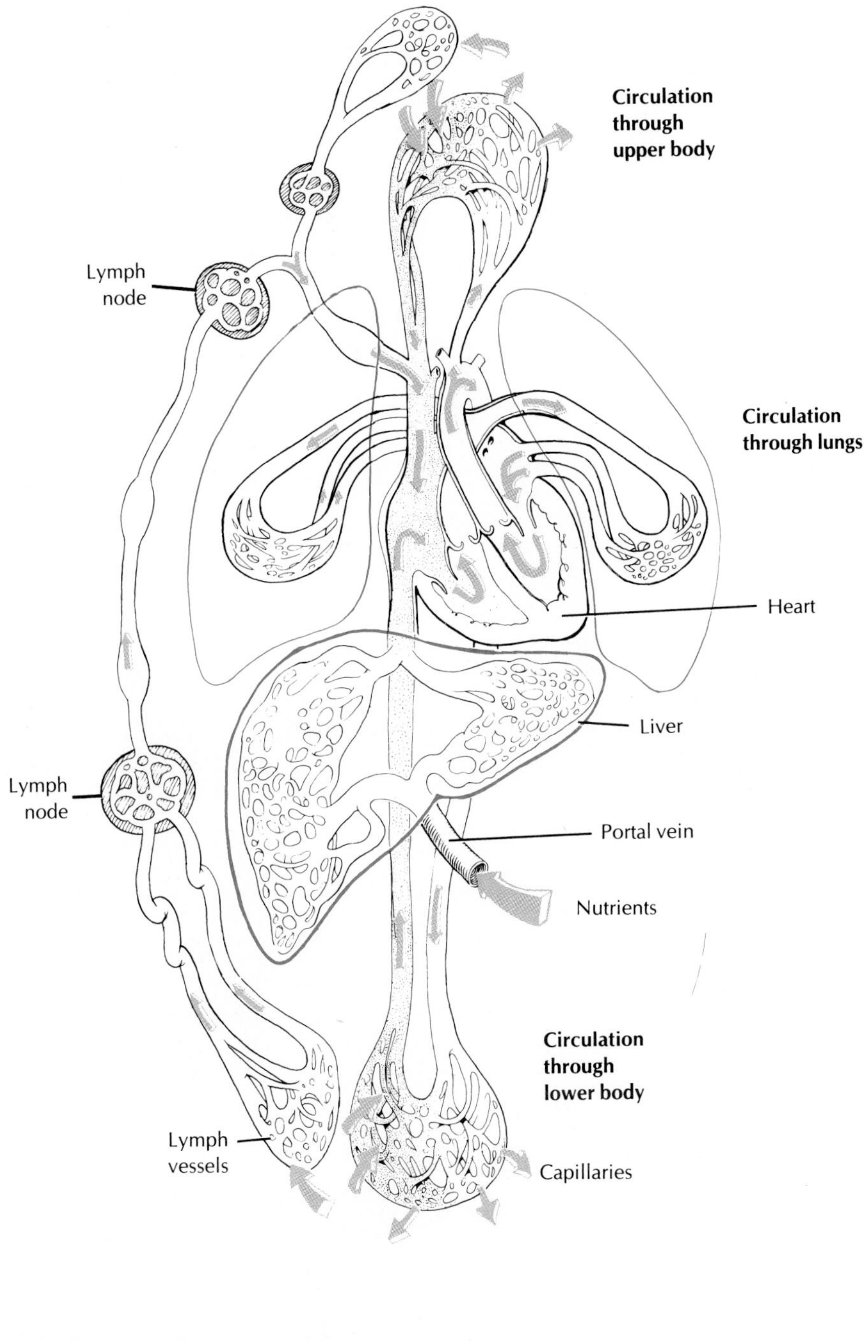

Figure 2-2 The relationship between the arteriovenous and the lymphatic circulatory systems. Nutrients enter the arteriovenous system primarily by way of the portal vein. In the circulatory system, nutrients are distributed through arteries and very small vessels (capillaries). Nutrients are then passed into extracellular fluid that surrounds capillaries. Some are reabsorbed into capillaries and veins; others enter the lymphatic system, bypass liver, and enter the arteriovenous system again in the neck before blood enters the heart.

it needs. In this case, the cell membrane acts as a selective barrier to regulate the entrance of material into the cell.

duodenum
The first segment of the small intestine

jejunum
The second segment of the small intestine, beyond the duodenum

ileum
The third and last section of the small intestine; between the jejunum and the large intestine

villi
Small fingerlike projections on the internal surface of the intestine

microvilli
Similar projections on the surface of the villi

The small intestine is divided into three segments: the **duodenum, jejunum,** and **ileum.** Besides being a long coiled tube, the small intestine has an inner surface that is structured to increase the area through which nutrients may be absorbed. The surface, especially in the duodenum and jejunum, has projections or circular folds that extend about halfway around the inner intestinal surface. These folds are 8 to 10 mm in height and increase surface area by at least three times. On the surface of these folds and on the rest of the inner surface are small projections called **villi.** Villi are from 0.5 to 1.5 mm high and are tightly packed at a density of 20 to 40/mm^2; they significantly increase the inner surface area of the intestine to about 15 times its original surface to enhance absorption.

Each villus in turn is covered with even smaller projections called **microvilli,** which are 1 μm high and are packed at a density of 200,000/mm^2; this further multiplies the absorptive surface, by a factor of 20, to an area of 300 times the original surface area. The surface of each villus is made of a layer of cells that is one cell thick. Some villi secrete mucus to protect the intestinal wall, but most function in digestion and absorption. Some produce hormones, and others produce immune substances that protect against toxins and infective substances in food.

The way in which the absorptive area is increased due to the structure of a villus is shown in Figure 2-3. Enzymes are embedded in the microvilli, where they carry out the final stage of digestion necessary for the absorption of nutrients. It is the epithelial (surface) cells of the microvilli that control absorption. They act either

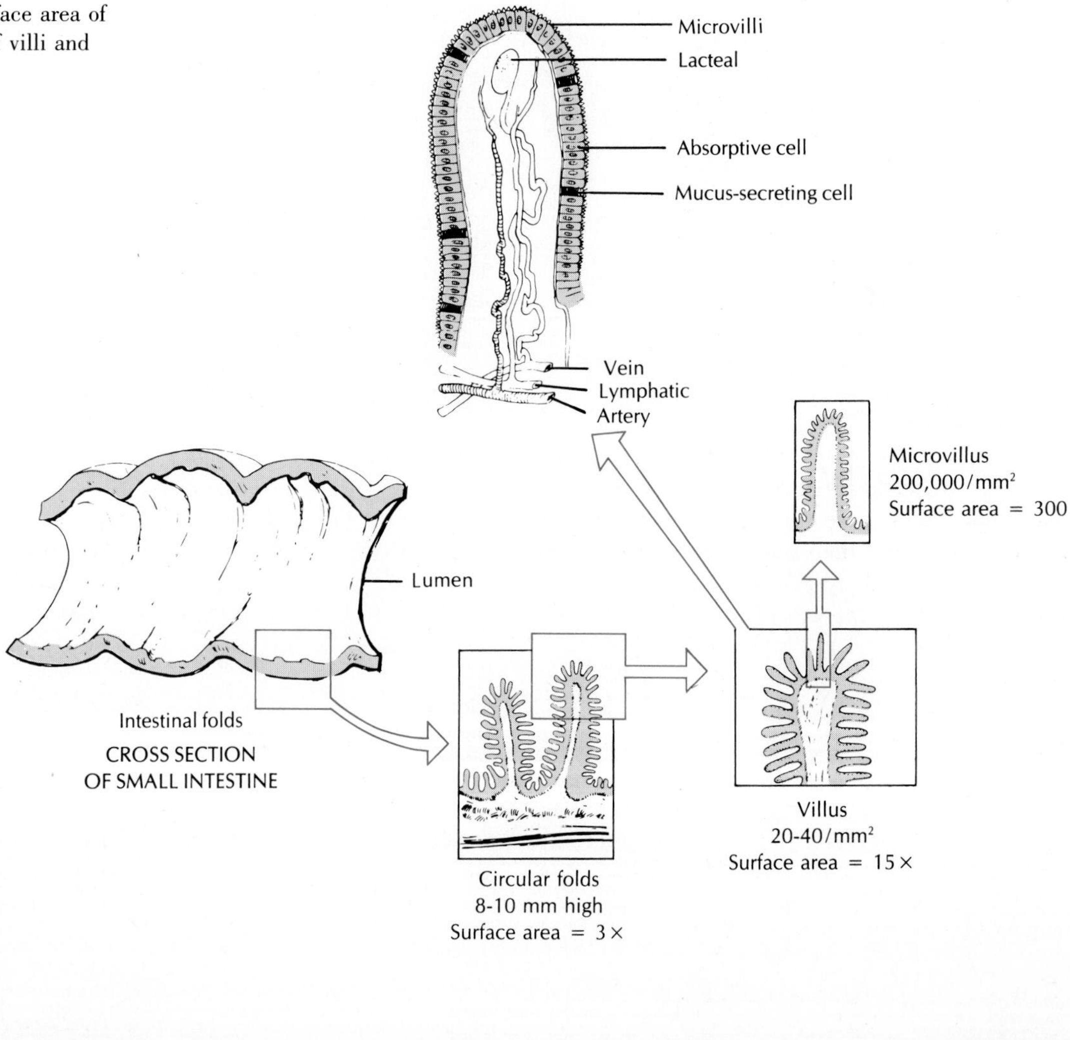

Figure 2-3 Increase in surface area of the intestinal wall because of villi and microvilli.

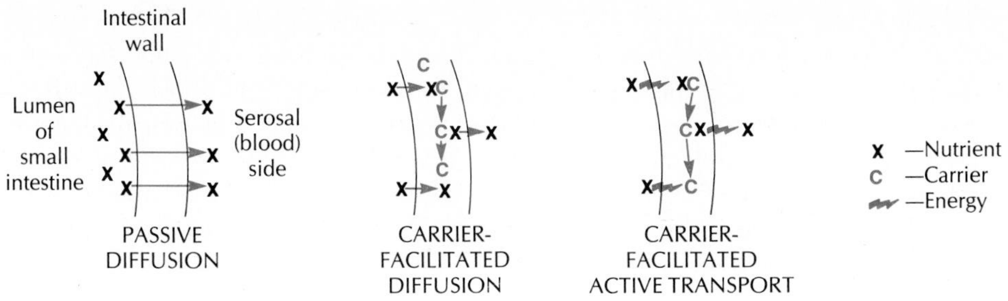

Nutrients are absorbed in three ways: passive diffusion, facilitated diffusion, or active transport.

by controlling the amount of the nutrient that is picked up from the digestive mass in the gastrointestinal digestive tract or the amount of the nutrient that is released into the blood. Some nutrients are transported rapidly and completely to the blood. In the case of many minerals and vitamins, the amount of the nutrient picked up and passed on is determined by the body's needs for the nutrient.The proportion in the diet that is absorbed is usually inversely related to the extent to which the body stores are satisfied, and vice versa.

Mechanisms of Absorption

Nutrients are absorbed in several ways: passive diffusion, facilitated diffusion, active transport, and osmosis. Only a small proportion of nutrients is absorbed by **passive diffusion,** the process by which nutrients travel from an area of higher concentration to one of lower concentration. Passive diffusion takes place when the concentration of the nutrient in the intestinal tract is higher than that in the blood; this occurs when the intake of a nutrient is especially high. Water is absorbed by **osmosis,** the process by which water is drawn across a cell membrane. (See Chapter 6.)

passive diffusion
Process by which a substance crosses a membrane from an area of high concentration to one of lower concentration; diffusion does not require energy or a carrier

osmosis
Process in which water enters or leaves a cell to establish equilibrium between the contents of the cell and its environments

facilitated diffusion or **active transport**
The process by which a substance is transported across a cell membrane using energy and usually a carrier protein specific to the nutrient

Most nutrients are absorbed either by **facilitated diffusion** or **active transport.** Both processes involve a carrier protein that picks up a nutrient on the outer (intestinal), or mucosal, side of an absorptive cell and transports it across the cell to release it on the inner, or serosal, side and from there to the blood. In addition, active transport usually requires energy and involves the exchange of sodium. Carrier proteins are used primarily for the absorption of a particular nutrient, as transferrin for iron, transmagnin for manganese, or retinol-binding protein for vitamin A. In some cases, two nutrients such as a pair of amino acids or iron and zinc may compete for the same carrier.

As nutrients are carried across the absorptive cells on the microvilli, most of them are released directly into the blood and carried in the portal vein directly to the liver. From there they go either to (1) cells that need them; (2) the kidneys, to be filtered and then either reabsorbed or excreted; or (3) storage sites such as the liver, the kidneys, and bone. Some nutrients—primarily lipids reformed in the absorptive cells and fat-soluble vitamin A—are released to the lacteals, or fat-collecting ducts. These ducts in turn merge into the secondary circulatory system, that is, the lymphatic system. From there they are dumped into the general circulation near the heart. In the blood, some of these fat-soluble nutrients are attached to carriers such as lipoproteins, which are produced in and released from the liver to make the nutrients more soluble in the aqueous medium of the blood. Others are taken up as fat globules or micelles with a thin protein layer to allow them to mix with water in the blood. They account for the milky appearance of blood after a high-fat meal. Other fat-soluble nutrients such as vitamin A attach to a protein; this makes them larger so they will not be filtered out by the kidneys.

The Large Intestine

ileocecal valve
The muscle separating the small intestine from the large intestine; it controls the passage of the digestive mass into the large intestine.

feces
The material, largely made up of dietary fiber and water, that is excreted through the anus from the large intestine

For discussion of diverticulitis, see Chapter 3

By the time the food mass passes through the **ileocecal valve** at the end of the small intestine to enter the large intestine, most nutrients have been absorbed. These include minerals and vitamins in addition to products of the digestion of carbohydrate, lipid, and protein. The remaining mass consists mostly of dietary fiber and water. Some of this is changed by the digestive action of microorganisms, in some cases producing gas as a by-product. As the mass continues through the 10-foot length of the large intestine, water is absorbed resulting in a progressively more solid mass until it reaches the anus as semisolid fecal matter, or **feces.** Dietary fiber retains some fluid, increasing the bulk of the stools and facilitating their passage through the colon. Lack of fiber results in hard, dry stools that are passed with difficulty, causing constipation and sometimes contributing to diverticulitis.

METABOLISM

anabolism
The metabolic process that causes the synthesis or formation of a new substance

catabolism
The metabolic process that causes the breakdown or destruction of a substance

waste products
End products of metabolism that need to be excreted from the body either in the feces, through the kidneys in the urine, or through the lungs

metabolism
All the chemical changes that occur in a nutrient once it is absorbed

epithelial cells
The cells on the outer surface of the body or lining all the internal passages in the body, including the gastrointestinal tract and respiratory tract

From the blood, nutrients are picked up by individual cells, where they undergo the biochemical changes known collectively as metabolism.

Metabolism of the energy-yielding nutrients carbohydrate, lipid, and protein includes two quite different processes: **anabolism,** in which the primary products of digestion are used to build body compounds and storage material; and **catabolism,** in which the products of digestion are broken down further, primarily as a source of energy. The metabolism of vitamins and minerals that are stored, built into essential body components, or used as part of enzymes or coenzymes will be discussed in the chapters that deal with each particular vitamin or mineral.

The **waste products** of cellular **metabolism**—that is, the products of the changes that occur once food is absorbed—and unused nutrients are released into the extracellular fluid. They enter the capillaries and then the veins of the bloodstream and are eventually excreted from the body, primarily through the lungs and kidneys.

Almost all of the carbon dioxide produced in the body and 10% of the water are excreted through the lungs. The kidneys act as an efficient and selective filtering system for the bloodstream. They are capable of concentrating waste products of metabolism in the urine and excreting them; they also allow excesses of nutrients such as water-soluble vitamins to leave the body. However, as the blood is filtered through them, the kidneys will reabsorb practically all of the glucose or protein, both of which the body must save or retain. For some other nutrients such as sodium, the kidney will reabsorb the amounts needed to maintain normal blood and tissue levels and will release the rest in the urine. The kidneys are extremely sensitive, regulating the nature and amount of the *metabolites*, or substances related to the nutrients, excreted in response to hormones and the body's need for particular nutrients.

Some nutrients are lost from the body through the skin—either in perspiration, as **epithelial cells** from the surface of the body, or as loss of hair and nails. Cells lining the intestinal tract are completely replaced every 3 to 4 days; the old cells that slough off are lost through the feces. The feces may also contain nutrients that are part of the digestive secretions, which are not reabsorbed. An analysis of the kinds and amounts of nutrients lost from the body in any of these ways can shed much light on the need for various nutrients and on the way in which they are changed in the body.

While the processes of digestion and absorption are much more complex than this discussion suggests, the student of nutrition can function quite adequately with this level of information. It is important to remember that food must enter through the mouth, but the products of digestion and metabolism are absorbed into the blood or are excreted, or leave the body, through the lungs (in the breath), the skin (as perspiration), the kidney (as urine), or the colon (as feces).

BY NOW YOU SHOULD KNOW

- Digestion of food takes place in the mouth, stomach, and small intestine and is accomplished by mechanical and chemical actions.
- All foods must be digested to be absorbed and used by the body for either anabolism or catabolism.
- Most absorption takes place in the small intestine.
- Enzymes and hormones respond to the presence of food in the gastrointestinal tract.
- The waste products of digestion leave the digestive tract through the large intestine.

STUDY QUESTIONS

1. Define and explain the following terms and their relationship to digestion: enzymes, duodenum, jejunum, ileum, liver, bile duct, portal vein, villi, and microvilli.
2. Compare and describe the difference between the small intestine and large intestine. Include in your comparison the size, shape, location, and function of the two organs.
3. How do the mouth and the small intestine differ in the way they mechanically digest foods?
4. What is the difference between anabolism and catabolism? Is digestion a catabolic or anabolic process?
5. What is the function of peristalsis? Where and when does it begin and end?
6. In your opinion which part of the intestinal tract is least essential? Why?

Applying What You've Learned

1. **Follow Your Food**

   Think about what you last ate. Trace what happened to that food from the time of ingestion to the time it became fecal waste.

2. **Hunger or Appetite?**

   Before you take your next bite of food ask yourself if you are eating out of hunger or appetite. If you were triggered to eat by the smell of food, sight of food, or even the time on the clock you were probably eating out of appetite. Begin now to become more aware of your reasons for eating. Make a simple Food/Mood Chart and record the foods you eat, time of day, where you were, who you were with, and what else you were doing. Over a few days you may see trends.

SUGGESTED READING

Fox SI: Human physiology, 2nd ed., Dubuque, IA, 1987, Wm C Brown.

This basic physiology text provides an introductory level overview of the human digestive system in a clear and succinct way. The descriptive material is well illustrated with simplified drawings to help in understanding even the most complex physiological processes. An excellent adjunct to the simple essentials presented in this chapter.

ADDITIONAL READINGS

Cashman MD: Principles of digestive physiology for clinical nutrition, Nutrition in Clinical Practice 1:241, 1986.

Crane RK: A perspective of digestive-absorptive function, American Journal of Clinical Nutrition 22:242, 1969.

Darby W: Nutrition: gastronomy, mythology or science? Nutrition Today, 2:4, Sept./Oct., 1986.

Friedman HI, and Nylund B: Intestinal fat digestion, absorption and transport, American Journal of Clinical Nutrition 33:1108, 1980.

Merhouf GM: Function of the gallbladder, Nutrition Today, p. 10, Jan./Feb., 1982.

Moog F: The lining of the small intestine, Scientific American, p. 154, Nov., 1981.

Phillips SF, and Stephen AM: The structure and function of the large intestine, Nutrition Today, p. 4, Nov., 1981.

FOCUS RDAs and U.S. RDA—What Do They Mean?

Throughout the text you will be seeing frequent reference to the Recommended Dietary Allowances, usually referred to as the RDAs. On a few occasions we will be referring to the proposed RDAs or dietary standards. In addition, if you look on food packages you will see the nutrient content expressed as a certain percentage of the U.S. RDA. This Focus is intended to sort out some confusion that may result from the use of these terms.

Since 1943 nutritionists have depended on the regular publication of the Recommended Dietary Allowances by the Food and Nutrition Board of the National Academy of Sciences as the "gold standard" to guide them in knowing the amount of essential nutrients to include in diets for their patients or for the public. They have come to expect to see revised tables and a book describing the rationale for the figures regularly every 5 years.

What are the "RDAs?" They are the best judgment of a group of nutrition scientists as to the amount of an essential nutrient that is needed on a daily average intake in the diet to meet the needs of almost all healthy people. They are more than generous for many people but can still be obtained from a carefully selected diet. When the first RDAs were published in 1943, standards were set for only energy and seven nutrients. Our knowledge of nutrition and nutrient requirements has increased to the point that we now have standards for energy and 17 nutrients. In addition, there is another group of 11 nutrients for which we know enough to now suggest "estimated safe and adequate intakes." We have been given a range of values for three age groups rather than a single value for each of 17 different age and sex groups. All of this information is taken into account when nutritionists set up a dietary guidance such as the "Basic Four."

What about the "U.S. RDA?" In 1974 the Food and Drug Administration was given the responsibility of finding a way of letting the public know the nutrient content of the food available in the grocery store. They decided to express it in relation to the RDAs with which people were already familiar as the goal to aim for. However, it soon become obvious that they could not list all 17 categories provided in the RDAs; thus, they decided to use one figure for each nutrient for everyone over 4 years of age who was not either pregnant or breastfeeding. For this they chose the highest recommendation for any age and sex group (almost always the recommendation for the adolescent male 15 to 18 years of age) and expressed the amount in the food as a percentage of that figure. Although the RDAs have changed twice since 1974, labeling has continued to be based on the 1974 RDAs. Since the changes have been minor for the adolescent male there would have been little impact on the label values had the standard changed. Any decision to change the standard every 5 years would impose a very heavy cost on the food industry in creating new labels and conducting new analyses, which would undoubtedly act as a deterrent to their using nutrient labeling. For current standards see Appendix C.

When the 1980 RDAs, the most recent ones (reprinted inside the front and back covers), were announced a new committee was appointed to prepare the 1985 RDAs (tenth edition). However, when the committee presented its report in 1985 the National Academy of Sciences found it unsatisfactory because it called for a lower allowance for vitamins A and C, which some people believed was not supported by the data. As of 1988 attempts were still being made to reconcile the differences to permit the publication of the new recommendations, which included many important and significant modifications beyond those in question. These included new age categories for infants and people over 50 years of age and an adjustment in the age categories for adolescent boys and girls, whose growth patterns differ between ages 10 and 18. Because we feel some of these are important to the interpretation of nutrient needs, and because there is a strong possibility that these will be released shortly after the publication of this text, we have included some of that information. Even if they are not published, it seems important for the reader to have the advantage of the thinking of this group, whose recommendations will at least be presented in other scientific publications. (Several reports on individual nutrients have been published in the *American Journal of Clinical Nutrition*, July, 1987.)

In addition to being used as goals for nutrient intakes of individuals, the RDAs have been used as a standard against which to compare actual nutrient intakes of individuals and populations to assess the probability that an intake is either adequate or inadequate. They are also used as criteria in setting standards for many of the food assistance programs in the United States and for feeding population groups such as the military, children in group care, and the elderly. As a result of these multiple uses the RDAs play a prominent role in both nutritional assessment and nutritional guidance. The RDAs have also been widely used by the 40 other countries who have established similar standards for their own populations.

In summary, the 1980 RDAs are the currently accepted standard. The proposed RDAs represent the recommendation of a more recent committee's evaluation of the nutrition science literature. The 1974 RDAs are the basis on which nutrient labeling standards (U.S. RDA) have been established.

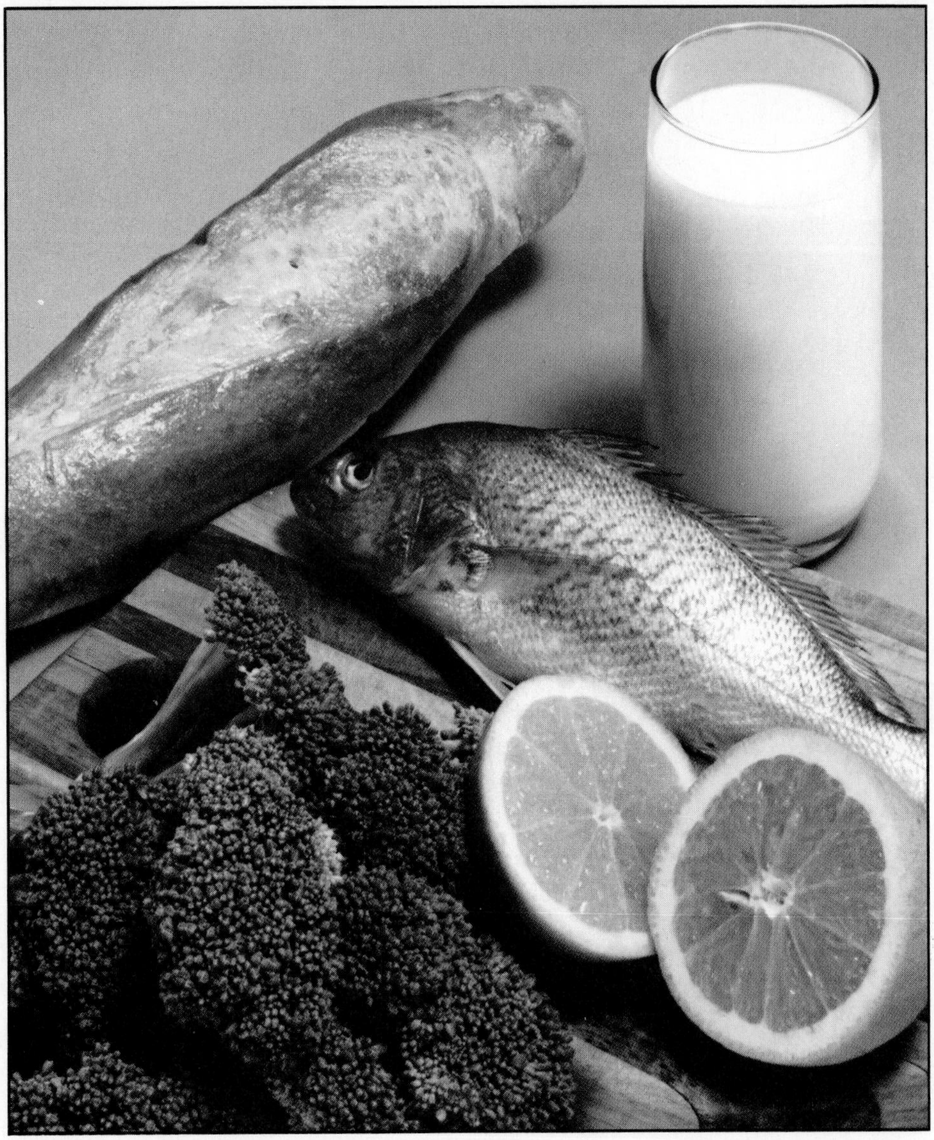

AWARENESS CHECK

Truth or Fiction?

- Healthy adults need at least 6 oz of meat or meat substitute a day.
- Eggs and butter are part of the milk or dairy group.
- Eliminating all fat from the diet is the best way to reduce one's risk for heart disease.
- One half cup of cottage cheese has the same amount of calcium as one half cup of milk.
- Everyone must take in 100% of their U.S. RDA for all nutrients to maintain good health.

Selection of an Adequate Diet

CHAPTER

3

Long before we had anything more than vague ideas of the dietary components and their relationship to health, we had some simple rules to guide us in making appropriate food choices. Today, with much more sophisticated knowledge about the need for vitamins and minerals and the interactions among them and concern about the balance of carbohydrate, lipid, and protein in the diet, dietary guidance has become a complex issue. Dietary guidelines are based on a consensus about our needs for various nutrients, the availability of good food-composition data, and knowledge of prevailing food practices and the influences supporting them. An ability to effectively communicate the information necessary to influence people's food behavior is essential.

An inventory of the references to nutrition in the media—radio, television, newspapers, magazines, and advertisements—gives convincing evidence of an increasing public interest in what should be eaten for optimal health. Interest in calories, sodium, calcium, cholesterol, fat, and sugar as they relate to health is widespread. Throughout this text, in addition to discussing why we need various nutrients, we will be concerned with three common questions: (1) How much of a particular nutrient do we need? (2) Where do we get this nutrient? and (3) How well do Americans select their foods to meet this nutritional need? To help you have a better understanding of discussions about these questions you will want to become familiar with major dietary standards, food guides, and surveys used in the United States.

DIETARY STANDARDS

Once it was established that nutrients were essential to human health, one of the important questions was, how much of a particular nutrient do we need? The first impetus to answer that question came with the threat of war in 1940, and a growing recognition that nutritional science, by giving us a scientific basis on which to make food choices, could make a contribution to national security. The United States had been appalled at the high rejection rate among young service recruits for reasons that could be attributed to suboptimal nutrition. Against this background, 25 scientists met in 1941 as the first Food and Nutrition Board of the National Research Council (NRC). They were asked to examine the available information on nutrient needs to decide if recommendations could be made to the public about the amount of various nutrients needed to maintain health in the majority of the population.

Once they had decided there was adequate information available, this group was charged with establishing dietary standards that could be used to evaluate the dietary intake of large population groups and to provide a rational guide for practical nutrition and for the planning of agricultural production. They agreed that they had insufficient information on nutritional needs to propose exact requirements and that the standard needed should reflect more than minimal needs. Board members believed that even if there were a good chance that the standards they proposed should later prove to be inaccurate, it was necessary to make the best possible estimate. Indeed, it was with the belief and hope that soon enough information would be available on which to revise them that they proposed the first standards.

RDAs
Recommended Dietary Allowances; see inside of front and back covers

Their deliberations resulted in the first **Recommended *Dietary* Allowances (RDAs),** published in 1943. They made recommendations regarding energy and eight nutrients for the healthy population. The term "recommended allowances" was purposely chosen (rather than "requirements") to emphasize that the RDAs are not final figures and need periodic updating as more data become available. Since its beginning, the RDAs have been revised eight times, with the most recent version released in 1980. These allowances represented the quantities of certain nutrients believed to be adequate to meet the known nutritional needs of practically all healthy persons in the United States. Because needs varied with age, sex, and body size, scientists classified the population into 17 age and sex categories, including pregnant and lactating women. The allowances did not represent average requirements, which would be adequate for only half the population, but were set approximately two standard deviations above the mean requirement, to take care of the needs of 97.5% of the population (Figure 3-1). These figures also included a margin of safety to take into account nutrient losses that might occur in cooking and storage of food and the range of requirements in the population, and to provide a buffer under stress conditions. Other factors considered were the stability of the nutrients, the body's ability to store the nutrient, the range of observed requirements,

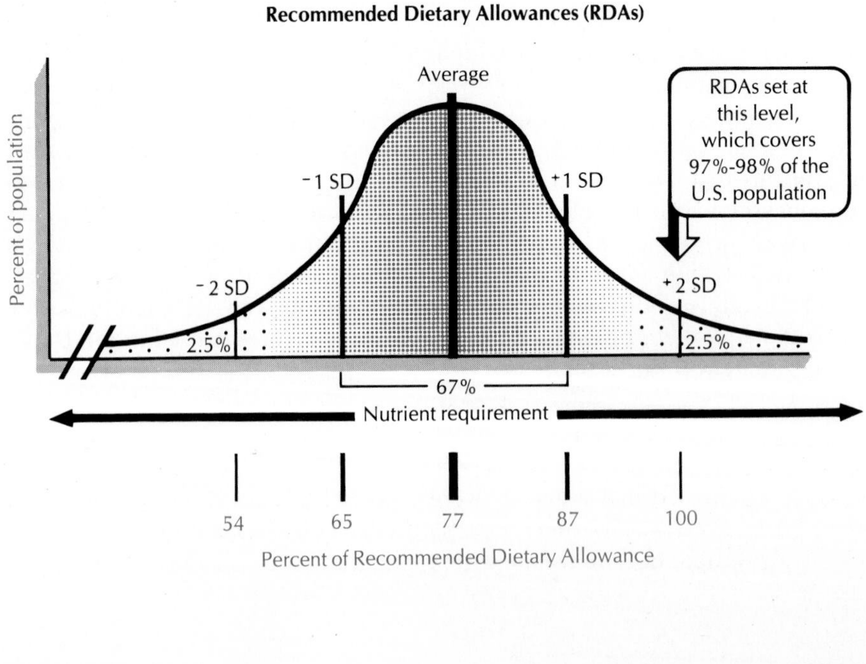

Figure 3-1 Distribution of actual nutrient requirements with coefficient of variation of 15% around the mean requirement.

RDA = Mean + (2 × Coefficient of variation, or SD [Standard Deviation])

RDA = Average requirement + (2 × SD [15%])

Average requirement = RDA × 100/130 = 77% RDA

the availability of the nutrient in the North American diet, the possible hazards from an excessive intake, and the difficulties involved in establishing precise requirements.

These allowances were used as goals in planning national food supplies and meals for large groups. Obviously, if the intake for a group met the RDAs, the amount available would be in excess of the needs of practically everyone in the group. Similarly, when they are used to assess the usual intake of an individual, it must be remembered that they are high for most people of a given age or sex. Thus a person who failed to have an intake at the recommended level would not necessarily be deficient in a nutrient. However, the more the intake falls below the RDA level, the greater the risk of suffering from a marginal or deficient intake. It is also possible that a small segment of the population will have needs *slightly* greater than the amounts suggested; however, this is infrequent unless there is a health problem causing increased need, increased losses, or poor absorption of a nutrient.

The task of determining dietary standards is still not an easy one. For some nutrients, very little information is available, especially to assess differing needs of different age and sex groups; for other nutrients, scientists are unsure about how to interpret the information we have; for still others there is such a wide range of apparent requirements that it is difficult to arrive at an acceptable figure. The data on which judgments are based are obtained from (1) surveys of food (and from that, nutrient) intake of large numbers of apparently healthy individuals, (2) surveys that included both food intake and nutritional status assessment, (3) controlled metabolic experiments with limited numbers of individuals, (4) relevant studies on several species of animals, and (5) epidemiological information about diet and disease in a population.

Improved analytical techniques and increased knowledge of the biological role of most nutrients have led to some change and to an increasing confidence in the recommended allowances. In addition, the number of nutrients considered has increased steadily. For instance, in 1980, for the first time scientists believed they had enough information to propose provisional dietary allowances expressed as estimated safe and adequate intakes for 12 additional nutrients for a restricted number of age and sex categories. The rationale by which the allowances are set is becoming more and more consistent from one nutrient to another. It is believed that the allowances provide a sufficient buffer in cases of nutritional stress but will not meet the additional requirements of persons whose reserves are depleted by disease.

For estimated safe and adequate intakes, see inside front cover

As a result, the RDAs as proposed in 1980 represented the best judgment of the committee for intakes of nutrients that would meet the needs of essentially all healthy people. There is no confirmed benefit from higher intakes. A coefficient of variation of 15% assumed for most biological measurements is used to arrive at an RDA that is believed will encompass the needs of essentially all healthy persons. If indeed it is set two standard deviations (30%) above the mean, then an intake of 77% (100/130) of the RDA would be an average requirement.

Originally it was emphasized that the allowances did not provide a criterion for judging the nutrient adequacy of an individual but only for a population group. They are now considered a reference point to judge the nutritional adequacy of individuals and the probability that any intake below the RDA will really be inadequate. Only when you have clinical, physical, or biochemical evidence of a nutrient lack is there a true deficiency. The lower the typical intake, the greater the probability that it will be inadequate for any one individual. Thus a major goal of the allowances is to encourage the development of food practices by the U.S. population that will provide the greatest dividends in health and resistance to disease.

Although the RDAs may represent neither a minimal nor an optimal level of intake, they have served several useful purposes. They provided a yardstick in planning diets for groups, and they have been widely used as a standard for evaluating individual diets. They have provided a nutrient guide for many nutrition-intervention programs, such as the school lunch, senior citizen congregate feeding, and Women, Infants, and Children (WIC) programs, and as a basis for formulating regulations governing the composition of foods, dietary supplements, and nutrient labeling. They are admittedly high for use under conditions of economic stringency or national emergencies, but under normal conditions they are a desirable and achievable goal.

DIETARY STANDARDS IN OTHER COUNTRIES

Many other countries have established dietary standards for their populations. Any appreciable difference in recommendations is usually explained by the criteria or philosophy used in establishing allowances rather than cultural differences in needs. For example, the Canadian standard is based on a sufficient excess above minimum requirements for the maintenance of health among the majority of Canadians. Variations are made for age, sex, body weight, and degree of activity. The **Recommended Nutrient Intakes for Canadians** are shown in Appendix D.

Recommended Nutrient Intakes for Canadians (RNI)
Estimates of nutrient needs of Canadians; see Appendix D

The British Medical Association, in establishing dietary standards for the United Kingdom, chose levels they believed represented the *average* needs of practically all healthy persons. United Kingdom standards tend to be lower for some nutrients than U.S. standards, although in a few instances they are the same, despite the differences in rationale behind them.

The Food and Agricultural Organization (FAO) of the United Nations, charged with devising a standard to meet the needs of fully active, healthy individuals that is equally applicable in all cultures, has worked with the World Health Organization (WHO) to assess available information. Thus far they have proposed *practical* allowances for energy (kilocalories), calcium, protein, thiamin, riboflavin, niacin, vitamin A, iron, vitamin C, folacin, vitamin D, and vitamin B_{12}. A comparison of the American, Canadian, United Kingdom, and FAO/WHO standards for adults is given in Table 3-1.

The terms *energy, kilocalories,* and *calories* are frequently used interchangeably in nutrition literature. Precise definitions will be provided in Chapter 7

DIETARY STANDARDS FOR LABELING FOOD PRODUCTS

As you develop a greater interest in nutrition, you will undoubtedly take a closer look at food labels. Thus, you will become familiar with the **U.S. RDA,** or **United States Recommended *Daily* Allowances,** a dietary standard seen on many food products used in the United States. It is frequently (and understandably) confused with the RDAs. Unlike the Recommended *Dietary* Allowance that proposes separate standards for 17 different age and sex groups, the U.S. RDA involves only one standard for everyone over age 4 except pregnant and lactating women. This system was proposed by the Food and Drug Administration (FDA) and is used solely for the nutrient labeling of processed food and drugs. In nutrient labeling, which is required only when a nutritional claim is made for a product on the label or in advertising or a nutrient has been added, the amount of the nutrient is expressed as a percentage of the U.S. RDA rather than in weights. For other foods, this labeling is voluntary. It would be not only utterly confusing but extremely cumbersome to list the separate standards for each age and sex group. In most cases the U.S. RDA is the highest of the RDAs for a particular nutrient (excluding the values for pregnant and lactating women). Because this standard is high for most people, it is not necessary for an individual to obtain 100% of the U.S. RDA to meet the appropriate RDA. In addition, because these standards are used by the FDA to identify any cases of mislabeling of food products, manufacturers have a tendency to "play it safe" by claiming amounts on the label that are somewhat below the amounts actually in the product. An example of the information provided on the label of food products is shown in Figure 3-2. The blocked area is the part that uses the U.S. RDA.

United States Recommended Daily Allowance (U.S. RDA)
Standards for nutrient intakes, used as the basis for nutrient labeling of foods and drugs; based on 1968 RDA (for details, see Appendix C)

The U.S. RDAs are listed in Appendix C.

Table 3-1 ◇ Comparison of United States (1980), United Kingdom (1980), Canadian (1983), and FAO/WHO (1957-1985) dietary standards for the adult male and adult female

Classification	Kcal	Protein (grams)	Calcium (grams)	Iron (mg)	Vitamin A (RE)	Thiamin (mg)	Riboflavin (mg)	Vitamin C (mg)
United States								
Female (55 kg, 1.63 m)	2000	44	0.8	18	800	1.1	1.3	60
Male (70 kg, 1.77 m)	2700	56	0.8	10	1000	1.4	1.6	60
United Kingdom								
Female	2150-2500	54-62	0.5	12	750	1.0	1.3	30
Male	2500-3350	63-84	0.5	10	750	1.0-1.3	1.6	30
Canada								
Female (55.8 kg)	2100	41	0.7	14	800	1.1	1.3	30
Male (71.1 kg)	3000	56	0.8	10	1000	1.5	1.8	30
FAO/WHO								
Female	2300	39	0.4-0.5	18	750	0.9	1.3	30
Male	3200	46	0.4-0.5	10	750	1.3	1.8	40

Nutrition information
(per serving)
Serving size = 8 oz
Servings per container = 2

Calories	**560**
Protein	**23 g**
Carbohydrate	**43 g**
Fat	**33 g**
Sodium (365 mg/100 g)	**810 mg**

Percent of kilocalories from fat = 53%

Polyunsaturated*	22 g
Saturated	9 g
Cholesterol* (18 mg/100 g)	40 mg

Percentage of U.S. Recommended Daily Allowance (U.S. RDA)

Protein	**35**	**Niacin**	**25**
Vitamin A	**35**	**Calcium**	**2**
Vitamin C	**10**	**Iron**	**25**
Thiamin	**15**	**Vitamin B_6**	**†**
Riboflavin	**15**	**Vitamin B_{12}**	**†**

*Information on fat and cholesterol content is provided for individuals who, on the advice of a physician, are modifying their total intake of fat and cholesterol.
†Contains less than 2% of the U.S. RDA for these nutrients.

Figure 3-2 Label format using U.S. RDA as standard (see Appendix C). Optional information in light type; mandatory information in boldface type.

Nutritional claims that Mandate Nutrient Labeling
- Lower in . . .
- Higher in . . .
- Less . . .
- Fortified with . . .
- No . . . added
- Reduced . . .

(where . . . is shown a nutrient is named)

Nutrient information is expressed as a percentage of the U.S. RDA, with amounts up to 10% being indicated in increments of 2% and amounts above 10% in increments of 5%. If any nutrition information is provided on the label, the label must then provide information on serving size and number per package and data on energy (calories) and weights of carbohydrate, fat, protein, and sodium. Data for protein, vitamin A, vitamin C, thiamin, riboflavin, niacin, calcium, and iron as a

Table 3-2 ◆ Interpretation of food label terms

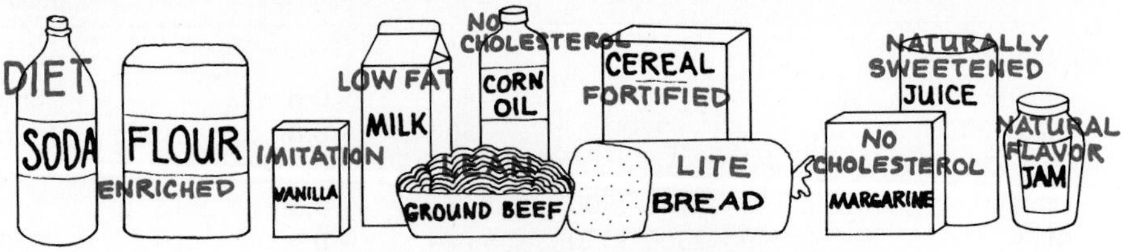

Label Terms	Meaning
Diet or dietetic	Contain no more than 40 calories per serving or have at least one-third fewer calories than the regular product
Enriched or fortified	Contains added vitamins and/or minerals
Imitation	Nutritionally inferior to the regular product
Substitute	Nutritionally equivalent to the regular product
Lean	Used for meat and poultry; means no more than 10% fat by weight
Extra lean	No more than 5% fat by weight
Light or lite	Can refer to light in color, sodium, calories, or fat
Low calorie	No more than 40 calories per serving or 0.4 calorie per gram
Low fat	For dairy products, between 0.5% and 2% milk fat; for meat, no more than 10% fat by weight
Natural	Meat and poultry, which are under control of the USDA, can have no artificial flavors, colors, preservatives, or synthetic ingredients of any kind if labeled "natural." For any other product, which is under the control of FTC and FDA, the term "natural" has no meaning
Naturally flavored	Essential oil, extract, or other derivative of a juice, spice, herb root, leaf, or other natural source; it does not mean there are no artificial colors, preservative, or other additives
Naturally sweetened	No regulation, but manufacturers use it when they use fruit or juice in place of sugar
New	Used for 6 months to indicate new or changed
No cholesterol	Indicative of only cholesterol. May contain saturated fats. Cholesterol is only found in animal foods; thus plant foods such as peanut butter or spaghetti are naturally without cholesterol.
Cholesterol free	Less than 2 mg cholesterol per serving
Low cholesterol	Less than 20 mg cholesterol per serving
Cholesterol reduced	Food product reformulated to reduce cholesterol by at least 75% (i.e. may not have more than 25% of cholesterol in food for which it is a substitute)
No preservatives	Only indicative of preservatives; can have other additives such as sweeteners, flavors, or colors
Organic	Used without any guidelines, thus no meaning
Reduced calorie	One-third fewer calories than the standard product; label must include comparison of the two products
Salt free	Less than 5 mg of sodium per serving
Very low sodium	No more than 35 mg of sodium per serving
Low sodium	Contains no more than 140 mg of sodium per serving
Reduced sodium	Sodium level is reduced by at least 75%
Unsalted, salt free, no salt added, without added salt	No salt added during processing, but product can contain naturally occurring sodium
Sugar free or sugarless	Cannot contain table sugar (sucrose) but can contain other sweeteners such as honey or corn syrup
Whole wheat or whole grain	Whole wheat should be first ingredient listed on the ingredient list

percentage of the U.S. RDA must also be supplied. Data may also be provided on 12 other nutrients—zinc, pyridoxine, magnesium, folic acid, vitamin D, vitamin E, vitamin B_{12}, phosphorus, iodine, biotin, copper, and pantothenic acid—as well as other dietary components such as cholesterol, dietary fiber, added sugar, and types of fatty acids. Since July 1975, any label information on nutritive value has conformed to the format shown in Figure 3-2. Nutrients for which the amount is less than 2% of the U.S. RDA can be identified by an asterisk and a footnote, indicating that they were present in this insignificant amount. Because this labeling standard is the highest amount recommended for any age group, it is generous for the majority of the population.

Nutrient labeling is applicable only to labeling foods whose composition can be carefully controlled, such as processed foods, bread, and milk. Because of the great variability in nutrient content of fresh foods, information may not yet be provided on fresh fruits and vegetables, meat, fish, poultry, or eggs at the point of purchase. The first test of providing information on these products was carried out in 1984, but so far there is no legislation permitting it. Currently, about half the processed foods in the grocery store carry nutritional information. Many manufacturers are adding this information, even though they do not need to, because it satisfies the consumer's right to know the nutritional value of food. Nutrient labeling information can be used to compare different brands or to choose among comparable products but not to assess the total nutrient content of meals. There is little information about how much of the mandatory information is understood by the consumer, but it appears that if the system is to be fully effective it must be accompanied by a constant education campaign.

Because it is now permissible to make nutrition-related claims on packages and in advertising, consumers must learn to recognize what some of these labels such as "low sodium" or "no cholesterol" actually mean (Table 3-2).

Selecting an adequate diet. Information on the nutritive value of available foods is essential to help us judge their contribution to nutritive needs and to help us select an adequate diet. As methods of food processing vary, as requirements of additional nutrients are proposed, and as fabricated foods (that is, man-made foods such as "meat" products from soybeans) appear on the market, the whole process of eating to achieve good nutrition becomes increasingly complex. In general we approach it either from a food base, with emphasis on selecting certain food groups, or from a nutrient base, with concern for achieving recommended levels of nutrients. Both play a role in helping us make appropriate food selections; clearly neither alone will be totally satisfactory.

FOOD-BASED GUIDANCE

Five Food Groups

Attempts to translate scientific knowledge of nutrient needs into food guides to help individuals and families select an adequate diet go back as far as 1916. By that year, belief that humans needed the five nutrient classes—protein, starch, carbohydrate, and fat for energy, and mineral substances, plus organic acids and sugars—led to assurances to the public that if these were included, a diet would provide not only the materials needed for body fuel and building and repair, but also the "unknown" essentials.

Later, as specific minerals and vitamins were identified as essential, the emphasis in food selection guides shifted from providing adequate calories and body-building protein to providing specific vitamins and minerals. This led to the designation of foods that provided these nutrients as **protective foods.**

protective foods
Those foods that provide significant amounts of vitamins, minerals, and protein, in addition to calories

Basic Seven

The importance of good nutrition in protecting the nation's health was recognized in 1941 through the publication of the first RDAs. To guide the public, which had little scientific knowledge of food composition, in selecting a diet that would meet the RDAs, the Bureau of Home Economics published a food guide in which it recommended that certain classes of foods be included in the diet in specified amounts. These recommendations formed the foundation for the Basic Seven, promoted as part of the National Wartime Nutrition Program of the Department of Agriculture in 1943. This familiar guide, presented in Table 3-3, was the basis of practically all nutrition education programs from 1943 until its revision in 1956.

While the United States was promoting the seven-group plan, many other countries were developing plans designed to accomplish the same educational objective using three, four, or five groups. All plans stressed the importance of variety and of balancing the proportion of nutrient-dense foods with those that provided primarily energy.

Basic Four

In 1956 the United States Department of Agriculture (USDA) recommended that the seven-group plan be replaced by a simpler, less detailed four-group plan, presented first as *Essentials of an Adequate Diet* but soon designated as the "Basic Four." This plan, shown in Table 3-3, differed from the Basic Seven only in that the three fruit and vegetable categories were grouped as one, and the fat group was eliminated entirely. The elimination of the fat group was justified on the grounds that the use of foods from the other groups usually led to the use of fat (butter, salad dressing, oil, etc.) to improve flavor and palatability. In addition, the change was made at a time of developing concern about the role of increased fat consumption in coronary heart disease. The USDA did not want to find itself encouraging the consumption of a food that might later prove to be the villain in a degenerative disease.

Table 3-3 ◇ Comparison of United States food guides—1916, 1943, 1956, 1979, and 1984*

Five Food Groups 1916†	Basic Seven 1943†	Basic Four 1956†	Hassle-Free Food Guide 1979†	Food Wheel, 1984‡
Milk, meat, fish, poultry, eggs, and meat substitutes	Milk and milk products (2) Meat, fish, etc. (2), eggs (4 per week)	Milk and milk products (2) Meat, fish, poultry, eggs (2)	Milk-cheese group (2-4) Meat, poultry, fish, beans, eggs (2)	Milk, cheese, yogurt (2) Meat, fish, poultry, eggs (2-3)
Fruits and vegetables	Green and yellow vegetables (1) Citrus fruit and raw cabbage (1) Potatoes, other fruit and vegetables (2)	Fruits and vegetables (4)	Fruits and vegetables (4)	Fruits (2-4) Vegetables (3-5)
Bread and other cereal foods	Bread, flour, cereal (enriched or whole grain) (3)	Bread, flour, cereal (enriched or whole grain) (4)	Whole grain bread and cereal (4)	Bread, whole grain cereals (6-11)
Butter and wholesome fats	Equivalent of 2 tablespoons butter or fortified margarine			
Simple sugars			Fats, sweets, alcohol (caution)	Fats, sweets, alcohol (moderation)

*Recommended number of servings per day in parentheses.
†Foundation diet.
‡Total diet.

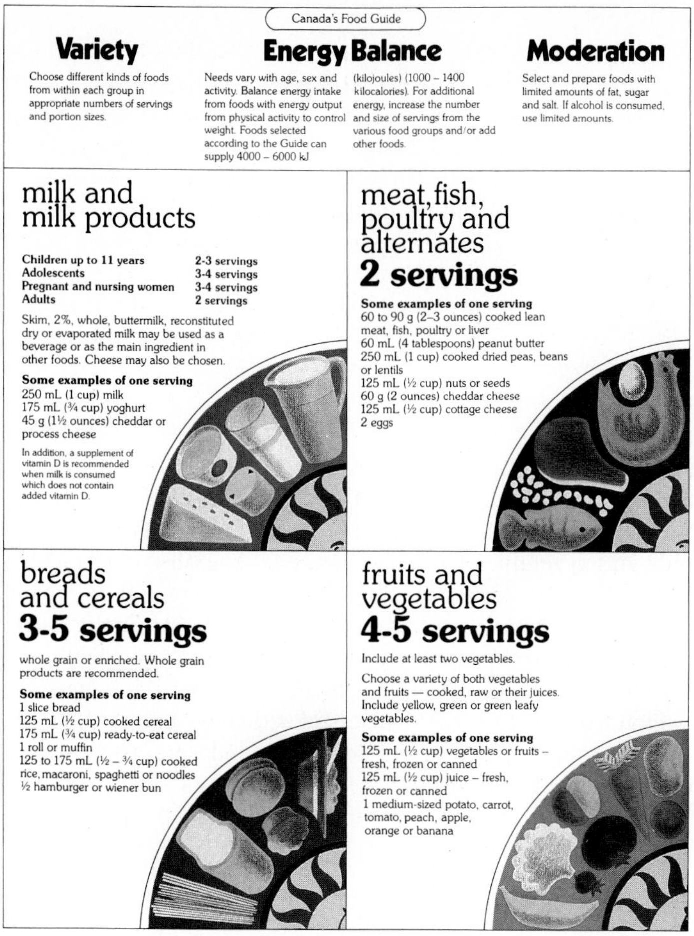

Figure 3-3 Canada's Food Guide.
From "Canada's Food Guide," Health and Welfare Canada, 1983, and reproduced with permission of the Minister of Supply and Services Canada.

The purpose of the Basic Four was "to translate what is known about nutritional requirements and the composition of foods into a workable plan that will help people select the kinds and amounts of foods that will give a nutritionally good diet." The plan, which provided approximately 1200 to 1400 kcal and 80% of the RDA for the eight nutrients for which standards had been published, allowed for diversity of food preferences and eating patterns because choices within food groups were unlimited. Similarly, the *Food Guide for Canada* (Figure 3-3) is based on information about needs and sources of nutrients, but it differs from the Basic Four mainly in the number of servings recommended.

In both cases it was assumed that the foods recommended would form the foundation of an adequate diet and that the foods chosen to provide additional calories would contribute some other nutrients, to bring the total close to recommended levels. Recent research has confirmed this assumption. It has shown that when all four groups are present in the recommended number of servings, resulting diets have a nutrient content over 80% of the RDA for over 80% of the population for the 12 nutrients for which standards and food composition data are now available. Even diets with all food groups represented, and half the number of recommended servings, provided 80% of the RDA in over 60% of the 21,000 diets analyzed. Based on 1980 RDAs, vitamin B_6, calcium, vitamin A, vitamin C, folacin, iron, zinc, and magnesium were most likely to be present in limited amounts in relation to needs.

Problem Nutrients in U.S. diet
Vitamin A
Vitamin C
Vitamin B_6
Folacin
Calcium
Iron
Magnesium
Zinc

Based on data from NFCS 1977-78, USDA, Washington, D.C., 1987.

Hassle-Free Guide

In 1979, in response to criticisms that the Basic Four did not reflect expanding knowledge about nutrient needs or prevailing food patterns, the USDA published a slighly modified version known as the Hassle-Free Guide. This plan emphasized whole-grain rather than enriched cereals and stressed legumes as a reasonable substitute in the protein group. In support of this plan, an attractive publication, *Food*, was prepared, emphasizing reduced sugar, fat, calories, and sodium, and increased fiber. The addition of a fifth group recognized that people use fats, sweets, and alcohol. This was done not to encourage their use but to draw attention to the need to consider them in dietary planning and use them only in moderation, if at all.

Food Wheel

In 1984 the American Red Cross, working in collaboration with the USDA, promoted a food guidance plan called the *Food Wheel, a Pattern for Daily Food Choices* (Figure 3-4) to meet total nutrient needs. It included five major food groups (Table 3-3) with fruits and vegetables treated separately. A sixth group, alcohol, fats, and sweets, was to be used in moderation. It was designed not only to provide adequate amounts of vitamins, minerals, and protein, but also to stress the use of fiber-rich whole grains, fruits, and vegetables and limit calories from fat to 35% of total energy. It was found that to accomplish these goals, an adult needed more than 2200 kcal, which exceeds the energy needs of sedentary adults. If sedentary adults choose to consume the upper level of recommended servings, they may need to increase their energy expenditure.

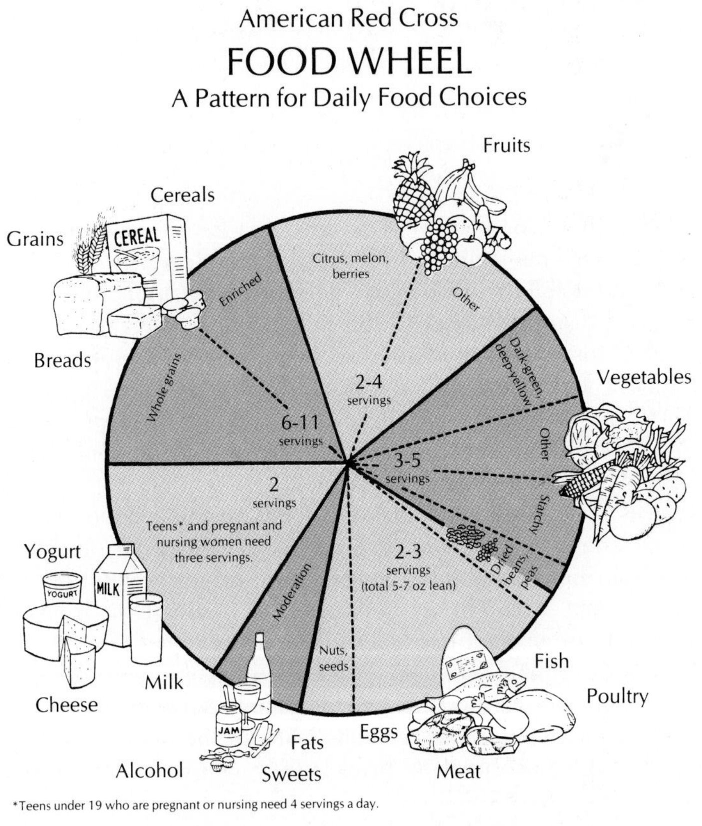

Figure 3-4 The Food Wheel—a pattern for daily food choices, developed in 1984 through the collaboration of the American Red Cross and the USDA.
From USDA, Human Nutrition Information Service, Administrative Report No. 377, Hyattsville, MD, 1985.

NUTRIENT-BASED GUIDANCE

Dietary Goals

About the same time (the late 1970s) that the USDA was issuing modifications of its food guidance material, the Senate Select Committee on Nutrition and Human Needs issued a document entitled *Dietary Goals for the United States*, focusing on the role of diet in several "killer" diseases—hypertension, coronary heart disease, obesity, diabetes, and cancer—and in the incidence of tooth decay. As a result they were primarily nutrient based, dealing with the distribution of calories from the macronutrients, carbohydrate, lipid, and protein and with the amount of saturated fat, cholesterol, sodium, and sugar in the diet. Their original recommendations were slightly modified 10 months later, as follows:

- **To avoid overweight, consume only as much energy (kilocalories) as is expended; if overweight, decrease energy intake and increase energy expenditure.**
- **Increase the consumption of complex carbohydrates and "naturally occurring" sugars from about 28% of energy intake to about 48% of energy intake.**
- **Reduce overall fat consumption from approximately 40% to 30% of energy intake.**
- **Reduce saturated-fat consumption to account for about 10% of total energy intake, and balance that with polyunsaturated and monounsaturated fats, which should account for about 10% of energy intake each.**
- **Reduce cholesterol consumption to about 300 mg a day.**
- **Reduce consumption of refined and processed sugars by about 45% to account for about 10% of total energy intake.**
- **Decrease consumption of salt and foods high in salt content to provide 5 grams or less.**

The following chapters will enhance your understanding of these recommendations

It is generally agreed that the goals suggest the following changes in food selection and preparation:

- **Increase consumption of fruits and vegetables and whole grains.**
- **Decrease consumption of animal fat and choose poultry and fish, which will reduce saturated fat.**
- **Decrease consumption of foods high in total fat and partially replace saturated fats with unsaturated fats.**
- **Except for children under 2, substitute low-fat and nonfat milk for whole milk and low-fat dairy products for high-fat dairy products.**
- **Decrease consumption of butterfat, eggs, and other high cholesterol sources. Some consideration should be given to easing the cholesterol-reduction goal for premenopausal women, young children, and the elderly to obtain the nutritional benefits of eggs in the diet.**
- **Decrease consumption of refined and other processed sugars and foods high in such sugars.**
- **Decrease consumption of salt and foods high in salt content.**

A comparison of the goals with current dietary practices is presented in Figure 3-5.

Almost simultaneously, a National Institutes of Health consensus group recommended a reduction in total intake of fat to 30% of calories, of saturated fat to 10% of calories, and of cholesterol to 250 to 300 mg/day to reduce the risk of coronary heart disease. Essentially the same recommendations have been made by the American Heart Association, the National Cancer Institute, and the American Diabetes Association. Another report from the National Academy of Sciences sug-

Recent Dietary Guidance

1977	Dietary Goals
1979	Dietary Goals (revised) Senate Select Committee on Food, Nutrition and Health Hassle-Free Diet (USDA) Healthy People (Surgeon General)
1980	Toward Healthful Diets (National Academy of Science)
1982	Diet and Cancer (National Academy of Sciences)
1984	Food Wheel—A Pattern for Daily Food Choices (USDA—American Red Cross)
1985	Nutrition and Your Health: Dietary Guidelines for Americans (USDA and DHHS), revised
1988	Surgeon General's Report (DHHS)
1989	Diet and Health (NAS)

cruciferous vegetable
Any vegetable in the cabbage family; includes cabbage, broccoli, and cauliflower

gested that 60% of cases of cancer were diet related. They urged increased consumption of fiber, complex carbohydrate, and **cruciferous vegetables** (broccoli and other members of the cabbage family) and a reduction in fat consumption from the current average of 43% to 35% of caloric intake. Another panel on the health implications of obesity concluded that obesity is clearly associated with hypertension, elevated blood cholesterol levels, diabetes, certain cancers, and other medical problems. This panel urged that weight be maintained at levels no more than 20% above desirable weight for height.

The implications of these recommendations are significant and far-reaching for nutrition intervention programs and for individuals. Thus they have been the subject of extensive and often acrimonious debate among nutrition scientists and educators. Some support these goals and recommendations, whereas others believe they were based on inadequate evidence, could not be implemented, or might even be counterproductive.

For a comparison of recommended dietary guidance from various government and health groups, see Chapter 21

The 1980 report, *Toward Healthful Diets*, from the Food and Nutrition Board of the National Academy of Sciences, urged Americans to consume a varied diet in moderation and maintained that there was inadequate information on the consequences of modifying the macronutrient intake to make specific recommendations.

These concerns about the relation of nutrition to health are not limited to the United States. In 1983 the British Health Education Council followed suit and published a paper, "Proposals for Nutritional Guidelines for Health Education," in Britain. The council suggested an average fat intake of 30% of calories, with saturated fat providing 10%; a reduction in sugar intake to 44 pounds per year; increased intake of fiber to 30 grams per day; and decreased intake of salt (3 grams per day) and alcohol (4% of calories); they made no recommendation for cholesterol.

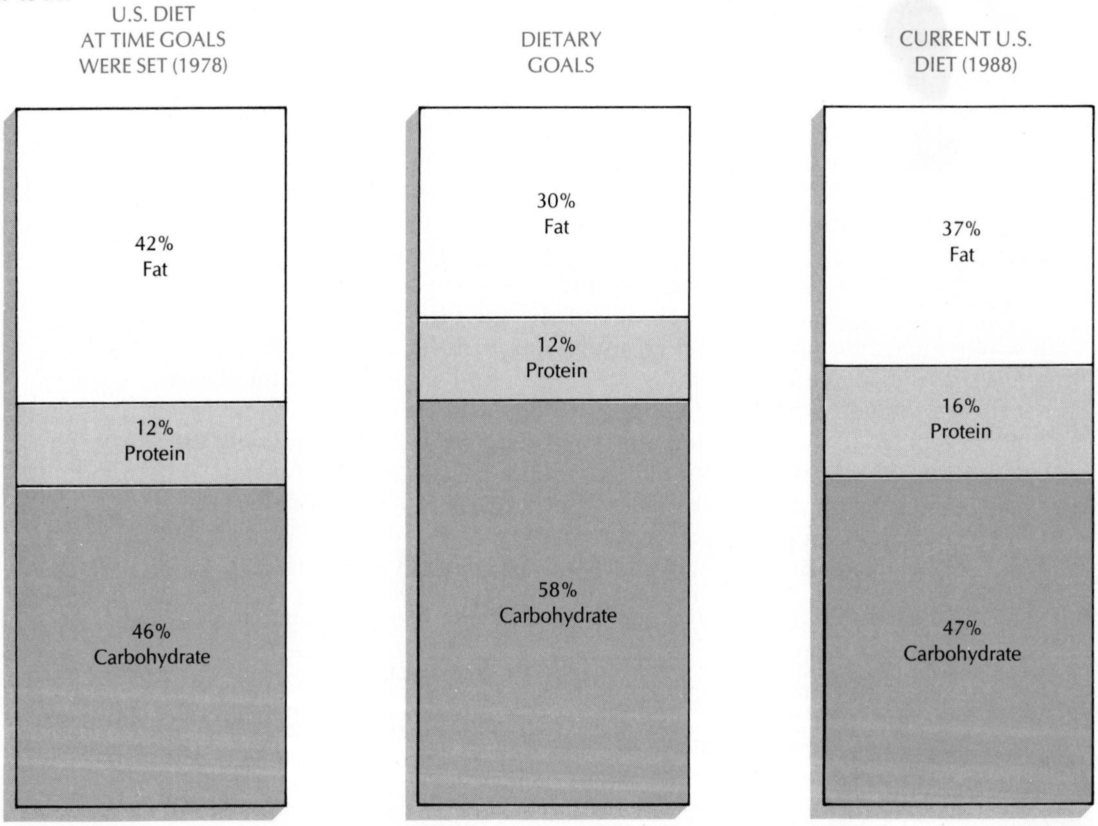

Figure 3-5 Comparison of current North American diet with the diet proposed in "Dietary Goals of the United States."

Like the U.S. plan, it stirred considerable debate as to whether there is sufficient information on which to base recommendations.

Following some debate surrounding the dietary goals and concern that they were overly specific, the Department of Health and Human Services (DHHS) and the USDA jointly published a new set of guidelines, *Nutrition and Your Health: Dietary Guidelines for Americans*. This document recommended certain dietary changes but did not provide specific numerical goals. It was a landmark document, representing the first time these two agencies had collaborated to provide nutritional guidance. An expert panel of nutritionists appointed in 1984 reviewed the guidelines and endorsed a slightly modified version, depicted in Figure 3-6. As is evident, these guidelines focus on macronutrients rather than on vitamins and minerals and reflect a growing concern that overnutrition is a significant health problem.

In 1987, the American Dietetic Association believed there were enough unique nutritional requirements for women to warrant the development of a set of guidelines to improve women's diets and decrease their risk of disease. Specifically, the American Dietetic Association recommended that women:

- **Eat a variety of foods from all the major food groups**
- **Maintain healthy body weight**
  - **—To lose weight safely and effectively: don't go below 10 calories per pound of present weight and don't skip meals; increase physical activity (exercise)**
  - **—To gain weight, increase calorie intake and exercise in moderation**
- **Exercise regularly**
- **Limit total fat intake to less than ⅓ of total calories per day**
- **Eat at least half of your daily calories from carbohydrates, with an emphasis on complex carbohydrates**
- **Eat a variety of foods rich in fiber**
- **Include 3 to 4 servings of calcium-rich foods per day**
- **Include plenty of iron-rich foods**
- **Limit intake of salt and sodium-containing foods**
- **If you drink alcohol, limit your intake to 1 to 2 drinks per day (the amount of alcohol in one drink is equivalent to 12 oz of beer, 5 oz of wine, or 1½ oz of distilled spirits)**
- **Avoid smoking**
- **If you have questions about the adequacy of your diet, see a registered dietitian**

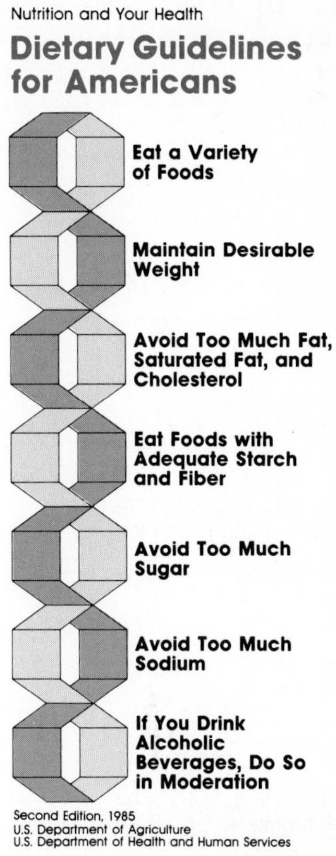
Nutrition and Your Health
Dietary Guidelines for Americans
Eat a Variety of Foods
Maintain Desirable Weight
Avoid Too Much Fat, Saturated Fat, and Cholesterol
Eat Foods with Adequate Starch and Fiber
Avoid Too Much Sugar
Avoid Too Much Sodium
If You Drink Alcoholic Beverages, Do So in Moderation
Second Edition, 1985
U.S. Department of Agriculture
U.S. Department of Health and Human Services

Figure 3-6 Nutrition and Your Health—Dietary Guidelines for Americans.
HHS/USDA, Washington, D.C., 1985.

NUTRITIVE CONTRIBUTION OF FOOD GROUPS

The selection of the food groupings used in the various food guides was based primarily on the unique nutritive contributions of the foods classified in each group. For instance cereals, which are fairly similar in their nutritive contribution, fall together as a natural food grouping. Similarly, fruits are dependable sources of some nutrients and poor sources of others, so it makes sense that we advise the public to include them in the diet for the nutrients that they provide in significant amounts. The following section provides an overview of the unique nutritional features of the usual food groupings. The details of food sources of specific nutrients and how stable they are under usual conditions of storage and food preparation will be discussed in the individual nutrient sections throughout the book. Slight differences in the number and size of servings recommended merely reflect various interpretations and objectives. Also, any small variations in food composition data from one table to another should not be cause for concern.

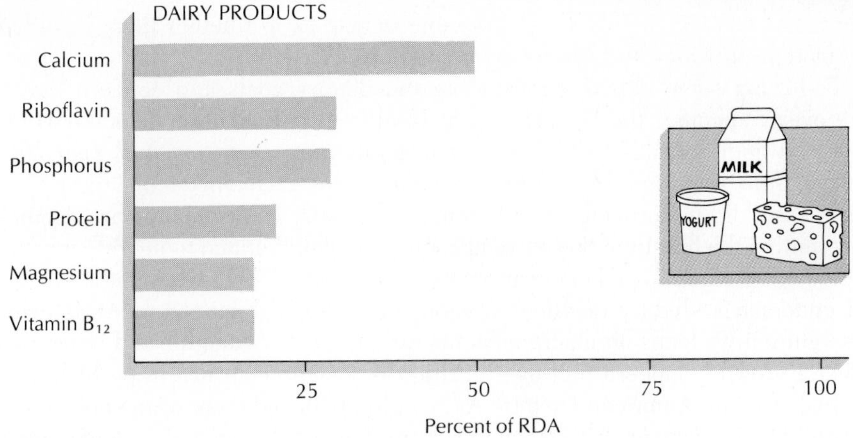

Figure 3-7 Major contributions of nutrients in the milk group to the RDAs.

Milk Products
Cheese
Yogurt
Cottage cheese
Ice cream

Whole milk	>3.2% fat
Low-fat milk	2.0% fat
Nonfat milk, Buttermilk, Skim milk	<0.5% fat

Milk and Milk Products

As shown in Figure 3-7, the major nutrient contributions of the milk group are calcium (which is almost impossible to obtain in sufficient amounts from other sources alone), riboflavin, phosphorus, high-quality protein providing all nine essential amino acids, magnesium, and vitamin B_{12}. Although exposure to sunlight reduces the riboflavin content of milk by as much as 50%, the use of opaque plastic containers and paper cartons has practically eliminated this loss, leaving milk as a dependable source. Milk is a poor source of iron and vitamin C.

The recommendation that the equivalent of at least 2 cups of milk be used by an adult can be satisfied in many ways. The use of low-fat or nonfat milk, with 2% and less than 0.5% fat, respectively, in place of whole milk, with at least 3.2% fat, will reduce its contribution of energy and saturated fat. Chocolate milk has a slightly higher caloric value than whole milk but otherwise has the same nutritive value. Chocolate drink has the same nutritive value as nonfat milk.

Cottage cheese may be an undependable source of calcium; good if it is made in a way that keeps the calcium in the curd and not if it is made so that calcium in the liquid whey, which is discarded. It is however a consistently good source of protein. Cheese has a nutritive value comparable to the milk from which it is made, but, depending on the method of processing, some nutrients may be lost in whey. With cheese (as with milk) the protein, calcium, and riboflavin contents increase as the fat content decreases. Ice cream, when substituted for milk as a source of calcium, contains only half as much calcium per kilocalorie. This energy increase is due to added sugar and a higher butterfat content. Commercially prepared yogurt often has the fat removed and replaced by nonfat milk, giving a product with high milk sugar and calcium content. Yogurt with fruit may have up to 50% of the milk replaced by the fruit and sugar, thus reducing calcium and other nutrients and increasing calories. Sour cream, cream, and butter do not qualify for this group because of the high fat content and low nutrient density.

The per capita consumption of dairy products has been declining slowly but steadily since 1960, despite an increase in the sales of yogurt, low-fat milk, and cheese. The decline has been attributed to concern about obesity and blood cholesterol levels, lack of understanding of the nutritive value of milk, competition from other beverages, and the development of dairy substitutes.

Fruits and Vegetables

The recommendation that the diet contain four servings of fruits and vegetables does not emphasize the choices to be made within this group. Because foods in this group vary so much in nutritional value, nutrition education programs promote the use of one serving of a citrus fruit or another fruit or vegetable high in ascorbic acid every day and a serving of dark green, yellow, or orange vegetables as a source of vitamin A every other day. Because of the low caloric content of this group of foods, they can be considered relatively good sources of vitamins C, A, and B_6 and iron. In addition, valuable amounts of folacin, magnesium, calcium, and dietary fiber will be contributed (see Figure 3-8).

Citrus Fruits
Oranges
Lemons
Grapefruit
Limes

A 6-oz serving of fruit juice is considered an average serving, although in practice many people use 4- or 8-oz servings. Citrus juices are generally rich sources of vitamin C, but other fruit juices provide varying amounts. Emphasis should be placed on those juices that provide at least 30 mg of vitamin C in a 4-oz portion, especially if the diet contains no other rich source. Many juices, such as apple and grape juice, that are naturally low in vitamin C are now fortified at this level. Fortification with acerola, a vitamin C–rich tropical fruit, has no advantage over fortification with synthetic vitamin C.

Other seasonal fruits rich in vitamin C are strawberries, cantaloupe, and cherries; among vegetables, broccoli, asparagus, spinach, and cabbage are important sources, especially when they are served raw or prepared in a way that minimizes nutrient losses.

Because relatively few of the dark green or yellow fruits and vegetables that are rich sources of vitamin A are used on a daily basis, and because the vitamin is stored in the body, a realistic approach to food guidance suggests the use of these foods every other day. This is additionally justified because of the stability of vitamin A and because foods that are rich sources usually provide more than the day's allowance in one serving. Thus a daily intake of foods high in vitamin A value, although desirable, is not absolutely necessary. The vitamin A value of typical dark green and yellow vegetables increases as the color becomes more intense. The practice of using butter, margarine, or salad oil to enhance the flavor of vegetables is desirable, because fat enhances the absorption of vitamin A.

Aside from the unique contributions of vitamins A and C, the fruit and vegetable group contributes about 25% of the day's requirement of iron. The amount of iron varies with the foods and parts chosen: iron content is higher in leaves than in stems, fruits, or underground portions. Calcium intake from fruits and vegetables is small compared with that from the milk group but will assume more importance if milk intake is low. The vitamin C in fruits and vegetables offers additional benefit by facilitating iron and calcium absorption.

The trace mineral content of fruits and vegetables depends on the amount present in the soil in which the plant was grown. The diverse geographical sources of fruits and vegetables and modern systems of transporting produce to market reduce the chance of a low intake. If peas or beans are chosen, a rich source of thiamin is provided, and if dark green leafy vegetables such as spinach are used, riboflavin intake will be high.

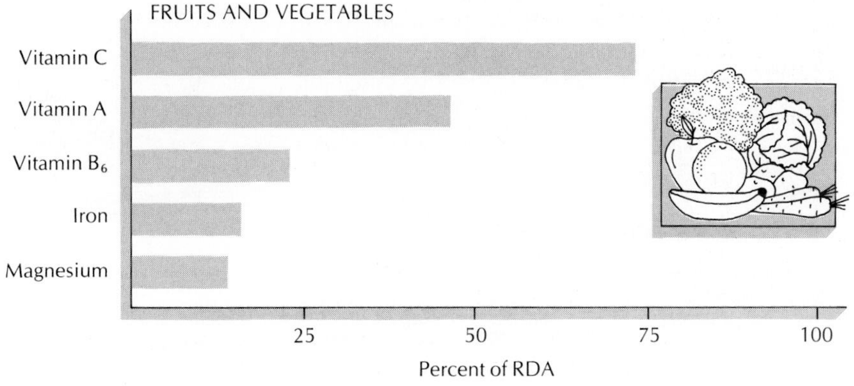

Figure 3-8 Major contributions of nutrients in the fruit and vegetable groups to the RDAs.

Generally fruits and vegetables are poor sources of protein, and that present is of poorer quality than protein in foods of animal origin. Roots and tubers contain 2% protein and 20% carbohydrate, whereas legumes such as peas and beans have 4% protein and 13% carbohydrate.

dietary fiber
The nondigestible portion of plant foods

The energy contribution of the fruit and vegetable group is generally low because of the high proportion of **dietary fiber** and water and low fat content. Immature seeds, such as peas and beans, and starchy tubers, such as potatoes, contribute two to eight times as many calories per serving as do celery, carrots, spinach, and cabbage, which are high in fiber and water but low in starch. One must remember, however, that the caloric contribution of a fruit or vegetable dish may be double or triple that of the basic food alone, depending on the way it is prepared.

How Method of Food Preparation Influences Amount of Energy

Baked potato	145 calories
Mashed potato (1C)	160 calories
French fries (10)	160 calories
Baked potato with sour cream and butter	270 calories

Another important nutritional benefit from the fiber in fruits and vegetables is the bulk provided. This promotes normal gastrointestinal motility and greatly facilitates the passage of food through the digestive tract, helping to prevent constipation. Recent evidence that low dietary fiber may be responsible for the increasing incidence of **diverticulosis** and that it may be associated with cancer of the colon is further reason to use fruits and vegetables.

diverticulosis
A condition in which there is a weakening in the wall of the large intestine; usually the result of pressure from hard stools (See Chapter 4)

Protein-Rich Foods—Meat, Fish, Poultry, and Eggs

This group contributes 75% of the vitamin B_{12} and over 50% of the protein recommended in the diet, as well as from 25% to 50% of the iron and 35% of the niacin. The nutritional profile of a typical selection of foods from the protein-rich food group for 1 day is shown in Figure 3-9. One average 3- to 4-oz serving of meat, fish, or poultry provides at least 20 grams of protein, but the amount will vary slightly with the type of meat.

The fat content of meat is variable, ranging from 1% in low-fat processed meat to 40% in prime beef; it depends on the type of animal and its diet, its condition at the time of slaughter, the cut, the extent to which the meat is trimmed, and the method of preparation. The higher the grade of meat, the more fat will be marbled throughout the muscle fiber and the higher the caloric value. The approximate composition of different meats shows wide variation in fat but much less variation in protein content (Table 3-4).

Legumes
Dried beans and dried peas
- Black-eyed peas
- Kidney beans
- Navy beans
- Lentils
- Lima beans

Meat substitutes, such as eggs, cheese, legumes, and peanut butter, contain somewhat less than 20 grams of protein per average serving. However, because they are usually consumed in combination with cereal protein, as in cheese or peanut butter sandwiches, macaroni and cheese, or eggs on toast, the combined protein values will approach that of a meat and will usually cost less.

Dried peas and beans, with a protein content ranging as high as 35%, and nuts, with 15% protein, are frequent meat substitutes in the protein group, but

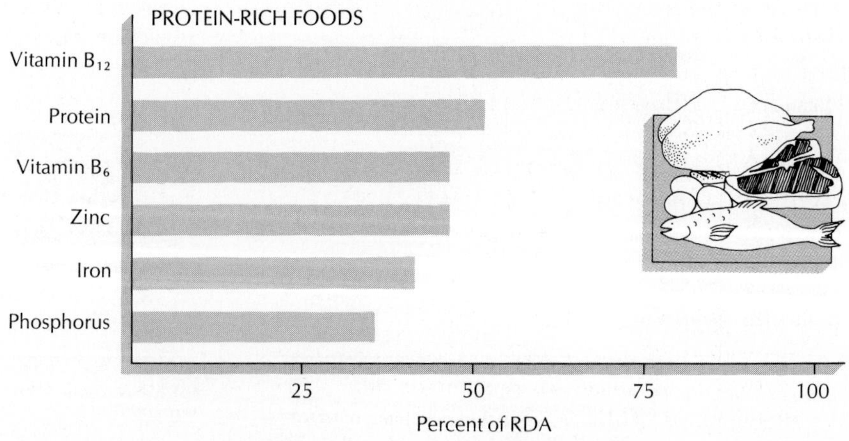

Figure 3-9 Major contributions of nutrients in the protein-rich group to the RDAs.

Table 3-4 ◆ The nutrient content of the four main types of meat and beef liver compared with nutrient allowance for 1000 kcal

	Nutrient Content for 1000 Kcal*					Nutrient Allowance for 1000 Kcal
Nutrient	Pork loin (25% Fat)	Beef Sirloin (24% Fat)	Lamb Loin (23% Fat)	Chicken (5% Fat)	Beef Liver	
Protein (gram)	57	60	61	186	142	25
Fat (gram)	84	82	82	30	27	—
Calcium (mg)	34	34	36	87	57	450
Iron (mg)	9	9	5	6	46	8
Vitamin A (RE)	0	170	0	108	49,250	1300
Thiamin (mg)	2.8	0.3	0.5	0.4	1.8	0.5
Riboflavin (mg)	0.7	0.6	0.8	0.8	23.3	0.6
Niacin (mg)	15	14	18	72	97	7
Vitamin C (mg)	0	0	0	0	128	15-30

Data from USDA, 1985.
*A food with a nutrient content in 1000 kcal that is greater than the nutrient allowance for 1000 kcal is considered a good source.

these foods have less protein per 1000 kcal. Although the protein is of lower quality than that of meat, legumes have the additional nutritional benefits of a low fat and a high fiber content. They are most effective if used in combination with cereal protein or as extenders of meat products. For example, chili con carne—beans with meat—features a legume (the beans) with animal protein (often beef).

The amount of iron depends on the meat or meat substitute chosen; it is low in chicken and fish but high in organ meats. Pork liver, the richest source of iron and also one of the least expensive, is unfortunately not very popular; in addition, like all liver, it is high in cholesterol. The iron in meat is more efficiently absorbed than iron from other food sources, such as legumes and vegetables.

Use of Meat, Fish, and Poultry in the United States
99% ate at least once in 3 days
81% ate every day
67% used beef
50% used pork
1.5% used lamb
2.3% used veal
43% used poultry
10% ate hamburgers
25% used fish
Source: Nationwide Food Consumption Survey, 1977-1978, USDA, Washington, D.C.

Meat is also a major source of zinc and phosphorus. If pork is chosen, the meat group becomes the major source of thiamin. Vitamin B_{12} (cobalamin), which is derived only from foods of animal origin, is provided by meat and milk products. Meat provides practically no calcium or vitamin C. Liver is a rich source of vitamin A, iron, and riboflavin and a fair source of vitamin C.

Meat is the most expensive single item in the average diet, often accounting for over a third of every food dollar; thus people frequently plan meals around the meat or protein dish. The cost of a serving of meat may range from a low of 12¢ for pork liver to a high of $1.60 for filet mignon or veal for a 3- to 4-oz serving (1988). Fish, which used to be a relatively low-priced protein source, is increasing in price as its popularity increases.

The use of the meat supply in the United States has been extended by a process of mechanically removing the flesh from the bone of both poultry and beef. This product contains the same high-quality protein, vitamins, and minerals of meat and some calcium and fluorine extracted from the bone. It is a nutritious, palatable, and economical product for use in processed meats. It has often been incorporated into other meat products, such as hamburgers, frankfurters, and luncheon meats. In these cases it must be labeled "tissue from ground bone" and "mechanically processed (species, e.g., chicken) product." Several million pounds are used annually in the United States.

In general, North American dietary patterns provide adequate intakes of protein. Thus there is little reason to promote the use of additional servings of foods from this group. The exclusion of meat from the diet, however, makes it increasingly difficult to obtain adequate intakes of vitamin B_{12} and zinc and has implications for the effectiveness of iron absorption.

Many ecologists still recommend that Americans eat "lower on the food chain," using more vegetable proteins, particularly legumes and seeds and fewer animal products, particularly meat. Their recommendations are based on the fact that energy yield per acre is greater when vegetable products are used directly—rather than being processed through an animal before being eaten. Much meat, however, is from animals raised on land that is suitable only for grazing.

Bread and Cereal Products

whole-grain cereals
Wheat, oats, corn, and other cereals from which a minimum portion of the outer husk has been removed

Cereal Products
Pasta
Oatmeal
Wheat flakes
Rice
Bread
Muffins
Flour products

The Hassle-Free Guide urges the frequent use of **whole-grain cereals** and does not mention the enriched cereals promoted in earlier guides, while the Food Wheel suggests use of half whole-grain and half enriched cereals. This reflects a growing recognition that enriched cereal products are not equivalent to their whole-grain counterparts, because the fiber, vitamin B_6, magnesium, and trace elements such as zinc and iron lost in milling are not returned to the cereal. For those labeled "enriched," specified levels of thiamin, riboflavin, niacin, and iron must be added so that for these nutrients levels are comparable to the original grain. One of the major justifications for the inclusion of cereal products in the diet is their contribution of many nutrients at minimum cost. The nutrient contribution of this food group to the food supply and the usual diet is shown in Figure 3-10.

This group contributes significantly to the total protein in the food supply. Although most cereal products are not meat substitutes, we use them so frequently with other proteins that the quality of the cereal protein is improved. Examples are macaroni and cheese, rice with chicken, poached egg on toast, or cereal and milk.

Nutrients Added to Enriched Cereals

Required	Optional
Iron	Calcium
Thiamin	Vitamin D
Riboflavin	
Niacin	

The belief that only such foods as bread, rice, macaroni, and dry or cooked cereal would satisfy the recommendation for four servings of cereal is not nutritionally defensible. Any product made primarily of flour is considered in the group. Although only 30 states require enrichment of bread and flour, over 90% of the flour now sold in the United States is enriched. (A 1987 proposal to permit addition of pyridoxine, magnesium, folic acid and zinc to flour, to create "superbreads," was turned down by the FDA.) Most products made from flour, including mixes, contain the B vitamins and iron. Therefore waffles, muffins, pancakes, pastries, cakes, and cookies can be counted in meeting the recommendation for cereal products. Because these products usually contain more fat and sugar, calories are higher but the nutrients from flour are still there. The use of milk or nonfat milk solids in many baked products increases the calcium to significant levels and supplements the cereal protein; it also further enhances the nutritional value of many foods in the cereal group.

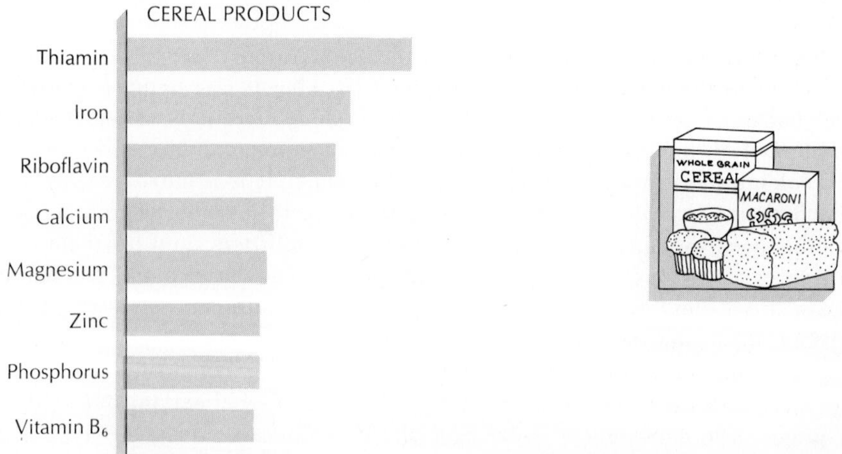

Figure 3-10 Major contributions of nutrients in the cereals groups to the RDAs.

Currently about 85% of ready-to-eat cereals are fortified, which means they have nutrients restored to the original level of the unmilled cereal, or fortified to higher levels. It can be readily seen from advertisements that the highly competitive breakfast cereal business is promoting cereal products enriched with any number of nutrients. There is little justification for adding vitamins A, C, D, and B_{12} to cereal products, because none of these are nutrients normally present in whole-grain cereal. The addition of excessive amounts of many nutrients helps sell the cereal but is not a nutritionally sound practice. On the other hand, the charge that most breakfast cereals are devoid of nutritional value is far from justified.

The addition of sugar to ready-to-eat cereals has become a highly controversial issue. Opponents question the value of having sugar added as an integral part of the product, often at excessive levels. Those in favor point out that the amount present is often less than most people would add to the cereal. Cereal with 1 tablespoon of sugar added per 1-oz serving is 50% sugar by weight; cereal with 1 teaspoon is 16% sugar. Both are widely available. Obviously, if a product is 50% sugar, it is only 50% cereal, so that 1 oz of presweetened cereal provides only ½ oz of cereal and a proportionately smaller amount of nutrients.

Converted rice is prepared by parboiling the rice kernels before polishing. During this process the nutrients normally concentrated in the outer husk are driven into the kernel, where they remain when the husk is removed. Thus a refined cereal that has been enriched with its own nutrients is produced. This process has been used in India for many years. It should be distinguished from quick-cooking rice, which does not retain the nutrients from the husk.

About the only persons who do not get the recommended number of servings from the bread and cereal group are young girls and people on weight-reducing diets, who tend to unadvisably avoid them.

Data from the Nationwide Food Consumption Survey (NFCS) show that adult men eat cereal products equivalent to 8 oz of flour per day, whereas women eat the equivalent of 5.5 oz per day.

Sugar Content of Breakfast Cereals

Shredded Wheat	1.0%
Cornflakes	7.8%
Raisin Bran	10.6%
Granola	14.5%
Team	16.0%
Familia	22.4%
Sugar Frosted Flakes	29.0%
Lucky Charms	50.4%

1 oz of cereal sugared with 1 tsp sugar is 16% sugar

Americans Using Specific Cereal Products at Least Once in 3 Days

Bread	94
Ready-to-eat cereals	43
Cookies	31
Crackers	26
Cakes	25
Cooked cereals	17
Pasta	11

From Nationwide Food Consumption Survey, 1977-1978

FOUNDATION OF AN ADEQUATE DIET

As can be seen from Figure 3-11, which combines the nutrients from the inclusion of 2 cups of milk or its equivalent, two servings of meat or meat substitutes, four servings of fruits and vegetables, and four servings of enriched or whole-grain cereals will make possible an intake close to the RDA of all nutrients, except kilocalories for adult men and iron for adult women. With this foundation diet you have little need for guidance in the selection of additional foods to provide the calories to meet your individual requirements. However, the greater the variety of foods you use, the greater the chance of providing adequate amounts of trace elements.

Often the calorie requirement will be at least partially met through additional servings of the four food groups. The use of the visible fats and oils, butter and salad dressings, which are natural accompaniments to the bread and vegetables and which constitute about a third of the total fat intake, will provide about 15% of the total kilocalories. The use of carbohydrate-rich foods, which are recommended as the least expensive way of obtaining the additional kilocalories, is questioned when simple sugars are used rather than complex carbohydrates, which also provide other nutrients. The use of whole-grain and enriched cereals and additional servings of fruits and vegetables has the advantage of providing both fiber and trace elements along with the additional kilocalories. Once the basic nutritional needs are met, there is no reason to avoid the use of foods of low nutrient density. In fact, the psychological advantages and enhanced palatability from their *limited* use should not be overlooked. Only when they replace foods that provide the nutritional foundation of the diet or add excessive kilocalories is there reason for concern.

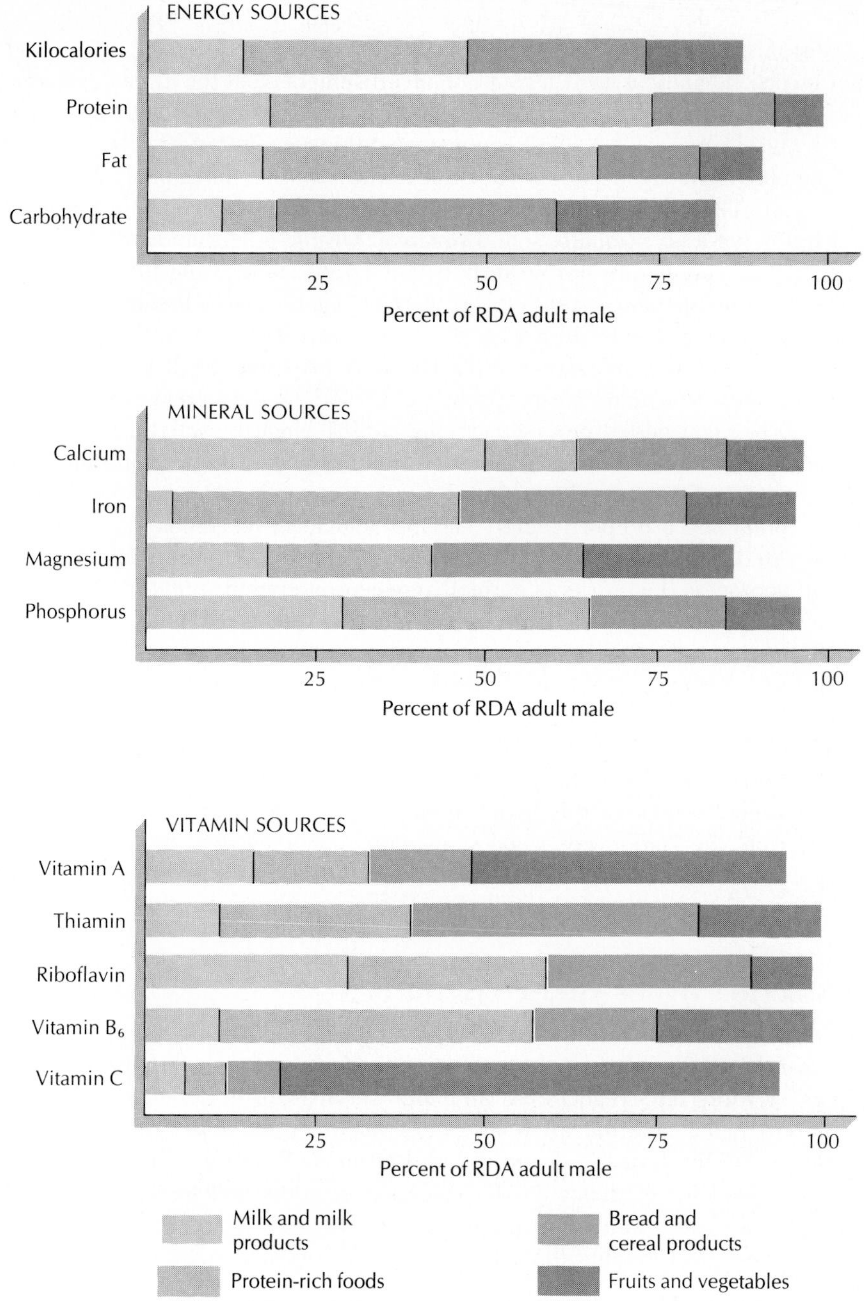

Figure 3-11 Major contributions of representative foods from all four food groups to nutrients in the diet.

Because women are very likely to have inadequate iron intakes, foods high in iron should be stressed as sources of the additional kilocalories. In addition, if the energy intake is less than 2500 kcal, an iron supplement is advised.

The number of kilocalories provided by the four basic food groups will depend on the selection of foods made within each category. To illustrate the range possible within the specifications of the four-group plan, the caloric value of two extremes is calculated in Table 3-5. Admittedly, differences will also exist in the level of other nutrients, but the selection does meet the requirements of the plan. The plan proposed in the *Food Wheel* calls for a minimum of an additional two servings of grains and one serving of vegetables.

The person interested in adjusting caloric intake either up or down has many trade-offs available. To help you in making choices among several options, some common trade-offs in various food groups are given in Table 3-6.

Table 3-5 ◇ Caloric value of two diet patterns meeting requirements of essentials of an adequate diet

Food Group	Diet I Foods	Kcal	Diet II Foods	Kcal
Milk	Nonfat milk (2 C)	160	Whole milk (1½ C)	290
			Ice cream (1 C)	145
Meat	Chicken, broiled (3 oz)	185	Chicken, fried (3 oz)	245
	Salmon, canned (3 oz)	120	Ham (3 oz)	340
Fruits and vegetables	Tomato juice (6 oz)	30	Sweet potatoes, baked	155
	Carrot (½)	22	Lima beans (½ C)	75
	Apple (1 medium)	70	Grape juice (6 oz)	93
	Green beans (½ C)	12	Figs (4)	190
Cereal	Puffed wheat (1 C)	50	1 waffle	240
	Bread, thin-sliced (3 slices)	135	2 cookies (3-inch diameter)	220
			Oatmeal (1 oz)	115
			Muffin	135
TOTAL		884		2243

Calculations are based on energy value of the food prepared and served without any flavor adjunct, such as butter, sugar, syrup, sauces, etc. Based on Nutritive value of foods, Home and Garden Bulletin, No. 72, Washington, D.C., 1985, USDA.

As the Food and Nutrition Board has emphasized ever since the publication of its first dietary standards, these nutritional goals can be met in innumerable ways by an unlimited combination of foods. The suggestions made in the Basic Four groups represent but one pattern that reflects dietary practices that are acceptable to a large number of persons in the United States. Following such a plan will usually ensure at least a minimal level of nutritional adequacy, but failure to do so does not necessarily result in inadequacy. Other cultures have eating patterns that are ostensibly different from ours but that result in quite adequate nutrient intake, because it is only the choice of foods within a group that accounts for the difference. The Basic Four food guide does provide an easy basis for evaluating the potential adequacy of a prescribed or popular diet. If the minimum recommendations are met, one can be reasonably confident that the diet has a sound nutritional basis.

TABLES OF FOOD COMPOSITION

In order to determine if the amount of the nutrient in the diet is adequate, it is necessary to make calculations using information on food intake and data in tables of food composition. Tables of food composition similar to that provided in Appendix F have been developed, using data provided from the chemical analysis of food by laboratories in government, universities, and food industries. Because it is feasible to provide only one figure per nutrient per food, the values in the table represent a weighted average from all the analyses available. A figure provided may not be precise for a particular food item you eat on a particular day, but it will be a good estimate of the average amount of the nutrient obtained for all the times you eat the food.

To use information in the food composition tables, you must first know the amount, kind of food you eat, and how it was prepared. This involves keeping an accurate record of all the food you consume during a specific period of time. This record must include butter, mayonnaise, ketchup, or beverages that are often overlooked. With your best estimate of the amount of food you eat, it is possible to go to tables of food composition and calculate the amount that your diet provided of any of the 17 to 24 nutrients usually included in these tables. The total amount can then be compared to the recommended dietary allowance for your age and sex. This is the least expensive and most widely used tool in estimating the nutrient intake of an individual or group.

For further instruction see Appendix E

Table 3-6 ◆ Trade-offs in food choices within various food categories

For Fruit

½ C frozen sweetened fruit = ½ C of fresh or frozen unsweetened fruit + 6 tsp sugar
½ C fruit, canned in heavy syrup = ½ C unsweetened fruit + 4 tsp sugar
½ C fruit, canned in light syrup = ½ C unsweeted fruit + 2 tsp sugar

For a Starchy Vegetable

10 French fries = 1 medium boiled potato + 2 tsp fat

For Meat Alternates

½ C cooked dried beans or peas + 1 tsp fat = 1 oz lean meat, fish, or poultry + 1 slice of bread
2 T peanut butter = 1 oz lean meat, fish, or poultry + 3 tsp fat
¼ C seeds = 1 oz lean meat, fish, or poultry + 4 tsp fat
⅓ C nuts = 1 oz lean meat, fish, or poultry + 5 tsp fat

For Meat, Fish, Poultry, and Eggs

2 oz bologna = 1 oz lean meat, fish, or poultry + 3 tsp fat
½ chicken breast, batter fried = ½ breast, roasted + 1 slice white bread + 2 tsp fat

For Milk, Yogurt, and Cheese

1 C whole milk = 1 C skim milk + 2 tsp fat
1 C 2% milk = 1 C skim milk + 1 tsp fat
1 C low-fat (2%) chocolate milk = 1 C skim milk + 1 tsp fat + 3 tsp sugar
8 oz plain low-fat yogurt = 1 C skim milk + 1 tsp fat
8 oz low-fat vanilla yogurt = 1 C skim milk + 1 tsp fat + 4 tsp sugar
8 oz low-fat fruit yogurt = 1 C skim milk + 1 tsp fat + 7 tsp sugar
1½ oz natural cheese = 1 C skim milk + 3 tsp fat
2 oz processed American cheese = 1 C skim milk + 4 teaspoons fat
Cottage cheese contains less calcium than other cheeses; ½ C of cottage cheese contains only as much calcium as found in ¼ C of milk, while providing considerably more kilocalories.

For Desserts and Snack Foods

½ C ice cream = ⅓ C skim milk + 2 tsp fat + 3 tsp sugar
½ C ice milk = ⅓ C skim milk + 1 tsp fat + 3 tsp sugar
½ C low-fat frozen yogurt = ⅓ C skim milk + 4 tsp sugar
1/16 of a white layer cake with chocolate frosting = 1 slice bread + 6 tsp sugar + 3 tsp fat
2 oatmeal cookies = 1 slice bread + 1 tsp sugar + 1 tsp fat
⅙ of 9″ apple pie = 2 slices bread + ⅓ medium apple + 6 tsp sugar + 3 tsp fat
18 potato chips = 1 medium boiled potato + 3 tsp fat

For Fats

1 tsp mayonnaise = 1 tsp margarine, butter, or oil
2 tsp Italian salad dressing = 1 tsp margarine, butter, or oil
3 tsp cream cheese = 1 tsp margarine, butter, or oil
4 tsp light cream = 1 tsp margarine, butter, or oil
5 tsp sour cream = 1 tsp margarine, butter, or oil

For Sweets

(These trade-offs are based on approximate kilocalorie content.)
1 tsp jam or jelly = 1 tsp sugar, syrup, or molasses
Chocolate bar, 1.05 oz = 5 tsp sugar + 2 tsp fat
12 oz noncarbonated fruit drink, ade, or punch = 12 tsp sugar
12 oz cola = 9 tsp sugar

From USDA Human Nutrition Information Service: Developing a food guidance system for "Better eating for better health," a nutrition course for adults, Admin. Report No. 377, Hyattsville, MD, 1985, U.S. Government Printing Office.

Available Revised Units of Handbook 8
8-1: Dairy and egg products
8-2: Spices and herbs
8-3: Baby foods
8-4: Fats and oils
8-5: Poultry products
8-6: Soups, sauces, and gravies
8-7: Sausages and luncheon meats
8-8: Breakfast cereals
8-9: Fruits
8-10: Pork products
8-11: Vegetables
8-12: Nuts
8-13: Beef
8-14: Beverages
8-15: Finfish and shellfish

It is important to understand how the tables were developed and to recognize their limitations in order to interpret the results intelligently. The food composition tables in Appendix F, which provide information on average servings or common household units, are based on values in the standard publication for food composition in the United States, the 1985 USDA Home and Garden Bulletin No. 72, *Nutritive Value of Foods*. These values in turn are based on data from the U.S. Department of Agriculture Handbook No. 8, *Composition of Foods—Raw, Processed, and Prepared*. This handbook was originally published in 1916 and revised in 1950 and 1963. It is now being revised in 21 segments, each segment being devoted to a particular food group. These segments will provide data on over 60 different nutrients, including vitamins, minerals, and amino acids. Altogether, data on 4000 foods will be included. In addition to providing information on the nutrient content of 1 pound as purchased (A.P.), 100 grams, and on average serving of a food (edible portion, E.P.), the tables indicate the number of analyses on which each piece of information was based and the range of values obtained. Differences in values for the same foods in different editions may reflect changes in marketing and processing techniques, as well as improved analytical techniques. For instance, selective breeding of poultry has produced animals with a reduced fat content; the use of dried milk solids in bread has led to an increase in its calcium content; the use of cooking oils with higher percentages of unsaturated fatty acids has changed the character of fat in many food products; and new analytical techniques have given us more precise information on the iron content of meat.

The USDA has now set up a computerized nutrient data bank that can be constantly updated to provide the kinds of nutrient information needed by those concerned with nutritional evaluation and counseling. The majority of independent data bases for nutrient analyses incorporate the same information. The requirement that industries using nutrient labeling provide analytical data to support their label claims has greatly increased available nutrient data.

Most of the data in food composition tables and in the data bank were obtained from analyses made by laboratories of government agencies, colleges, universities, and private industry. Only data on adequately identified food samples were used. In some instances few reports or only a single analytical report was available. In other cases data were available on several varieties of the same food at several seasons of the year and from various geographical areas. An example is the vitamin C in oranges. The single value appearing in the table represents a weighted average obtained by making use of marketing information on the extent to which each variety was consumed, the percentage of the domestic production coming from each geographical area, and the size of the crop in each season. Thus, although the value may not be accurate for any one specific orange, it does provide a value representative of all oranges consumed in the United States.

Similarly, values for other foods and nutrients take into account varietal, seasonal, and geographical differences in the nutrient content of foods; loss or gain of nutrients through harvesting, handling, commercial processing, packaging, storage, home practices of preparation, cooking, and serving; and consumption statistics. The factors that affect the amount of the nutrient in a food vary with the food and the nutrient. As an example, the vitamin A value of sweet potatoes varies with the variety; the vitamin C in potatoes varies with the maturity and conditions of storage; the vitamin A in butter varies with the season; the vitamin C in oranges varies with the site of production and the time of harvesting; and the vitamin A in plants varies with the part used.

There are many other widely used food composition tables that include additional sound analytical data. The beginnning student is cautioned not to be concerned over slight differences between values from different tables. Usually the differences are small when one considers the errors in the methods of collecting food intake data. As a general rule, values that differ by 10% or less can be considered essentially the same.

Details on the way in which data for the various nutrients are determined can be found in the preface and appendix of each section of *Handbook No. 8,* available from the Government Printing Office.

Niacin values in food composition tables reflect only preformed niacin and not that converted from tryptophan (amino acid) and thus they underestimate the niacin in any protein-rich food (see Chapter 12 for further discussion). Similarly, vitamin C values are only for reduced ascorbic acid and thus do not include the dehydroascorbic acid in some fruits and vegetables, which is also available to the body. Thus vitamin C value may be underestimated (see Chapter 13).

In spite of their recognized limitations, the food composition tables allow estimates of the nutritive content of diets that are comparable to those determined by direct chemical analysis but at a much lower cost in time, equipment, and money. These tables represent an indispensable tool for persons concerned with evaluating national food supplies, developing programs of food distribution, planning and evaluating food consumption surveys, and estimating the nutritive intake of individuals. The availability of the information from food composition tables on disks and magnetic tapes for storage in computers has greatly facilitated the use of this information in menu planning, in the analysis of dietary intake, and as a basis for nutrition counseling and has tremendously increased the scope of calculations that can be reasonably made with this information.

engineered or **novel food**
A food made by modifying food ingredients and combining them into a product resembling a natural food; examples are Tang and Surimi

Advances in biotechnology, and with them the apppearance of **engineered** or **novel foods,** have compounded the problem of keeping tables of food composition up to date. As the character of the food supply changes, the USDA attempts to make available information that will help the public assess the nutritive quality of diets.

NUTRIENT DENSITY

On the basis of the information provided in tables of food composition, it is possible to judge which of several sources of a nutrient will provide the most in an average serving. Many times, however, people who must watch their energy or calorie intake want to know which source is best in relation to the number of calories per serving.

To provide some guidance, nutritionists have developed the concept of an index of nutrient quality (INQ). This is an expression of the nutrient density of a food—the relationship between the extent to which it meets the requirements for a specific nutrient compared to the extent to which it meets the needs for energy. Thus the definition of an INQ becomes:

$$\frac{\text{Percent RDA of a nutrient for an individual}}{\text{Percent energy requirement for an individual}}$$

As an example, from Appendix F we see that 8 oz of low-fat milk provides 180 kcal, 284 mg calcium, and 4 mg vitamin C. In checking the RDA for a woman 23 to 50 years old, we find she needs 2000 kcal, 800 mg calcium, and 60 mg vitamin C. Thus milk provides 180/2000 = 9% of her total energy intake, 284/800 = 35% of her calcium need, and 4/60 = 7% of her vitamin C needs. For this person, then, milk has a nutrient density or INQ of 35/9 = 4.0 for calcium and 7/9 = 0.8 for vitamin C.

A food that has an INQ of 1 or more for a nutrient is making as great a contribution to the needs for that nutrient as for energy. If that particular food were the sole source of energy in the diet, the food would provide the full day's requirement for all nutrients for which it has an INQ of 1 or more. Thus milk is considered a very good source of calcium and a fair source of vitamin C on the basis of nutrient density.

It has been proposed that if a food has an INQ of 1 or more for four nutrients or an INQ of 2 or more for two nutrients, it makes a significant contribution to the nutrient intake and may be identified as nutritious. Most foods that have traditionally

Nutrient Density or Index of Nutrient Quality (INQ)

	Amount provided in 8 oz milk	RDA* for Woman Age 23-50 yrs	Percentage of RDA Provided by 8 oz Milk
Calories (energy)	180 kcal	2000 kcal	$\frac{180}{2000} \times 100 = 9\%$
Calcium	284 mg	800 mg	$\frac{284}{800} \times 100 = 35\%$
Vitamin C	4 mg	60 mg	$\frac{4}{60} \times 100 = 7\%$

Nutrient density

$$\text{For calcium} = \frac{\%\ \text{RDA}}{\%\ \text{Energy}} = \frac{35}{9} = 4.0$$

$$\text{For vitamin C} = \frac{\%\ \text{RDA}}{\%\ \text{Energy}} = \frac{7}{9} = 0.8$$

*RDA used varies with age and sex. Therefore, INQ will be different for different people. If calculating the INQ for a population rather than a specific age/sex group, use the U.S. RDA for both nutrient and an appropriate energy value (usually 2000 kcal for women and 3000 kcal for men).

been considered wise choices meet these nutritional criteria. Those that do not are foods with a high caloric density, usually as a result of the addition of sugar, starch, or fat in preparation. In Figure 3-12, representing nutrient profiles for three foods, food *A* qualifies as nutritious because of the four nutrients with an INQ greater than 1, and food *B* on the basis of two nutrients with an INQ greater than 2. Food *C* does not qualify, since it provides no nutrients in greater amounts than it does energy. Many such foods may make a significant nutritional contribution for one nutrient or a small contribution for several nutrients. Thus a food that does not qualify as "nutritious" is not necessarily of no nutritional merit.

As a general rule, a food is considered a source of a nutrient if it has an INQ of 1 and if one serving provides at least 2% of the U.S. RDA for the nutrient. To qualify as a good or excellent source, it must have an INQ of 1.5 and provide 10% of the U.S. RDA in each serving.

U.S. DIETARY SURVEYS

Most of the information that we have on how well Americans eat has been obtained from two major surveys. One, the NFCS, is conducted every 10 years by the USDA. In 1977-1978 they obtained data on the food intake of about 34,000 individuals in 15,000 households for 3 consecutive days. This information was used to calculate the nutrient intake of each individual in the household. From this information it is possible to assess how closely the nutrient intake of a certain age and sex group corresponds to the appropriate RDAs for that age and sex group. It is also possible to determine the effect of various factors such as income, education, geographical location, size of household, and meal patterns on dietary adequacy. In 1985, the USDA began surveying the food intake of women, 23 to 50 years old, and their children, 1 to 5 years old. These surveys will be carried out continuously, except in the years when the regular 10-year survey of households and individuals is being

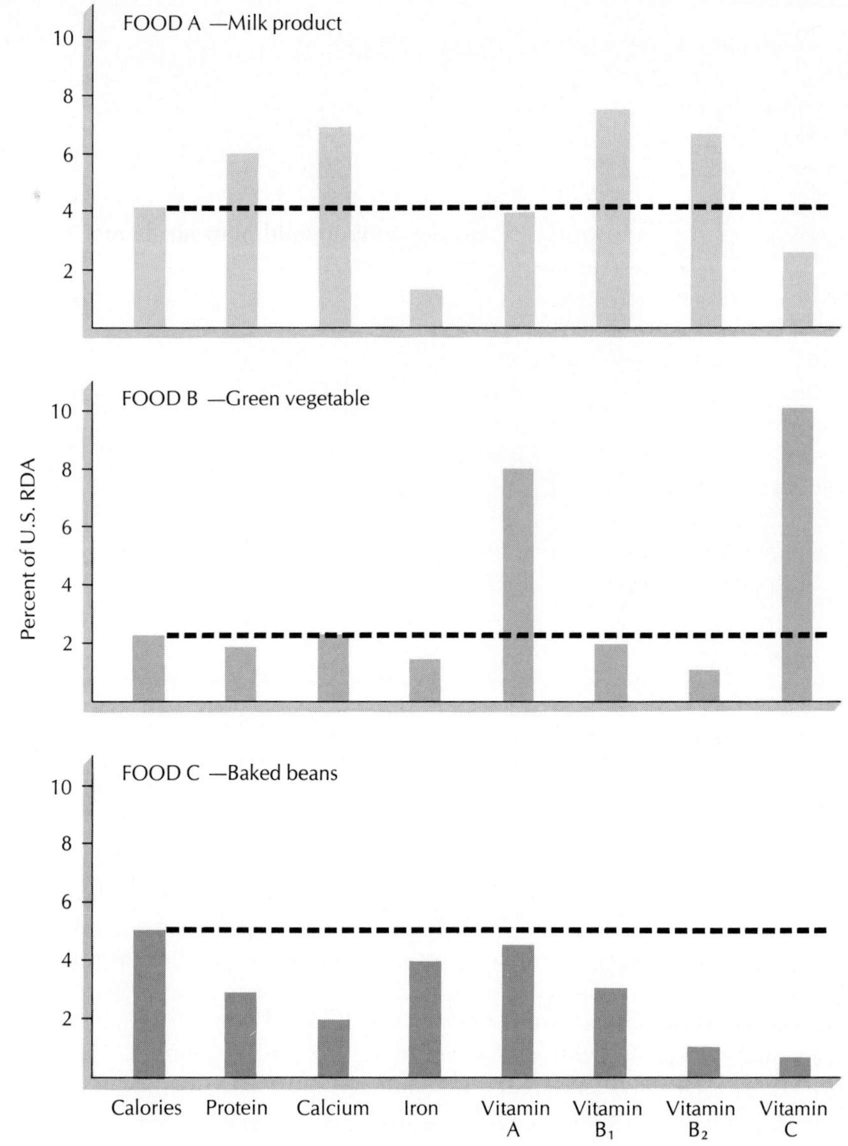

Figure 3-12 Nutrient profiles. Food A has an INQ > 1 for four nutrients; food B has an INQ > 2 for two nutrients; food C has no nutrients with INQ > 1. INQ = 1 when percent U.S. RDA for nutrient = percent U.S. RDA for calories, which is represented by a dotted line. These graphs are based on calculations using the U.S. RDA. They will be slightly different for specific age and sex groups.

conducted. Results of both the NFCS and the Continuing Survey of Food Intake of Individuals (CSFII) will be used throughout the text in discussions of the adequacy of the U.S. diet. Data were collected in 1988 for the next NFCS survey.

A second major study usually referred to as NHANES, or the National Health and Nutrition Examination Survey, is conducted approximately every 5 years on a random sample of the American population by the National Center for Health Statistics (NCHS). They obtain information on the food intake of about 20,000 people for a 24-hour period. They also collect data on the health status of the participants and do blood and urine analyses so that it is possible to relate dietary patterns to evidence of health problems. Information from this study will also be used throughout this book. It should be noted that, because of day-by-day variability in food intake, it is more difficult to judge usual nutrient intake on the basis of the 24-hour food record used in this study than it is using the 3-day records of the NFCS. Plans call for closer coordination between NFCS and NHANES in future surveys. NCHS in 1985-1986 conducted a survey of the Spanish speaking population. This survey is referred to as the Hispanic HANES. The next NHANES is scheduled for 1988-1989.

BY NOW YOU SHOULD KNOW

- The RDAs are used as a tool in planning diets for groups and evaluating individual diets.
- Based on the Recommended Dietary Allowances, the U.S. Recommended Daily Allowances are used for labeling food products.
- Dietary standards have been set not only in America but also in Canada, in the United Kingdom, and for the FAO/WHO.
- Food guides were developed so that the public could plan meals around certain food groups with the assurance that a person would be obtaining the nutrients needed to prevent deficiencies.
- The first food guide had five food groups, the second had seven, and the food guide most commonly used today has four food groups.
- The major nutrients in the milk and milk products group are protein, calcium, and riboflavin; in the protein-rich food group protein, vitamin B_{12}, vitamin B_6, zinc, and iron; in the fruit and vegetable group vitamins C and A; in the bread and cereal product group vitamin B_1, riboflavin, and iron.
- Information on food groups identifies foods included in the group, the serving sizes, and the number of servings to be eaten in one day. Food preparation and selection can be adjusted to meet individual needs.
- The USDA/American Red Cross Food Wheel is the most recently developed food guide. It is based on six food groups.
- The Dietary Goals and the Dietary Guidelines were developed to give guidelines for Americans to choose foods to promote a high level of health.
- The nutrient density of a food can be determined by calculating the INQ for any food.
- Food composition tables can be used to estimate the nutrient intake of an individual's or a group's diet.

STUDY QUESTIONS

1. Define: RDA, U.S. RDA, INQ, and nutrient density. What do all of these terms have in common?
2. Why do dietary standards differ from one country to another?
3. Where do the data in food composition tables and in computer data banks come from?
4. How is the Food Wheel different from the Basic Four?
5. Name the Dietary Goals for Americans. Explain how they differ from the current food intake.
6. Name foods that are considered meat substitutes.

Applying What You've Learned

1. **Find your RDAs**

   Locate and list the RDAs that apply to you. (See the inside front and back covers of textbook.)

2. **Food Selection Check Sheet**

   Keep a record of the foods you eat in a 24-hour period. Using the Food Selection Check Sheet, determine your daily score. If you did not achieve a score of 100, explain what foods you would need to add or subtract from your diet. Are these changes realistic based on your food preferences, budget, and foods available to you at this time?

Food selection check sheet

Food		Maximum Score	Daily Score					
Milk		30						
One cup of milk or equivalent	10							
Second cup of milk	10							
Third cup of milk or more	10							
Fruits and Vegetables		30						
One serving of green or yellow vegetables	10							
One serving of citrus fruit, tomato, or cabbage	10							
Two or more servings of other fruits and vegetables, including potato	5 each							
Breads and Cereals		15						
Three servings of whole-grain or enriched cereals or breads	5 each							
Protein-Rich Foods		25						
One serving of egg, meat, fish, poultry, or cheese (or dried beans or peas)	15							
One or more additional servings of egg, meat, fish, poultry, or cheese	10							
TOTAL		100						

Dietary score*

	Score Each Time Food is Mentioned	Maximum Score
Milk and milk products	2	4
Protein foods—meat, fish, poultry, eggs	2	4
Fruits and vegetables	1	4
Cereals	1	4
TOTAL		16

*An alternative system gives an additional point for one serving of legumes, for a total score of 17.

3. **Converting %U.S. RDAs to Absolute Values**

   Choose a food label. Using the % U.S. RDA and Appendix C of this text, determine the number of milligrams of iron in the serving. For example, if the label reads 5% the U.S. RDA for iron, you would first find the U.S. RDA for iron in Appendix C; it is 18 mg. Now find 5% of 18 (0.05 × 18 = 0.9). You know that one serving of this food provides 0.9 mg iron.

4. **Testing for Nutrient Density**

   Choose five foods that have nutrition information on the label. Using the nutrition information, determine the INQ for four nutrients. Determine which of the five foods you have chosen would be considered nutrient dense. (HINT: The label will provide the %U.S. RDA, but not the percent energy requirement. Because the % U.S. RDA does not change with calorie needs, you will want to select a standard for calories. For the sake of this exercise, use 2000 calories. Therefore, if a food were to provide 30% of the U.S. RDA for iron and the calories per serving were 120, you would first need to determine the percent energy requirement provided by the food. For example, 120 ÷2000 is 6%. Now apply the formula for determining the INQ: 30%/6% =5. The INQ is 5. Therefore, you could conclude that [because 5 is greater than 1] this food is nutrient dense in iron. However, to be "nutritious" the food must have an INQ of 1 or more for four nutrients.)

5. **Becoming Familiar with Food Composition Tables**

   Using your 24-hour food record, from activity 2, and Appendix F, locate the foods you ate. Could you find them all? How many were missing? What category were they listed under? What was the suggested size of an average serving? How was the food measured (cups, ounces, grams, slices)?

SUGGESTED READINGS

Food and Nutrition Board, National Academy of Sciences. Recommended Dietary Allowances. Washington, D.C., 1980.

This publication, which accompanies each edition of the Recommended Dietary Allowances, provides the rationale for the figures presented in the tables as well as a discussion of the state of our knowledge of the need for other nutrients for which there is not enough evidence on which to set a precise standard. This discussion helps the nutritionist understand the strengths and limitation of the data for the various nutrients.

Haughton B, Gussow JD, and Dodds JM: An historical study of the underlying assumptions for United States food guides from 1917 through the Basic Four Food Group guide, Journal of Nutrition Education 19:169, 1987.

This article is a historical review of the assumptions underlying the construction of the United States food guides up to and including the Basic Four. The five categories of assumptions are related to food and nutrient needs, economics, food habits and taste, food supply, and food and nutrition education.

Rosenberg IH: Behind and beyond the recommended dietary allowances, American Journal of Clinical Nutrition 41:139, 1985.

This symposium report includes a paper by A.E. Harper, G.M. Beaton, H.M. Munro, and H.J. Kamin, all of whom have been closely involved in setting the recommended allowances for the United States and Canada. They deal with the historical perspective, the conceptual base, and the process by which the standards are set, the data on which they are based, the limitations in the available data, and the current state of our knowledge of requirements. This series of papers is one of the most comprehensive, clearly written, and authoritative presentations of the RDA available for persons who wish a good basic knowledge of this important nutritional tool.

Smith J, and Turner JS: A perspective on the history and use of the recommended dietary allowances, Currents 2:1, 1986.

This article was prepared form the perspectives of nutritional science and public policy. Historically, it summarizes the changing definitions, targeted populations, and aims and objectives of the RDAs. It discusses how the RDAs are determined, the uses and limitations of the RDAs, and the need to keep the RDAs in alignment with today's social and health concerns.

ADDITIONAL READINGS

Food Selection Guides

Cronin F, Shadou A, Krebs-Smith S, Marsland P, and Light L: Developing a food guidance system to implement the dietary guidelines, Journal of Nutrition Education 19:281, 1987.

Department of Health, Education, and Welfare: Healthy people: the Surgeon General's report on health promotion and disease prevention, No. 79-55071, Washington, D.C., 1979, DHEW Public Health Service.

Food and Nutrition Board, National Research Council: Toward healthful diets, Washington, D.C., 1980, National Academy of Science.

Guthrie H: Concept of a nutritious food, Journal of the American Dietetic Association 71:14, 1977.

Guthrie H: Principles and issues in translating dietary recommendations to food selection: a nutrition educator's point of view, American Journal of Clinical Nutrition 45:1394, 1987.

Hansen RG, and Wyse BW: Expression of nutrient allowances per 1,000 kilocalories, Journal of the American Dietetic Association 76:223, 1980.

Harper AE: Dietary guidelines for Americans, American Journal of Clinical Nutrition 34: 121, 1981.

Harper AE: Transitions in health status, implications for dietary recommendations, American Journal of Clinical Nutrition 45: 1094, 1987.

Health Education Council, the National Advisory Committee on Nutrition Education: Proposals for nutritional guidelines for health education in Britain, Lancet, p. 719, Sept. 24, 1983.

Hertzler AA, and Anderson HL: Food guides in the United States, Journal of the American Dietetic Association 64:19, 1974.

Light L, and Cronin FJ: Food guidance revisited, Journal of Nutrition Education 13:57, 1981.

National Institutes of Health: Health implications of obesity, Annals of Internal Medicine 103:147, 1985.

Pao EM, and Mickle SJ: Problem nutrients in the United States, Food Technology 32:58, 1982.

Pennington JAT: Considerations for a new food guide, Journal of Nutrition Education 13:53, 1981.

Peterkin B, and others: Changes in dietary patterns: one approach to meeting standards, Journal of the American Dietetic Association 78:453, 1981.

U.S. Department of Agriculture and U.S. Department of Health, Education and Welfare: Nutrition and your health: dietary guidelines for Americans, Home and Garden Bulletin No. 232, Washington, D.C., 1985, U.S. Department of Agriculture.

Wolf, ID, and Peterkin BB: Dietary guidelines: the USDA perspective, Food Technology, p. 80, July 1984.

Dietary Standards

Department of National Health and Welfare: Recommended nutrient intake for Canadians, Ottawa, Canada, 1982, Departement of National Health and Welfare.

Food and Agricultural Organization/World Health Organization/U.N. University: Energy and protein requirements, Rome, 1985, Food and Agricultural Organization.

Food and Nutrition Board: recommended dietary allowances, ed. 9, Washington, D.C., 1980, National Academy of Sciences.

Food and Nutrition Board: recommended dietary allowances: scientific issues and process for the future, Journal of Nutrition 116:482, 1986.

Hegsted DM: Dietary standards: guidelines for prevention of deficiency or prescription for total health? Journal of Nutrition 116:478, 1986.

Olsen JA: Vitamin A. Recommended nutrient intake, American Journal of Clinical Nutrition 45:704, 1987.

Recommended daily amounts of food energy and nutrients for groups of people in the United Kingdom, Report on Health and Social Subjects No. 15, HMSO, London, 1979, Committee on Medical Aspects of Food Policy.

Young VR, and others: Genetic and biological variability in human nutrient requirements, American Journal of Clinical Nutrition 32: 486, 1979.

Tables of Food Composition

Food and Agricultural Organization: Amino acid content of foods, Nutrition Study No. 24, 1967, FAO.

Freeland JH, and Cousins RJ: Zinc content of selected foods, Journal of the American Dietetic Association 68:526, 1976.

Freeland-Graves JH, Ebangit ML, and Bodzy PW: Zinc and copper content of foods used in vegetarian diets, Journal of the American Dietetic Association 77:648, 1980.

Hepburn FN: The USDA National Nutrient Data Bank, American Journal of Clinical Nutrition 35:1297-1301, 1982.

Hertzler, AA, and Hoover IW: Development of food tables and use with computers, Journal of the American Dietetic Association 70:20, 1977.

Institute of Food Technologists: The effects of food processing on nutritional values, Nutrition Reviews 33:123, 1975.

McNeill DA, Ali PS, and Song VS: Mineral analysis of vegetarian, health, and conventional foods: magnesium, zinc, copper, and manganese content, Journal of the American Dietetic Association 85:569, 1985.

Murphy EW, Willis BW, and Watt BK: Provisional tables on the zinc content of foods, Journal of the American Dietetic Association 66:345, 1975.

Nazir DJ, Moorecroft BJ, and Mishkel MA: Fatty acid composition of margarines, American Journal of Clinical Nutrition 29:331, 1976.

Pantothenic acid, vitamin B_6, and vitamin B_{12} in foods, USDA Home Economics Research Report No. 36, Washington, D.C., 1969, U.S. Government Printing Office.

Toepfer E, and others: Folic acid content of foods, Agriculture Handbook No. 29, Washington, D.C., 1951, U.S. Department of Agriculture.

Truesdell DD, and Whitney EN: Nutrients in vegetarian foods, Journal of the American Dietetic Association 84:28, 1984.

Walsh, JH, Wyse BW, and Hansen RG: Pantothenic acid content of 75 processed and cooked foods, Journal of the American Dietetic Association 78:140, 1981.

Wyse BW: Nutrient analysis of exchange lists for meal planning, Journal of the American Dietetic Association 75:238, 1979.

FOCUS Computers—Tools for Nutritionists

The era of computers has brought to nutrition the same opportunities and challenges that it has brought to such disciplines as engineering and linguistics. Although a tremendous amount of time may eventually be saved by turning over routine computational tasks to computers, it is essential to know what the machine is programmed to do with the information it is given. Of course, the quality of the data output can be no better than the data input. In addition, the user must understand the concepts and information well enough to be able to judge whether the message delivered by the machine makes sense.

Students of nutrition and their families and friends will probably first encounter the application of computer technology in relation to dietary analysis—indeed a promising and legitimate application. These analyses may be a part of a classroom assignment or may be offered free in shopping malls, at health clinics, or at science exhibits.

In a slightly different context, they may be used in physicians' offices as part of routine medical assessments; at the far end of the continuum, such analyses are available through the mail at prices ranging from modest to exorbitant. In almost all cases the individual is given a computer printout that represents a nutrient analysis of his or her diet. The accompanying material may or may not attempt to interpret the printout. If the computer analysis compares your intake to the recommended dietary allowances and makes some suggestions about foods that might be substituted for those already in the diet or those that should be added, you can be reasonably certain that the service is educational and not a business enterprise. On the other hand, if the analysis indicates that your diet is severely lacking in one or more nutrients, is characterized by imbalances of nutrients that may have health consequences, and suggests that you correct the problem by purchasing a particular food, taking a nutrient supplement, or using a prescribed diet plan, you should be skeptical.

What can such an analysis tell you? The answer depends on many things. First, how good the information that you receive is depends on how good the information was that you provided. If in your questionnaire you described a food intake

ITEM	FOOD NAME	PORTION	SERVING	AMOUNT
366	BREAKFAST-OATMEAL	1 CUP	100%	240.0 GM
50	MILK-FLUID WHOLE-3.3% FAT	1 CUP	50%	122.0 GM
307	RAISINS-SEEDLESS	1 CUP	10%	14.5 GM
278	ORANGE JUICE-FROM FROZEN	1 CUP	100%	249.0 GM
358	BREAD-WHEAT-SOFT-16/LOAF	1 SLICE	200%	56.0 GM
524	PEANUT BUTTER	1 TBSP	200%	32.0 GM
235	BANANA-WITHOUT PEEL	1 BANANA	100%	119.0 GM
654	POTATO CHIPS	10 CHIPS	100%	20.0 GM
50	MILK-FLUID WHOLE-3.3% FAT	1 CUP	100%	244.0 GM
210	CHICKEN-BREAST-FRIED	1/2 BREAST	100%	79.0 GM
486	RICE-WHITE-PARBOILED-CKD	1 CUP	75%	131.2 GM
573	SNAP BEANS-GREEN-FRENCH	1 CUP	50%	65.0 GM
460	PIE-CHERRY	1/7 PIE	100%	135.0 GM
731	COFFEE-BREWED	6 FL OZ	100%	180.0 GM

NUTRIENT VALUES (%RDA)

KCALORIES	1710 KC (85%)	RIBOFLAVIN	1.27 MG (105%)
PROTEIN	70.5 GM (160%)	NIACIN	25.1 MG (193%)
CARBOHYDRATE	237 GM (- %)	VITAMIN B6	2.41 MG (120%)
FAT	59.5 GM (- %)	FOLACIN	265 UG (66%)
FIBER	6.24 GM (- %)	VITAMIN B12	1.57 UG (52%)
CHOLESTEROL	119 MG (- %)	PANTO- ACID	6.15 MG (111%)
SATURATED FA	18.2 GM (- %)	CALCIUM	660 MG (82%)
OLEIC FA	21.2 GM (- %)	PHOSPHORUS	1212 MG (151%)
LINOLEIC FA	14.8 GM (- %)	TRYPTOPHAN	786 MG (482%)
SODIUM	1970 MG (89%)	THREONINE	2566 MG (589%)
POTASSIUM	2766 MG (73%)	ISOLEUCINE	3211 MG (491%)
MAGNESIUM	333 MG (110%)	LEUCINE	5229 MG (600%)
IRON	9.5 MG (52%)	LYSINE	4155 MG (636%)
ZINC	7.73 MG (51%)	METHIONINE	1393 MG (418%)
VITAMIN A	2243 IU (56%)	CYSTINE	885 MG (418%)
VITAMIN D	153 IU (76%)	PHENYL-ANINE	3029 MG (645%)
VITAMIN E	15.6 MG (195%)	TYROSINE	2585 MG (645%)
VITAMIN C	148 MG (246%)	VALINE	3632 MG (476%)
THIAMIN	1.25 MG (125%)	HISTIDINE	1776 MG (- %)
		ALCOHOL	0 GM (- %)

PERCENTAGES BY CALORIE (4:4:9:7)

PROTEIN: 16% CARBOHYDRATE: 54% FAT: 30% ALCOHOL: 0%

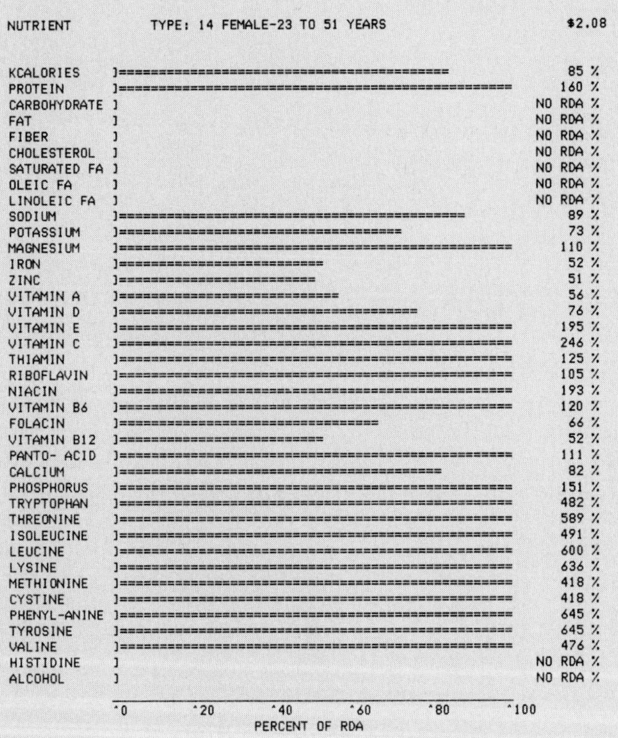

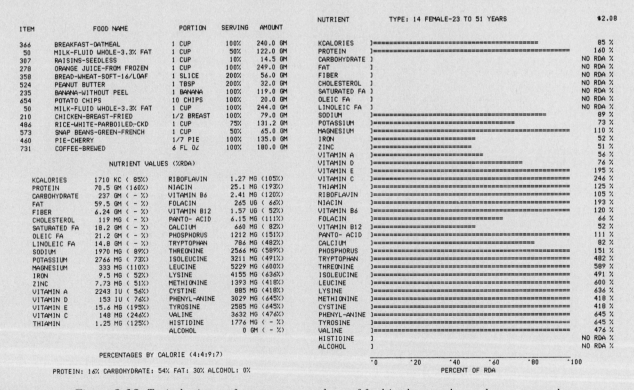

Figure 3-13 Typical printouts from computer analyses of food intake records; results are reported in relation to the 1980 Recommended Dietary Allowances.

that was typical of your usual intake, the analysis will be much more accurate and useful than if you gave it a 1-day food intake record that does not represent your usual food habits. The longer the period over which you describe your food intake, the more useful the computer analysis can be to you. But if in trying to cover a longer period of time you provide less accurate information, then there are no advantages to giving more but poorer information. The second thing that is important, and this is often much more difficult for you to know, is what the computer does with the information you gave it before it gives you back some information. Usually the computer is programmed to do exactly what you did or would do if you kept a record of your food intake and then looked up the nutrient content of each of the foods, calculated the total for each nutrient, and compared it to a dietary standard. How well the computer is able to do that depends on where the information on the nutrient content of food came from, how many foods and how many nutrients it has information on, and what it is told to do with the information. You can get this information on what is called the "data base," from documentation provided, or rely on the recommendation of a recognized professional group. The cost of the analysis or the price of the program may bear little relationship to the quality of the data analysis.

Examples of reports from dietary analyses are shown in Figure 3-13.

Another efficient use of computers is in nutrition education. This can be informal education of the public in which people are taught about snacks or fast foods, or how to put together a balanced diet, or about the energy expenditure of various forms of exercise. Such computer programs are available for home use but are also being used extensively in public education. There are computer programs that can be used by persons who, because of health problems such as diabetes or kidney disease, must modify their diet as part of the treatment. These programs effectively teach the principles of dietary practices and help the patient learn appropriate and inappropriate food choices. By having such a program available for use on a home computer, a patient is able to get immediate answers to questions without the cost and inconvenience of contacting a professional nutritionist or dietitian. Many of the programs are set up to take advantage of learning theories involving reinforcement of learning experiences. Before computers were widely used, this was possible only on a one-to-one teaching-learning basis.

In a more formal educational setting, computers as essential components of "computer assisted instruction" (CAI) have made it possible to reach a large number of students, often in geographically separated settings, with an effective, low-cost instructional approach. Most programs are set up to allow the student to proceed at his or her own pace, repeat difficult material, and have the capability of scheduling his or her own learning program. In elementary school programs in which students are being introduced to the use of computers, nutritionists have a golden opportunity to introduce nutrition concepts as part of the child's learning experience.

The uses of computers in research and evaluation of program effectiveness are beyond the concern of most students of introductory nutrition, but they should be aware of the extent to which they have made possible much more extensive and comprehensive analyses of available data on a much more timely basis. Throughout this book we make extensive use of data collected in the Nationwide Food Consumption Study (NFCS). Had it not been possible to analyze that data by computer, we would have been very limited in the amount of information that we could have extracted from the vast amount of information collected. Similarly, investigators involved in laboratory nutrition studies have the capability of more timely, sophisticated, and rapid analyses of the research data as a result of computer capability.

One of the dangers of writing for textbooks on such a rapidly advancing topic as nutrition and computers is that the material may be superseded or obsolete before it reaches the reader. One thing is certain, however: computers will continue to be used as an educational, diagnostic, and therapeutic tool. What kinds of advances are made is open to speculation. Current predictions that the majority of homes will have their own computer capabilities and that the potential for cable television viewers to interact with educational programs will soon be exploited reinforces the urgency for nutritionists to move to capitalize on this emerging technology. We can only caution the reader that as the potential for legitimate uses increases, so does the possibility of fraud. And past experience would suggest that we are more vulnerable to fraud in the more personal aspects of our lives. Nutrition is certainly one of these personal facets.

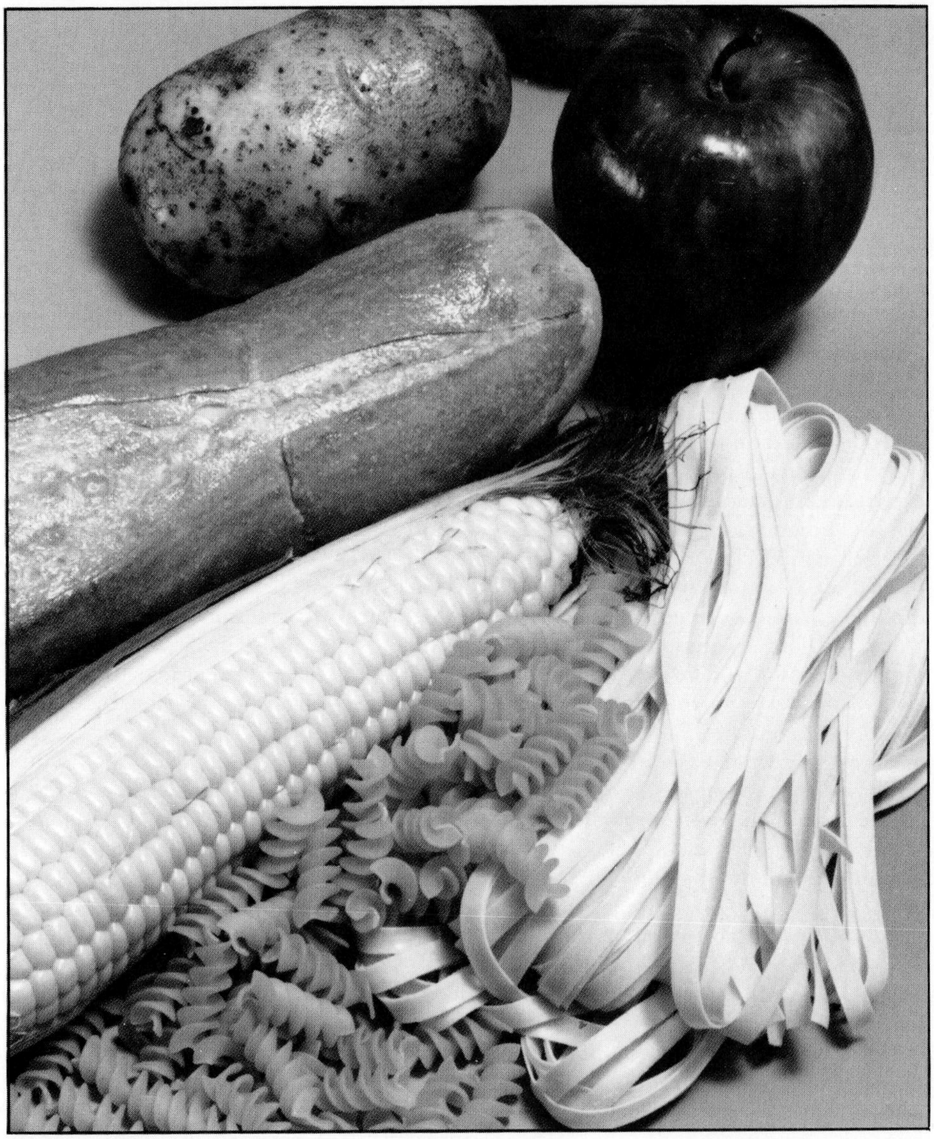

AWARENESS CHECK

Truth or Fiction?

- Carbohydrates are fattening.
- Sugar causes diabetes.
- People should avoid sugar and use sugar substitutes whenever possible.
- A person who is lactose intolerant can never eat dairy products.
- Carbohydrate loading is recommended for the weekend athlete.
- Dietary fiber may reduce one's risk of colon cancer.
- Low-carbohydrate diets are one of the most successful ways to lose weight and keep the weight off.

Carbohydrate

CHAPTER 4

The three major sources of dietary carbohydrate are starch, sugar, and fiber. Many people identify starch and sugar as "fattening and to be avoided," sugars as the cause of hyperactivity in children, and fiber as something to consume to avoid constipation. Although there is some basis for each of these beliefs, none is entirely supported by fact. Carbohydrate is an essential dietary component; only when it is used in excess of energy needs does it lead to weight gain. Only a very few of the many children considered hyperactive are sensitive to sugar. While a certain amount of fiber is good, there are problems associated with too high an intake. Health authorities in almost all developed countries are encouraging people to increase their intake of starch, to use sugar in moderation, and to include adequate but not excessive fiber in their diet. The kind and amount of carbohydrate in the diet play a role in the prevention and treatment of tooth decay, diabetes, hypoglycemia, and some other health problems.

Although carbohydrate was just about the first nutrient to be identified chemically, it was only recently recognized as an essential nutrient. Carbohydrate is a term that has quite different meanings for different people. To most people it means "starch and sugar," which in turn is too often erroneously considered synonymous with "fattening." To the diabetic, carbohydrate is a part of the diet that must be constantly monitored. To the chemist, it is a compound composed of carbon, hydrogen, and oxygen. To the botanist, it is the form in which plants store energy trapped from the sun. Finally, to the nutritionist, carbohydrate is an essential nutrient provided almost entirely by plant foods. It is the only source of dietary fiber and the major source of energy in most diets.

Carbohydrates include starch, which is found in both whole-grain and refined cereals and vegetables; cellulose or fiber in whole grains, fruits, and vegetables; and various sugars found in fruits, vegetables, milk products, and sweeteners.

Aside from water, carbohydrate is the single largest component in the diet. Over half of the energy needed by the American adult, who requires at least 2000 **kilocalories,** or kcal, a day, is usually provided by carbohydrate. Because 1 gram of carbohydrate provides 4 kcal, 300 grams (⅔ pound) of carbohydrate will be

kilocalorie
A measure used to express the energy value of food

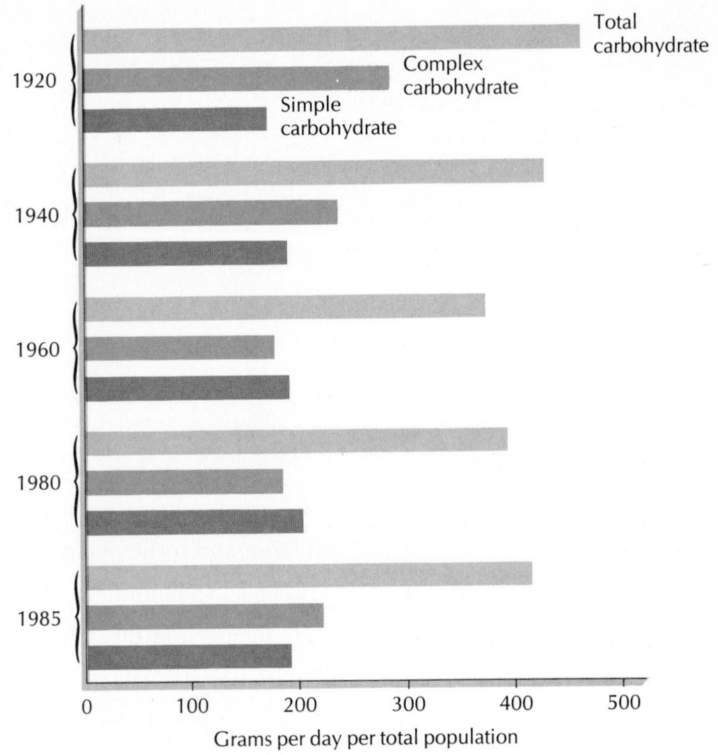

Figure 4-1 Trends in total, complex, and simple carbohydrate available in the U.S. food supply, 1920-1985.
Derived from data from the USDA.

needed to provide 1200 kcal (that is, the recommended 60% of the daily energy requirements). Although we could get this from about 1½ cups of sugar (which is 100% carbohydrate) or 3 cups of flour (which is 88% carbohydrate), we normally get most of it in a more palatable form, disguised in fruits, vegetables, and cereal products.

1 pound = 454 grams
1 ounce = 28.5 grams
1 gram = 0.036 ounce

In some parts of the world—particularly developing countries where inexpensive and locally grown carbohydrate-rich cereals such as rice, corn, or millet and root crops such as cassava, or sweet potatoes are dietary staples—many diets contain over a pound of carbohydrate that provides 80% or more of energy intake. These diets tend to be much less varied than diets in developed countries. At the other extreme are Eskimos, who live where animals are the major source of food and where plant life is limited. They get only 8% of their energy from carbohydrate.

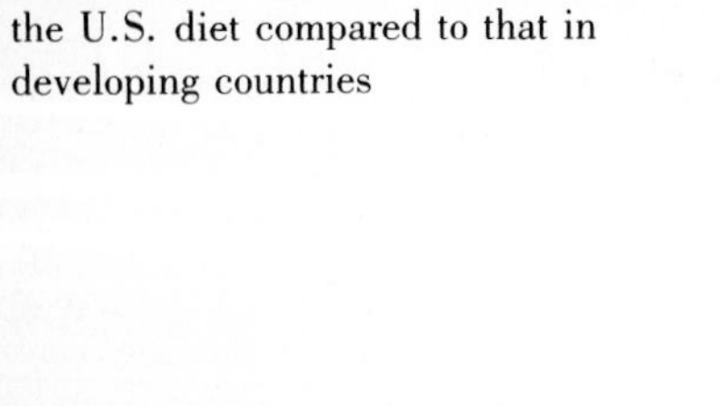

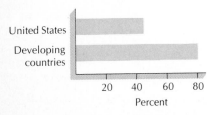

Percent of energy from carbohydrate in the U.S. diet compared to that in developing countries

Since 1920 we have seen some interesting trends in the type of carbohydrate available in the North American diet (Figure 4-1). The total amount of carbohydrate in the food supply has declined by about 20%, from over a pound to slightly less than a pound (413 grams per person per day). The use of starches has declined by one third, primarily because of a drop in the use of potatoes. The use of sugar and sweeteners, which dipped to its lowest level during World War II, has stabilized at 204 grams (almost half a pound) per day. Since 1970 part of this trend has reflected the growing use of other sweeteners, particularly corn syrup and high-fructose corn syrup, calculated at 60 grams per day in 1985 or about one third of all dietary sugar. As a result of these trends, the proportion of total carbohydrate provided by sugar has increased. All added sugars account for 12% of an average American's daily calorie intake. The health implications of these trends have been the subject of some research and much speculation and discussion in the popular press. Current dietary guidelines suggest that of 60% of total calories from carbohydrates, no more than 10% should come from added sweeteners.

Our changing life-styles have led to a shift from home-prepared food to com-

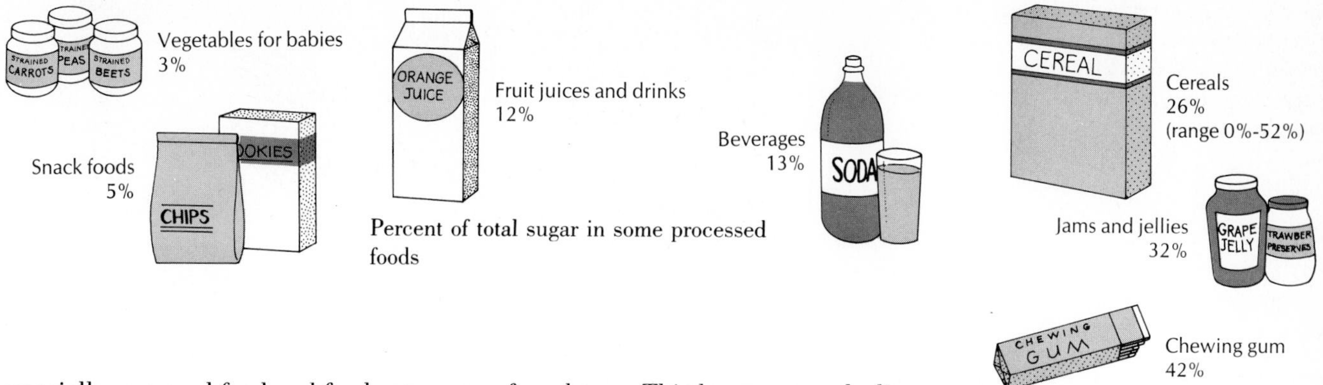

Percent of total sugar in some processed foods

mercially prepared food and food eaten away from home. This has meant a decline, until now only one fourth of the 9 million tons of sugar marketed in the United States is sold directly for home use. Almost all of the rest is used commercially by the food industry, either as a preservative and as a sweetener to enhance the palatability of food. Beverages alone account for 28% of the sugar used in the United States; other processed foods—with 3% to 42% added sugar—account for 43% of U.S. sugar used (Figure 4-2). The amount of sugar added to any food may vary considerably—it may be less but will never be more than the amount declared on the label. The amount of naturally occurring and added sugar in some representative foods is shown above.

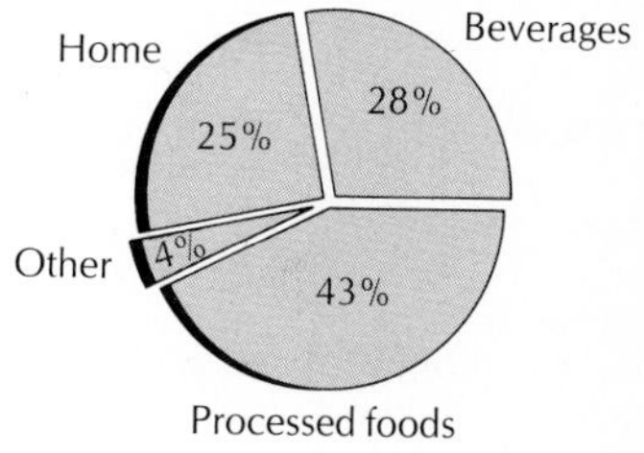

Figure 4-2 Use of sugar in the United States.

SYNTHESIS

Carbohydrates are the most abundant organic chemicals found on earth. All have their origins in plants with green leaves. Through a process known as **photosynthesis,** plants are able to trap the radiant energy from the sun and store it as chemical energy in carbohydrates. As shown in Figure 4-3, carbon dioxide from the atmosphere and water from the soil are picked up by the plant and combined in the presence of **chlorophyll,** the green pigment in leaves. An energy-rich simple carbohydrate, usually glucose, is formed. This carbohydrate is then stored in the plant as sugar or more complex starch, which ultimately provides energy for the animals or humans who eat the plants. It is estimated that 100 billion tons of carbohydrate are formed each year through photosynthesis. There is some concern that changes in the ozone layer above the earth may interfere with photosynthesis and reduce the amount of carbohydrate produced.

photosynthesis
The process by which plants, using the green pigment chlorophyll in their leaves, are able to trap energy from the sun and store it in the form of carbohydrate

chlorophyll
The green, magnesium-containing pigment in leaves

In some plants such as potatoes, wheat, and rice the carbohydrate is stored in the form of starch. In others such as sweet peas, bananas, cherries, and sugar beets, it is stored in the form of sugar. In vegetables such as peas and corn carbohydrate that is stored initially as sugar is changed to starch as the seed matures. Similarly the sweetness of carrots declines with age as the sugar in the root is

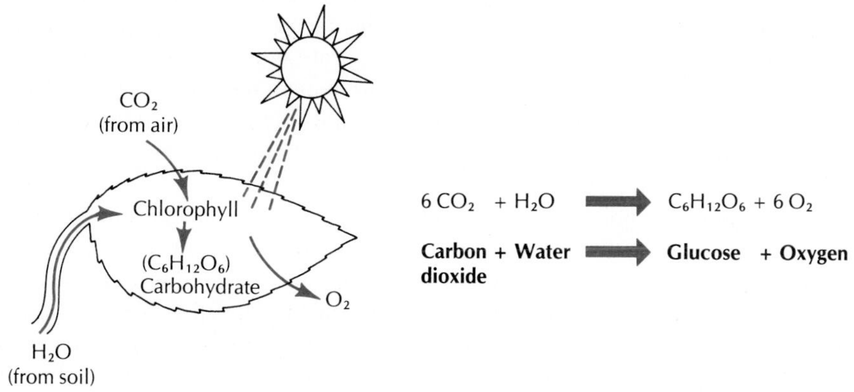

Figure 4-3 Process of photosynthesis. Carbon dioxide (from the air) is combined with water (from the soil) in the chlorophyll-containing cells of the plant leaf to trap energy from the sun in the form of a simple carbohydrate (usually glucose). This process involves six molecules each of CO_2, H_2O, and O_2 because glucose is a six-carbon hexose.

Foods such as bananas develop sugar and become sweeter as they ripen. Vegetables such as peas and beans develop more starch as they mature and become less sweet.

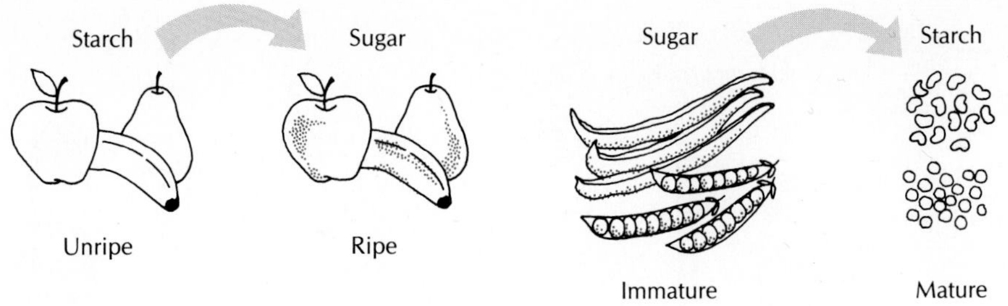

converted into starch. On the other hand, the starch in immature fruits such as bananas, apples, and pears is converted to sugar during the ripening process to produce a sweeter, more palatable product. On further ripening, this sugar changes to acid, as is found in overripe fruits, or is fermented to alcohol.

CLASSIFICATION

monosaccharide
A simple sugar unit (mono = one; sacchar = sugar)

disaccharide
Combination of two monosaccharides (di = two)

polysaccharide
Combination of many monosaccharides (poly = many)

As we see from photosynthesis, carbohydrate is composed of only three elements: *carbon, hydrogen,* and *oxygen*. The ratio of hydrogen to oxygen in almost all carbohydrates is 2 to 1, the same as in water ("hydro"); hence the name *carbohydrate*. The plant may store the carbohydrate in three major forms: **monosaccharides** and **disaccharides,** known as simple sugars; and **polysaccharides,** known as complex carbohydrates, which include starch, cellulose or fiber, and some related compounds.

In the simplest of these, the *monosaccharides*, there are equal numbers (usually six) of carbon atoms and water molecules: $[C_6(H_2O)_6]$. For complexes of two simple carbohydrates, known as *disaccharides*, there are 11 water molecules for each 12 carbon atoms $[C_{12}(H_2O)_{11}]$, because one water unit must be released or separated off when the two monosaccharides are chemically joined:

$$\underset{\textbf{Monosaccharide}}{C_6H_{12}O_6} + \underset{\textbf{Monosaccharide}}{C_6H_{12}O_6} \longrightarrow \underset{\textbf{Disaccharide}}{C_{12}[H_2O]_{11}} + \underset{\textbf{Water}}{H_2O}$$

In starch, which is a *polysaccharide* (or combination of many monosaccharides), the number of simple carbohydrate units reaches several hundred. Each time another glucose unit is added, another unit of water is released in the same way as when two glucose or monosaccharides were joined.

Monosaccharides

Hexoses

The simplest form of carbohydrate is the monosaccharide, one sugar unit. This is the chemical unit from which almost all the more complex carbohydrates are built. Most of the monosaccharides are also known as hexoses because chemically the carbon atoms form a six-carbon chain or ring (*hex* means *six*). Hydrogen and oxygen atoms are attached to this chain or ring as separate atoms or as a hydroxyl (OH) group. There are three monosaccharides of importance in nutrition: *glucose, fructose,* and *galactose*. A fourth, *mannose*, is present in only a few foods and therefore has little significance in human nutrition. Note that the names all end in "-ose."

All hexoses contain the same number and kinds of atoms: six carbon atoms, 12 hydrogen atoms, and six oxygen atoms. They differ from one another only in the way that the hydrogen and oxygen atoms are arranged around the carbon atoms. The differences in the four monosaccharides are evident in the formulas in Figure 4-4. These differences in arrangement of atoms are responsible for differences in sweetness, solubility, and other properties that distinguish one monosaccharide from another.

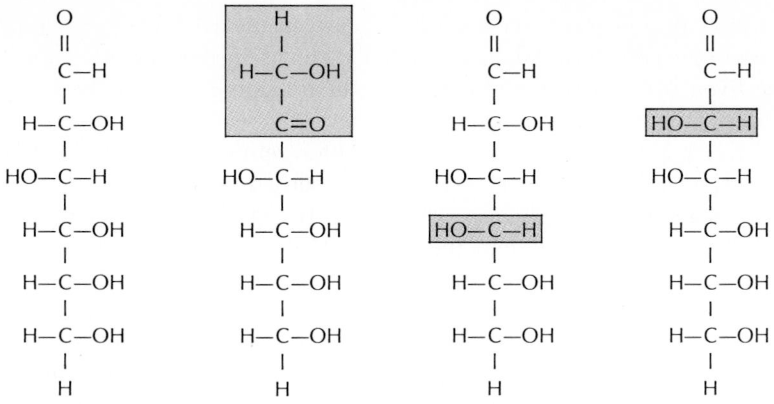

Glucose Fructose Galactose Mannose

Figure 4-4 Comparison of the chemical structure of the four monosaccharides. (Boxed and shaded areas are where structure differs from glucose.)

These simple, naturally occurring monosaccharides, found primarily in fruits, vegetables, and milk make up approximately 10% of dietary carbohydrate.

Glucose

Glucose, also known as dextrose or blood sugar, is found free in fruits, vegetables, and honey. However, these foods provide only about 18 grams of glucose per day, which is only a small fraction of the glucose used daily by the body. Glucose is the main source of energy for the central nervous system (CNS), which includes the brain and nerve fibers. The CNS uses about 140 grams (9 tablespoons) of glucose per day. Red blood cells need about 40 grams, or 3 tablespoons. This extra glucose comes from the breakdown of more complex carbohydrates or from some amino acids.

Glucose is the only form in which carbohydrate can be transported in the blood to all the tissues such as muscles, heart, and lungs. Hence it is sometimes called **blood sugar.** These tissues also rely on glucose to serve as a major source of energy. Usually the body tries to keep at least 100 milligrams (1 mg = 0.001 gram) of glucose per deciliter of blood by converting carbohydrate stores or some amino acids into glucose. (A **deciliter,** or dl, is 100 ml.) This is sometimes referred to as the **fasting glucose level.** After a meal, however, when the carbohydrate in the diet is digested and the monosaccharides are absorbed, the amount of glucose in the blood will rise and then gradually fall as the glucose is removed from the blood by the tissues to meet their immediate energy needs or to be stored for future use.

Whenever the amount of glucose in the blood increases above 160 mg/dl, a person is described as having **hyperglycemia,** or too much sugar in the blood. Hyperglycemia occurs most often in people suffering from diabetes when the hormone **insulin** is not produced fast enough by the pancreas to help the cells remove glucose from the blood. Under these circumstances the blood glucose levels get so high that the kidneys, which usually reabsorb glucose so that it will not be lost, cannot keep up. The result is that some sugar spills over into the urine. When this loss of glucose occurs, more urine must be produced to dilute the glucose being excreted and urination is more frequent. A person who urinates more frequently feels thirsty because of the need to replace the fluids that are being lost. As a result, the symptoms of diabetes are high blood glucose levels, glucose in the urine, thirst, and frequent urination.

When blood glucose levels fall below 60 mg/dl, the condition is known as **hypoglycemia.** In addition to feeling hungry, people with low blood glucose levels often experience weakness, sweating, and light-headedness. Hypoglycemia is not a disease but rather a symptom (like fever) by which other diseases can be diagnosed.

A mild form of hypoglycemia, sometimes called reactive hypoglycemia, occurs from time to time in almost everyone. Sometimes reactive hypoglycemia merely

blood sugar
Another name for glucose, the only form in which carbohydrate can be transported in blood

deciliter (dl)
100 ml; measure in which most blood values are reported. Most adults have 5 liters, or 50 deciliters, of blood.

fasting glucose level
100 mg, or 0.100 gram, of glucose per deciliter of blood; the usual glucose level that the body tries to maintain

hyperglycemia
A condition in which the level of sugar in the blood is elevated above normal (hyper = too much; gly = sugar; emia = blood)

insulin
A hormone secreted by the pancreas that regulates the rate at which cells take up glucose from the blood

hypoglycemia
A condition in which the level of glucose in the blood is below normal (hypo = too little)

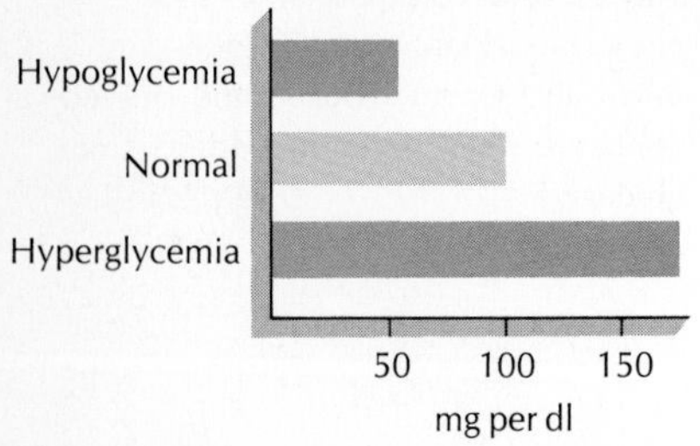

Blood glucose levels in hypoglycemia and hyperglycemia compared to normal levels

neuromotor coordination
The integration of the stimulus from the nerve with the contraction of the muscles; when this is lacking a person has trouble controlling movements

sorbitol
A reduced form of glucose that has one additional hydrogen atom

flatulence
Gas produced in the colon

cariogenic
Capable of producing tooth decay (cario = tooth decay; genic = giving rise to)

means that a person has waited too long between meals. Reactive hypoglycemia results when the cells have taken up the blood glucose faster than it can be replaced from the liver, where reserves of carbohydrate are stored. It tends to occur several hours after eating and lasts only a short time.

Reactive hypoglycemia may also occur after eating a diet very high in carbohydrate, especially simple sugars that are absorbed very rapidly. This causes a sudden increase in blood glucose, which in turn signals the pancreas to produce more insulin and release it into the blood. The insulin travels to the cells and stimulates them to take up more glucose from the blood quickly. Sometimes the pancreas overreacts and continues to produce insulin longer than necessary. This overreaction causes the cells to take up too much glucose, which causes the blood glucose levels to fall to a very low level. Symptoms usually include a lack of **neuromotor coordination.** Because this form of hypoglycemia occurs after eating, it is sometimes known as *postprandial* (post = after, prandium = meal) *hypoglycemia*.

Very few of all those who believe themselves to be hypoglycemic have *spontaneous hypoglycemia*, which is characterized by chronically low blood glucose levels because the pancreas constantly puts out too much insulin. This occurs whether or not there has been a surge of glucose into the blood to stimulate the pancreas. The symptoms are the same and indicate that the brain and nerves, which can use only glucose as a source of energy, are literally starved and are reacting by sending out distress messages.

Because symptoms such as anxiety, weakness, and dizziness are common to both reactive and spontaneous hypoglycemia, it is not surprising that many people are misdiagnosed as having true hypoglycemia when they do not.

Sorbitol is a reduced form of glucose—that is, it has had one hydrogen atom added. Sorbitol is found in fruits such as apples, pears, and peaches and in several vegetables. Because it is absorbed from the intestine into the blood at about one third the rate of glucose, sorbitol permits blood glucose levels to remain above fasting levels for a longer time following a meal, thus delaying the onset of hunger sensations. It may be included as an ingredient in weight-reducing aids. However, in some people sorbitol causes **flatulence** and diarrhea, which greatly reduce its acceptance. Sorbitol is also used extensively in chewing gum because it is less likely to lead to dental cavities.

Fructose

Another monosaccharide, fructose is also known as fruit sugar or levulose. It occurs naturally in many fruits and berries and makes up over one third of the sugar in honey. Recently we have been able to use enzymes to produce crystalline fructose and a high fructose corn syrup (HFCS) from cornstarch or from sucrose. Crystalline fructose and HFCS are sweeter per calorie than sugar and were first used commercially in the early 1970s. They are now being used in a large number of processed foods, especially beverages. If the price of sugar is high relative to that of corn, the use of HFCS will usually increase. If the price of sugar is lower and competitive, less HFCS is used. The growing popularity of HFCS is evident from Figure 4-5. Current use amounts to 30 pounds per person each year.

Although fructose does not cause a rise in blood sugar in the diabetic because insulin is not required for it to be taken up by the cell, we have not had enough experience with diets high in fructose to be sure that it is entirely safe as a sugar replacement for diabetics. We do know that it is less likely to be **cariogenic** (tending to cause tooth decay) than other sweeteners. Caries are produced when bacteria in the mouth act on carbohydrate to produce acid. Acid production depends on the type of carbohydrate available.

Despite what some ads suggest, there is no merit associated with the use of fructose as an "animal sugar" produced by bees. When fructose is sold in crystalline form, it must be considered a processed rather than a natural food product. Honey

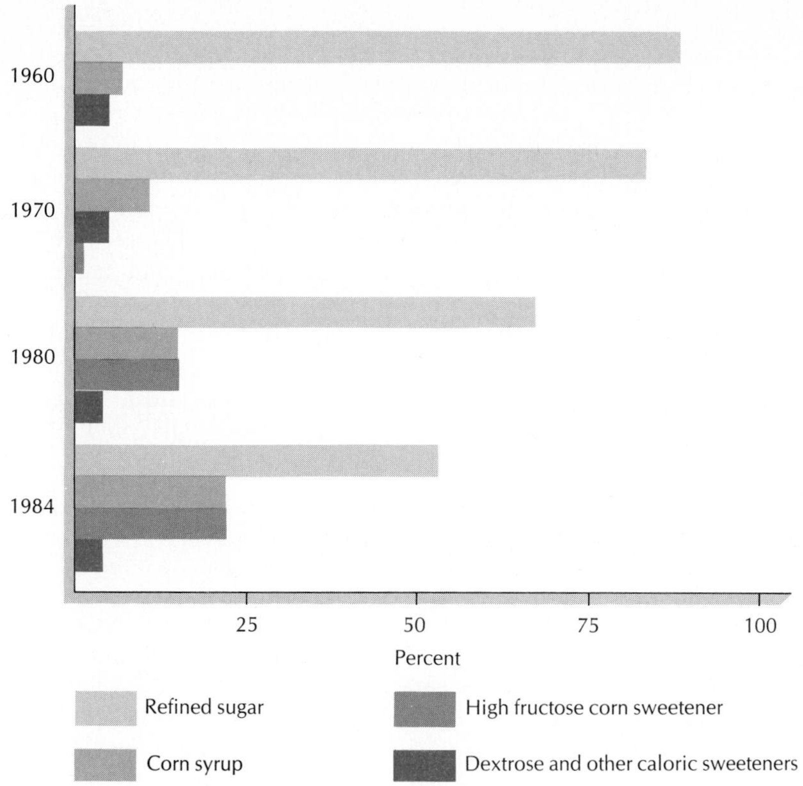

Figure 4-5 Percent of population in the United States using various nutritive sweeteners, 1960-1984.
USDA data.

has been advertised as a natural food high in fructose. As far as we know, however, aside from its pleasant flavor there is no reason to promote the use of fructose over other carbohydrates. On the negative side there is growing evidence that it may increase the need for copper.

The sugar in honey is predominantly fructose. Thus it provides sweetness with half the calories of sugar. It does not make any significant contribution of other nutrients.

Galactose

Galactose, the third monosaccharide, occurs only as the result of the digestion, or hydrolysis, of the disaccharide lactose, which is the sugar in milk. Galactose is the only monosaccharide obtained primarily from animal foods. Too much galactose was found to be associated with cataracts in animal studies, but at levels usually consumed it is unlikely to present any problem in human beings, except for the few people with a genetic metabolic defect known as galactosemia (too much galactose in the blood).

Pentoses

In addition to the hexoses just described, which are the major monosaccharides in food, there are several five-carbon sugars known as **pentoses.** One, ribose, is part of the vitamin *riboflavin* (or B_2) and the coenzymes made from it and part of RNA, or ribonucleic acid, which is an essential link with DNA (deoxyribonucleic acid) needed for the synthesis of protein. Because ribose can be produced in the body from glucose, however, it is not essential to have it provided in food.

pentose
A five-carbon sugar (pento = five; ose = sugar)

Xylose, another pentose, is now being produced commercially from cellulose and hemicellulose, which are found in many types of wood, particularly birch. Xylitol, the alcohol sugar derived from xylose, is being used to provide the sweetness and texture we want in candies and gum without contributing to tooth decay. As little as 1 oz slows the emptying time of the stomach by 50% and reduces caloric intake by one fourth. There is no concern about its safety at the levels usually consumed.

Disaccharides

SUCROSE = **GLUCOSE** + FRUCTOSE

LACTOSE = **GLUCOSE** + GALACTOSE

MALTOSE = **GLUCOSE** + GLUCOSE

The three *disaccharides* found in food—*sucrose*, *lactose*, and *maltose*—are formed when one unit of the monosaccharide glucose is combined with one unit of either fructose, galactose, or glucose. Sucrose and maltose are made in plant cells, and lactose is produced in the mammary gland of animals. When the two molecules (units) are joined together or condensed to form a disaccharide, one molecule of water is split off. The water molecule forms when an "H" of one monosaccharide combines with an "OH" from the second monosaccharide. The resulting sugars, all with the same formula $[C_{12}(H_2O)_{11}]$, are sucrose, lactose, and maltose (again, note the names that end in "ose").

After we eat these sugars, the process of synthesis must be reversed to break them into their original monosaccharide units so they are small enough to be absorbed through the intestinal wall. This process of **digestion,** or **hydrolysis** requires that one molecule of water be split into "H" and "OH" and added back to reform the monosaccharide units. This can occur either when the disaccharide comes into contact with acid or when an enzyme facilitates the split. The reversible reactions of synthesis and digestion are shown in Figure 4-6.

digestion (hydrolysis)
Process by which foods are broken down into smaller units until they are small enough to be absorbed through the intestinal wall

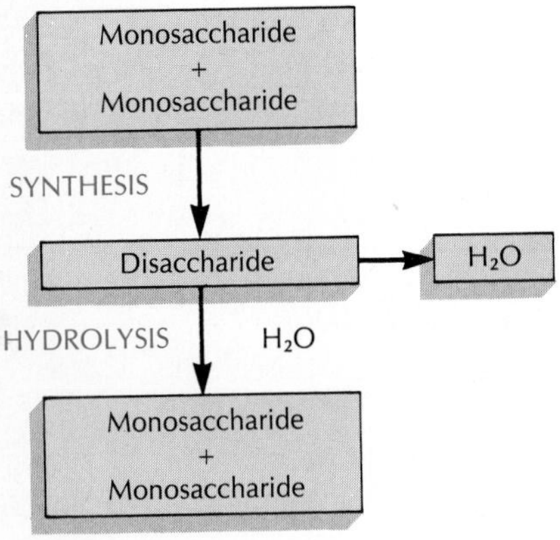

Figure 4-6 Synthesis and hydrolysis (digestion) of disaccharides.

Sucrose

Sucrose is the most common disaccharide; it is a combination of glucose and fructose. It is obtained commercially from both sugar cane and sugar beets to produce the familiar granulated and powdered sugars, which are both 100% sucrose. Brown sugar, with its more distinctive flavor, is 97% sucrose and is made by adding some molasses to white sugar. Because both sugar beets and sugar cane yield far more calories per acre of land than any other food, sugar is our least expensive food source of energy. Although sugar does not provide other nutrients, it does much to enhance the palatability of foods.

The average amount of added sucrose consumed in the United States per person per day is 81 grams (about 3 ounces, or 6 tablespoons). This is only 10 grams more than was consumed in 1909. There is some concern that the increase in total sweetener (sucrose plus HFCS) to 125 grams per person may have adverse health consequences.

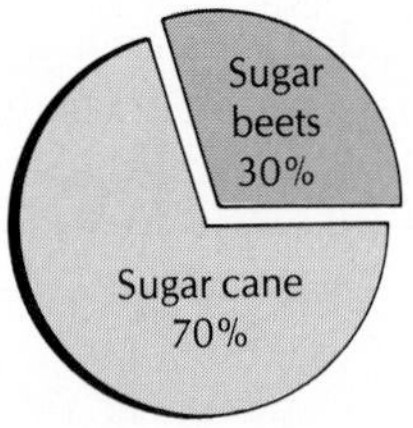

Two major sources of sucrose in the food supply

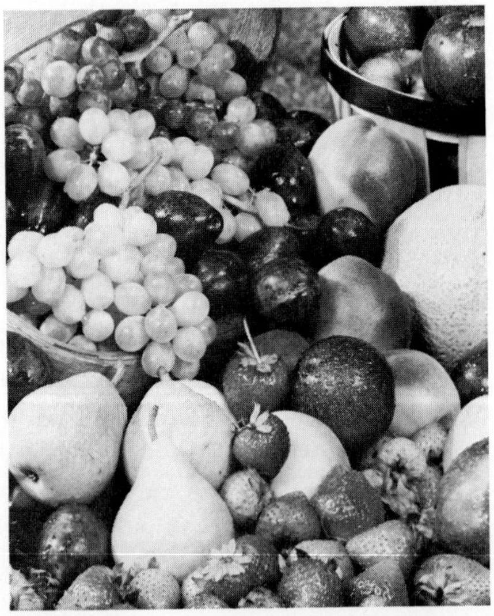

Most fruits contain the simple carbohydrates—sucrose, glucose, and fructose

Lactose

Lactose accounts for 25 grams total dietary sugar. It is a combination of glucose and galactose and is found exclusively in milk. Lactose serves to enhance the absorption of calcium. It is interesting that milk, which is our major source of lactose, is also the most dependable source of calcium in our diets.

lactose = milk sugar

Many adults, especially those of Asian or black ancestry, suffer from a deficiency of the enzyme *lactase*, which is produced normally in the wall of the intestine and is essential for the conversion of dietary lactose to glucose and galactose. This **lactase insufficiency** results in **lactose intolerance;** in this case, undigested lactose, which is too large to be absorbed, remains in the gastrointestinal tract, where it serves as food for microorganisms that thrive there. Some of these organisms produce a large amount of gas, resulting in symptoms of flatulence, bloating, and abdominal cramping. In addition, because lactose has an **osmotic effect** (a tendency to attract water), its presence in the colon leads to retention of water with resulting watery stools or diarrhea.

lactase insufficiency/lactose intolerance
A lack of the enzyme lactase, which is needed to convert lactose to glucose and galactose

osmotic effect
The tendency to attract water, usually to dilute some constituent of a fluid

Although people with lactose intolerance experience a lot of discomfort from eating lactose-containing dairy products, they can eat fermented dairy products such as cheese because much of the lactose has been changed to lactic acid, which does not cause a problem. Yogurt contains lactose, but it is tolerated because it also provides enzymes that are activated and digest the lactose when the yogurt is warmed in the stomach. Many people are also able to tolerate small amounts of lactose and can therefore consume some milk products. Although they may never start to produce lactase, they seem to build up a lactose tolerance and are able to take increasing amounts over time.

It appears that all young infants have the appropriate enzymes to allow them to use milk without any discomfort. However, milk intolerance does develop in early childhood in people who lack the gene that triggers the production of lactase. Therefore many have questioned the wisdom of providing milk in school feeding programs when the children are primarily of black ancestry. There have also been questions about the use of milk in feeding programs for world population groups that are likely to have lactase deficiency.

The availability of enzymes produced by yeasts and molds makes it possible for lactose-intolerant people to drink milk. When these enzymes, which are available in tablet form, are mixed with the milk, they split lactose into glucose and galactose before the milk is even consumed. Thus, the lactose never reaches the colon.

Maltose

The third disaccharide, maltose, is found only in germinating cereals. During germination the cereal starch is being broken down into maltose units of two glucose molecules. These are then further broken into single glucose units to nourish the developing seed. The production of beer and other malt beverages requires the fermentation, rather than hydrolysis or digestion, of maltose into alcohol.

All sugars contribute sweetness to food, but the relative amount of sweetness varies with the sugar used. In general, the more easily the sugar dissolves, the greater its sweetening power. For example, fructose is 75% sweeter than other sugars; it is very soluble in water, difficult to crystallize, and as a result very expensive. It is useful in syrups and is the type of sugar used in soft-centered candies. At the other extreme is the least sweet, least soluble sugar—lactose. Lactose is seldom if ever used as a sweetener because it is almost impossible to dissolve in the food to be sweetened. A comparison of various physical properties of some carbohydrates is presented in Table 4-1.

Polysaccharides

The third class of carbohydrates, the *polysaccharides*, which include starch and dietary fiber, is much more complex than the other two groups. Polysaccharides are considered complex carbohydrates rather than sugars.

Table 4-1 ◆ Comparison of physical properties of carbohydrates (relative values)

	Sweetening Power	Soluble	Rate of Absorption	Rate of Acid Production*
Monosaccharides				
Hexoses				
Fructose	170	Yes	30	80-100
Glucose	70	Yes	**100**	**100**
Galactose	32	Yes	110	
Mannose			10	
Alcohol sugars				
Sorbitol	60	Yes		10-30
Mannitol	70	Slightly		0
Maltitol	90			10-30
Zylitol	90-100			0
Lactitol	35			10-30
Pentoses				
Ribose	—	Yes	15	
Xylose	40	Yes	9	
Arabinose	—	Yes		
Disaccharides				
Sucrose	**100**	Yes		100
Lactose	20	Yes		40-60
Maltose	40	Yes		
Polysaccharides				
Starch		No		
Glycogen		No		
Dextrin		Slightly		
Cellulose		No		
Other Sweeteners				
High fructose corn syrup	100-500	Yes		
Sugar Substitutes				
Cyclamate	3-8000	Yes		0
Aspartame	10-20,000	Yes		0
Saccharin	30-70,000	Yes		0

Boldface = standard for comparison; blanks indicate that data are unavailable.
*Relative rate at which carbohydrate is fermented to acid.

amylose
A starch in which the glucose units are linked together in one long chain (amyl = starch)

G—G—G—G—G—G—G—G—G_n

amylopectin
A starch in which the glucose units are linked together in a branched arrangement

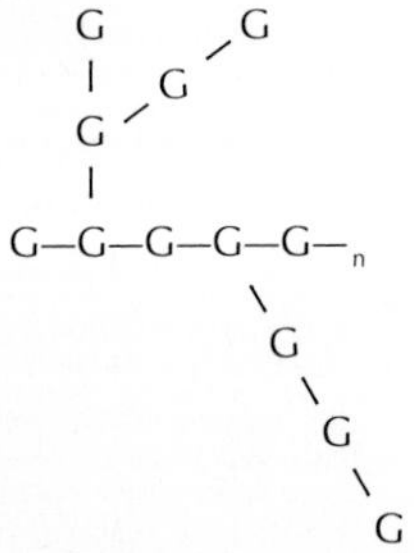

Starch

Starches represent about half of dietary carbohydrate and are composed solely of glucose units linked together. A polysaccharide may contain as many as 2000 glucose units (one with 26,000 units has been identified). These units may be in one long chain (an **amylose**) or in a branched arrangement (an **amylopectin**).

Each plant produces its own characteristic starch determined by the number of glucose units and their arrangement within the molecule. Granules of potato starch can thus be distinguished from granules of rice, wheat, cassava, corn, or any other starch by microscopic examination of the shape and size of the granule. In addition, each of these starches has unique characteristics of solubility, thickening power, and flavor. Nutritionally the body does not discriminate among starches; it is able to break down all cooked starches into their component glucose units for absorption and use by the body cells.

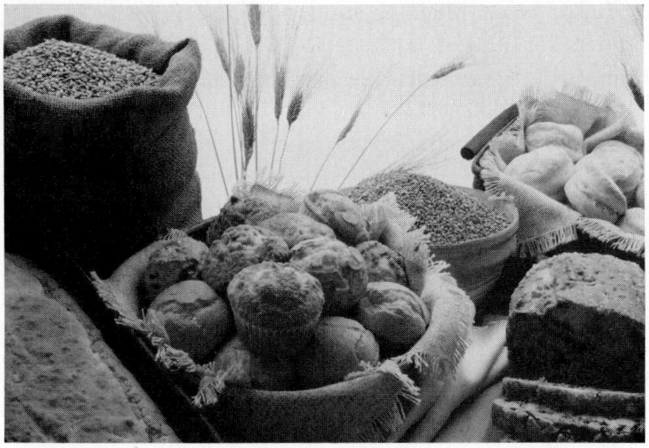

These grains and grain products are composed of carbohydrates that are more complex than the carbohydrates found in fruits. Unrefined grains are sources of dietary fiber.

Glycogen

The animal stores a limited amount of carbohydrate as the polysaccharide **glycogen,** primarily in the liver and in muscle. These are the only two animal tissues besides milk and blood that contain carbohydrate. The adult human stores only about 340 grams of glycogen—one third as liver glycogen and two thirds as muscle glycogen. The energy stored in glycogen represents only enough energy to last an adult human about half a day.

glycogen
A polysaccharide; a carbohydrate that is stored in the muscle or liver; sometimes known as animal starch

When it is used as food, liver or muscle contains no glycogen because most is converted into lactic acid at the time of slaughtering.

The capacity of the liver and muscles to store glycogen may be increased 100% by manipulating the diet in association with exercise. This procedure, known as **carbohydrate loading,** was popular with athletes such as soccer players or long-distance runners who need a large amount of energy derived from muscle glycogen for a period of 30 minutes or more of continuous exercise. However, because of some adverse side effects, athletes are abandoning carbohydrate loading in favor of a diet high in complex carbohydrates.

carbohydrate loading
Process by which athletes increase their stores of glycogen in the liver; for further discussion, see Chapter 19

Dextrin

Dextrin, another nutritionally important polysaccharide, is the slightly soluble product that results when very long glucose chains are split into shorter chains by the removal one at a time of maltose units made up of two glucose units. This process may be accomplished by enzymes, as occurs during digestion; by the action of dry heat on starch, as when bread is toasted; or during production of the dry bread, **zweibach,** for infants. In all of these the resulting dextrin is sweeter and more soluble than the original starch.

Fiber

There are two types of fiber found in food—crude fiber and dietary fiber. Cellulose, the major component of crude fiber, is another polysaccharide. It provides the structural framework for all plant material; that is, it gives the shape to a carrot, a bean, or a squash. Cellulose is the most abundant organic compound in the world, being found in fruits, vegetables, and whole-grain cereals as well as wood and leaves. Like starch, it is composed of many glucose units. Unlike starch, however, these units are linked together in such a way that human digestive enzymes are unable to break them apart to form separate glucose units. Nor can the chemist digest them with acid in the laboratory.

zweibach
Dextrinized, easily digested bread, often fed to babies; its texture is hard, crisp, and more similar to crackers than the texture of many other breads

In addition to cellulose or **crude fiber** there are several other complex carbohydrates and related compounds, pectins, hemicelluloses, and lignins that also resist digestion in the human digestive tract. Together these are known as **dietary fiber.**

crude fiber
Portion of a plant that resists chemical breakdown

dietary fiber
Any material that remains undigested in the intestine

Dietary fiber can be further classified as soluble and insoluble fiber. Soluble

To add oat bran to homemade foods for all recipes that call for flour, substitute for each cup of flour—⅓ cup of oat bran for ⅓ cup flour.

Dietary Sources of Fiber
>4 grams/serving
- Oat bran*
- Kidney beans*
- Split peas*
- Raisins
- Pear*
- Prunes
- Figs

3-4 grams/serving
- Oatmeal*
- Kale
- Corn*
- Peanuts

2-3 grams/serving
- Tomato
- Carrot*
- Wheat bran
- Orange*
- Banana
- Peach

*Soluble fiber; all others insoluble

diverticulosis
A condition in which there is a weakening in the wall of the intestine; usually the result of pressure from hard stools

diverticulitis
An inflammation in the wall of the intestine; usually the result of an irritation following diverticulosis

fiber found in fruits, some legumes, and grains, such as oats, rye, and barley dissolves in water to form a gel. This gel serves to slow the rate at which digested food passes through the large intestine and thus increases the rate of absorption. Soluble fiber also binds cholesterol from the bile and prevents its reabsorption and recirculation in the blood, accounting for its effectiveness in controlling or lowering blood cholesterol levels. Alternatively, soluble fiber may act by binding the bile acids that normally promote the absorption of dietary cholesterol, thus causing less to be absorbed. Oat fiber appears to be more effective than fibers from other cereals in reducing cholesterol absorption.

In contrast, the insoluble fiber found in vegetables and wheat bran that consists of cellulose, hemicellulose, and lignins does not dissolve in water. Instead, it tends to absorb water and increase in bulk, contributing to the volume of the stools. This helps maintain normal gastrointestinal motility (i.e., it keeps food moving through the gastrointestinal tract, especially the colon) and prevents constipation and diverticulosis.

As indicated in Chapter 3, health authorities continue to recommend that Americans increase their fiber intake. This has led some food processors to add fiber to their foods, primarily in the form of bran or wood fiber. There is now concern that some people will be getting too much fiber and develop a condition known as irritable bowel syndrome. It is also possible that too much fiber may lead to a decreased absorption of some mineral elements, either by binding them or by speeding the passage of food through the intestinal tract, so that the time for absorption of nutrients may be reduced. Currently, it appears that an intake of 18 to 35 grams of dietary fiber, considerably higher than current intakes, will provide maximum benefits while minimizing the possibility of adverse effects of either too much or too little fiber.

Interest in the role of fiber in the diet has been stimulated by the observation that in other cultures, where the consumption of fiber is high, there is a much lower incidence of cancer of the colon and **diverticulosis.** Cancer of the colon causes 52,000 American deaths annually. Diverticulosis affects 30 million Americans and is characterized by a weakening of the intestinal wall caused by pressure from hard stools. The weakened intestinal wall then develops small outpouchings in which fecal material becomes trapped (Figure 4-7). As these outpouchings are irritated or become infected, a condition known as **diverticulitis** develops; it afflicts many adults. Dietary treatment involves a diet with 18 to 35 grams of fiber to help prevent the formation of hard stools.

Comparison of crude and dietary fiber

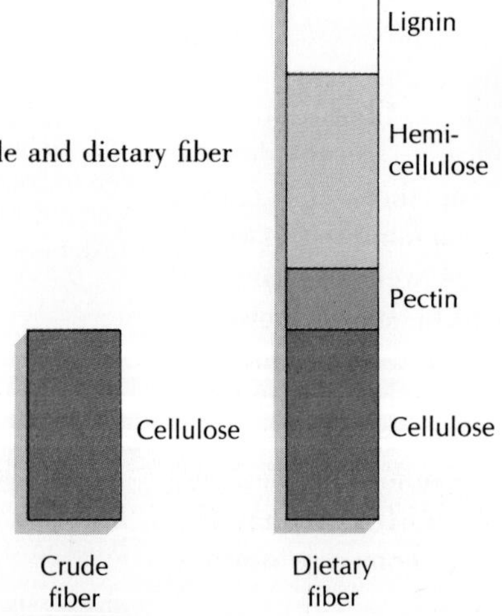

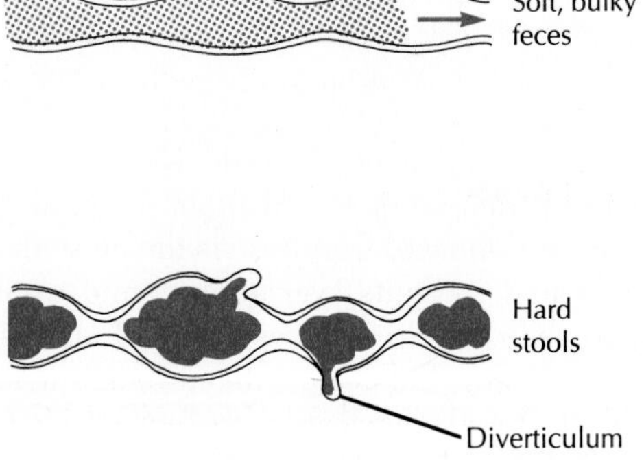

Figure 4-7 Development of diverticulosis and associated diverticulitis.

The relationship between lack of dietary fiber and cancer of the colon has been attributed to changes in the microorganisms in the gastrointestinal tract or in the decreased time in which food residue remains in the colon. Scientists postulate that the microorganisms associated with low dietary fiber favor the formation of cancer-producing substances, or **carcinogens.** These microorganisms may also prevent or limit the breakdown of carcinogens that are normally destroyed when dietary fiber is higher. Another theory is that dietary fiber exerts its beneficial effect by speeding the passage of the feces through the large intestine so that carcinogens are in contact with the intestinal wall for a much shorter period of time. Additionally, the bulk and water of the feces may dilute the carcinogen to a nontoxic level.

carcinogens
Cancer-producing substances

The data on fiber recorded in tables of food composition have traditionally been for crude fiber or cellulose, which resists digestion by strong acid or alkali in the chemistry lab. From a nutritional standpoint we are interested in data on dietary fiber that includes all fiber that remains undigested in the intestine. In addition to crude fiber, this includes pectins, hemicelluloses, and the noncarbohydrate lignins. Values for dietary fiber in Table 4-2 (p. 85) may be up to 10 times higher than those for crude fiber. Dietary fiber is found only in foods of plant origin such as legumes, cereals, nuts, seeds, fruits, and vegetables.

Because of the limited data we have on dietary fiber in foods, it is difficult to recommend a desirable intake. Current intakes of 6 to 8 grams of crude fiber are associated with lack of symptoms. This is probably equivalent to 20 or more grams of dietary fiber. USDA data show that the amount of fiber available in the food supply has declined throughout this century, as has the intake by individuals. Current recommendations and advertising of fiber-rich foods is reversing this trend among the health-conscious segment of the population. Experience has shown that a diet providing four daily servings of fruits and vegetables and four servings of cereal (at least two of which should be minimally processed or whole grain) will provide enough fiber.

Related Carbohydrates

Mucopolysaccharides and *mucoproteins,* groups of compounds that are chemically related to carbohydrates, do not occur in food but are normal constituents of the body. The most common mucopolysaccharides are found in the fluid lubricating the joints; in the vitreous humor of the eye; in the cartilage, skin, and bone; as an anticoagulant in the blood; and in hard structures such as nails.

Modified starches, which have been changed to give them properties such as stability in acid and at high temperatures and different textures that are important in the processing of foods, are usually considered food additives. They seldom make up more than 5% of a food. *Sugar alcohols* such as sorbitol, xylitol, and mannitol are derived from monosaccharides. They are used in some foods largely because of special properties, such as rate of absorption or effect on dental health.

Sugar-free on a label does not always mean low in calories or low-carbohydrate. If sorbitol or mannitol is used to sweeten a dietetic product, there will still be calories.

FUNCTIONS

Source of Energy

The major function of carbohydrate is as a source of energy. This function is not unique to carbohydrate, but at a cost of as little as one penny per 100 kcal carbohydrate is the least expensive source of energy. Glucose is the major source of energy for both nervous tissue and the lungs. In addition to obtaining glucose from dietary carbohydrates, the body can produce glucose from part of a protein or fat molecule in a process called **gluconeogenesis,** or the formation of new glucose. Therefore even these tissues can get along without dietary carbohydrate for a short period of time. Glucose is the most usual source of energy for muscles. However, they can use fatty acids, although somewhat less efficiently.

gluconeogenesis
The formation of glucose from substances other than carbohydrate

1 gram carbohydrate provides 4 kcal
1 teaspoon sugar weighs 4 grams
1 teaspoon sugar provides 16 kcal

Check ingredient labels on food products for clues about the sugar content. If sugar appears first, the product is relatively high in sugar.

Terms on a label that mean sugar:

sucrose	galactose
dextrose	corn syrup
glucose	invert sugar
lactose	honey
fructose	molasses
maltose	maple syrup

The amount of energy provided is almost constant for all forms of carbohydrate. One gram of carbohydrate provides 4 kcal, regardless of whether the carbohydrate is starch or sugar, monosaccharide or disaccharide. In 1987 carbohydrate provided 45% of the calories in a typical U.S. diet; the figure was higher—56%—at the beginning of the century. The proportion of carbohydrate in the diet coming from complex carbohydrates has declined by more than 30% since the early 1900s, and that from sugar has increased proportionately.

The current dietary goals of the United States recommend a reversal of this trend to increase the energy provided from carbohydrate, back to 55% to 60% of the calories, of which less than 10% should be from added sugar. Thus, on a 2000-kcal diet, an intake of 275 to 300 grams (1100 to 1200 kcal) of carbohydrate is recommended with only 30 grams from added sugar.

Dietary Essential

Although carbohydrate can be replaced as a source of energy by fat or protein, a series of undesirable symptoms appear when there is none in the diet. The symptoms are similar to those that develop with starvation. There is an unexplained loss of large amounts of both sodium and body water. This accounts for the rapid loss of body weight that occurs in people on a low or carbohydrate-free diet. The loss of sodium is usually followed by a loss of potassium from the cells, and this usually leads to symptoms of weakness. At the same time the body is unable to prevent the breakdown of body protein, except at very high protein intakes; this contributes further to weight loss. Even more seriously, the use of fat as a source of energy is blocked in the middle of the process, leading to the accumulation of intermediary product of fat metabolism known as *ketones*. As ketones build up, they appear as abnormal constituents of the blood and urine. Because they change the hydrogen ion concentration or acid-base balance of tissues, they interfere with normal body functioning. People with this problem are said to have **ketosis** and usually suffer from symptoms of fatigue, dehydration, and loss of energy. All these undesirable results of a lack of carbohydrate in the diet are reversed by the addition of carbohydrate, an indication that it is a dietary essential.

ketosis
A condition in which ketones, or abnormal products of fat metabolism, accumulate in the blood

These facts help us to see that low (less than 60 grams) carbohydrate or starvation diets are a dangerous and unsuccessful way to try to lose weight. Fortunately, because a low-carbohydrate diet is very unpalatable, the dieter often soon abandons it and regains the lost water and weight.

The notion that carbohydrate is not only "not bad" but also actually essential runs counter to long-held popular beliefs that have led people to try to avoid carbohydrate (or at least talk about avoiding it). Carbohydrate is, indeed, an essential part of the diet. The importance of including more complex carbohydrate, which often involves foods containing fiber, and less simple carbohydrates or sugar is being constantly stressed.

Source of Sweetness

One of the major roles of carbohydrate is to contribute sweetness to food and in many cases make it more palatable. Whether the desire for sweetness is innate or acquired is a question that has puzzled scientists for a long time. Recent studies indicate that, even **in utero** (in the womb) and immediately after birth, the fetus and the newborn baby respond favorably to a stimulus from a sweet substance and unfavorably to a bitter substance.

in utero
Latin, "in the womb"

DIGESTION AND ABSORPTION

Before carbohydrate can fulfill its role in the body, it must be converted into monosaccharide units that are small enough to pass through the wall of the intestine and into the bloodstream. These changes are brought about by the action of certain enzymes: *amylases*, which act on starch; and the specific disaccharide-splitting enzymes *sucrase*, *lactase*, and *maltase*, which act on sucrose, lactose, and maltose to convert them into glucose, fructose, and galactose. Amylase is present in the saliva and in the pancreatic juice. The enzymes that digest disaccharides are found in the wall of the intestine.

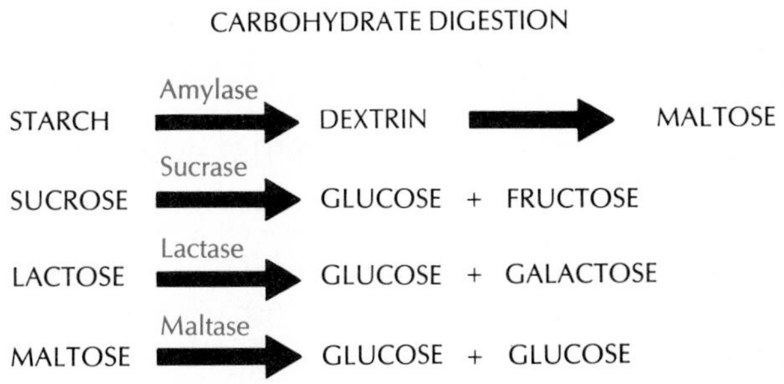

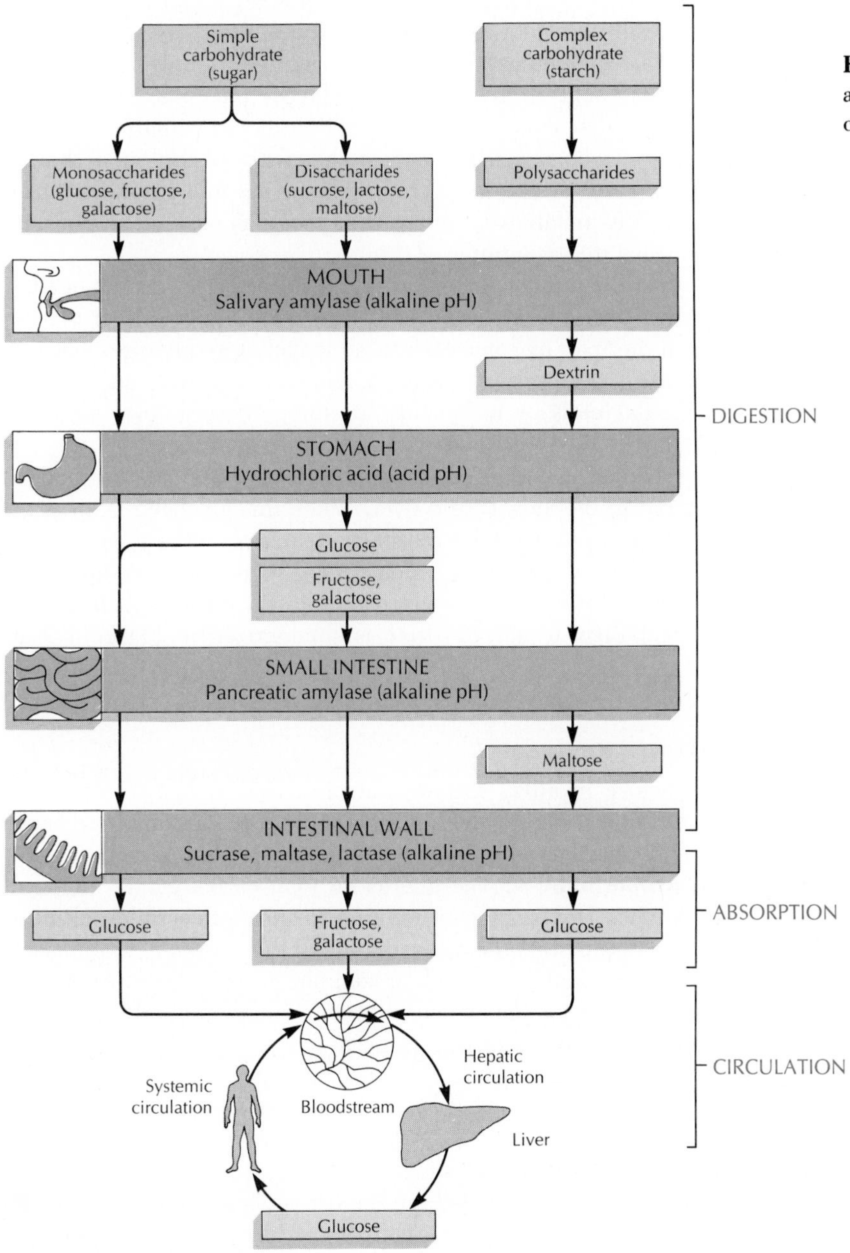

Figure 4-8 Summary of digestion, absorption, and circulation of carbohydrate.

Some disaccharides are split apart by hydrolysis in the presence of hydrochloric acid in the stomach. Once in their simplest form, the three monosaccharides pass through the intestinal wall and are carried in the blood through the portal vein to the liver. These digestive changes and absorption of carbohydrates are presented in Figure 4-8. Once in the liver fructose and galactose are converted to glucose, which is then released to the blood.

METABOLISM

As soon as glucose is in the bloodstream, it is carried to the individual cells. There it is used in one of three ways:

1. It is metabolized or oxidized immediately as a source of energy. The first steps are known collectively as **glycolysis** (from the Greek *-lysis*, to break). The changes involve breaking glucose, which has six carbons, into two three-carbon compounds of pyruvic acid. The changes are anaerobic, which means that they do not require oxygen. Two molecules of the energy-rich compound **ATP (adenosine triphosphate)** are also required for glycolysis. As a result of glycolysis, which produces 4 units of ATP, there is a net gain of 2 ATP molecules. This amount represents only a small portion of the potential energy stored within the glucose molecule, which yields a total of 38 ATP units. However, even 4 ATP units are valuable for athletes such as sprinters, who may have very high energy needs for a short period. The pyruvic acid formed in glycolysis enters the mitochrondrion of the the cell, where it is metabolized along with products of digestion of fat and protein to release the remaining ATP units.
2. When the amount of glucose available exceeds the amount needed for energy, it is converted to glycogen and stored in either the liver or muscle tissue.
3. When the liver and muscle can no longer store glycogen because they have saturated their storage capacity, glucose is converted into fat and stored in regular cells or in special fat storage cells known as adipose cells or adipocytes.

glycolysis
The breakdown of carbohydrate in metabolism (glyco = sugar; lysis = to break)

For more information on energy (ATP) see Chapter 7.

ATP (adenosine triphosphate)
Compound in which energy is stored when the third phosphate is added and released as it is taken away

ADP + energy ⇆ ATP

For more information on cell structure see Appendix A.

Later, if the intake of energy is less than the requirement, the body will use the glycogen stored in the muscle and liver. When this glycogen is almost all used up, the body will switch to using fat reserves. At this time the blood glucose level will have fallen to the fasting level, which usually stimulates the appetite and causes the individual to eat so that the glycogen and fat reserves will not be used. The digestion metabolism of carbohydrate is summarized in Figure 4-9 and in Table 4-2.

FOOD SOURCES

Except for lactose in milk, carbohydrate is found almost exclusively in foods of plant origin. Table 4-3 provides information on the carbohydrate content of foods most frequently used in the United States and foods generally considered to be good carbohydrate sources. The figures for total carbohydrate include the amount of usable starches and sugars in addition to the indigestible cellulose and fiber. The difference between total carbohydrate and the sum of fiber and sugar or simple carbohydrates represents the starch or complex carbohydrate. As reflected in Table 4-4, many processed foods have considerable amounts of added sugar, which contributes appreciably to the energy value of foods.

Some foods such as sugar and cornstarch have little or no water and are over 80% carbohydrate. Other foods that are known for their carbohydrate content, such as potatoes and cooked rice, have a fairly high water content and are actually less than 20% carbohydrate.

Sugar is added to baked goods for flavor, tenderness, and crispness. Most recipes that call for sugar can be modified by reducing the sugar to ⅓ to ½ without affecting the quality.

Most of the calories in foods from the cereal, fruit, and vegetable groups listed in Table 4-3 are contributed by carbohydrate. It should be remembered, however,

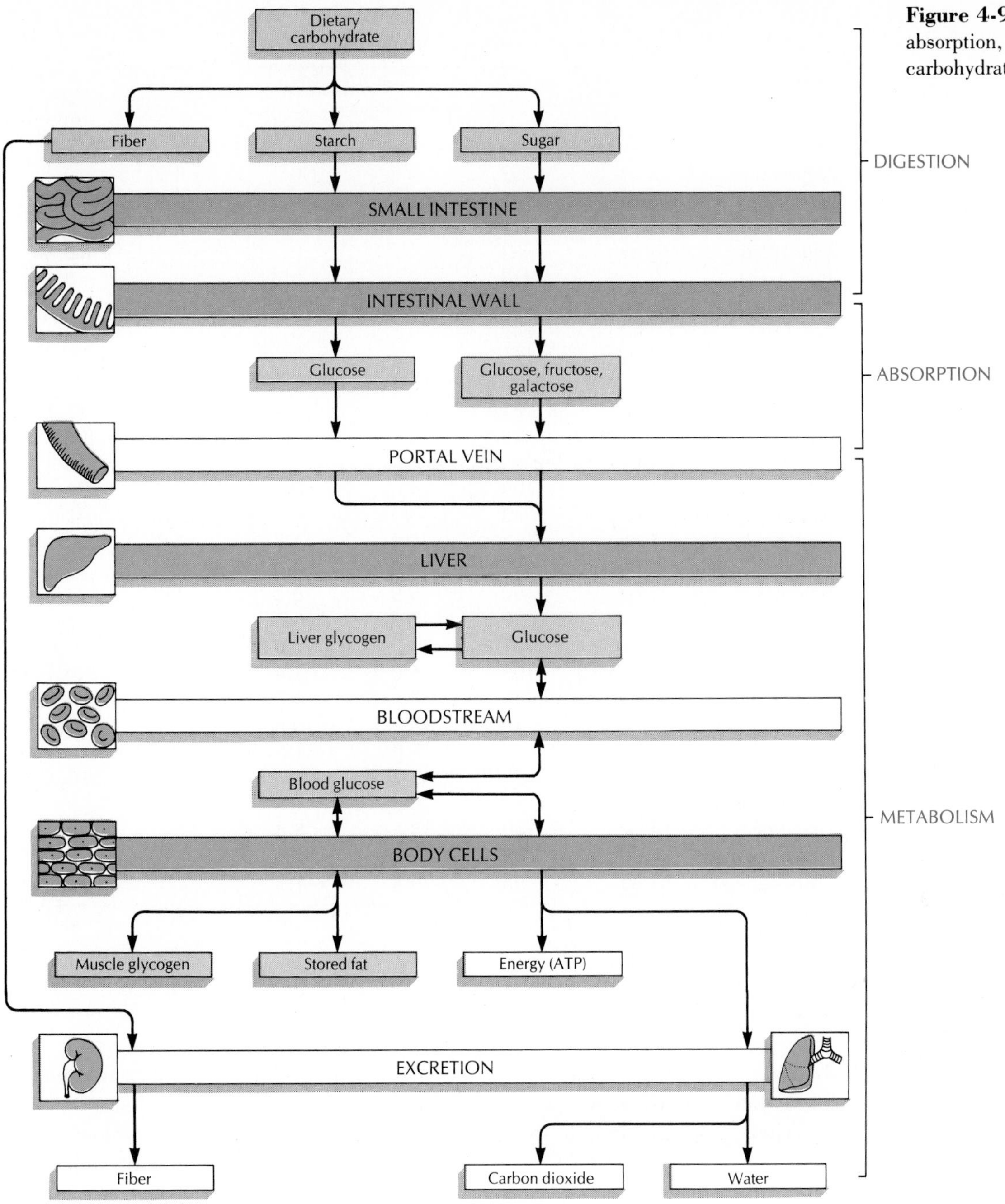

Figure 4-9 Summary of digestion, absorption, and metabolism of carbohydrate.

Table 4-2 ◆ End products of digestion and metabolism of carbohydrate

Nutrient in Food	End Product of Digestion*	End Products of Metabolism† Anabolism	Catabolism
Carbohydrate →	Monosaccharides Glucose Fructose Galactose	Glycogen (muscle, liver) Fat	CO_2 H_2O Energy (ATP)

*Changes occur within lumen digestive tract or in cells lining tract.
†Changes occur within individual body cells.

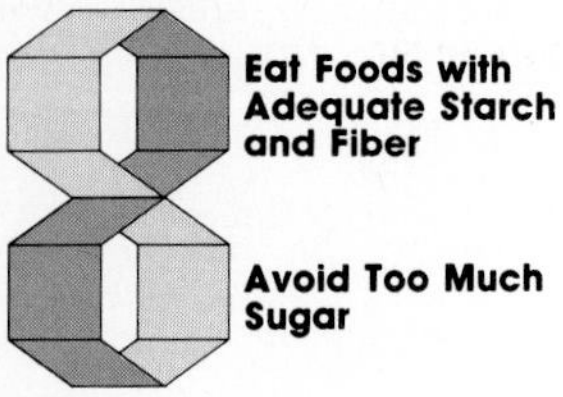
Eat Foods with Adequate Starch and Fiber
Avoid Too Much Sugar

Table 4-3 ◆ Carbohydrate content of the most frequently used foods in the United States and selected carbohydrate sources

Food	Amount	Kcal	Total Carbohydrate (in grams)	Dietary Fiber (in grams)*	Sugar (in grams)†	Starch (in grams)
Whole milk	8 oz	157	4.7	0	4.7	0
2% milk	8 oz	121	5.0	0	5.0	0
Cheddar cheese	1 oz	114	7.2	0	7.2	0
Eggs, fried	1 egg	83	1.2	0	1.2	0
Beef, roast	3 oz	318	0	0	0	0
Hamburger	3 oz	285	0	0	0	0
Chicken	3 oz	242	0	0	0	0
Tuna fish	3 oz	170	0	0	0	0
Peanut butter	2 T	178	5.4	2.1	5.4	0
Bread, white	1 slice	81	15.0	0.8	1.0	13.2
Bread, whole wheat	1 slice	73	130	2.4	1.0	9.6
Rice	1 oz	109	24.0	0	1.0	23
Saltine crackers	4 crackers	43	7.0	0	0	7
Corn flakes	1 oz	114	25.0	2.8	1.9	20.3
Shredded wheat	1 biscuit	105	26.0	3.0	0.1	23
Bran flakes	1 oz	90	25.0	8.2	3.4	13.4
All Bran	1 oz	70	22.0	10.0	5.0	7.0
Apple	1 apple	81	21.0	2.6	18.0	0.4
Banana	1 banana	105	26.0	1.4	24.6	0
Orange juice	4 oz	56	15.0	0.5	14.0	0.5
Peach	1 peach	40	10.0	0.6	9.0	0.4
Lettuce	¼ head	8	3.0	1.1	1.9	0
Tomatoes	1 tomato	25	5.3	1.0	4.3	0
Green beans	4 oz	30	10.0	1.8	8.2	0
Green peas	4 oz	110	18.0	5.4	12.6	0
Potato, baked	1 potato	95	21.0	1.4	1.5	18.1
Corn, canned	4 oz	98	19.8	1.3	2.3	14.2

USDA data, 1984, 1987.
*Includes all fiber not digested by human.
†Naturally occurring monosaccharides and disaccharides.

that very few of these foods are eaten without the addition of a fat or oil such as butter, salad dressing, or a sauce to enhance the flavor, and add calories.

There is a considerable range in the amount of carbohydrate in various fruits. Diabetics who must regulate the amount of carbohydrate in their diet are well aware of the classification of fruits and vegetables on the basis of their carbohydrate content. They know that foods are classified into six major exchange lists, which include lists of foods with equivalent amounts of carbohydrate. As shown in Table 4-5, these equivalencies permit the diabetic to make appropriate food choices. The diabetic exchange list is summarized in Appendix I. Exchange lists are also used extensively by people on weight control diets to recognize foods of approximately equal caloric value.

Until very recently we thought that the quickly digested simple sugars would enter the bloodstream rapidly and cause an immediate increase in blood sugar levels. It was also thought that foods containing complex carbohydrates would be digested much more slowly and as a result would cause a slower and steadier rise in blood sugar levels. However, this long-standing theory has now been challenged. There is now convincing evidence that questions the necessity of advising diabetics to avoid foods with simple carbohydrate and eat foods with more complex carbohydrate to stabilize blood glucose levels. Table 4-6 shows the blood glucose re-

Table 4-4 ◆ Added sugar in processed foods

Product (Serving Size)	Total Calories in Product	Teaspoon Sugar in Serving	% Calories from Added Sugar
Coke (12 oz)	150	9	100%
Tonic water (8 oz)	88	5.5	100%
Club soda/seltzer water (8 oz)	0	0	0%
Jello (½ cup)	83	4.5	87%
Vanilla pudding (½ cup)	90	4	71%
Cranberry sauce (½ cup)	200	12	96%
Catsup (1 T)	16	0.6	61%
Yogurt, fruited (8 oz)	260	6.5	40%
French dressing (2 T)	134	1.5	18%
Instant cocoa powder (1 T)	83	2	38%
Instant oatmeal (1 package)	170	4	38%
Regular oatmeal (¾ cup)	110	0	0%
Cheerios (1¼ cup)	110	0.2-.3	4%
Granola (⅓ cup)	133	1.5	18%
Frosted Flakes (¾ cup)	110	2.7	40%
Fruit drink (8 oz)	120	7	93%
Kool-Aid (8 oz)	96	6	100%
Tang (8 oz or 3 rounded tsp)	122	7.6	100%

Sugar values taken from resources at the Penn State Nutrition Center

Metric measurements are still unfamiliar; 4 grams of sugar equal 1 teaspoon sugar.

Table 4-5 ◆ Food sources providing equivalent amounts (10 grams) of carbohydrate

¾ C milk	1 apple	⅓ C bran flakes
⅚ C yogurt	½ banana	½ C cooked rice
1 C asparagus	½ grapefruit	2 C popcorn
1 C spinach	12 grapes	2 rye wafers
1 C cabbage	2 T raisins	4 saltines
2 C bean sprouts	⅓ C mashed potatoes	10 potato chips
1 C mushrooms	⅔ slice bread	⅔ waffle
1 C tomatoes	2 T bread crumbs	

Table 4-6 ◆ Glycemic index for selected foods*

Milk products		Grains	
Yogurt	36	Cornflakes	80
Ice cream	36	Whole-wheat bread	72
Whole milk	34	White rice	72
Sugars		Shredded wheat	67
Maltose	105	Sweet corn	59
Glucose	**100**	Oatmeal	49
Honey	87	Vegetables	
Sucrose (table)	59	Carrots	92
Fructose	20	Potatoes	70
Fruits		Potato chips	51
Bananas	62	Peas	51
Orange juice	46	Baked beans	40
Apples	39	Peanuts	13

From Jenkin DJA, and others: The glycemic index of foods: a physiological basis for carbohydrate exchange, American Journal of Clinical Nutrition 34:362, 1981.

*The blood glucose response following the feeding of a test dose of the food relative to glucose (glucose = 100).

glycemic index
The relative rate at which glucose appears in the blood following the ingestion of various carbohydrate rich foods; standard for comparison is the response of glusoce fed alone

Lactose Content of Milk Products

	grams
Whole milk (1 cup)	12
Nonfat milk (1 cup)	11
Buttermilk (1 cup)	9
Acidophilus milk (1 cup)	6
Fruit yogurt (1 cup)	8
Cheddar cheese (1 oz)	1
American cheese (1 oz)	2.7
Cottage cheese (1 cup)	4.6
Ice cream (1 cup)	10
Milkshake (1 cup)	14

legumes
Vegetables such as peas and beans

sponse, or **glycemic index** (that is, the relative effect of different individual foods on blood glucose levels), compared to the response from glucose fed alone. It is evident that vegetables such as carrots and complex carbohydrates such as white rice, potatoes, and whole-wheat bread have a more rapid effect than table sugar (that is, sucrose). Fructose has practically no effect, and many fruits have less effect than previously believed. (Two different forms of the same food—for example, mashed and boiled potatoes—do not necessarily have the same effect.) These effects are observed when foods are fed singly. We need to learn whether they have the same effect when fed as part of a meal.

Milk, a major source of lactose, is the only animal food that makes a consistent contribution of carbohydrate to the diet. Eggs have a very small amount of carbohydrate, and scallops and oysters (hardly dietary staples) are the only other animal foods with any carbohydrate. Human milk has about 1½ times as much lactose as cow's milk.

A group of starch-related polysaccharide gums has a variety of uses in food processing. Their names in a list of food ingredients may be puzzling. They include *agar* and *carrageenan,* which are both derived from algae and are used in fruit fillings, gels, icings, and baked goods where they function as fat stabilizers and jelling agents. *Pectin,* which comes from citrus peel, and *guar gum,* which comes from a legume, are both used as jelling agents. (**Legumes** are vegetables such as peas and beans.) *Methylcellulose,* a synthetic material, is used in low-calorie cookies, mayonnaise, and candy to help provide bulk without calories.

Fluffy cellulose is a newly developed product made from nonwoody plants that can be used as a noncaloric flour, replacing up to 50% of the flour used in baked goods. It does not affect the taste, but it is responsible for a sizable reduction in the caloric value of the products. Because it absorbs more water than the flour it replaces, it results in cakes with greater volumes than those made with flour.

MILLING OF CEREALS

endosperm
The center of the cereal grain

The cereals, corn, wheat, and rices are the major sources of carbohydrate in our diets. From the diagram of a typical cereal grain (Figure 4-10), it is evident that the **endosperm,** or center, makes up the largest portion. The endosperm, composed primarily of starch, is where the plant stores energy. Although some other nutrients

Figure 4-10 Diagrammatic representation of a cereal grain.

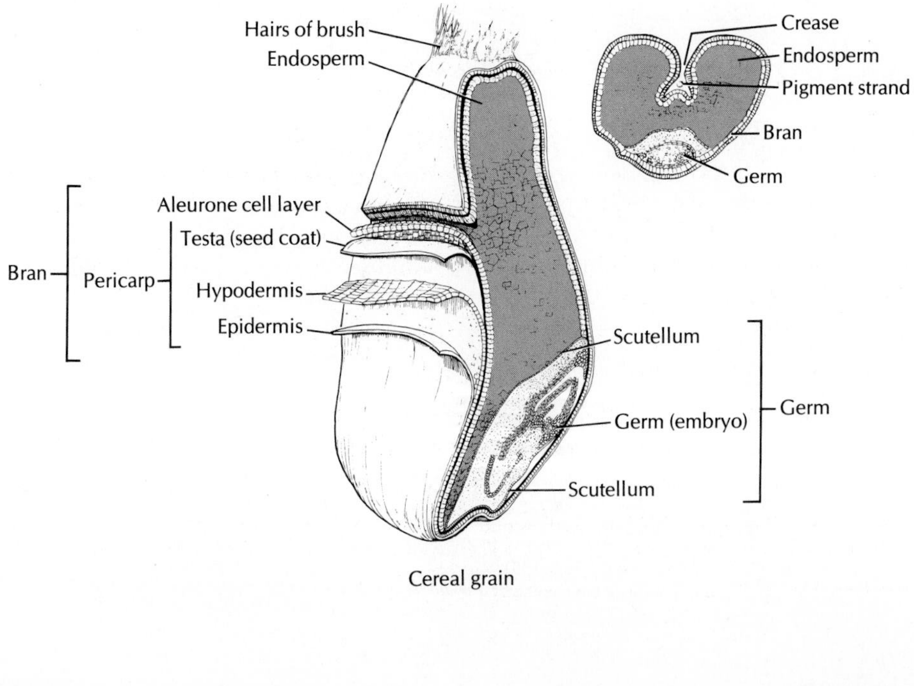

Table 4-7 ◆ Distribution of nutrients in cereal grain (percent of total content)

			B Vitamins				
	Protein	Total Mineral	Thiamin	Riboflavin	Niacin	Pyridoxine	Pantothenic Acid
Endosperm	72	20	3	32	12	6	43
Bran							
Pericarp	4	7	1	5	4	12	9
Aleurone	15	61	32	37	82	61	41
Germ (embryo)	3	4	2	12	1	8	3
Scutellum	5	8	62	14	1	12	4

are provided in the endosperm, most occur in higher amounts in the **bran** layers (primarily the aleurone and pericarp) and the **germ** (Table 4-7). As a result, the nutritive value of any cereal product depends largely on the amount of the bran that is retained when a cereal is milled. The lower the *extraction* (that is, the higher the percentage of the wheat kernel remaining after milling), the more bran retained and the higher the nutrient content. The wheat germ, which includes the scutellum between the germ and the endosperm, contains large portions of the vitamins B_1 and E of the grain. The wheat germ is usually removed during milling because it contains oil, which becomes rancid very quickly and results in "off" flavors and spoilage. Wheat germ sold alone is usually marketed in vacuum-packed containers that reduce spoilage but markedly increase the price.

bran
The four outer layers of the cereal grain

germ
The small fat-containing portion of cereal grain needed for its germination

Choose breads, cereals, and crackers made from the "whole grain."

For discussion of cereal enrichment, see Chapter 12.

DIETARY REQUIREMENTS

We know that the body can function on much less carbohydrate than we usually consume, but we have practically no information to establish a minimum dietary standard. Diets that are low in carbohydrate or have none at all are so unpalatable, not to mention expensive, that they probably won't be followed for very long. In addition, the fact that carbohydrate is the most economical source of calories leads to its use in sufficient quantities to ensure at least a minimum intake. The Food and Nutrition Board recommends an intake of 100 grams a day to prevent ketosis, excessive use of body protein as an energy source, and other undesirable metabolic consequences. Because most diets contain 200 or more grams, a lack of carbohydrate will not be a problem. There is concern only when a person makes a very conscious effort to restrict carbohydrate intake.

CARBOHYDRATE IN THE U.S. DIET

An analysis of the U.S. food supply shows that through the years carbohydrate has provided a decreasing proportion of energy intake, reaching a current low of 45% as shown by the USDA dietary survey in 1977 and 1978. Less than 5% of the population got less than 30% of their kilocalories from carbohydrate, and only 2% of the population got more than 60% of their kilocalories from carbohydrate. Compared to earlier surveys, there was an increase in the percentage of calories from carbohydrate and in the use of fiber-rich foods.

Carbohydrate and Brain Function

Recent research suggesting that the kind and amount of carbohydrate in the diet can influence brain function, particularly in regulating food intake and mood, has been widely reported in the popular press. The findings are based largely on animal studies that show that when carbohydrate intake is very high—70% to 80% of

neurotransmitter
Substance that transfers messages from one nerve to the next

serotonin
A neurotransmitter produced by the brain; some research findings suggest that it triggers the desire to consume more carbohydrate

kilocalories—the brain produces more of a **neurotransmitter** called **serotonin** than is needed. Serotonin causes a craving for and the consumption of more carbohydrate, which in turn stimulates the brain to produce more serotonin. This makes a person sleepy and sluggish. Those who have been identified as "carbohydrate cravers" may suffer from this problem. They gain weight because they have an irresistible urge to eat carbohydrate, and they have great difficulty adhering to a low-carbohydrate diet.

Fermentable Carbohydrate and Dental Caries

Carbohydrate is one of the major factors implicated as a cause of dental caries, or tooth decay. Before a tooth erupts it is nourished through the bloodstream; therefore, carbohydrate has no direct effect on tooth health. Carbohydrate has an indirect and adverse effect on the tooth before eruption only when the diet contains simple carbohydrates to the exclusion of foods providing nutrients such as calcium, vitamin D, and vitamin C, all of which, along with fluoridated water, ensure the health of the developing tooth.

After erupting, the tooth is exposed to the oral environment and has only limited connection to the blood supply. Carbohydrate, both sucrose and starches, begins to assume importance in tooth health. Tooth decay occurs when both microorganisms and carbohydrate, which serves as food for them, are present. Carbohydrates in solution do not adhere to the tooth surface and therefore cause relatively little harm. However, sucrose-rich foods such as caramels and gummy starches tend to adhere to the tooth surface and provide ample food for bacteria. The bacteria are able to convert this food into polysaccharides known as **dextrans,** which adhere to the tooth surface and form dental plaques. The plaques in turn tend to attract sucrose. Once it is in the plaque, a microorganism called ***Streptococcus mutans*** acts on the sucrose to produce acid. As the acid accumulates, it causes the tooth enamel to dissolve and the tooth to decay.

dextrans
Polysaccharides that adhere to the tooth surface as the results of changes in dietary carbohydrate by microorganisms in the mouth; also referred to as *dental plaque*

Streptococcus mutans
A microorganism that acts on sucrose to produce acid; this causes tooth enamel to dissolve and leads to tooth decay

Carbohydrate and Behavior

Interest in the relationship between nutrition and behavior has focused on many nutrients, including the kind and amount of carbohydrate in the diet. Many unconfirmed anecdotal accounts suggest that children exhibit a shortened attention span and a high level of activity inappropriate for their age after eating sugar. However, it is good to keep in mind that this behavior often follows the use of ice cream or candy, often eaten on special occasions that might alone be stimulating to a child. Controlled studies have failed to show that sugar has an adverse effect on behavior in any appreciable number of children.

ALCOHOL

Although alcohol, or ethanol, is chemically related to fats, it is produced from carbohydrate and will therefore be discussed in this chapter. Alcohol is produced by the fermentation of glucose in foods such as sugar, fruit, or cereal grain. For this fermentation to happen, certain enzymes in yeast must be present and oxygen must be absent.

It is very difficult to get estimates of the amount of alcohol consumed. Data based on the sale of alcohol suggest an intake of about 1 oz of pure alcohol per person per day. These data assume that one third of all people over 14 years of age do not use alcohol. Reports from surveys of individuals and households, however, show daily intakes of 0.2 oz of alcohol consumed per person in the home. This suggests either that most alcohol is consumed outside the home or that people do not provide accurate data on alcohol consumption. For most people, alcohol contributes from 42 to 200 kcal a day. For the 3% of the population over 15 years of age who report consuming more than 150 grams of alcohol, however, it contributes over 1000 kcal daily.

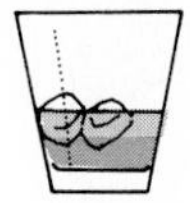

1 oz liquor
84 kcal
100 proof—50% alcohol

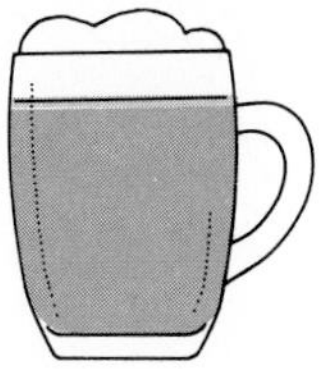

12 oz 4% beer
150 kcal
4% alcohol

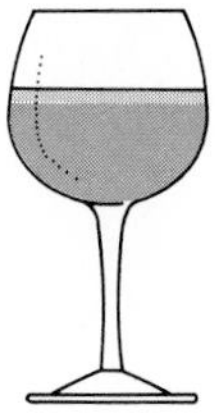

4 oz dry wine
80 kcal
12% alcohol

Percentages of alcohol in beer, wine, and liquor

Absorption and Metabolism

Ethanol is a small, water-soluble molecule that does not require digestion. It is absorbed quickly throughout the length of the gastrointestinal tract; as much as 80% of alcohol is absorbed into the small intestine immediately after leaving the stomach. Because alcohol is water soluble, it immediately disperses throughout the body fluids. Its concentration in any one tissue is similar to the water concentration in that tissue. Thus a large amount of absorbed alcohol is found in the blood, but very little in fat or bone. Practically no alcohol is excreted; less than 5% is lost in the breath and urine. However, because these amounts are in equilibrium with amounts in the blood, they are used as a legally valid measure of the latter. A blood concentration of 0.1% is evidence of intoxication—one of 0.4% is usually fatal.

The metabolism of alcohol begins in the liver, which has the enzyme *alcohol dehydrogenase*. This enzyme is necessary to convert alcohol into a form in which it can be used as a source of energy. Once this is accomplished, muscles can use alcohol as an energy source. Although alcohol could be converted to fat and stored, it is usually used immediately as a source of energy in preference to fatty acids and glucose; it therefore spares other energy sources and indirectly contributes to fat storage. The brain has enough alcohol dehydrogenase to keep alcohol levels from getting too high. This is important because the brain is very sensitive to increases in the amount of alcohol in the blood.

1 gram alcohol provides 7 kcal

Alcohol provides 7 kcal of energy/gram, or 200 kcal/oz of 200-proof alcohol (100% alcohol). Because alcohol seems to stimulate metabolism, however, the net result of alcohol use as a source of energy may be somewhat less than the amounts given, with the remainder being lost as heat. Most people are able to use from 45 to 90 mg of alcohol/pound of body weight/hr (or 100 to 200 mg of alcohol/kg of body weight/hr). This is equivalent to the alcohol in 800 ml (one fifth) of 100-proof whiskey or 3.5 liters (or quarts) of wine per day for a 154-pound (70-kg) man.

The absorption of alcohol can be modified by other drugs; contrary to popular belief, however, metabolism is not affected by physical exercise, vitamin supplementation, thyroid hormone, or caffeine.

Effect on Nutrition

The effect of alcohol on nutritional status is felt in a variety of ways. Alcohol may depress appetite and therefore food intake; it may displace food in the diet, thus lowering the intake of nutrients; it may affect the gastrointestinal tract so that digestion and absorption are impaired; or, through its effect on the liver, it may alter the transport, use, and storage of nutrients. In addition, the money spent on alcohol reduces money available for food, which may be a problem in low-income families.

If You Drink Alcoholic Beverages, Do So in Moderation

Some alcoholic drinks contribute small amounts of nutrients in addition to kilocalories. Beer, in which only half the kilocalories come from alcohol, retains some of the nutrients in the malt from which it was made. Therefore it can contribute reasonable amounts of magnesium, phosphorus, and some vitamins. Wine, with 12% alcohol, retains smaller amounts of these nutrients; hard liquors such as gin, rum, or whiskey, which have been made by distilling the ethanol produced by natural fermentation, contribute nothing but calories.

After the body has suffered from malnutrition it is less able to counteract the toxic effects of alcohol, which compounds its effect on nutritional status. There is convincing evidence that fatty livers and other forms of liver disease are the direct result of excessive alcohol consumption. An otherwise adequate diet does not protect against these problems.

Table 4-8 ◊ Caloric, carbohydrate, and alcohol content of alcoholic beverages

Beverage	Amount (oz)	Alcohol (grams)	Carbohydrate (grams)	Energy (kcal)
Beer				
Regular	12	13	14	150
Light	12	10	6	90
Extra light	12	8	3	70
Near	12	2	12	60
Distilled				
Gin, rum, vodka, whiskey	1.5	15	—	105
Brandy, cognac	1.0	11	—	75
Wine				
Red	4	12	1	85
Dry white	4	11	0.5	80
Sweet	4	12	5	103
Sherry	2	9	1.5	75
Port, muscatel	2	7	7	95
Vermouth, sweet	3	12	14	141
Vermouth, dry	3	13	4	105
Manhattan	3	21	2	165
Martini	3	19	1	140
Old-fashioned	3	21	1	180

The caloric content of some commonly used alcoholic beverages is presented in Table 4-8.

Fetal Alcohol Syndrome

For further discussion of fetal alcohol syndrome, see Chapter 15

In the past 15 years we have recognized a condition known as "fetal alcohol syndrome." This is the result of a mother ingesting as little as 3 oz of alcohol (or 6 oz of a 100-proof beverage) per day or indulging in a single alcohol binge at a critical period during pregnancy. Fetal alcohol syndrome is characterized by slow infant growth, a small head, distorted facial features, and mental retardation. It is estimated that at least 5000 babies a year are born suffering from one or more symptoms of fetal alcohol syndrome. Clearly, pregnant women should be warned of the potential damage to the fetus from alcohol consumption during pregnancy.

BY NOW YOU SHOULD KNOW

- Carbohydrates include simple sugars and complex carbohydrates such as starches and fiber.
- Carbohydrates are composed of the elements carbon, hydrogen, and oxygen.
- There are three classes of carbohydrates: monosaccharides, disaccharides, and polysaccharides.
- Monosaccharides vary in sweetening power, rate of absorption, acid production, and degree of solubility.
- Carbohydrates contribute about 50% of the calories in the typical American diet, but up to 80% of the calories in diets in developing countries.
- Sugar occurs naturally in fruits, vegetables, and milk, but much is ingested in the form of added sucrose.
- Sugar and starch that adhere to teeth can cause dental caries.

- Diabetes develops when insulin is not produced fast enough by the pancreas to allow cells to remove glucose from the blood. It is *not* caused by overconsumption of sugar.
- Lactose intolerance is caused by a lactase insufficiency.
- Cereals and bread products that are refined are low in fiber.
- Fiber is provided in whole-grain products, fruits, and vegetables.
- Insoluble fiber enhances gastric motility and decreases the incidence of colon cancer. Water-soluble fiber can help lower blood cholesterol levels.
- There is no RDA set for carbohydrate, but a minimum of 100 grams per day should be included in the diet.
- Alcohol is derived from the fermentation of naturally occurring sugars.
- Alcohol does not need to be digested but is quickly absorbed. Its metabolism is dependent on the enzyme alcohol dehydrogenase.
- Alcohol abuse can have a negative effect on nutrition.
- Dietary guidelines urge Americans to avoid too much sugar; to eat foods with adequate starch and fiber; and if they drink alcoholic beverages, to do so in moderation and not drive.

STUDY QUESTIONS

1. What is the primary function of carbohydrate in the body?
2. In what form and where is glucose stored in the body?
3. Differentiate between hypoglycemia and hyperglycemia. Describe symptoms that are characteristic of each of these conditions.
4. If you were to go on a low-carbohydrate diet for a prolonged period, what symptoms might you experience?
5. Trace the pattern of carbohydrate consumption in the United States since 1900.
6. How does milling alter the nutritive value of cereals? Name three milled cereal products you eat regularly in your diet.
7. What is the relationship between crude fiber and dietary fiber? What foods would you choose to eat if you wanted to increase your fiber intake? Do the foods you have listed contain water-soluble or insoluble dietary fiber? What difference would these choices make on levels of blood cholesterol?
8. What are the conditions associated with a lack of dietary fiber?
9. What causes lactose intolerance? Give three symptoms that are characteristic of this disorder. What specific foods must be avoided?
10. Name the enzymes that are specific for the digestion of the polysaccharides and disaccharides.
11. What happens to the monosaccharides after they are absorbed from the small intestines and into portal circulation?
12. If you had more kilocalories than you needed, how would the fate of an extra teaspoon of sugar differ from that of sugar that was not extra?
13. How is alcohol absorbed and metabolized? Discuss why an alcoholic may suffer from malnutrition.

Applying What You've Learned

1. **Finding the Carbohydrates in Your Diet.**

   List the foods you have eaten today or yesterday. Circle all the food sources of carbohydrates. Now divide these carbohydrate foods into three groups: 1) simple sugars naturally occurring in fruits, vegetables, and milk; 2) added sugars, such as refined sucrose—table sugar and corn syrup; and 3) complex carbohydrates, such as starches and fiber found in vegetables, grains, and cereals. Of the total number of foods providing carbohydrates did you have more from naturally occurring sugars, refined sugars, or starches and fiber?

2. **Your Carbohydrate Consumption and The Dietary Guidelines.**

   Think about the two Dietary Guidelines for Healthy Americans that pertain to carbohydrate consumption (that is, Avoid Too Much Sugar and Eat Adequate Starch and Fiber). Do you think you follow these guidelines? If not what changes should you make?

3. **Find the Percentage of Calories from Carbohydrates in Food Products.**

   Select several different types of packaged foods and look for carbohydrate information on the label. How many grams of carbohydrate are in one serving? With the number of calories and the grams of carbohydrate per serving you can calculate the percent of calories from carbohydrate in this food. Since each gram of carbohydrate has 4 kcal, simply multiply the grams of carbohydrate times 4 to find the number of carbohydrate calories per serving. Now divide the carbohydrate calories by the total number of calories per serving. Multiply the quotient times 100 to get the percentage of carbohydrate calories.

4. **Carbohydrates in Breakfast Cereals.**

   Compare several cereal box nutrition labels. Find the labels that provide additional carbohydrate information listed at the bottom of the nutrition information panel. Is the carbohydrate predominantly in the form of sugar, starch, or dietary fiber? We don't always visualize sugar in terms of grams but instead in teaspoons. To determine how many teaspoons of sugar are in your favorite breakfast cereal all you need to know is the conversion factor—4 grams of sugar equals 1 teaspoon. Therefore, if you divide the grams of sucrose and other sugars, as listed on the label, by 4 the quotient will be the number of teaspoons per serving of cereal. Does this amount surprise you? Do you add even more sugar at the table?

5. **Evaluating Alcohol Consumption.**

   If you consume alcoholic beverages, count the number of drinks you have in one weekend. Use Table 4-8 to calculate the number of calories consumed from these beverages. Now evaluate your food intake. When drinking do you continue to eat as you would throughout the week or do you cut back on food to compensate for the calories from alcohol? In either case what outcome would you expect?

SUGGESTED READINGS

Greenwald P, Lanza E, and Eddy GA: Dietary fiber in the reduction of colon cancer risk, Journal of the American Dietetic Association 87:1178, 1987.

As a result of their research, these authors conclude that an inverse relationship exists between a fiber-rich diet and colon cancer. Therefore, a prudent increase in mean fiber intake among the U.S. population is recommended. The authors also point out that fat and/or meat is positively associated with colon cancer, and therefore the causes of colon cancer involve more than just low-fiber diets.

Slavin JL: Dietary fiber: classification, chemical analyses and food sources, Journal of the American Dietetic Association 87:1164, 1987.

This article defines dietary fiber, its classes and chemical components, and food sources and their physiological effects. Some of the limitations in measuring dietary fiber are included. Recommendations for amounts and ways to increase dietary fiber are presented.

ADDITIONAL READINGS

Carbohydrate

Anderson TA: Recent trends in carbohydrate consumption, Annual Review of Nutrition 2:113, 1982.

Crapo P: Simple versus complex carbohydrate use in diabetic diet, Annual Review of Nutrition 5:95, 1985.

Evans WJ, and Hughes VA: Dietary carbohydrates and endurance exercise, American Journal of Clinical Nutrition 41:1146, 1985.

Food and Drug Administration Sugar Task Force: Evaluation of health aspects of sugar, Journal of Nutrition (Supp) 117: 51, 1987.

Franz MJ: Diabetes mellitus: considerations in the development of guidelines for the occasional use of alcohol, Journal of the American Dietetic Association 83:147, 1983.

Jenkin DJA, and others: The glycemic index of foods: a physiological basis for carbohydrate exchange, American Journal of Clinical Nutrition 36:362, 1981.

Levine R: Monosaccharides in health and disease, Annual Review of Nutrition 6:211, 1986.

Lieberman HR: Sugars and behavior, Clinical Nutrition 6:195, 1985.

Macdonald I: Metabolic requirements for dietary carbohydrate, American Journal of Clinical Nutrition 45:1193, 1987.

Scheinin A: Dietary carbohydrates and dental disorders, American Journal of Clinical Nutrition 45:1218, 1987.

Shafer RB, Levine AS, Marlette JM, and Morley JE: Effects of xylitol on gastric emptying and food intake, American Journal of Clinical Nutrition 45:744, 1987.

Sharon N: Carbohydrates, Scientific American 243:90, 1980.

Woteki CE, Welsh SO, Raper N, and Marsten RM: Recent trends and levels of dietary sugars and other calorie sweeteners. In Reiser S, editor: Metabolic effects of utilizable dietary carbohydrates, New York, 1982, Marcel Dekker, Inc.

Fiber

American Dietetic Association: Position paper: dietary fiber, Journal of the American Dietetic Association 88:216, 1988.

Anderson JW: Fiber and health: an overview, Nutrition Today 21:6(22), 1986.

Bingham S: Definitions and intakes of dietary fiber, American Journal of Clinical Nutrition 45:1226, 1987.

Burkitt DP: Dietary fiber and cancer, Journal of Nutrition 118:1152, 1988.

Burkitt DP, Walker ARP, and Painter NS: Dietary fiber and disease, Journal of the American Medical Association 229:1068, 1974.

Jacobs LR: Dietary fiber and cancer, Journal of Nutrition 117:1319, 1987.

Klurfeld, DM: The role of dietary fiber in gastrointestinal disease, Journal of the American Dietetic Association 87:1172, 1987.

Lanza E, and Butrum R: A critical review of food fiber analysis and data, Journal of the American Dietetic Association 86:732, 1986.

Von Borstel RW: Metabolic and physiologic effects of sweeteners. Clinical Nutrition 6:215, 1985.

Walhqvist ML: Dietary fiber and carbohydrate metabolism, American Journal of Clinical Nutrition 45:1232, 1987.

Sweeteners

ADA Reports: Position of the American Dietetic Association: Appropriate use of nutritive and non-nutritive sweeteners, Journal of the American Dietetic Association 87:1689, 1987.

Alfin-Slater RB, and Pi-Sunyer FX: Sugars and sugar substitutes, Postgraduate Medicine 82:18, 1987.

Council on Scientific Affairs, American Medical Association: Aspartame, review of safety issues, Journal of the American Medical Association 254:400, 1985.

Institute of Food Technologists Expert Panel on Food Safety and Nutrition: Sweeteners: nutritive and non-nutritive, food technology, p. 195, Aug., 1986.

National Academy of Sciences: Sweeteners, issues and uncertainties, Washington, D.C., 1975, National Academy of Sciences.

Stegink LD: Aspartame: Review of safety issues, Food Technology p. 119, Jan. 1987.

Xylitol as a sucrose substitute: relation to dental caries, Nutrition Reviews 39:368, 1981.

Alcohol

Halsted CH: Alcoholism and malnutrition: introduction to the symposium, American Journal of Clinical Nutrition 33:2705, 1980.

Iosub SL, and others: Fetal alcohol syndrome revisited, Pediatrics 68:475, 1981.

Lieber CS: The influence of alcohol on nutritional status, Nutrition Reviews 46:241, 1988.

Roe D: Nutritional concerns in the alcoholic, Journal of the American Dietetic Association 78:17, 1981.

Windham CT, Wyse BW, and Hansen RG: Alcohol consumption and nutrient density of diets in the Nationwide Food Consumption Survey, Journal of the American Dietetic Association 82:364, 1983.

FOCUS Sweetness Mania

The past 10 years have seen a continual and steady decline of about 2% per year in the use of sugar, and a comparable increase in the use of nonnutritive sweeteners or other sugar substitutes. We still eat about 70 pounds of sugar a year, which accounts for 18% of our calories. Because the only health consequence of a high intake of sugar in the diet relates to its adverse effect on dental health, these trends seem to reflect our inate desire for sweetness without wanting to pay the price of the calories associated with the use of sugar. The result has been an ongoing search for a calorie-free substance with an intensity of sweetness such that it can be used in very small amounts as a sugar substitute. It must also be proved safe enough to meet the standards of the Food and Drug Administration imposed by the Delaney Amendment. This legislation requires convincing evidence that the sweet substance will not cause cancer in any animal at any level of use.

Although a great many substances have been proposed and tested as potential sugar substitutes, most of the interest has focused on saccharin, cyclamates, and aspartame. Saccharin has been in use since 1879, while aspartame was discovered only in 1965.

Saccharin, which is derived from a by-product of the petroleum industry, is a relatively stable substance that is 300 times as sweet as sugar. Because it is not changed in the body, it is excreted unchanged in the urine. Based on the fact that some animals develop bladder tumors when fed saccharin at high doses, there is still some question about its safety for use in human beings. Its use was permitted only in beverages and as a table-top sweetener in the United States while it was under review. In 1987 this review concluded that saccharin was likely safe and that its continued use should be permitted as the review continues. Up to that time, it was allowed to be used as a table-top sweetener in Canada. Some people find that it has an undesirable metallic aftertaste, which limits its acceptance. Some authorities suggest that it is wise to restrict the use of saccharin by pregnant women and young children until we have more information on its possible effects on the fetus.

Aspartame, which is 180 times as sweet as sugar, was first approved in 1974 but immediately banned in 1975, only to be approved again in 1981 after more testing established its safety. It has been approved for use in beverages, in a variety of food products, and as a table-top sweetener. Aspartame consists of two amino acids, phenylalanine and aspartic acid, that occur in almost all protein-rich foods at appreciably higher levels than could possibly be provided from aspartame-sweetened products. Only the 1 in 15,000 people who have the genetic defect, known as phenylketonuria (PKU), that prevents them from metabolizing phenylalanine in excess of the amount that they need for growth need worry about limiting the amino acid in their diet. Similar fears about possible toxicity from the methanol that is formed when aspartame is digested or when aspartame-containing liquids are stored for a long time at a high temperature should be allayed by the fact that foods such as grape and tomato juices have up to twice as much naturally occurring methanol as is produced from the aspartame in a 12-oz beverage sweetened with aspartame.

In assessing the safety of food products, the FDA uses the level of the acceptable daily intake (ADI), which is a 1/100 of the amount a person could safely consume every day of his or her life. For aspartame, the ADI of 50 mg per kilogram of body weight represents the amount of aspartame in 18 cans of sweetened beverage per day for a 60-kg (132-pound) person! Concern about the effect of aspartame on the developing fetus revolves around the fact that the fetus concentrates phenylalanine at twice the level in maternal blood. Although aspartame has been ruled safe for use in food products—over 160 of which now use it as a sweetener—there are frequent questions about its safety and requests that the FDA reevaluate its decision. Students of nutrition should remain alert to the status of the safety of aspartame, which is sold under the brand name, Nutrasweet.

There are a great many other sugar substitutes that are being tested. One of these (Acesulfame K) that has no aftertaste received FDA approval in 1988, particularly for use in products for patients with diabetes. Sugars known as L-sugars because they are "left-handed" (that is, rotate a beam of light to the left) compared to the naturally occurring D-sugars (right-handed) have potential because they taste like sugar, are noncaloric (the body cannot use this form of sugar), are noncariogenic (do not produce tooth decay), are stable in the presence of heat (useful in the preparation of baked products), and are suitable for diabetics. A ruling by the FDA is expected soon. Among the other sweeteners currently being developed are naragin, found in the rind of grapefruit; the amino acid trytophane; xylitol, derived from cellulose; and bioflavinoids, many of which come from oranges and grapefruits.

Cyclamates, the other widely used nonnutritive sweetener, were discovered in 1937, but have been banned in the United States since 1969 because it had not been clearly established that they were not carcinogenic. They have, however, been allowed for use as a table-top sweetener and in drugs in Canada and 40 other countries. Cyclamates are available as calcium cyclamate and sodium cyclamate. Current evaluations conclude that cyclamates are not carcinogenic, but the FDA is awaiting further information on their safety in human beings before granting approval for their use.

It is inevitable that the quest for the ultimate sugar substitute will continue as long as we maintain our taste preference for sweetness and continue to have health problems with obesity. Doubtlessly, there will continue to be questions regarding the safety of any product that is consumed regularly by a certain segment of the population. Because no one sweetener is likely to meet the needs of every individual, we will continue to rely on a mixture of nutritive and nonnutritive sweeteners to satisfy our desire for sweetness.

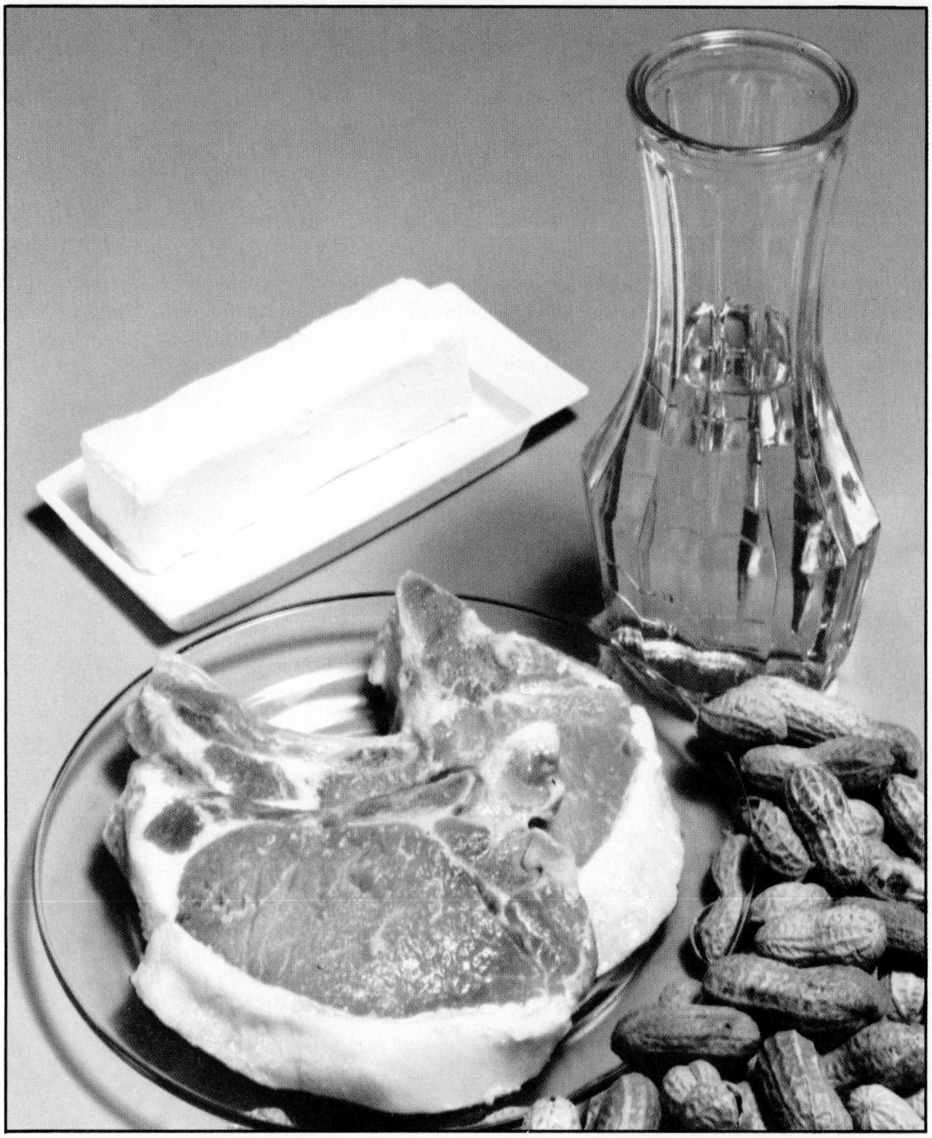

AWARENESS CHECK

Truth or Fiction?

- All fats should be eliminated from the diet.
- Butter and margarine have the same number of calories per serving.
- Prime quality meat has less fat than a less expensive cut.
- A fat is either totally saturated or totally unsaturated.
- Avoiding all cholesterol is the most important dietary change to reduce the risk for cardiovascular disease.
- A food product that claims to be cholesterol-free is a safe food for persons modifying their fat and cholesterol intake.

CHAPTER 5

Lipid

Until recently nutritionists considered the lipid (mostly fats and oils) component of the diet important only as a concentrated source of energy. They now recognize that at least two fatty acid components of lipid are dietary essentials and that some lipids are essential for cell membrane structure. The type of fat—animal, vegetable, saturated, unsaturated, monounsaturated, polyunsaturated, or highly unsaturated—has important health implications. Although recommendations remain somewhat controversial, dietary guidelines encourage Americans to reduce the amount of fat in their diets and to substitute vegetable fat for part of the animal fat consumed. Body lipids that can be synthesized from dietary carbohydrate and protein, as well as from dietary lipids, are essential for normal body functioning. Lipids include fat-related substances such as cholesterol, phospholipids, and prostaglandins, which play essential roles in maintaining health.

The term "fat," or the more inclusive term "lipid" (from Gr. *lipos* meaning fat), means different things to different people. To most people lipid means the fats and oils that make many foods taste better but also add calories to the diet. To the middle-aged man working under stress it means the threat of heart disease. To the biochemist it is an energy-rich molecule made up of carbon, hydrogen, and oxygen. To the nutritionist it is a dietary essential and a concentrated source of calories. To many women it represents ugly and unwanted deposits under the skin that they believe detract from appearance. To the epidemiologist it is linked to obesity and heart disease, major health problems in the developed world.

After water and carbohydrate, the most plentiful nutrient in the American food supply is lipid. Some sources of lipid are easily recognized as visible fats and oils such as the fat surrounding meat, butter, margarine, and salad oils. These sources, however, account for less than half of the lipid in the diet; the rest is invisible fat. Invisible fat includes fat that is marbled throughout meat fibers, dispered in finely divided form in egg yolk or homogenized whole milk, and found in whole-grain cereals and nuts.

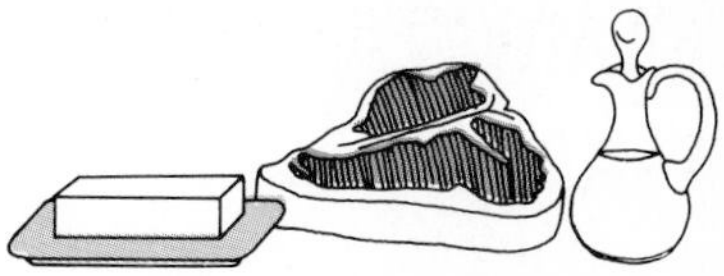

Visible fat in foods makes up 40% of dietary fat

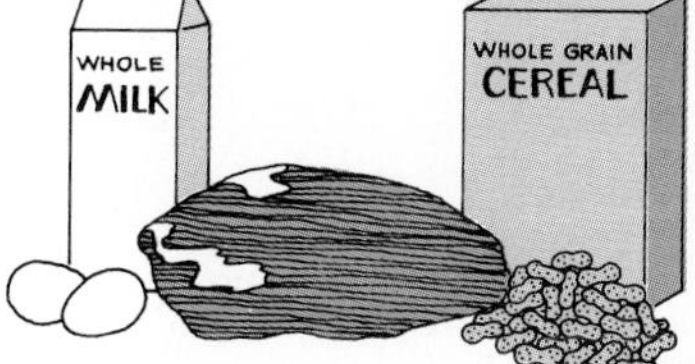

Invisible fat in foods makes up 60% of dietary fat

Foods with visible and invisible fats

TRENDS IN AVAILABILITY AND USE OF DIETARY FAT

Fat Intake = 30% of Total Kilocalories

Kcal	Grams of Fat
1200	40
1500	50
1800	60
2100	70
2400	80
2700	90
3000	100

As indicated in Figure 5-1, throughout this century there has been a steady increase in the amount of fat available for consumption. At the same time there has been a gradual increase in the use of fats from vegetable sources, particularly vegetable oils. This increase is the result of a shift form the use of butter, lard, and cream to margarine, cooking oils, and nondairy creamers made from vegetable oils. Also, there has been a slight decrease in the use of animal fats from meat, poultry, eggs, and milk products. Nevertheless over half of the fat available continues to come from animal sources. Fat in the American diet continues to provide about 43% of total calories, compared to a dietary goal of 30% to 35% of calories.

In spite of a rise and at best a plateau in the amount of fat available in the food supply there seems to be a decline in the amount of fat consumed. This is largely a result of a shift from the use of whole milk to 2% and nonfat milk and from the marketing of leaner meat animals and more closely trimmed cuts of meat. Although the equivalent of 6 oz (¾ cup) oil is available in the food supply, the average person consumes only 2.4 oz (>⅓ cup) per day. This suggests that there is considerable waste of dietary fat or that people are making a conscious effort to limit their intake of fat.

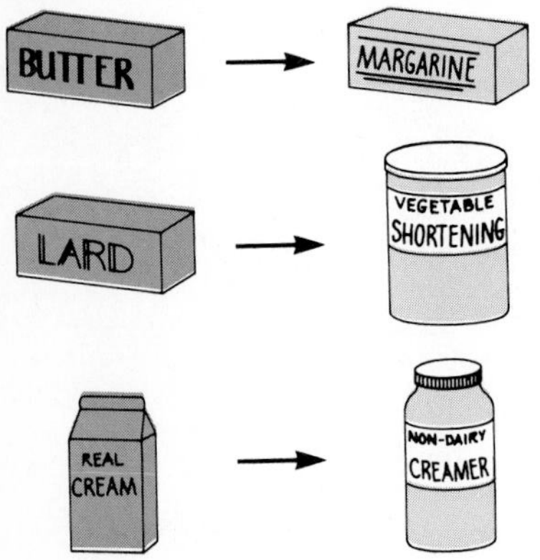

Shift from animal fat to vegetable fat

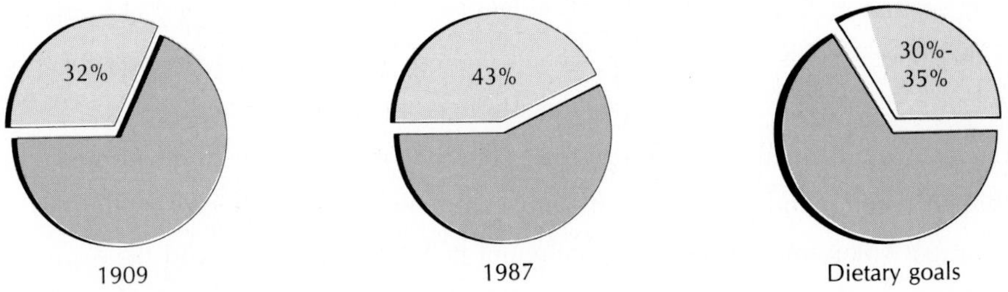

Percent kilocalories from fat in the U.S. food supply.
National Food Review 37:1987.

Figure 5-1 Trends in the availability of animal and vegetable fat in the U.S. food supply, measured in grams.
National Food Review 37, 1987.

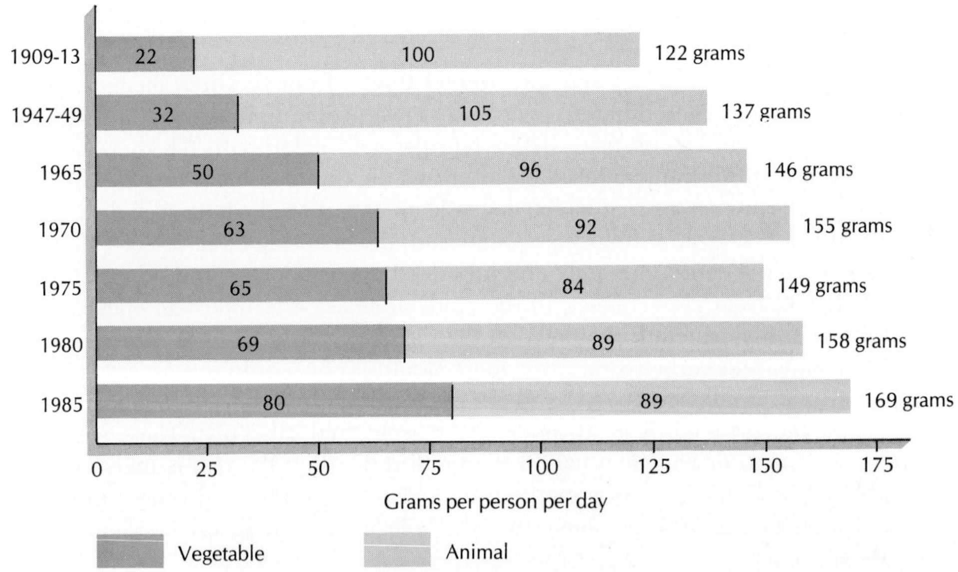

In the 1977-1978 Nationwide Food Consumption Survey (NFCS) over half the population had diets in which over 40% of total calories came from fat. By 1985 when there was a follow-up survey of women (23 to 50 years old), children (1 to 5 years old), and men (19 to 50 years old), the percentage of calories from fat had dropped from 42% and 43% for women and men to 37% and 36% respectively. In 1985 the actual intake of fat averaged 65 to 67 grams per day for women and 106 grams for men. This compares to an average intake of 72 grams for women and 112 grams for men in 1977-1978. In light of the fact that the available fat had not declined, these figures represent a conscious effort on the part of individuals to reduce their intake of fat.

Average Daily Fat Consumption, 1985

	Grams	% Kcal
Men	106	36
Women	66	37
Children	65	35

U.S. Dept. of Agriculture, NFCS-CSF11, 85-1, 2, 3, 1986.

Total lipid intake in developed countries is considerably higher than in the developing world; in general the amount of fat in the diet increases with a country's affluence. It is important to remember that fat is a dietary essential, but both very high and very low intakes have undesirable health consequences.

The kind and amount of fat in the diet are influenced as much by social, cultural, geographical, and economic factors as by nutritional concerns. For example, the Japanese diet is traditionally low in fat while that of the Italians, who make considerable use of olive oil, is high. In the United States the type of fat or oil used in processed foods is determined by price as long as it has no effect on the quality of the final product.

Avoid Too Much Fat, Saturated Fat, and Cholesterol

In spite of concerns about the consequences of animal fat use, many Americans still prefer it. They pay a high price for prime-quality meat with fat marbled throughout it, cover desserts with whipping cream, add butter to vegetables and fish, and consider ice cream, sour cream, and whole milk to be dietary staples. As anyone who has tried knows, it is impossible to eliminate all fat from the diet for long. If we did succeed, we might become deficient in fat-soluble vitamins, essential fatty acids, and calories. In addition, we would probably grow to dislike a diet that is very unpalatable to most Western tastes and lacks satiety. The Dietary Goals urge us to reduce our use of fat—not to cut out its use completely.

CHEMICAL COMPOSITION

Fat, like carbohydrate, is composed of the three elements carbon, hydrogen, and oxygen. However, in fat the ratio of oxygen to carbon and hydrogen is much lower than in simple carbohydrates. The lower amount of oxygen in relation to the other two elements results in fat being a more concentrated source of energy than carbohydrate.

Formation of Triglyceride

Dietary fat is composed of two major components: a three-carbon molecule known as **glycerol,** with one to three compounds called **fatty acids** (FA) attached to it. The most common fats both in food and stored in the body are **triglycerides,** in which three fatty acids are attached to the glycerol core. These fats have long been known as *triglycerides* but are now correctly referred to as *triacylglycerol*. They provide about 95% of the energy from dietary fat.

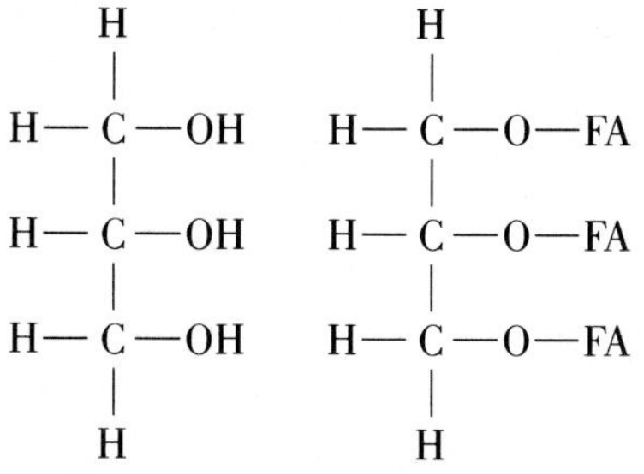

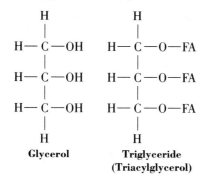

Glycerol **Triglyceride (Triacylglycerol)**

glycerol
A three-carbon molecule that occurs as part of all fats

fatty acid
A compound made up of a chain of even-numbered carbon atoms, with a methyl group at one end and a carboxyl group at the other

triglycerides (triacylglycerol)
Class of lipids with two major components: glycerol and three fatty acids

If all three fatty acids in a fat molecule are the same, which is rare, the fat is referred to as a simple triglyceride. If the fatty acids differ from one another, as is most often the case, the fat is called a mixed triglyceride. When only two fatty acids are attached to the glycerol molecule the resulting fat is known as a **diglyceride** or diaclyglycerol, and when only one is attached (usually in the middle position) the fat is known as a **monoglyceride** or monoacylglycerol.

diglyceride (diacylglycerol)
Class of lipids with glycerol and two fatty acids

monoglyceride (monoacylglycerol)
Class of lipids with glycerol plus one fatty acid

When the fatty acid joins the glycerol molecule the H of the carboxyl (COOH) end attaches to the hydrogen (OH) end on the glycerol. Water (H_2O) separates and the fatty acid becomes firmly attached, thus forming a monoglyceride.

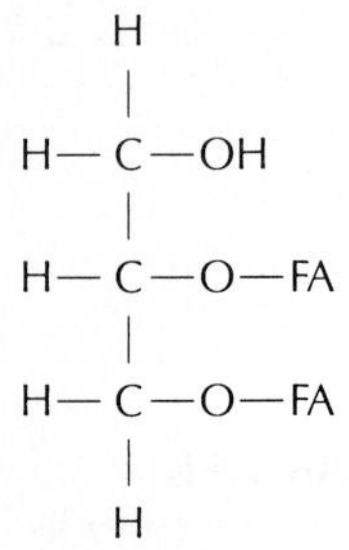

Diglyceride (Diacylglycerol)

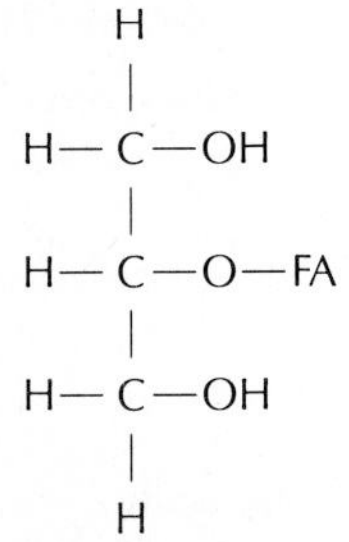

Monoglyceride (Monoacylglycerol)

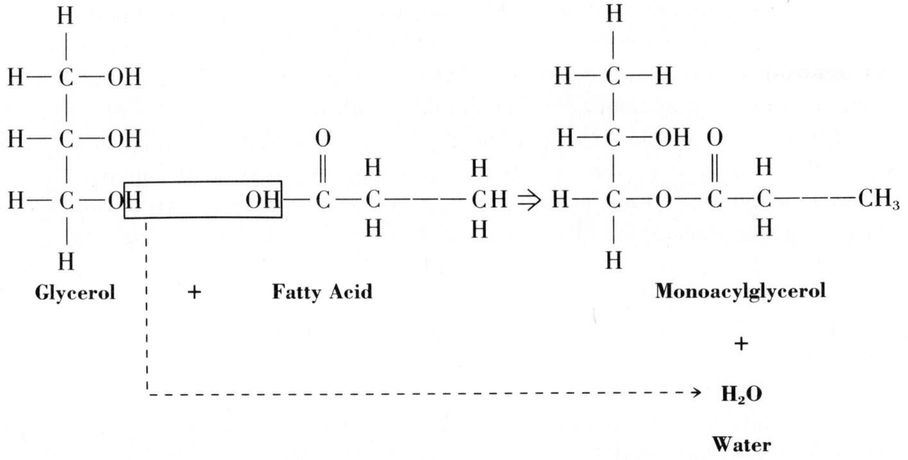

Monoglycerides and diglycerides are often listed on food labels because they are used in very small amounts as additives in many processed foods to give the desired texture and consistency.

There are many different kinds of fatty acids in food fats. They vary according to many features, one of which is the number of carbon atoms linked together in their fatty acid chain.

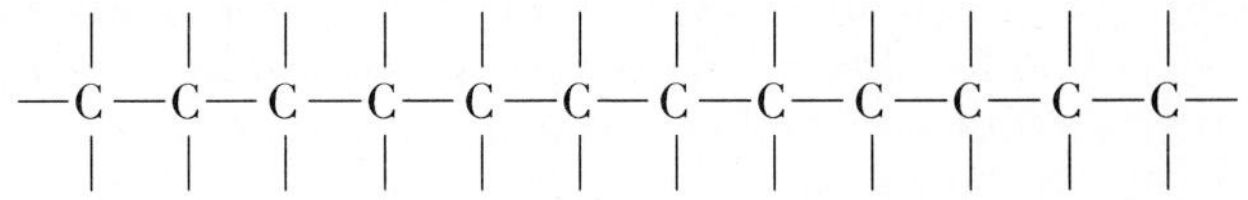

Methyl group = CH_3

Carboxyl group = $\overset{\overset{O}{\|}}{C}$—OH

The fatty acids in foods almost always have an even number of carbon atoms, ranging from 4 to 22. All fatty acids have a methyl group, CH_3, at one end and a carboxy group, $\underset{\underset{O}{\|}}{C}$—OH, at the other. Thus a fatty acid has this structure.

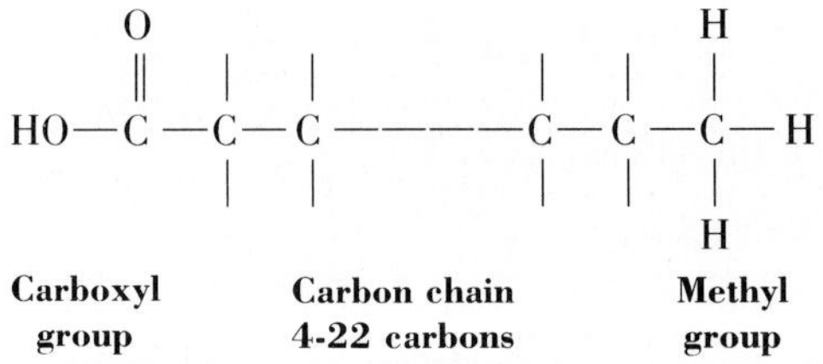

For more discussion of chemistry of carbon compounds see Appendix A.

Because carbon atoms always have four bonds attached to the bond of another atom, each of these carbon atoms normally has either a hydrogen atom, another carbon atom, or a hydroxyl (OH) attached to each of the four bonds.

Fatty acids are classified on the basis of the length of the carbon chain. Fatty acids with 12 or fewer carbon atoms are called short-chain fatty acids and those with 14 or more carbon atoms, long-chain fatty acids. The long-chain fatty acids predominate in food. Fatty acids with 8 to 12 carbon units are sometimes grouped as medium-chain fatty acids, and they account for 4% to 10% of the fatty acids in food. Medium-chain fatty acids are more soluble and more easily absorbed than fatty acids with longer carbon chains. Truly short chain fatty acids are relatively rare. Very long-chain fatty acids with 20 or more carbon atoms are found in rape seed or mustard seed and in fish oils.

The kind of fat formed when fatty acids attach to the glycerol depends not only on the length of the fatty acid chain but also on the number of hydrogen atoms attached to the carbon atoms. This characteristic is referred to as *saturation*.

Saturation

In fatty acid chains each carbon atom between the methyl end and the carboxyl end has the capability of holding or having two hydrogens attached to it. When every carbon atom has two hydrogen atoms attached, the maximum number possible, the fatty acid is called a **saturated fatty acid.** Butter has 51% saturated fatty acids, mainly butyric.

saturated fatty acids
Fatty acids that have two hydrogen atoms (the maximum number possible) attached to each carbon in the chain

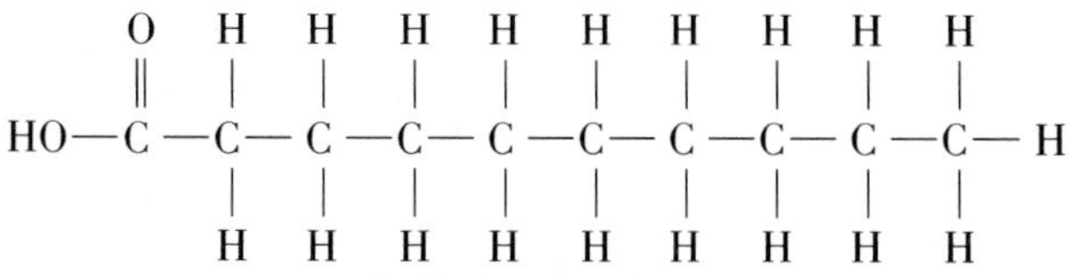

Saturated fatty acid

Some fats found in foods however do not have the maximum number of hydrogen atoms attached to their carbon chain. They are known as **unsaturated fatty acids.**

In some unsaturated fatty acids two adjacent carbon atoms each lack a hydrogen atom. To make up for the missing hydrogens they form a double bond between themselves. Fatty acids in which this occurs at one spot are called **monounsaturated fatty acids.** Olive oil has a predominance (77%) of oleic acid, a monounsaturated fatty acid.

unsaturated fatty acids
Fatty acids that have fewer than the maximum number of hydrogen atoms attached to the carbon chain

monounsaturated fatty acids
Fatty acids in which one hydrogen atom is missing from each of two adjacent carbons, resulting in a double bond between the two carbons

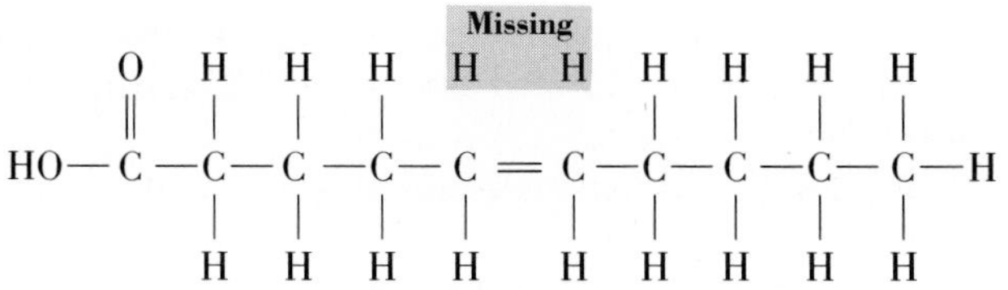

Monounsaturated fatty acid

When four or more hydrogen atoms are missing, two each from two pairs or more of carbon atoms, two or more double bonds are formed and the fatty acid is said to be **polyunsaturated (PUFA).** Corn oil has a predominance (59%) of linoleic acid, a polyunsaturated fatty acid.

polyunsaturated fatty acids
Fatty acids in which double bonds between carbon atoms appear in two or more places

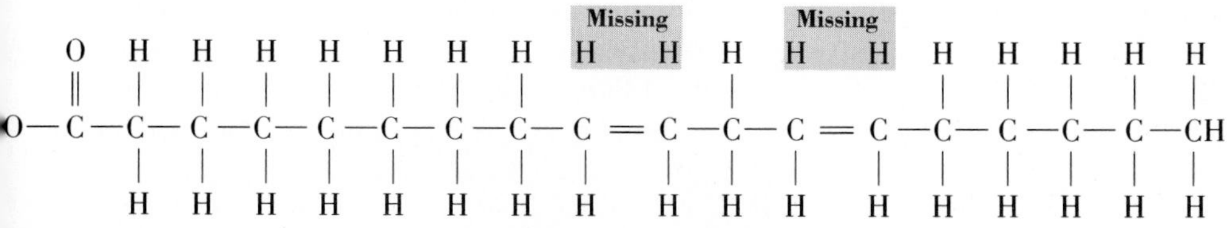

Polyunsaturated fatty acid

Table 5-1 ◆ Name and sources of fatty acids most commonly found in food

Name	Number of Carbon Atoms	Number of Double Bonds	Food Source
Saturated			
Short-chain			
Butyric	4		Butter
Caproic	6		Butter
Caprylic	8		Coconut oil
*Capric	10		Palm oil
*Lauric	12		Coconut oil
*Myristic	14		Butterfat, nutmeg, coconut oil
Long-chain			
Palmitic	16		Animal fat and vegetable oil
Stearic	18		Animal fat and vegetable oil
Arachidic	20		Peanut oil and lard
Unsaturated			
Long-chain			
Palmitoleic	16	1	Butter and seed oils
Oleic	18	1	Most fats and oils
Linoleic	18	2	Seed fats—corn, cottonseed
Linolenic	18	2	Soybean oil
Arachidonic	20	4	Peanut oil, lard
Eicosapentaenoic acid (EPA)	20	5	Fish oil
Docosahexaenoic acid (DHA)	22	6	Fish oil

*Sometimes classified as medium-chain fatty acids.

Recently the recognition of the dietary importance of some very long-chain (22 to 24 carbon atoms) fatty acids, with five or six double bonds, has introduced another classification called **highly unsaturated fatty acids (HUFA).**

highly unsaturated fatty acids
Long chain fatty acids in which double bonds occur in five or six places

The chemical nature and sources of common dietary fatty acids are shown in Table 5-1.

The degree of saturation is often expressed as the **P/S ratio**—that is, the ratio of polyunsaturated fatty acids to saturated fatty acids after monounsaturated fatty acids have been excluded.

P/S ratio
The ratio of polyunsaturated to saturated fatty acids in a fat

With the current evidence that monounsaturated fatty acids also have beneficial health effects, the P/S ratio may soon be replaced by a **P-M/S ratio,** in which the ratio of polyunsaturated fatty acids plus monounsaturated fatty acids to saturated fatty acids is used to express the health value of a fat.

P-M/S ratio
The ratio of polyunsaturated plus monounsaturated fatty acids to saturated fatty acids in a fat

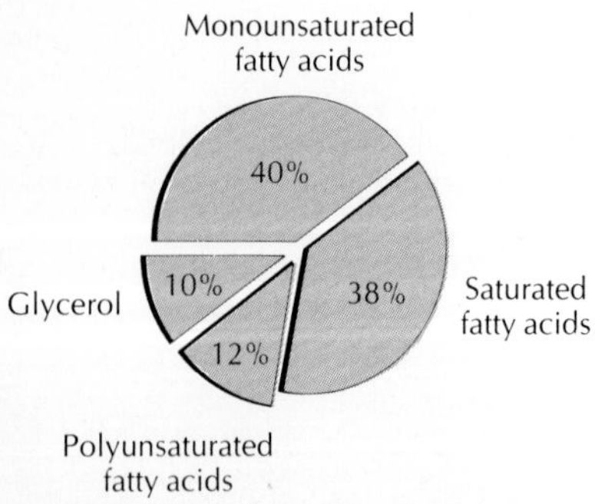

Distribution of different fat components to total fat in the American diet

Dietary triglycerides contain a mixture of fatty acids with varying degrees of saturation and varying chain lengths. Because glycerol is common to all triglycerides, differences among them are the result of the number and kind of fatty acids, their order on the glycerol core, or their place of attachment to it. The characteristics of each type of fat reflect these differences. A fat that predominates in fatty acids with one double bond (that is, lacks two hydrogen atoms) is called a monounsaturated fat even though it may contain some saturated and polyunsaturated fatty acids. A fat that predominates in fatty acids with two or more double bonds is called a polyunsaturated fat. The more unsaturated fatty acids in a fat the more likely it is to be a liquid at room temperature. The more saturated fatty acids in a fat the more likely it is to be a solid at room temperature. There are exceptions to this rule. Coconut and palm oils, except palm kernel, sometimes called tropical oils, consist predominately of saturated fatty acids, yet they are liquid at room temperature because they have many short-chain fatty acids, which keep fat liquid.

Table 5-2 ◇ Classification and dietary sources of unsaturated fatty acids

Family	Fatty Acid	Number of Carbon Atoms	Number of Double Bonds	Food Source*
Omega-3	Linolenic (18:3ω3)†	18	3	Soybean oil (6.8%) Canola (11.1%) Nuts (10%)
	Eicosapentaenoic acid (EPA) (20:5ω3)	20	5	Fish
	Docosahexaenoic acid (DHA) (22:6ω3)	22	6	Fish
Omega-6	Linoleic (18:2ω6)	18	2	Vegetable oils (>50%)
	Arachidonic (20:4ω6)	20	4	Animal tissue
Omega-9	Oleic (18:1ω9)	18	1	Vegetable oils (24%-39%)

*Values in parenthesis indicate the percentage of the oil that is composed of the designated fatty acid.
†18:3ω3 means that the fatty acid has 18 carbons in its chain and 3 double bonds, the first of which is located 3 carbons from the methyl end (ω = omega = end).

canola
Oil extracted from rapeseed; high in polyunsaturated fatty acids; sold and first produced in Canada; allowed in the United States since 1986, where it is a major source of oil

Polyunsaturated fatty acids are further classified on the basis of their chemical structure and the position of the first double bond in relation to the methyl (CH_3) end of the molecule. Those in which the first double bond occurs between the third and fourth carbon atom are called omega-3 (omega-end or sometimes designated as N-3) fatty acids. Fatty acids in which the first double bond is between the sixth and seventh carbon atoms are classified as belonging to the omega-6, or N-6, family of fatty acids, and those in which it occurs between the ninth and tenth carbon atoms as omega-9, or N-9, fatty acids. The members of these families and food sources are shown in Table 5-2.

Ingredients high in saturated fatty acids
- Beef fat
- Butter
- Cream
- Lard
- Cocoa butter
- Coconut oil
- Palm oil
- Hydrogenated vegetable oil

Ingredients high in monounsaturated fatty acids
- Olive oil
- Peanut oil
- Avocado oil

Ingredients high in polyunsaturated fatty acids
- Corn oil
- Cottonseed oil
- Safflower oil
- Sesame oil
- Soybean oil
- Sunflower oil

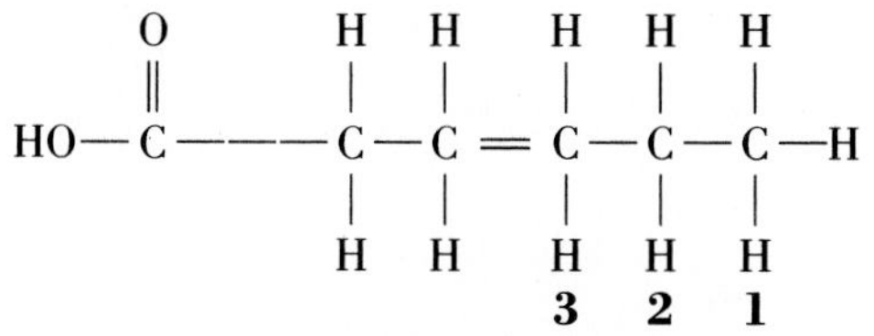

omega-3 fatty acid

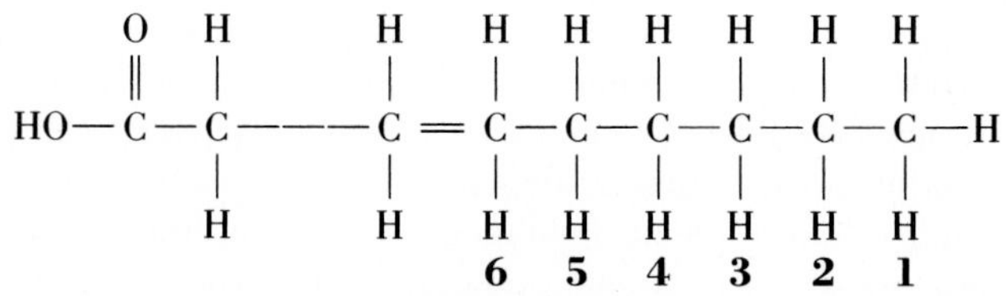

omega-6 fatty acid

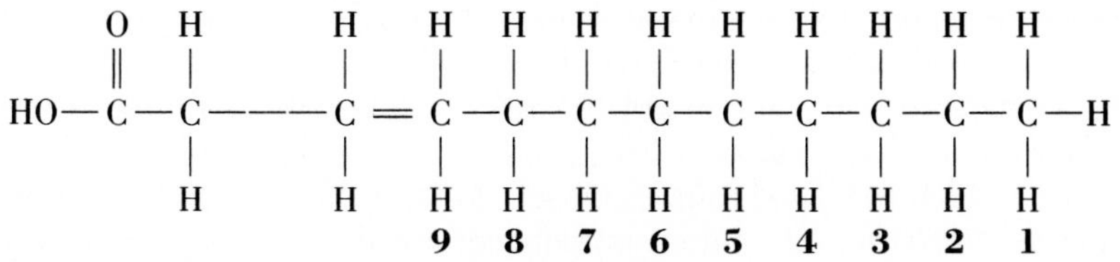

omega-9 fatty acid

A fatty acid such as linolenic acid, which is a major fatty acid in the omega-3 series, is designated 18:3ω3, indicating that it has 18 carbon atoms in its chain and that it has three double bonds, the first of which occurs between the third and fourth carbons from the methyl end of the chain. Using the same system, linoleic acid becomes 18:2ω6 and oleic acid is 18:1ω9.

The other two omega-3 fatty acids are EPA (20:5ω3) and DHA (22:6ω3). The conversion of linolenic to eicosapentaenoic acid (EPA) and docosahexaenoic acid (DHA) can occur in humans but does so very slowly because the conversion of linoleic (18:2ω6) to arachidonic acid (20:4ω6) requires the same enzyme for which the two conversions compete. The production of arachidonic acid usually wins out and very little EPA and DHA are produced.

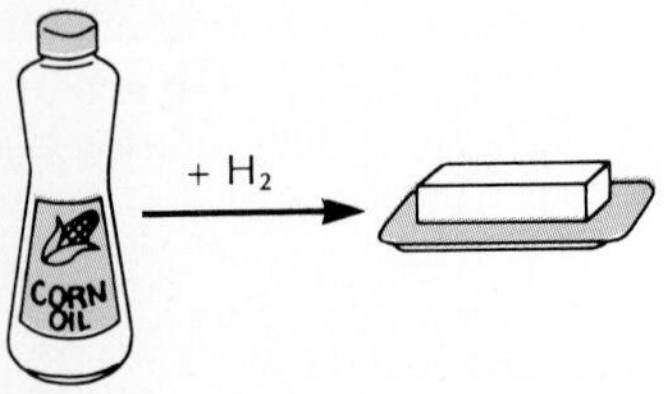

hydrogenation
The process by which hydrogen is added to an unsaturated fatty acid to make it more solid at room temperature

Modification of Fatty Acid Composition of Foods

Hydrogenation. Although hydrogen cannot be removed to make unsaturated from saturated fatty acids, it is possible to convert unsaturated fatty acids to saturated by the addition of hydrogen. This process, called **hydrogenation,** is used commercially to change less expensive oils such as cottonseed, soybean, and sunflower into fats that resemble the more expensive animal fats, particularly in regards to spreadability. For example, margarine and shortening, which are similar to butter and lard in consistency and texture, are produced by the hydrogenation of vegetable oils. In the process it is possible to keep many but not all of the unsaturated fatty acids and still have a fat with the desired characteristics. How much the fatty acids are actually changed in processing depends on the stage at which the process is stopped. In most hydrogenated fats about 30% of the fatty acids have been hydrogenated. However, many double bonds that remain unsaturated are changed from a "cis" to a "trans" configuration. In the "trans" form they are folded so that the hydrogen atoms on adjacent carbon atoms are on opposite sides of the chain and the total chain length is shortened. In "cis" fatty acids the molecule is stretched out instead of being folded at the double bond and the hydrogens on adjacent carbon atoms are on the same side of the chain. This is the naturally occurring form.

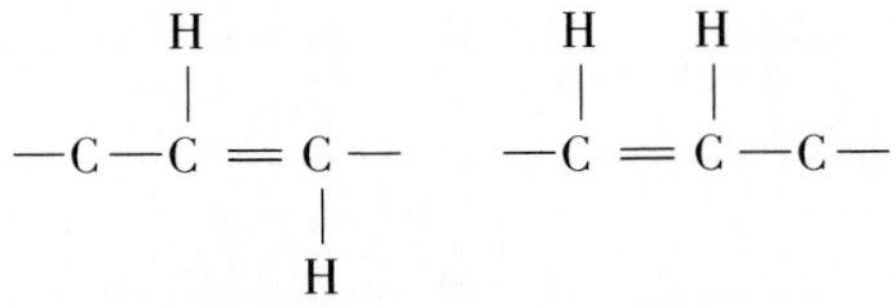

"Trans" **"Cis"**

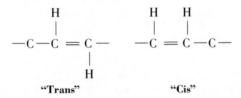

"Trans" fatty acids account for 8% to 70% of the bonds in hydrogenated fats but only 5% to 8% in the U.S. diet. They are also found in milk as the result of the action of microorganisms in the rumen of the cow. Since they function in much the same way as saturated fatty acids it has been proposed that in labeling food saturated fatty acids and trans fatty acids be combined. It has only been in the last 40 years that hydrogenated fats such as margarine have been dietary staples, and even more recently that we have known about the change of "cis" to "trans" unsaturated fatty acids. As a result, we are not yet sure about the long-term physiological effects of "trans" fatty acids, especially as they affect young infants.

Although an animal tends to produce a fat characteristic of its own species—for example, pork fat is very different from beef or lamb—it is possible to modify the composition of the fat by modifying the diet of the animal. This technique was used by animal producers to control the type of product according to consumer wants. They are now more likely to use growth hormones that allow them to produce an animal in which the proportion of muscle to fat is higher. This practice yields an animal in which the fat content is reduced and the efficiency with which the animal utilizes food energy is increased.

Table 5-3 ◇ Interrelationship of essential fatty acids

Fatty Acid	Structure	Biological Role	Sources
Linoleic (N-6) ↓	18 carbons 2 double bonds	Growth factor Antidermatitis factor	Vegetable oils Seed oils
Arachidonic (N-6)	20 carbons 4 double bonds	Antidermatitis factor	Animal fat
Linolenic (N-3)	18 carbons 3 double bonds	Growth factor	Soybean oil

ESSENTIAL FATTY ACIDS

The term **essential fatty acids,** or EFAs, has traditionally been used to refer to three long-chain fatty acids: *linoleic, linolenic,* and *arachidonic*. These fatty acids are known to cure **dermatitis,** or inflammation of the skin, and to restore the growth of young animals that have been fed a diet very low in fat.

essential fatty acid (EFA)
A fatty acid that must be provided in the diet; the three EFAs are linoleic, linolenic, and arachidonic acids

dermatitis
A condition characterized by inflammation of the skin

Linoleic acid, an 18-carbon fatty acid with two double bonds, cannot be produced by the body. It has been clearly shown both to restore growth and prevent dermatitis. Because it must be provided in the diet, linoleic acid is considered an EFA. Linolenic acid, an 18-carbon fatty acid with three double bonds, cannot be synthesized by mammals. It has no antidermatitis effect but does promote growth; as a result, it is considered essential.

Arachidonic acid is a 20-carbon polyunsaturated fatty acid with four double bonds. It prevents dermatitis but does not promote growth. Unlike linolenic acid arachidonic acid can be formed in the human body by the conversion or change in linoleic acid involving the addition of more double bonds. Thus it is not strictly considered an essential fatty acid; it is said to have partial EFA activity.

The relationship among these fatty acids is shown in Table 5-3. All three EFAs serve as precursors of a large group of hormone-like substances called **prostaglandins** that may be responsible for some of the functions previously attributed to EFAs.

prostaglandins
Hormone-like substances produced in the body from fatty acids, particularly arachidonic acid

Deficiency

EFA deficiency occurs almost exclusively in infants who are fed a nonfat milk formula. They suffer from poor growth and dermatitis. For infants the EFA requirement has been set at 3% of total calories; this is easily met by breast milk, in which 6% to 9% of the calories come from linoleic acid.

EFA deficiency is practically unknown among adults, although cases of reproductive failure, impaired fetal development, and lactation failure have been reported. Adult needs for essential fatty acids are usually met when 2% of the total calories are provided by linoleic acid. Most diets provide many times the minimum EFA requirements.

It is believed that meeting the requirements for linoleic acid will also provide for linolenic acid because they are found in the same food sources.

RELATED LIPIDS

In addition to the monoglycerides, diglycerides, and triglycerides, foods also contain small amounts of fat-related substances known as **phospholipids** and **sterols**.

phospholipid
A lipid-related compound composed of glycerol, a phosphate molecule, and other chemical groups; helps to emulsify many fats

sterol
A lipid-related compound in which the carbon, hydrogen, and oxygen atoms are arranged in rings

Phospholipids

In phospholipids, one of the fatty acids is replaced by a phosphate (PO_4) group and either a nitrogen-containing or a carbohydrate-like substance. Because the phos-

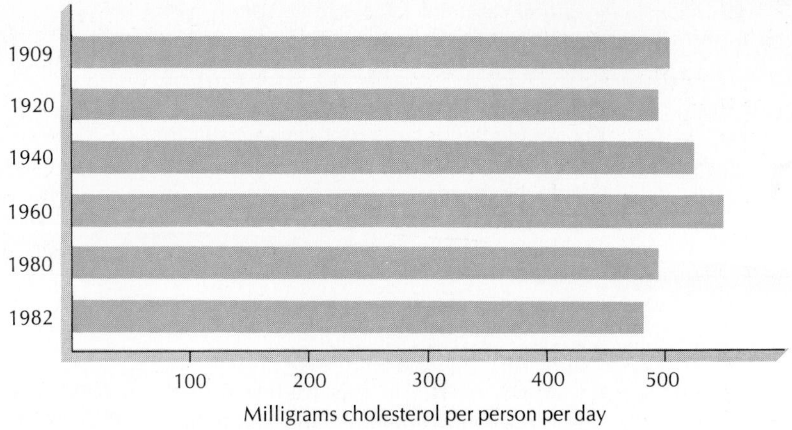

Figure 5-2 Trends in the amount of cholesterol in the American food supply.

phate groups are more water soluble than fatty acids, phospholipids serve to increase the solubility of the lipid and keep fats in a finely divided, or **emulsified,** form. The best known of the phospholipids is **lecithin,** in which choline, a vitamin-like substance, is the nitrogen-containing portion.

Lecithin serves as a natural emulsifier in eggs and is present in cell membranes of the human body. It has achieved popularity recently as a dietary supplement that (supporters say) prevents the accumulation of fat in artery walls. However, there is no evidence that lecithin should be provided in the diet because it is synthesized, or created from other substances, in the liver. In fact, many dietary sources are digested before being absorbed. This makes dietary lecithin supplements useless and unnecessary.

emulsified
Finely divided; refers to fat particles that are broken up into many small units and coated with protein film to prevent them from forming one large molecule (coalescing) again

lecithin
A phospholipid, found in food and in the body, in which choline is attached to the phosphate group

Sterols

Cholesterol. **Cholesterol** belongs to another lipid group called sterols. It is an alcohol lipid that is present in all animal fats and absent in vegetable fats. Cholesterol is necessary for the formation of many essential substances in the body such as sex hormones and bile salts. It is also an integral part of all the body membranes including myelin, which forms a protective sheath around nerve fibers and contains about 30 grams of cholesterol that is seldom interchanged with other cholesterol in the body. The adult body usually contains about 0.2% cholesterol or 130 grams. Cholesterol is not a dietary essential because it can be synthesized in the body, primarily in the liver and in the cells lining the small intestine. The amount synthesized depends on the quantity needed by the body and what is available in the diet but is usually between 600 and 1500 mg (compared to 300 to 500 mg usually provided in the diet).

Although there has been an increase in cholesterol-containing meat in the diet, this has been offset by the substitution of cholesterol-free vegetable fats for many animal fats. As a result the cholesterol content in the American diet—480 mg per person—has not changed appreciably in the last 10 years (Figure 5-2).

Phytosterols. **Phytosterols** are a group of related lipids found in plants. One of these, sitosterol, apparently competes with cholesterol for absorption, thus causing a decreased absorption of cholesterol. Another, ergosterol, is found in yeast and is a **precursor** of vitamin D—that is, vitamin D is formed from it.

Proposed Cholesterol Labeling Standards (FDA, 1988)

Cholesterol-free	<2 mg/serving
Low cholesterol	<20 mg/serving
Cholesterol reduced	Food reformulated to reduce cholesterol to ≤25% original product

cholesterol
A sterol that is found in animal fats and in the blood and is part of many essential body compounds

phytosterol
A group of sterols found in plant foods; sometimes cause decreased absorption of cholesterol

precursor
A substance that serves as the source of another substance

OTHER FAT-LIKE SUBSTANCES

Another class of fatlike substances, *hydrocarbons,* are by-products of petroleum refining and have physical characteristics such as texture and taste that are similar to true lipids. Hydrocarbons contain carbon and hydrogen, as lipids do, but they lack oxygen. Because they are not affected by digestive enzymes, they cannot be absorbed to contribute calories and are therefore sometimes used in place of oils to make low-kilocalorie foods such as salad dressings. Because hydrocarbons, of which mineral oil is the most commonly used, pass through the digestive tract unchanged, and because of their oily characteristics, they act as a lubricant or laxative. Unfortunately, they also pick up fat-soluble vitamins, which are excreted along with the undigested hydrocarbons.

A new synthetic product known as *sucrose polyester (SPE)*, which is a combination of sucrose and fatty acids, is being developed as a possible fat substitute under the trade name Olestra. It has many of the characteristics of hydrocarbons but it has the acceptable taste and texture of food fat. Because it cannot be digested, it is not a source of calories. However, it does reduce the absorption of valuable fat-soluble vitamins, as well as cholesterol in the colon. As a result of tests to show that sucrose polyester is an acceptable food ingredient with only minor side effects, it will be introduced in reduced-calorie foods in place of fats and oils as soon as it has received FDA approval. Similarly, a product, **Simplesse,** with flavor and texture characteristics similar to fat, is under review by the FDA. It is made from the protein in egg or milk, which has been physically changed into very small particles, and provides 1.3 kcal/gram.

PHYSICAL PROPERTIES

Fat is insoluble in water but soluble in solvents such as ether, chloroform, and benzene. Fats are less dense than water and will rise to the surface of any mixture such as oil and vinegar.

In foods such as egg yolk the fat is in finely divided particles surrounded by a thin layer of phospholipid-protein complex. This layer keeps the particles from joining together, or *coalescing*, to form visible fat globules. These fats are known as *emulsified fats*. Because they are in fine particles, emulsified fats have a much larger surface area and are therefore digested more rapidly than unemulsified fats. For example, homogenized milk is whole milk with the fat globules broken up mechanically and dispersed so that they no longer rise to form a layer of cream. Another example is the oil in mayonnaise, which is mechanically emulsified and stabilized by a thin layer of egg protein.

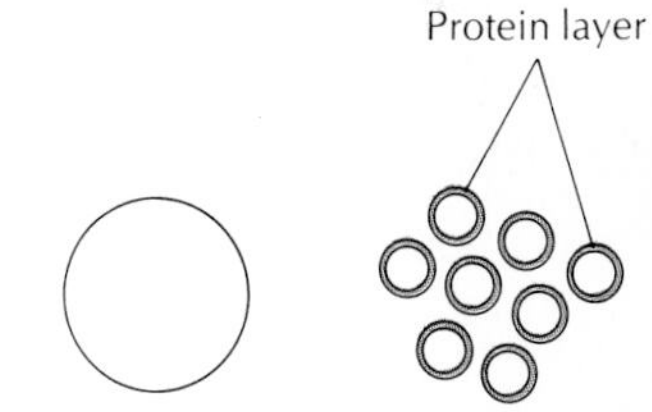

Emulsified fats have fat globules in finely divided form.

Other than melting when it is heated, fat is not affected by temperatures normally used in food preparation. However, heating at high temperatures (above 400° F) leads to the decomposition of fatty acids and the production of *acrolein* from glycerol. Acrolein has a very pungent, acrid fume that is extremely irritating to the nasal passages and gastrointestinal tract. It is responsible for the coughing spell you may have if you burn fat when frying food.

The double bonds of unsaturated fatty acids explain why they spoil easily. The double bond reacts with atmospheric oxygen in a process called **oxidation,** which produces peroxides that are responsible for the rancidity and "off" flavors in some fats. It is often necessary to add **antioxidants**—substances that oppose oxidation—to unsaturated oils if they are to be kept for long periods without deterioration. Vitamins C or E, BHT (butylated hydroxytoluene), and BHA (butylated hydroxyanisole) are the most common antioxidants. They are listed on the label whether they are added to the food or to the packaging material. Another problem in storing fats is their tendency to absorb odors and flavors. This is an advantage in distributing flavors in cooking, but a disadvantage when uncovered stored fats pick up unwanted flavors. For instance, we want butter to take on the flavor of onion in the frying pan—not in the refrigerator.

$$\text{Unsaturated fatty acids} + O_2 \rightarrow \text{Rancid fat}$$

oxidation
Reaction between oxygen and unsaturated fatty acids that produces peroxides, which result in rancidity of some fats

antioxidant
Substance that prevents the (usually undesirable) oxidation of another substance by taking up oxygen themselves

Common Antioxidants in Food
Vitamin E
C
BHT-butylated hydroxytoluene
BHA-butylated hydroxyanisole

Table 5-4 ◆ Summary of fat digestion

Site	Enzyme	Substrate	End Product
Mouth	Lingual lipase	Emulsified fat	Diglycerides Fatty acids
Stomach	Gastric lipase	Emulsified fat	Diglycerides Monoglycerides Fatty acids
Small intestine	Bile*	Unemulsified fat	Emulsified fat Diglycerides
	Pancreatic lipase	Emulsified fat	Monoglycerides Fatty acids Glycerol

*Not an enzyme—synthesized in liver, stored and secreted by gallbladder.

Figure 5-3 Summary of digestion, absorption and circulation of lipids.

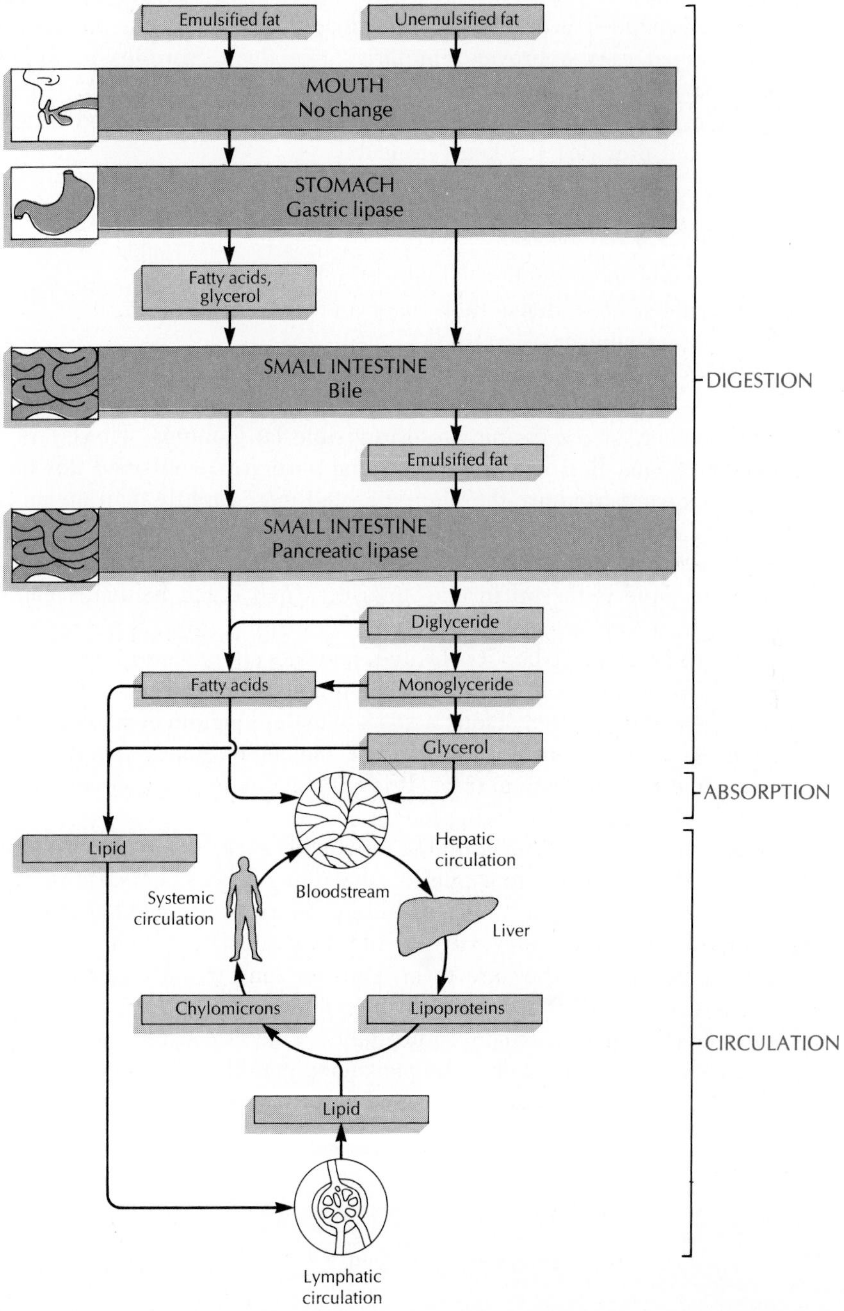

DIGESTION

Before fat can be absorbed across the intestinal wall and then transported to various tissues, it must be broken down chemically into units that are small enough to be taken up by the cells lining the intestinal tract. Emulsification, essential for the fat digestion process, breaks fat into small particles after which a series of reactions involving fat-splitting enzymes, **lipases,** split fatty acids from glycerol. Most dietary fat is triglyceride, with stearic and palmitic being the most common saturated fatty acids and oleic and linoleic the most common unsaturated fatty acids. About half of the dietary triglycerides are broken down completely to fatty acids and glycerol. The remainder are split into diglycerides, monoglycerides, and fatty acids, but mainly monoglycerides.

lipase
An enzyme that hydrolyzes fat (Gr. *lipos* = fat; -ase = enzyme)

The digestion of fat is initiated by the action of lingual lipase, an enzyme secreted at the base of the tongue, which mixes with the chewed food to split some fatty acids from triglycerides to form diglycerides as the food travels down the esophagus to the stomach. After entering the stomach some of the emulsified fat in the food mass is changed by the action of gastric lipase, which splits off one or two fatty acids from diglycerides or triglycerides, leaving monoglycerides, diglycerides, and free fatty acids. From the stomach the food mass passes into the small intestine, where the presence of fat stimulates the release of the hormone cholecystokinin. This triggers the release of **bile,** which is synthesized in the liver and stored and released from the gallbladder. Bile acts on unemulsified fat from the food to break it into water-soluble globules known as **micelles** of small size and greater surface area. This step prepares fat for the action of pancreatic lipase secreted from the pancreas into the small intestine. This enzyme splits fatty acids from the glycerol core, forming diglycerides, monoglycerides, fatty acids, and glycerol, all of which can be absorbed by the cell lining of the small intestine. The digestion of fat is summarized in Table 5-4 and graphically in Figure 5-3.

bile
Substance made in the liver and stored in the gallbladder

micelle
A very small particle of lipid and bile salts

ABSORPTION

Short-chain fatty acids (4 to 6 carbon atoms), which are relatively soluble in water, and some glycerol are absorbed through the cells lining the intestine and enter the portal vein to be taken directly to the liver. In the liver they are reformed into fat molecules and incorporated into lipoproteins to be carried to various body tissues. When the monoglycerides, diglycerides, medium- and long-chain fatty acids, and glycerol have entered the cells lining the intestinal wall, the majority recombine to form triglycerides, which are secreted into the lacteals or fat-collecting ducts in the villus of the intestinal cells. From there they enter the lymphatic circulation as **chylomicrons**—particles composed of about 85% triglyceride, some cholesterol, some phospholipid, and enough protein to allow them to be transported in the aqueous blood. These chylomicrons are responsible for a milky appearance in the blood, which lasts about 1 hour after a meal.

lymph
The fluid in the circulatory system of the body that collects extra fluids

chylomicron
A very small fat particle surrounded by a thin layer of protein to make it more soluble in the blood

METABOLISM

In the liver lipids are built into **lipoproteins,** combinations of fat and protein that are synthesized to help carry fat to various tissues. Most of the lipid is then carried to the cells in these very low–density lipoproteins, or VLDL, which carry as much as 55% to 65% lipid.

lipoproteins
Combinations of lipid and protein that are more readily transported in the blood than lipid alone; for more discussion, see Chapter 3

Fatty Acids and Glycerol

Dietary lipid is composed of 95% triglycerides. After being absorbed, these triglycerides are carried to the liver as small fat globules called chylomicrons. From there they go to all the body's cells as lipoproteins. The fat portion of the lipoprotein is split off from the protein portion before entering the cell; once within the cell,

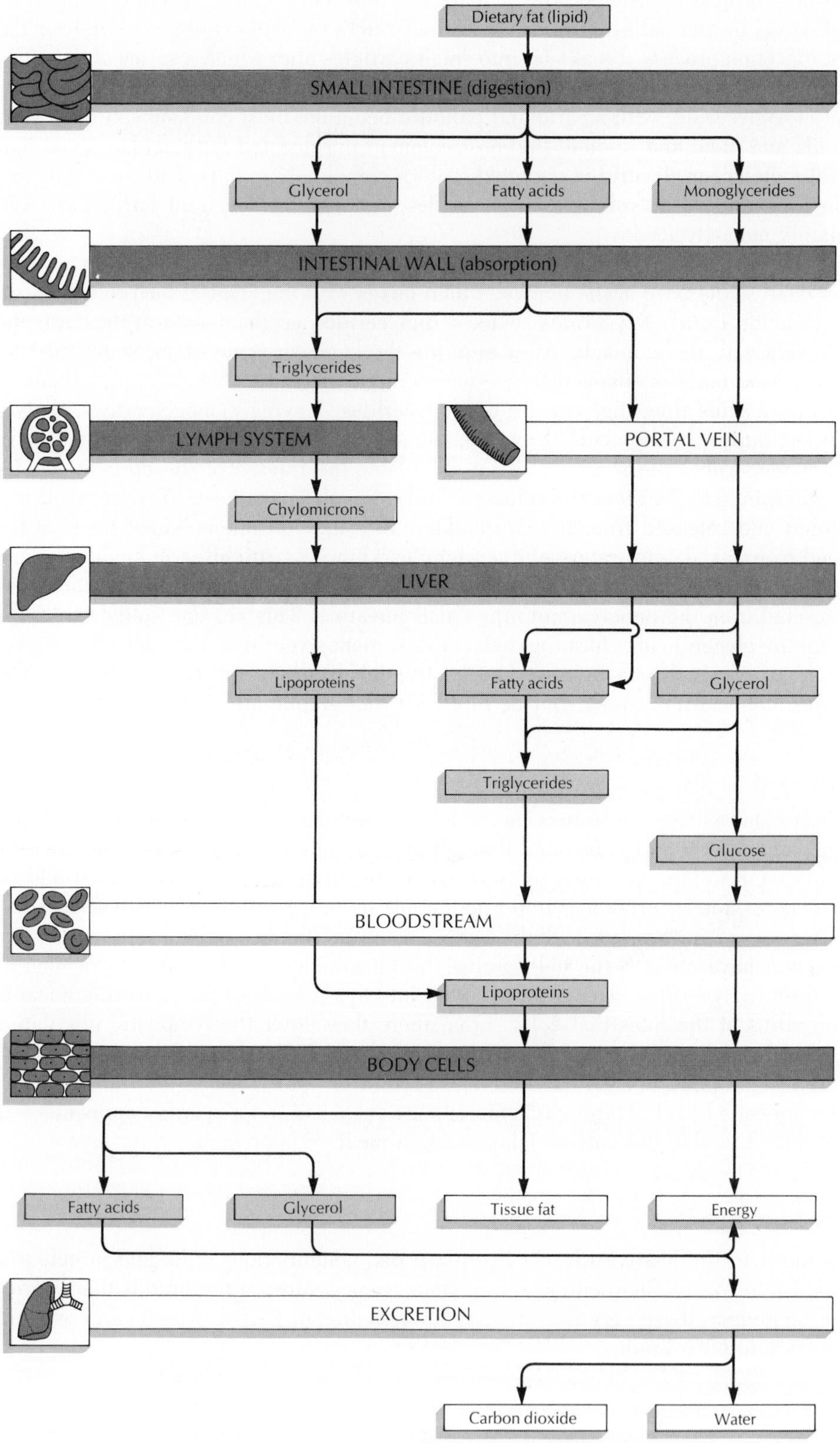

Figure 5-4 Summary of metabolism of lipid.

the fat portion is split again into glycerol and fatty acids before being metabolized in one of four ways:

1. **They are used immediately as a source of energy.**
2. **They are stored in the form of lipid as an energy reserve in regular or special adipose cells.**
3. **They are incorporated into cell structures.**
4. **They are used in the synthesis of essential body compounds.**

The metabolism of lipid is depicted in Figure 5-4.

The lipid stored in **adipocytes (adipose cells),** which can hold up to 90% fat, is mostly triglyceride. This may be the result of (1) a resynthesis of fat when fatty acids combine with glycerol that is synthesized within the cell or (2) **lipogenesis,** that is, formation of new fat from carbohydrate and protein present in excess of the body's need for energy or growth. Adipose cells tend to form beneath the skin and create a layer of subcutaneous fat. They are found in all parts of the body, however.

adipocyte or **adipose cell**
Special cell designed to store fat

lipogenesis
Formation of fatty acids from carbohydrate

Cholesterol

Because **hypercholesterolemia,** a high cholesterol level in the blood (>240 mg/dl), is considered a risk factor in coronary heart disease, there is a great deal of interest in how the body uses cholesterol. The study of cholesterol is complicated by the fact that although some blood cholesterol comes from animal foods in the diet, much is synthesized in cells from both lipid, especially saturated fatty acids, and carbohydrate.

Food cholesterol is absorbed into the lymphatic system along with additional cholesterol that is secreted in the bile or results from the loss of cholesterol-containing intestinal cells. The amount absorbed is controlled by the cells in the intestinal wall. Once absorbed, cholesterol is incorporated into the chylomicrons (4% cholesterol) and VLDLs (very low–density lipoproteins, which are 19% cholesterol). After the fat is removed to be used as a source of energy by various tissues, the chylomicrons become proportionately richer in both free and **esterified cholesterol,** first as VLDLs then as LDLs (low-density lipoproteins), which are 45% cholesterol. Most extra cholesterol is transported to the cells in the form of LDLs. High-density lipoproteins, or HDLs, are over 50% protein and carry relatively small amounts of cholesterol away from the cells. They predominate when there is

hypercholesterolemia
A blood cholesterol level > 240 mg/dl

esterfied cholesterol
Cholesterol bound to another substance rather than existing free in the blood

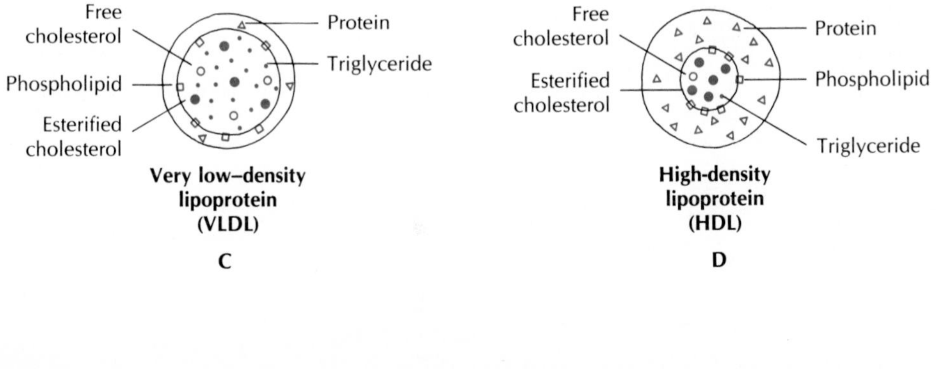

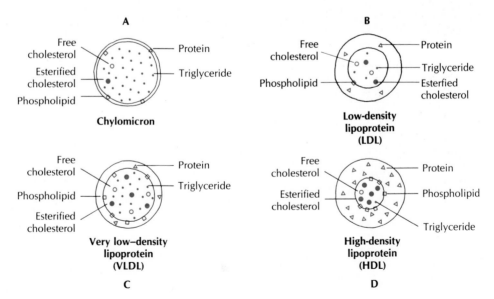

Diagrammatic representation of various forms in which lipid is carried in the blood

Figure 5-5 Composition of chylomicrons, very low–density lipoproteins, low-density lipoproteins, and high-density lipoproteins.

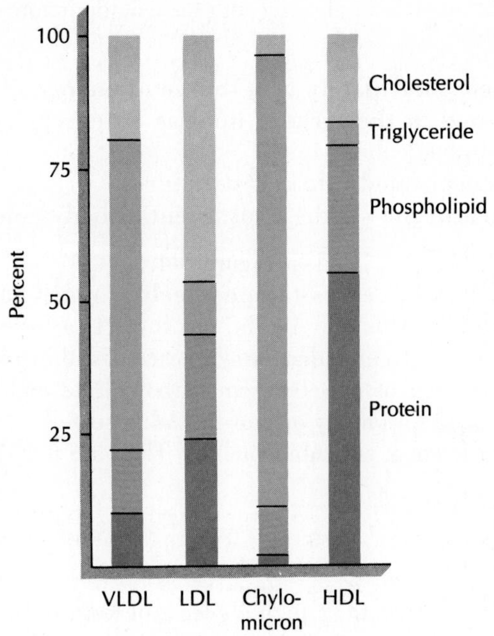

Table 5-5 ◆ Cholesterol and energy (kcal) content of common measures of selected foods*

Food	Amount	Kcal	Cholesterol (mg)
Milk (skim, fluid, or reconstituted dry)	1 cup	90	5
Cottage cheese, uncreamed	½ cup	62	5
Yogurt, frozen	½ cup	95	6
Lard	1 T	116	12
Cottage cheese, creamed	½ cup	116	17
Milk, 2%	1 cup	125	18
Cream, light table	2 T	58	20
Cream, half and half	¼ cup	80	24
Ice cream (regular, approximately 10% fat)	½ cup	135	28
Cheese, cheddar	1 oz	114	30
Milk, whole	1 cup	150	33
Butter	1 T	102	31
Oysters	3 oz, cooked	56	42
Tuna	3 oz, cooked	83	55
Chicken, turkey (light meat)	3 oz, cooked	147	72
Lamb, pork, chicken (dark meat)	3 oz, cooked	180	80
Crab	3 oz, cooked	86	85
Shrimp	3 oz, cooked	100	130
Heart, beef	3 oz, cooked	190	230
Egg	1 yolk or 1 egg	80	274
Liver, beef, calf, pork, lamb	3 oz, cooked	195	370
Kidney	3 oz, cooked	180	680
Brains	3 oz, raw	150	More than 1700

From Human Nutrition Information Service: Provisional table on the fatty acid and cholesterol content of selected foods, USDA, 1984.

*Fruits, vegetables, cereals, and margarines contain no cholesterol.

little surplus cholesterol, as blood leaves the cell. The composition of various carriers of cholesterol in the blood is shown in Figure 5-5.

The amount of circulating cholesterol depends on three factors: (1) the amount synthesized in the liver, (2) the amount of dietary cholesterol absorbed by the intestine, and (3) the amount of cholesterol secreted in the bile, which is reabsorbed rather than excreted in the feces. There is an elaborate interaction among these factors, with the amount synthesized determined by the amount present in the blood. High blood cholesterol levels do not necessarily mean a person is likely to suffer from coronary heart disease. It does mean, however, that the chances are greater, especially if LDL cholesterol is high relative to HDL cholesterol. Data on the cholesterol and kilocalorie contents of representative foods are shown in Table 5-5.

ROLE OF FAT IN THE DIET

Source of Energy

Fat is a concentrated source of energy. Each gram of fat, whether animal or vegetable, liquid or solid, provides 9 kcal—2¼ times as much energy as an equal weight of either carbohydrate or protein. Fat is the form in which the animal stores excess energy; thus the amount of fat in an animal that we use for food is determined by the way the animal is fed. Practically all animal foods contain some fat. Even relatively lean steak has 28% fat, which contributes 77% of the food's calories, while the 51% fat in cheddar cheese provides 73% of its calories. Any fat in plant foods is mainly in the form of oil. In cereals such as corn or in legumes such as soybeans, this oil is either in the germ or the starchy endosperm. Most fruits and vegetables have practically no fat. Fats such as butter, sour cream, or salad oil, routinely added to enhance the flavor of foods such as bread, potatoes, or salad greens, increase the caloric value of food two- to threefold.

1 gram fat	9 kcal
1 tablespoon fat	123 kcal
1 oz fat	246 kcal

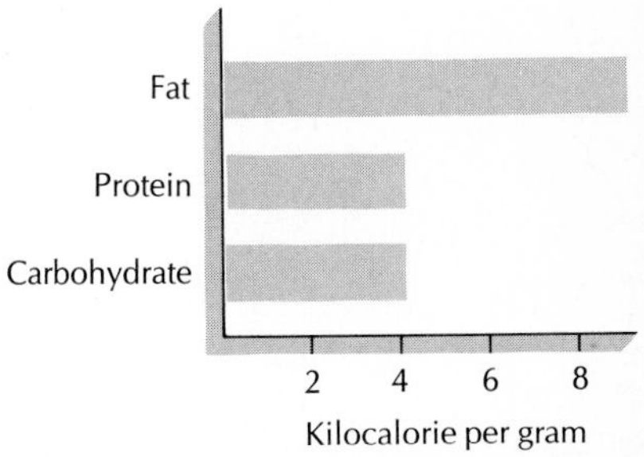

One unit of fat provides 2¼ times as many kilocalories as an equal amount of either carbohydrate or protein.

Satiety Value

Fat tends to leave the stomach relatively slowly. It is released up until 3½ hours after being eaten, depending on size and composition of the meal. This delay in the emptying time of the stomach helps to delay the onset of hunger pangs and contributes to a feeling of satiety after a meal. Because of its high caloric value, fat is frequently reduced or eliminated from diets suggested for weight control. However, current research shows that including some fat—low-fat milk, butter on vegetables and bread, or oil on salads—increases the satiety value of low-calorie diets and makes it easier for most people to stick to them. This strategy more than compensates for the concentrated caloric content of the fat. Currently, moderate-fat reducing diets are considered more successful than low-fat diets.

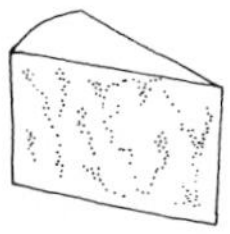

Cheddar cheese
51% fat provides
73% of kilocalories

Low-fat cheese
16% fat provides
54% kilocalories

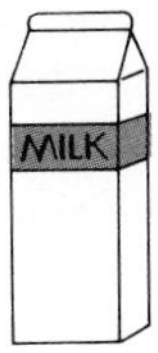

Milk
3.5% fat provides
50% of kilocalories

Low-fat milk
2% fat provides
38% kilocalories

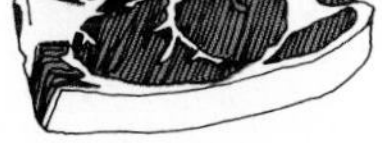

Steak
28% fat provides
77% of kilocalories

Fat content and kilocalories from fat in various foods

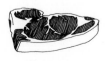

Carrier of Fat-Soluble Vitamins

Among the dietary essentials are four fat-soluble vitamins: A, D, E, and K. Dietary fat serves as a carrier of these nutrients; thus eliminating fat from the diet leads to reduced intake of them. In addition, fat at a level of at least 10% of total energy intake appears to be necessary for the absorption of vitamin A precursors from nonfat sources such as carrots. Anything that interferes with the absorption or use of fat, such as obstruction of the bile duct or rancidity of fat, depresses the availability of the fat-soluble vitamins.

Palatability

1 teaspoon margarine, butter, or oil is equivalent to:

5 teaspoons	sour cream or whipped cream
4 teaspoons	light cream
3 teaspoons	mayonnaise-type salad dressing or cream cheese
2 teaspoons	Italian or French salad dressing or imitation margarine
1 teaspoon	mayonnaise

The presence or addition of fat to food is responsible for much of its flavor. The marbling of fat throughout the lean muscle tissue of a steak contributes to its tenderness and flavor. Conversely, the removal of skin and fat from chicken may detract from its flavor. Using fat to fry food, to enhance the flavor of vegetables, as a spread, and as a base for salad dressing greatly improves taste appeal. Many substances that are responsible for the flavors and aromas of food are fat soluble. It has also been suggested that fat in the diet stimulates the flow of digestive juices. The role of fat in increasing the palatability of food is appreciated best by those who must eat a low-fat diet.

ROLE OF FAT IN THE BODY

Energy Reserve

Body fat is the primary form in which energy is stored in the body. It is an essential constituent of the cell membrane, and all tissues contain some of it. The size of most cells increases in adults with the need to store more fat. In addition, the body has a group of specialized adipocytes whose main function is the storage of fat. For some time we believed that the number of adipocytes was solely determined within the first few years of life. We now know that the body can at any time increase the number of fat cells to meet demands for storing excess fat.

Normal Body Fat
15% to 18% in men
18% to 24% in women

Once fat has been formed and deposited in the adipose tissues, the body has no way of excreting it. Therefore body fat can be reduced only by oxidizing, or burning, it as a source of energy. This use of fat occurs only when caloric intake is less than caloric expenditure. A certain amount of body fat, about 18% to 24% of body weight for women and 15% to 18% for men, is considered normal and desirable. People with reserves of fat in excess of these percentages are considered overweight. In extreme cases (that is, when the percentages are very high) they are considered obese with all the associated physical, physiological, aesthetic, and psychological disadvantages.

Although most body fat is described as white fat, a small portion known as brown fat (so named because of its generous blood supply) is distributed in small amounts in the upper part of the body. Infants have a much higher proportion of fat in brown adipocytes compared to adults. (There is some reason to believe that the amount of brown fat in an adult's body is the same as when he was a child.) Brown fat can be oxidized or used as a source of heat at a much faster rate than can that in white fat. In addition, brown fat never leaves the cell but is regenerated in a process requiring energy. This process occurs when the body temperature needs to be regulated as the result of exposure to cold or when energy intake from the diet is excessive and energy must be used at a faster rate to prevent the formation of more fat (body weight). This increase in rate of metabolism is known as **thermogenesis** and can be initiated by either cold temperatures, which cause shivering, or by diet. The same conditions stimulate the formation of more brown fat, so that the body's capacity to produce heat or regulate body weight is increased. This

thermogenesis
The process by which the body produces extra heat, usually by speeding up metabolism or shivering

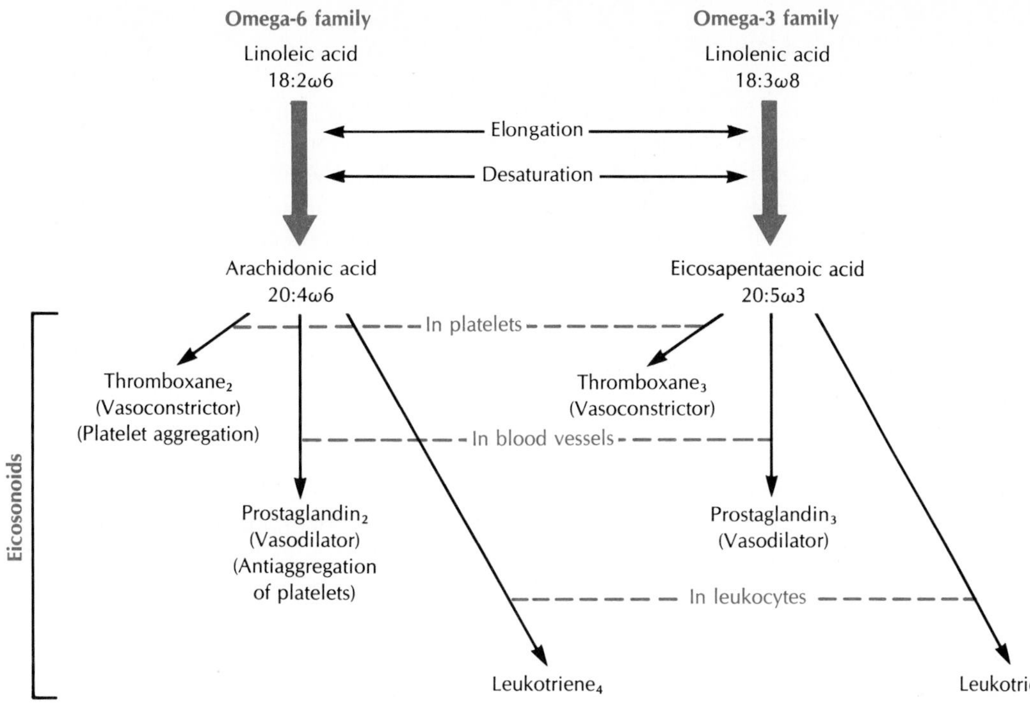

Figure 5-6 Production of eicosonoids from omega-3 and omega-6 fatty acids.

phenomenon has been well demonstrated in animals and is assumed to be a factor in weight control in humans.

Regulator

As an essential constituent of the membrane of each individual cell and as a precursor of prostaglandins, fat indirectly helps to regulate the uptake and excretion of nutrients by the cell and to control many vital body functions.

Precursor of Prostaglandins

In 1962 a group of hormone-like substances were identified as **prostaglandins.** Since then the study of these substances has led to the identification of a vast number of related compounds that fulfill many physiological functions. Most of these compounds are synthesized from the fatty acid arachidonic acid, which is either provided in the diet from animal foods or produced from linolenic acid found in several vegetable oils, such as soybean and canola, also known as low erucic acid rapeseed (LEAR), or EPA (eicosopentaenoic acid) or DHA (docohexanenoic acid) in fish oils. As shown in Figure 5-6, EPA and arachidonic acid can both be metabolized into a variety of these important physiological compounds—prostaglandins (PG), leukotrienes (LT), and thromboxanes (TX)—which are all classified as **eicosonoids.**

Prostaglandins act on the brain, the wall of blood vessels, certain blood cells, and blood platelets. Another group of substances, **leukotrienes,** derived from arachidonic acid, act mostly on white blood cells. The results of excessive production of some of these hormones may cause excessive clotting of the blood and the accumulation of material in the wall of the artery to cause blood clotting. The possibility of these undesirable consequences of the overproduction of prostaglan-

prostaglandins
Hormone-like substances produced by various body cells from HUFA
- Leukotrienes
- Prostacyclins
- Thromboxanes

eicosonoids
Hormone-like prostacyclins with a 20-carbon structure

leukotrienes
A special group of hormone-like substances produced in white blood cells from HUFA

dins can be regulated by EPA and DHA, both 20-carbon omega-3 fatty acids found in fish oil. EPA and DHA act to decrease the stickiness of blood platelets. It is this stickiness that causes platelets to adhere to each other and to form a clot, thus EPA and DHA reduce the possibility of a heart attack. On the other hand too much EPA may lead to asthma or to blood that does not clot enough.

For further discussion of prostaglandins see Focus section.

Prostaglandins also perform many important and varied functions such as promoting conception, inducing labor, effecting spontaneous abortions, regulating transmissions of nerve impulses, and regulating blood pressure. Prostaglandins are synthesized and used in the same tissue rather than being synthesized in one tissue and transported to act on another, as are hormones from endocrine glands. As a result they have become known as *local* hormones. They also differ in that they are quickly destroyed if not used.

Insulator

Deposits of fat beneath the skin, or subcutaneous fat, serve as insulating material for the body, protecting it against changes in environmental temperature. A certain minimal layer of fat is desirable to prevent excessive heat loss from the body, but too thick a layer slows down the rate of heat loss during hot weather, causing physical discomfort.

Protector

Fat deposits surround certain vital organs such as the kidneys and heart, serving to hold them in position and shield them from physical shock. These fat deposits are the last to be reduced when there is a caloric deficit.

FOOD SOURCES

The total fat and fatty acid composition of some commonly used foods is shown in Figures 5-7 and 5-8 and Table 5-6, which includes amounts of saturated and unsaturated fatty acids, and the P/S ratio, and the P-M/S ratio. As shown, special margarines now on the market have a P/S ratio of 0.3 to 4.9, compared with 0.2 to 0.5 for regular margarines. In the hydrogenation of polyunsaturated fatty acids some fatty acids may be converted into monounsaturated fatty acids and even saturated fatty acid. A comparison of the composition of commonly used fats is shown in Figure 5-7. The polyunsaturated fatty acid linoleic acid is the predominant essential fatty acid (EFA) in dietary fats. From Table 5-6 and Figure 5-7 it is evident that coconut, olive, and palm kernel oil contain no EFA, while safflower and corn oil contain large amounts. Poultry and game also provide large amounts. There is considerable interest in determining how much of the omega-3 fatty acids should be consumed. Approximately 1 gram was found to be adequate for a 6-year-old girl. The ratio of 5:1 of omega-6 to omega-3 fatty acids in human milk was considered adequate but may change with age. A ratio between 4:1 and 10:1 appears desirable. A major source of omega-3 fatty acids is fish, such as salmon, mackerel, and eel. The amount of omega-3 fatty acid in fish and oils is shown in Table 5-7.

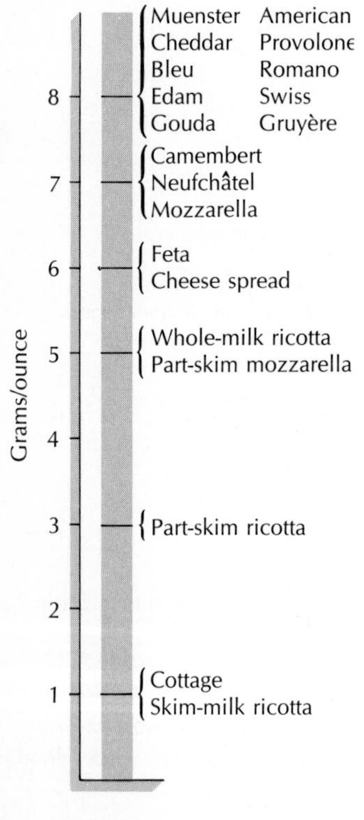

Fat content of cheese

It is difficult to present precise data on the fatty acid composition of animal fats because of differences resulting from variation in each animal's diet. The methods used to process and store food may also affect the fatty acid composition of the food as it is consumed. Food producers are responding in many ways to the public's interest in foods of lower fat content. An example of the efforts of animal breeders is shown in Figure 5-9.

The percentage of calories contributed by fat tends to be relatively high in most foods from animal sources. Whole milk has 3.2% fat, which contributes 50% of milk's total calories. Frankfurters are 27% fat, and this fat accounts for 70% of

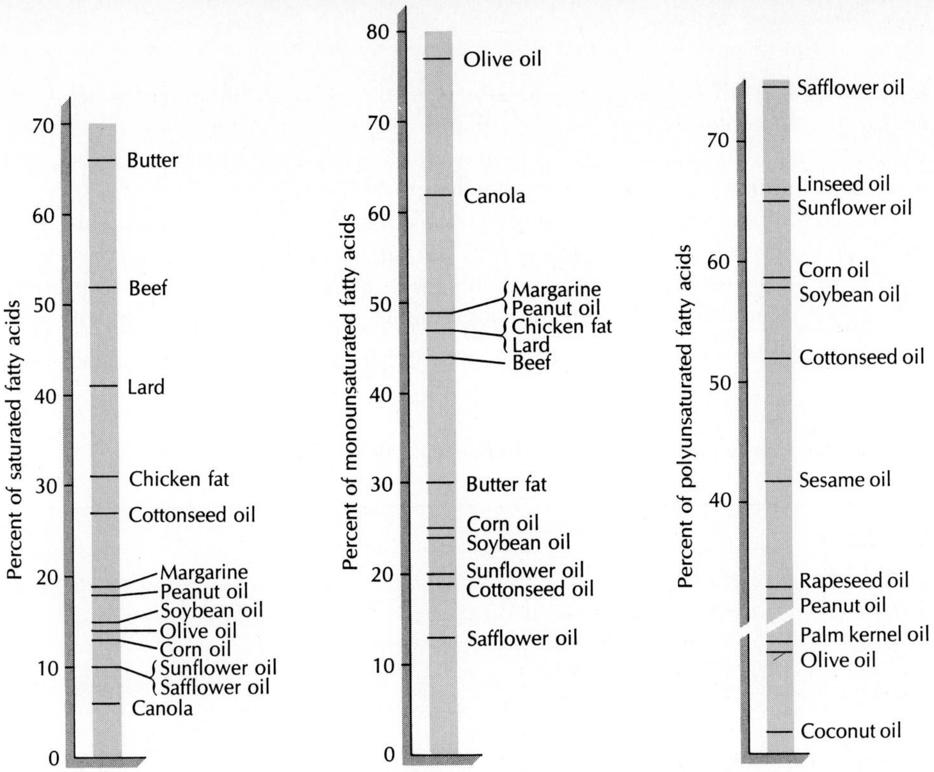

Figure 5-7 The relative saturated, monounsaturated, and polyunsaturated fatty acid composition of commonly used oils and fats.

Based on data from USDA Handbook 8-4, Nutrient Composition of Fats and Oils, Washington, D.C., 1983.

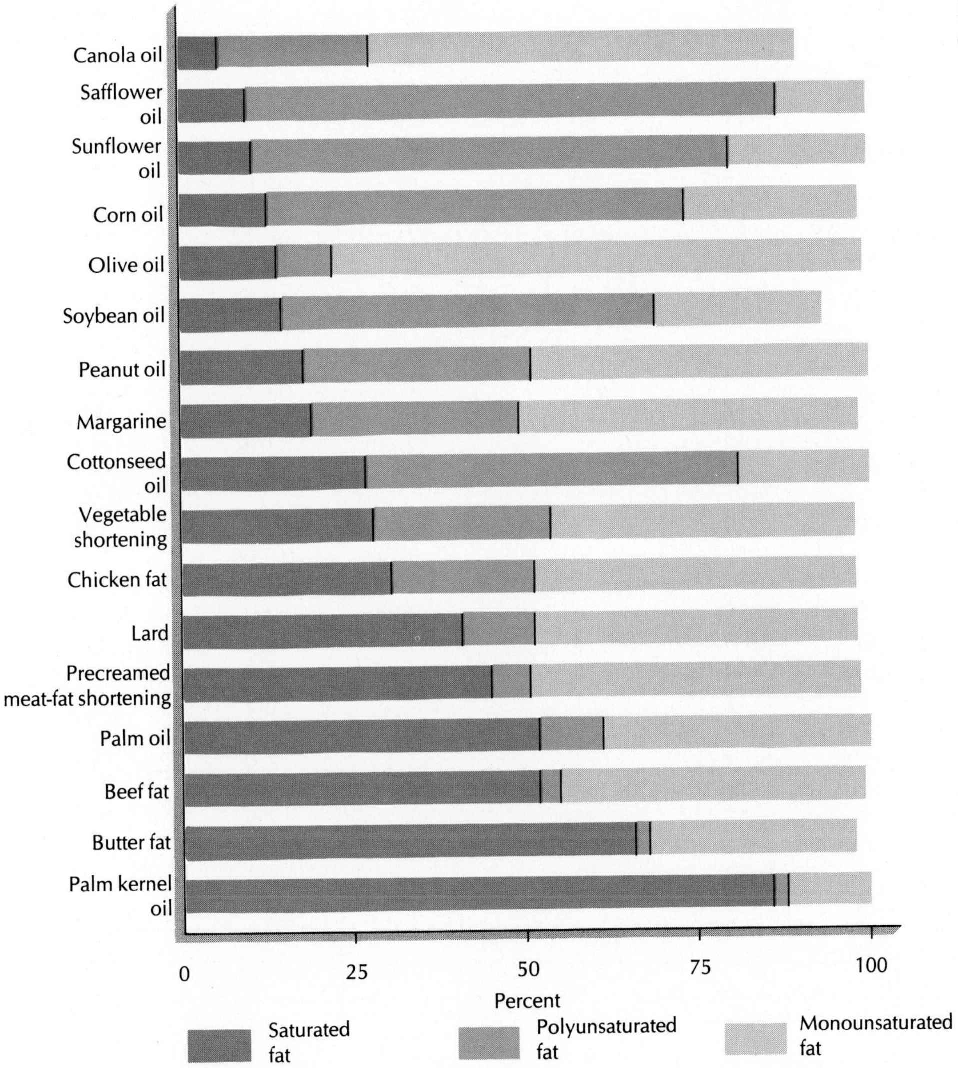

Figure 5-8 Profiles of fatty acids and commonly used fats and oils.

total calories. Half of the fat in chicken is in the skin or directly beneath it. In cheese the fat content varies from less than 5 grams per serving in low-fat cheeses such as cottage, ricotta, and part-skim mozarella to 8 grams in cheddar, swiss, and colby to 10 grams in cream cheese, which is 33% fat.

Vegetable foods, however, usually contain less fat. Whole-grain cereals have from 2% to 9% fat, mainly in the germ. The fat in seed varies, from 4% in corn to 17% in soybeans. Nuts such as peanuts, with 50% fat, and pecans, with 68%, have more. The only fruits with any appreciable fat are avocados with 16% and ripe olives with 30%.

Table 5-6 ◆ Fat content and major fatty acid composition of selected foods (in decreasing order of linoleic acid content within each group of similar foods)

		Fatty Acids*				
			Unsaturated			
Food	Total Fat (%)	Saturated (%)	Mono-unsaturated (%)	Poly-unsaturated (Linoleic) (%)	P/S Ratio†	P-M/S Ratio‡
Salad and cooking oils						
Safflower	100	9	12	74	8.2	9.5
Wheat germ	100	19	15	62	3.3	4.1
Corn	100	13	24	59	4.5	6.4
Soybean	100	14	23	58	4.1	5.8
Cottonseed	100	26	18	52	2.0	2.7
Sesame	100	14	40	42	3.0	5.9
Peanut	100	17	46	32	1.9	4.6
Rapeseed (canola)	100	7	56	33	4.9	12.7
Olive	100	14	74	8	0.6	5.9
Palm	100	49	37	9	0.2	1.0
Coconut	100	87	6	2	0.02	0.09
Palm kernel	100	81	11	2	0.02	0.16
Butter	81	51	23	3	0.05	0.51
Margarine, first ingredient on label						
Safflower oil—tub	80	9	23	44	4.9	7.4
Corn oil (liquid)—tub	80	14	32	31	2.2	4.5
Soybean oil—stick	80	17	39	21	1.2	3.5
Corn oil—stick	80	13	46	18	1.4	4.9
Lard	100	39	45	11	0.3	1.4
Animal fats						
Poultry	100	30	37	20	0.7	1.9
Beef, lamb, pork	100	50	36	3	0.06	0.78
Fish, raw						
Salmon	9	2	2	4	2.0	3
Mackerel	13	5	3	4	0.8	1.4
Herring, Pacific	13	4	2	2	0.5	1
Tuna	5	2	1	1	0.5	1
Nut						
Walnuts, English	64	9	23	63	7.0	9.5
Brazil	67	13	32	17	1.3	3.8
Peanuts or peanut butter	51	17	46	32	1.9	5.6
Pecan	65	4-6	33-48	9-24	—	—
Egg yolk	33	10	12	4	0.4	1.6
Avocado	16	3	7	2	0.6	3

From USDA Handbook 8-4: Composition of fats and oils, 1979.
*Total is not expected to equal total fat.
†Polyunsaturated fatty acids: saturated fatty acids (excluding monounsaturated fatty acids).
‡Polyunsaturated fatty acids plus monounsaturated fatty acids: saturated fatty acids.

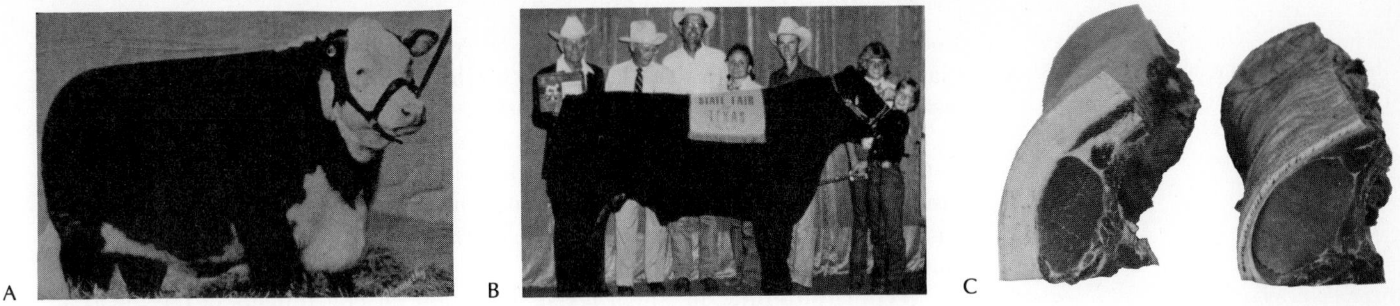

Figure 5-9 The change in the physical features of these animals being prepared for the U.S. market reflects the attempts of animal breeders to respond to public interests in lowering fat in the diet. Notice the difference in body fat of the prize-winning animals in 1956 **(A)** and 1984 **(B)**. **C,** Advances in biotechnology have made it possible to produce leaner, more nutritious pork loin *(right)*. Treating pigs with recombinant porcine growth hormone does not affect taste and is completely safe for the consumer.

A and **B** courtesy Dr. Bridenstein, National Meat and Livestock Board, Chicago, IL. **C** courtesy Dr. Terry Etherton, Pennsylvania State University.

Table 5-7 ◇Food sources of omega-3 fatty acids

Food	% of Total Lipid as Omega-3	
Oils		grams/oz*
Menhaden	23	6.9
Salmon	22	6.6
Cod liver	20	6.0
Canola	10	3.0
Soybean	7	2.1
Butter fat	2	0.6
Corn	1	0.3
Fish		grams/4 oz
Cod	42	0.3
Shrimp	38	0.5
Tuna	30	2.3
Pink salmon	29	1
King crab	20	0.6
Mackerel	17	1.8-2.6
Herring	6	1.0-2.0

*1 oz = 2 tablespoons; 1 oz provides 246 kcal.

Based on its nutrient composition, bacon is correctly designated as a fat food rather than a protein food. Raw bacon is over two-thirds fat; cooked bacon has considerably less, depending on the extent of cooking.

The contribution of various food groups to the total fat in the American food supply is shown in the margin. Average daily fat consumption reported in the USDA surveys is 68 grams below the 172 grams available in the food supply, and reflecting a relatively large waste of fat in food preparation.

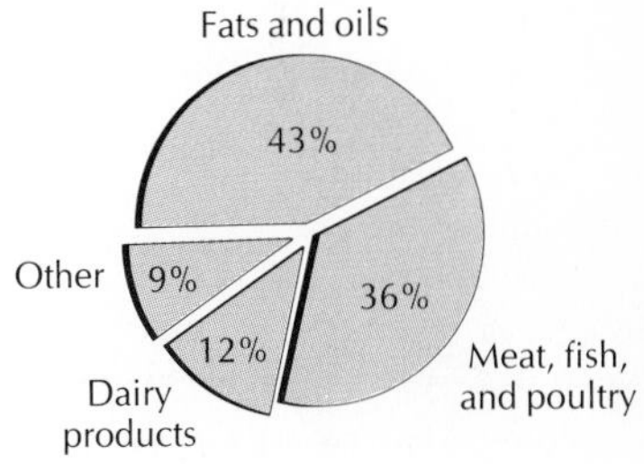

Contribution of various food groups to the fat content of the American diet

DIETARY REQUIREMENTS

Aside from the need for a dietary source of linoleic acid, humans do not require fat. A diet providing 2% of kilocalories from linoleic acid (about 5 grams [2 tsp]) meets this requirement. Fat is a concentrated source of energy and therefore allows us to meet energy requirements without eating large quantities of food. However, the current practice of obtaining as much as 43% of kilocalories from fat is being questioned because of the prevalence of excessive energy intake and the possibility of adverse effects from high-fat diets contributing to cardiovascular diseases and cancer. Nutritionists suggest that an intake of fat providing 25% to 35% of kilocalories is more compatible with good health; this amount will provide essential fatty acids and facilitate the absorption of fat-soluble vitamins.

To get needed nutrients without too much fat and cholesterol:
- Choose low-fat dairy products
- Eat lean meats
- Use low-fat cooking methods (steaming, broiling, baking, stir-fry)
- Use little butter or margarine on breads and vegetables
- Use little or low-fat salad dressing

Modifications in Dietary Fat

steatorrhea
The presence of fat in the stools

Modification of dietary fat intake may be necessary in several conditions. For example, in gallbladder disease, in which bile cannot be stored, fat intake may be restricted to as little as 10% of kilocalories, or emulsified fats may be substituted for nonemulsified ones. For the treatment of excess fat in the stools, or **steatorrhea,** medium-chain and short-chain fatty acids are absorbed better than long-chain and can be used without requiring reduction in the total amount of fat in the diet. The recommendation to restrict fat intake in such conditions as hepatitis, cirrhosis, and jaundice is now being questioned.

hyperlipidemia
High amounts of lipid in the blood

Hyperlipidemia, in which levels of certain fat constituents of the blood are elevated, may call for a modification of the kind and amount of total dietary fat. Some types of hyperlipidemia do not respond to dietary changes and can be treated only with drugs.

Lipids and Degenerative Diseases

Dietary factors may be involved in degenerative diseases in several ways. Nutrients in food can act to either promote or inhibit the initiation or continuation of the disease.

Coronary heart disease. Our first inkling of a relationship between diet and heart disease came with the observation that persons who suffered heart attacks almost always had above-normal levels of blood cholesterol. Cholesterol was shown to be a major constituent of the plaques that form on the inside of some blood vessels. As these plaques continue to increase in size, they narrow the passage in some major blood vessels to the point that if a clot forms, it closes the vessel entirely. If this occurs in the blood vessels to the heart, as it usually does, the person suffers a heart attack. If it occurs in the blood vessels to the brain, a stroke is the result.

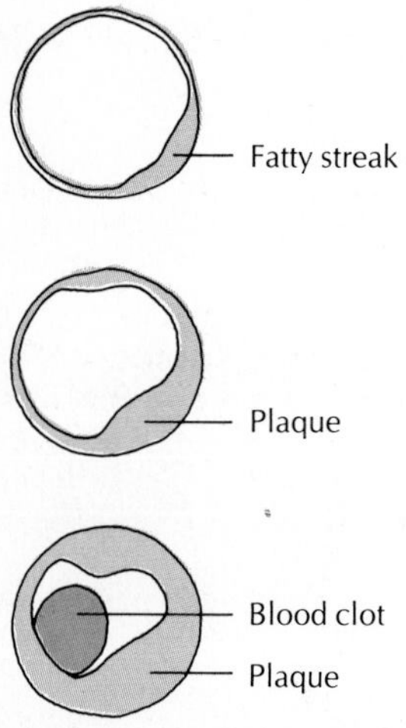

Buildup of atherosclerotic plaque in blood vessel—starts with fatty streaks; addition of cholesterol forms plaque, which narrows the lumen and causes a blood clot.

Studies on rabbits showed that a restriction of dietary cholesterol resulted in lower levels of cholesterol in the blood. In humans, however, restriction of the amount of cholesterol-containing foods such as eggs, meat, and liver in the diet did not consistently result in lowered blood cholesterol levels. The reason for this became clear when we learned that the liver can synthesize as much as 2000 mg of cholesterol a day. This amount is considerably more than the 500 mg of cholesterol provided from a normal diet.

People who consumed liquid fats or oils had lower blood cholesterol levels than those who ate more solid, primarily saturated, animal fats. Because liquid fats differ from solid fats primarily in the proportion of PUFA they contain, we shifted our emphasis toward an increased use of vegetable oils high in PUFA such as corn oil or safflower oil. We found that when PUFA provided about half the dietary fat, blood cholesterol levels were reduced, but heart disease was not. Among the unsaturated fatty acids, those with 16 to 18 carbon atoms had the greatest effect in lowering blood cholesterol.

Until very recently, it was believed that all saturated fats stimulated cholesterol synthesis and caused a lowering of HDL levels. It now appears that stearic acid, found in cocoa butter, hydrogenated soybean oil, and beef fat, not only does not increase LDL cholesterol levels but also does not decrease the protective HDL cholesterol level. The effect of diet on blood cholesterol levels depends on how high the blood cholesterol levels were initially. When levels are elevated above 260 mg/dl, it is almost impossible to bring about a drop sufficient to reduce the risk of heart disease by diet alone. The use of the drug cholestyramine, which prevents the absorption of cholesterol, is effective. Unfortunately it is very expensive and so unpalatable that people have difficulty using it. Fortunately there are new drugs on the market, such as Levostatin, which act to reduce plasma cholesterol levels. It is possible that if they prove successful, the need for dietary restriction among individuals at high risk of heart disease because of elevated blood cholesterol will be reduced.

The search for dietary factors that will most reduce the risk of coronary heart disease has led to studies that assess the effect of substituting complex for simple carbohydrates to reduce serum triglycerides; increasing fiber, especially oat bran fiber, to reduce the absorption of cholesterol; increasing the intake of highly unsaturated fatty acids such as EPA and DHA from fish oils to enhance the production of thromboxanes, which inhibit the tendency of blood platelets to adhere to each other and to the side of the arterial wall; and following diets high in monounsaturated fatty acids such as oleic acid to inhibit the receptors of LDL, particularly on liver cells.

Knowledge of the role of various dietary factors and of the balance that exists among these factors in the development of atherosclerosis is still inconclusive. It is believed that any drastic modification of the American diet on the basis of current information is unnecessary. However, professional groups suggest that many people would benefit (1) if the amount of fat in the diet were reduced from the present level of 43% to less than 30% of total calories, (2) if the amount of dietary cholesterol were restricted to less than 300 mg, (3) if polyunsaturated fats were substituted for some of the saturated fat in the diet so that the distribution among polyunsaturated, monounsaturated, and saturated fatty acids would be about equal, (4) if saturated fat were limited to 10% of total calorie intake, and (5) if caloric intake were adjusted to maintain desired body weight. The American diet seems to be shifting in these directions; at the same time there is a reassuring reduction in mortality from coronary heart disease. The extent to which these two facts are related is unknown. However, for those people who are most likely to suffer from atherosclerosis, adherence to a prudent diet as just described is strongly recommended. These include people with several risk factors, for example, overweight persons, middle-aged men with high blood cholesterol and triglyceride levels, people with a family history of heart disease, those working under emotional tension, persons who smoke, or people who have elevated blood pressure.

It must also be recognized that diet is not the only life-style factor that influences the risk of coronary heart disease. Exercise and stress both significantly affect the ratio of HDL cholesterol to LDL cholesterol. Stress and lack of exercise have the undesirable reverse effect of increasing LDL cholesterol and reducing HDL cholesterol. Smoking, through its effect on the vascular system, is an additional risk factor.

Although drugs may eventually reduce the need for dietary modification to control cholesterol levels, the need to control body weight will continue to call for dietary modification.

Cancer. Food may also serve as a carrier of carcinogens or substances that are responsible for the initiation of the tumor. These are usually substances that have been added to food or have been produced in the food as a result of the conditions of processing. They may, however, occur naturally.

Epidemiological data demonstrating a relationship between the amount of fat in the diet and the incidence of certain type of cancers, particularly breast and prostate cancer, have stimulated extensive research to determine if dietary lipid is a factor. Presently it appears that it may be the total calories in the diet that are responsible rather than fat per se, although the two are closely related. Large intervention studies to see if the incidence of breast cancer in women could be reduced by limiting dietary fat to 20% to 30% of total calories was abandoned when it was discovered that although women could adhere to such a low-fat diet for about 6 months, they all lost weight in excess of a desirable amount. When they needed an increase in calories they found it impossible to continue the dietary modification because they could not get enough calories without increasing fat. At the same time experimental data were failing to show that fat was responsible for growth of cancers. Intervention studies in connection with heart disease suggest that very high intakes of polyunsaturated fatty acids are associated with increased cancer deaths.

National Cholesterol Education Program for Adults

GOAL: Total blood cholesterol <200 mg/dl
LDL cholesterol <160 mg/dl
or <130 mg/dl with 2 or more risk factors

If total blood cholesterol is >200 mg/dl and individual has 2 or more of the following risk factors:

- Family history of CHD
- Smokes cigarettes
- Diabetes
- Obesity
- Hypertension
- Low HDL cholesterol
- Male

Test for LDL cholesterol

If LDL cholesterol >130 mg/dl:
Reduce saturated fat intake to 10% of total kilocalories
Reduce total fat intake to 30% of total kilocalories
Reduce cholesterol intake to 300 mg/day
For 6 months

If unsuccessful (that is, LDL cholesterol >130 mg/dl)
Reduce saturated fat intake to 7% of total kilocalories
Reduce cholesterol intake to 200 mg/day
For 6 months

Use drug therapy only on physician's advice.

American Heart Association Dietary Guidelines for Healthy American Adults

Total fat	<30% calories
Saturated fat	<10% calories
Polyunsaturated fat	≤10% calories
Carbohydrate	≥50% calories
Protein	Remainder of calories
Cholesterol	≤300 mg/day
Sodium	<3 grams/day
Ethanol	≤1-2 oz/day
Total calories	Sufficient to maintain recommended body weight

Eat a wide variety of foods
Circulation 77:721A, 1988.

BY NOW YOU SHOULD KNOW

- Lipids, or fats, are made up of glycerol and fatty acids.
- Lipids are classified or identified on the basis of 1) length of carbon chain, 2) degree of saturation, and 3) position of double bond.
- Triglycerides in foods are either predominately saturated, monounsaturated, or polyunsaturated fatty acids.
- Lipids are essential body or dietary components.
- In the diet lipids provide satiety and palatability and serve as a source of energy, as a carrier for fat-soluble vitamins, and as a source of essential fatty acids.
- In the body, fat serves as a reserve of energy, as a source of essential fatty acids from which prostaglandins are synthesized, as an insulator to help regulate body temperature, and as protection for vital body organs.
- Almost all animal foods contain fat, but among plant foods only nuts, seeds, and avocados contain fat.
- Lecithin and cholesterol are fat-related substances found in foods. Both are manufactured by the body, but neither is considered a dietary essential.
- Lipids must be emulsified in order to be digested; bile is an emulsifying agent.
- Lipids are insoluble in water; they are carried throughout the circulatory system as soluble lipoproteins.
- Lipid is digested by enzymes known as lipases.
- The small intestine, gallbladder, and liver all play important roles in the digestion, absorption, and metabolism of fats.
- Lipid provides 9 kcal/gram of fat; therefore 1 pound of body fat, which is 20% water, represents 3500 kcal of stored energy.
- Excessive fat in the diet has been implicated as a cause of several degenerative diseases, particularly coronary heart disease and cancer. However, it is not known whether the kind or the amount of fat is important.
- Linoleic acid, a polyunsaturated fatty acid, is essential and should represent at least 2% of dietary fat.
- Many vegetable fats such as corn, cottonseed, and soybean oil are liquid at room temperature and are changed into solid and semisolid fats by a process called hydrogenation.

STUDY QUESTIONS

1. How have the total consumption and sources of fat changed in the U.S. diet from 1909 to present?
2. What is the relationship between fat consumption and health problems such as cancer or heart disease?
3. Give examples of food sources of saturated, monounsaturated, and polyunsaturated fatty acids.
4. What food products are produced by the hydrogenation of vegetable oils?
5. What is the significance of the P/S ratio?
6. Why are fats a more concentrated source of energy than carbohydrates?
7. Describe why certain fatty acids are essential in the diet.
8. List some important roles of cholesterol in the body.
9. What foods should be avoided on a low-cholesterol diet?
10. Will lowering dietary cholesterol prevent heart disease?
11. What specific dietary recommendations would you make for someone at high risk of developing heart disease?
12. What are some important functions of prostaglandins?

Applying What You've Learned

1. Food Intake Record

Write down everything you have eaten today or yesterday.

a. Circle all the food sources of fats and categorize the fats according to their predominate fatty acids—saturated fats, monounsaturated fats, and polyunsaturated fats. Using Appendix F, look up the foods you have circled, and total the amounts of the different forms of fat.
   How many grams of saturated fatty acids?
   How many grams of monounsaturated fatty acids?
   How many grams of polyunsaturated fatty acids?
   What is your total fat intake from these foods?
   Would you say you have equal distribution of the three types of fatty acids in your diet? What would you say are the major sources of fat in your diet? What are low in fat? If you could make any changes, what would they be?

b. Now put a box around the foods on your list that are sources of cholesterol. Rank order these foods from what you believe will be highest to lowest in cholesterol. Check your ranking by using Appendix F or Table 5-5.

2. Reading Labels

a. Look for information on content (grams of fat) on several food labels. It is often hard to visualize the grams of fat in a food. To make this an activity in which you can visualize the grams of fat, try converting the grams to pats of butter. Each pat of butter (approximately 1 teaspoon) equals 4 grams of fat. Therefore if you discovered that 1 serving of the snack food contained 8 grams of fat, by dividing by 4 you would know that a serving of this food has fat equivalent of eating 2 pats of butter.

b. Next, look at the list of ingredients on the same food labels. What are the ingredients that contribute fat to this food? Are the fats at the beginning or the end of this ingredient list? If they are at the beginning, the fat content is greater than if the fats are listed at the end. Are the fats predominantly saturated or unsaturated?

c. The Dietary Guidelines for Healthy Americans recommend a maximum fat intake of 30% of our total calories. One way to work toward this goal is to choose individual foods that provide 30% or less of the calories from fat. By using the nutrition information on the label you can determine the percent calories from fat. For example: In potato chips with 150 kcal and 10 grams of fat per serving 60% of the calories come from fat. To determine the percent of calories, first convert fat grams to kcal by simply multiplying the grams of fat times 9 (since each gram of fat = 9 kcals). Once you know the calories from fat you simply divide those kilocalories by the total number of kcal and multiply the quotient times 100 for the percentage of fat kilocalories. Try this simple calculation on foods you regularly eat. You can use food labels or Appendix F to find calories and grams of fat. Do your choices meet the Dietary Guidelines?

3. Controlling Fats when Dining Out

Think about some of your favorite meals eaten away from home. Write down five of the menu items you most often order. Ask yourself: How are these foods prepared? Are these foods fried? Are these foods in a creamy rich sauce? Do these foods require extra butter, sour cream, or a dressing that will add additional fats? Do you choose foods with added fat? Next time you go out to eat read the menu. Look for broiled, baked, or grilled items. Look for foods without cream sauces. What are the choices? Will you make low-fat choices? Why or why not?

SUGGESTED READING

Grundy SM: Monounsaturated fatty acids, plasma cholesterol, and coronary heart disease, American Journal of Clinical Nutrition 45:1168, 1987.

This article lends support to the growing recognition that, when substituted for saturated fatty acids, monounsaturated fatty acids found in vegetable oils such as olive oil and canola have as great an effect as polyunsaturated fatty acids in lowering total blood cholesterol and LDL cholesterol. In contrast, however, they do not cause a decrease in HDL cholesterol, which is a protective against heart disease (CHD).

Lands WEM: Renewed questions about polyunsaturated fatty acids, Nutrition Reviews 44(6)189, 1986.

This brief historical overview presents a summary of polyunsaturated fatty acids and examines a few aspects of defining essential fatty acids.

Leaf A, and Weber PC: Cardiovascular effects of n-3 fatty acids, New England Journal of Medicine 318:549, 1988.

The authors present a succinct review of our knowledge of the effect of n-3 fatty acids on coronary heart disease. They point out the possibility that the protective effect of fish may be the result of some factor other than their HUFA content, or that benefits from long-term fish consumption providing small amounts of n-3 fatty acids may be the same as short-term benefits of much higher doses.

ADDITIONAL READINGS

Anderson K, Castelli MW, and Levy D: Andosterol and mortality: 30 years follow-up from the Framingham study, Journal of the American Medical Association 257:2176, 1987.

Beynen AC, and Katan MB: Why do polyunsaturated fatty acids lower serum cholesterol? American Journal of Clinical Nutrition 42: 560, 1985.

Consensus Conference: Treatment of hypertriglyceridemia, Journal of the American Medical Association 251:1196, 1984.

Dyerberg J: Linolenate-derived polyunsaturated fatty acids and prevention of atherosclerosis, Nutrition Reviews 44(4): 125, 1986.

Expert Panel. Report of the National Cholesterol Education Program Expert Panel on Detection, Evaluation, and Treatment of High Blood Cholesterol in Adults, Archives of Internal Medicine 148:36, 1988.

Friedman HI, and Nylund B: Intestinal fat digestion, absorption, and transport: a review, American Journal of Clinical Nutrition 33:1108, 1980.

Glomset JA: Fish, fatty acids, and human health, New England Journal of Medicine 312:1253, 1985.

Grundy SM: Comparison of monounsaturated fatty acids and carbohydrates for lowering plasma cholesterol, New England Journal of Medicine 314:745, 1986.

Grundy SM: Mono-unsaturated fatty acids, plasma cholesterol, and coronary heart disease, American Journal of Clinical Nutrition 45:1168, 1987.

Harper AE: Coronary heart disease—an epidemic related to diet? American Journal of Clinical Nutrition 37:69, 1983.

Himms-Hagen J: Brown adipose tissue thermogenesis, Nutrition Reviews 41:261, 1983.

Lipid Research Clinics Program: The lipid research clinics primary prevention trial results, Journal of the American Medical Association 251:351, 1984.

Mattson FH, and Grundy SM: Comparison of the effects of dietary saturated, monounsaturated and polyunsaturated fatty acids on plasma lipids and lipoproteins in man, Journal of Lipid Research 26:194, 1985.

Multiple Risk Factor Intervention Trial Research Group: Multiple risk factor intervention trial, Journal of the American Medical Association 248:1465, 1982.

Neuringer M, and Connor WE: N-3 Fatty acids in the brain and retina: evidence for their essentiality, Nutrition Reviews 44: 285, 1987.

Nestel PJ: Polyunsaturated fatty acids (N-3, N-6), American Journal of Clinical Nutrition 45:1161, 1987.

Nutrition Committee, American Heart Association: Dietary Guidelines for Healthy American Adults, Circulation 77:721A, 1988.

Phillipson BE, and others: Reduction of plasma lipids, lipoproteins, and apoproteins by dietary fish oils in patients with hypertriglyceridemia, New England Journal of Medicine 312:1210, 1985.

Rosenberg I, and Schaeffer EJ: Dietary saturated fatty acids and blood cholesterol, New England Journal of Medicine 318:1270, 1988.

Simoupoulos A: ω-3 fatty acids in growth and development and in health and disease, Nutrition Today 23:10, 1988.

Theuson L, Hennikson LB, and Engby B: One year experience with low-fat, low-cholesterol diet in patients with coronary heart disease, American Journal of Clinical Nutrition 44:212, 1986.

Walker WJ: Changing U.S. life-style and declining vascular mortality—a retrospective, New England Journal of Medicine 308:649, 1983.

Willett WC, and others: Dietary fat and the risk of breast cancer, New England Journal of Medicine 315:22, 1987.

FOCUS Fish Oils and Health

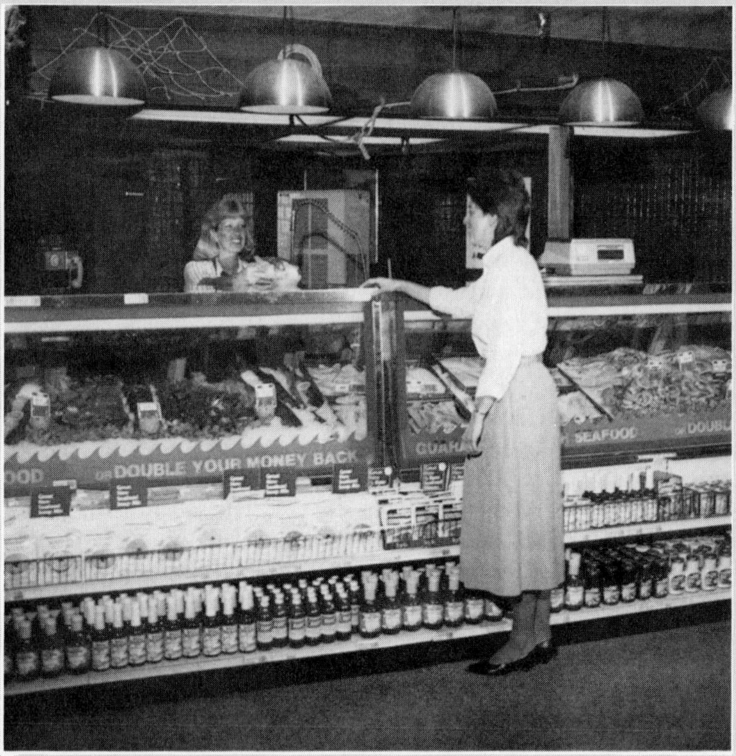

Interest in the possibility of health benefits associated with the use of fish—and in particular fatty fish—began in the early 1960s. It was the result of the observation that Eskimos living in Greenland had a remarkably low incidence of heart disease, despite the fact that their diets contained very high amounts of cholesterol, which at that time was believed to be a major dietary risk factor for coronary heart disease (CHD). Since then we have learned that although elevated plasma cholesterol is a risk factor, dietary factors other than cholesterol intake are more important determinants of CHD. We have also learned a lot about the fatty acid composition of fish oils and the physiological results of including them in the diet.

The unique feature of fish oils is its high content of EPA, a 20-carbon, highly unsaturated fatty acid that is metabolized in various cells to a wide range of physiologically potent substances, all of which belong to a class of compounds known collectively as eicosonoids. Within this broad grouping are substances identified as thromboxanes, prostaglandins (or prostacyclins), and leukotrienes. These are synthesized in blood platelets, blood vessels, and white blood cells respectively. Each of these groups of substances has a unique physiological role, with the function of one group often being completely antagonistic to that of the other. For instance thromboxanes produced in the platelets are vasoconstrictors, meaning that they cause a narrowing of the blood vessels, while the prostacyclins produced in the blood vessels are vasodilators, meaning that they cause an expansion of the size of the blood vessels. Our understanding of the role of fish oils in all these effects is further complicated by the fact that substances which are chemically very similar can be produced from arachidonic acid, another 20-carbon fatty acid that comes primarily from linoleic acid, the major fatty acid in vegetable oils. Although the effects of any one group of compounds are similar whether the compounds originated from fatty acids, from vegetable oils, or from fish oils, the size of the effect differs.

As if the relationship among these were not involved enough, it appears that the biochemical changes involved in making eicosonoids from either source require the same enzymes. Thus there is competition as to which reaction will have priority. As far as nutritionists are concerned, all this means that it is difficult to give firm dietary advice because the laboratory scientists are still trying to untangle all the relationships, which at this point seem to be getting more, rather than less, complicated.

In spite of many uncertainties regarding the benefits of fatty acids from fish versus those from vegetable sources, we are fairly confident that fish, presumably due to the nature of their oils, do have a beneficial effect in several disease states, particularly heart disease, vascular disease, cancer, and immune function. It is, however, premature to recommend the use of fish oil supplements because fish oil itself has not been tested and proven clinically effective in coronary heart disease prevention.

Heart disease. Fish oils act in combatting heart disease by (1) decreasing the tendency for blood platelets to clot, which eventually could block a major blood vessel, (2) decreasing the synthesis of the precursor of very low–density lipoproteins (VLDL), which are associated with an increased incidence of coronary heart disease, (3) decreasing the production of triglycerides especially in persons suffering from hyperlipidemia, and (4) increasing the synthesis of high-density lipoproteins (HDL), which are associated with a decreased risk of CHD.

In influencing the incidence of heart disease the ratio of linoleic acid (omega-6) to EPA (omega-3) is as important as the actual amount of omega-3 fatty acids from fish oil. As little as 1.8 grams of omega-3 fatty acids, providing less than 1% of the calories in a diet, may be effective in reducing triglycerides. Other studies, however, suggest that as much as 8 grams providing 4% of calories may be necessary for any benefits. A ratio of 5:1 of omega-6 to omega-3 is currently being recommended.

Vascular disease (hypertension). The value of fish oils in vascular disease is the result of the fatty acids stimulating the production of vasodilators rather than vasoconstrictors. This permits a free flow of blood through the vessels. Fish oils also cause a decrease in the production of the thromboxanes that cause platelets to clump together.

Inflammatory reactions and immune response. The overall effect of the EPA, which predominates in fatty fish, is to enhance the antiinflammatory response. As a result there is hope that EPA may be beneficial for people with rheumatoid arthritis and with asthmatic problems. In this connection, however, there is concern that too much EPA may lead to excessive production of eicosonoids. The natural immune response might then be suppressed, increasing the risk of infection.

Cancer. The evidence that omega-3 fatty acids may delay the progression of tumor growths suggests it would be beneficial in cancer control.

It is obvious that our current knowledge of the metabolism of the omega-3 fatty acids from fish oil suggests that (1) they may have a positive effect on health status, (2) there may be a critical balance between desirable amounts and excessive amounts that have deleterious effects, and (3) the balance between omega-6 fatty acids and omega-3 fatty acids may be critical in relation to health benefits. For instance, it is suggested that if fish is breaded and cooked in vegetable oil, high in omega-6 fatty acids, the ratio of the two groups of fatty acids is shifted so that the benefits from the fish are counteracted by the way in which it is prepared.

Although we may be unsure of the health ramifications of a shift to a greater use of fish in the diet, anyone who has monitored the price of fish in recent years will recognize that a shift to greater consumption of fish has had major economic impact on the fish industry. The industry has responded to the demand by enhancing the market value of previously relatively unpopular fish.

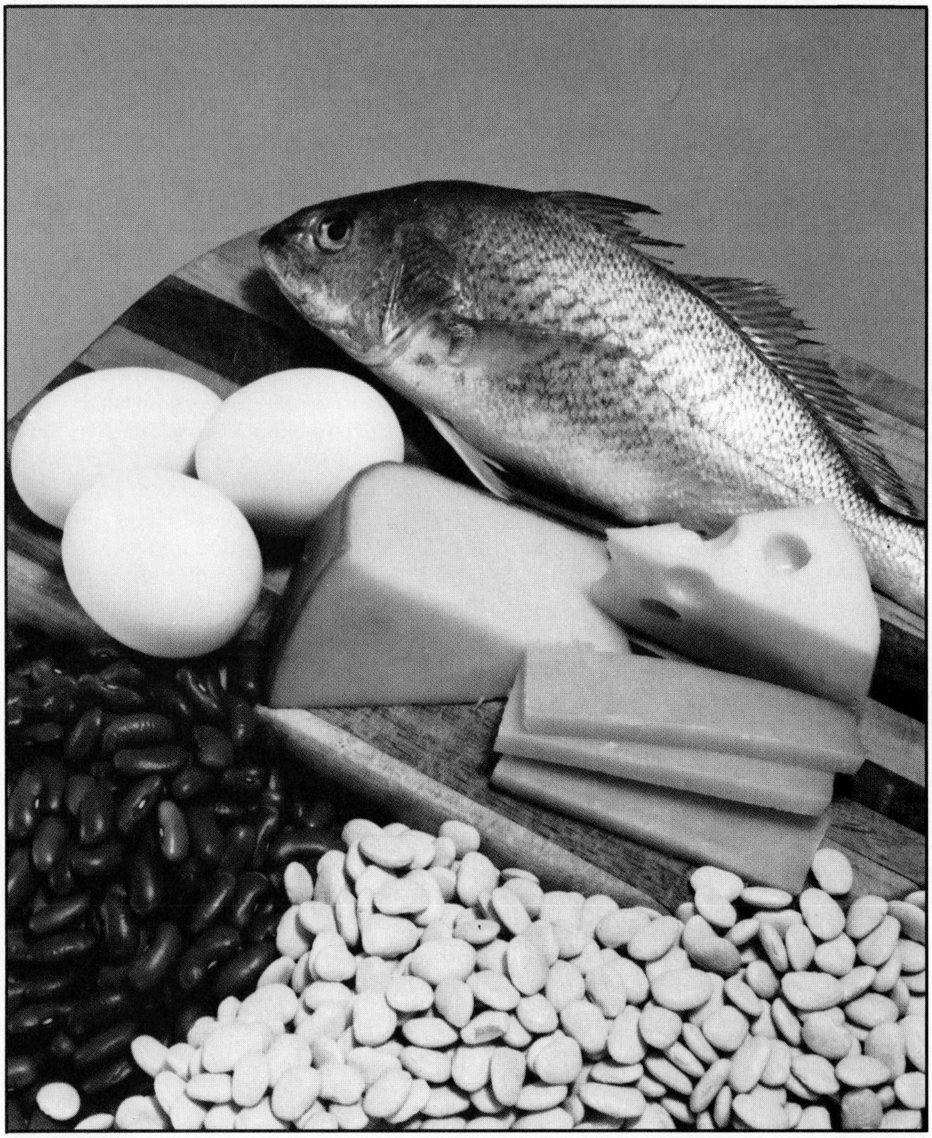

AWARENESS CHECK

Truth or Fiction?

- Protein malnutrition is a major concern in the American diet.
- Excess dietary protein is stored as muscle or lean body tissue.
- Dietary protein eaten in amounts greater than needed for growth, maintenance of cells, or energy is converted to fat.
- Protein is necessary to produce antibodies that will fight off foreign substances such as bacteria.
- Lipoproteins will be manufactured regardless of the amount of protein in the diet.
- Amino acid supplementation is recommended to ensure nutritional well-being even in healthy individuals.

Protein

CHAPTER

6

Protein has been recognized as a dietary essential for at least a century. Proteins fill many roles: as structural components of body tissues; as enzymes, hormones, and carriers for nutrients; and as regulator of fluid balance. These functions account for long-standing and continued interest in protein. Dietary protein's ultimate role—as a source of the amino acids and nitrogen needed to synthesize body tissue and essential body compounds—makes it especially important during periods of growth and recovery from disease. Excessive protein intake is discouraged, however, because any excess is an expensive source of energy—economically, ecologically, and metabolically.

In contrast to carbohydrate and lipid, which have caught the public's attention because of their perceived negative features, protein has an almost totally positive "press." To the young child it means he or she will grow; to the adolescent, it promises shiny hair and strong nails; to the pregnant woman, it helps assure a healthy baby; to the athlete, it promotes strong muscles and gives a competitive edge; to the chemist, it presents a never-ending challenge to understand its mysteries; and to the nutritionist, it is an essential nutrient with many roles.

Protein is seen as essential and beneficial; as a result, to many people any notion that it is either possible or undesirable to eat too much of it is unacceptable. Those who are concerned about the cost of animal protein may advocate using vegetable rather than animal sources, but they seldom suggest limiting the total amount.

The term protein, meaning "to take first place," was first introduced by Mulder, a Dutch chemist, in 1838. He defined protein as a nitrogen-containing constituent of food and believed it to be of such importance in the functioning of the body that, without it, life would be impossible. Today it is difficult to maintain that protein is more important than other nutrients. However, it is unlikely that Mulder had

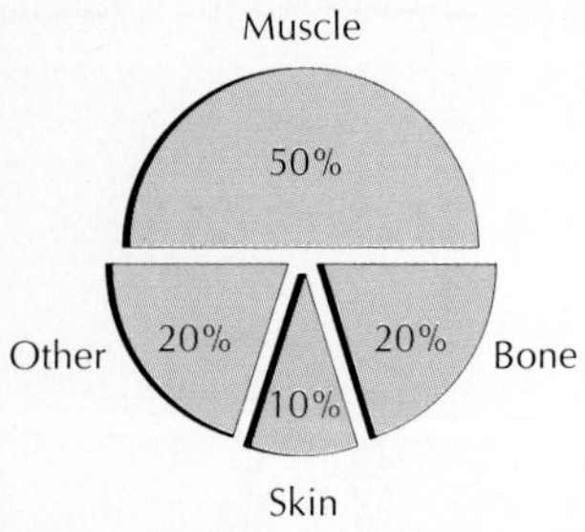

Distribution of protein in the body

any conception of the number or complexity of protein components in the body and in food.

We now know that protein is a constituent of every living cell. One fifth of an adult's total weight, that is, 20 to 35 pounds, is protein. Almost half of this protein is in muscle, a fifth is in bone and cartilage, a tenth is in skin, and the rest is in other tissues and body fluids such as blood, glands, and nervous tissue. All enzymes are proteins. Many hormones are either protein or protein derivatives. Genetic information for cell reproduction often occurs in combination with protein as *nucleoproteins*. The only body constituents that normally contain no protein are urine and bile.

Protein is needed for growth, maintenance, and repair of tissue. As part of every enzyme and many hormones, proteins are vital in the regulation of body processes. After these needs have been met, any remaining protein is used as a source of energy. Therefore protein performs all three of the functions of nutrients: it provides energy, promotes growth, and regulates body processes.

CHEMICAL COMPOSITION

amino acids
The units from which protein is synthesized and into which it is broken down during digestion

Protein is synthesized from basic units called **amino acids,** which are made up of carbon, hydrogen, oxygen, and nitrogen. It is nitrogen that is characteristic of protein and distinguishes it from lipid and carbohydrate. Protein is converted into

Table 6-1 ◇ Amino acids in food and body tissue

Classification	Amino Acid
Naturally occurring amino acids	
Essential for all humans	Isoleucine
	Leucine
	Lysine
	Methionine
	Phenylalanine
	Threonine
	Tryptophan
	Valine
	Histidine
Nonessential	Glycine*
	Glutamic acid
	Arginine†
	Aspartic acid
	Proline
	Alanine
	Serine
	Tyrosine
	Cysteine
	Asparagine
	Glutamine
Related compounds sometimes classified as amino acids	Hydroxyglutamic acid
	Hydroxylysine
	Hydroxyproline
	Thyroxine
	Norleucine
	Cystine
	Taurine
	Carnitine

*Essential for chicks.
†Essential for birds and rats.

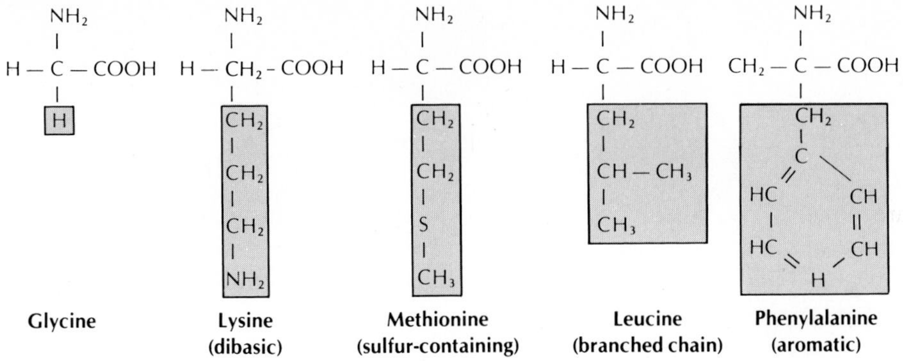

Figure 6-1 Representative formulas for classes of amino acids. *Boxed portion* is unique to the specific amino acid and is often designated by the letter *R* in general formulas of amino acids.

amino acids as end products of digestion or during catabolism, the breakdown of body tissue. Protein molecules, which contain up to hundreds of amino acids, are much larger than either carbohydrate or lipid molecules. Some have molecular weights as high as 40 million, compared to glucose's molecular weight of 180. The twenty different naturally occurring amino acids that have been identified as the building blocks for body protein are listed in Table 6-1.

Chemically, amino acids are composed of a carbon atom to which is attached a carboxyl group (COOH), a hydrogen atom (H), an amino group (NH_2), and an amino acid radical (R), as shown below:

Carboxyl group = A chemical unit (COOH) in an amino acid

Amino group = A chemical unit (NH_2) in an amino acid

R group = A chemical entity unique for each amino acid

H (hydrogen)
|
(**Amino group**) H_2N—C—COOH (carboxyl group)
|
R (amino acid radical)

The carboxyl group, the amino group, and the hydrogen atom are the same for all amino acids. The R group, however, distinguishes one amino acid from another. R varies from a single hydrogen atom (H) as is found in glycine, the simplest amino acid, to longer carbon chains of up to seven carbon atoms. Those amino acids in which the carbon atoms are arranged in a hexagon rather than a straight line are called **aromatic amino acids:** tyrosine, tryptophan, and phenylalanine are examples. Other amino acids, such as cysteine and methionine, also contain small amounts of sulfur as part of the R portion. Lysine, arginine, and histidine, which contain a second nitrogen atom, are called **dibasic amino acids.** Examples of the classes of amino acids are shown in Figure 6-1. Because nitrogen almost always comprises 16% of protein, most studies of protein metabolism can be based on nitrogen determinations.

aromatic amino acids
Amino acids in which the carbon atoms are arranged in a ring; include tryptophan, phenylalanine, and tyrosine

dibasic amino acids
Amino acids that contain a second nitrogen atom; include lysine, arginine, and histidine

SYNTHESIS

Proteins can be synthesized by both plant and animal cells if the plant has available nitrogen or the animal has amino acids. Without being able to synthesize proteins, neither plants nor animals can survive and grow. Plants obtain essential nitrogen through the soil. The nitrogen is provided either by chemical fertilizers or is released from nitrogen-containing organic fertilizers by the action of bacteria. Plants use both forms of nitrogen equally well. In addition, some plants such as legumes have small nodules of bacteria on their roots that are capable of **fixing,** or **trapping,** atmospheric nitrogen. Some nitrogen from the atmosphere is made available through the action of lightning, which also fixes nitrogen. Animals obtain most of their nitrogen in the form of amino acids from either plant or other animal sources; they are also able to synthesize a few amino acids in their gastrointestinal tract, using

fixing, or **trapping**
In chemistry, the conversion of a gas into solid or liquid form by chemical reactions, either with or without the help of living tissue

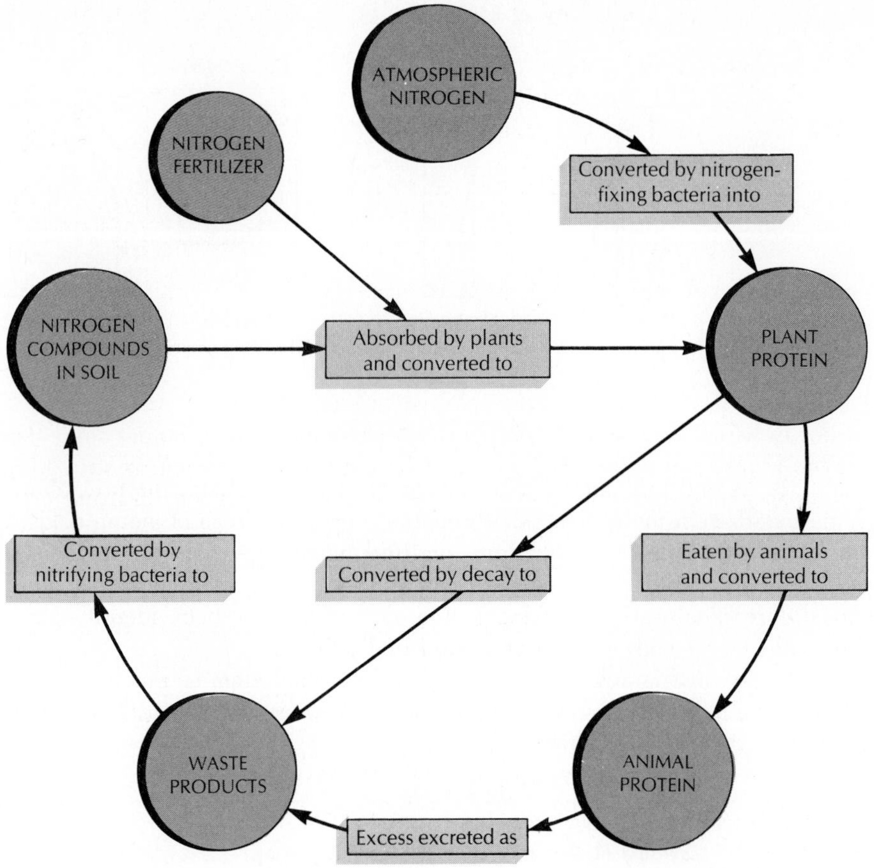

Figure 6-2 Nitrogen is cycled from the atmosphere or soil, then to the plant, then to the animal, and back to the plant. Most nitrogen is used for protein synthesis; some is used for nucleic acids.

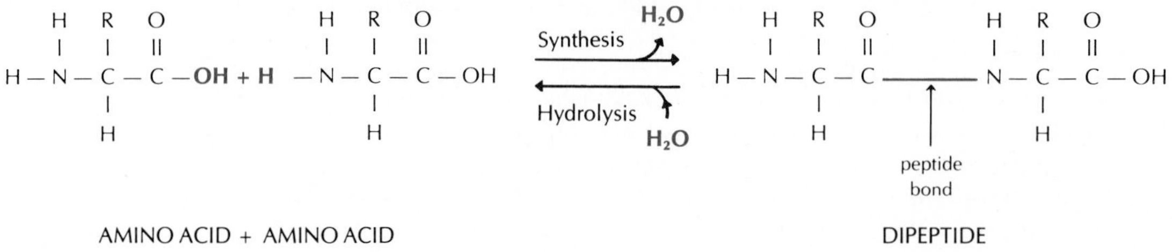

Figure 6-3 Synthesis and hydrolysis of a dipeptide—reversible reactions involving either the addition or loss of water.

peptide bond
A chemical link that joins two amino acids together, such as in CO—NH (CO comes from one amino acid and NH from another; in this example, water is split off)

dietary nitrogen. The cycling of nitrogen from plant to animal to plant sources is depicted in Figure 6-2.

In both plants and animals, protein synthesis involves the formation of long chains of amino acids called *peptide chains*. These chains are so named because the chemical bond that holds two amino acids together is called a **peptide bond.** In forming the chain, a hydrogen from the amino group of one amino acid joins with the OH from a carboxyl group of the adjoining amino acid. In this process one molecule of water is formed and the remaining CO and NH are joined through a peptide bond (CO—NH). When the peptide linkage is broken, water must be added before the amino acids can be split apart either by acid or by digestive enzymes. This is illustrated in Figure 6-3.

The characteristics of a particular protein are determined by the types of amino acids that are used, the number of times they are repeated, and the order in which they are joined together. Because each amino acid may be used any number of times in relation to other amino acids, the number of different proteins that can be formed becomes enormous. This number can be compared to the number of combinations of 50 or more letters that could be made from an alphabet of 20 letters,

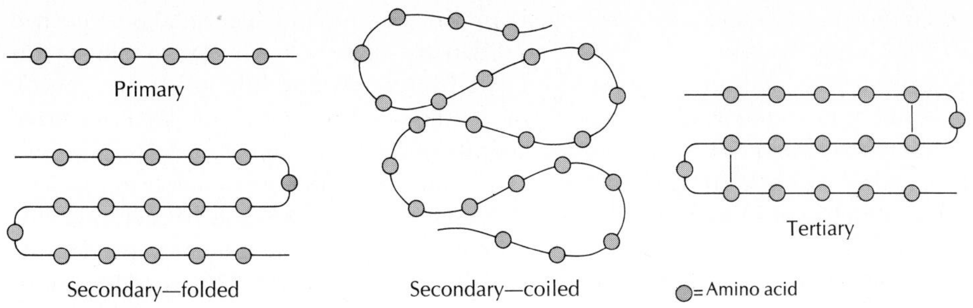

Primary, secondary, and tertiary structures of protein molecules

with practically no limitations on the number of times each letter could be used or the order in which letters could be joined. This sequencing of amino acids determines the *primary* structure of the protein. In addition, the *secondary* structure, or shape, of the amino acid chain influences the properties of the resulting protein and the possibilities of the number of proteins. This secondary structure may be either coiled, folded, or straight. Additional links between the R groups of the amino acids determine the *tertiary* structure, the three-dimensional shape which determines the function of the protein.

The shape of a protein molecule and therefore its function can be changed by heat, light, acid, or ultraviolet light. The changed protein is called a **denatured** protein and has different physical and physiological properties from the original protein. Perhaps the most obvious example of this type of change is seen in an egg, which changes from runny transparent fluid when raw to an opaque solid as it coagulates when heated. Denatured body proteins are unable to carry out their normal biological functions.

denatured
Changed; a denatured protein is one in which the shape of the protein has been changed

Although it is unlikely that there are actually anywhere near the number of proteins theoretically possible, a great many do exist. The human body contains at least 30,000 different proteins, some containing as many as 300 amino acids. Only 2% of these proteins have been identified. It is estimated that a liver cell alone contains 1000 different enzymes, each a protein. In addition, every animal builds many unique proteins. For example, hemoglobin, a protein in the blood of a horse, resembles hemoglobin in a duck or a dog or a human, but they all differ sufficiently so that they cannot be interchanged with one another. In fact, the protein of one species is frequently toxic to another. Because of these differences, blood transfusion from one species to another is impossible. However, an advantage in protein differences is that the type of hemoglobin can be the basis for identifying the source of a blood sample, an invaluable tool in criminal investigations.

Another example of the importance of the exact structure of a protein is seen in **sickle cell anemia.** In this condition, hemoglobin is incapable of carrying oxygen because one glutamic acid unit in the chain of 300 amino acids is replaced with one valine unit. As simple an exchange as this changes the shape—and therefore the function—of the hemoglobin molecule.

sickle cell anemia
A genetically transmitted disease in which one amino acid in a long chain of 300 is displaced

In 1961 **myoglobin,** a protein found in muscle, was the first protein to have its complete composition and structure identified. Although myoglobin consists of 150 amino acid units, representing 19 different amino acids, it is considered a relatively simple protein. The amino acid composition and sequence of many other proteins have now been determined.

myoglobin
An iron-containing protein that is found in muscle

Once the composition of a protein was known, it was not surprising that 8 years later two groups of scientists were able to announce the synthesis of an enzyme, **ribonuclease.** Since then, the synthesis of other enzymes has opened up many new approaches to clinical medicine and has allowed nutritionists to study the way in which nutrients are absorbed and transported.

ribonuclease
An enzyme that splits ribonucleic acid; one of the first proteins for which the amino acid composition was known

One of the goals for biologists, nutritionists, and biochemists studying protein was to determine how the cells "know" which protein to build and the kind, order, and number of amino acids to use when building new protein. This goal was reached in 1962 when Watson and Crick showed that the pattern for protein synthesis was present, or encoded, in the substance **DNA (deoxyribonucleic acid),** the genetic material in the nucleus of the cell. It was learned that the directions are transferred to the **ribosomes,** or protein-synthesizing **organelles** in the cytoplasm of the cell, by another **nucleic acid** called RNA (ribonucleic acid), specifically messenger RNA, which is a mirror image of DNA. Using this message, the ribosome is able to pick up, in the proper order, the required amino acids, which are carried to the ribosome by yet another form of RNA, called transfer RNA. This process builds the amino acids into a protein molecule in a prescribed order, dictated indirectly from DNA through messenger RNA. The sequence of the amino acids in the protein determines how the chain folds and coils.

DNA (deoxyribonucleic acid)
The genetic material in the nucleus of the cell

ribosomes
Protein-synthesizing organelles in cytoplasm of cell

organelle
Distinctive structures within a cell that carry out a specific function

nucleic acids
The chemicals within the nucleus of the cell that provide the code for the synthesis of thousands of body proteins

For more details on cell structure and function, see Appendix A

The codes for specific amino acids contained in DNA have been identified. Thus we know that the code is sent to the ribosome by messenger RNA, which directs it to incorporate a particular amino acid such as glutamic acid. The amino acid will be brought to the ribosome by transfer RNA. After glutamic acid has been attached to the growing amino acid chain, the ribosome will read the next code, perhaps telling it to add one molecule of the amino acid threonine to the chain. This process continues until all the amino acids of a particular protein have been joined together in a prescribed order. This process of protein synthesis is depicted in Figure 6-4.

If the amino acid needed is not available or cannot be synthesized immediately and brought to the cell, the synthesis of the protein ceases. In addition, that part of the protein already formed will be broken down into its component amino acids because it cannot be stored, only synthesized, until the missing amino acid is available. As we will see later, this is the reason that it is so important to have a diet that provides all of the amino acids at the same time.

cytoplasm
Substance enclosed within cell membrane exclusive of the organelles

nucleus
A body within the cell that contains relatively large quantities of DNA

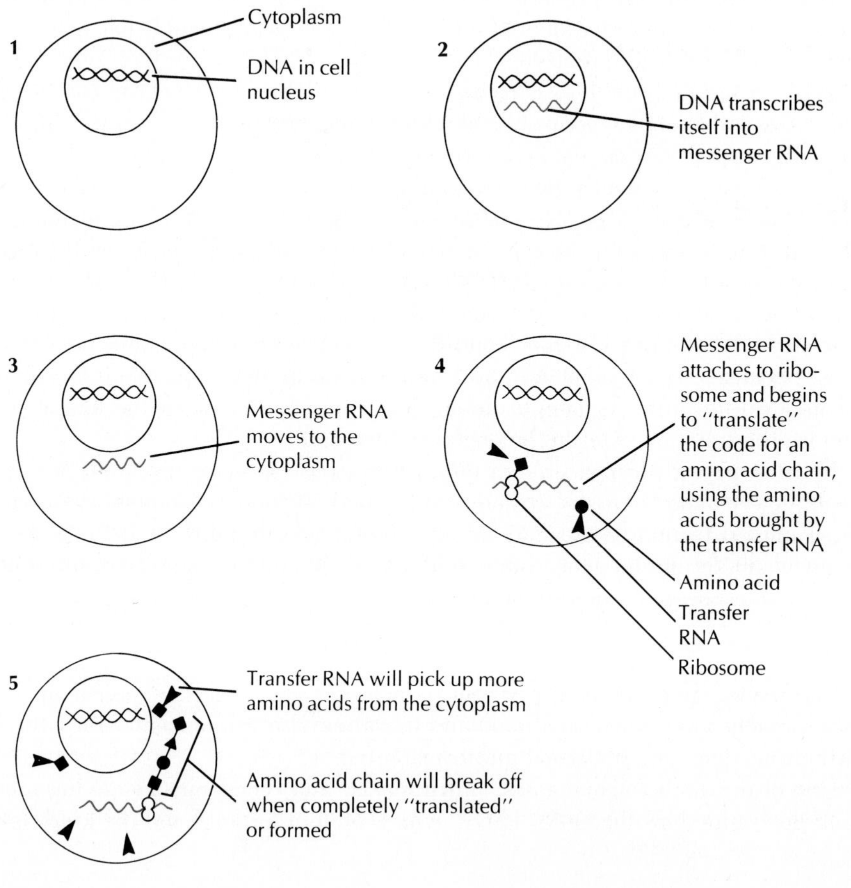

Figure 6-4 The process of protein synthesis on the ribosomes in the cytoplasm of the cell. Messenger RNA tells the ribosome the order in which amino acids must be joined. Transfer RNA brings the correct amino acid to the ribosome to be added to the growing amino acid chain.

With the level of understanding we now have about protein synthesis, geneticists have the capability of changing the code in DNA and therefore the resultant protein. This offers great promise in the control of genetic diseases that result from the production of a defective protein, usually an essential enzyme. In addition, it opens the possibility of producing a protein or a living organism (such as a virus) with specific or perhaps unknown characteristics. The awesome implications of this have led to heated debates about the ethics of what is known as **recombinant DNA** research. This involves the production of new genetic material to direct the synthesis of a protein we want. In addition, there is the possibility that we might produce a protein we don't want. Most gene splicing is done in bacteria.

recombinant DNA
Genetic material that has been produced or changed in the laboratory by splicing together various parts of the DNA molecule

CLASSIFICATION OF AMINO ACIDS

From a physiological standpoint, amino acids are classified into two groups: **essential** (indispensable) and **nonessential** (dispensable). An essential amino acid is one that cannot be synthesized by the body at a rate sufficient to meet the needs for growth and maintenance. In the classifications in Table 6-1, we see that 9 of the 20 amino acids are essential and as such must be provided by the diet. Only recently have we learned that adults are incapable of producing enough histidine to meet their needs over a long period of time and must rely on getting it from food. If sufficient nitrogen is available in the form of amino acids, we can synthesize the other 11 amino acids, the nonessentials, needed to build body proteins. **Indispensable nitrogen** is the nitrogen needed by the body to synthesize any nitrogen-containing substances, including amino acids, not provided in the diet. The nitrogen used in the synthesis of nonessential amino acids may come as an amino group (NH_2) from other nonessential amino acids or from an excess of essential amino acids. Like many animals, we can make use of a limited portion of nitrogen provided by a nonprotein nitrogen such as urea.

Before amino acids from food can serve as a source of nitrogen for the synthesis of nonessential amino acids, they must undergo a process called **transamination.** In this process, the amino group is transferred to another substance, often a carbohydrate, to form the needed amino acid. Because the body must obtain this nitrogen from food, extra nitrogen over and above that in essential amino acids becomes a dietary essential. Transamination requires vitamin B_6.

essential amino acids
Amino acids that cannot be manufactured within the body and must be provided in the diet

nonessential amino acid
An amino acid that can be synthesized by body cells as long as enough nitrogen is available

indispensable nitrogen
The nitrogen needed by the body to synthesize amino acids not provided in the diet

transamination
The transfer of the NH_2 group of amino acid to another substance, usually to make a different amino acid

PROTEIN QUALITY

The quality of a protein is determined by the kind and proportion of amino acids it contains. Proteins that contain all essential amino acids in proportions capable of promoting growth when they are the sole source of protein in the diet are described as complete proteins, good-quality proteins, or proteins of high biological value. Most complete proteins are made up of one third essential and two thirds nonessential amino acids. All animal proteins except gelatin, which has limited amounts of both tryptophan and lysine, are complete proteins.

The pattern of amino acids in animal proteins is best able to meet human needs because it closely resembles the pattern of human amino acid requirement. Therefore, if animal foods are used as the sole source of protein, they usually provide enough of all the essential amino acids. Extra amounts of essential amino acids can be used to synthesize nonessential amino acids. The amino acid profile of a high-quality protein (protein A) compared to the adult requirement is illustrated in Figure 6-5.

Incomplete proteins, also known as poor-quality proteins or proteins of low biological value, are those that lack or have limited amounts of one or more essential amino acids. Even in these proteins, however, about one fourth of the amino acids are essential. In contrast to complete proteins, if these low-quality proteins (such as *protein B* in Figure 6-5) were used as the sole source of protein in the diet, they could not support growth.

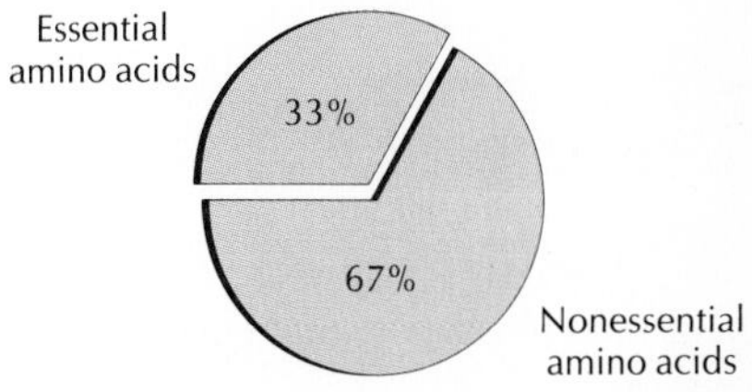

Proportion of essential amino acids and nonessential amino acids in good-quality protein

Classification of Proteins
Complete proteins contain all the essential amino acids
Incomplete proteins are lacking in one or more essential amino acids
Partially complete proteins have a limited amount of one or more essential amino acids

Animal Protein Sources	**Vegetable Protein Sources**
Milk	Legumes—Beans
Eggs	—Peas
Cheese	Cereals—Rice
Meat	—Wheat
Fish	—Oats
Poultry	

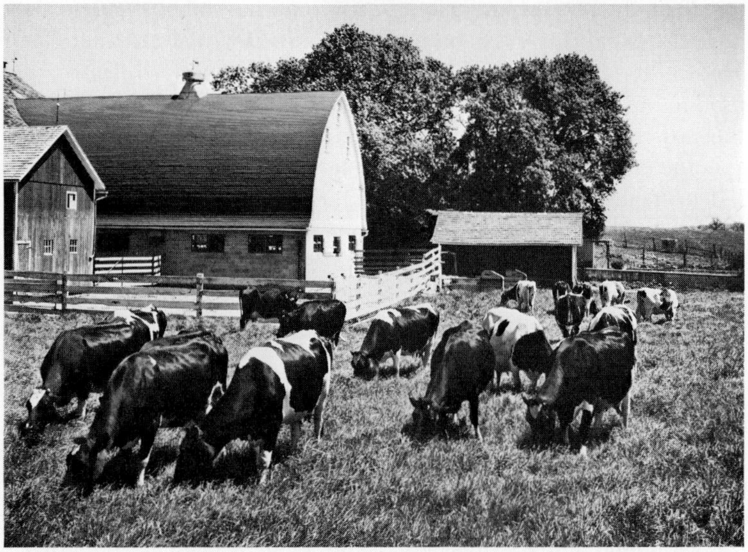

Animal proteins, such as beef from cattle, are complete proteins because they contain all the essential amino acids; in contrast, vegetable proteins, such as wheat proteins, are considered incomplete because they lack one or more essential amino acids

limiting amino acid
The amino acid in a protein that is present in the lowest amount relative to the amount needed for growth

Some proteins that contain all the essential amino acids but a relatively small amount of one of them have sufficient amino acids to repair body tissue but not enough to promote growth. The amino acid present in the smallest amount relative to the amount required for growth is called the **limiting amino acid.** Methionine is the limiting amino acid in legumes, as is lysine in cereal protein. Vegetable proteins such as soybeans and nuts contain some of all the essential amino acids, but they do not have enough of one or more of them to make them effective in meeting the needs for growth.

An understanding of the concept of limiting amino acids helps us to understand why it is important to have a combination of several different vegetable proteins rather than just one in a meal.

By combining two proteins that are limited in different amino acids, it is possible to simulate a complete protein. In this way, vegetarians can have a diet as adequate in protein as that of people who eat both animal and vegetable proteins. For example, when wheat, which has ample methionine but lacks lysine, is combined with soybeans, which have ample lysine but are limited in methionine, we have a mixture that is quite capable of promoting growth. Moreover, adding a small amount of milk—which has all the essential amino acids—to a wheat cereal provides enough of the missing lysine to greatly enhance the ability of the wheat protein to promote growth. We practice this type of supplementation constantly when we serve macaroni and cheese, put milk on cereal, spread peanut butter on bread, or prepare an egg sandwich. The use of very small amounts of animal protein with cereal protein is much more meaningful in areas of the world where people consume a diet based on a dietary staple such as rice or corn. In this case, even small amounts of fish or meat used as a flavor enhancer increase protein quality. Figure 6-6 illustrates how the amino acid pattern of the one protein complements that of another and how the combination more closely meets the adult requirements for all amino acids. Mixtures of two vegetable proteins or small amounts of animal proteins with vegetable proteins can provide high-quality protein less expensively than animal protein can by itself.

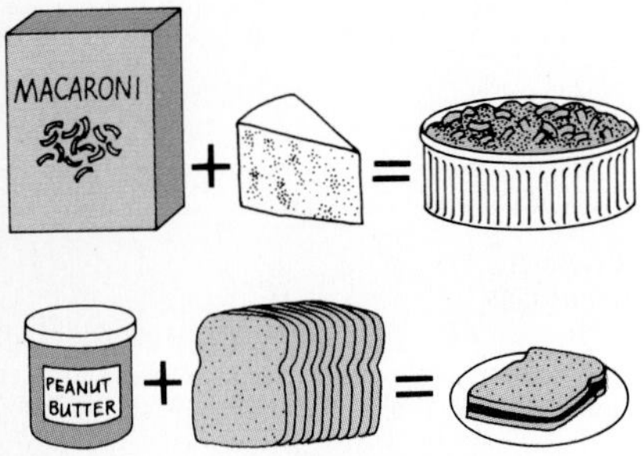

Examples of complementary protein sources

The growth curves in Figure 6-7, which show the almost immediate growth response of rats when they are fed proteins of different quality, provide convincing evidence of the importance of amino acid balance to growth.

When choosing a balanced diet, people need only to be concerned with providing a source of protein and seldom need to think of the amino acids that are

Figure 6-5 Comparison of the amino acid pattern of a good-quality *protein A* and poor-quality *protein B* with patten of amino acid requirement of adult male. Methionine is limiting amino acid in *protein B*.
Courtesy Dr. Barbara Shannon, Pennsylvania State University.

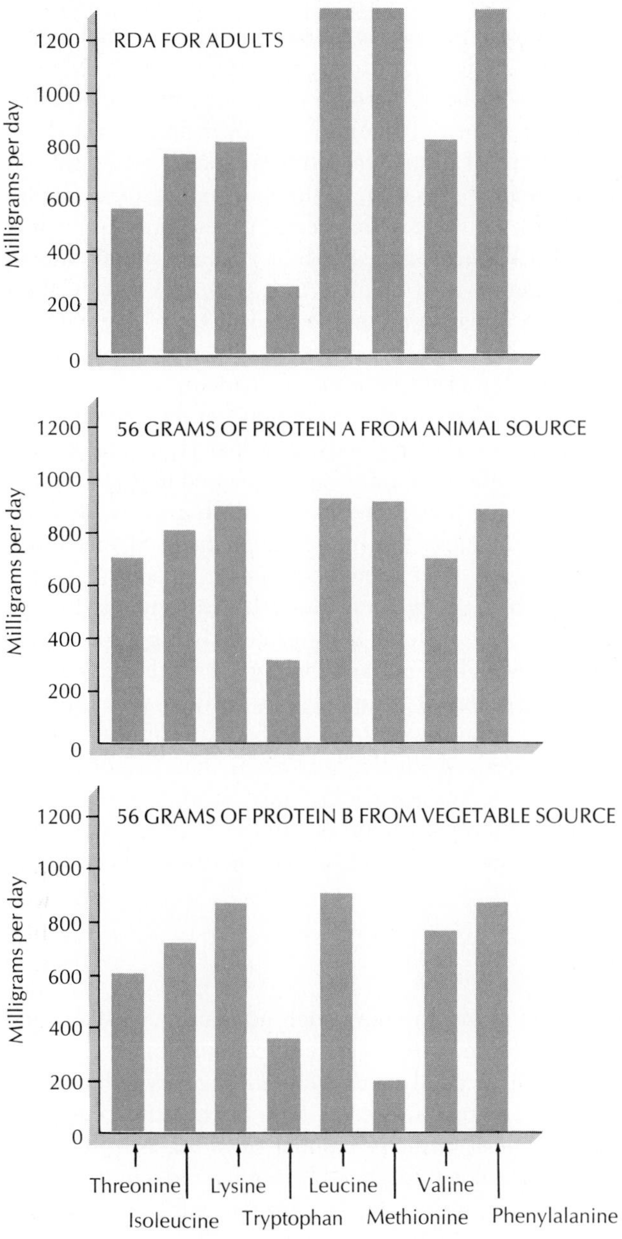

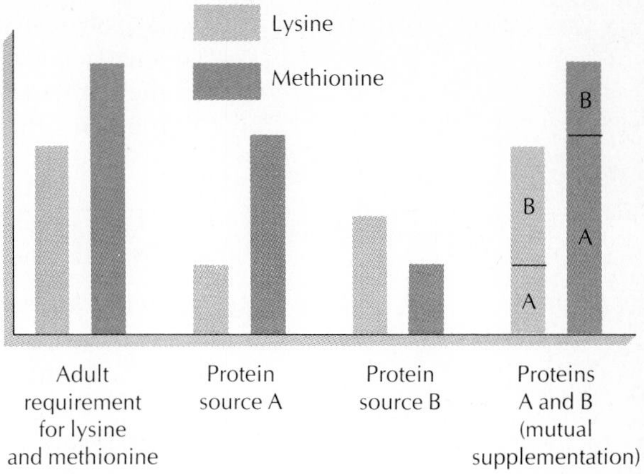

Figure 6-6 Mutual supplementation of low-quality *protein A* (such as wheat) lacking in lysine and low-quality *protein B* (such as beans) lacking in methionine. They complement each other to provide a good-quality protein.
Courtesy Dr. Barbara Shannon, Pennsylvania State University.

Figure 6-7 Growth pattern of weanling rats fed an incomplete protein (gelatin) as 18% of diet, a partially complete protein (casein) as 4% of diet, and a complete protein (casein) as 18% of diet; also, the effect of reversing the last diet.

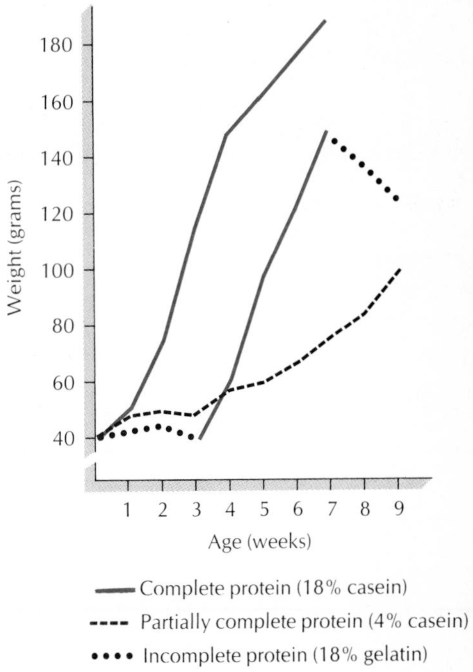

provided, even though it's been established that the amino acids are the essential nutrients and not the protein. It is, however, ultimately the amount and balance of the amino acids that determine how effectively the body can perform the various functions that the amino acids, as part of protein, make possible.

FUNCTIONS

Growth and Maintenance of Tissue

Before cells can synthesize any new protein, they must have all the essential amino acids available simultaneously plus sufficient nitrogen or amino groups (NH_2) to form the nonessential amino acids. Growth or increase in muscle mass is possible only when there is an appropriate mixture of amino acids over and above those needed for the maintenance and repair of tissue. In addition, some tissues call for larger amounts of specific amino acids. The hair, skin, and nails, for example, require larger amounts of the sulfur-containing amino acids. (These are responsible for the characteristic pungent odor of burnt skin and hair.) Some animals are so sensitive to the importance of an amino acid balance that they will reduce their food intake or even refuse to eat an unbalanced amino acid mixture. Humans do not have the same kind of instinct, but a person eating a diet with poor protein quality soon experiences symptoms related to the nutrient inadequacy.

Cell division and growth are dependent on the availability of protein as is the synthesis of much of the structural material of the body. The matrix, or framework, for bones and teeth, in which calcium and phosphorus are deposited to give strength and rigidity to these tissues, is a protein. This same protein, **collagen,** is the main protein in tendons and ligaments and is also the intercellular material that binds the cells together. Actin and myosin are other proteins found in muscles.

collagen
The protein that forms the structural material of tissues

The protein of the body is in a constant dynamic state. It is alternately broken down and resynthesized, with about 3% of total body protein being turned over each day. The wall of the intestine, which is replaced every 4 to 6 days, requires the synthesis of 70 grams of protein a day. Fortunately the body is very efficient in conserving protein and reuses the amino acids from the breakdown of tissues to build more of the same or other tissues. About the only times that loss of protein occurs are when cells are lost from the surface of the body or when some of the intestinal cells that are constantly being replaced are lost in the feces without being digested and reabsorbed from the intestine. Failure to replace any of these losses will be reflected in loss of body weight.

Formation of Essential Body Compounds

Since the body produces all the digestive enzymes required, it is unnecessary and even useless to buy them in pills because these ingested enzymes are digested before they can act.

Hormones produced by various glands in the body, such as insulin, gastrin, and growth hormone, are proteins. In addition, every body cell contains many different enzymes, all of which are protein. These catalyze or facilitate digestive changes in food and the many biochemical changes that are essential to the health of cells and tissues. RNA and DNA account for most of the remainder of nitrogen in the cell.

Hemoglobin, the pigment in the blood responsible for its red color and its capacity to carry both oxygen and carbon dioxide, is a protein substance. So are almost all of the many substances involved in blood clotting. The photoreceptors in the eye that are responsible for vision are among the many other vital body compounds that are proteins. The catecholamine, adrenaline or epinephrine, is produced from tyrosine. The amino acid tryptophan serves as a precursor for the vitamin niacin and for serotonin, a neurotransmitter responsible for carrying messages from one nerve cell to another.

During a protein deficiency, the synthesis of these vital body compounds seems to have priority over less important uses for protein, such as hair and nail formation.

Regulation of Water Balance

Fluid in the body is contained in two different compartments: the *intracellular* (within the cell) and the *extracellular* made up of *intercellular* (between cells) and *intravascular* (within blood vessels). These compartments are separated from one another by cell membranes. The distribution of fluid among them must be kept in balance. This balance is achieved through a complex system of controls involving both protein and electrolytes, primarily sodium and potassium. Protein in the blood that is too large to pass out of the bloodstream exerts an **oncotic pressure,** which draws fluid from the intercellular compartment back into the blood. When blood proteins are low, the oncotic pressure of the protein pulling fluid back into the circulation is not as strong as the **hydrostatic pressures** pushing it out of the bloodstream. This results in an accumulation of fluid in the tissues that makes them soft and spongy and gives a somewhat bloated appearance. This condition, known as **edema,** has several other causes but is recognized as an early sign of a protein deficiency. The balance between the forces pushing the fluid out of the blood and pulling it back in is depicted in Figure 6-8.

hydrostatic pressure
Pressure on fluid in blood vessels (arteries and capillaries) from pumping action of heart

oncotic pressure
Pressure drawing intercellular fluid back into blood vessels; usually due to higher concentration of protein in blood

edema
Condition caused by protein deficiency in which fluid collects in body tissues

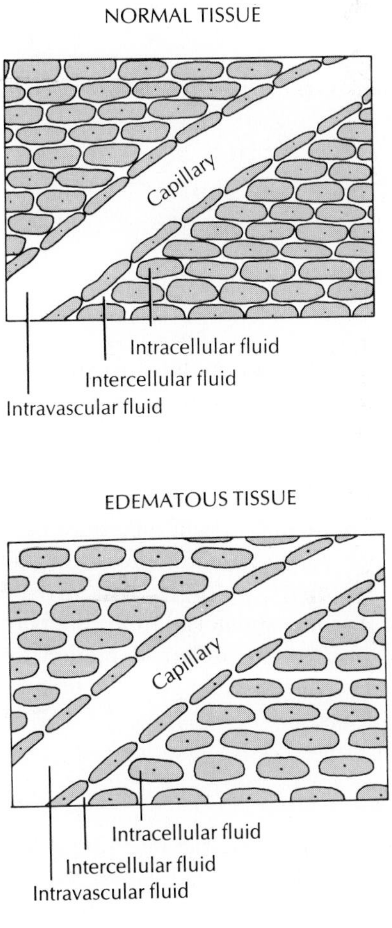

Distribution of intracellular, intercellular, and intravascular fluid in normal and edematous tissue

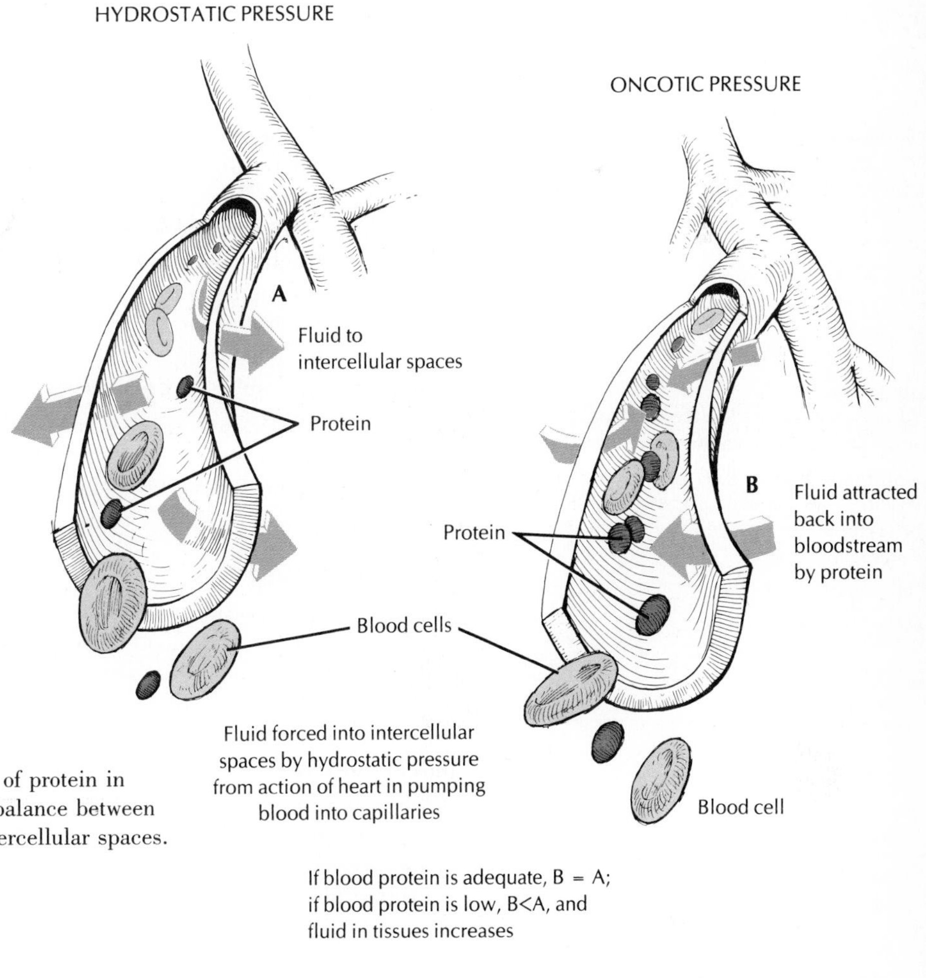

Figure 6-8 Role of protein in maintaining fluid balance between capillaries and intercellular spaces.

Maintenance of Body Neutrality

buffers
Substances in the body that are capable of reacting with either acid or base to neutralize them

pH (hydrogen ion concentration)
A measure of the relative acidity or alkalinity of a solution

1 — 14
Acid — pH — Alkaline

Proteins in the blood serve as **buffers**—substances capable of reacting with either acid or base to neutralize them. This is an extremely important function because most body tissues cannot function when the **hydrogen ion concentration** (high = alkaline; low = acid), or **pH,** of the blood and intercellular fluids deviates by even a very small amount. By reacting with any excess acid or base (alkali), proteins in the blood represent one of several ways in which the body ensures that there is no change in the pH of the blood.

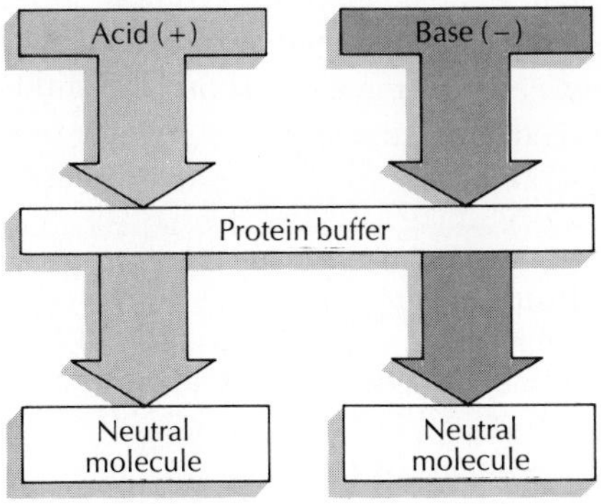

Buffering effect of protein

Antibody Formation

antibodies
Proteins produced by the body to fight off foreign substances such as bacteria

The body's ability to fight infection depends on its ability to produce **antibodies,** proteins that react with particular infective organisms or foreign substances that may enter the body. Because the body must produce an antibody specific to each organism or foreign substance, the need for protein for this purpose may be extensive. In fact, the lowered resistance to infection that accounts for the high infant mortality rate among malnourished children, who are unable to fight infections such as measles, is attributed to their failure to produce adequate antibodies—in turn due to a protein deficiency.

detoxify
To remove or destroy the toxic properties of a substance; usually occurs in the liver

Similarly, the ability to **detoxify,** or remove poisonous material from, the body is controlled by enzymes located primarily in the liver. In protein depletion the ability to counteract the toxic effect of chemicals is reduced. This makes a protein-deficient person more susceptible to poisons or drugs.

Transport of Nutrients

Protein plays an essential role in the transport of nutrients from the intestine across the intestinal wall to the blood, from the blood to the tissues, and across the cell membrane into the cell. Most substances necessary to transport specific nutrients are proteins. These protein carriers are usually specific to one nutrient such as retinol-binding protein, which carries only vitamin A; sometimes they carry several different nutrients, which compete with each other to be carried; or they may carry a whole group of substances, which is what lipoproteins do. If there is a lack of protein, less carrier will be synthesized, and either the absorption or transportation of some nutrients will be reduced.

Protein in excess of needs for other functions is used as a source of energy or stored as fat.

DIGESTION

All dietary proteins that consist of complex units of amino acids joined together are too large to pass through the intestinal wall. They must be broken down in the digestive tract to simple units of one, two, or three amino acids to be absorbed. Digestion is accomplished by the action of specific protein-splitting enzymes known as **proteases,** which are available in the stomach, small intestine, and intestinal wall. Digestion involves breaking the peptide linkages joining the amino acids.

The digestibility of protein ranges from 78% for vegetables to 97% for meats and eggs. In some foods, amino acids are bound in a way that resists being broken by gastrointestinal enzymes. Undigested protein is excreted in the feces.

There is no chemical or enzymatic digestion of protein in the mouth. The chewing that reduces food particle size and the lubrication of the food that occurs as food is mixed with saliva prepare the food for digestion after it reaches the stomach.

In the stomach, the release of hydrochloric acid (HCl) decreases the pH of the food mass, so that the several **pepsinogens** (inactive protein-splitting enzymes) can be converted to the active form **pepsin.** Pepsin acts on the protein in the wall of the cells in food to hydrolyze, or break apart, some of the peptide bonds to form smaller units or single amino acids. This allows the hydrochloric acid to enter the cell to denature the protein so that it can be acted on by the protein-splitting (or **proteolytic**) enzymes in the intestine.

The food mass then enters the small intestine, where the bicarbonate from the pancreatic juice neutralizes acidity in the food mass to allow intestinal enzymes to digest the denatured protein. The juices secreted from the pancreas contain many inactive proteolytic enzymes that become activated and attack very specific peptide bonds, either in specific locations on the peptide chain or those involving specific amino acids. Examples are elastase, collagenase, trypsin, and carboxypeptidase. The final digestion of protein to individual amino acids or to dipeptides and tripeptides is accomplished by enzymes available from the mucosal cells lining the small intestine, which act either within the mucosal membrane or within the mucosal cells. Final release of individual amino acids from the peptides occurs within the mucosal cell.

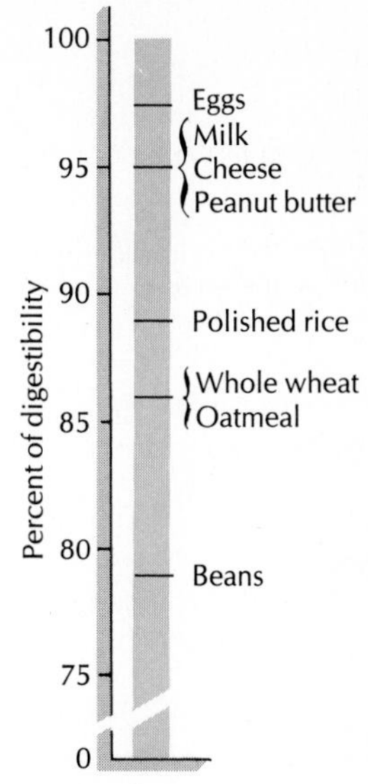

Digestibility of protein

pepsinogens
Inactive form of protein-splitting enzymes in the stomach

pepsin
Proteolytic enzyme formed when pepsin is activated; also known as gastric protease

proteolytic enzymes
Protein-splitting enzymes of the small intestine

Examples of Proteolytic Enzymes
Elastase
Collagenase
Trypsin
Carboxypeptidase

ABSORPTION

The amino acids, **dipeptides,** and **tripeptides** (and possibly chains of five amino acids) formed in the process of digestion are in a simple enough form chemically to pass from the wall of the intestinal tract directly into the bloodstream. Absorption of amino acids is dependent on the carrier capable of transporting one of five particular classes of amino acids. Surprisingly, peptides are absorbed more rapidly than amino acids. Once the amino acids reach the liver, through the portal vein, some are synthesized into plasma proteins. The remainder are released into the general circulation to be transported to the individual cells of the body to make the unique proteins that the cells need.

dipeptide
Two amino acids linked together

tripeptide
Three amino acids linked together

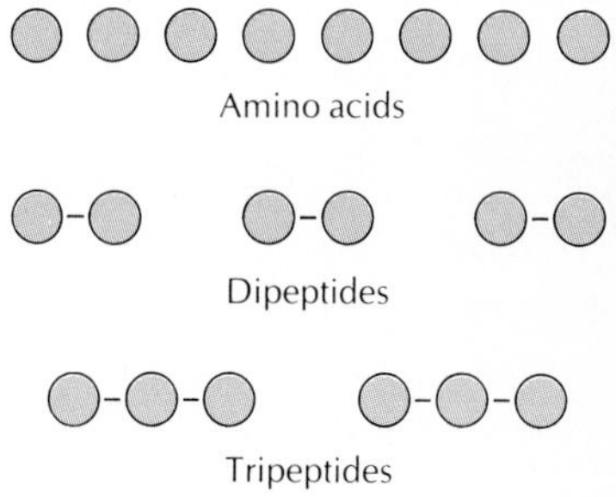

METABOLISM

Early ideas about protein metabolism maintained that body proteins were relatively static, changing slowly, if at all. However, when radioactive isotopes became available, we soon learned that body proteins are in a dynamic state; that is, there is a constant interchange of nitrogen from one tissue to another and between newly absorbed amino acids and body proteins. Tissue proteins are continually being broken down and resynthesized, contributing to and taking away from the pool of amino acids to which dietary proteins also contribute. Although there is no major storage site for extra protein, the liver will increase in size when protein is available. Some tissue proteins such as plasma albumin make up small **labile,** or easily

labile
Easily mobilized

globulin
A protein found in the blood

mobilized protein reserves. In a deficiency of either quantity or quality of dietary protein, "storage" protein is broken down to provide amino acids for more vital uses in the body. In the blood, levels of **globulin,** one major protein, are maintained even when levels of albumin, the other main protein, are being depleted.

In adults there is very little change in the total amount of protein in the body, but the rate of turnover varies from tissue to tissue. Some proteins such as those in the gut (or intestinal tract), pancreas, and liver turn over very rapidly, whereas muscle and collagen turn over their amino acids more slowly. The rate of synthesis of protein in the adult male is estimated at 0.3 gram/kg of body weight per day, or about two thirds of an ounce.

deamination
The removal of the amino group (NH_2) from an amino acid

urea
A nontoxic compound made from two molecules of toxic ammonia; produced when amino acids are deaminated

glucogenic
Capable of producing glucose

When the energy intake is adequate, the amino acids derived from dietary protein are used first for synthesizing body proteins. However, those amino acids in excess of needs for growth and maintenance undergo **deamination** and lose their characteristic NH_2 group and the remaining nitrogen-free portion enters the same metabolic pathways as carbohydrate and lipid, to be used as a source of energy. These amino acids can enter the metabolic pathway in many places, the exact place being determined by the chemical structure of each amino acid. The amino portions are released as ammonia, a poison, but two of the ammonia units are quickly combined to produce **urea,** a much less toxic substance. Urea in turn is excreted by the kidneys.

About half of the amino acids, including alanine, serine, glycine, cysteine, methionine, and tryptophan, are called **glucogenic** amino acids because after deamination they serve as potential sources of glucose.

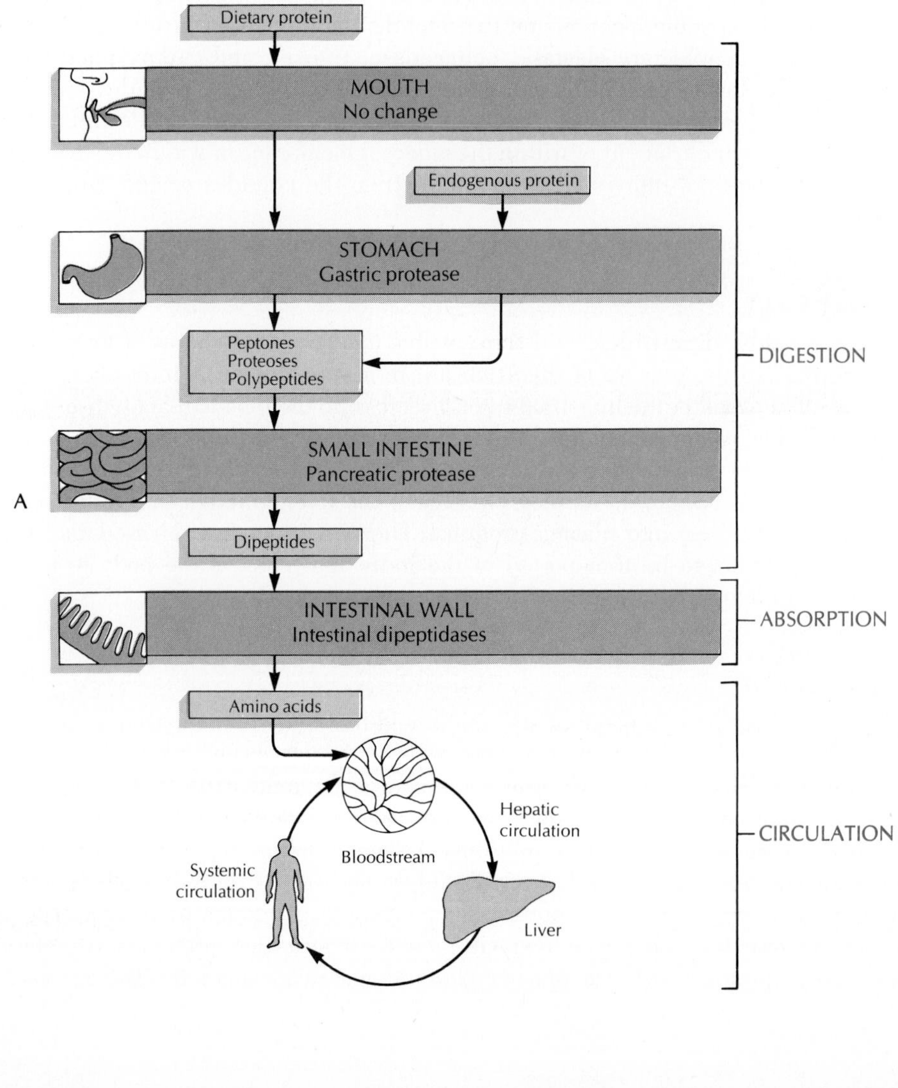

Figure 6-9 A, Summary of digestion, absorption, and circulation of protein.

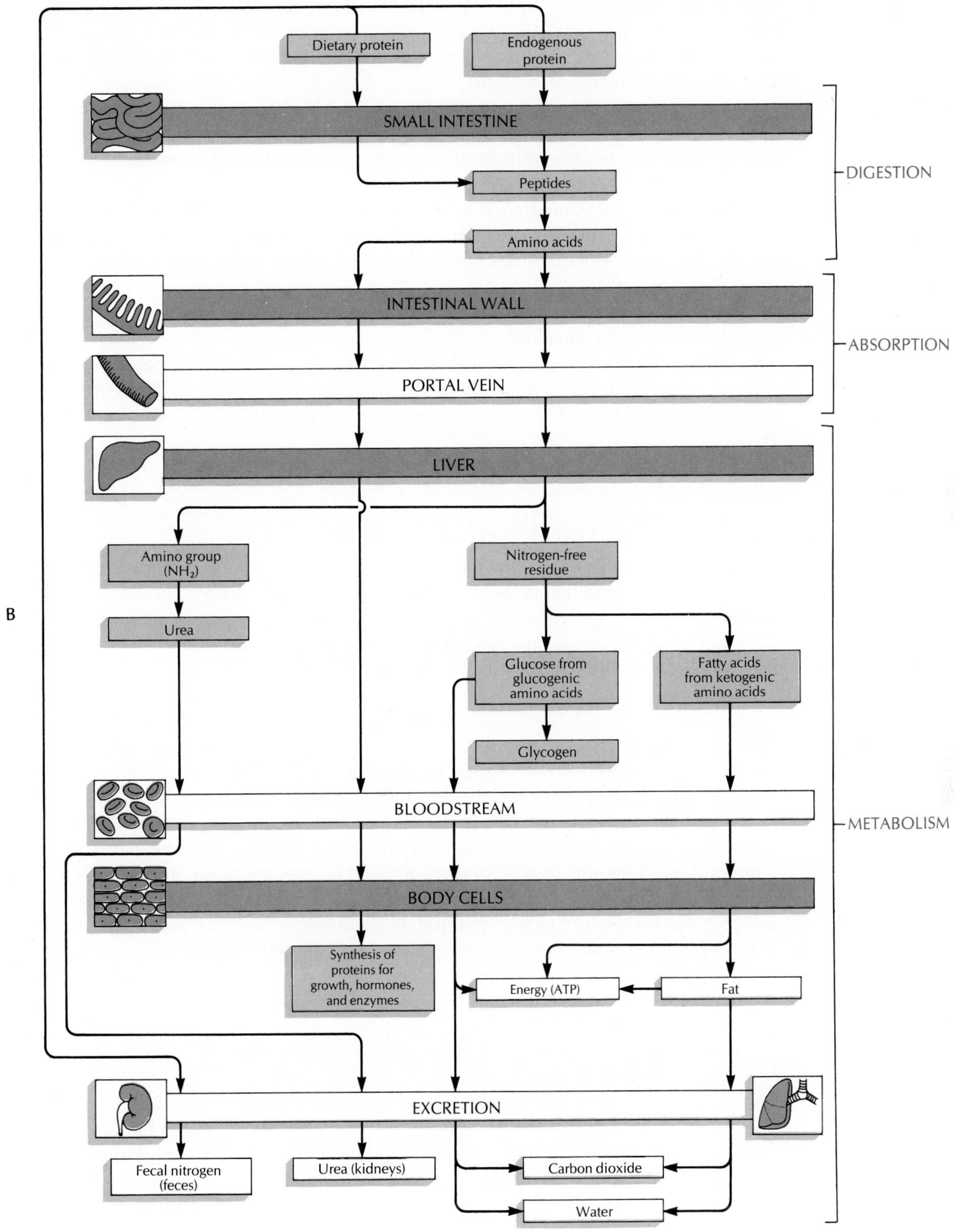

Fig. 6-9, cont'd B, Summary of digestion, absorption, and metabolism of protein.

About half of the remaining amino acids, including phenylalanine, tryosine, leucine, isoleucine, and lysine, can be deaminated (lose their NH_2 group) and broken down like fat into the 2-carbon fragments that eventually form acetyl coenzyme A (CoA). Like fat, these amino acids are able to form compounds called ketones, which can be used as a source of energy by the brain. They are therefore known as **ketogenic** amino acids.

ketogenic
Capable of producing ketones

Of the remaining amino acids, all but aspartic acid are converted into glutamic acid, deaminated, and used as an energy source immediately. Aspartic acid that is not used in protein synthesis is deaminated and enters the metabolic cycle directly.

Amino acids are deaminated to be used as an energy source when

1. Inadequate fat and carbohydrate are present to meet immediate energy needs
2. There are inadequate amounts of essential amino acids to synthesize required protein, or
3. The diet provides more amino acids than are needed for growth and synthesis of essential compounds

The end products of protein metabolism are the same carbon dioxide, water, and energy that result from the metabolism of carbohydrate and fat. In addition, however, the body must get rid of the leftover nitrogen, which it does by excreting urea in the urine.

The digestion and metabolism of protein are summarized in Figure 6-9.

FACTORS AFFECTING PROTEIN UTILIZATION

Factors Affecting Protein Utilization
Amino acid imbalance
Caloric inadequacy
Immobility
Injury
Emotional stress

Whether the amino acids from the breakdown of endogenous protein within the body or from the digestion of dietary protein are retained and used for the synthesis of new protein, or the repair of worn-out tissue protein, or are deaminated to be used for energy depends on a variety of conditions. An increase in the amount of urea in the urine indicates an increased loss of body protein.

Amino Acid Balance

It is now recognized that not only do actual amino acid requirements vary with age, but also that amounts of one relative to another change. Thus the value of a specific food in promoting growth will vary depending on how closely its **amino acid pattern** (i.e., the relationship of one amino acid to the other) in the food compares to the pattern of requirements, which in turn, depend on the age of the person eating it.

amino acid pattern
The amount of one amino acid relative to another either for requirements or in food sources

It is the ratio of the amino acid to nitrogen in a food relative to the ratio of the need for that amino acid to nitrogen that determines how useful a particular protein is in meeting the protein requirement. Therefore a protein may have an amino acid pattern that meets the needs of one age group but is relatively limited in meeting the needs of another.

Caloric Inadequacy

The protein content of the diet cannot be evaluated without consideration of the adequacy of the caloric intake. When the caloric intake drops below a certain critical point, protein will be deaminated and used as a source of energy. This will happen in low-carbohydrate/high-protein weight reduction diets, in which the food you eat is really providing you with a very expensive source of energy.

Immobility

The ability to synthesize protein is greatly reduced among people who are immobile. Older people who are bedridden lose protein mass even when dietary protein and caloric intake seem adequate. There has been a similar problem among astronauts, who lose protein as a result of both weightlessness and immobility during a space flight.

Injury

An increase in nitrogen loss after injury is well documented. High protein intakes either before or after injury do not prevent this loss. However, losses are recovered more rapidly once healing begins.

Emotional Stress

Emotional stresses such as fear, anxiety, or anger increase the secretion of epinephrine from the adrenal gland, which in turn causes a series of changes that result in the loss of nitrogen. Students lose nitrogen under the stress of exams. Other stressors that can result in nitrogen loss are severe pain, emotional anxiety, reversal of biological rhythms caused by night shift work, extreme cold, and jet travel across time zones.

ESTIMATING PROTEIN/AMINO ACID NEEDS

The need for protein and amino acids can be estimated in one of three ways. For young infants the amount of protein and the pattern of amino acids available daily in breast milk are considered to be appropriate for optimal growth. Recommendations are thus based on the total protein and amino acid pattern in the average 750 ml of milk produced daily. For children the factorial method is used; this involves an estimate of the amount of all the unavoidable nitrogen losses through urine, feces, and skin plus an allowance for growth needs. For adults nitrogen balance, measured at various levels of intake, has given us most of our information on which to estimate needs.

Nitrogen Balance

Because practically all proteins contain 16% nitrogen, we have been able to use the relatively simple analysis for nitrogen to study protein. We convert nitrogen to protein values by multiplying nitrogen by 6.25 ($^{100}/_{16}$).

Nitrogen balance involves a comparison of the intake of nitrogen in food with the loss of nitrogen from the body in the urine, in feces, and from the surface of the skin. Urinary losses include nitrogen from the breakdown of body tissue (**endogenous** nitrogen) plus nitrogen from the deamination of absorbed dietary protein in excess of what is needed to build and repair body tissue (**exogenous** nitrogen). Exogenous nitrogen will also appear in the urine when kilocalorie intake has been so low that some of the absorbed amino acids have been deaminated so that the rest of the molecule can be used for energy or when the diet does not provide all of the essential amino acids simultaneously. Fecal losses (which are both endogenous and exogenous) include 8% of dietary protein that is not absorbed plus a small amount lost with the loss of intestinal cells. The other losses of nitrogen, which amount to about 5 mg/kg, include the loss of cells from the surface of the skin and in hair, saliva, and perspiration. These are so difficult to measure that they are usually omitted in nitrogen balance studies.

nitrogen balance
The relationship between the amount of nitrogen taken into the body and the amount excreted

endogenous
Originating inside the body; for example, serum proteins and muscles

exogenous
Originating outside the body; for example dietary protein

Nitrogen Equilibrium

When nitrogen intake equals nitrogen loss, a person is in *nitrogen equilibrium*, indicating that the intake of protein is sufficient to replace any lost tissue but that no growth is taking place. Nitrogen equilibrium will occur in adults who are receiving as much or more protein than they need.

Nitrogen Equilibrium Intake = Loss

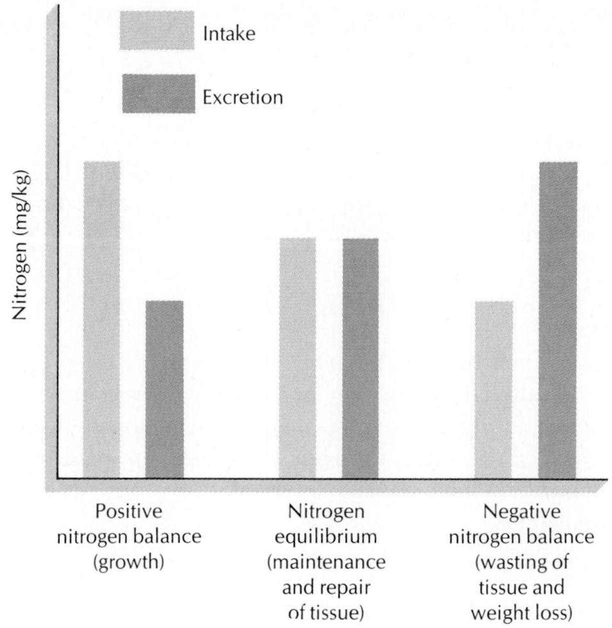

Figure 6-10 Diagrammatic representation of nitrogen balance, dependent on the relationship between intake (of food) and excretion (of urine and feces) with small losses through the skin.

Positive Nitrogen Balance

Positive Nitrogen Balance Intake > Loss

When nitrogen intake exceeds nitrogen losses, an individual is in *positive nitrogen balance*, indicating that growth is occurring. This positive balance should occur throughout infancy, childhood, and adolescence and during pregnancy. It will also occur during recovery from an illness in which protein has been lost. A positive nitrogen balance, sometimes known as *adult growth*, occurs in adults for no obvious reason.

Negative Nitrogen Balance

Negative Nitrogen Balance Intake < Loss

Negative nitrogen balance indicates that nitrogen losses are greater than nitrogen intake. This occurs when the tissues of the body are being broken down at a faster rate than they are being replaced. Prolonged negative nitrogen balance will show up as loss of body weight. This occurs most often when there is a severe calorie deficit, especially when the protein intake is very low. People who are immobile, under emotional stress, or who have suffered an injury are especially prone to loss of body protein, which is reflected in negative nitrogen balance.

Nitrogen balance studies give information on changes in body protein mass but provide no indication of the shift in body proteins from one tissue to another. For example, plasma albumin levels may drop even though a person is in nitrogen equilibrium, indicating that this person's labile protein pool has been depleted to meet the needs of other tissues.

The concept of nitrogen balance is presented graphically in Figure 6-10.

PROTEIN REQUIREMENTS

The need for protein has always been considered to be just below the lowest level of intake at which the body is in nitrogen equilibrium and just above the highest level at which it is in negative nitrogen balance. The nitrogen equilibrium point can be closely defined by a series of nitrogen balance studies in which the amount of dietary protein is reduced step by step until negative balance occurs. The intake is then increased in another series of experiments, each of which usually takes 1 to 3 weeks, until positive balance is restored. The real need lies between these two levels of intake, the point at which balance is achieved, or is essentially at zero. This conforms to the definition proposed by the FAO/WHO/UNU Committee on Protein and Energy Requirements that the "requirement for protein is the intake needed to prevent loss of body protein and to allow for adequate deposition or production of protein during growth, pregnancy, or lactation."

FAO/WHO/UNU = Food and Agricultural Organization/World Health Organization/United Nations University

Based on both long-term and short-term balance studies, the protein requirement for adults appears to be 0.75 gram of high-quality protein per kilogram of body weight. This provides a 25% margin of safety, representing two standard deviations above the mean of 0.63 gram/kg body weight. It is assumed that this will take care of the needs of essentially all healthy adults. However, because the total North American diet can be assumed to include some low-quality protein, it is important to increase these figures to sufficiently compensate for it.

For current Recommended Dietary Allowances for the United States, see inside front cover and Table 6-2

Because the quality of protein depends on the pattern of amino acids in the diet compared to the pattern of amino acid requirements, the quality or biological score for the North American diet will vary slighly from one age to another. This is determined by comparing the amino acid pattern of the typical diet of a country to the recommended amino acid pattern. For the United States the amino acid pattern was computed for diets as reported in the Nationwide Food Consumption Study (NFCS). After making further correction for the fact that protein is about 92% digestible (85% digestible in a vegetarian diet), it is possible to arrive at a figure representing the need for protein.

There is now growing evidence that the requirement should be set slightly higher, recognizing that even high-quality protein will be used immediately for energy.

Table 6-2 shows the calculation of protein needs, using the approach recommended by the International FAO/WHO/UNU committee responsible for recommending protein and energy standards. Average weights and food quality scores appropriate to the United States are used. (These values are more recent and slightly different from the 1980 RDAs.)

Recommended Protein Intakes

Infant	9-12 mo	1.4 gram/kg/day
Child	1-2 yr	1.2 gram/kg/day
	5-6 yr	1.03 gram/kg/day
	9-10 yr	1.00 gram/kg/day

Although we traditionally have assessed and continue to assess the adequacy of the diet in terms of protein, many nutritionists feel that we should be considering amino acid requirements rather than protein requirements. This would, of course, be a much more complex task because we would be dealing with nine requirements instead of one. However, we do have the information available to estimate amino acid requirements. The information has been obtained in the same way that we estimate protein requirements, that is, by eliminating one amino acid from the diet and adding progressively larger amounts of it until the negative nitrogen balance caused by the lack of the amino acid changes to nitrogen equilibrium in most adults or a positive balance if growth is occurring. For those who have reason to use amino acid requirements, estimates for the United States based on the recommendations of FAO/WHO/UNU are presented in Table 6-3. From this table it is evident that amino acid requirement patterns vary with age. Experience has shown that, in addition to the need for essential amino acids, there is a need for nitrogen for the synthesis of the nonessential amino acids. It is also evident that the only amino acids that are likely to be limiting in the diet are lysine; the two sulfur-containing amino acids cystine and methionine, threonine, and tryptophan. However, few natural diets are low in essential amino acids.

Throughout growth, the proportion of the total protein intake needed for growth decreases and that needed for maintenance of the body increases, as depicted in Figure 6-11.

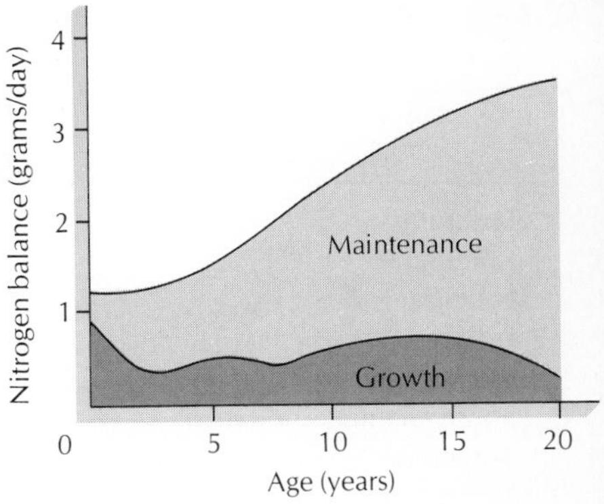

Figure 6-11 Protein needs for growth and maintenance of the body throughout the life cycle.

Modified from Allison, JB: Transactions of the New York Academy of Science 25:293, 1963.

FOOD SOURCES

The protein content of the most frequently used foods within the major food groups is shown in Table 6-4, and relative amounts of protein per serving are shown in the margin on p. 151. In assessing the amount of protein in a food, it is important to keep in mind that foods containing all the essential amino acids are more useful

Table 6-2 ◇ Derivation of the Recommended Allowances of the U.S. dietary protein

Age	Weight (kg)	Safe Allowance of Reference Protein g/kg	Safe Allowance of Reference Protein g/day	Score*	Estimated NPU†	Recommended Allowance (g/day)
Infant						
0-2.9 m‡	4.5	2.00	9.0	1.00	0.90	10†
3-5.9 m	6.6	1.73	11.0	0.81	0.73	16†
6-11.9 m	8.8	1.51	12.0	0.78	0.70	18
Children						
1-1.9 yr	11	1.21	13.0	0.82	0.74	18
2-3.9 yr	14	1.12	16.0	0.99	0.90	18
4-5.9 yr	18	1.05	19.0	0.99	0.90	21
6-7.9 yr	22	1.02	22.0	1.00	0.90	25
8-9.9 yr	28	1.00	28.0	1.00	0.90	31
Males						
10-11.9 yr	36	0.98	35.0	1.00	0.90	39
12-17.9 yr	57	0.93	53.0	1.00	0.90	59
18-24.9 yr	73	0.75	55.0	1.00	0.90	61
25-49.9 yr	79	0.75	59.0	1.00	0.90	66
50-69.9 yr	77	0.75	58.0	1.00	0.90	64
70+ yr	74	0.75	56.0	1.00	0.90	62
Females						
10-14.9 yr	44	0.96	42.0	1.00	0.90	47
15-17.9 yr	56	0.83	47.0	1.00	0.90	52
18-24.9 yr	58	0.75	44.0	1.00	0.90	48
25-49.9 yr	62	0.75	47.0	1.00	0.90	52
50-64.9 yr	65	0.75	49.0	1.00	0.90	54
70+ yr	64	0.75	48.0	1.00	0.90	53
Pregnancy						
1st trimester			+1	0.70	0.63	+ 3
2nd trimester			+6	0.70	0.63	+10
3rd trimester			+11	0.70	0.63	+17
Lactation						
1st 6 months			+16	0.70	0.63	+22
2nd 6 months			+11	0.70	0.63	+18

Adapted from Energy and protein requirements, FAO/WHO/UNU, 1985. Courtesy Dr. Peter Pellett, Amherst, MA.
*Amino acid score based on comparison of intake pattern for various ages in U.S. to requirement.
†NPU = Net protein utilization = Amino acid score × Coefficient of digestion of 0.9.
‡Breast milk consumption assumed.

Table 6-3 ◇ Pattern of amino acid requirements at various ages compared to the pattern of amino acids in beef, wheat, and the U.S. food supply (milligrams of amino acid per gram of protein)

	Infant	Preschool (2-5 yr)	Child (10-12 yr)	Adult	U.S. Food Supply	Beef	Wheat
Histidine	26	20	18	16	30	34	19
Isoleucine	46	30	29	13	49	48	37
Leucine	93	70	46	19	87	81	61
Lysine	66	62	46	16	68	89	25
Methionine and cysteine	42	26	23	17	35	40	36
Phenylalanine and tyrosine	72	66	23	19	90	80	74
Threonine	43	36	29	9	42	46	31
Tryptophan	17	12	9	5	12	11	11
Valine	55	37	26	13	55	50	43
Total							
with Histidine	460	359	244	127	468	479	337
without Histidine	434	339	226	111	438	445	318

Source of values: requirement values (mg/gram protein): FAO/WHO/UNU, 1985. Values (mg/gram N) can be calculated from these using N = Protein × 6.25.
U.S. food supply: Calculated from FAO Food Balance Sheets (FAO, 1980) using a simplified diet structure.
Beef and Wheat: Amino acid content of foods and biological data on proteins (FAO, 1970).

than those with low or limiting amounts of one or more amino acid. Thus, as a general rule, proteins from animal sources are better suited to the amino acid requirements of humans than proteins from vegetable sources. Within each group, however, the proteins have a wide range of biological value.

Because protein-rich foods are usually the most expensive items in the diet, it is useful to have information on the relative costs of equal amounts of protein from various food sources. This is especially helpful if someone is trying to plan nutritionally adequate meals on a limited food budget. A comparison of the costs of protein in various food, is shown in the margin below.

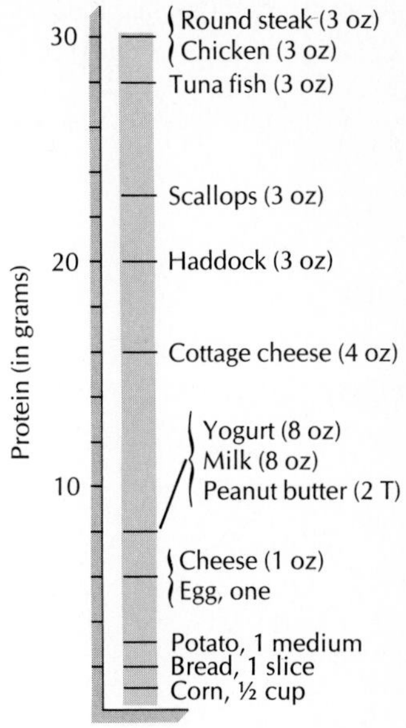

Relative amount of protein in average serving of various food sources

Table 6-4 ◇ Protein in average servings and per 100 kcal of foods most frequently reported in surveys and other recommended sources

Food	Amount	Kcal	Per Serving (grams)	Per 100 kcal (grams)	INQ*
Eggs, Meat, Poultry, Fish, Nuts					
Egg, fried	1 large	95	6	6	2.6
Beef, roast	3 oz	315	19	6	2.8
Hamburger	3 oz	230	21	9	4.0
Chicken	3 oz	140	27	19	8.5
Tuna	3 oz	65	24	14	6.4
Peanut butter	2 T	190	10	5	2.2
Bacon	3 slices	110	6	5	2.2
Pork†	3 oz	295	23	7.7	2.5
Cereal Products					
Beans, kidney†	½ cup	115	7.5	6.5	2.0
Cornflakes	1 cup	110	2	2	0.6
Shredded wheat	1 biscuit	100	3	3	0.9
Saltines (10 grams)	4 crackers	50	1	2	0.6
Rice	1 oz dry (½ cup cooked)	109	2	2	0.6
White bread	1 slice	65	2	3	0.9
Whole-wheat bread	1 slice	70	3	4	1.2
Dairy Products					
Whole milk	8 oz	150	8.0	5	2.2
2% fat milk	8 oz	120	8.0	7	3.0
Cheddar cheese	1 oz	115	7.0	6	2.6
Fruit					
Apple	1 medium	80	0.3	0.4	0.1
Banana	1 medium	105	1.1	1.0	0.3
Orange juice, frozen	4 oz	55	0.8	1.4	0.4
Peach	1 medium	35	0.6	1.7	0.5
Vegetables					
Corn, canned	4 oz (½ cup)	82	2.5	3	1.1
Green beans	4 oz (½ cup)	22	1	5	1.5
Green peas	4 oz (½ cup)	62	4	6	1.8
Lettuce	¼ head	20	1	5	1.5
Tomatoes	1 medium	25	1	4	0.8
Potato, baked	1 medium	130	3	2	0.7

*INQ = % RDA for protein (45 grams animal protein or 65 grams vegetable protein)/% Energy requirement (2000 kcal).

†Other recommended sources.

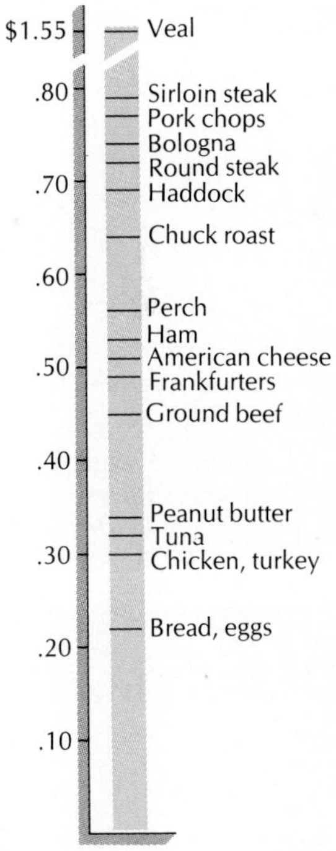

Relative cost of 20 grams of various protein sources. Actual prices will vary at different times in different places, but they will tend to remain in approximately the same relationship to each other.

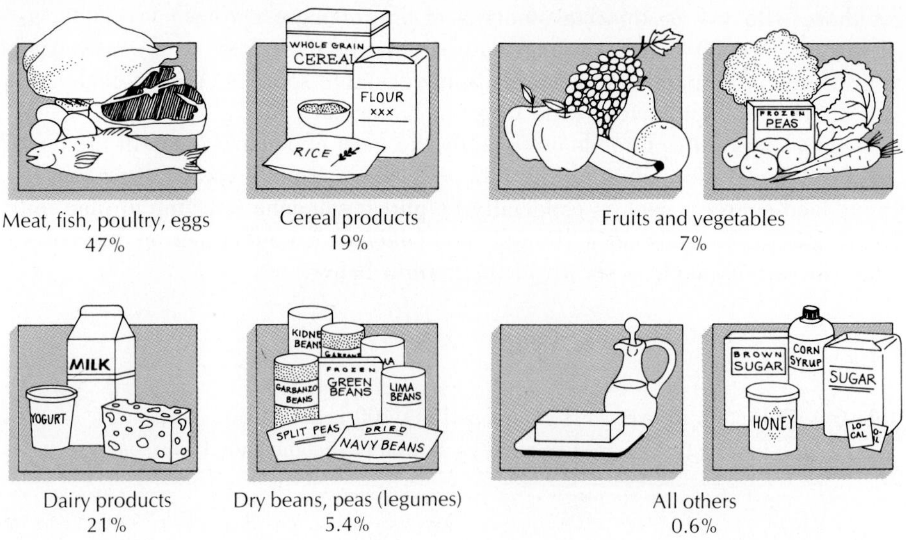

Figure 6-12 Contribution of various food groups to the protein in the U.S. food supply in 1984.
From National Food Review, USDA, Winter, 1986.

The relatively high cost of protein may be part of the reason we describe a meal in terms of the major protein component (for example, ham dinner, chicken casserole, or beef tenderloin). It may also be part of the reason why we plan a meal around a protein item rather than starting with the less expensive dessert or salad item.

In assessing the adequacy of protein in a diet, it is important to look at the protein sources. Although a knowledgeable person can plan a diet with protein of high biological value using foods of vegetable origin alone, it is usually recommended that about one third of the protein come from foods of animal origin. As seen in Figure 6-12, about three fourths of the protein in the American diet is of animal origin. These foods must, however, be distributed in such a way that each meal contains all the essential amino acids. The increasing use of dried milk solids in many bread products, which belong to the cereal group, means that the bread products have a protein content of enhanced biological value. Similarly, flour products made with eggs or milk have good-quality protein.

Protein and Fat in Alternate Protein-Rich Food Sources

	Sirloin (3 oz)	Cheddar Cheese (1 oz)	Navy Beans (1½ cup)
Protein (grams)	24	7	23
Fat (grams)	10	9	2
Calories	195	112	314

Seeds such as pumpkin, sunflower, or sesame are often promoted as rich protein sources. They do indeed have a high percentage of protein but are not a practical source because they are also high in fat and in the cost per gram of protein. Also, some people find that seed fiber causes intestinal irritation.

The efforts of some entrepreneurs to promote the addition of limiting amino acids, especially lysine and methionine, to cereals and legumes to enhance protein quality are not justified in the Western world, where there is absolutely no deficiency of protein or protein quality. In addition, if supplementation with one amino acid creates an amino acid imbalance, the quality of the protein is decreased rather than improved. Amino acid supplementation may be appropriate when the diet is composed primarily of a cereal staple and very little animal protein. This supplementation is feasible, however, only in countries where dietary staples are processed in relatively few centers so that the addition of nutrients can be monitored and controlled.

ADEQUACY OF THE U.S. DIET

The analysis of data from both the NHANES II and the NFCS surveys showed that there was no deficiency of protein for over 50,000 people in the United States. In the NHANES II, mean intakes of 92 grams of protein per day for males and 60 grams per day for females were considerably above the RDA. Serum albumin levels, which are indicative of protein status, were all above standard values. In the NFCS,

88% of the participants reported intakes meeting 100% of the RDA, and only 2% had diets providing less than 80% of the RDA. Almost all of those with low intake had very low kilocalorie intakes as well.

EVALUATION OF PROTEIN QUALITY

At present, several biological and chemical measures are used to measure protein quality. The most commonly used are the biological value (BV), net protein utilization (NPU), the protein efficiency ratio (PER), and chemical scores.

Measures of Protein Quality
Biological value (BV)
Net protein utilization (NPU)
Protein efficiency ratio (PER)
Chemical score

Biological Value

The *biological value*, or *BV*, of a food is measured as the percentage of absorbed nitrogen that is retained (i.e., not excreted) for growth or maintenance. This indicator is based on the assumption that more nitrogen will be retained when the essential amino acids are present in sufficient quantity to meet the needs for growth. Determination of the BV of a protein involves controlled animal feeding studies. As a result, it is a costly and time-consuming procedure. A food or diet with a BV of 70 or more—meaning that 70% of the absorbed nitrogen is retained—is considered capable of supporting growth, assuming that the diet provides adequate kilocalories.

$$\text{BV} = \frac{\text{N retained}}{\text{N absorbed}} \times 100 = \frac{\text{N intake} - \text{N excretion}}{\text{N intake} \times \text{digestibility}} \times 100$$

Foods with BV Greater Than 70

Egg	Chicken
Rice	Corn
Fish	

Net Protein Utilization

Net protein utilizaton, or *NPU*, another index of protein quality, is the measure of nitrogen ingested that is retained. Since it does not take into account differences in digestibility, a poorly digested but good-quality protein will have a false low value.

$$\text{NPU} = \frac{\text{N retained}}{\text{N intake}} \times 100 = \frac{\text{N intake} - \text{N excretion}}{\text{N intake}} \times 100$$

Protein Efficiency Ratio

The *protein efficiency ratio*, or *PER*, is the simplest measure of protein quality, but it still has some limitations. It is based on the weight gain per gram of protein ingested in young rats. Casein, a high-quality protein in milk, has a PER of 2.5 and is considered the standard used for nutrient labeling purposes. The PER is based on the unproven assumption that weight gain in a growing animal is proportional to the gain in body protein.

$$\text{PER} = \text{weight gain (grams)} \div \text{protein intake (grams)}$$

Chemical Methods

Chemical methods of assessing protein quality require information on the amino acid composition of the food or the diet. The chemical score is usually expressed as the ratio of milligrams of an amino acid per gram of protein in the food compared to the amino acid requirement per gram of protein for the age and sex group whose diet is being evaluated. The protein score for the food is the lowest ratio for any amino acid for the food to the amino acid requirement. Using this method, a particular amino acid has a different score for each age and sex group. From the information in Table 6-3 it can be seen that the score for wheat, in which lysine is the limiting amino acid, will be 54 (25/46) for a 10- to 12-year-old child but will exceed 100 (25/16) for an adult. Therefore wheat, with a chemical score of over 100, could support growth or repair of tissues in an adult. However, its score of 54 for a child indicates that this protein source alone is not adequate for children. The use of whole egg or milk as a standard, formerly used by FAO, has been abandoned.

The fact that we have so many different approaches to assessing protein quality indicates that it is a complex task. Although the chemical score is the easiest to compute, we unfortunately have little evidence that the animal uses protein as predicted by the score.

ENERGY-PROTEIN MALNUTRITION

kwashiorkor
A protein deficiency disease affecting young children

marasmus
A condition resulting from a lack of kilocalories and (usually) also protein

During the late 1940s and early 1950s, interest in protein nutrition was stimulated by the observation that protein deficiency was a major factor in the high infant mortality of developing countries, where starchy roots such as cassava were dietary staples. A protein-deficiency condition that affected young children between the ages of 2 and 5 became known as **kwashiorkor.** This term was coined by Ghanaians to describe a sickness that struck the firstborn child when a second child was born. (The literal translation of the word is appropriately "first-second.") Once it was recognized that the condition developed within 3 to 4 months after the older child was abruptly weaned from the breast, which was its only source of good-quality protein, the condition was identified as a protein deficiency. Children suffering from kwashiorkor lose weight or fail to gain, becoming apathetic, listless, withdrawn from their environment, and (most importantly) increasingly susceptible to infection. Conditions such as fever and measles, which are only temporarily disruptive in the lives of well-fed children, are severely debilitating and often fatal for a child with kwashiorkor.

It was not long before it was recognized that kwashiorkor was closely related to another condition known as **marasmus,** which comes from the Greek word for "wasting." Marasmus is caused by a chronic lack of kilocalories. When energy intake is insufficient, protein is diverted from its role in growth to be used as a source of energy, essentially causing a protein deficiency. As a result of our increasing knowledge of the complex interrelationship between protein deficiencies and kilocalories, the syndrome previously known as protein-calorie malnutrition (PCM) is now referred to as energy-protein malnutrition (EPM) or energy-protein deficits (EPD). The use of these terms acknowledges the fact that lack of kilocalories is likely to be more common than lack of protein. With either deficit, the problem is a major one that affects as many as half the children in third world countries. There is even recent speculation that kwashiorkor is the result of an exposure to aflatoxin rather than a protein deficiency.

Regardless of whether the primary deficit is kilocalories, protein, or protein quality, there are several clinical symptoms associated with EPM:

1. Failure to grow both in height and weight accompanied by thin, weak, and wasting muscles
2. Behavioral changes, ranging from the irritability of kwashiorkor to the apathy of marasmus
3. Edema, which is the accumulation of fluid in the tissues, causing them to be soft and spongy (especially in the lower abdomen, arms, and legs)
4. Skin changes including changes in color, lack of color, drying, peeling, and the eventual formation of ulcers that heal slowly (if at all) and permit a point of entry for other infective organisms
5. Changes in the hair, which becomes dry and sparse and either loses its pigmentation or takes on a characteristic red color
6. Loss of appetite, vomiting, and diarrhea, all of which result in severe dehydration and loss of sodium and potassium
7. Enlargement of the liver
8. Anemia
9. Increased susceptibility to infections and fever, with much more devastating consequences than normal

The effect of this severe undernutrition is evident from the child with kwashiorkor pictured in Figure 6-13, *A*. This is in contrast to child with marasmus, an energy deficit (Figure 6-13, *B*). Children who survive to age 5 years, when they can compete more effectively for food from the family supply and are able to forage for themselves, do reasonably well. However, they are seldom able to make up the growth deficit of the earlier years.

A

B

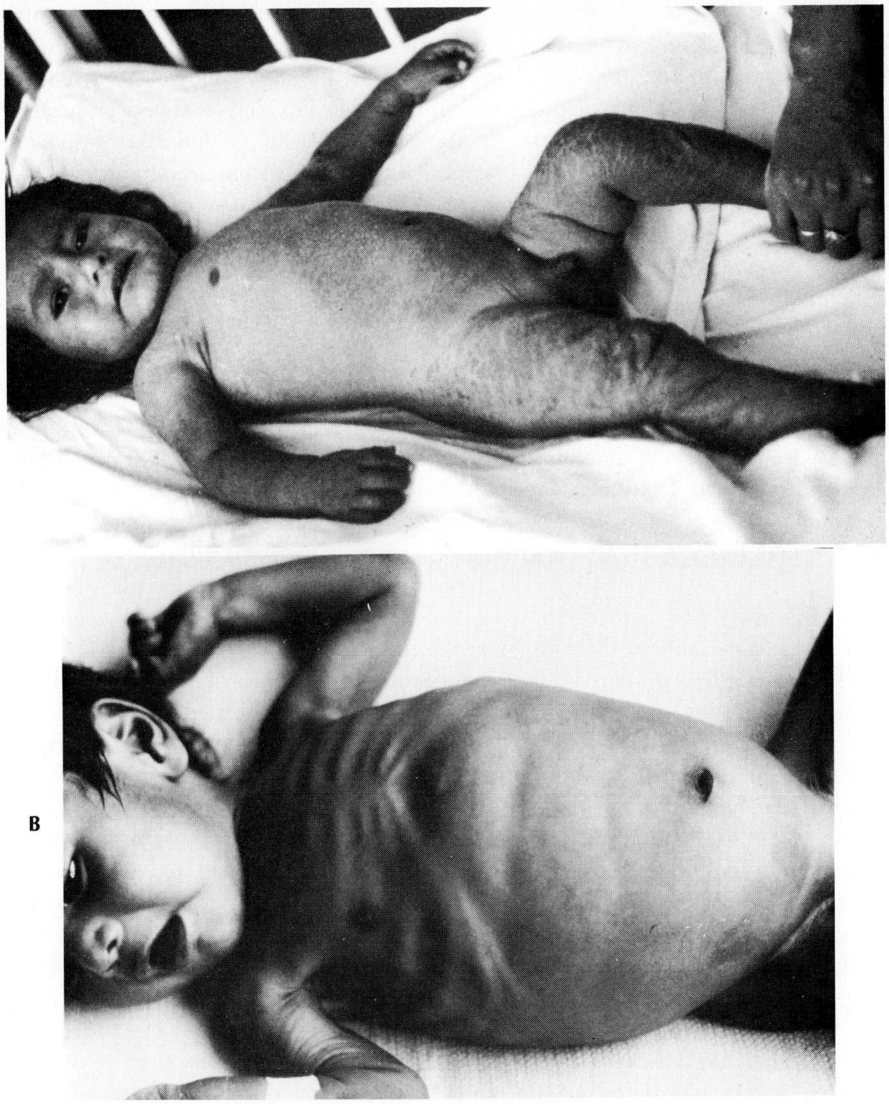

Figure 6-13 **A,** Child suffering from kwashiorkor. **B,** Child suffering from marasmus as the result of an inadequate energy intake.
Courtesy Dr. John Beard, Pennsylvania State University.

Protein Malnutrition in Developing Countries

Although for some time it was believed that the malnutrition of early childhood had a permanent and stunting effect on mental development, evidence now suggests that deficits in brain size and brain cell number have few behavioral consequences that cannot be overcome by environmental stimulation. Unfortunately, those who suffer from nutritional deficits are more often than not deprived of environmental stimulation as well. They also may live in a very poor hygienic environment in which they are constantly exposed to sources of infection; the high fever accompanying many infections can have severe consequences on brain functioning.

In some cases, malnutrition is caused by illness rather than the reverse. Diarrhea and vomiting lead to the loss of nutrients, fever and infection cause increased needs, and gastrointestinal disease results in a secondary undernutrition caused by poor absorption of many nutrients. The combined result of these various forms of malnutrition is a very high mortality rate in developing countries: 1 in 4 to 5 children before the age of 5 years. (This can be compared to 1 in 50 to 90 children in developed countries.)

Causes of Energy/Protein Malnutrition
Lack of kilocalories
Lack of protein—inadequate animal protein
Poverty
Lack of access to land
Poor marketing systems
Inequitable distribution of food within the family
Poor sanitation
Lack of water

The causes of severe undernutrition and malnutrition in developing countries are many and varied. Poverty and the resulting lack of money for adequate food are obvious factors. In countries where the monthly family income may be as low as $20 for a large segment of the population, it is often impossible for parents to provide even enough kilocalories, let alone worry about the quality of the diet. Shortages of water; lack of access to arable land; lack of money for fertilizer and the other materials necessary to grow food; and problems of insect infestation, plant and animal diseases, and theft are all deterrents to the home production of food in developing countries. High rates of population growth only increase the pressure on the land to provide adequate food. For families with no reserves, natural disasters such as floods, soil erosion, and droughts have consequences that further limit their access to food. Moreover, poor environmental sanitation contributes to high rates of infection and illness, which reduce the capacity of the family to work, earn money, grow food, or hunt for it. Even after food is produced, the marketing and transportation systems of the country are often so poorly developed that it is difficult to distribute it to those in greatest need. Under these circumstances, there is little incentive to raise food for sale to others, with the result that most marketing is done at a very basic subsistence level. The extensive use of arable land by wealthy landowners to produce nonfood cash crops such as rubber and **copra** (dried coconut from which oil is extracted) is the result of inequitable land tenure arrangements, which make it even more difficult for a family to raise food or animals.

copra
Dried coconut from which oil is extracted; often exported to developed countries as a cash crop

All of these deterrents to solving the problems of malnutrition are complicated by many cultural beliefs and practices that prohibit or discourage the use of certain foods. Young children and pregnant and lactating women are, from a nutritional standpoint, the most vulnerable groups. Customs that dictate feeding the men and elderly first decrease food access to those who have the greatest need.

The magnitude and severity of the problems of kilocalorie-protein malnutrition are great. Much effort is being directed toward finding solutions to these problems. Attempts to slow population growth are essential, especially as our resources to deal with illness improve so that more people survive conditions that previously were fatal. Progress toward the goal of zero population growth is slow and at best a long-range solution to the problem. Research to develop new strains of food crops with higher yields, resistance to natural pests and plant diseases, enhanced nutritional qualities, and better storage qualities are ongoing. The success of these efforts will depend on the extent to which they can be used by the individual farmer, whose available resources are limited, and on the extent to which the final product is acceptable from both palatability and cultural standpoints.

indigenous
Occurring naturally in a particular area

The development of appropriate weaning foods for infants from **indigenous** food, or food that occurs naturally in a particular area, is a goal of many projects. The weaning foods must be reasonable in price; available in native markets; sufficiently palatable so that babies will eat them; not so pleasing to adult tastes that they are eaten by adults; compatible with cultural beliefs; and available on a regular basis. Ideally they should be foods that can be produced in the community or home, that do not require sophisticated food technology, and that do not rely on commercial production methods. Foods based on a mixture of plant proteins or that involve the addition of small amounts of available animal protein, such as fish, fish pastes, or vegetable staples, are most likely to be acceptable. The critical criteria are that they reach young children in the lower socioeconomic classes, where the need is greatest, and that they be culturally acceptable.

The availability of health services, directed toward preventive rather than crisis care, can be an important factor in the prevention of EPM. One of the very early signs of malnutrition is a slowing of growth rate; this can be detected very early if the child is weighed and measured on a regular basis and the growth compared to standards. In developing countries, infants who are breast-fed exhibit a growth that is comparable to the growth of infants in developed countries up to the age of 5 or 6 months. After that, growth begins to drop off if the diet is not supplemented. This lack of proper growth may have no obvious consequences until children are subjected to infection; at that time they lack the resistance of normal children and will suffer much more severe and often fatal consequences. Sometimes it is the infection that triggers the decline in growth. In any case, careful monitoring of growth progress appears to be an effective and economically sound approach in identifying nutritionally vulnerable young children in developing countries. Mothers should be encouraged to continue breast feeding as long as possible; in addition, they should be advised to add solid foods to the baby's diet at 4 months of age to avoid the likelihood of various degrees of malnutrition.

Although most of the emphasis in the study of energy-protein malnutrition has been on children, there is some evidence of deficiencies occurring among other age groups. In these cases, kilocalorie deficits are usually the problem rather than protein, which assumes more importance when a person is still in the process of growing.

BY NOW YOU SHOULD KNOW

- Protein is essential for the growth of all body tissues, for all enzymes, and for many hormones.
- Dietary protein is made up of 20 different amino acids.
- It is the nitrogen molecule that makes protein chemically different from carbohydrate and fat.
- The amino group gives each amino acid its uniqueness.
- There are nine essential amino acids that cannot be synthesized by the body and therefore must be provided in the diet.
- There are 11 nonessential amino acids that can be synthesized by the body, as long as there is sufficient nonessential nitrogen and adequate calories in the diet.
- Protein needs are determined by nitrogen balance studies, which involve measuring the intake of dietary nitrogen in relation to the excretion of nitrogen in the urine and feces and other necessary losses of nitrogen.
- Protein functions in the growth and maintenance of tissue, the formation of essential body compounds, the regulation of water balance, the maintenance of body neutrality, antibody formation, and the transporting of nutrients.
- Protein digestion begins in the acid environment of the stomach.
- Amino acids are absorbed in the small intestine.
- If calorie intake is sufficient, amino acids will be used for protein synthesis. If calorie intake is insufficient to meet energy needs or if amino acids are in excess of needs, the amino acids must be deaminated. The carbon and hydrogen atoms are oxidized for energy or converted and stored as fat.
- Protein requirements are 0.75 gram per kilogram body weight for maintenance of body tissue.
- Additional protein is needed for growth during childhood, adolescence, pregnancy, and for milk production during breast-feeding.
- Sources of dietary protein are meat, fish, poultry, eggs, cereals, legumes, seeds, and nut products.
- There is no evidence of a protein deficiency in the North American diet.
- Kwashiorkor and marasmus are energy-protein deficiency diseases that occur most often in young children in developing countries.

STUDY QUESTIONS

1. How is the chemical composition of protein different from that of carbohydrate or fat? How does this difference affect the biological function of protein?
2. How is nitrogen cycled from plants to animals?
3. Why are some amino acids considered essential? Why is it necessary to consider the amino pattern when determining protein requirements?
4. Under what conditions will protein be broken down and used for energy?
5. How does animal protein differ from vegetable protein?
6. What is meant by protein complementation?
7. What is meant by nitrogen balance? Describe the situations that alter nitrogen balance.
8. Trace the digestion and absorption of a protein-rich meal.
9. How is protein quality evaluated?
10. Differentiate between kwashiorkor, marasmus, and energy-protein malnutrition.
11. Suggest some possible solutions that may decrease the incidence of energy-protein malnutrition in developing countries.

Applying What You've Learned

1. **Sources of Protein**

   List everything you have eaten today or yesterday. What were the sources of animal protein? What were the sources of plant protein? How do your food choices of protein influence your saturated fat and complex carbohydrate intake?

2. **Determining Your Protein Requirement**

   Calculate your protein requirement based on your body weight in kilograms. To convert pounds to kilograms, divide the pounds by 2.2 (2.2 pounds = 1 kilogram). To calculate the recommended intake of protein, multiply your weight in kilograms by 0.75:

   (0.75 gram protein/kilogram body weight = grams of protein)

   Now that you know your recommended protein intake, determine if your dietary intake of protein was adequate to meet this need. Using Appendix F, total your protein intake. How does it compare to the recommended intake?

$<\frac{2}{3}$ RDA	Possible protein deficiency
$\frac{2}{3}$ to 2 × RDA	Normal
>2 × RDA	No known benefit; no known harm

3. **Plan a Menu**

   Plan a 2-day menu for yourself, using complementary proteins with no animal sources of protein to contribute to the protein quality.

4. **Investigate Food Labels**

   Read a food nutrition label for protein in grams and for %U.S. RDA for protein. Then read the ingredient list to identify the source of protein.

SUGGESTED READINGS

Benevenga NJ, and Steele RD: Adverse effects of excessive consumption of amino acids, Annual Review of Nutrition 4:157, 1984.

This article deals with the possibility of toxicity from excess consumption of the amino acids phenylalanine, tryptophan, histidine, and methionine, all of which are now being sold over the counter to the general public. It is a fairly technical article, but it provides the reader with the documentation necessary to decide on the wisdom of using individual amino acids.

Crim M, and Munro HN: Protein. In Present knowledge of nutrition, Washington, D.C., 1984, Nutrition Foundation, Inc.

This chapter contains a comprehensive review of the current knowledge of protein nutrition and metabolism. Munro is considered the foremost authority in the field of protein nutrition.

Sampson DA, and Jansen GR: Protein and energy nutrition during lactation, Annual Review of Nutrition 4:43, 1984.

This review pulls together the information now available on the roles of both protein and energy in the success or failure of lactation. It includes some discussion on how the mammary gland functions to use the nutrients provided in the maternal diet.

Timmons KH, Pace R, Anderson SD, and Svacha AJ: Protein quality and the cost of selected protein supplements, Journal of the American Dietetic Association 78:606, 1984.

This article provides information on the cost of a wide range of nutrient supplements available on the market. It questions their value in normal nutrition.

ADDITIONAL READINGS

Food and Agriculture Organization: Energy and protein, Rome, 1985, World Health Organization and United Nations University.

Garza C, Scrimshaw NS, and Young VR: Human protein requirements: the effect of variations in energy intake within the maintenance range, American Journal of Clinical Nutrition 29:280, 1976.

Gersovitz M, and others: Human protein requirements: an assessment of the adequacy of the current recommended dietary protein in elderly men and women, American Journal of Clinical Nutrition 35:6, 1982.

In what forms are digested proteins absorbed from the small intestine? Nutrition Reviews 39:380, 1981.

Irwin MI, and Hegsted DM: A conspectus of research on amino acid requirements of man, Journal of Nutrition 101:539, 1971.

Laidlaw SA, and Kopple JD: Newer concepts of indispensable amino acids, American Journal of Clinical Nutrition 46:593, 1987.

Mortimore GE: Mechanisms of cellular protein metabolism, Nutrition Reviews 41:1, 1982.

Spencer H, Kramer K, and Dosis D: Protein and calcium cause calcium loss, Journal of Nutrition 118:657, 1988.

Visek WJ: An update of concepts of essential amino acids, Annual Review of Nutrition 4:137, 1984.

Young VR, and Bier DM: Amino acid requirements in the adult human: How well do we know them? Journal of Nutrition 117:1484, 1987.

Young VR, and Bier DM: A kinetic approach to the determination of human amino acid requirements, Nutrition Reviews 45:289, 1987.

FOCUS Vegetarianism

vegan
A person who will eat no food of animal origin

ovolactovegetarian
A person who will eat only milk and eggs from animals

ovo-lacto-pollovegetarian
Vegetarians who include the use of milk, eggs, and poultry in their diet

pescovegetarian
A person who will eat fish but no other food of animal origin

oxalic acid
Organic acid in spinach that binds calcium

phytic acid
Substance in outer husk of grain that binds calcium and other mineral elements

Yin Foods	Yang Foods	Neutral Foods
Pork	Beef	Rice
Potatoes	Tomatoes	Noodles
Grains	Peanuts	Sugar

Vegetarianism, or the reliance on foods of vegetable origin for nourishment, has been practiced throughout recorded history by a wide variety of groups for a number of reasons, primarily on the basis of health beliefs and religion. In the latter half of this century, a growing number of people have also become vegetarians because they are concerned about our ability to feed the world's population if we continue to eat animals that depend on other animals or forage crops for food; their concerns are ecological, political, economical, and ethical.

While a great many people (several million in the United States alone) call themselves vegetarians, a very small number actually can be considered **vegans,** or true vegetarians. Vegans avoid all products of animal origin, including milk and eggs. Much more common are the **ovolactovegetarians.** They avoid eating any food obtained by slaughtering an animal but have no objection to consuming milk (Latin, *lacto*) and eggs (Latin, *ovo*). This is because they do not consider these foods to be animal parts but rather products of the animal that are designed to be given away. **Ovolactopollovegetarians** eat poultry in addition to milk and eggs, while **pescovegetarians** consider fish an acceptable food. At the farthest end of the spectrum are the *fruitarians*, who not only avoid foods of animal origin but also those classified as vegetables and cereals. This leaves them with a diet of fruit, honey, and nuts.

Macrobiotic diets are vegetarian diets based on a balance of foods with "yin" (female) and "yang" (male) characteristics. Macrobiotic diets consist mostly of whole grains and vegetables but include the use of special teas, herbs, seaweed, and fermented soybean products. Most adherents to this diet participate in a variety of spiritual rituals and eat at least one daily meal in a communal setting. An extreme form is the Zen macrobiotic diet, which requires its followers to proceed in 7 to 10 steps to reduce the number and kinds of foods in the diet until only brown rice is consumed or a balance of "strong" and "weak" foods is achieved. Followers believe that any disease can be cured with this diet, because it theoretically rids the body of toxins. Although such a diet is lacking in vitamins, calcium, and high-quality protein, the lack of vitamin C is the first deficiency to be recognized. Scurvy, a vitamin C-deficiency disease, has been reported among those who adhere to the regimen, especially pregnant women and young children. The restricted fluid intake designed to "spare" the kidneys represents an additional hazard because this diet is high in sodium, which increases thirst and a need for fluid. The use of seawater (with its high salt content) to alleviate thirst only serves to make the problem worse.

In the Nationwide Food Consumption Survey, respondents were asked if they were vegetarians. Of the 2% to 3% who responded that they were, 90% reported eating animal foods over a 3-day period. These data suggest that the term "vegetarian" is not well understood by many people.

What are the nutritional consequences, if any, of eating a vegetarian diet rather than the omnivorous diet (animal and vegetable) diet consumed by most Americans? The answer depends on what degree of vegetarianism we are talking about and the age of the vegetarian.

The true vegetarian diet probably poses the greatest risks to the young growing child and to the pregnant woman. It *is* possible to put together a diet for a young child composed entirely of foods of vegetable origin that will supply nutrient needs except for calcium and vitamin B_{12}. However, such a diet is so bulky that it is unlikely that enough food would be consumed to meet the energy needs of a young child. As we discussed earlier, if the diet does not provide adequate energy, some of the protein that would normally be used for growth gets diverted to be used as an energy source. This is even more of a problem when the quality of the protein is marginal.

Thus we find that many young vegetarian children are at about the 5th percentile in weight and height for their age and sex; this means that 95% of the children in their age bracket are taller and heavier. Part of the growth retardation noticed in vegetarian children may reflect the low calcium content of their diet and the fact that calcium is poorly absorbed from vegetable foods, particularly those such as spinach and collards that contain **oxalic acid. Phytic acid** in whole-grain cereals also depresses calcium absorption. Because calcium is essential for bone and skeletal growth, it is easy to understand why there might be decreased stature among vegetarian children. The role of vitamin D in bone growth cannot be overlooked either. Studies in Boston have actually found cases of rickets, a vitamin D-deficiency disease, among vegetarian children who are not allowed to drink milk. In a northern city such as Boston, where exposure to ultraviolet rays of the sun, a nondietary source of vitamin D, is limited, fortified milk may be the only significant source of vitamin D.

In a vegetarian diet zinc, which is obtained primarily from animal foods, will be present in inadequate amounts; so will vitamin B_{12}, which comes only from animal foods. It is possible that a breast-fed child may build up a substantial store of vitamin B_{12} during the nursing period, enough to last through the first few postweaning years.

A lack of vitamin B_{12} could be a partial explanation for the "anemia" observed in certain people after relatively short periods on a meatless diet. Another factor contributing to anemia is the bulk or fiber content of the vegetarian diet, which tends to bind iron and other trace minerals and greatly reduces the amount absorbed. In addition, fiber stimulates the passage of food through the gastrointestinal tract, further reducing the absorption of trace elements and other nutrients. The total amount of iron in the vegetarian diet, which almost certainly falls below the 18 mg per day recommended for an adult woman, and the absence of meat, which normally enhances iron absorption, increase the possibility that a vegetarian diet will contribute to anemia in both women and children.

Why, then, do vegetarians feel that there are nutritional benefits that justify such a diet? For children, the disadvantages clearly seem to outweigh nutritional advantages. For adults, a concern over the relationship of cholesterol to heart disease frequently is the motivation to avoid meat products. Because cholesterol does not occur at all in foods of plant origin, it stands to reason that if no animal products are consumed, no cholesterol is being consumed either. For the mature individual, it is undoubtedly possible for the body to synthesize sufficient cholesterol to produce hormones and bile acids that require cholesterol.

In addition to being devoid of cholesterol, the vegetarian diet is often low in fat, with the only fat coming from whole-grain cereals, nuts, and the occasional use of avocados. If, however, vegetable salad oils and margarines are used to enhance palatability and increase the caloric density of vegetarian meals, the fat content will increase. Except for hydrogenated oils in margarines and the unlikely use of coconut oil or palm oil, the fatty acids in a vegetarian diet will be primarily unsaturated. Although there has been a general recommendation that the P/S (polyunsaturated to saturated fats) ratio of the diet should be close to 1, we know very little about the consequences of eating a diet in which the ratio is above that. There is now some evidence, however, that health problems may be associated with a very high P/S ratio because of the tendency of unsaturated fatty acids to oxidize to substances of unknown safety. This theory offers a possible explanation of the reported increase in colon cancer among those with very low serum cholesterol levels.

For adults, the advantages of a vegetarian diet are that it is low in calories, fat, and cholesterol; that it has a high P/S ratio; and that it has adequate fiber. These advantages must be weighed against the disadvantages of a decreased zinc content, poor availability of trace elements, almost no vitamin B_{12}, and low available calcium. In most cases the advantages and disadvantages more or less counterbalance one another.

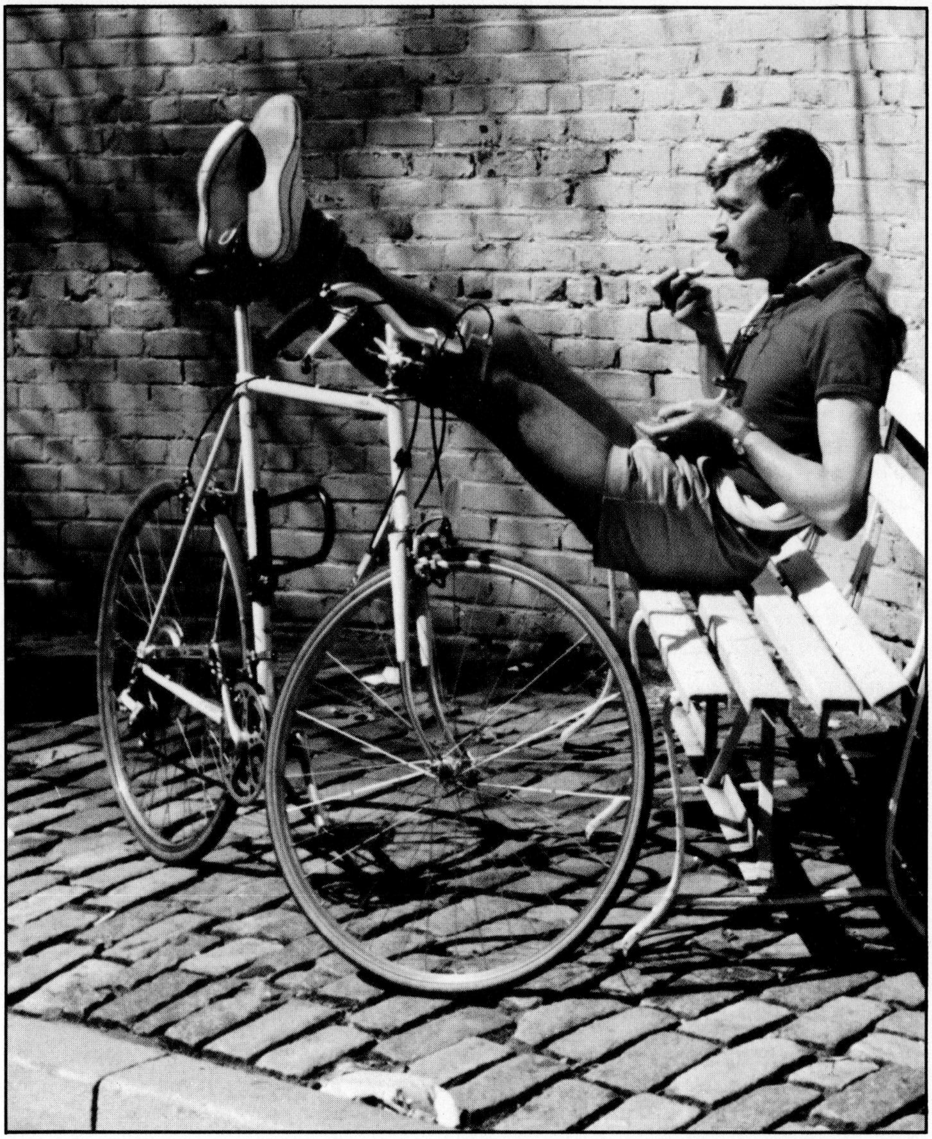

AWARENESS CHECK

Truth or Fiction?

- Calories have no function in the body; they only make people gain weight.
- Two people who weigh the same and are the same height will have the same basal energy requirement.
- Most people who are overweight have an underactive thyroid gland.
- Men usually have a higher caloric need than women.
- Studying very intently requires more calories than just reading for pleasure.
- Breast-feeding women have higher energy needs than pregnant women.

Energy Balance

CHAPTER 7

Energy and calories, or more correctly kilocalories, as they influence body weight, are among the nutrition topics that most concern the public. Moreover, there seem to be more "instant experts" on this subject than on any other in nutrition. Scientists are working to understand why there are differences in the energy requirements of apparently similar people and how people use energy. Meanwhile, however, the public is being bombarded with advice and help from many sources in solving their problems of energy balance. It isn't likely that researchers will find that the law of conservation of energy (that energy can be neither created or destroyed) can be repealed, but it is possible that their findings about energy metabolism will help us understand the complexities of adjusting energy intake to energy expenditure. With sedentary life-styles, there is concern that the decreased need for kilocalories will result in an intake of food that is deficient in other nutrients. There is also growing recognition that we should encourage moderate exercise programs to increase kilocalorie needs, so that they correspond more closely to our desire for food.

Although the terms *energy* and *calories* are synonymous, we find that the notions conjured up by these terms are quite different for different people. To the nutrition scientist, they represent the potential of a food to produce heat and the ability to do work; to most people, energy means pep and vitality; to the mother of the young child, calories give the child energy for growth and activity; to the athlete, they represent the "winning edge"; and to those who fear weight gain, calories are the food villains to be avoided.

As discussed in the previous three chapters, the carbohydrate, protein, lipid, and alcohol components of the diet are responsible for its energy content. In fact, they are the only energy sources that can be used by human beings. These four components account for different proportions of foods, varying from 4% in lettuce to 100% in sugar, salad oil, and dry gelatin. The remaining portion of the food consists of water, cellulose, minerals, and vitamins. None of these contributes energy, but they do influence the texture, bulk, and nutritional merits of food.

In the typical North American diet, carbohydrate provides 43% to 58% of the energy, protein provides 12%, and fat provides 30% to 45%. Figure 7-1 shows that the use of fat as a source of energy has increased constantly since the turn of

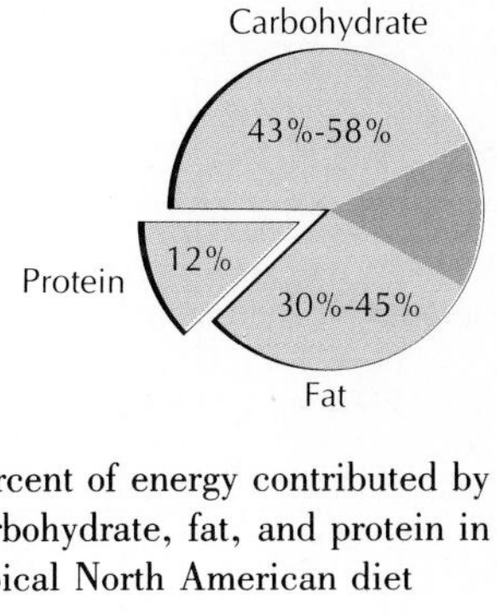

Percent of energy contributed by carbohydrate, fat, and protein in the typical North American diet

Figure 7-1 Trends in dietary sources of energy in the United States.

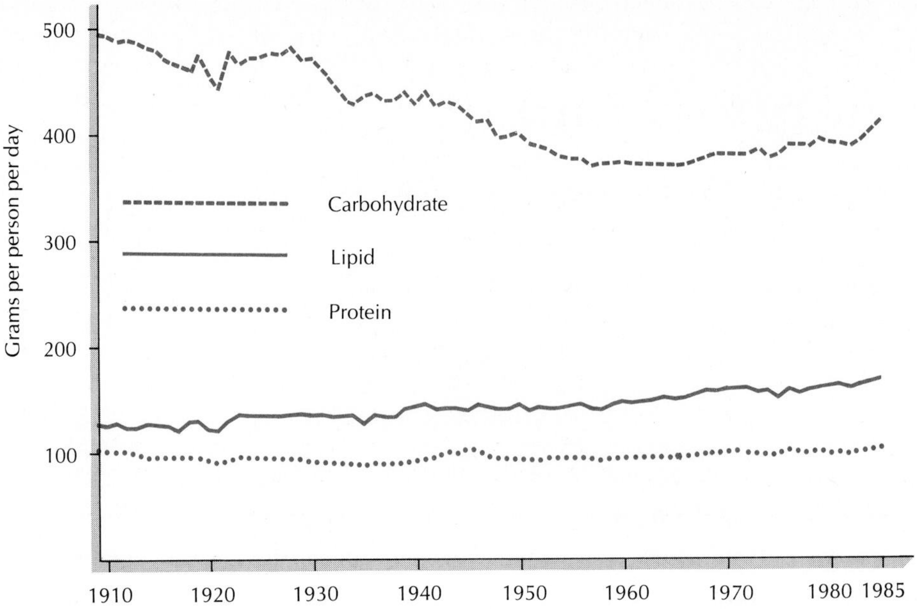

the century, while the use of carbohydrate has declined. Protein, however, has remained essentially constant.

The source of energy in diets varies, not only from one individual to another, but also among varying ethnic and socioeconomic groups. For example, in rice-eating countries carbohydrate makes a large contribution to the energy intake. In countries with an emphasis on dairying, protein assumes greater importance. In Italy, with the extensive use of cooking oil, more energy is derived from fats. In the United States the amount of money available for food has increased over the years, resulting in a greater use of protein and fat and a decreased use of complex carbohydrate. More recently, however, a growing concern about the potential of the world food supply and its ability to meet the needs of an expanding population has led many North Americans to reduce their intake of animal protein and substitute cereal grains. Similarly, those concerned about the relationship between fat and health problems such as cancer and heart disease are reducing their fat intake.

MEASURING ENERGY

kilocalorie (kcal)
Amount of heat required to raise the temperature of 1 kg of water 1° C (from 15° to 16° C)

1 kilocalorie = 1000 calories
1 calorie = 0.001 kilocalories

The energy value of a food is currently expressed in terms of a unit of heat, a **kilocalorie** (abbreviated as *kcal*). A kilocalorie represents the amount of heat required to raise the temperature of 1 kg (slightly over 1 quart) of water 1° C (from 15° to 16° C). This unit, often referred to as a *Calorie*, is correctly designated as a kilocalorie to distinguish it from a smaller unit, the *calorie*, which is equal to 0.001 kcal. However, most nutrition sources use the terms calorie, Calorie, and kilocalorie interchangeably, assuming that they are common enough in nutrition literature that no distinctions need to be made. We will use the term kilocalorie when referring to a specific number of kilocalories.

kilojoule (kJ)
Unit representing the amount of energy needed to move 1 kg of weight 1 meter, by a force of 1 Newton

1 kilocalorie = 4.18 kilojoules = 0.004 megajoules
1 kilojoule = 0.24 kilocalories

There is a growing trend, especially in Europe and Canada, to use the unit **kilojoule** to replace kilocalories. One kilojoule is defined as the energy involved in physically moving a 1 kg (2.2 lb) weight 1 meter (39 inches) by 1 Newton (a unit of force). If the kilojoule is ever universally adopted, we will have to multiply all values currently given in kilocalories by 4.18 or 4.2 (1 kcal = 4.18 kJ). Thus a 2000 kilocalorie diet would become an 8360 kilojoule diet. Some food scientists have suggested that we use a larger unit, the megajoule (mJ), which is equivalent to 1000 kilojoules. If this suggestion is accepted, we will use much smaller units of energy (2000 kcal = 8.36 megajoules).

Although the acceptance of the term kilojoules in American publications has been slow, if not nonexistent, it has been more widely used in British and European journals. It will undoubtedly be some time before the term calorie, as used in popular literature or in food labeling, is replaced by the more correct kilocalorie. It will probably be even longer before the concept of the kilojoule receives popular acceptance. It is important, however, for the nutrition student to be aware of the relationship between these two measurements of energy because many scientific publications are already reporting energy values in both calories (or kilocalories) and joules.

Energy available from food. An appreciation of the amount of energy or heat available from foods can be reached by noting that 2 tablespoons of sugar provide 100 kcal, which is enough heat to raise the temperature of slightly over 4 cups of water from 0° C (freezing) to 100° C (boiling). One tablespoon of fat or 4½ cups of shredded cabbage have a similar energy potential. In human beings as much as 80% of the energy obtained from food is converted into heat; the rest is used to support biochemical changes, shifts in body fluids, and other energy-requiring processes necessary for life.

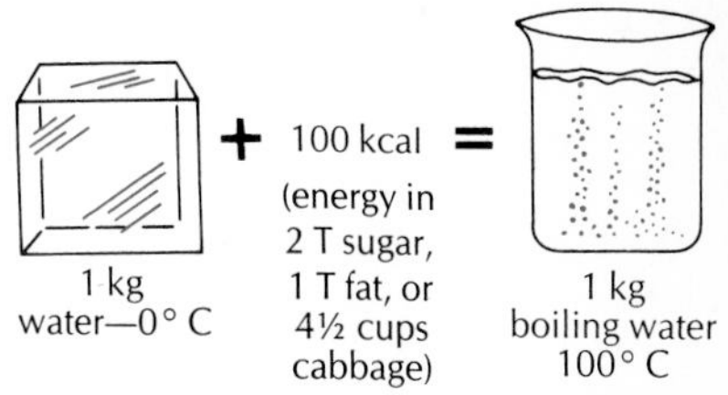

100 kcal provides enough heat to raise the temperature of 1 quart (1 kg) of water from freezing to boiling temperature

Direct Calorimetry

Much of our information about how much energy is in foods is obtained by a technique called **direct calorimetry,** or the direct measurement of heat. Direct calorimetry involves an instrument known as a *bomb calorimeter*, which is a highly insulated, compact, boxlike container, about 1 cubic foot in size. The essential features of a bomb calorimeter are shown in Figure 7-2. A precisely weighed dried sample of food is completely burned within the container, and the heat produced is absorbed by the water surrounding the chamber. By measuring the change in temperature of the known amount of water in the container, it is possible to calculate the number of kilocalories of heat produced by burning the sample. Because the bomb is well insulated, there is no exchange of heat with the surrounding air. Thus any change in the temperature of the water is due to the heat produced by the burning or oxidizing of the food sample.

direct calorimetry
The direct measurement of heat by recording the change in temperature of a known volume of water

Heat of Combustion

The energy value of a sample of food determined in a bomb calorimeter is known as the **heat of combustion,** that is, the maximum amount of energy that the sample is capable of yielding when it is completely burned or oxidized. When samples of carbohydrate, fat, and protein are burned, the amount of heat produced is always the same for each of these nutrients. Values of 4.1 kcal/gram of carbohydrate, 9.45 kcal/gram of fat, and 5.65 kcal/gram of protein are generally considered representative for foods in the North American diet.

heat of combustion
The maximum amount of heat that can be produced by burning a substance

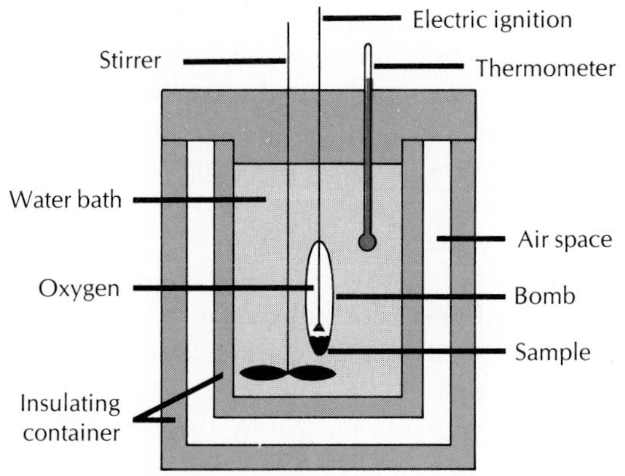

Figure 7-2 Cross section of a bomb calorimeter showing essential features. Food sample is completely burned in the inner section; heat produced is absorbed by the known volume of water in the surrounding section. Change in temperature provides measure of heat produced.

Energy stored in nitrogen is not available to the body

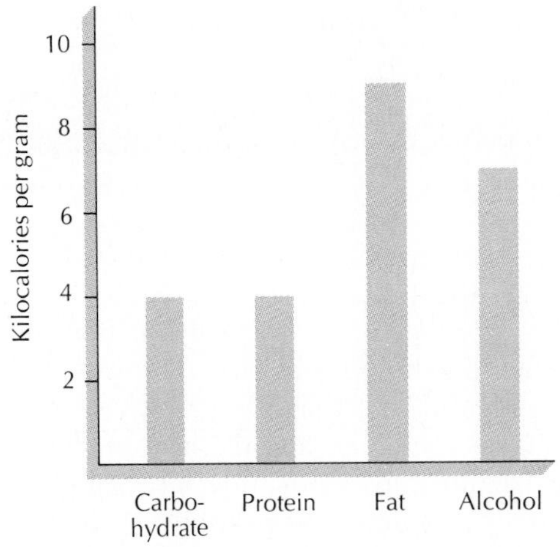

Amount of energy stored per gram of energy-yielding nutrients

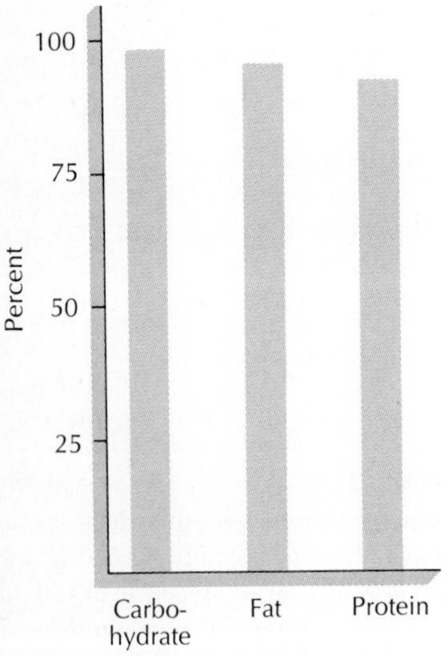

Coefficients of digestibility of energy sources

coefficient of digestibility
Percentage of a nutrient that is ultimately available for absorption and use by the body cells

However, the net heat of combustion in the human body is slightly different than that in the bomb calorimeter. In the calorimeter the heat of combustion comes from the energy produced by the oxidation of carbon to carbon dioxide, hydrogen to water, and nitrogen (from protein) to nitrous oxide. The body is capable of releasing the energy potential of carbon and hydrogen. It cannot, however, use the energy of nitrogen. Therefore the heat measured in the bomb calorimeter from the oxidation of nitrogen cannot be considered available to meet our energy needs. Because the oxidation of nitrogen accounts for 1.3 kcal of the 5.65 kcal/gram of protein, a potential of only 4.3 kcal/gram of protein remains available to the body.

Coefficient of Digestibility

Once food has been taken in, the body is not 100% efficient in digesting (preparing food for absorption) or absorbing nutrients. We must therefore take into account how much of the nutrients consumed actually become available to the cells. The extent of digestion varies from one nutrient to another and is further influenced by the food in which a nutrient is found. For example, the protein of egg, meat, or milk is more readily digested (or is more bioavailable) than protein from plant sources such as wheat, rice, and vegetables.

To calculate the potential energy from carbohydrate, fat, and protein representative **coefficients of digestibility** are used to express the percentage of the nutrient that is ultimately available. For carbohydrate, fat, and protein, the coefficients of digestibility are 0.98, 0.95, and 0.92, respectively, showing that 98%, 95%, and 92% of each is available for use by the body cells.

Table 7-1 ◇ Calculation of physiological fuel value of nutrients (kcal/gram)

	Carbohydrate	Fat	Protein	Alcohol
Heat of combustion	4.15	9.45	5.65	7
Energy from combustion of nitrogen unavailable to the body	—	—	1.30	—
Net heat of combustion	4.15	9.45	4.35	7
Coefficient of digestibility	0.98	0.95	0.92	1.00
Physiological fuel value (in kilocalories)	4.0	9.0	4.0	7
Physiological fuel value (in kilojoules)	17	38	17	30

Table 7-2 ◇ Calculation of energy value of 100 grams (¾ cup of ice cream) from proximate analysis (percentage composition)

Nutrient	Percent* in Food	Amount in 100 grams (grams) A	Energy Value/gram (kcal) B	Energy Value of 100 grams (kcal) A × B
Carbohydrate	24	24	4	96
Fat	10	10	9	90
Protein	4	4	4	16
TOTAL ENERGY				202

*Remaining 62% is made up of water, which does not provide energy.

Physiological Fuel Value

It is the **physiological fuel value,** or the amount of potential energy available, that is important in human nutrition. Calculations that combine information on the heat of combustion and the digestibility of a nutrient are summarized in Table 7-1. The factors 4, 9, 4, and 7 kcal, representing the amount of energy available to the body per gram of carbohydrate, fat, protein, and alcohol, respectively, are widely used in nutrition and dietetics to plan and evaluate diets.

physiological fuel value
The maximum amount of heat that the body can receive from oxidizing the energy components in food: carbohydrate, lipid, and protein

ENERGY VALUE OF FOODS

In addition to using calorimetry to determine the fuel value of a food, scientists are able to determine the energy-rich components in food. The amount of fat is determined directly by extracting and measuring the lipid chemically. Protein is estimated from an analysis for nitrogen and water by drying the food and comparing the dried weight to the wet weight. Carbohydrate is determined by the difference between the total weight of the food and that accounted for by lipid, water, protein, and crude fiber. Because carbohydrate values include some nonutilizable dietary fiber, they may be overestimated and hence be less accurate than the values for lipid and protein.

By knowing the amount of each of these components in a food and the physiological fuel value of each, it is possible to calculate the energy value of the food. For most foods, analytical data on the **proximate (approximate) composition**— the percentage of carbohydrate, fat, protein, fiber, and water in a typical sample— are included in tables of food composition such as those in Appendix F. Of these, neither fiber nor water is a source of calories.

proximate (approximate) composition
Expression used to describe the percentage of the macronutrients (lipid, carbohydrate, protein, fiber, and water) in a particular food

As the example in Table 7-2 shows, we may learn from tables of food composition that 100 grams of ice cream contains 4 grams of protein, 10 grams of fat, and 24 grams of usable carbohydrate—the only energy-yielding nutrients in food. Using

Calculation of Percent of Total Calories Contributed by One Nutrient Group

Problem

Given the information that a diet provides 2000 kcal and contains 200 grams of carbohydrate and 100 grams of fat, calculate the amount of protein and the percentage of calories from carbohydrate, protein, and fat in the diet.

Solution

Carbohydrate provides 200 × 4 = 800 kcal.

Fat provides 100 × 9 = 900 kcal.

Because protein is the only other component in food to provide calories, the remaining kilocalories were provided by protein.

2000 − (800 + 900) = 300 kcal

Because 4 kcal are provided by each gram of protein, 300 kcal would be provided by 300/4 = 75 grams protein.

The determination of the percentage of calories from a nutrient involves the following equation: $\frac{\text{Kcal from a nutrient}}{\text{Total kcal}} \times 100$

The percentage of kilocalories from carbohydrate is 800/2000 × 100 = 40%.

The percentage of kilocalories from fat is 900/2000 × 100 = 45%.

The percentage of kilocalories from protein is 300/2000 × 100 = 15%.

the physiological fuel values of 4, 9, and 4 kcal per gram, it is then a simple matter to calculate the energy value of a 100-gram sample of food. From the information that this food sample provided—202 kcal/100 grams or 2.0 kcal/gram—it is easy to calculate the energy value in any amount of this particular food (e.g., 30 grams of the food would have 2.0 × 30 = 60 kcal).

By knowing the total carbohydrate, fat, or protein content of the diet, one can determine the percentage of total calories contributed by any one nutrient group. In fact, as illustrated in the box above, by knowing any three of the four variables—carbohydrate, fat, protein, and total energy—one can calculate the unknown factor. This kind of information is used by dietitians, as well as those with special dietary needs such as diabetics, in prescribing or following certain diet restrictions.

Variation in Energy Value

The energy value of a serving of a particular food is determined by the amount of carbohydrate, fat, and protein composition it contains. The relation of these to the water and cellulose in a food determines its nutrient density, i.e., the relative amount of energy in a given volume of food. Foods with a high percentage of fat or foods of high caloric density such as mayonnaise are concentrated sources of kilocalories, as are foods with a low water content such as cheese. Because small amounts of such foods yield a relatively large number of kilocalories, they are often erroneously considered "fattening" foods. Although it is indeed easier to eat excess kilocalories from foods low in water or high in fat content, the foods themselves should not be condemned as fattening. Only the total diet can be described as fattening—and only then if its energy value exceeds the energy need of the person consuming it.

From Table 7-3, we can see the amounts of various foods required to provide 100 kcal and the size and caloric value of an average serving. It is clear that foods from the bottom of the list, such as butter, mayonnaise, or salad oil, will increase our caloric intake. These items with their concentrated calories are often used to enhance the palatability of foods relatively low in both fat and calories. On the other hand, foods such as apples or carrots from the top of the list will provide fewer calories but enough satisfaction by producing bulk in the stomach and requiring more chewing. Examples of the effects of methods of food preparation on the caloric value of foods are shown in Table 7-4.

The relationship between the weight of a food and its caloric value is evident in Table 7-5, showing relative energy in foods of the same weight. Foods low in water and high in fat are at the bottom of the list and have a high caloric density. Foods low in fat but high in water and cellulose are at the top of the list and are lower in calories.

The major contributions of various food groups to energy in the U.S. food supply are shown in the margin.

Contribution of Various Food Groups to the Energy Content of the U.S. Food Supply

Meat, fish, poultry, and eggs	22%
Cereal products	20%
Fats and oils	20%
Sugar	18%
Dairy products	10%
Vegetables	5%
Fruits	3%
Other	1%

Marston RM, and Raper NR: Nutrient content of the U.S. food supply (1984), National Food Review, Winter, 1985.

Table 7-3 ◇ Size and caloric value of an average serving of food and the amount of food needed to provide 100 kcal

Food	Average Serving	Kcal/Serving	Amount to Provide 100 kcal
Lettuce	⅛ head	10	1¼ heads
Cabbage	½ cup	10	5 cups, shredded
Asparagus	4 spears	15	25 spears
Carrots	1 medium	30	3½ medium
Sugar	1 tablespoon	50	2 tablespoons
Bread	1 slice	70	1½ slices
Apple	1 medium	80	1¼ apples (7 cm in diameter)
Egg	1 large	80	1¼ large
Potato	1 medium	85	1⅓ medium
Nonfat milk	1 cup	90	1+ cup
Pear	1 medium	100	1
Dates	4	100	4
Butter	1 tablespoon	100	1 tablespoon
Mayonnaise	1 tablespoon	100	1 tablespoon
Banana	1 medium	105	1 small
Salad oil	1 tablespoon	120	⅚ tablespoon
Whole milk	1 cup	150	⅔ cup
Chicken breast	one	160	1.7 oz
Pork chop	one	305	0.9 oz

From Nutritive value of foods, Home and Garden Bulletin No. 72, Agriculture Research Service, Washington, D.C., 1985, U.S. Department of Agriculture.

Table 7-4 ◇ Effect of method of preparation on energy value of an average serving of a single food

Food	Kcal	Food	Kcal
Apple	80	Potato (1 medium)	
Applesauce	195	Boiled	120
Baked apple	225	Baked with skin	150
Apple pie	330	French fried (10 strips)	160
Apple crisp	350	Mashed with 1 tsp butter	170
Apple pie à la mode	440	Baked (served with 1 pat butter)	195
		Creamed	210

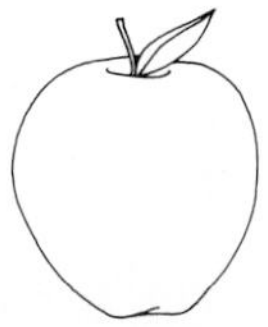

Apple
80 kcal

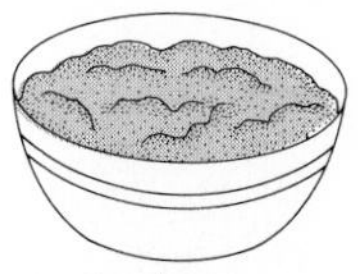

Apple crisp
350 kcal

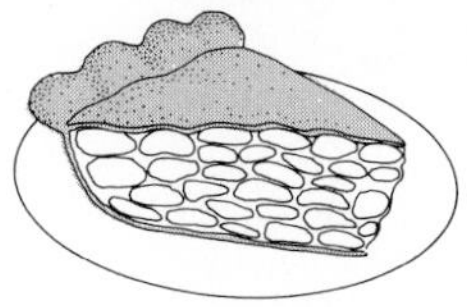

Apple pie
330 kcal

Method of food preparation influences the amount of energy in a food

Table 7-5 ◇ Caloric value and measure of 100-gram (3.5-oz) portions of food

Food	Serving Size	Caloric Value/100 grams
Lettuce	½ head	14
Asparagus	6 spears	20
Cabbage	1½ cups, shredded	24
Carrots	1½	42
Nonfat milk or buttermilk	⅖ cup	36
Milk	3.7% fat; ⅖ cup	66
Peas	⅝ cup	68
Potato	1 small	90
Lamb	1 serving	197
Chicken	1 serving	208
Pork	1 serving	236
Bread	4 slices	250
Dates	10	274
Sugar	½ cup	400
Butter	7 T	716
Mayonnaise	7 T	718
Salad oil	7 T	884

From Adams C: Nutritive value of American foods, USDA Handbook No. 456, Washington, D.C., 1975, USDA, updated with values from Handbook Nos. 8-1 to 8-16, 1976-87.

Table 7-6 ◇ Proximate analysis of diabetic food exchange groups (1986)

Exchange	Carbohydrate (grams)	Protein (grams)	Lipid (grams)	Energy (kcal)
Nonfat milk	12	8	0	80
Vegetables	5	2	0	25
Fruit	15	0	0	60
Bread	15	3	0	80
Lean meat	0	7	3	55
Fat	0	0	5	45

With permission of the American Diabetes Association and the American Dietetics Association, 1986.

Exchange Lists

Because diabetics must regulate their caloric, carbohydrate, fat, and protein intake, the American Diabetes Association and the American Dietetic Association have developed exchange lists so that they do not need to constantly calculate their intake of energy and nutrients. This exchange system is also useful to nondiabetics and people on other therapeutic diets to help them regulate their energy intake or to know the approximate amount of carbohydrate, lipid, or protein in their diets. Exchanges are for six major food groupings. Within each group, the foods are similar in carbohydrate, lipid, protein, and energy content. The approximate content of each group is shown in Table 7-6; the complete exchange lists can be found in Appendix I.

THE BODY'S NEED FOR ENERGY

The body needs energy for a wide range of interrelated functions: for growth involving the synthesis of muscle, hormones, and the body's structural materials; for activity; and for internal work such as respiration, circulation, digestion, the secretion of hormones, and the maintenance of body temperature. A person's need for energy, however, can be grouped into three distinct categories, each of which can be estimated separately. These needs are for basal metabolism, activity, and the thermic effect of food. All of these in turn are a function either directly or indirectly of a person's size; a larger person always has higher total requirements than a smaller person with similar activity. In general, the requirement for energy is the average amount required over time to balance expenditure, maintain appropriate body weight in adults, promote adequate growth in children or contribute to adequate development of the fetus, and facilitate milk production in pregnant and lactating women. If there is a consistent pattern of imbalance between energy intake and expenditure over long periods of time (i.e., intake is always in excess of expenditure or vice versa), there will be a change in body weight and composition. With extra energy intake there will be a gain in weight and usually fat; with too little energy intake, there will be a loss of both weight and fat. With an increased energy expenditure and decreased intake there may be a loss of body fat but an increase in muscle.

TOTAL ENERGY NEED =
BASAL METABOLISM
+
ACTIVITY NEED
+
THERMIC EFFECT OF FOOD

Basal Metabolism

Basal metabolism is a measure of the minimum amount of energy needed to carry on the vital body processes, without which life is impossible. The basal metabolic energy need includes the amount of energy for the minimum rate of respiration to provide sufficient oxygen to maintain life; it also includes energy for a minimum rate of circulation to carry oxygen and nutrients to the cells and waste products away from the cells. As long as there is life, glands such as the thyroid, the adrenals, the pancreas, and the pituitary produce and secrete hormones that control cellular metabolism. The synthesis and secretion of these substances into the bloodstream require energy.

basal metabolism
The minimum amount of energy needed to carry on the vital body processes; basal energy needs include needs for respiration, circulation, glandular activity, and muscle tonus

No matter how relaxed a person may be, the body is still in a state of muscular contraction or muscular elasticity. Without this muscle tone, the body would become a shapeless mass of protoplasm. The energy required to maintain muscle tonus is also included when basal metabolic needs are assessed. In addition, metabolic processes such as the uptake of nutrients, the synthesis of new compounds, the excretion of waste, and the maintenance of the internal environment of the cells are constantly going on as long as the cell is living. The minimum amount of energy to maintain this cellular activity is also included in basal metabolism, as is energy needed to maintain the nervous system.

Measurement of Basal Metabolism

Basal metabolism can be measured in the same way that we measure the energy in food—by direct calorimetry. More common, however, is **indirect calorimetry,** which measures oxygen used rather than heat produced to assess energy used. A third test, which is a clinical evaluation of T_3 and T_4 (thyronine and thyroxine) in a blood sample, will give relative but not exact energy costs.

indirect calorimetry
The measurement of energy need by calculating the energy equivalent of the amount of oxygen used

Direct calorimetry to measure basal metabolism involves the measurement of the heat given off by the body in a human calorimeter or respiration chamber, a small insulated room that operates on the same principle as the bomb calorimeter. By measuring the change in temperature of a known volume of water circulating in pipes in the top and walls of the chamber, it is possible to determine the amount of heat produced by a subject inside it.

direct calorimetry
The measurement of energy need by measuring the heat produced

In addition, the exchange of carbon dioxide and oxygen that takes place is often measured. This allows the calculation of a **respiratory quotient (RQ),** which is the ratio of CO_2 produced to O_2 consumed. From the RQ, we can determine whether carbohydrate, fat, or protein was used for energy. If carbohydrate is the sole source of fuel, the RQ is 1. Fat has an RQ of 0.7. Protein has an RQ of 0.8, depending on the amino acid mixture. Under basal conditions, in which both fatty acids and glucose are being used as energy sources, the RQ is usually 0.82. Because the cost of operating a respiration calorimeter is high and there are few available,

respiratory quotient (RQ)
The ratio of CO_2 exhaled to O_2 inhaled

A

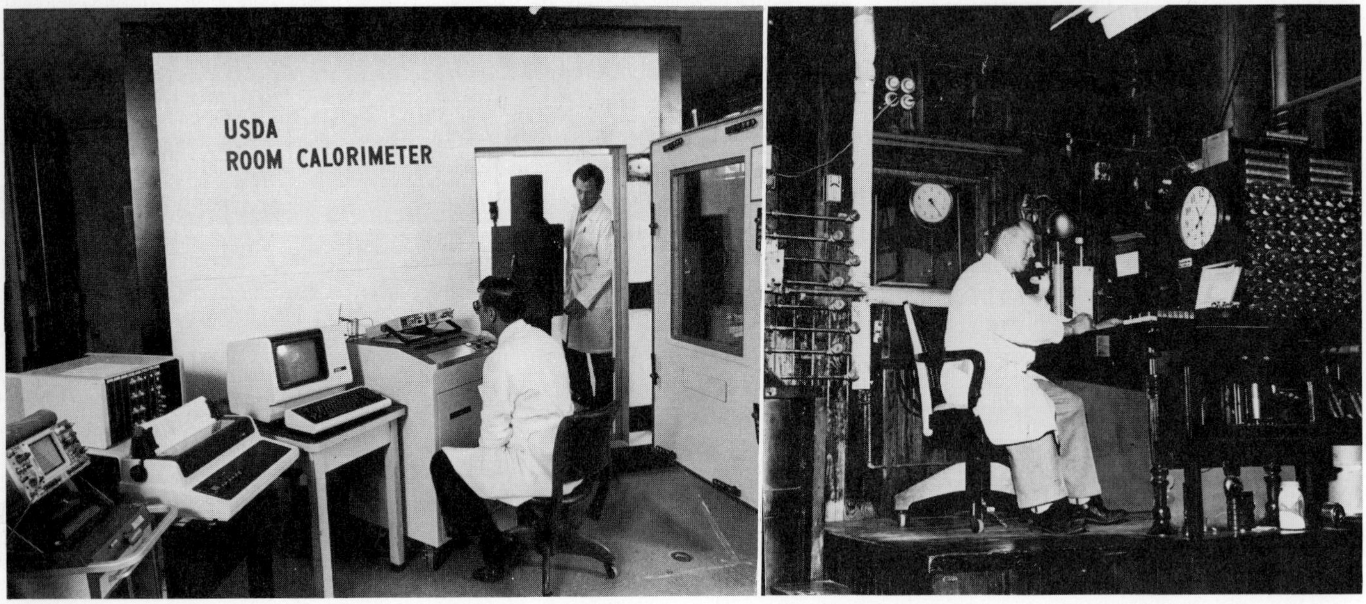

B

Figure 7-3 **A,** New room calorimeter at the USDA in Washington, D.C. **B,** Armsby calorimeter at the Pennsylvania State University.
A, courtesy USDA, Beltsville, MD; photo by Fred S. Witte.

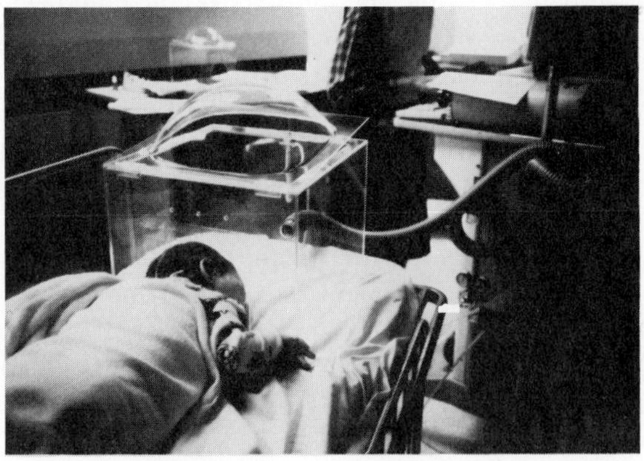

Figure 7-4 Indirect calorimetry using the dilution technique. Air is drawn past a person's head while under a canopy, allowing long periods of comfortable testing.
Courtesy Dr. V. Stallings and J. Tomezsko, Children's Hospital of Philadelphia.

they are used only under carefully controlled experimental conditions. Figure 7-3 shows the newest calorimeter, built in 1983 at the USDA Nutrition Center in Beltsville, Maryland, and the Armsby Calorimeter, built at the Pennsylvania State University at the turn of the century. Although the USDA chamber is more modern in appearance and many of its functions are automated and computerized, it is no more sensitive in measuring energy output than the earlier models.

A modification of the respiration chamber, the metabolic chamber, measures the heat given off by the subject with thermocouples and heat-exchange disks attached to the skin. Any changes in temperature are recorded on instruments outside the chamber. Both types of chamber can be used for determinations of basal energy needs, and they also are used to assess the energy costs of activities that can be performed in a limited space. Figure 7-4 illustrates the use of one type of metabolic chamber.

Indirect calorimetry is a much simpler, less costly method in which energy needs are determined by measuring oxygen consumption. For many years the Benedict Roth respiration apparatus was the standard machine used for this purpose. This apparatus is a closed-circuit system in which the subject receives oxygen only

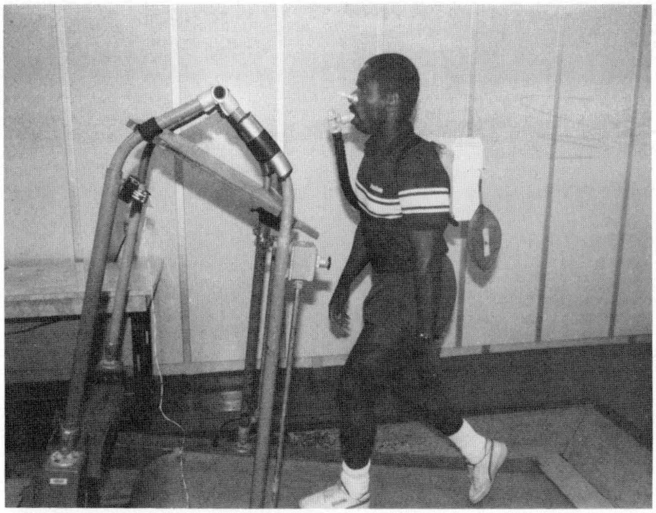

Figure 7-5 Respiration meter used to measure energy expenditure during mild exercise. Subject breathes room air; total expired air volume is measured; aliquot or sample is analyzed for CO_2 and O_2.
Courtesy Joseph Loomis.

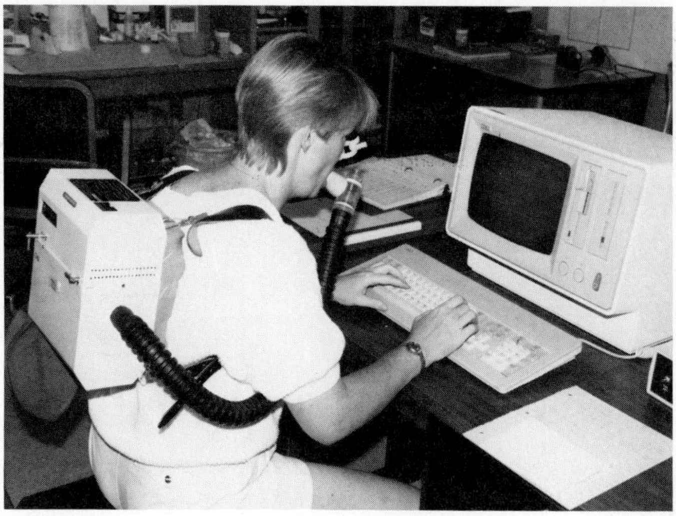

Figure 7-6 Open-circuit respirometer used to measure energy expenditure in sedentary activity.

from a measured source of oxygen-rich air and exhales into a container in which the carbon dioxide and water are removed and the remaining oxygen and nitrogen are recirculated. By measuring the volume of oxygen in the air mixture before and after the standard 6-minute test, the amount of oxygen consumed can be readily calculated. Because the use of 1 liter of oxygen represents 4.82 kcal when the RQ under basal conditions is 0.82, it is possible to calculate the caloric equivalent of a known volume of oxygen.

Open-circuit indirect calorimetry, which involves the use of room air and a determination of the amount of carbon dioxide produced from it during a test period, is an equally good way to determine oxygen used. From this information, the energy used during a specific period can be calculated. The open-circuit method is even less expensive and reduces the possibility of stimulation in metabolism from the use of oxygen-rich air. Typical instruments used in this test are shown in Figure 7-5 and Figure 7-6. Again, these can be used to determine both basal and activity energy costs.

Measurements of Basal Metabolism
Direct—heat production
Respiration calorimeter
Metabolic chamber
Indirect—O_2 intake/CO_2 expenditure

The actual measurement of basal energy requirements by either direct or indirect calorimetry must be done under basal conditions, which require that the subject be awake, lying down, and both emotionally and physically relaxed and have not eaten for at least 12 hours. Data from many actual basal metabolic tests have given us enough information to predict basal energy needs from measurements of body height and weight and other measurements derived from these. There are four formulas (illustrated in Table 7-7) that are appropriate for estimating energy costs of basal activities. The first and simplest (Method A) is most appropriate for persons of average body build and hence body composition. It involves a factor of 1 kcal/kg body weight/hr for men and 0.9 kcal/kg body weight/hr for women. When this formula is applied to someone whose body build is either more fat or muscular than average, it is increasingly less satisfactory, apparently because the simple measurement of body weight does not reflect body composition, which influences energy needs.

More precise formulas developed in 1909 by Harris and Benedict (Method B), using information on height, weight, age, and sex, are still considered one of the

Table 7-7 ◇ Comparison of methods of estimating basal metabolic needs*

Method	Subject A	Subject B
A. Body weight 1 kcal/kg/hr	1440	2400
B. Harris-Benedict equation (for males)† 66.5 + [13.5 × wt (kg)] + [5.0 × ht (cm)] − [6.75 × Age]	1968	2643
C. Metabolic body size 70 × wt in $kg^{3/4}$	1694	2212
D. FAO/WHO/UNU equation (for males)‡ 11.6 × wt (kg) + 879	1691	2039

* *A* and *B* are both 50-year-old men and are 5′10″ (178 cm) tall. *A* weighs 154 lb (70 kg) and *B* weighs 220 lb (100 kg).
† For females: Resting energy expenditure (REE) = 655.1 + [9.56 × wt (kg)] + [1.85 × ht (cm)] − [4.68 × age (yr)].
‡ For females: 8.7 × w + (kg) + 829 (Table 7-8).

Table 7-8 ◇ FAO/WHO/UNU equations for predicting basal metabolic rate from body weight (W)

Age Range (Years)	Kcal/Day	Age Range (Years)	$Kcal_{th}$/Day
Males		**Females**	
0-3	60.9 W − 54	0-3	61.0 W − 51
3-10	22.7 W + 495	3-10	22.5 W + 499
10-18	17.5 W + 651	10-18	12.2 W + 746
18-30	15.3 W + 679	18-30	14.7 W + 496
30-60	11.6 W + 879	30-60	8.7 W + 829
>60	13.5 W + 487	>60	10.5 W + 596

From report of a joint FAO/WHO/UNU Expert Consultation: Energy and protein requirements, Technical Report Series 724, Geneva, 1985.

best predictors of basal energy needs. The Harris-Benedict formulas are for males over 10 years of age and for females of all ages. Although it has been used for almost one century, it is still considered one of the most valid predictors available.

Metabolic body size = Body weight in $kg^{3/4}$ (1 kg = 2.2 lbs)

Basal metabolism = 70 × Metabolic body size (wt in $kg^{3/4}$)

Estimates based on body surface area, which is believed to reflect body composition but which requires a chart involving height and weight measurements in its determination (in square meters), has been largely replaced by a formula based on metabolic body size, or biological body weight (Method C). Biological body size is represented by body weight in $kg^{3/4}$. Basal metabolism is predicted to be 70 × metabolic body size (equivalents of some body weights are given in Table 7-9). Values for energy needs obtained this way are remarkably applicable for quite different body builds and can be applied to almost all animals.

After an extensive evaluation of both energy and protein requirements, an expert committee of FAO/WHO/UNU (Food and Agricultural Organization, World Health Organization, and the United Nations University) developed a set of formulas (Method D) based on body weight for estimating the energy requirements of six age groups for both males and females (Table 7-8). As seen from Table 7-7, however, estimates based on these various methods may differ by as much as 30%.

Table 7-9 ◆ Body weights in pounds, kilograms (kg), and metabolic body size $(kg)^{3/4}$

Pounds	Kilograms	Metabolic Body Size $(kg)^{3/4}$	Pounds	Kilograms	Metabolic Body Size $(kg)^{3/4}$
11	5	3.3	100	45	17.4
22	10	5.6	110	50	18.8
33	15	7.6	332	60	21.6
26	20	9.5	154	70	24.2
31	25	11.2	176	80	26.7
35	30	12.8	198	90	29.2
77	35	14.4	220	100	31.6
88	40	15.9			

To calculate metabolic body size—wt$(kg)^{3/4}$ (D):

1. Calculate A = wt in kg = wt in pounds/2.2
2. Calculate B = A × A × A
3. Calculate C = square root of B
4. Calculate D = square root of C

Factors Affecting Basal Energy Needs

Body Composition

All body tissues are metabolically active, being constantly broken down and repaired and participating in vital functions. However, they do this at different rates. Muscle, the brain, glands, and organs such as the liver are relatively active metabolically, consuming large amounts of oxygen per unit of weight and producing more heat. On the other hand, bones and adipose tissue, although far from static, are relatively inactive tissues and require less oxygen per unit of weight to maintain normal metabolic activity. Energy requirements per unit of body weight are higher when weight is made up of a higher proportion of muscle tissue; they are lower when fat or bone predominate.

Body Condition

A person in good physical condition has usually developed more muscle tissue than someone who has not had much exercise. Let us compare two men, both the same height and weight. One of them is an accountant in an essentially sedentary occupation. The other is a construction worker whose work requires much physical activity. The weight of the less active person represents less muscle and more fat than that of the physically active person. Therefore the accountant's basal metabolic needs are lower.

Sex

Differences in body composition between men and women of the same age, height, and weight have been documented. Women characteristically develop more adipose tissue and less musculature than men. This is reflected in basal metabolic rates for women, which are 5% lower than those for men.

Hormone Secretions

Hormones are synthesized by various glands of the endocrine system that secrete them into the bloodstream within the body, to be carried to various tissues to help control and maintain balance among many body functions. The secretions of the adrenal and thyroid glands have more influence on basal energy needs than any other single factor. Both glands have a stimulating effect. The secretion of the adrenal gland, which is called epinephrine or adrenaline, is produced in response to intense emotional stimuli such as anger or fear. The stimulation in metabolism that results from the production of more epinephrine is intense but of short duration, with metabolism returning to normal levels in 2 or 3 hours.

hypothyroidism
Undersecretion of thyroxin

hyperthyroidism
Oversecretion of thyroxin

parathyroidectomy
Removal of part of the thyroid gland

exophthalmic goiter
Hyperthyroidism; high basal metabolic rate because of excess secretion of thyroxin (in contrast to simple goiter, which is the enlargement of the thyroid gland because of lack of iodine to produce thyroxin)

Although it is not the only possible cause, any marked deviation from predicted basal energy needs is usually attributed to oversecretion or undersecretion of the thyroid gland. **Hypothyroidism** results from the below-normal secretion of thyroxine, the iodine-containing hormone of the thyroid gland, and may be reflected in a basal metabolic rate that is depressed as much as 30%. This means that the energy required for vital body functions is 30% below the energy needed by a person with normal thyroid activity. People with hypothyroidism have low energy needs and gain weight easily. The depressed secretion can be counteracted by the careful use of thyroxin pills, which are available only under medical supervision. Conversely, **hyperthyroidism** is characterized by an above-normal thyroxin secretion and may elevate basal metabolism as much as 50% to 75%. This means that the energy available for basal needs alone is 50% to 75% above predicted levels. Hyperthyroidism is more difficult to correct because the drugs that interfere with the production of thyroxin or the uptake of iodine, which is needed to synthesize an essential part of thyroxin, are very difficult to control. Alternative approaches to treatment are **parathyroidectomy** (removal of part of the thyroid gland) or a limitation in iodine intake to reduce the amount available. Deviations in basal metabolism that exceed 20% of predicted levels almost always indicate some problem in thyroid functioning. People with hyperthyroidism, also known as **exophthalmic goiter,** have high energy requirements and have trouble gaining weight.

Sleep

Measurements and estimates of basal metabolism are made when a subject is awake but muscularly and emotionally relaxed. During sleep both muscular and emotional relaxation is even greater, which causes a further drop in energy needs. However, these energy savings may be counteracted by the energy expended in tossing and turning during sleep.

Age

Changes in Basal Metabolic Needs with Age for Men (1.8 m, or 5 ft 10 in, tall)

18-30 yr	24.8 kcal/kg/day
30-60 yr	23.9 kcal/kg/day
>60 yr	20.3 kcal/kg/day

The basal metabolic rate changes with age. The rate is high at birth, increases until the subject is 2 years of age, and then gradually declines except for a rise at puberty. The decline in basal energy needs between ages 25 and 35 amounts to only 35 kcal/day for a 132-pound (60-kg) person, but between ages 35 and 55 there is a more significant decline of 145 kcal/day. Those who fail to adjust their caloric intake to reflect reduced basal energy needs will experience a slow and insidious gain in weight.

Pregnancy

During the sixth to ninth months of pregnancy, basal metabolism increases to 20% above normal. This is caused either by the high metabolic activity of the fetus and placenta or by an increase of metabolic activity in maternal tissues.

Undernutrition

After prolonged caloric undernutrition, basal energy use may be as low as 20% below predicted levels. This apparently reflects the body's adaptive efforts to conserve energy when kilocalories are restricted. This adaptation may explain the ability of persons in areas of chronic undernutrition to maintain their body weight on caloric intakes below predicted needs. Because starvation is not experienced by many North Americans, this adaptation is seldom seen in the United States, but it is common in developing countries.

Body Temperature

Because heat acts as a catalyst to almost all chemical reactions, it is not surprising to find that basal metabolism increases with an increase in body temperature. A rise of 1° F in body temperature leads to an average increase of 7% in basal

Table 7-10 ◇ Factors affecting basal metabolism

Factors That Increase Basal Metabolism	Factors That Decrease Basal Metabolism
Increase in muscle mass	Increase in body fat
Good physical condition	Poor physical condition
Being a male	Being a female
Hyperthyroidism	Hypothyroidism
Pregnancy	Sleep
Puberty	Aging
Extremes of environmental temperature	Undernutrition

metabolism (13% for 1° C), although increases as high as 15% have been observed. It is obvious, then, that a person with a fever has an increased need for energy.

Environmental Temperature

Lowest basal metabolism readings are obtained at an environmental temperature of 78° F (26° C), with higher readings reported at both higher and lower environmental temperatures. A temporary decrease in environmental temperature, not compensated for by additional clothing, will cause shivering and a temporary **thermogenesis,** or heat production, which increases basal metabolic needs as the body attempts to produce more heat to counteract the effect of lower temperatures. This is known as *cold-induced thermogenesis*. Infants who have proportionately higher amounts of the type of fat known as brown fat are able to produce heat to maintain body temperature through a process of metabolic stimulation called *nonshivering thermogenesis*.

thermogenesis
The production of heat

Smoking

Recent research indicates that the reason people who stop smoking have a tendency to gain weight can be attributed to the fact that the nicotine associated with smoking tends to increase the basal metabolic rate by approximately 10%. This dispels a widely held belief that this phenomenon is due to the depression of appetite by nicotine.

In summary, many factors such as body composition, hormonal secretions, sleep, and previous nutritional status influence basal metabolism; for most persons, however, an accurate estimate of needs can be made on the basis of body weight, or metabolic body size. The effects of various factors on basal energy needs are summarized in Table 7-10. For many individuals, especially those engaged in sedentary or moderate activity, basal energy needs account for 50% to 70% of their total caloric requirements.

Resting Energy Expenditure

The term **resting energy expenditure,** often referred to as **REE,** is being used increasingly in place of basal metabolism. Instead of representing just the bare minimum of energy needed to maintain vital body processes, resting energy expenditure includes, in addition, sufficient energy for sedentary activities and the energy needed for the digestion of food. REE is usually considered to be 10% above basal energy needs. The terms *resting metabolic rate* (RMR) and *resting metabolic expenditure* (RME) are used interchangeably with REE.

resting energy expenditure (REE)
The energy needed for vital body processes plus the small amount needed for sedentary activities (sedentary = "sitting")

The FAO/WHO/UNU committee came up with a slightly higher estimate for the energy cost of maintenance activities such as washing, dressing, and short periods of standing. They term this *baseline energy need* or *survival requirement*. They assume that these activities have an energy cost of 1.4 × basal needs, and that the individual spends two thirds of his or her time in these activities and

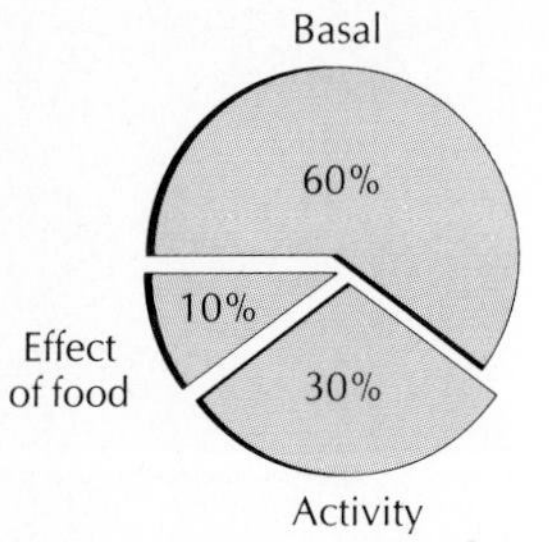

Distribution of energy needs

one third sleeping, to arrive at a requirement of 1.27 × basal [(⅔ × 1.4) + (⅓ × 1.0)]. In either case, there is agreement that the cost of taking care of minimal body activities is greater than the cost of maintaining the body in a resting, postabsorptive state.

Activity

Energy costs for activity include the amount of energy needed for all the muscles involved in the activity plus a small amount of energy to take care of the increase in heart rate and breathing that takes place during strenuous activity. For many activities, energy costs depend on body size and the relative severity of the exercise.

The actual cost of various activities has been determined by a series of tests that measure the amount of oxygen consumed and therefore the energy used in performing a specific activity (Figure 7-7). This information has been used to compile tables such as Table 7-11, which includes the average energy cost per kilogram of body weight per hour for a wide range of activities. If you want to

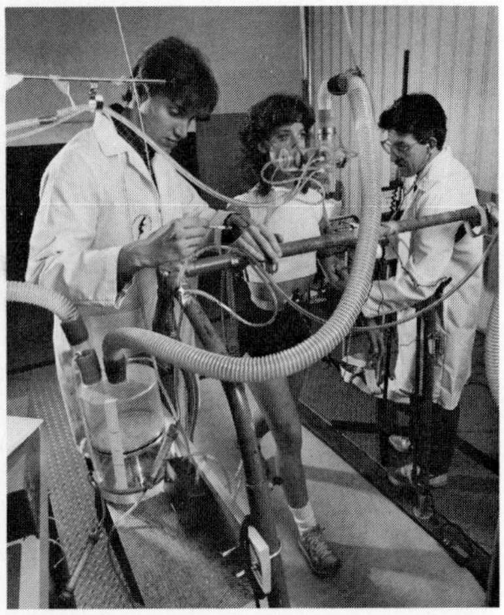

Figure 7-7 Energy cost of activity is determined by measuring the amount of oxygen used and the carbon dioxide excreted as a subject is walking on a treadmill. Other tests are being made at the same time.

Courtesy Dr. E. Buskirk and J. Loomis, Human Performance Laboratory, Pennsylvania State University.

Table 7-11 ◇ Energy cost of activities exclusive of basal metabolism and influence of food

Activity	Kcal/kg/hr	Activity	Kcal/kg/hr
Bicycling (century run)	7.6	Piano playing (Liszt's "Tarantella")	2.0
Bicycling (moderate speed)	2.5	Reading aloud	0.4
Bookbinding	0.8	Rowing in race	16.0
Boxing	11.4	Running	7.0
Carpentry (heavy)	2.3	Sawing wood	5.7
Cello playing	1.3	Sewing, hand	0.4
Crocheting	0.4	Sewing, foot-driven machine	0.6
Dancing, foxtrot	3.8	Sewing, motor-driven machine	0.4
Dancing, waltz	3.0	Shoemaking	1.0
Dishwashing	1.0	Singing in a loud voice	0.8
Dressing and undressing	0.7	Sitting quietly	0.4
Driving automobile	0.9	Skating	3.5
Eating	0.4	Standing at attention	0.6
Fencing	7.3	Standing relaxed	0.5
Horseback riding, walk	1.4	Stone masonry	4.7
Horseback riding, trot	4.3	Sweeping with broom, bare floor	1.4
Horseback riding, gallop	6.7	Sweeping with carpet sweeper	1.6
Ironing (5-pound iron)	1.0	Sweeping with vacuum sweeper	2.7
Knitting sweater	0.7	Swimming (2 mph)	7.9
Laundry, light	1.3	Tailoring	0.9
Lying still, awake	0.1	Typewriting rapidly	1.0
Organ playing (30% to 40%	1.5	Violin playing	0.6
of energy hand work)		Walking (3 mph)	2.0
Painting furniture	1.5	Walking rapidly (4 mph)	3.4
Paring potatoes	0.6	Walking at high speed (5.3 mph)	9.3
Playing ping-pong	4.4	Walking downstairs	*
Piano playing (Mendelssohn's	0.8	Walking upstairs	†
songs)		Washing floors	1.2
Piano playing (Beethoven's	1.4	Writing	0.4
"Apassionata")			

From Taylor CM, and McLeod G: Rose's laboratory handbook for dietetics, ed. 5, New York, 1949. The Macmillan Co., p. 18.

To estimate energy costs of activities not listed here, choose one that involves a comparable amount of muscular activity.

*Allow 0.012 kcal/kg for an ordinary staircase with 15 steps without regard to time.

†Allow 0.036 kcal/kg for an ordinary staircase with 15 steps without regard to time.

estimate the energy cost of an activity that is not listed, you can substitute for it an activity in the table that involves similar muscles and a similar degree of exertion. This table is fairly accurate for activities such as walking and running, in which moving the whole body accounts for 75% of energy costs; on the other hand, it probably overestimates energy costs for activities like knitting or piano playing, which involve moving only a small portion of the total body mass and for which energy costs are not proportional to body size. Alternative tables such as Table 7-12, which provides information on the energy cost of an activity only in terms of the time spent on it, are more accurate for activities in which energy costs are not directly proportional to body size. In addition, this table will underestimate the energy cost for a large person when the activity involves moving the whole body, as in playing tennis. The usefulness of either table depends on the accuracy of the record of the kinds of activities and of the amount of time spent on each.

Before using the tables, it is important to recognize their limitations. Although the energy costs do represent the best average estimates available, they do not reflect the differences in efficiency when various people perform the same task. We also know that while a 198-pound (90-kg) man requires more energy to walk a mile than a 132-pound (60-kg) man does, the increase is not 50% more, as would be predicted from the use of the tables. Because the energy costs recorded in the tables were derived from very few observations, they should not be considered "precise" measures of the energy cost of an activity each and every time it's done, any more than the values for apples in tables of food composition should be thought to represent all apples. In addition, it is important to know if the person engaged in the activity did it constantly or only intermittently. For example: is someone who reports swimming for an hour actually in motion the whole time or resting a good portion of it? Discrepancies such as this have been found to account for the differences in energy expenditure in the obese and nonobese, who both report being involved in the same activity for the same time.

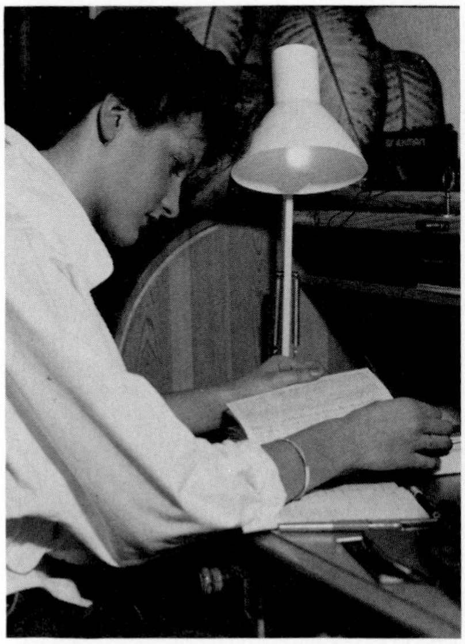

Although you work hard studying in college, this mental "energy" unfortunately does not burn any more calories than daydreaming, reading for pleasure, or watching TV

Many people are dismayed to learn how few kilocalories are actually involved in some activities that they consider relatively strenuous. For example, the energy cost of walking 3 miles in an hour is only 2 kcal/kg of body weight/hr more than that of merely being awake. Thus a 132-pound (60-kg) woman will only use 120 kcal during that walk. Even skating for 1 hour will only require 210 kcal for this person, and bicycling uses only 150 kcal. Even more disturbing is the fact that intense mental work requires practically no more energy than daydreaming. Any extra energy cost could be attributed to tension in the muscles, associated with mental stress.

Before we can estimate the energy needs of an individual, we must have an accurate record of all activities for a day and the time spent on each. That information combined with information on the energy costs of various activities make it possible to calculate total energy costs. Total energy costs will vary in proportion to body size and time if the table of energy costs per kilogram of body weight (Table 7-11) is used. They will vary only in proportion to the time involved if the table of energy costs per minute (Table 7-12) is used. Estimates using these two methods will be quite similar when the individuals are of normal body size, but they will differ as a person's actual size deviates from usual weight for height.

Thermic Effect of Food

It is well known that sufficient food to meet the combined needs for basal metabolism and for activity is inadequate to meet total energy needs and leads to weight loss. The reason for this is a phenomenon called the *specific dynamic effect of food*, or the **thermic effect of food.** The thermic effect of food refers to the stimulation in metabolism and therefore the production of heat that occurs from 1 to 3 hours after a meal as the result of the presence of food in the stomach and intestine and nutrients in the bloodstream. The increase in energy cost because of this thermo-

thermic effect of food
Stimulation in metabolism resulting from the availability of food for digestion, absorption, and metabolism within the cell; also known as the specific dynamic effect or specific dynamic action of food

Table 7-12 ◇ Energy expenditure in specified activities, including basal energy and the effect of food

	Kcal/min	KJ/min
Man (65 kg, or 143 pounds)		
In bed asleep or resting	1.1	4.52
Sitting quietly	1.4	5.82
Standing quietly	1.7	7.32
Walking 3 miles/hr (4.9 km/hr)	3.7	15.5
Walking 3 miles/hr (4.9 km/hr) with a 10-kg load	4.0	16.7
Office work (sedentary)	1.8	7.5
Domestic work		
Cooking	2.1	8.8
Light cleaning	3.1	13.0
Moderate cleaning (such as polishing and window cleaning)	4.3	18.0
Industry		
Garage work (repairs)	4.1	17.2
Carpentry	4.0	16.7
Electrical and machine tool industry	3.6	15.1
Laboratory work	2.3	9.6
Construction work	6.0	25.1
Bricklaying	3.8	15.9
Driving tractor	2.4	10.0
Feeding animals	4.1	17.2
Planting	4.7	19.7
Sawing—hand saw	8.6	36.0
power saw	4.8	20.1
Shoveling	6.5	27.2
Recreation		
Sedentary	2.5	10.5
Light (playing pool, bowling, golf, sailing)	2.5-5.0	10.5-21.0
Moderate (such as dancing, horseback riding, swimming, and tennis)	5.0-7.5	21.0-31.5
Heavy (such as athletics, football, and rowing)	7.5+	31.5
Woman (55 kg, or 110 pounds)		
In bed asleep or resting	0.9	3.7
Sitting quietly	1.2	4.8
Standing quietly	1.4	5.7
Walking 3 miles/hour (4.9 km/hr)	3.0	12.6
Walking 3 miles/hour (4.9 km/hr) with 10-kg load	3.4	14.2
Office work (sedentary)	1.6	6.7
Domestic work		
Cooking	1.7	7.1
Light cleaning	2.5	10.5
Moderate cleaning (such as polishing and window cleaning)	3.5	14.6
Light industry		
Bakery work	2.3	9.6
Laundry work	3.2	13.4
Machine tool industry	2.5	10.5
Recreation		
Sedentary	2.0	8.3
Light (playing pool, bowling, golf, sailing)	2.0-4.0	8.3-16.7
Moderate (such as canoeing, dancing, horseback riding, swimming, and tennis)	4.0-6.0	16.7-25.1
Heavy (such as athletics, football, rowing)	6.0+	25+

Modified from Durnin JVGA, and Passmore R: Energy, work and leisure, London, 1967, as reported in Energy and protein requirements, FAO/WHO Technical Report No. 522, 1973.

genesis amounts to about 10% of the total for basal metabolism and activity. Therefore, to estimate total energy needs, it is necessary to add an additional 10% so that there will be sufficient kilocalories available to meet total needs. The thermic effect was originally called the specific dynamic effect because it was believed that the stimulation of heat production was greater when the diet had a high proportion of calories specifically from protein. Indeed, there is considerable evidence that a diet very high in protein does increase energy costs of maintaining the energy needs of the body.

More recently the concept of a long-term effect on energy use called **luxus consumption** has been introduced. However, it has not yet been proven in humans. This theory maintains that when the intake of calories is greater than the need, some people adapt by using more calories and therefore prevent the storage of as much fat as would have been predicted. This use of calories may involve "futile" or unproductive metabolic activity that does nothing other than waste calories or energy. This certainly would help to explain why some people on some occasions can eat well beyond reasonable needs without any increase in body weight. Conversely, many people on restricted caloric intakes illustrate the **privo conservation** phenomenon; that is, they are able to decrease their energy expenditure—basal, activity, or both—to maintain their body weight on many fewer calories than would be predicted. This phenomenon explains why some people on weight-reducing diets hit plateaus in weight loss on intakes below their estimated expenditures and why people in food-deficient countries are able to maintain body weight on intakes that should lead to progressive weight loss. The ability to adapt by increasing or decreasing energy expenditure in times of caloric excesses or deficits may be partly an inherited or genetically determined trait and partly the result of the environment.

luxus consumption
The metabolism of energy yielding nutrients for no obvious purpose; apparently an automatic adjustment that helps prevent the accumulation of fat when extra food is eaten

privo conservation
The maintenance of body weight on fewer calories; apparently an automatic adjustment that keeps some people from a progressive weight loss

ESTIMATION OF TOTAL ENERGY NEEDS

Methods

So far we have seen that the total energy requirement of an individual is made up of three main components: basal, or resting, metabolism; activity; and thermic effect of food. All of these components vary depending on a variety of factors. To estimate energy needs, it is therefore possible to calculate each of these three components separately, adjust for as many factors that influence need as possible, and then add them together. This will give the most precise estimate possible short of using direct calorimetry.

Some methods for estimating total energy needs follow.

1. Rule of thumb—For those who want a quick answer, there is a rule of thumb that works quite well for many people of relatively normal body weight:

   Energy need = Body wt (lb) × 12 (for a sedentary woman)
   × 14 (for a sedentary man)
   × 15 (for a moderately active woman)
   × 17 (for a moderately active man)
   × 18 (for an active woman)
   × 20 (for an active man)

2. Factorial method (basal metabolism + activity + thermic effect of food)
   a. Calculate basal metabolism using one of the following methods:

      Method 1: kcal/kg/hr
      Males: Basal energy = Body weight (kg) × 1.0 × 24
      Females: Basal energy = Body weight (kg) × 0.9 × 24
      Method 2: Harris-Benedict Formula (p. 174)
      Method 3: Metabolic body size—70 × wt in $kg^{3/4}$
      Method 4: FAO/WHO/UNU Equation (p. 174)

b. Calculate activity costs based on a record of all activity over a 24-hour period. For example:

Activity	Time (hr) (A)	Energy Cost: Kcal/kg/hr (B)	Energy Cost: Kcal/kg (A) × (B)
Dressing	1.5	0.7	1.05
Sitting	6.0	0.4	2.4
Skating	0.5	3.5	1.7
Walking (3 mph)	2.0	2.0	4.0
Standing	1.0	0.5	0.5
Typing	4.0	1.0	4.0
Sleeping	8.0	—	—
Playing piano	0.5	2.0	1.0
Eating	0.5	0.4	0.2
TOTAL	24		14.85

Energy cost = Body weight (kg) × 14.85 = B (depends on body weight)

c. Add basal energy costs and activity costs.
d. Calculate thermic effect of food: Total of basal plus activity × 10% (D)
e. Basal energy (A) + Activity (B) + Thermic effect (D) = *Total energy needs*

3. Recommended energy intake (see table inside back cover)
4. FAO/WHO/UNU (1986)

Activities are classified as light (75% sitting or standing), moderate (25% sitting or standing, 75% moderate activity), and heavy (40% sitting or standing, 60% heavy activity). To estimate total energy needs per day, multiply the basal metabolic rate (BMR) by the following factors:

	Type of Activity: Light	Moderate	Heavy
Energy cost during activity			
Men BMR ×	1.7	2.7	3.8
Women BMR ×	1.7	2.2	2.8
Total energy cost per day			
Men BMR ×	1.6	1.8	2.1
Women BMR ×	1.5	1.6	1.8

5. Canadian Dietary Standards

Age (yr)	Kcal/kg Body Weight: Men	Women
13-15	57	46
16-18	51	40
19-24	42	36
25-49	36	32
50-74	31	29
75+	29	23

Almost all of these estimates are for moderately active healthy individuals living at comfortable environmental temperatures. Estimates should be adjusted upward for people living in very cold temperatures and for those who are appreciably larger than the reference man (69 kg) and woman (59 kg) used as references. Estimates are revised downward for people over 50 years old and for those smaller than the average man or woman. Perhaps the best estimate of energy need is the intake that maintains body weight at the desired level. A person who is neither gaining or losing weight has achieved a fine balance between intake and need. Those who are either obese or underweight to begin with should have an intake that will permit them to either lose or gain weight.

Reference Man (25-50 yr)
69 inches 152 pounds
176 cm 69 kg

Reference Woman (25-50 yr)
64 inches 130 pounds
163 cm 59 kg

Energy Needs of Special Groups

Pregnant Women

The additional energy needs of pregnancy represents the energy in the developing fetus, which is calculated to be approximately 40,000 kcal over the 9 months of pregnancy, with most of it accumulating during the latter part of pregnancy. As a result, it is suggested that the energy intake of the expectant mother be increased by 250 kcal/day to permit the growth of the fetus and the accumulation of sufficient maternal fat stores (2 kg) for the production of breast milk.

Breast-feeding Women

Assuming an average milk production of 750 ml/day, which is equivalent to 520 kcal, with an efficiency of production of 80% to 90%, the added energy cost for lactation is 600 to 650 kcal. Of this amount, up to 200 kcal will be provided for during the baby's first 6 months by the fat accumulated during pregnancy, leaving a net requirement of 400 to 600 kcal extra each day.

Infants

The energy requirement at birth is approximately 110 kcal/kg of body weight. This requirement declines to 95 kcal/kg by the time the baby is 6 months old and then rises again to 100 kcal during the first year to meet the needs related to the very high growth rate at this time. From age 2 years on, the energy need per kilogram of body weight continues to decline. Most of the estimates of the needs of infants and children have come from studies of the reported intakes of infants and children who are growing at very satisfactory rates. A child whose growth consistently follows one developmental line on the growth curves, whether it is the 5th or 95th percentile, is assumed to be getting adequate calories. As soon as energy intake is inadequate or excessive, growth will deviate from the normal pattern.

Children and Adolescents

After age 10 years, estimated energy needs are based on REE × a factor of 1.7 for girls or REE × a factor of 1.8 for boys to include needs for activity. The needs for growth represent an increase of less than 3% over basal needs plus activity needs. This increase gradually decreases to adult levels of 1.6 for young men and 1.5 for young women by age 17 years. The wide variation in activity needs throughout childhood and adolescence makes it difficult to estimate energy need. The pattern of growth is the most sensitive measure of adequacy or inadequacy of intake. Children who show a tendency toward obesity should be encouraged to increase their activity and practice moderation in intake until the weight is adjusted to expected levels; they should seldom be encouraged to lose weight but rather to stabilize it until they "grow into it."

Estimated energy needs for age and sex groups, based on the formula prepared by the FAO/WHO/UNU and applied to average weights and heights in the United States, are presented in Table 7-13. It should be stressed that in contrast to the allowances for other nutrients, these are sufficiently high to meet the needs of most people. The recommended energy intakes are *average* requirements for people engaged in light activity at a comfortable environmental temperature. To reinforce

Table 7-13 ◆ Mean heights, weights, and estimated daily energy allowances*

	Weight		Height		Resting Energy Expenditure (Kcal/day)	Mean Activity Factor	Estimated Energy Allowance (with Range)		
	Kg	Lb	Cm	In			Kcal/day	Kcal/kg	MJ/day
Infants (mo)									
0-2.9	4.5	10	55	22	—	—	500 (400-700)	110	2.1
3-5.9	6.6	15	64	25	—	—	650 (500-850)	100	2.7
6-8.9	7.9	17	69	27	—	—	750 (600-1000)	95	3.1
9-11.9	9.0	20	73	29	—	—	900 (700-1200)	100	3.8
Children (yr)									
1-1.9	11	24	82	32	600	2.0	1200 (900-1600)	105	4.8
2-3.9	14	31	96	38	700	2.0	1400 (1100-1900)	100	5.9
4-5.9	18	40	109	43	830	2.0	1700 (1300-2300)	92	7.1
6-7.9	22	49	121	48	930	2.0	1800 (1400-2400)	83	7.5
8-9.9	28	62	132	52	1050	1.8	1900 (1400-2500)	69	7.9
Males (yr)									
10-11.9	36	79	143	56	1200	1.8	2200 (1700-2900)	61	9.2
12-16.9	57	126	169	67	1580	1.7	2700 (2000-3600)	47	11.3
17-24.9	70	155	177	70	1750	1.6	2800 (2400-3200)	40	11.7
25-49.9	69	152	176	69	1620	1.6	2600 (2200-3100)	38	10.9
50-69.9	68	149	173	68	1440	1.6	2300 (1900-2700)	34	9.6
>70	66	146	171	67	1310	1.5	2000 (1600-2400)	30	8.4
Females (yr)									
10-13.9	42	96	155	62	1300	1.7	2200 (1700-2900)	50	9.2
14-16.9	56	123	162	64	1410	1.6	2200 (1700-3000)	41	9.6
17-24.9	58	128	163	64	1420	1.6	2300 (1900-2700)	39	9.6
25-49.9	59	130	163	64	1350	1.6	2200 (1800-2600)	37	9.2
50-69.9	59	130	160	63	1220	1.6	2000 (1600-2400)	34	8.4
<70	59	130	158	62	1140	1.5	1700 (1300-2100)	30	7.1
Pregnancy	1st trimester							+300	+1.3
	2nd trimester							+300	+1.3
	3rd trimester							+300	+1.3
Lactation	1st 6 months							+400	+1.7
	2nd 6 months							+600	+2.5

*Adapted from Energy and protein requirements, FAO/WHO/UNU, Rome and Geneva, 1985, for use with U.S. population. Courtesy Dr. Peter Pellett, Amherst, MA.

the notion of wide individual differences, a range of intakes for each age and sex category is included. From the table it is obvious that energy requirements per unit of body weight decrease with age. For children and adolescents, the energy allowances are sufficiently high to permit appropriate growth. The Nationwide Food Consumption Study showed an average intake of 84% of the RDAs (1980), with only one fourth of the respondents reporting that they ate the amount recommended. This may be explained by a failure to report all food intake, lower-than-anticipated energy expenditure, or unrealistically high recommended intakes. This raises the question why there may be a high incidence of obesity in a population that eats less than suggested.

FOOD AS A SOURCE OF ENERGY

So far in this chapter we have been concerned with the way in which the body uses energy; in the previous chapters we have focused on the three macronutrients—carbohydrate, protein, and lipid—as sources of energy. We have seen that car-

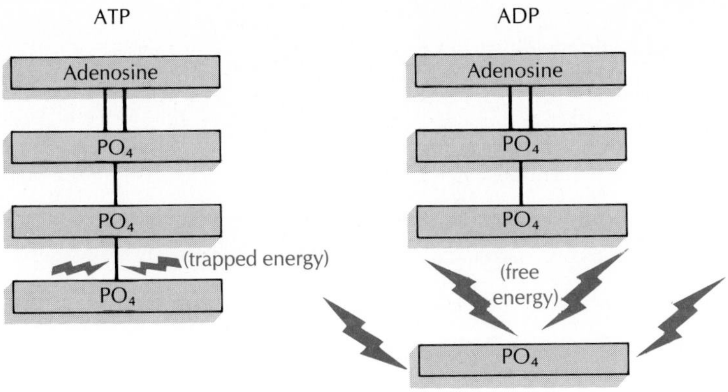

Figure 7-8 Energy from metabolism is trapped ("held") in ATP (adenosine triphosphate). When energy is needed by body cells, one phosphate (PO_4) is split off, freeing the trapped energy for use by the cell.

bohydrates are reduced to monosaccharides, which are absorbed into the bloodstream and transported to individual cells. Similarly, dietary protein is digested to its constituent amino acids, and lipids to fatty acids and glycerol.

As we have seen, animals (including humans) get glucose and fatty acids from food sources containing sugar, starch, and fat, or they make glucose and fatty acids from protein. Their ability to release energy from these products depends not only on the presence of oxygen but also on the availability of minerals, vitamins, and enzymes. These substances facilitate the many complex chemical changes involved in converting energy into ATP (adenosine triphosphate), a high-energy compound. Energy is trapped in this form and is released in slowly regulated amounts for use within the cell. ATP is used in virtually all organelles of the cell for the synthesis of complex substances from simple nutrients and for the many physical changes and metabolic reactions that require energy. When energy is needed, one molecule of phosphate splits off from the ATP, releasing the energy that held it to the ATP and leaving ADP (adenosine diphosphate) (Figure 7-8). If energy could not be stored as ATP it would all be released at once, as it is when wood burns as heat. Much would be wasted because it would not be needed immediately.

• • •

The following section may present more detail of metabolism than many students need. It is included for those who are intrigued by the complexity of releasing energy from various food sources.

METABOLISM

From the blood, nutrients are picked up by individual cells, where they undergo the biochemical changes known collectively as metabolism.

Metabolism of the energy-yielding nutrients carbohydrate, lipid, and protein includes two quite different processes: **anabolism,** in which the products of digestion are used to build body compounds and storage material; and **catabolism,** in which the products of digestion are broken down further, primarily as a source of energy.

anabolism
The metabolic process that causes the synthesis or formation of a new substance

catabolism
The metabolic process that causes the breakdown or destruction of a substance

This section presents an overview of how the cells use the products of digestion of carbohydrate, lipid, and protein to extract the energy stored in these products or store excess as body fat and some glycogen. The discussion will focus on the fate of four products of digestion: glucose, fatty acids, glycerol, and the amino acids. Together, they are the metabolic material used by the cell as energy sources. Some energy from carbohydrate is available even if there is no oxygen. However, most of the energy from carbohydrates and all energy from fat requires the release of oxygen. That is, it is an aerobic reaction.

Figure 7-9 Changes in glucose, fatty acids, glycerol, and amino acids during metabolism to yield carbon dioxide, water, and energy.

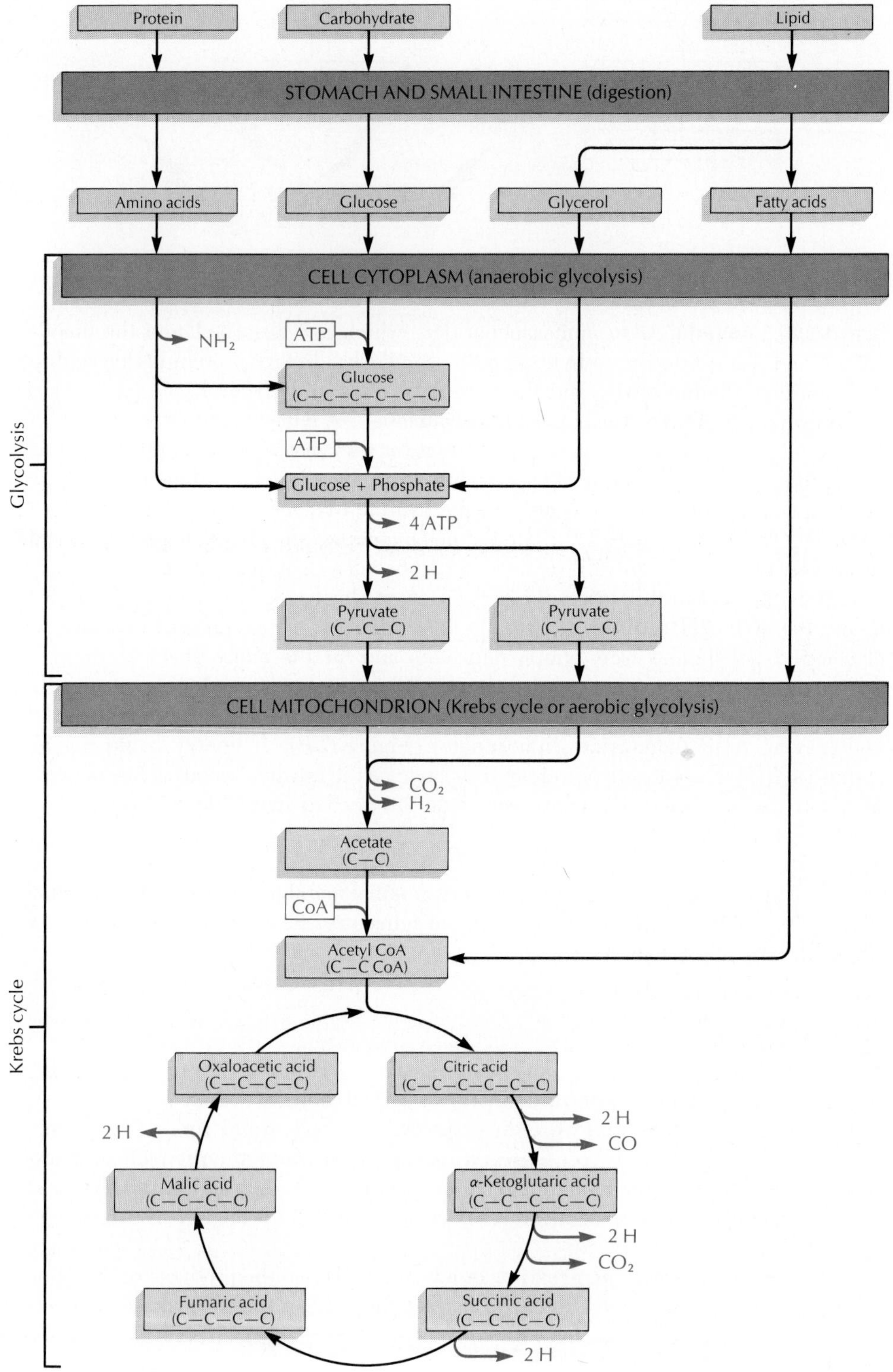

Metabolism of Glucose

The carbohydrate glucose is either derived directly from the digestion of any of the three disaccharides: sucrose, maltose, or lactose; produced in the liver from the other two monosaccharides, galactose and fructose; or derived from stored glycogen. The first steps in the breakdown of glucose occur in the cytoplasm of the cell and are known collectively as **glycolysis.** The changes involve breaking glucose, which has 6 carbons, into two 3-carbon compounds of pyruvic acid. The changes are **anaerobic,** which means that they do not require oxygen. Two molecules of the energy-rich compound ATP (adenosine triphosphate) are also required for glycolysis.

As a result of glycolysis, which produces 4 units of ATP, there is a net gain of 2 ATP molecules. This amount represents only a small portion of the potential energy stored within the glucose molecule, which yields a total of 38 ATP units.

However, even 4 ATP units are valuable for athletes such as sprinters, who may have very high energy needs for a short period. Glycolysis is represented in the top portion of Figure 7-9. The pyruvic acid loses a CO_2 to become acetic acid, which immediately unites with coenzyme A (CoA) to become acetyl CoA.

glycolysis
The breakdown of carbohydrate in metabolism (glyco = sugar; lysis = to break)

anaerobic
In the absence of oxygen

Metabolism of Fatty Acids and Glycerol

Dietary lipid is composed of 95% triglycerides. After being absorbed, these triglycerides are carried to the liver as small fat globules called **chylomicrons.** From there they go to all the body's cells as **lipoproteins.** The fat portion of the lipoprotein is split off from the protein portion before entering the cell; once within the cell, the fat portion is split again into glycerol and fatty acids before being metabolized.

The glycerol portion of the fat molecule can be readily changed to pyruvic acid, which can be used either to form glucose or to provide energy.

The fatty acid portion of the fat molecule is split apart into 2-carbon fragments. These fragments unite with CoA to produce acetyl CoA. This acetyl CoA cannot be distinguished from that produced from the pyruvic acid that comes from glucose. Although this may sound rather simple, it should be recognized that the breakdown of an 18-carbon fatty acid into nine 2-carbon units includes 45 different reactions involving three vitamins: riboflavin, niacin, and biotin; and four minerals: magnesium, copper, iron, and potassium. Fatty acids cannot be converted to glucose, but they can be resynthesized into fat if not used immediately for energy.

chylomicrons
Very small fat particles; for more discussion, see Chapter 5

lipoproteins
Combinations of lipid and protein that are more readily transported in the blood than lipid alone; for more discussion, see Chapter 5

Metabolism of Amino Acids

When the energy intake is adequate, the amino acids derived from dietary protein are used first for synthesizing body proteins. However, those amino acids in excess of needs for growth and maintenance lose their characteristic NH_2 group and enter the same metabolic pathways as carbohydrate and lipid, to be used as a source of energy. These amino acids can enter the metabolic pathway in many places, the exact place being determined by the chemical structure of each amino acid. The amino portions are released as ammonia, a poison, but two of the amino groups are quickly combined to produce **urea,** a much less toxic substance. Urea in turn is excreted by the kidneys.

Some amino acids can be converted to pyruvate and then can be used to make glucose. These include alanine, serine, glycine, cysteine, methionine, and tryptophan, which are called **glucogenic** amino acids because they are used this way.

About half of the remaining amino acids, including phenylalanine, tyrosine, leucine, isoleucine, and lysine, can be deaminated (lose their NH_2 group) and broken down like fat into the 2-carbon fragments that eventually form acetyl CoA. Like fat, these amino acids are able to form compounds called ketones, which can be used as a source of energy by the brain. They are therefore known as **ketogenic** amino acids.

urea
A nontoxic compound made from two molecules of toxic ammonia; produced when amino acids are deaminated

glucogenic
Capable of producing glucose

ketogenic
Capable of producing ketones

Of the remaining amino acids, all but aspartic acid are converted into glutamic acid, an amino acid, deaminated, and used as an energy source immediately. Aspartic acid that is not used in protein synthesis is deaminated and enters the metabolic cycle directly.

Amino acids are deaminated to be used as an energy source when

1. Inadequate fat and carbohydrate are present to meet immediate energy needs
2. There are inadequate amounts of essential amino acids to synthesize required proteins, or
3. The diet provides more amino acids than are needed for growth and synthesis of essential compounds

For details on the structure of cells, see Appendix A

Once these nutrients have been changed to the pyruvate or acetate (acetyl CoA) stage, they move from the cytoplasm to the mitochondrion of the cell. The number of mitochondria in a cell varies greatly; there are as many as 2000 in metabolically active cells such as liver cells. The location of the mitochondria within a cell reflects the needs of that cell at a particular time. Therefore in a cell that is busy synthesizing protein, mitochondria will concentrate near the ribosome, or protein-synthesizing organelle. If the cell functions mainly in absorption and needs energy to transport substances in and out, mitochrondria are located near the cell membrane.

In the mitochondrion, a reaction known as oxidative decarboxylation takes place, requiring the vitamin, thiamin. In this reaction, 1 of the 3 carbon atoms in pyruvic acid is oxidized to carbon dioxide, and the hydrogen atoms are removed. The hydrogen atoms attach themselves to the riboflavin- and niacin-containing coenzymes FAD and NAD to produce FADH and NADH. The carbon dioxide is released through the lungs. The 2-carbon compound, acetic acid, remains. Acetic acid combines with coenzyme A, which includes the vitamin pantothenic acid. This combination produces acetyl CoA which cannot be distinguished from the acetyl CoA formed from two-carbon fat fragments (Figure 7-9).

Alcohol is metabolized to acetate and therefore is used in the same way as acetate that is produced from either carbohydrate or fatty acids.

Krebs Cycle (Citric Acid Cycle)

The Krebs cycle, the TCA cycle, and the citric acid cycle are all names for the same set of metabolic changes that occur when energy is released from glucose, fatty acids, and amino acids within the mitochondrion of the cell

After glucose, fatty acids, glycerol, and some amino acids have been converted into acetyl CoA, they are all processed through the same series of metabolic changes. The process is known by several names: the Krebs cycle, named after the scientist who discovered it; the tricarboxylic acid (TCA) cycle, because it involves acids with three carboxyl (COOH) groups; and the citric acid cycle, because citric acid with 6 carbons is the first substance formed after the entrance of the 2-carbon fragment attached to CoA—that is, acetyl CoA—into the cycle. This series of reactions is identified as a cycle because the changes lead back to the starting point. It involves eight enzyme-controlled steps.

The Krebs cycle begins when 1 molecule of acetyl CoA joins with oxaloacetic acid, the 4-carbon compound available as the last compound in the previous cycle to make a 6-carbon compound. The removal of CO_2 and 2 hydrogen atoms results in a 5-carbon compound. This compound loses CO_2 and 2 more hydrogen atoms, making a 4-carbon compound. The CO_2 is released into the blood and excreted from the lungs. The hydrogen atoms, which carry a high amount of energy, attach to either the riboflavin-containing or niacin-containing coenzyme to join other hydrogens later; they will then transfer their energy to ATP molecules. The 4-carbon compound next loses 4 more hydrogen atoms and emerges as the 4-carbon compound that began the cycle. Some amino acids such as proline, lysine, arginine, histidine, and hydroxyproline are converted to glutamic acid and enter cycle at the 5-carbon stage. They are referred to as glucogenic amino acids. Phenylalanine and tyrosine enter either at the 4-carbon stage or throughout the fat sequence and referred to as ketogenic amino acids. Aspartic acid enters at the end of the cycle.

As a result of the changes within the mitochondrion, 6 molecules of carbon dioxide and 20 atoms of hydrogen are released from every molecule of glucose or from every 2 molecules of pyruvic acid. Although no energy is released as a result of these changes, the hydrogen atoms pick up and "store" energy as they are split from the carbon atoms and attach to coenzymes containing the vitamins riboflavin and niacin.

Electron Transport System

Once the hydrogen atoms have been attached to niacin-containing and riboflavin-containing enzymes (forming NADH and FADH, respectively), they are carried to the mitochondrion membrane, where they enter into another series of reactions known as the electron transport system. This system is responsible for a process known as **oxidative phosphorylation.** At the end of this sequence, water is formed. The electrons from the hydrogen atoms pass from one series of electron carriers (cytochromes) to another, losing some of their energy at each stage as ADP (adenosine diphosphate) is converted to ATP (adenosine triphosphate). This conversion traps some of the energy from the original glucose. Eventually the hydrogen, which has returned to a low-energy state, combines with oxygen to form water. If the hydrogen were transferred directly to the oxygen without cycling through the electron transport system and its cytochromes, a great deal of energy would be lost as heat. This would not only be wasteful but also would make it necessary for the body to have alternative ways of releasing heat to prevent the body temperature from rising.

oxidative phosphorylation
The addition of a phosphate molecule to ADP to form ATP, using the energy from the release of hydrogen (from NAD attached to NAD and FAD in the Krebs cycle)

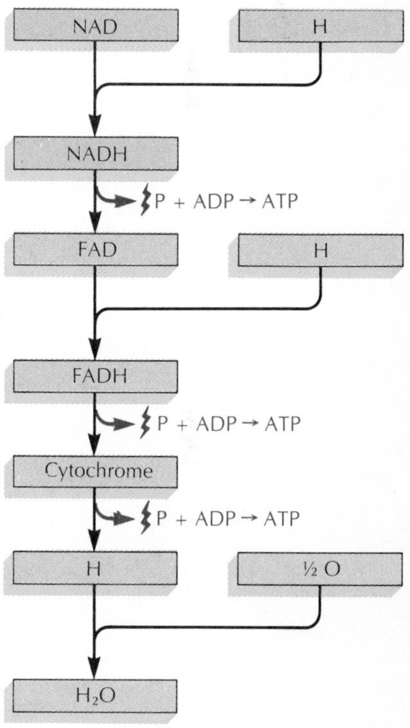

ATP is the form in which energy is stored until it is needed for the energy-requiring processes of the body. These include many processes such as the mechanical work of muscle contraction and chemical processes such as the synthesis of essential body compounds, the transport of nutrients across cell membranes, and the secretion of hormones. About 40% of the potential energy of dietary nutrients is extracted and stored as ATP; the remainder is converted to heat. Some of this heat is required to maintain body temperature, and the rest is released through evaporation of moisture from the skin or by direct heat loss.

The processes described above are all summarized in Figure 7-9. The system is much more complex than this presentation suggests, but the illustration demonstrates how all three major dietary nutrients interact in the energy-releasing process.

The end products are disposed of as follows: carbon dioxide is excreted through the lungs, and water is lost through the skin, lungs, and kidneys. Urea, produced from amino groups, is an additional end product of protein catabolism and is released as urea through the kidneys.

OVERNUTRITION

The changes described so far are those that result when carbohydrate, fat, and protein provide sufficient energy to meet the body's needs, with no surplus or deficit of kilocalories. It is important to understand how these processes change when caloric intake does not balance with caloric expenditure.

When food intake provides kilocalories in excess of need, the metabolism of all three nutrients is altered (Figure 7-10). First, extra glucose will be converted into the storage carbohydrate glycogen in the liver and muscle. Because the capacity to store glycogen is relatively small, it will soon be necessary to divert the extra glucose somewhere else. Under these conditions, the extra glucose will be metabolized to pyruvate and some of it changed to glycerol, the 3-carbon base of the fat molecule. Because only a small amount of glycerol is needed, pyruvate is quickly changed to acetyl CoA. From this point on, instead of entering the Krebs cycle,

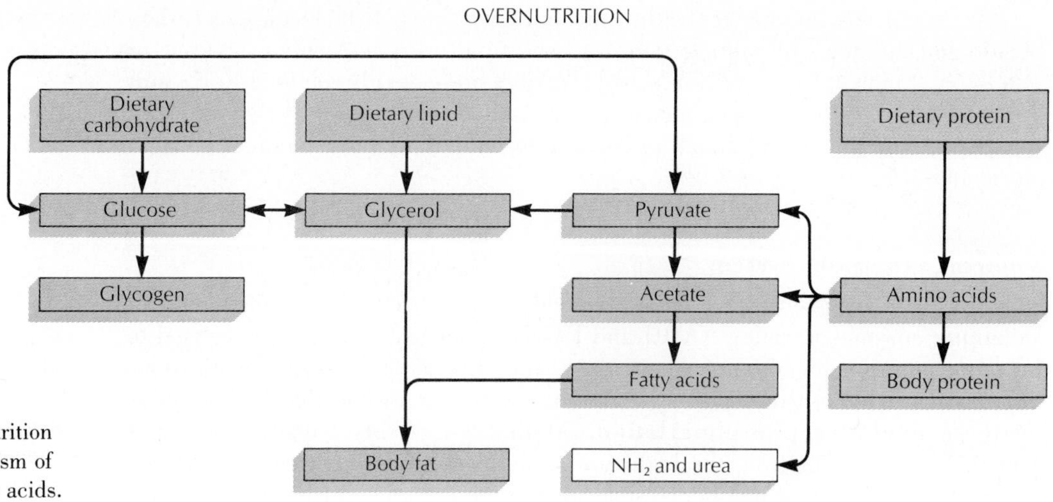

Figure 7-10 Effect of overnutrition (excess energy) on the metabolism of glucose, fatty acids, and amino acids.

1 μm = 0.001 milligram
1 μm = 0.000001 gram

extra carbohydrate derived originally from glucose is synthesized into fatty acids. These fatty acids then combine with glycerol to form a fat store within special adipose cells. The adipose cells can store up to 7 μg of fat each; once they are filled to capacity, new fat cells are formed to accommodate the fat.

Similarly, extra protein can be converted through pyruvate to glycerol if the amino acids are glucogenic and through acetate to fatty acids if the amino acids are ketogenic. In either case, the extra nutrients have lost their original identity but not their energy potential. From this information, it is evident that fat can be derived from any of the three nutrients, but only when more calories are consumed than are needed. Because there is no way to get rid of the surplus energy—that is, energy over and above that needed for immediate energy needs—it must and will be converted into fat.

UNDERNUTRITION

When energy intake is inadequate to meet immediate energy needs, the glucose, fatty acids, glycerol, and amino acids from the digested food are used first for energy. Once they are used, the body has several alternative energy sources—stored glycogen (carbohydrate), stored lipid, and finally the breakdown of body protein (Figure 7-11). First, the energy reserve in glycogen will be used. Then, if the diet provides enough carbohydrate to meet the needs of the brain for glucose, fat will be mobilized from adipose and other cells to provide fatty acids and glycerol as energy sources for other tissues. There will then be a steady loss of weight proportional to the amount of fat used.

If, however, the diet is very low in carbohydrate (less than 100 grams/day), once the glycogen stores have been depleted (usually within 1 day), metabolism changes to help provide alternative sources of glucose for the brain. These can be obtained by the conversion of glycerol or glucogenic amino acids to pyruvate and then to glucose. However, because glycerol, which represents only 5% of the fat molecule, is a potential source of glucose, there is a problem in getting rid of the acetate formed from fatty acids fast enough. This problem is usually handled by uniting 2 molecules to form another energy source: ketones. After a period of adaptation, some ketones can be used as an alternative fuel source by the brain. An excess of ketones change the pH of the blood, but it also affects the functioning of enzymes and depresses the appetite. These changes, caused primarily by a lack of carbohydrate in the diet, can be reversed by including some carbohydrate. Excess

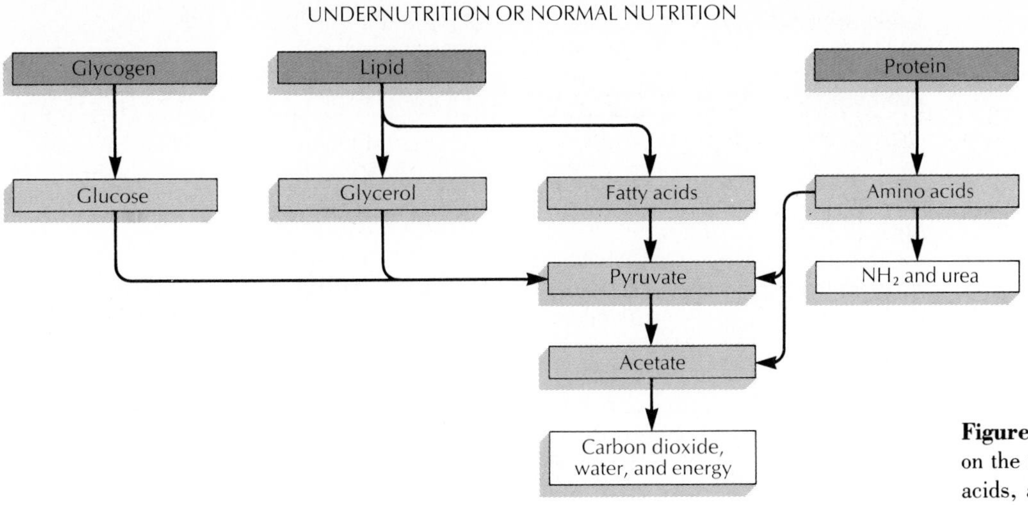

Figure 7-11 Effect of undernutrition on the metabolism of glucose, fatty acids, and amino acids.

ketones must be excreted, which requires a large volume of fluid. Thus people following low-carbohydrate diets, who must metabolize fat to provide fuel for the brain, produce ketones and experience the high weight loss associated with water loss, as well as loss of fat tissue.

Other sources of glucose as fuel for the central nervous system are certain amino acids. These also have drawbacks, however. To get the glucogenic amino acids, nonglucogenic amino acids are released in large amounts, causing a depletion of body protein. The large amount of water stored with body protein and the minerals (particularly potassium) that are lost as muscle is broken down contribute to a rapid loss of weight and the muscle weakness associated with starvation or low-carbohydrate diets. The leftover ketogenic amino acids contribute to the formation of ketones.

From this it is evident that in a calorie deficit, the body can draw on stored carbohydrate and lipid. When carbohydrate is too low to meet the needs for glucose, the use of fat or glucogenic amino acids leads to a loss of body water (as ketones and protein are broken down and excreted) and a rapid weight loss. However, when some carbohydrate is supplied in the diet, stored fat is mobilized and weight loss is proportional to the use of stored fat.

THE ROLE OF MINERALS AND VITAMINS

The changes necessary to convert food nutrients into energy can proceed only when minerals and vitamins are available as catalysts, either in conjunction with or as part of the enzymes involved. In the absence of any of these elements, the metabolic pathway may be blocked, resulting in the accumulation of the intermediate product. Depending on the point at which such blockage occurs, the intermediate product may be shifted to an alternative pathway, or it may continue to accumulate.

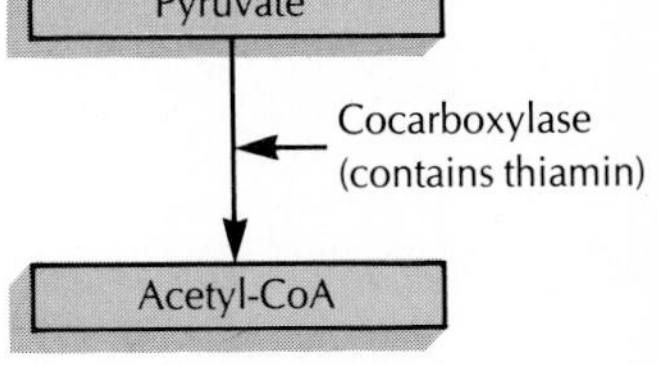

The accumulation of an intermediate product almost always interferes with cellular functioning and always results in a failure to produce the normal end product of metabolism. For example, thiamin, a vitamin, is a necessary part of the enzyme cocarboxylase, which is needed to change pyruvic acid to acetyl-CoA. A lack of thiamin therefore inhibits the entrance of glucose into the Krebs cycle, resulting in an accumulation of pyruvic acid in the blood.

There are a great number of reactions in the body in which vitamins and minerals play a vital role in the metabolism of the three major energy-yielding nutrients (Table 7-14).

Table 7-14 ◇ Requirements of vitamins and minerals in catalyzing processes of digestion, absorption, and metabolism

Process	Vitamin	Mineral
Digestion		Chloride Zinc*
Absorption		Sodium
Anabolism		
Glycogenesis	Riboflavin Niacin Pyridoxine	Magnesium Manganese Cobalt
Catabolism		
Glycolysis	Niacin Lipoic acid Thiamin Panthothenic acid	Potassium Magnesium
Krebs cycle	Pantothenic acid Niacin Lipoic acid Thiamin Riboflavin	Manganese Iron Mangesium
Electron transport	Niacin Riboflavin	Iron* Copper

*Functions as an essential part of the enzyme.

Although many of the terms and concepts used throughout the text have been identified in this chapter, a glossary to help the student to interpret other concepts is included in the back of the book. For students with a high degree of curiosity and a desire for more in-depth understanding of the physiology of the body, an elementary physiology text or a high school biology text may prove helpful, especially if they are unable to enroll in other college science courses.

BY NOW YOU SHOULD KNOW

- The energy content of the diet is provided by carbohydrate, lipid, protein, and alcohol.
- Food energy is measured in kilocalories (kcal) or kilojoules (kJ).
- Energy needs are divided into three main groups: those for basal, or resting metabolism; those for activity; and those for the thermic effect of food.
- Energy content of food can be determined directly in a bomb calorimeter or indirectly by calculating from the proximate analysis, either by the use of physiological fuel values for carbohydrate, lipid, and protein or of tables of food composition.
- Energy requirements for basal resting metabolism can be determined by direct calorimetry; obtained indirectly in a respiration calorimeter; or calculated from metabolic body size or the Harris-Benedict equation, which involves height and weight measurements.
- Energy expended for activity varies with the duration of the activity, the severity of the activity, and the amount of weight being moved.
- Energy needs for activity are calculated from tables of energy cost of activity and from records of activity patterns.

- Energy intake beyond the body's needs is stored as body fat. When intake is insufficient to meet needs, body fat is metabolized to yield 3500 kcal/pound.
- Within the mitochondrion of the cells, nutrients are metabolized to yield energy.
- Glucose, glycerol, and some amino acids are converted to pyruvate. Pyruvate is broken down to acetyl CoA, which is used for energy or stored as fat, a potential source of energy.
- Minerals and vitamins serve as catalysts to many of the metabolic reactions within the cell.

STUDY QUESTIONS

1. What is the difference between calorie, Calorie, kilocalorie, and kilojoule?
2. Explain why the heat of combustion for protein is 5.65 kcal/gram but the net heat of combustion is 4.35 kcal/gram.
3. How are the physiological fuel values of carbohydrate, lipid, and protein determined?
4. What are the three components of energy expenditure?
5. Explain the relationship between direct and indirect calorimetry.
6. Name the factors involved in determining basal metabolism and how they affect basal metabolism.
7. Differentiate between BMR and REE.
8. If you had more kilocalories than you needed, how would the fate of an extra teaspoon of sugar differ from that of a teaspoon of sugar that was not extra?
9. How could you use the Exchange System to help you plan your food intake?
10. Compare the energy needs of certain special groups of people to the needs of normal healthy adults.

Applying What You've Learned

1. **Calculate Your Own Basal Metabolism**

   Use at least three of the different methods shown on page p. 174. How do the results compare? Can you explain any differences in the calculated basal metabolic needs?

2. **Personal Basal Metabolic Need**

   Name five specific factors that affect your personal basal metabolic need.

3. **Compare Your Intake to Expenditure to Energy Balance**

   Record your activities (energy expenditure) and your food and beverage intake (energy intake) for 1 day. Use Table 7-12 to calculate energy expenditure of your activities. Use Appendix F to calculate your total kilocalorie intake. Compare your intake to expenditure to energy balance. Do you take in more energy than you expend, or do you expend more than you take in? What would you expect to happen if you followed this pattern of eating and activity daily for 1 month?

4. **Total Energy Needs vs. RDAs**

   Calculate your total energy needs, using the factorial method on p. 181. How does this method compare to the RDA found on the back inside cover of this text? Can you explain any differences?

5. **Evaluate Source of Energy**

   Select several food labels with nutrition information. Determine the number of calories per serving. Now look at the distribution of energy-yielding nutrients. Is it carbohydrate, fat, or protein that contributes the greatest number of kilocalories? Remember, 1 gram of fat has twice as many calories as 1 gram of carbohydrate and protein.

6. Record Everything You Eat and Drink For 1 Day

Use Appendix F to find the kilocalories and grams of carbohydrate, fat, protein, and alcohol in these foods. Determine the percent of calorie distribution for each of these energy-yielding compounds. Compare your distribution to the Dietary Goals (58% carbohydrate, 12% protein, and 30% fat).

1. Convert grams to kilocalories

$$\text{grams carbohydrate} \times 4 = \text{kcal from carbohydrate}$$
$$\text{grams protein} \times 4 = \text{kcal from protein}$$
$$\text{grams fat} \times 9 = \text{kcal from fat}$$
$$\text{grams alcohol} \times 7 = \text{kcal from alcohol}$$

2. Find the distribution of calories

$$\frac{\text{Kilocalories from carbohydrate}}{\text{Total kilocalories}} \times 100 = \%\ \text{Calories from carbohydrate}$$
$$\frac{\text{Kilocalories from protein}}{\text{Total kilocalories}} \times 100 = \%\ \text{Calories from protein}$$
$$\frac{\text{Kilocalories from fat}}{\text{Total kilocalories}} \times 100 = \%\ \text{Calories from fat}$$
$$\frac{\text{Kilocalories from alcohol}}{\text{Total kilocalories}} \times 100 = \%\ \text{Calories from alcohol}$$

SUGGESTED READINGS

Beaton GH: Energy in human nutrition: perspectives and problems, Nutrition Reviews 41:325, 1983.

Dr. Beaton encompasses a wealth of information in one paper. He discusses the basis for controversial points of view regarding ways in which the human energy requirement should be determined.

Hegsted DM: Energy requirements. In Present knowledge of nutrition, ed. 5, Washington, D.C., 1984, Nutrition Foundation.

This succinct review deals with some of the problems we still have in estimating energy requirements. Hegsted argues that it may not always be possible to predict energy needs from body size and activity and points to evidence of a high degree of adaptation that occurs when energy supplies are limited.

Himms-Hagen J: Brown adipose tissue thermogenesis, Nutrition Reviews 41:261, 1983.

This paper presents an update of the metabolism of brown fat—a relatively new concept in energy balance. It makes the transition from our information on animals to its application in human energy balance.

Joint FAO/WHO/UNU Expert Consultation: Energy and protein requirements, Geneva, 1985, World Health Organization.

This report represents the consensus of an international group of experts who first met in 1981 to evaluate the research on the energy and protein requirements of human beings to propose requirements for these nutrients that would be applicable across different cultures and various age and sex groups. Although these estimates are designed primarily for groups, they may be applied to the needs of individuals with the understanding that they represent the probability of a specific intake being either adequate or inadequate for a particular individual.

Stricker EM: Biological basis of hunger and satiety, Nutrition Reviews 42:333, 1984.

Discussions of the need for food, the stimulus for eating, the site of action of satiety and hunger symptoms provide the basis for the section on the therapeutic implications. The deemphasis on the theory that a total control rests in the hypothalmus is discussed with the recognition that there is no generally accepted theory to replace it.

ADDITIONAL READINGS

Cunningham JJ: A reanalysis of the factors influencing basal metabolic rate in normal adults, American Journal of Clinical Nutrition 33:2372, 1980.

FAO/WHO: Energy and protein requirements, Rome and Geneva, 1985, World Health Organization.

Henson LC, Poole DC, Donahoe CP, and Heber D: Effects of exercise training on resting energy expenditure during calorie restriction, American Journal of Clinical Nutrition 46:893, 1987.

Mahalko JR, and Johnson LK: Accuracy of predictions of long-term energy needs, Journal of the American Dietetic Association 77:557, 1980.

Oliver ED, and others: A reappraisal of calorie requirements of men, American Journal of Clinical Nutrition 46:875, 1987.

Owen OE, and others: A reappraisal of the calorie requirements of men, American Journal of Clinical Nutrition 46:875, 1987.

Ravussin E, and others: Reduced rate of energy expenditure as a risk factor in body-weight gain, New England Journal of Medicine 318:467, 1988.

Rothwell NJ, and Stock MJ: Regulation of energy balance, Annual Review of Nutrition 1:235, 1981.

Sukhatme PV, and Margen S: Auto-regulatory homeostatic nature of energy balance, American Journal of Clinical Nutrition 35:355, 1982.

FOCUS Weight for Height—What Does it Mean?

The mother of the young infant who finds her child at the 95th percentile on the growth charts reacts with pride—she has produced a bigger and (to her at least) obviously better child than 95% of other mothers! As the child approaches early adulthood, more often than not this same mother's pride changes to consternation if her offspring remains at the top of the weight charts. As an adult, this person will probably seek ways to drop from the top of the chart to the middle or will protest that his weight problem is beyond his control because he was fat from birth.

Most of us enjoy comparing ourselves to norms, whether they reflect average income, average IQ, or average weight for height. Sometimes, however, we don't seem to fit where we want to or think we should. Some people become skilled at manipulating the data so that they come closer to getting the "right" message. When interpreting height and weight tables, they take the option of deciding that their frames are really medium or large, not small; that their heel height is different from that used in the charts; that their clothing weighs more or less than the standard; or that they have not correctly measured their heights, weights, or both.

For those who were told by the 1959 Metropolitan Desirable Weight Tables that they were on the verge of obesity, the revised 1983 Metropolitan Height and Weight Tables brought almost instant relief. The short male with a small frame found that he could appropriately weigh 15 pounds more with the newer tables; however, the less fortunate tall female with a small frame was given only 1 pound's grace. For others, the differences in two standards fell between these two extremes. If we intend to use height and weight standards, it's important to know where they came from and what they tell us.

Before 1942, the only tables available gave information on the average weight for height or age but no information on what was good or bad for our health. In 1942, the Metropolitan Life Insurance Company (as a public service) published a set of tables that they called "Ideal Weight Tables." These tables gave information on the weights for height that the insurance company found were associated with the lowest mortality rates. In almost all cases, the weights were lower than the average weights used previously and provided guidance to people who wanted to know which weight range would give them the best chance of living longer. Because the tables were based on information obtained only from people who bought insurance, however, they did not necessarily represent the whole population.

These tables were replaced in 1959 by "Desirable Weight Tables" based on the experience of 26 insurance companies, who followed 4 million insured people for 20 years. After eliminating those who had major diseases such as diabetes, heart disease, and cancer, these tables also showed that people who weighed somewhat below the average for their height were likely to live longer. These tables were set up in such a way that people had to make a judgment as to whether they had small, medium, or large frames, but they were given no help in making that decision. For each height and frame size, a range of weights was presented.

Because it was decided that the terms "ideal" and "desirable" only confused people, the most recent tables released in 1983 are simply called "The 1983 Metropolitan Height and Weight Tables." They are based on an analysis of the records of more than 4 million people followed up over a 22-year period. Although these tables showed that the weight for height associated with the lowest mortality had increased, they showed also that this weight was still below the average weight. The new weights are essentially the average weights for men 27 years old and women 23 years old. In presenting the new tables with their increased weights, the company made it clear that they should not be used as a license to gain more weight but that overweight people might perhaps have less to lose than they previously thought.

Regardless of which tables you use, it is important to read the footnotes and the fine print. For example, the current tables usually tell you that heights and weights were measured with subjects wearing "ordinary indoor clothing." This means that 1-inch heels and 5 pounds of clothing for men and 1-inch heels and 3 pounds of clothing for women are assumed. In preparing the table in this book, heel height and clothing weight have been subtracted to give nude weight for barefoot heights. Tables are also provided based on the breadth of the elbow to help you decide what your frame is. The directions for making this measurement, however, leave considerable room for error! For that reason, we have chosen to omit the standards from this text.

It is interesting to note that, during the same time period in which there was a weight increase relative to lowest mortality, average weights for height were also increasing. This increase was greatest for taller men and for men who were 25 to 44 years of age. For women, the increase was considerably smaller; in fact, for women over 25 years old there was actually a decrease in average weight over a 30-year period.

Average weights are still more than 20 pounds heavier for men of all ages and 17 pounds heavier for women over 50 than the figures in the new tables. This suggests that there is still a large segment of the population that would be well advised to decrease food intake or increase exercise level to bring their weight into line with the weights found to lead to greatest longevity.

In contrast to tables published earlier, the 1983 tables have attracted a great deal of public interest, appearing in almost all popular magazines and in newspaper supplements instead of being buried in college textbooks. This is just one of the many manifestations of a growing concern about fitness and health in our world today.

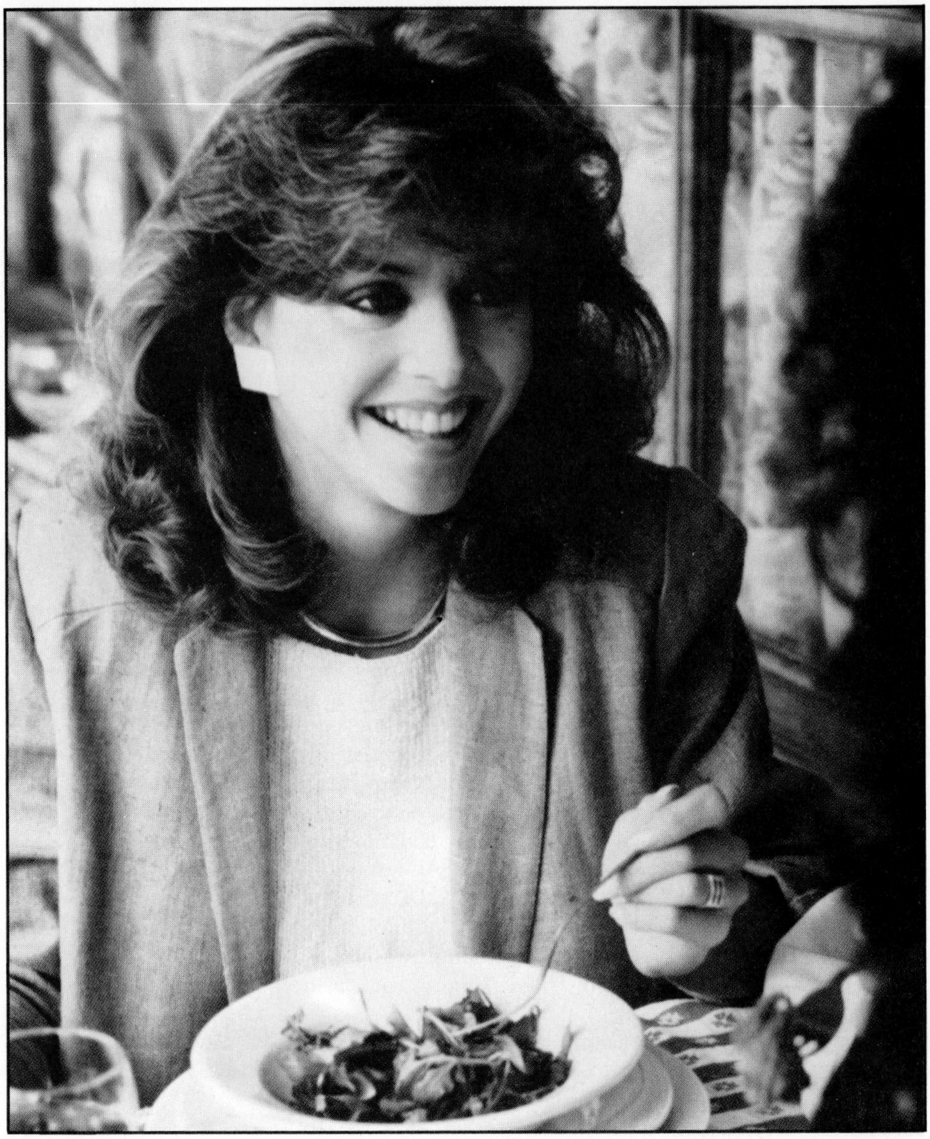

AWARENESS CHECK

Truth or Fiction?

- Obesity occurs when energy intake exceeds energy expenditure.
- Fat weighs more than muscle.
- The number and sizes of fat cells vary in people.
- People who skip breakfast and lunch and overeat at night may actually store more fat than people who eat at regular intervals throughout the day.
- Except in the case of extreme obesity, it is best to lose only 1 to 1½ pounds per week.
- High-protein diets are the quickest and best way to lose excess body fat.
- Weight loss can reduce the risk for heart disease and high blood pressure.

CHAPTER 8

Weight Control

Both obesity and its predecessor, overweight, are considered major health problems in the United States, affecting 34 million Americans representing from 10% to 40% of the population in any age group. Both have serious health consequences and therefore present a challenge to nutritionists, who are now enlisting the help of psychologists and exercise physiologists to deal with the behavioral aspects of prevention and treatment. Because very small discrepancies between intake and expenditure of energy over time result in large changes in weight, it is truly amazing that so many people are able to maintain their weight at a consistent level. Weight control, although difficult, is very important to many people for reasons of appearance as well as health. Unfortunately, misinformation abounds; entrepreneurs everywhere are ready to capitalize on any approach that sounds plausible, regardless of whether there is any evidence of its effectiveness. Although problems of undernutrition are not as prevalent as obesity and do not arouse as much concern, they too represent a health hazard and deserve attention.

Maintain Desirable Weight

Just as different people view carbohydrate, lipid, and protein differently, excesses and deficits in body weight are viewed quite differently under varying social and cultural conditions. Through the centuries, some cultures have given higher status to those with excess body weight; other cultures and subcultures have put an emphasis on slimness. Only in the last 50 years, however, has weight control become a national preoccupation in developed and affluent countries. This is evident in the media, in grocery stores, in the physician's office, in bookstores, in magazines, and in the recently popular diet centers, health clubs, and exercise spas. Ambitious businesspeople are catering to and possibly creating the market for a vast array of diet and calorie-controlled foods, diet books, diet pills, and diet aids, along with exercise devices, cooking pans, psychological aids, hot baths, clothing, and creams all designed to ease the pain of weight loss. Many of these aids promise an easy solution to a problem for which there *is* no easy solution. In general, they are more likely to ensure success for the seller rather than the buyer.

Overweight = >110% of desirable weight for height
Obese = >120% of desirable weight for height

It is estimated that about one tenth of the population of the United States—that is, 13 million people—are truly obese; that is, they weigh more than 120% of the desirable weight for their height. Another 19 million people are overweight;

that is, their body is more than 110% above the level considered desirable but is not high enough to represent an excess of body fat. Overweight individuals, of course, may become obese unless preventive measures are taken to stop or reverse weight gain as soon as the trend is recognized. Of less concern are the many others who only think they are overweight. It seems that most people are either on a diet now, have been on a diet recently, or think they should be on a diet to control body weight. Some people do need to control their weight, but many who "diet" do not.

bariatrics
The science of weight control

Weight control is a term applied to efforts made to maintain or adjust body weight within the limits associated with optimal health and minimal health risks, while **bariatrics** is the science that studies weight control. For the vast majority of adults, weight control is achieved with little or no conscious effort. This is especially impressive because most people consume 1 million kcal/yr and a daily error of 10 kcal, or 0.5% of the energy needs of a sedentary woman, will accumulate to produce a change in body weight either gain or loss of 1 pound (0.45 kg) per year. Similarly, an error of 100 kcal (the energy in 1 tablespoon of butter or one apple) would result in a change of 11 pounds (5 kg) per year. The cumulative effect of such a deviation over a 10-year period is significant. There may be some adjustments made by the body in energy use as fat accumulates or is lost, but initially the relationship that 1 pound fat = 3500 kcal holds. There is a limit to the amount one can lose without severe wasting of the body, but there is no apparent upper limit to the amount that can be gained. The hazards do, however, increase in proportion to the amount gained above a certain critical point, usually more than 40% overweight. Although health professionals are as concerned about the underweight as the overweight individual, they direct considerably more attention to research on the problems of obesity than those of undernutrition.

OBESITY

Obesity is defined as a condition that is marked by an excessive amount of fat in the body. For men, this is considered to be 20% of body weight or more, compared to the normal values of 15% to 18%. For women, obesity is present when body weight consists of 28% to 30% fat or more, compared to the normal values of 18% to 24%. As the amount of fat in the body increases, the individual cells that usually hold up to 20% fat increase in size, two to three times, and become saturated, holding all the fat they can. At this time additional special fat cells known as adipocytes are formed. These cells, which hold up to 62% fat, can be formed in any part of the body. However, the majority of them form beneath the surface of the skin, forming what is known as **subcutaneous fat.** Subcutaneous fat cells appear to be formed any time they are needed, but they tend to increase in number primarily in early infancy and again in adolescence. Once formed they are never lost, they may, however, shrink in size during weight loss (Figure 8-1).

subcutaneous fat
Fat located just beneath the surface of the skin

Figure 8-1 Change in number and size of fat cells with weight gain and weight loss.

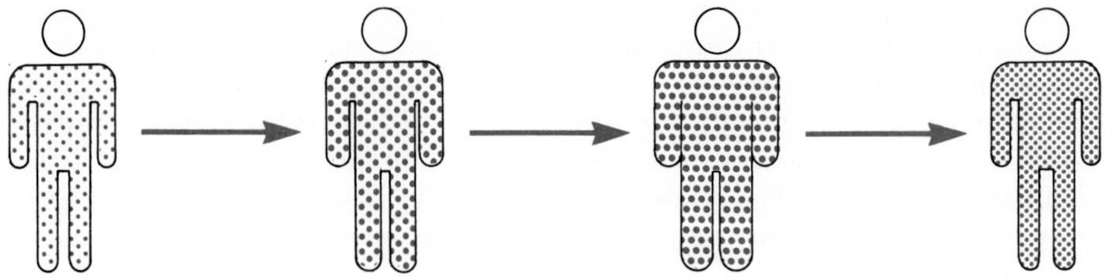

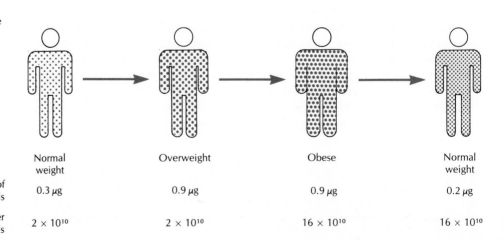

	Normal weight	Overweight	Obese	Normal weight
Size of cells	0.3 μg	0.9 μg	0.9 μg	0.2 μg
Number of cells	2×10^{10}	2×10^{10}	16×10^{10}	16×10^{10}

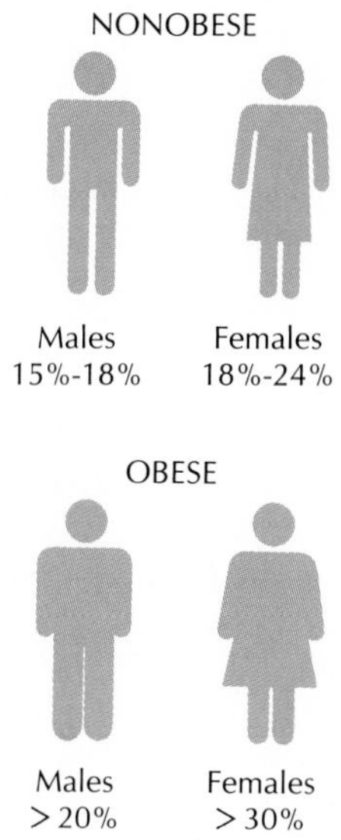

Percentage of body fat in obese vs nonobese people

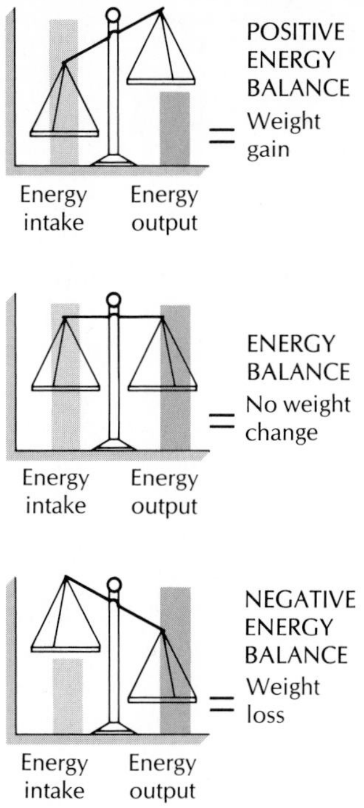

Effect of relative intake and output of energy on body weight

There is a general consensus that weight gain and eventual obesity can occur only when energy intake exceeds energy expenditure. As a result of this easily understood theory, obesity was originally described as *simple obesity*. However, it is now recognized that obesity is a complex condition with a range of causes: physiological, psychological, environmental, and pathological. Treatment is multifaceted to reflect multiple causes and individualized responses.

Incidence

The National Center for Health Statistics estimates that 18% of North American men and 28% of North American women are obese, but it recognizes that there is considerable variation in different regions of the country. The incidence of obesity is high in those parts of the country where people have a sedentary life-style. Of those who are obese about 90% are mildly obese, 9% are considered moderately obese, and only 0.5% are considered severely obese. The incidence of overweight increases throughout adulthood and peaks for men in their mid-50s and women in their mid-60s. After these ages it declines, possibly because of the higher mortality rate among middle-aged obese adults. Figure 8-2, which is based on the application of the body mass index (weight [kg]/height [m]^2) to data on over 36,000 participants in the Nationwide Food Consumption Study, shows the incidence of obesity in 1977-1978. Data from the NHANES studies (1976-1980) show a comparable incidence, based on measurements of subcutaneous fat in triceps (back of upper arm) and subscapular (beneath the shoulder blade) skinfolds. Because almost twice as many people consider themselves overweight or obese as are actually found to be so by weighing or measuring, it is important not to rely on asking people about their weight. The incidence of obesity is considerably higher (up to 7 times) among the lower socioeconomic classes than among the more affluent, who are less likely to continue to gain weight after age 35. At 1 year of age, infants are now 50% heavier than they were a generation ago. The reported weight gain among women between

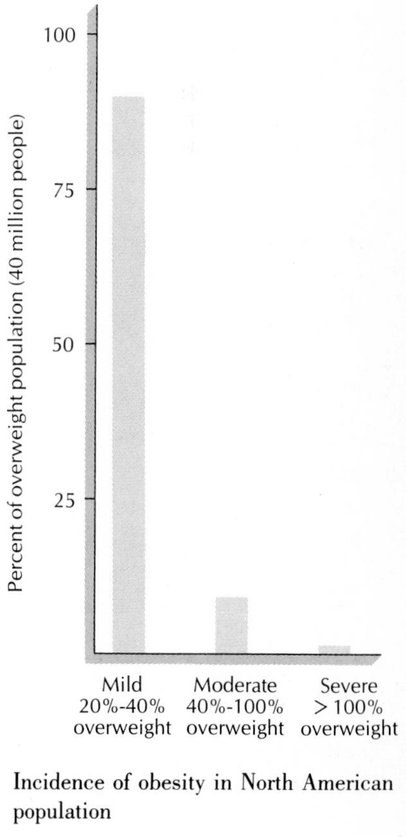

Incidence of obesity in North American population

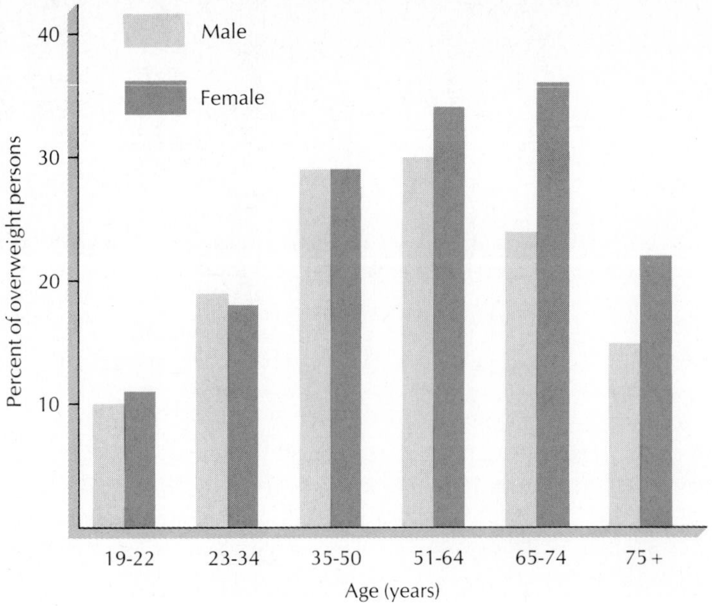

Figure 8-2 Incidence of overweight in the United States by age and sex, based on Nationwide Food Consumption Study. Overweight = BMI (body mass index) > 28, BMI being weight/height^2.

Values of BMI

<18	Underweight (Increased risk for death)
22-27	Normal weight (Minimum risk)
28-30	Mild obesity
30-40	Moderate obesity
>40	Severe obesity (Morbid)

pregnancies appears to be no higher than that among nonpregnant women of the same age. Among children, the incidence of obesity is reported to be about 5% to 15%. One longitudinal study of 5- to 14-year-old children showed a dramatic increase from 15% to 24% in the prevalence of overweight in the 11 years between 1973 and 1984. Some studies have suggested that this increase parallels the increase in the time children spend in sedentary activities, such as watching television. Similarly there has been an increase of almost 40% in obesity in adolescents since 1970. It now affects 22% of 12- to 17-year olds. Adolescent obesity is more likely to persist into adulthood than is childhood obesity.

See Chapter 17 for more discussion of childhood and adolescent obesity

Diagnosis

Because obesity has been defined as a condition in which there is an excess of body fat, its diagnosis must depend on methods of estimating body fat. As you will see, direct methods for measuring body fat are expensive, require considerable technical skill, and are often uncomfortable for the subject. As a result, the most commonly used measures involve indirect assessment of body fat using primarily height, weight, and skinfold thickness.

Direct Methods

Underwater weighing. The relative amount of body weight as fat, compared to more dense or heavy muscle and bone, influences body density. Therefore body density is the standard for determining body fat. Measuring body density involves a comparison of the weight of subjects submerged in a water tank to their weight in air (Figure 8-3). When the proportion of fat to the rest of body weight is approximately 15%, the specific gravity will be about 1. As the fat portion, which has specific gravity of 0.92, increases, the specific gravity of the body decreases (that is, the weight underwater is lower than the weight in the air), and the body is more likely to float. Underwater weighing, which requires subjects to expel all air from the lungs and hold their breath while being weighed, is often frightening. Until recently it was used only for research purposes. The underwater weighing that is now popular in health spas seldom accounts for air in the lungs and is therefore not completely accurate.

$$\text{Specific gravity} = \frac{\text{Weight in water}}{\text{Weight in air}}$$

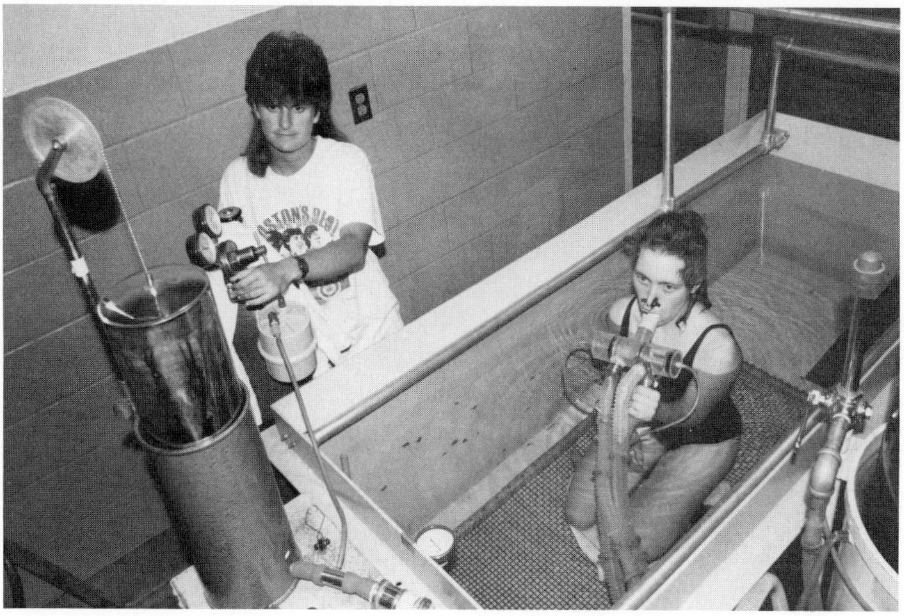

Figure 8-3 Underwater weighing to determine body fatness. Weight is taken with subject completely submerged and all air expelled from the lungs; this weight is compared to subject's weight in air.
Photo courtesy Jos. Loomis, The Pennsylvania State University.

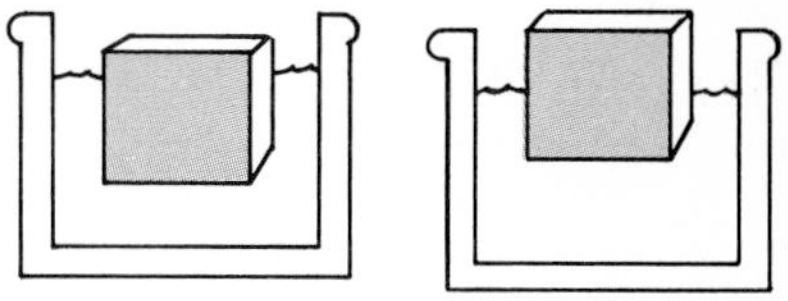

Relative density of fat and muscle tissue

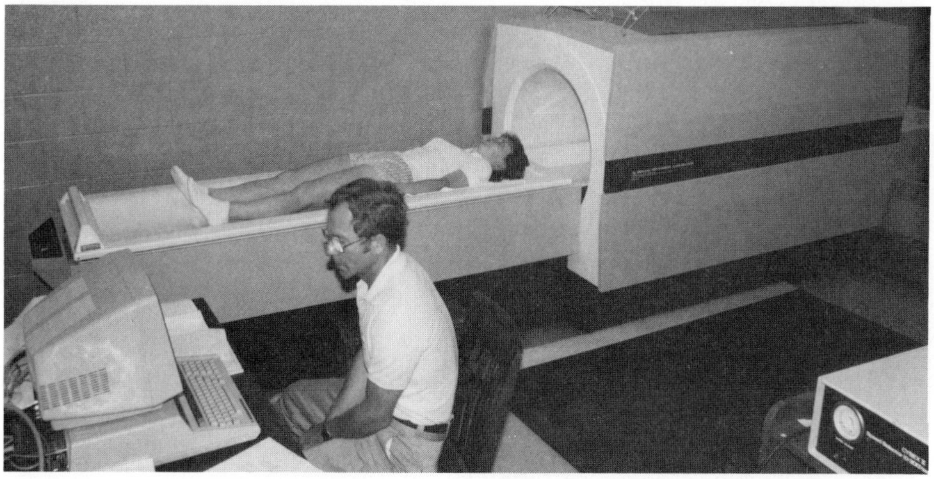

Figure 8-4 TOBEC, or total body electric conductivity, involves moving a body through a tunnel-like apparatus that can measure the amount of body fat based on the change in the magnetic field surrounding the body.
Photo courtesy Jos. Loomis, The Pennsylvania State University.

Other techniques. Several relatively new and sophisticated techniques, such as isotope dilution or total body water determination, ultrasound, TOBEC (total body electric conductivity) (Figure 8-4), computed tomography, magnetic resonance imaging, whole body counter, and neutron activation, allow researchers to get good estimates of total body fat and its distribution. However, because of their complexity and high cost of operation they are not feasible even in clinics. One relatively simple technique known as bioelectric impedance is inexpensive and simple to use (Figure 8-5). It is based on the principle that an electric current travels at a different rate through fat than through water. This technique is being promoted for use in physicians' offices and health spas where there may be an interest in body composition.

In spite of the promise of these recently available techniques for assessing body composition, we still rely heavily on standards based on the anthropometric tools of skinfold thickness, height, and weight.

Methods of Assessing Body Composition
Direct
- Underwater weighing
- Whole body counter
- Isotope dilution
- Ultrasound
- TOBEC
- Computed tomography
- Magnetic resonance imaging
- Neutron activation
- Bioelectric impedence

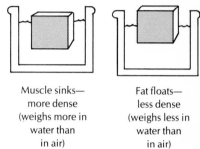

Indirect
- Skinfold
- Height and weight

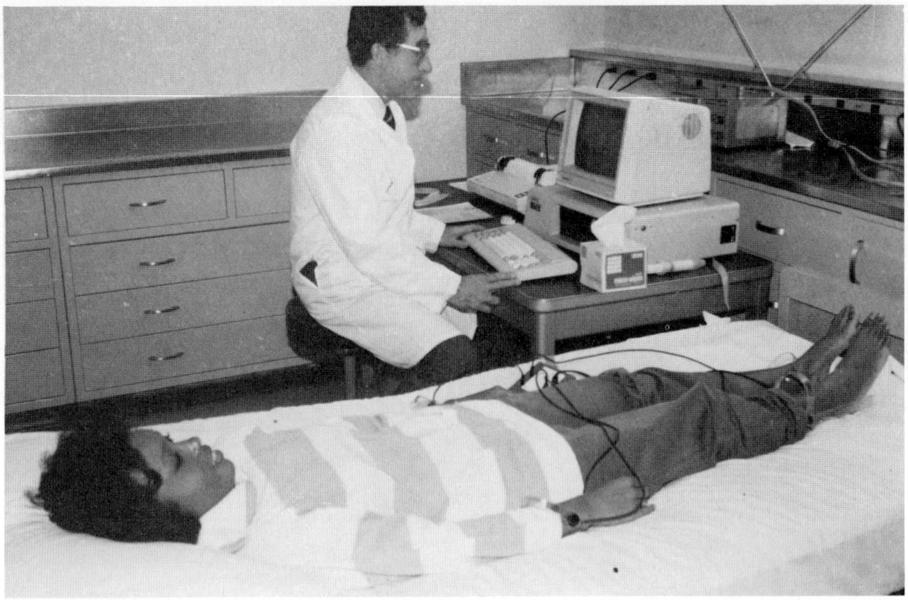

Figure 8-5 Bioelectric impedence is a method of measuring body fat that involves determining the flow of small electric current sent through the body from electrodes attached to the ankles and wrists. The flow is influenced by the amount of water in the body. Since only fat-free tissue contains water, it is possible from this information to calculate the amount of fat.
Photo courtesy Jos. Loomis, The Pennsylvania State University.

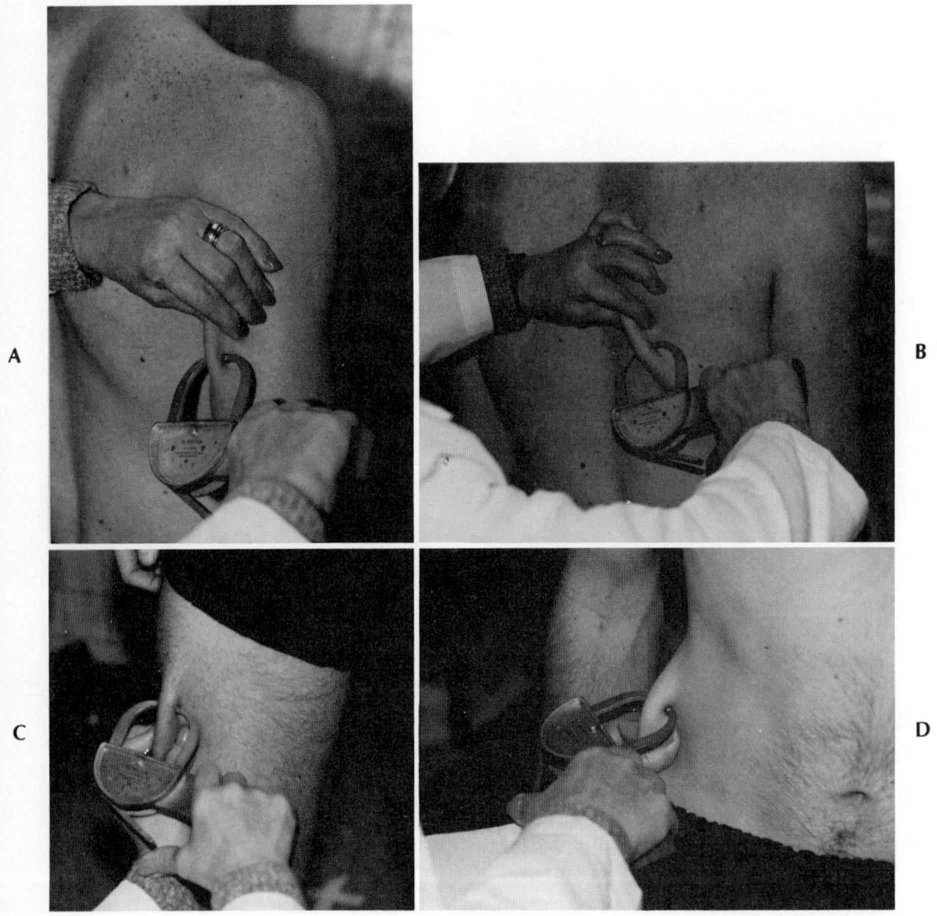

Figure 8-6 Measuring skinfold with calipers. Skin is pinched with fingers to separate fat from muscle; calipers are applied just beneath fold. **A,** Triceps—halfway between shoulder and elbow on back of arm. **B,** Subscapular—below shoulder blade. **C,** Thigh. **D,** Abdomen.
Photos courtesy Jos. Loomis, Human Performance Laboratory, The Pennsylvania State University.

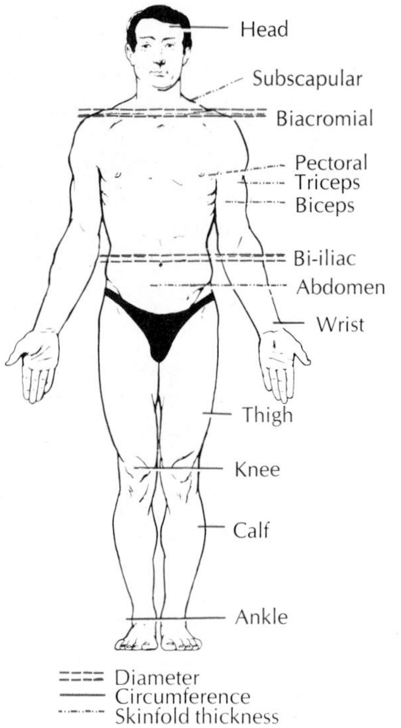

Figure 8-7 Anthropometric measurements used to assess nutritional status.

Indirect Methods

Skinfold thickness measurement. The usefulness of skinfold thickness, which provides a measure of subcutaneous fat, depends on the skill of a professional using a caliper (Figure 8-6). Measurements most frequently involve the thickness of the skin, or fatfold, over the triceps muscle on the outside back of the arm; the biceps on the inside of the arm; or the subscapular region, which is beneath the shoulder blades. Usually an average of several measurements is then compared to standards, such as those for triceps in Appendix M, for the appropriate age and sex or are incorporated into formulas to predict the percentage of body fat. Some formulas require measurements for as many as 10 sites (Figure 8-7), but these are not practical for routine assessment. Although the subscapular is the most useful single measurement, the single triceps skinfold has an advantage because subjects willingly permit this measurement, whereas they are less enthusiastic about others that require undressing.

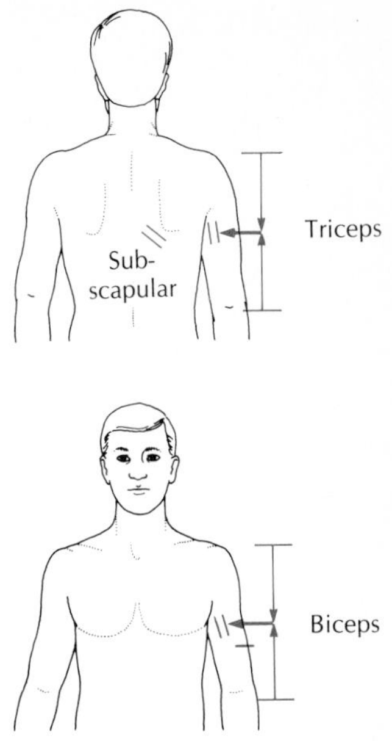

Skinfold measurements: biceps, triceps, and subscapular

Weight and height measurement. Because of the difficulties in measuring skinfolds in infants and young children and the lack of appropriate standards for some other groups used in one of many available formulas, we still rely almost totally on the interpretation of height and weight data to assess body fat. For infants and children, standards are based on data from the National Center for Health Statistics from several large surveys (see Figures 16-2, 16-3, 17-4, and 17-5, presenting growth curves for infants and children). The use of these growth grids, in which periodic measures of height and weight or weight for height are plotted, makes it easy to detect trends toward either undernutrition or obesity before a serious problem develops. For adults, the standards are based on data from the 1979 Body Build and Blood Pressure Study, which in turn was based on data from insurance companies showing the weight for height associated with lowest mortality. Individuals with body weights in excess of 110% of the midpoint of the standard for age, sex, and height (after care is taken to make necessary adjustments for clothing or heel height) are considered overweight. Those with weights in excess of 120% are considered obese (see inside back cover for current standards). We stress that these are arbitrary standards and are most appropriate for assessing incidence of obesity and overweight in a population. Those in the borderline area should be assessed individually, taking into account apparent body composition and patterns of weight over time. Some standards require a judgment about the person's body build or frame size. Sometimes subjective judgments are made by the person being measured; more objective judgments can be obtained by comparing either wrist circumference or elbow width to available standards.

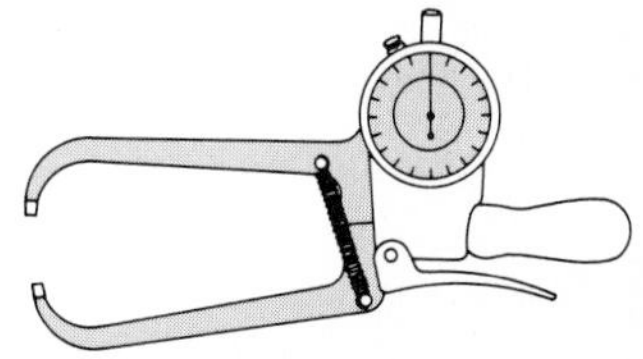

Caliper—instrument used to measure skinfold thickness

A very quick standard to check to see how your weight relates to a desirable weight is:

For men

105 pounds plus 6 pounds/inch over 60 inches, *or*
105 pounds minus 6 pounds/inch under 60 inches

For women

100 pounds plus 5 pounds/inch over 60 inches, *or*
100 pounds minus 5 pounds/inch under 60 inches

These standards can be increased 10% for people with large frames and decreased 10% for small frames.

When obesity is severe, merely looking in the mirror will suffice; however, when obesity is marginal, such subjective measures are of limited value. A simple ruler test suggests a weight problem when a ruler, placed on the chest and abdomen of a subject lying down, is slanted upward toward the feet.

Other standards using information on height and weight have been developed for specific uses. These include the **ponderal index** and the **body mass index (BMI)** also known as the Quetelet index. The ponderal index is the ratio of height to the cube root of weight. The body mass index, which is increasingly popular, is the ratio of weight (kg) to height^2 (m) for both men and women. An index greater

ponderal index <13 = Obesity
Height (inches)/$\sqrt[3]{\text{Weight (pounds)}}$

A person 5 ft 5 in tall weighing 216 pounds has a ponderal index of 65/6 = 10.8.

A person 5 ft 5 in tall weighing 125 pounds has a ponderal index of 65/5 = 13.

body mass index or **Quetelet index**
Weight (kg)/Height^2 (m)

To Determine Your BMI:

1. Divide your weight in pounds by 2.2 to convert it to kilograms.

   A = Weight (kg) = Weight (pounds)/2.2
2. Multiply your height in inches by 2.54 and divide by 100 to convert height to meters.

   B = Height (m) = Height (in) × 2.54/100
3. Multiply B × B.

   C = Height (m) × Height (m)
4. Divide A by C to determine BMI.

   BMI = Weight (kg)/Height^2 (m)

than 27.8 for males and 27.3 for females is indicative of obesity. The simple ratio of weight to height is most appropriate for assessing undernutrition in children, where weight gain will be slowed before the effects of undernutrition are seen in depressed height.

Disadvantages

Before people can be motivated to treat or prevent obesity, they must be convinced that the advantages of weight loss are sufficiently great to warrant the self-discipline involved. Weight reduction calls for willpower, family support, and perseverance over a long period of time, and it is often marked by disappointment and setbacks.

In addition to the well-recognized health hazards, there are many subtle physical, psychological, economic, and social disadvantages to obesity.

Health Hazards

Although the health problems associated with obesity have been evident for a long time, there is still considerable uncertainty about the stage at which obesity becomes a risk factor for morbidity and mortality. The relationship is complicated by the effect of smoking and the coexistence of other diseases. However, when the ponderal index falls below 13.0 or the BMI approaches 28, the mortality rate rises very quickly. Until weight exceeds desirable weight by 20%, there is little increased risk of many of the degenerative diseases. As evident from Figure 8-8, the risk of hypertension, diabetes, and hypercholesterolemia (heart disease) is considerably higher among those overweight or obese. Obese males, regardless of smoking habits, have higher mortality from cancer of the colon, rectum, and prostate than nonobese males. Similarly mortality from cancer of the breast, uterus, ovaries, gallbladder, and bile duct is higher in obese females than in nonobese females. On the other hand, the risk of tuberculosis and other respiratory diseases is less for the overweight or obese person, presumably because of the added protection against changes in

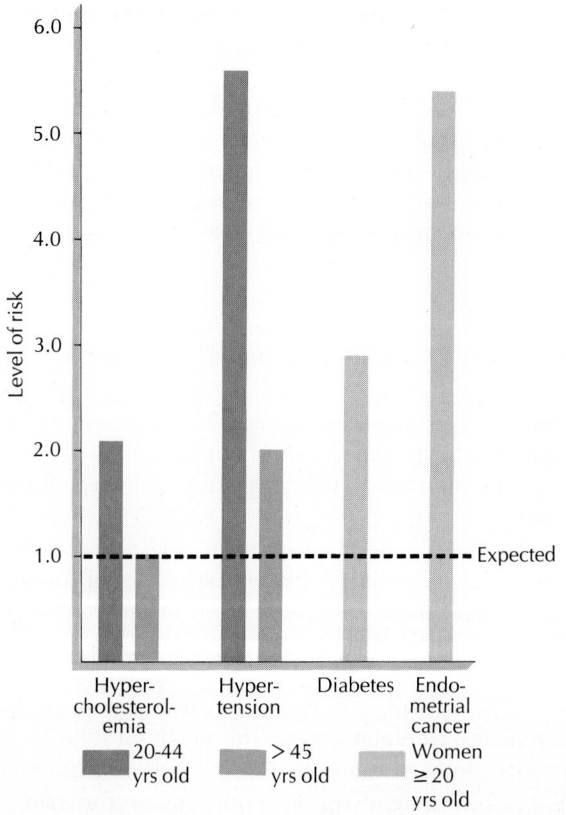

Figure 8-8 Risk of degenerative diseases among overweight individuals (that is, those more than 10% over desirable weight for height) as compared to those of normal weight.

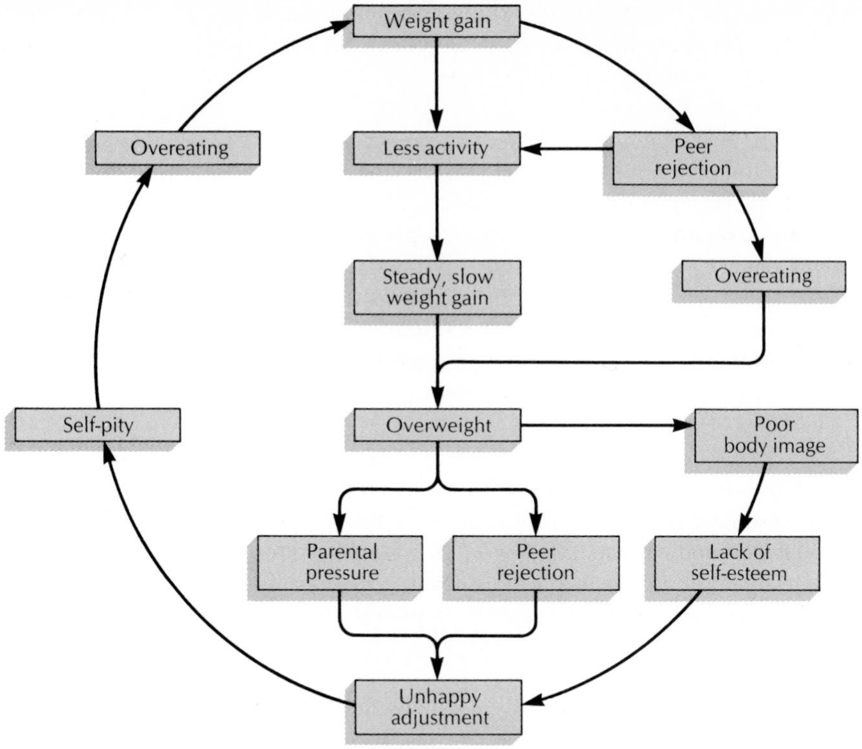

Figure 8-9 Pattern of obesity in adolescence follows vicious cycle of rejection and overeating.

environmental temperature that results from an additional subcutaneous fat layer. The relationship between diabetes and obesity may not be one of cause and effect; rather, obesity may be an early sign of diabetes. Women who are overweight when they become pregnant are greater obstetrical risks because of hypertension, diabetes, and postpartum infections. However, restriction of weight gain in these individuals may cause complications during pregnancy and is therefore not recommended.

The health hazards of obesity vary depending on the distribution of body fat. Fat on the top part of the body, particularly the abdomen, is associated with higher health risks than fat on the lower part of the body (thighs). Similarly, a ratio of waist and hip measurement (W/H) of >1.0 for men and >0.8 for women is associated with higher risk of cardiovascular disease, even within normal BMI range.

Psychological Hazards

The social and psychological costs of obesity may be high. Obese persons are surrounded by subtle and overt pressures from movies, television, and ads for weight-reducing aids that promote thinness and are subject to demands from relatives, friends, and doctors to lose weight. Obese children are teased and excluded from social and physical activities. Not only does this affect the child's self-image, but often it also initiates a vicious cycle of eating, and often sedentary life-style, to compensate for the unhappiness associated with being socially rejected. This in turn leads to greater obesity and perpetuates and increases social isolation and psychological insults (Figure 8-9). Obese girls have been found to have personality characteristics of self-blame, withdrawal, and feelings of inferiority that are also often found in other groups rejected by society.

Many obese people have a preoccupation with weight and a tendency to blame all failures and disappointments on their weight. There is, however, evidence of outright discrimination against the obese in college admissions and in selections for many jobs. This is especially true for jobs that involve contact with the public

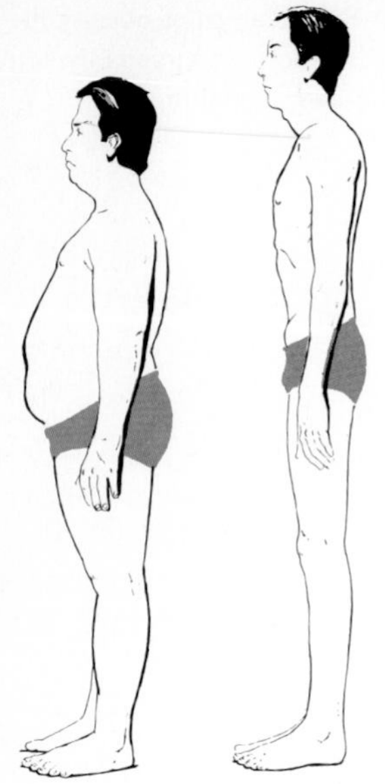

Physical characteristics of individuals with endomorphic features (tendency to obesity) and ectomorphic features (tendency to thinness)

or jobs in the health professions where it is important for people to serve as good role models. Whether or not the cause of obesity is psychological, the obesity itself has profound psychological implications.

Economic Hazards

In addition to being denied access to many jobs and to encountering discrimination in job advancements, the obese individual is subjected to many other economic pressures. In severe cases of obesity, it is necessary to buy clothes at higher prices in stores catering to the overweight. Special furniture, customized automobiles, wider first-class seats on airlines, increased insurance rates because of health risks, extra food consumed, and the weight-reducing aids associated with obesity are only a few of the things that contribute to a higher cost of living.

Causes

The underlying cause of all obesity is the persistence of a positive energy balance (that is, an intake of calories in excess of expenditure for any one individual) over a prolonged period of time. However, this simple statement does little to explain why some people have so much more trouble maintaining a desirable body weight than others do. Differences in genetics and activity levels are major explanations.

Causes of Obesity
Increased energy intake
Decreased activity
Genetic predisposition

Genetics

The role of genetics in obesity will be evident if you look at members of one family with very similar body builds. Obese people usually have predominantly endomorphic features that contribute to a short, stocky stature. Less evident is the impact of genetics on the ways individuals use food and the satisfaction they get from a given amount of food. There is convincing evidence that many obese people or those who gain weight easily eat less food than those who maintain easy weight control and are not obese. The reason appears to be that the obese group uses food more efficiently, has a tendency to store food quickly in the form of fat, and has much more difficulty mobilizing fat to meet energy needs. This does not mean that individuals who are unfortunate enough to inherit a tendency to obesity are doomed to be obese forever. It usually means, however, that they will be faced with a constant and often difficult struggle to overcome the strong tendency to accumulate fat. These people are more likely to produce more fat cells **(hyperplasia)** and to have larger fat cells **(hypertrophy)**, or both. Many genetically obese people have more of an enzyme called **lipoprotein lipase,** which is the enzyme that allows their cells to be more efficient in picking up lipid carried in the blood. These people show a marked taste preference for fat and dislike sweet-tasting solutions.

hyperplasia
Increase in the number of fat cells

hypertrophy
Increase in the size of fat cells

lipoprotein lipase
The enzyme that releases lipid from lipoprotein in the blood to be taken out by the cells

As early as 3 months of age there is a lower energy expenditure in infants born to obese mothers compared to those born to lean mothers. Infants who become overweight by 1 year of age also show lower energy expenditure compared to those who do not become overweight. Overweight adults also have a lower energy expenditure, both total and basal, than predicted. Since metabolic energy expenditure is controlled genetically, the trait is often inherited.

Activity

There is considerable evidence that the obese may gain weight because their activity level is low rather than because their food intake is excessive. The energy cost of many activities may seem quite small. However, 1 hour of tennis uses 350 kcal, and 3 miles of walking costs 140 kcal. For a 154-pound man, 15 minutes of tennis daily for a year would account for 9 pounds (4 kg) of body fat and half a mile of walking every day for a year would account for 2½ pounds of body fat. Almost all effective weight control programs involve exercise, as well as diet.

The energy costs of various activities for people of varying weights are shown in Table 8-1, whereas Table 8-2 gives some examples of the activity equivalents of some common foods.

Table 8-1 ◆ Kilocalories expended for 10 minutes of physical activity

	Body Weight				
Activity	125 Pounds	150 Pounds	175 Pounds	200 Pounds	250 Pounds
Personal Necessities					
Sleeping	10	12	14	16	20
Sitting (reading or watching television)	10	12	14	16	18
Dressing or washing	26	32	37	42	53
Locomotion					
Walking downstairs	56	67	78	88	111
Walking upstairs	146	175	202	229	288
Walking—2 mph	29	35	40	46	58
Walking—4 mph	52	62	72	81	102
Running—5.5 mph	90	108	125	142	178
Running—7 mph	118	141	164	187	232
Cycling—5.5 mph	42	50	58	67	83
Housework					
Domestic work	34	41	47	53	68
Washing windows	35	42	48	54	69
Preparing a meal	32	39	46	52	65
Shoveling snow	65	78	89	100	130
Light gardening	30	36	42	47	59
Mowing grass (power)	34	41	47	53	67
Sedentary Occupation					
Sitting and writing	15	18	21	24	30
Light office work	25	30	34	39	50
Light Work					
Assembly work in factory	20	24	28	32	40
Carpentry	32	38	44	51	64
Heavy Work					
Chopping wood	60	73	84	96	121
Recreation					
Badminton or volleyball	43	52	65	75	94
Basketball	58	70	82	93	117
Bowling (nonstop)	56	67	78	90	111
Dancing (moderate)	35	42	48	55	69
Golfing	33	40	46	53	68
Horseback riding	56	67	78	90	112
Racquetball/squash	75	90	104	117	144
Skiing (Alpine)	80	96	112	128	160
Skiing (cross country)	98	117	138	158	194
Swimming (crawl—20 yd/min)	40	48	56	63	80
Tennis	56	67	80	92	115

From Brownell KD: The partnership diet program, New York, 1980, Rawson, Wade Publishers, Inc.

Table 8-2 ◇ Energy equivalents of food kilocalories expressed in minutes of activity

Food	Kcal*	Activity				
		Walking† (min)	Riding a Bicycle‡ (min)	Swimming§ (min)	Running‖ (min)	Reclining¶ (min)
Apple (large) or banana medium)	101	19	12	9	5	78
Bacon (2 strips)	96	18	12	9	5	74
Beer (1 glass)	114	22	14	10	6	88
Bread and butter	78	115	10	7	4	60
Cake (1/12, 2-layer)	356	68	43	32	18	274
Carbonated beverage (1 glass)	106	20	13	9	5	82
Cereal, dry (1/2 cup) with milk and sugar	200	38	24	18	10	154
Cheese, cheddar (1 oz)	111	21	14	10	6	85
Chicken, fried (1/2 breast)	232	45	28	21	12	178
Cookie, chocolate chip	51	10	6	5	3	39
Doughnut	151	29	18	13	8	116
Egg, fried	110	121	13	10	6	85
Ham (2 slices)	167	32	20	15	9	128
Ice cream (2/3 cup)	193	37	24	17	10	148
Malted milk shake	502	97	61	45	26	386
Mayonnaise (1 tbsp)	92	18	11	8	5	71
Milk, whole (1 cup)	150	32	20	15	9	128
Orange juice (1 glass)	120	23	15	11	6	92
Pie, apple (1/6)	377	73	46	34	19	290
Pizza, cheese (1/8)	180	35	22	16	9	138
Pork chop, loin	314	60	38	28	16	242
Potato chips (1 serving)	108	21	13	10	6	83
Sandwiches						
Club	590	113	72	53	30	454
Hamburger	350	67	43	31	18	269
Tuna fish salad	278	53	34	25	14	214
Sherbet (2/3 cup)	177	34	22	16	9	136
Spaghetti (1+ cup)	396	76	48	35	20	305
Steak, T-bone	235	45	29	21	12	181

From Konishi F: Food energy equivalents of various activities, Journal of the American Dietetic Association 46:186, 1965.
*To convert to kilojoules, multiply by 4.2; to joules, by 4200.
†Energy cost of walking for 70 kg individual equals 5.2 kcal/min at 3.5 mph.
‡Energy cost of riding bicycle equals 8.2 kcal/min.
§Energy cost of swimming equals 11.2 kcal/min.
‖Energy cost of running equals 19.4 kcal/min.
¶Energy cost of reclining equals 1.3 kcal/min.

Theories of Obesity

Fat Cell Theory

adipocytes
Special cell in the body in which fat can be stored

It is well known that fat can be stored in regular cells or in special fat cells known as **adipocytes.** One theory, maintaining that the number of fat cells is determined early in life to provide space to store fat, was generally accepted. Another accepted theory was the concept that, once they have been formed, fat cells have a tendency to remain full of fat. It was also believed that the total number of fat cells was set early in life, supporting the notion that juvenile-onset obesity was caused by an increase in the *number* of fat cells whereas adult-onset obesity was caused by an increase in the *size* of fat cells.

We now know that the number of fat cells can increase in adult life with the likelihood varying from one part of the body to another. There is still evidence, however, that people with a large number of fat cells have more difficulty maintaining body weight than do those with fewer fat cells; they seem to be able to lose weight up to the point where cell size reaches a "normal level" but because of the larger number of cells, it is difficult to reduce beyond that point. Additionally, the increase in the activity of the enzyme lipoprotein lipase, which is produced in increasing amounts by the fat cells as the body loses weight, makes the fat cell more efficient in taking up and storing energy as fat. Ninety-five percent of severely obese persons regain weight after weight loss compared to 66% of moderately obese persons. This is because, in part at least, "reduced-obese" persons have lower energy needs than a person of the same weight who was never obese.

Set Point Theory

The set point theory maintains that each person has an ideal biological weight, or set point. Once body weight reaches this point, a whole set of signals is produced that influences the person's food intake to maintain this weight. The set point weight seems to be controlled in the brain in response to the fatty acid level in the blood. There is reason to believe (or at least hope) that this set point can be reset by a program of exercise and reduced food intake so that the biologically determined weight is a more acceptable one. Otherwise, this theory could provide obese individuals with a rationale for their failure to achieve desirable body weight.

Dietary Theory

The dietary theory maintains that people overeat and therefore gain weight more readily when foods are available and when they are encouraged to eat them. In American society we use food and beverages as expressions of friendship and hospitality in almost all social situations, from the morning coffee break to the late-evening buffet. The more important the occasion, the more food is frequently offered and the more unacceptable it is to refuse the food. Even in very poor societies people feel compelled to save and borrow to provide an acceptable "feast" for a special occasion such as a wedding or baptism.

The influence of the availability of food can be seen in many obese families. For them, obesity appears to be the result of a family environment in which more food than needed is served at each meal, fostering the intake of excessive amounts. This practice may stem from an era when families had much more strenuous activity patterns and therefore ate much larger quantities of food than are needed now.

Another dietary explanation for obesity is found in a fairly common practice known as the "night-eating syndrome," in which a person eats relatively small amounts of food during the day but eats excessive amounts throughout the evening. This eating pattern stimulates the storage of fat for use during the period when intake is lower. Unfortunately, this fat is often very resistant to being mobilized and contributes to the accumulation of more body fat.

Environmental Theory

Much of the problem of weight control can be attributed to our changing life-style, in which we do less and less for ourselves because we are surrounded by labor-saving devices. These include thermostatically controlled rooms that keep us at a comfortable temperature, telephones in each room or those that we carry with us to reduce walking around the house (by as much as 52 miles, or 100 km, a year), electric typewriters and word processors that reduce the energy cost of writing, power steering on automobiles, and electric door openers. Several studies have shown that obese people are much more successful than nonobese people in finding ways to reduce their energy expenditure; they tend to plan their time more efficiently to eliminate unnecessary activities and choose a life-style that is more sedentary than that of the nonobese.

External Environment Theory

A series of innovative studies has shown that many obese people are more likely to respond to external cues to eat rather than to internal hunger signals. They will eat food as long as it is in front of them but will not make an effort to get it. They

External Stimuli to Eat
Time of day
Sight of food
Aroma of food
Availability of food
Companions to share a meal
Money available for food

will buy or consume food immediately after having eaten, in contrast to the nonobese, who are comparatively disinterested in food immediately after eating. According to these studies, obese people eat in response to the clock rather than to internal hunger sensations. It is not clear, however, if the obese are less responsive to internal satiety signals.

Hunger and Satiety

Theories of Appetite Control
Glucostatic (relating to the use of glucose)
Lipostatic (relating to body fat)
Thermic effect
Presence of food

hypothalamus
Area at the base of the brain that controls hunger, appetite, and satiety

Although there has been much research to try to identify the ways in which the body senses hunger and satiety, there is still no agreement on which of the many theories are correct. It is probably true that there is short-term and long-term regulation. Perhaps the oldest theory is the *glucostatic theory*, which is a short-term regulation theory. It maintains that there are receptors in the **hypothalamus** of the brain that are sensitive to the glucose level in the blood. According to this theory, when the glucose level increases following a meal, the hypothalamus responds by sending out satiety signals that cause the individual to stop eating. It now appears that under normal circumstances the level of glucose in the blood as it reaches the brain is not allowed to drop sufficiently low to trigger hunger, nor does it rise sufficiently to cause satiety. However, because it is well established that the ingestion of glucose leads to satiety, scientists now propose that the tongue, the stomach, the intestine, and the liver or a combination of these organs may have receptors that respond to the presence of glucose and send out signals to depress the appetite. In the obese, these signals may be inadequate or the response may be delayed, allowing the person to overeat before the message to stop is received. With either of these theories, glucose ingestion seems to be involved in the short-term regulation of appetite.

lipostat
The body's regulator of appetite that responds to fat; it is located in the hypothalamus of the brain

In contrast, the *lipostatic theory* applies to a more long-term regulation. It is based on the assumption that once body weight reaches a certain point, reflecting either an excessive or an undesirably low percentage of body weight, desire for food intake will either be decreased or increased until the body fat and body weight return to the physiologically desired level. Currently it is assumed that the **lipostat,** which is the body's regulator of appetite that responds to fat, is located in the hypothalamus in the brain and is sensitive to the amount of fatty acids in the blood. Other theories suggest that the lipostat may be sensitive to how full the fat cells are or to the amount of room they have to store more fat. This would support the notion that the obese have trouble regulating their weight because they have more fat cells, "begging" to be filled with fat. How the message is conveyed is not yet understood.

thermic effect (or heat-producing effect)
Changes in body temperature that reflect the composition of the diet; temperatures are higher when protein is eaten and lower when carbohydrate and fat are eaten

Another theory of appetite regulation suggests that the brain responds to temperature changes. These temperatures reflect the composition of the diet, being higher when more protein is eaten and lower when more carbohydrate and fat are eaten. These changes are called the **thermic,** or **heat-producing, effect.**

Still another theory, which is very old, affirms that the stomach responds to the volume of food present and that a person stops eating when the stomach is full. It is now known that the stomach empties food into the small intestine at a fixed rate of a certain number of kilocalories per minute. It has been suggested that the brain can respond to information about the volume of food in the stomach and the rate at which it is emptied, determining the number of kilocalories eaten. Therefore the brain can signal that eating should cease. This signal is reinforced by the secretion of the hormone cholecystokinin, released in the small intestine when food passes into it from the stomach.

Regardless of which, if any, of these theories turns out to be correct, we do know that people of normal body weight can regulate their intake to match their needs more closely than the obese can. An understanding of the mechanism for appetite control does offer hope that before long we may be able to identify a substance to help the obese control their weight.

Weight Control

It is a well-established principle that weight gain occurs when the intake of energy, or kilocalories, exceeds the expenditure for the combined energy costs of basal (or resting) metabolism, activity, and the thermic effect of food. In general, a deficit or an excess of 3500 kcal represents a loss or gain of 1 pound of body fat. To change body weight, therefore, it is essential to create a change of 3500 kcal for every 1-pound adjustment wanted. When calorie intake is below needs, body weight will change much faster if it is muscle or fat-free body mass rather than fat that is being broken down to make up for the deficit in calories. Fat-free tissue, which is about 70% water, represents only 580 stored calories. The loss of any muscle is undesirable, and the loss of any appreciable amount is dangerous, especially because it affects vital muscles such as the heart. In general, weight that is lost rapidly (more than 1 to 2 pounds per week) is gained back more rapidly than that lost more gradually.

1 pound fat = 3500 kcal

Nevertheless, Americans spend over $10 billion every year for quick weight reduction treatments. These treatments and aids include special foods and aids, exercise devices, appetite suppressants, formula diets, health clubs and spas, camps for children, behavior modification, individual counseling, and surgery. What they have in common is failure; of those trying to lose weight, less than 5% maintain the weight loss for more than 3 years.

Contrary to the claims in many ads, there have been no breakthroughs and there are no easy solutions to weight control. In fact, there is increasing evidence to explain why it is so difficult for many people to achieve and maintain their desired body weight. In general, approaches that combine increasing energy expenditure with decreasing energy intake have the greatest likelihood of succeeding. Because it is impossible for this text to deal individually with each of the many approaches to weight control, only the most common will be discussed here.

Changing Treatment Techniques for Weight Control

1977
- Diet and exercise
- Behavior modification
- Starvation
- Appetite suppressants
- Thyroid hormone
- Jejunoileal bypass

1987
- Diet and exercise
- Behavior modification
- Very low calorie diets
- Appetite suppressants
- Serotonin-like drugs
- Thermogenic drugs
- Jaw-wiring
- Gastric restriction

Criteria for Successful Diets

Almost every day you can find headlines in several magazines proclaiming new diets that promise instant and continuing success. Practically all of these, however, are reruns of diets that have been promoted repeatedly over the years. If these diets had lived up to original claims and testimonies, they would have survived. The Focus section of this chapter provides a summary of the features of the most common classes of diets and points out the hazards and advantages associated with each of them.

Be wary of any diet, device, or pill that promises quick and easy weight loss. There is none. Weight loss is a slow and tedious process.

Any diet that meets the following seven criteria is one that will probably be nutritionally adequate and will lead to a steady and reasonable weight loss and a good possibility of long-term success.

Success in Weight Reduction is More Likely if the Individual is
- Young
- Single
- Of higher socioeconomic status
- Making a first attempt
- Less than 60% overweight
- Emotionally well adjusted

1. The diet must be deficient in kilocalories. This can be determined only by comparing the caloric value of the diet with a reasonable estimate of each person's needs. A diet that shows a deficit for one person does not necessarily do so for another. A daily deficit of 500 kcal, leading to a deficit of 3500 kcal/week, should result in the loss of 1 pound of body weight. Unfortunately, the tendency of the body to replace this fat temporarily with water is discouraging to the reducer. However, if the regimen is continued long enough—sometimes as long as 4 or 5 weeks—the total predicted loss eventually occurs, often all at once.

2. The diet should be adequate in all other nutrients except kilocalories. Although this is difficult to check precisely, a fairly good indication can be made by checking the diet to see that it includes servings from each of the four major food groups, each of which must be present if a diet is to approach adequacy in most nutrients. There should be as least two servings from each of the following four groups: milk and dairy products; fruits and vegetables; cereal products; and meat, fish, poultry, and eggs. At a level of 1400 kcal it is possible, with a careful choice of foods, to achieve a diet that meets the RDAs for all nutrients. As the number of kilocalories drops, it is increasingly difficult to choose an adequate diet.

If energy intake is restricted to less than 1000 kcal, the diet should be supplemented with protective, but not excessive (>100% RDAs), levels of the minerals and vitamins that will probably be lacking in the diet.

isocaloric
With the same number of calories (*iso* = the same)

3. The diet should have satiety value. Diets containing some fat and relatively high levels of protein delay the onset of hunger pangs longer than **isocaloric** diets (that is, diets with the same number of kilocalories) composed primarily of carbohydrate. It is easier to adhere to a diet of high satiety value than to one with foods that leave the stomach rapidly or have little bulk.

4. The diet should be one that can be adapted readily from family meals or obtained in public eating places. Any diet that sets reducers apart from others with whom they eat or that imposes extra work on the person preparing meals is less likely to be followed than a diet that allows people to eat inconspicuously with family or friends in all social situations.

5. The diet must be reasonable in cost. If it makes use of seasonal foods and staple dietary items, it will be more acceptable than a diet that calls for expensive, out-of-season, unfamiliar foods.

6. The diet should be one that can be adhered to for a sufficient period of time to achieve the desired weight loss. It is recommended that, except in extreme obesity, the rate of weight loss not exceed 1 to 1½ pounds (0.5 to 0.7 kg) a week. Therefore a person wishing to lose 20 pounds (9 kg) should try to accomplish this over a period of at least 15 weeks. Crash diets that limit dieters to a restricted list of foods such as "cottage cheese and peaches" or "steak, eggs, and tomatoes" are not only nutritionally inadequate but also so monotonous that their psychological appeal lasts only a short time. It is almost impossible for a person to remain on such a limited selection of foods long enough to achieve the desired weight loss.

7. Most important of all, if dieters are to achieve long-term success, the diet chosen should represent a sufficient departure from former eating patterns. Dieters need to be retrained in a new set of eating habits that they can expect to adhere to, with slight modifications, as a maintenance diet for a lifetime. The liquid formula diets fail largely because they do not lead to any permanent weight loss. This can be attributed partly to the fact that they do not substitute a new, socially acceptable, and satisfying pattern of eating for the old one that led to the weight gain.

It is obvious that a diet that meets these criteria, as summarized below, will lead to success only if it is followed long enough to effect the weight loss and to establish a new pattern of eating.

Criteria for Assessing Weight Reducing Diets

- **Must be deficient in kilocalories**
- **Must have adequate amounts of all other nutrients**
- **Must have sufficient fat or bulk to provide satiety**
- **Must be able to be adapted from family meals or when eating out**
- **Must be reasonable in cost**
- **Must be a diet that can be adhered to for a sufficient time to lose weight**
- **Must retrain the individual in a new set of eating habits**

It is important to caution prospective dieters about the characteristics of some diets that are almost certainly doomed to failure.

1. There is no single food that will facilitate weight loss either by "burning fat," stimulating metabolism, or causing fat to "melt away." Any diet composed of a single food will certainly cause weight loss, even during the short period of time

in which it is usually used. Unfortunately, it almost always results in a deficiency of one or more other nutrients, with potentially negative health consequences.

2. A diet that promises to allow you to eat as much as you want is almost certainly made up of foods that are so unpalatable that you will want only small amounts of them.

3. Total fasting is appropriate only for the severely or morbidly obese; even then it should be undertaken only under strict medical supervision and guidance. Protein sparing fasts following 400-calorie diets of approximately 50% protein are much more satisfactory.

4. Extremely low kilocalorie diets of less than 500 kcal not only are deficient in kilocalories and fail to establish new eating habits, but they may also lead to ketosis, a condition in which abnormal products of fat metabolism appear in the blood and urine. This condition results in a change in acid-base balance and abnormalities of metabolism. Low-calorie diets also cause problems with irregular heart rhythms. It is important that diets contain about 50% protein of good quality. The poor quality of the protein in liquid protein (from gelatin) was likely responsible for the many deaths on those diets.

Weight cycling (Yo-Yo dieting). The problem of rather large swings in body weight, as the result of successful dieting followed by a relapse and weight gain, often to an even higher level, has been around for a long time. We now know that many people who lose considerable body weight experience a decrease in energy requirements so that the period required to lose the same amount of weight is much longer on the second attempt at weight loss than on the first, and the period to regain lost weight is comparably shorter. As weight is lost muscle is lost. As weight is gained fat is gained. The reason for this effect has not yet been identified.

Behavior Modification

Behavior modification as an approach to weight control was introduced in the early 1970s. It includes an analysis of the conditions under which people eat, including both physical and emotional environments. This analysis involves keeping a record for at least 1 week of when and where a person eats and more importantly how he feels at the time—for example, angry, happy, or lonely. Following this, he is encouraged to set reasonable goals for modifying food intake, and a schedule of reinforcement for achieving these goals is established. In some cases it is appropriate to have negative consequences for failure to comply rather than positive rewards for compliance. The success of this method depends on the sensitization of the subjects to aspects of their behavior that are contributing to overeating. Achievable, stepwise goals for changing behavior that has been identified as a problem are set and achievement is rewarded. Examples of behavioral changes that may be recommended are eating more slowly, seldom eating alone, eating at specified times or places, putting down the fork between bites, reducing the amount and frequency of use of foods that were often eaten in excess, and resisting opening the refrigerator between meals.

Conservative treatments. As a result of experience with behavior modification an approach designated as "conservative" has been developed. This individualized dietary approach recommends a weight loss of approximately 1% of total body weight per week and includes a diet providing approximately 50%, and never less than 40%, of energy needs for maintenance of body weight. This minimizes the loss of lean body mass, which even under these conditions amounts to 1 gram for every gram of fat lost. Since this approach results in a slow weight loss over a long period of time, the possibility of achieving and maintaining a significant weight loss is enhanced. Conservative treatment has been shown to be cost effective. It involves seven elements

1. Self-monitoring or keeping records of behavior to be changed
2. Control of stimuli that precede eating
3. Development of techniques to control eating

4. Reinforcement of prescribed behaviors
5. Cognitive restructuring of expressed views toward positive expectations of success
6. Nutrition education
7. Increased physical activity

Self-Help Groups

Groups such as TOPS (Taking Off Pounds Sensibly), Overeaters Anonymous, or Weight Watchers have provided the group support that has made it possible for many to accomplish what they were unable to do by themselves in achieving weight control. In TOPS, participants are provided with encouragement; those who succeed each week are applauded, those who did not are helped to recognize where they had a problem. TOPS offers little dietary advice or guidance. Overeaters Anonymous is based on the same principle as Alcoholics Anonymous. Although the support system itself is beneficial, participants are encouraged to seek medical advice on nutrition. The nutritional quality of the program then depends on what advice, if any, is obtained. In Weight Watchers, group support is reinforced by a prescribed diet that nevertheless permits members to make choices within categories to suit their own preferences. This group also makes available portion-controlled low-calorie entrees and other menu items that can be used as the basis for a diet plan and as an aid to learning new eating habits. For children and some adult groups, summer camps and spas providing a program of activity and a controlled eating environment have helped establish a new life-style conducive to weight control.

Commercial Plans

Over the last 10 years, a large number of diet plans at all price ranges have been designed to provide complete dietary control. Some of these plans have been based on a liquid formula diet or on a complete line of packaged foods. Some include a residence program that combines controlled food intake with exercise. Others are largely exercise programs with general dietary advice. The creators of these plans are motivated by profit, with income obtained from the sale of foods, services, and dietary aids. Very few of the plans have survived profitably for any appreciable length of time. However, so many people are turning to such enterprises that failed programs are rapidly replaced by others with the same or similar appeal and promises.

Obviously, the programs that are attempting to provide overweight individuals with quick, easy, and painless ways to control weight are many and varied. At present, however, there is no substitute for a steady intake of calories below energy expenditure. In spite of large sums of money and the motivation of scientists to untangle the mysteries of appetite regulation, there is little hope that a panacea is forthcoming. When and if the breakthrough does come, it will be heralded in scientific literature; it won't come in the form of a "revolutionary product" announced in a newspaper or magazine advertisements. Criteria for assessing advertised weight-control plans are given in the box on p. 217.

Among the current commercial plans are Optifast, a formulated powdered meal replacement appropriately supplemented with vitamins and minerals that usually contains about 400 kcal. It is available only for use under medical supervision. Diet Center provides a four phase program based on an intitial diet of 915 kcal for women and 1045 kcal for men, in which dairy products are forbidden and starches greatly restricted. The initial diet is followed by a maintenance diet of 1500 kcal (women) and 1700 kcal (men). Nutri-System participants eat prepackaged entrees of about 100 kcal and flavor sprays for snacks. Residential spas focus on weight loss, healthy living, socially oriented programs, and "pampering" at a cost of $50 to $350 per day. Many spas require some fasting, which leads to a weight loss that is hard to maintain after leaving the controlling environment. Immune Power Diet of 800 to 1200 calories attributes obesity to hypersensitivity to certain foods. This supposedly can be determined by cytotoxic testing, but it is of unproven value.

Activity

Although our discussion so far has focused on the intake side of the energy equation, energy balance is determined as much by the output as by intake of calories. With growing concern that diets that are drastically restricted in calories may be associated with less than adequate intakes of other nutrients, much more attention has been directed toward recommending an increase in energy expenditure rather than relying solely on decreasing intake to balance the equation. A fringe benefit of a regular exercise program is the gradual increase in lean body mass and muscle tonus.

Guidelines for Evaluating Commercial Weight-Loss Promotions

Avoid commercial weight-loss or control programs which:

1. Promise or imply dramatic, rapid weight-loss (that is, substantially more than 1% of total body weight per week).

2. Promote diets that are extremely low in calories (that is, below 800 calories per day; 1200 calories per day diets are preferred) unless under the supervision of competent medical experts.

3. Attempt to make clients dependent upon special products rather than teaching how to make good choices from the conventional food supply (this does not condemn the marketing of low-calorie convenience foods which may be chosen by consumers).

4. Do not encourage permanent, realistic life-style changes including regular exercise and the behavior aspects of eating wherein food may be used as a coping device (that is, programs should focus upon changing the *causes* of overweight rather than simply the *EFFECTS*, which is the overweight itself).

5. Misrepresent salespeople as "counselors" supposedly qualified to give guidance in nutrition and/or general health. Even if adequately trained, such "counselors" would still be objectionable because of the obvious conflict of interest that exists when providers profit directly from products they recommend and sell.

6. Require large sums of money at the start or require that clients sign contracts for expensive, long-term programs. Such practices too often have been abused as salespeople focus attention upon signing up new people rather than delivering continuing, satisfactory service to consumers. Programs should be on a pay-as-you-go basis.

7. Fail to inform clients about the risks associated with weight-loss in general, or the specific program being promoted.

8. Promote unproven or spurious weight loss aids such as human chorionic gonadotrophin hormone (HCG), starch blockers, diuretics, sauna belts, body wraps, passive exercise, ear stapling, acupuncture, Electric Muscle Stimulating (EMS) devices, spirulina, amino acid supplements (e.g., arginine, ornithine), glucomannan, and so forth.

9. Claim that "cellulite" exists in the body.

10. Claim that use of an appetite suppressant or methylcellulose (a "bulking agent") enables a person to lose body fat without restricting accustomed caloric intake.

11. Claim that a weight-control product contains a unique ingredient or component unless it is unavailable in other weight-control products.

Courtesy National Center Against Health Frauds, Loma Linda, Calif.

The effectiveness and feasibility of increasing the level of activity to achieve weight control have been alternately underrated and overrated. The 3500 kcal stored in 1 pound of body fat is sufficient energy for many hours of vigorous activity—in fact that is enough to discourage many people from even considering exercise as a viable alternative. These people tend to lose sight of the fact that weight control is not a short-term solution but a lifetime commitment. Although a 132-pound (60 kg) woman may consider walking 90 miles to be a totally unreasonable way to lose 1 pound of weight, walking a short one fourth of a mile every day for a year is usually acceptable. These two methods will bring about the same results and will be sufficient to ensure that weight does not accumulate at a gradual but insidious rate as energy needs slowly but steadily decline with age. The importance of establishing a life-style that involves consistent mild exercise cannot be overstressed.

There are additional benefits in terms of enhanced vitality associated with a moderately active exercise program. Strenuous exercise initially leads to a loss of appetite; after the adjustment period, however, the appetite usually returns and counterbalances some of the benefits of a vigorous program. Efforts to cope with impending obesity among schoolchildren have been quite successful when the approach taken has been to increase activity and reduce intake to match requirements rather than attempt to have growing children actually reduce their weight. In this way, children solve their weight problem by "growing into" their weight.

It is relatively easy to calculate the energy cost of any activity over and above the amount needed for sedentary activities from the information in Table 7-11. We have also included Table 8-2, in which the energy cost of activity is related to the energy provided by some commonly eaten foods. With this information, it is possible to assess trade-offs in terms of food and activity. Table 8-1 provides essentially the same information from the perspective of the kilocalorie cost of 10 minutes of a variety of activities. The importance of a combined diet and exercise program is being recognized by a growing number of health clubs, spas, executive health programs, and programs on the work site that are providing instruction in both exercise and diet. Many worksite programs are also providing nutrition information in company cafeterias and a host of education opportunities to ensure that employees have a complete picture of the combined effect of diet and exercise on body weight, fitness, productivity, and work attendance.

Surgical Approaches

Lipectomy is the surgical removal of excess fat primarily from the abdominal area. Liposuction, which involves suctioning off subcutaneous fat, is practiced primarily during cosmetic surgery. These two methods were introduced relatively recently but are considered of questionable value and involve significant risk.

Jejunoileal bypass, which requires a surgical procedure to connect the beginning of the jejunum to the terminal portion of the ileum reduces the length of the absorptive surface of the intestine by as much as 20 feet. This approach is based on the theory that less carbohydrate, protein, and fat will be absorbed and hence fewer calories will be available to the obese individual. Even though this procedure may lead to a substantial weight loss of 60 to 100 pounds, the serious metabolic, biochemical, and surgical side effects mean that it should be used only under extreme circumstances.

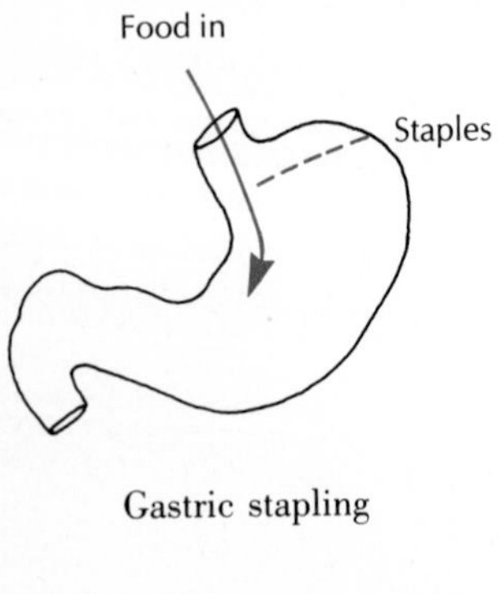

Gastric stapling

Gastric stapling, or gastroplasty, closes off most of the stomach, leaving only an opening large enough to hold a very small amount of food. This procedure results in considerable weight loss and involves fewer complications than bypass surgery. Much the same effect is obtained by inserting a balloon into the stomach and inflating it to reduce the capacity of the stomach, which makes the person feel less hungry and more satisfied with less food.

Jaw-wiring, which limits a person to a liquid diet, is used primarily to bring about some weight loss prior to other surgical procedures. Its other use for 6 to 9 months is a very drastic measure, appropriate only for extreme cases.

Diet Aids

Diet aids fall into two main categories: those that are reported to suppress the appetite and those that stimulate metabolism or energy expenditure. A third category—that of "useless" diet aids—might well be added. Many products on the market are part of the multimillion-dollar diet business but are not helpful as diet aids.

Appetite suppressing foods. The most common appetite suppressants are glucose and the more complex sugar, sucrose. Several diet aids are merely candy to which has been added the equivalent of vitamin-mineral supplement; this allows claims that they are balanced products. If taken about half an hour before mealtime, these suppressants do introduce a feeling of satiety as a result of the presence of glucose. The same effect could be obtained by eating ½ teaspoon of sugar or 3 jelly beans or by drinking ½ cup of grape, apple, or any other fruit juice.

Drugs. Difficulties and failure in dietary control of body weight have led to the use of a variety of drugs with little or no success. Drugs used include tranquilizers, which are supposed to reduce anxiety and therefore nibbling; phenylethylamines, which act by depressing the appetite but have serious side effects; bulking agents such as methylcellulose, used to give a feeling of fullness, but which cause flatulence; and adrenalin and thyroxin, which increase metabolism but *must* be used only under medical supervision.

Some other drugs currently marketed for dietary control of weight, which are described below, vary in effectiveness and have at least some limitations.

Growth hormone releasers, largely proteins with high levels of arginine, are sold under a wide variety of names. They are to be taken at night when they will stimulate the secretion of growth hormone and increase metabolism and hence calorie use. They are promoted for older people in whom growth hormone secretion is low. Because growth hormone releasers are taken at night, they are sometimes marketed under such names as "Dream Away" or "Nite-Time."

Amphetamines, which are available only by prescription (Benzadrine, Dexadrine), dull the appetite but are also addictive and have adverse effects on the heart and nervous system.

Human chorionic gonadotropin (HCG), a hormone from the urine of pregnant women, is given by injection and is neither safe nor effective for weight loss. This drug does not reduce hunger nor "melt" fat.

Phenylpropanolamine (PPA), the active ingredient in many cold remedies and over the counter (OTC) products, is considered a safe and effective appetite suppressant by the FDA but should not be taken by people with high blood pressure, diabetes, or thyroid or kidney problems. Almost all diet-control products based on phenylpropanolamine guarantee results *if* the subject follows the accompanying instructions, which invariably involve restricting caloric intake and increasing energy expenditure.

Fenfluramine is an appetite depressant that, in contrast to most others, does not cause central nervous system (CNS) stimulation. It does, however, have side effects, which cause drowsiness, lethargy, and depression.

Starch blockers, now considered as illegal drugs, were formerly promoted to block the digestion of starch and thus reduce the number of calories available for absorption.

Dehydroepiandrosterone (DHEA), which is the breakdown product of a hormone normally excreted in the urine, is unproven as a weight reducing aid and therefore not approved by the FDA.

Cholecystokinin (CCK) is a polypeptide hormone normally secreted in the small intestine in response to the presence of fat. It stimulates the pancreas and gallbladder to increase the flow of digestive enzymes. As a dietary drug, it has not been proven to meet the claim of causing sudden and dramatic weight loss. There is some evidence that as it normally functions in the body, CCK may act on the brain to depress the appetite. Because CCK is a protein, if taken orally, it would be digested to amino acids and would not reach the brain as CCK.

Arginine and ornithine, both amino acids, are promoted for their ability to stimulate the production of the growth hormone, which then causes the body to "burn" fat. They are of no proven benefit.

In spite of all the claims there is no drug on the market that is totally safe and effective in assisting in weight control for all people.

Low-calorie foods are foods with less than 40 kcal/serving
Reduced-calorie foods have less than one third the calories of the foods they replace

Other products. Other products on the market that are designed to promote weight loss are low-calorie foods with less than 40 kcal/serving; reduced-calorie foods with at least one third fewer calories than the foods they replace; diuretics, which bring about temporary and sometimes dangerous weight loss by causing the loss of body water; bulk-producing substances that tend to swell in the stomach and give a sense of satiety; and premeasured foods such as frozen entrees that help eliminate any error in judgment when estimating serving sizes. Some of these are useless and harmless, some are useless and harmful, and—fortunately—some are useful and harmless.

Foods sweetened with noncaloric sweeteners, such as aspartame, saccharin, and cyclamates, are designed to help control calorie intake. Fat-modified products, high-fiber foods, and foods containing bulking agents all have the same purpose of assisting calorie control.

Spirulina, a protein powder produced from the growth of algae, is sold as an appetite suppressant based on its high content of the amino acid, phenylalanine.

Glucomannan, sold as an "Oriental weight loss secret," comes from a Japanese root, konjac, does nothing more than create a sense of fullness.

Pectin, a polysaccharide with the ability to attract and hold water, has surfaced as a weight control substance undoubtedly in the belief that if it attracts water and increases in bulk it will be more filling in the stomach and hence depress the appetite. To obtain a significant amount of pectin from food a person would have to consume large amounts of fruits and vegetables, which in themselves would likely depress the appetite.

Benzocaine, a surface anesthetic used in many diet gums and candies, numbs the surface of the tongue to destroy the sense of taste.

Aerosol sprays with many popular food flavors are promoted as a way to control the "munchies" without the hazard of calories. They have been used as part of the commercial Nutri-System approach.

Among the worthless devices that the public has been duped into buying are eyeglasses that reflect an image supposed to dampen the desire to eat; electrical muscle stimulators, which provide a risk of electrical shock and burns if misused; wraps and garments that along with special creams "burn" fat; belts and sweatsuits that induce sweating and hence temporary weight loss from water loss. No doubt creative entrepreneurs will continue to devise imaginative ways to get those with weight problems to waste money.

Prevention

From a public health point of view, the most feasible solution to the problem of obesity is prevention. As our knowledge of the epidemiology of obesity increases, it should be possible to identify the groups and points of access to these groups that would increase the likelihood of preventing obesity. The best programs would probably include both exercise and dietary approaches and would capitalize on our knowledge of the responsiveness of various groups to alternative approaches.

Since the tendency toward obesity is genetic, pediatricians are in a key spot to alert parents to the problem. They can encourage the parents to promote eating patterns that will encourage caloric restriction and activity patterns that will encourage energy expenditure. Similarly, school authorities with access to school growth records can identify students at risk and guide them into appropriate preventive programs.

For women, obstetricians and gynecologists have the opportunity to sensitize their patients to the risk of weight gain both during pregnancy and at menopause. Physicians dealing with middle-aged men who are working under emotional stress also have an excellent opportunity; they can provide them with nutritional guidance to prevent a weight gain that will increase the risk of coronary heart disease and other degenerative diseases.

With increasing recognition that problems of weight control stem as much from low energy expenditure as from excessive food intake, the importance of creating opportunities for nutritionists and exercise physiologists to work together in planning preventive programs becomes more and more evident.

UNDERWEIGHT

Underweight = <85% desirable weight for height

People whose weight is more than 15% below the desirable weight for their height are not subjected to the same social pressures as are overweight people. Nevertheless, they are confronted with health problems that may be just as severe. Although they have a lower risk of hypertension, diabetes, and cardiovascular problems, they are much more susceptible to respiratory problems, ranging from the common cold to tuberculosis. In addition, they have difficulty conserving heat and maintaining a comfortable body temperature as environmental temperatures fluctuate. They usually do not have the deposits of brown fat that permit nonshivering thermogenesis (heat production), which is important in maintaining temperature. Unfortunately, there is not as much profit to be made from marketing a weight-enhancing product or gimmick. Therefore people who suffer from undernutrition tend to be a neglected segment of the population.

Treatment

The treatment of underweight people involves creating a positive energy balance by increasing intake to exceed expenditure. It is just as important to determine the underlying cause of undernutrition as it is to determine the cause of overnutrition. Because underweight people usually have a low caloric intake, there is the increased possibility that they will have only marginal intakes of many nutrients. (For discussions of anorexia nervosa and bulimia, which are eating disorders associated with weight loss, see Chapter 17.)

The use of smaller, more frequent meals will in some cases help increase the total food intake, as will the addition of calorie-dense foods such as butter, cheese, sugar, cream sauces, and gravies. These high-calorie foods are better used at the end of a meal because it is undesirable to create a feeling of satiety too early in the meal. Many of the commercial food products designed for use by postoperative patients and calorie-dense foods such as butter, cream sauces, dried fruits, granola, and nuts are reasonable foods to encourage underweight people to eat to increase caloric intake. Since many foods with high nutrient density are the same ones people should avoid to reduce the risk of cardiovascular disease, we should caution underweight people about the risks of long-term use of foods high in saturated fats and encourage periodic checks of their blood cholesterol levels.

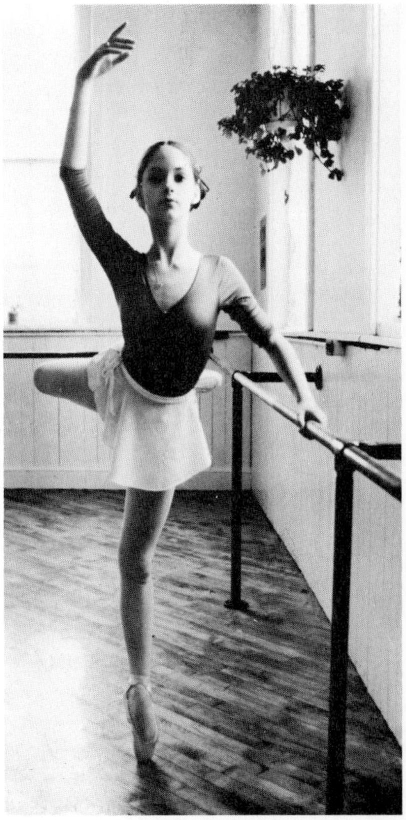

Some activities or occupations, such as ballet or modeling, require participants (who are often women) to maintain below-normal amounts of body fat. This can lead to health problems.

In gaining weight, it is important both that the adjustment be made gradually and that the weight gain be the result of a diet that is nutritionally balanced, as well as calorically dense.

Although discussions of weight gain do not usually include the role of exercise, it is as important here as in weight control for obesity. Not only does moderate exercise stimulate the appetite (strenuous exercise depresses appetite), it also fosters the development of muscle at the same time that extra energy is stored as fat.

BY NOW YOU SHOULD KNOW

- One fourth to one half of the North American population is either overweight or obese.
- Obese males have >20% body weight as fat and obese females have >30%.
- Subcutaneous fat is located just beneath the surface of the skin; this fat can be measured with calipers to predict an individual's total body fat.
- Because overweight leads to obesity, it is a health risk for degenerative diseases such as coronary heart disease, hypertension, adult-onset diabetes, cancer, and gout.
- The regulation of appetite and weight control is not clearly understood, but many theories are now being studied.
- Set point theory maintains we all have an ideal biological weight, it may, however, be reset through exercise and diet.
- A gain of 1 pound in body fat results from an excess of 3500 dietary kcal and a loss of 1 pound of body fat requires a deficit of 3500 dietary kcal or an expenditure of 3500 kcal over total energy needs.
- The ultimate goal in weight control is to adjust energy expenditure and/or energy intake so that intake is less than expenditure.
- There are specific criteria for assessing weight reducing diets.
- People who are considered underweight are <85% their desirable weight for their height.

STUDY QUESTIONS

1. Differentiate between overweight and obesity.
2. Compare direct and indirect methods of diagnosing obesity.
3. List the disadvantages of being obese.
4. List the health hazards of obesity.
5. Name and explain the theories of obesity.
6. Differentiate between hyperplasia and hypertrophy.
7. Your friend tells you he has gained 3 pounds in the past 2 weeks. How many extra kilocalories must he have eaten to gain this much weight?
8. If an individual drank 2 beers (240 kcal) every day in addition to the kilocalories necessary to maintain their weight, how much weight would he or she gain in 1 year?

Applying What You've Learned

1. **Evaluating Popular Diet**

   Locate a popular weight-loss diet in a magazine or from a book. Evaluate the diet based on the guidelines provided on pp. 213-215 and p. 217.

2. **Describing Eating Patterns**

   For the next 48 hours write down: what time you eat, where you eat, with whom you eat, what else you do while eating, your mood while eating, why you decided to eat. Do you deduce that you eat out of hunger or from a response to external stimuli? List the external stimuli cues that invited you to eat.

3. **Helping Others**

   If an overweight friend asked you advice about dieting, how would you respond, based on what you have learned in the Chapter 7: Energy Balance and Chapter 8: Weight Control?

4. **Analyze Advertisements**

   Collect information on diets and dietary aids from magazines or newspaper ads. Try to analyze their appeal and the physiological or psychological basis on which they might lead to success or failure. Use the chart on p. 217.

5. **Menu Planning**

   Using the table of kilocalories for food in Appendix I make up a 1200 kcal meal plan for 1 day. Be sure the meals include a variety of foods that will make dieting appealing and satisfying. Now reduce diet to the 1000 kcal. What foods would you take away or change? Now reduce diet to 500 kcal. What foods would you take away or change? Knowing that many low-calorie diets are 800 kcal or less, what conclusions can you draw from this reduction in food intake?

6. **Planning Energy Balance**

   Plan a meal using a variety of foods listed in Table 8-2. Now equate that meal to the type and amount of exercise you would need to undertake to achieve energy balance. What additional exercise would you add to expend another 200 kcal? (You may use Tables 7-11 or 7-12 to help you.)

7. **Genetics and Weight**

   Take a good look at yourself, your mother, your father, and any brothers or sisters. Which are endomorphs? Which are ectomorphs? What conclusions can you draw on your tendencies to gain weight based on your genetic makeup?

8. **Compute Your Ideal Weight**

   Using the quick standard method described on p. 205, compute your ideal weight. Be careful that you have an accurate reading of your correct height and weight.

SUGGESTED READINGS

National Institutes of Health Consensus Development Conference Statement: Health implications of obesity, Annals of Internal Medicine 103:147, 1985.

This paper presents the conclusions of a 14-member committee asked to examine the research findings relating obesity to health and to prepare a consensus statement on the topic. They examined the effect of obesity in coronary artery heart disease, cancer, and life expectancy and reviewed the uses and limitations of height and weight tables and the body mass index. They identify the conditions under which weight reduction should be recommended and the needs for further research.

Rock CL, and Coulston AM: Weight control approaches: a review by the California Dietetics Association, Journal of the American Dietetic Association 88:44, 1988.

This paper identifies criteria for an acceptable weight reduction diet as (1) satisfy all nutrient needs except energy, (2) meet individual tastes and habits, (3) minimize hunger and fatigue, (4) be readily obtainable and socially acceptable, (5) favor the establishment of changed eating pattern, and (6) be conducive to improvement of overall health. They summarize the major classes of dietary approaches to weight control as well as the use of drugs, exercise, and behavior modification.

Simopoulos A: Dietary control of hypertension and obesity and body weight standards, Journal of the American Dietetic Association 85:419, 1985.

This article reviews the use of weight standards to evaluate nutritional status and to set goals for weight control. It relates longevity and absence of disease to body weights that are somewhat below the average weights for appropriate age and sex; it related increased mortality with weights above these standards.

Stricker EM: Biological basis of hunger and satiety, Nutrition Reviews 42:333, 1984.

Discussions about the need for food, the stimulus for eating, the site of action of satiety, and hunger symptoms provide a basis for the section on therapeutic implications. The deemphasis on the theory that total control rests in the hypothalamus is discussed, along with the recognition that there is no generally accepted theory to replace it.

Vasselli JR, Cleary MP, and Van Itallie TB: Modern concepts of obesity, Nutrition Reviews 41:361, 1983.

This review presents data from animal and human studies that are advancing our knowledge of the etiology (cause) and treatment of obesity. It gives special attention to the role of diet and exercise in the control of body weight. It describes the "ratchet effect," in which an irreversible increase in fat cells results in high fat stores that are very resistant to reduction.

ADDITIONAL READINGS

Apfelbaum M, Fricker J, and Igoin-Apfelbaum L: Low and very low calorie diets, American Journal of Clinical Nutrition 45:1126, 1987.

Atkinson, RL: Very low calorie diets: getting sick or remaining healthy on a handful of calories, Journal of Nutrition 116:918, 1986.

Brown MJ, and Vetter FJ: Cardiac complications of protein-sparing modified fast, Journal of the American Medical Association 240:120, 1978.

Bray GA: Obesity—a disease of nutrient and energy balance, Nutrition Reviews 45:33, 1987.

Brownell KD: Obesity and weight control: the good and bad of dieting, Nutrition Today 22(3):4, 1987.

Burton BJ, and Foster WR: Health implications of obesity: A NIH Consensus Development Conference, Journal of the American Dietetic Association 85:1118, 1985.

Clausen JD, and others: Relationship of dietary regimens to success, efficiency, and cost of weight loss, Journal of the American Dietetic Association 77:249, 1980.

Committee on Nutrition of Mothers and Preschool Children, The Food and Nutrition Board: Fetal and infant nutrition and susceptibility to obesity, American Journal of Clinical Nutrition 31:2026, 1978.

Danforth E: Diet and obesity, American Journal of Clinical Nutrition 41:1132, 1985.

Dietz WH, Jr: Childhood obesity: susceptibility, cause, and management, Journal of Pediatrics 5:676, 1983.

Drenick EJ, and others: Excessive mortality and causes of death in morbidly obese men, Journal of the American Medical Association 143:443, 1980.

Garn SM: Family-line and socioeconomic factors in fatness and obesity, Nutrition Reviews 44:361, 1986.

Himes JH: Infant feeding practices and obesity, Journal of the American Dietetic Association 75:122, 1979.

Himms-Hagen J: Determinants of human obesity, American Journal of Clinical Nutrition 1:4, 1982.

Hirsch J, and Leibel RL: New light on obesity. New England Journal of Medicine 318:509, 1988.

James WPT, Lean MEJ, and McNeill G: Dietary recommendation after weight loss: how to avoid relapse to obesity, American Journal of Clinical Nutrition 45:1135, 1987.

Keys A: Overweight, obesity, coronary heart disease and mortality, Nutrition Reviews 38:297, 1980.

National Center for Health Statistics, Public Health Service: Obese and overweight adults in the United States, vital and health statistics, Series 11, No. 230, DHHS Pub. No. (PHS) 83-1680, DHHS, Hyattsville, MD, 1983, U.S. Government Printing Office.

Shear CL, and others: Secular trends of obesity in early life: the Bogalusa heart study, American Journal of Public Health 78:75, 1987.

Simopoulos A: Health implications of overweight and obesity, Nutrition Reviews 43:33, 1985.

Society of Actuaries: Body build and blood pressure study, Chicago, 1979, Society of Actuaries.

Stewart AL, and Brook RH: Effects of being overweight, American Journal of Public Health 73:171, 1983.

Stricker EM: Biological bases of hunger and satiety, Nutrition Reviews 42:333, 1984.

Stunkard AJ: Appetite suppressant medication lowers a body weight set point, Life Sciences 30:2043, 1982.

Stunkard AJ: Conservative treatments for obesity, American Journal of Clinical Nutrition 45:1142, 1987.

Volkmar FR, and others: High attrition rates in commercial weight reduction programs, Archives of Internal Medicine 141:426, 1981.

Weigley E: Average? Ideal? Desirable?: A brief overview of height-weight tables in the United States, Journal of the American Dietetic Association 84:417, 1984.

Wirth J: Hunger and satiety, American Journal of Clinical Nutrition 1:19, 1982.

Young CM: Some comments on the obesities, Journal of the American Dietetic Association 45:134, 1963.

FOCUS Diets—Past, Present, and Future

At any given time it is easy to find several magazines with headlines proclaiming yet another diet discovery. Similarly, many fashion magazines publish a January issue announcing some sort of breakthrough for those who want to make it to the Easter parade in trim shape. Almost all of these "new" diets promise instant success with a minimum of stress and self-control on the part of the dieter. Some diets claim that they are based on "medical discoveries" that have been kept from the public. Others report that a magic food combination has been found that "melts away" the excess pounds. A few take a more realistic approach, recommending a slow steady weight loss based on a diet program that includes all of the major food groups coupled with a regular exercise routine. These diets stress the merits of behavior modification and the importance of support from family and associates.

Are there really that many new approaches to weight control? How can the public be expected to evaluate them? Can people be helped in their efforts to select those diets that might conceivably be the answer to their problems and to reject those that will most certainly cause nothing but grief? In this section we will provide broad general outlines of diets (see the table on pp. 226-227) that have come and gone over the years. These fall into several major categories and account for the vast majority of diets that have appeared or are likely to appear. Although the individual diets are and will continue to be hailed by a whole array of names, their general descriptions are readily recognizable and not as changeable.

There are many variations on these diets. The most extreme are total starvation diets that should be undertaken only under strict medical supervision in a hospital—under no circumstances should they be self-prescribed. Other diets are falsely credited to responsible medical units such as the Mayo Clinic or Johns Hopkins University.

The success rate for dieters is discouraging; there are estimates that less than 5% of dieters have been able to sustain their weight loss for more than a year. This large percentage of failure can be explained by a combination of genetics, psychological, and environmental factors; all of these may hinder success.

The potential dieter should be warned against miracle pills and potions even if they come with complete money-back guarantees. The promoters can make these offers because they know that even after paying fairly substantial prices, buyers will probably not admit defeat or gullibility by asking for a refund.

When judging diet aids for weight reduction, several clues should serve as warning signals:

Is the product a new "scientific discovery"?

Is it promoted with testimony from doctors?

Is it sold with a money-back guarantee?

Is it sold in 3-month or 6-month quantities?

Can you eat all you want as the pounds "slip away"?

Is it unavailable in stores?

Is it based on "enzymes" or "endocrines"?

Does it involve buying an expensive book or other paraphernalia?

Does it fail to include exercise?

Does it promise that fat will "melt away"?

If the answer to any of the above questions is "yes," the diet aid may be suspect and should be investigated further.

It is highly unlikely that any major breakthrough is going to be announced initially by scientists through a commercial enterprise (such as a paperback book) or in a magazine "scoop." It is also very unlikely that the "Law of Thermodynamics," which states that energy can be neither created nor destroyed, will ever be repealed. In the last analysis, weight loss will always be accomplished by expending more energy than is taken in. Future breakthroughs will probably supply ways to help people make this adjustment. Whether the help comes from behavioral scientists, the psychologists, or physiologists remain to be seen.

Continued.

FOCUS Diets—Past, Present, and Future—cont'd

Type of Diet	Advantages	Disadvantages	Examples
High-Protein, Low-Carbohydrate Diets Usually include all the meat, fish, poultry, and eggs you can eat Occasionally permit milk and cheese in limited amounts Prohibit fruits, vegetables, and any bread or cereal products	Rapid initial weight loss because of diuretic effect Very little hunger	Too low in carbohydrate Deficient in many nutrients—vitamin C, vitamin A (unless eggs are included), calcium, and several trace elements High in saturated fat, cholesterol, and total fat Will result in ketosis because the major energy sources are protein and fat—both dietary and body. Extreme diets of this type could cause death Impossible to adhere to these diets long enough to lose any appreciable amount of weight Dangerous for people with kidney disease Weight loss, which is largely water, is rapidly regained Diet does not develop a new and useful set of eating habits Expensive Unpalatable after first few days Difficult for dieter to eat out	Dr. Stillman's Quick Weight Loss Diet Calories Don't Count by Dr. Taller Dr. Atkin's Diet Revolution Scarsdale Diet Air Force Diet
Low-Calorie, High-Protein Supplement Diets Usually a premeasured powder to be reconstituted with water or a prepared liquid formula	Rapid initial weight loss Easy to prepare—already measured Palatable for first few days Usually fortified to provide recommended amount of micronutrients Must be labeled if >50% protein	Usually prescribed at dangerously low kilocalorie intake of 300 to 500 kcal Will result in ketosis Do not retrain dieters in acceptable eating habits Overpriced; initially, users are often urged to buy several large cans of different flavors of the diet food (which is usually nonfat dried milk) Low in fiber and bulk—constipating in short amount of time Frequently cause loss of potassium with resultant weakness and heart arrhythmias Often certain poor quality protein	Metracal Diet Cambridge Diet Liquid Protein Diets Last Chance Diet Oxford Diet
High-Fiber, Low-Kilocalorie Diets	High satiety value Provide bulk	Irritating to the lower colon Decrease absorption of trace elements, especially iron Nutritionally deficient Low in protein	Pritikin Diet F Diet Zen Macrobiotic Diet

Type of Diet	Advantages	Disadvantages	Examples
Protein-Sparing Modified Fats <50% protein: 400 kcals	Safe under supervision High quality protein Minimize loss of lean body mass	Decreases BMR Monotonous Expensive	Optifast Medifast
Premeasured Food Plans	Provide the prescribed portion sizes—little chance of too small or too large a portion Total food programs Some provide adequate kilocalories (1200) Nutritionally balanced or supplemented	Expensive Do not retrain dieters in acceptable eating habits Preclude eating out or social eating Often low in bulk Monotonous Low long-term success rates	Nutri-System Carnation Plan
Limited Food Choice Diets	Reduce the number of food choices made by the users Limited opportunity to make mistakes Almost certainly low in calories after the first few days	Deficient in many nutrients, depending on the foods allowed Monotonous—difficult to adhere to Eating out and eating socially are difficult Do not retrain dieters in acceptable eating habits Low long-term success rates No scientific basis for these diets	Banana and milk diet Grapefruit and cottage cheese diet Kempner rice diet Lecithin, vinegar, kelp, and vitamin B_6 diet Beverly Hills Diet Fit for Life
Restricted-Calorie, Balanced Food Plans	Sufficiently low in kilocalories to permit steady weight loss Nutritionally balanced Palatable Include readily available foods Reasonable in cost Can be adapted from family meals Permit eating out and social eating Promote a new set of eating habits	Do not appeal to people who want a "unique" diet Do not produce immediate and large weight losses	Weight Watchers Diet Prudent Diet (American Heart Association) The I Love New York Diet UCLA Diet Time-calorie Displacement (TCD)
Fasting/Starvation Diet	Rapid initial loss	Nutrient deficient Danger of ketosis >60% loss is muscle <40% loss is fat Low long-term success rates	ZIP Diet
High-Carbohydrate Diet	Emphasizes grains, fruits, vegetables High in bulk Low in cholesterol	Limits milk, meat Nutritionally very inadequate for calcium, iron, and protein	Beverly Hills Diet Quick Weight Loss Diet Pritikin Diet Carbohydrate Cravers

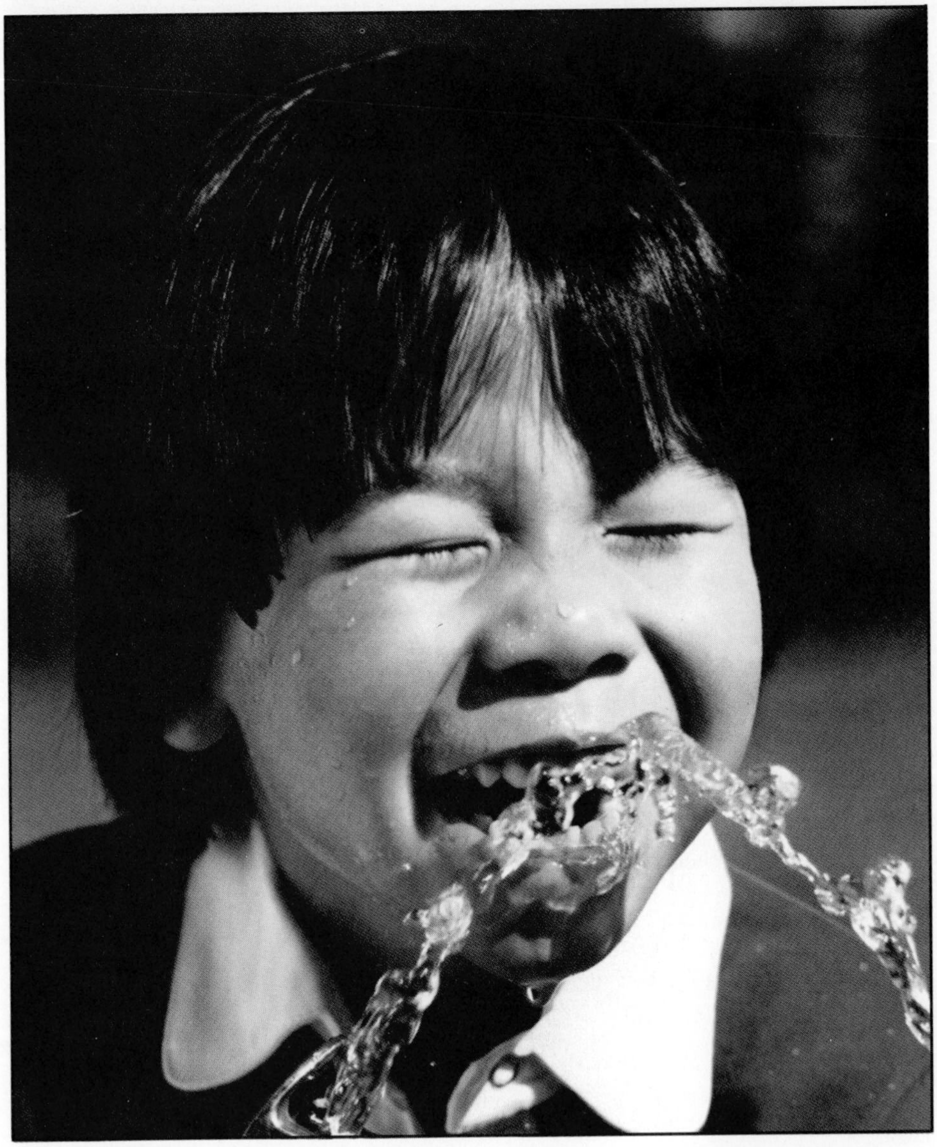

AWARENESS CHECK

Truth or Fiction?

- Water is not an essential nutrient.
- Lettuce is composed almost entirely of water.
- A low-sodium product is the same as a product with no salt added.
- Pregnant women should restrict their salt intake.
- Persons living in areas with a fluoridated water supply have protection against loss of skeletal calcium.

Water, Fluorine, and Electrolytes

CHAPTER

9

Body functions are regulated to a large extent by the amount of water that is available and the way in which it is distributed throughout the body. In addition to the water that we consume in the form of beverages, we receive much of our water from food and some from the metabolism of energy-yielding nutrients. The distribution of water within and between the cells depends on two mineral elements, sodium and potassium, which along with chloride are generally known as electrolytes. In spite of the fact that we take water for granted and seldom make a conscious effort to obtain it, our thirst sensation is so finely regulated that we instinctively know when water intake and water loss are out of balance. In contrast, electrolytes may be out of balance for some time before we are aware of a problem.

Human beings can live for weeks or even years without other essential nutrients, but they will survive only a few days without water. The longest time a person has been known to survive without water is 17 days, but 2 or 3 days is the usual limit. Because the need for water is so critical, the body has rather involved **homeostatic mechanisms** for conserving it when the supply is short. These involve the functions of the kidneys, lungs, and skin and the secretion of several hormones, all of which help maintain a consistent and desirable water composition in tissues.

homeostatic mechanisms
Series of adjustments that act to prevent change in the internal environment in the body

WATER

In the adult body, 6% of the water is replaced each day; in the infant's body 15% is replaced. Although up to 4 quarts (3.8 liters) of water may be taken into the body and another 4 quarts may be lost each day, homeostatic mechanisms are so sensitive that the variation in body weight from change in body fluids seldom exceeds ⅓ pound (150 grams) daily.

Water is a constituent of every cell of the body. As shown in Figure 9-1, it is present in varying amounts in different tissues. The total amount of body water is

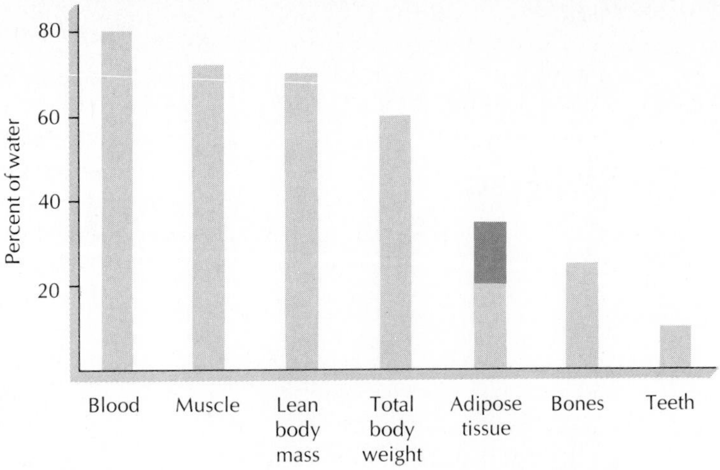

Figure 9-1 Water content of various body tissues. (NOTE: Water content of adipose tissue varies from 20% to 35%.)

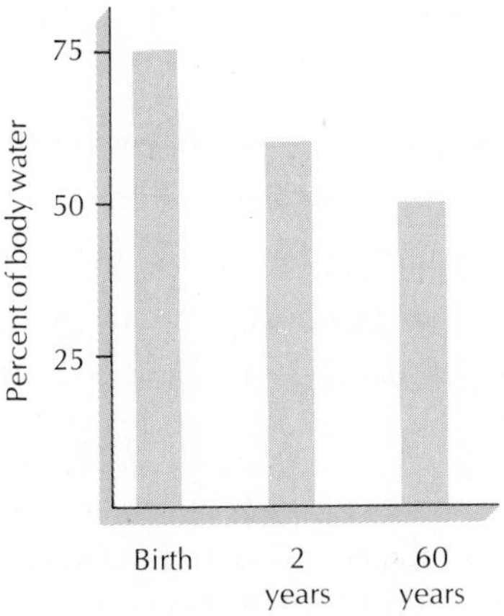

Decline in the percentage of body water with age

Table 9-1 Changes in body composition with age (by percent body weight) for females

	Birth	10 Years	30 to 60 Years
Fat	14	19	28
Lean body mass	3	26	42
Intracellular water	24		31
Extracellular water	44		23

Fat-Free Body Mass
Lean body mass/muscle
Bones
Teeth

a function of age and body composition. In most adults, water makes up about 60% of total body weight and 70% of lean body mass (or fat-free tissue). More muscular people have a higher proportion of body water because muscle contains almost three times as much water as adipose (fat) tissue. Males have a higher amount of body water than females because they have proportionately more lean tissue and less fat. People lose water as they age, with a decline from 80% body weight at birth to 50% in old age, largely caused by a loss of extracellular water (Table 9-1).

Distribution

intracellular
Within the cells

Water comprises 70% of the fat-free weight of the body and 60% of total body weight. It is present in two major compartments: the **intracellular** (within the cells) and the **extracellular** (outside the cells), as shown in Figure 9-2. These two compartments are separated by a semipermeable membrane that allows water to pass through readily. Some electrolytes or ions—particularly sodium, potassium, and chloride—can cross the membrane. The extracellular fluid can be further divided into the intravascular and intercellular compartments. The **intravascular** compartment includes the fluid in all parts of the vascular system: arteries, veins, and capillaries. It is separated from the **intercellular** (between cells) compartment (also called **interstitial** or **extravascular**) by the walls of these blood vessels. It is the intercellular fluid that is responsible for carrying the nourishment to the individual cells and collecting any waste products to be taken back to the bloodstream.

The intercellular compartment acts as a buffer area; its volume will adjust to prevent changes in the volume of either the intravascular or intracellular fluid. A third (transcellular) compartment includes the fluid that lubricates the joints and the fluid in the eyeball. The transcellular compartment represents a very small portion of total body water and is not usually involved in fluid shifts.

The movement of fluid from one compartment to another is controlled to a large extent by the concentration of minerals on either side of the membrane separating the compartments. Mineral elements in body fluids occur primarily as salts. These salts in solution separate into their component **ions;** one ion has a positive charge **(cation)** and the other a negative charge **(anion)**. The charged ions are known as **electrolyes.** They account for the **osmotic pressure** that causes water to move from one compartment to another to establish a balance in the concentration of electrolytes on either side of the membrane. As the concentration of electrolytes increases, the osmotic pressure increases. When the osmotic pressure of fluid in one compartment becomes higher than that in the adjacent compartment, fluid is moved from the side with the lower concentration of electrolytes to that with the higher concentration until the pressure, or ion concentration, on each side of the membrane is equalized. When this occurs, the same number of molecules and ions per volume of fluid are present on either side of the membrane, the osmotic pressures are the same, the amount of fluid on either side remains relatively constant, and no fluid shifts back and forth.

Under most circumstances, the body is able to prevent an unfavorable shift in electrolyte concentrations so that there is no significant change in water balance among compartments. However, shifts do occasionally occur as the result of changes in electrolyte concentration in one of the fluid compartments. These shifts will be discussed further in the section on sodium (p. 243).

extracellular
Outside the cells—includes extravascular (intravascular and intercellular)

intravascular
Within the bloodstream (arteries, veins, and capillaries)

intercellular/interstitial/extravascular
Between the cells and outside the blood vessels

ion
Electrically charged particle

cation
A positively charged ion, such as sodium (Na^+) and potassium (K^+)

anion
A negatively charged ion, such as chloride (Cl^-)

electrolyte
Any substance that splits into charged ions when dissolved in water

osmotic pressure
Pressure in a fluid caused by charged ions that causes water to move across body membranes

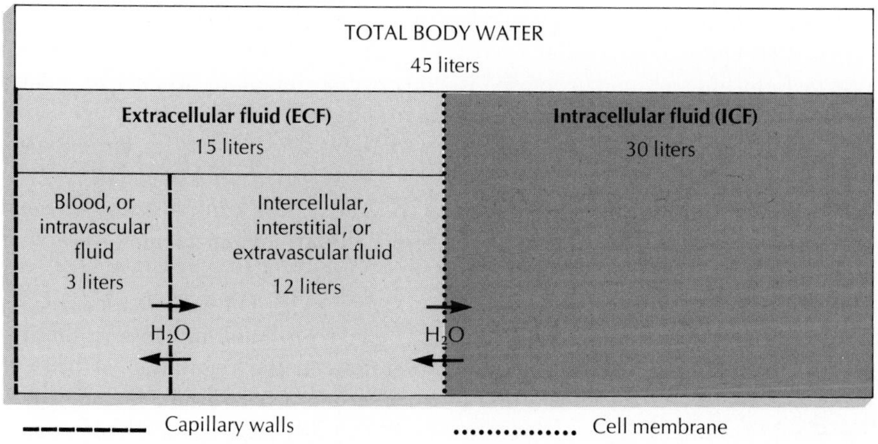

Figure 9-2 Diagrammatic representation of the two major fluid compartments of the body. A third division, the transcellular fluid compartment, is a subdivision of extracellular fluid and includes water in collagen, connective tissue, bone, synovial fluid, vitreous humor, and digestive secretions.

Functions

Functions of Water
Solvent
Growth promoter
Catalyst
Lubricant
Temperature regulator
Source of minerals

The reason that we can only survive a short time without water becomes evident as we consider the many functions of water in vital body processes. The importance of a constant source of water is even more apparent when we consider the large amount of fluid that can be lost from the body in a very short period of time.

Solvent

The average male has a blood volume of approximately 5 liters (or quarts). This intravascular water acts as a solvent for monosaccharides, amino acids, fats (in the form of lipoproteins), vitamins, and minerals. These nutrients as well as many hormones must be carried to all parts of the body for the individual cells to be adequately nourished and to function properly. Water in the intravascular fluid also acts as a solvent to transport the waste products of metabolism, including carbon dioxide, urea, and **metabolites,** which must be carried from the cells to the lungs, skin or kidneys to be excreted.

metabolite
A form of a nutrient that is created during the metabolism of the nutrient

The 12 liters of fluid in the spaces between cells (intercellular) carry nutrients that have left the blood vessels into close proximity with cell membranes. This fluid also collects waste products and hormones or other substances that may be secreted by the cell. Most of the fluid between the cells is pulled back into the capillaries when the oncotic pressure (which is built up by the blood proteins that do not leave the bloodstream) exceeds the hydrostatic pressure (from the heartbeat, forcing fluid out of the blood). Any remaining intercellular fluid is collected by the lymphatic system and is eventually returned to the bloodstream. The amount of water in the intercellular spaces fluctuates considerably and serves as a buffer zone between the cells and the blood, both of which need to maintain a fairly constant fluid level.

For a review of oncotic and hydrostatic pressure, see Chapter 6, Figure 6-8

Within the cell, water acts in much the same way as it does between cells. It serves as a solvent for nutrients that must be transported from one organelle to another and for the waste products that must be eliminated.

Growth Facilitator

Water as a part of all tissues is essential for growth. Glycogen, the form in which carbohydrate is stored in the liver and muscle, is about two-thirds water. Fat tissue is one-fifth water, and muscle is close to three-fourths water. Obviously, growth would be impossible if water were not available.

Catalyst

Water acts as a catalyst in many biological reactions within the cell, as well as in the stomach and small intestine, where digestion of food occurs. Water is necessary for the reactions required to break apart, or **hydrolyze,** complex nutrients into their simpler component parts. One example of a hydrolytic reaction is the digestion of sucrose to form two monosaccharides. In this reaction, water (H_2O) is split into hydrogen (H) and hydroxyl (OH) groups, which are added to the sucrose as it breaks down to form glucose and fructose. In the reverse reaction, when two monosaccharides unite to form a disaccharide, water splits off.

hydrolyze
(hydro- = water; -lyze = to break)
To break down a complex substance into two or more component parts, with the addition of H and OH (from water) to the parts; the process is called *hydrolysis*

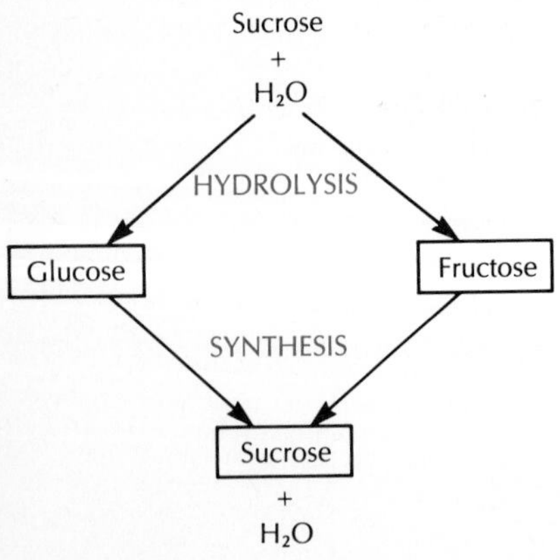

Lubricant

In the synovial fluid of the joints, such as the knee, the prime function of water is to act as a lubricant. This is part of the transcellular compartment.

Temperature Regulator

Because of its ability to conduct heat, water plays an important role in the distribution of heat throughout the body and therefore in the regulation of body temperature. Some of the heat from the metabolism of carbohydrate, fat, and protein is required to maintain body temperature at 98.6° F (37° C). This is the temperature at which all enzymes operate most effectively. But the metabolism of the nutrients, which provide energy in the form of ATP (adenosine triphosphate) for chemical, muscular, and osmotic work in the body, yields more heat (as a by-product) than is necessary to maintain normal body temperature. If this heat were not released promptly, the body temperature would increase to such a point that all cellular enzymes would be inactivated.

Some heat is lost by radiation and conduction, especially at low temperatures. However, the most effective way by far to rid the body of extra heat is through the evaporation of water from the surface of the body. The evaporation of 1 liter or quart of fluid from the skin requires 600 kcal of energy in the form of heat. The body constantly cools itself by causing water to be lost through evaporation. The loss of heat through the skin accounts for about 25% of the basal caloric expenditure. The accompanying water loss, which amounts to 350 to 700 ml/day at normal environmental temperature and humidity, is referred to as **insensible perspiration** loss. The greater the body surface area, the greater the amount of heat that can be lost through the skin. Subcutaneous fat acts as an insulating material, reducing the speed with which heat can be lost; this is an advantage in winter and a disadvantage in summer. Heat loss may also be affected by how close the blood comes to the surface of the skin. The blood vessels near the surface of the skin expand to promote heat loss in hot weather; in cold weather, they contract to minimize the possibility of heat loss. The distance between the blood vessels and the skin is the reason that obese people suffer more in hot climates than nonobese people do.

insensible perspiration
Water lost as the body cools itself by means of evaporation from the surface of the skin.

Source of Minerals

Although water itself is made up of only two elements (hydrogen and oxygen), depending on its origin, water may be a significant source of minerals such as fluorine, zinc, and copper. Up to 50 mg of calcium and 120 mg of magnesium per liter may be present in hard water but are removed in the ion exchange processes used to soften the water supply. Two quarts or liters of hard water may provide as much as 240 mg of magnesium, two thirds of the recommended intake. The use of hard water has been associated with decreased risk of cardiovascular disease. In contrast, soft water may contain up to 250 mg of sodium per quart, with high intakes a risk factor for hypertension. Because water is such a good solvent, it may also be the source of toxic elements such as lead or cadmium, pesticides, herbicides, and industrial wastes. Constant monitoring of the water supply is therefore essential to safeguard the health of the public.

People considering installing a water softener can reduce any adverse health consequences from increased sodium intake by attaching it only to the hot water line.

Water and Work Performance

Studies to determine limiting factors in the work output of people suggest that a lack of water has a much more profound effect on work production than a lack of food. A reduction as small as 4% to 5% of body water (6 cups, or 1.5 liters) will result in a decline of 20% to 30% in work performance. For athletes in good physical condition, a loss of 3% body water is reflected in poorer performance; those in prime condition may be able to tolerate up to 5% water loss. This finding is especially significant for wrestlers. Too often some wrestlers lose weight by dehydrating themselves in an attempt to "make weight," or qualify for competition in a lower weight class. Because it takes well over 5 hours to restore water loss, athletes who do this usually enter a match at a competitive disadvantage. In addition, if water loss exceeds 10% of body weight, there is a possibility of circulatory failure.

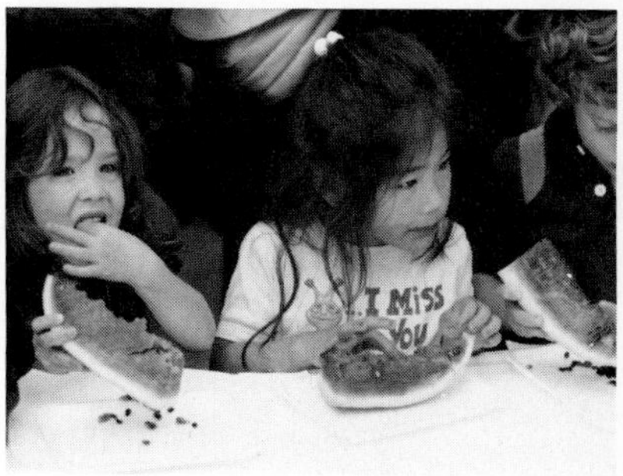

You may not think of foods as being a source of water. However, some foods such as watermelon are composed almost entirely of water

Water Balance

Sources of Body Water

In contrast to all other nutrients, which can be provided by food and beverages alone, water is available to the body as an end-product of metabolism.

Beverages. The major sources of water are fluids consumed as beverages. Tap water makes up half of the beverages consumed. In general, infants take in more per unit of body weight than do adults; people living in the tropics, where there is greater evaporation from the skin, take in more than those in temperate climates;

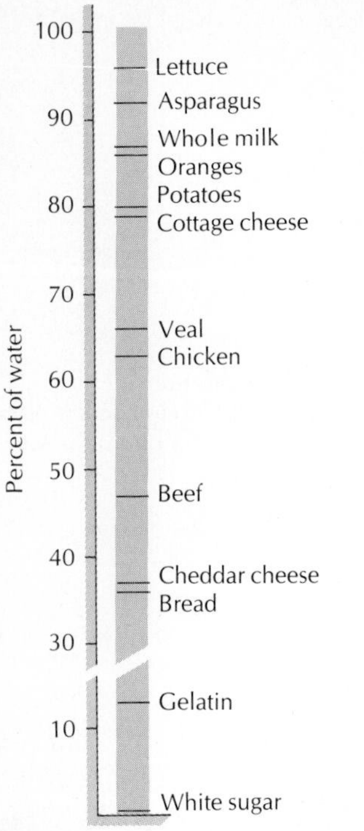

Figure 9-3 Water content of various foods and beverages (percent of total weight).

Table 9-2 ◆ Water released in the metabolism of carbohydrate, fat, and protein

Nutrient	Water Produced (ml/gram)	ml/100 kcal
Carbohydrate	0.6	15.0
Protein	0.42	10.5
Lipid	1.07	11.1

Table 9-3 ◆ Calculation of water of metabolism produced on a 2000 kcal diet

Source of Kcal	Percent of Kcal Provided	Distribution of Kcal in 2000-kcal Diet	Weight of Nutrient (grams)	Water of Metabolism (ml/gram)	Total Water of Metabolism (ml/2000 kcal)
Carbohydrate	50	1000	250	0.6	150
Fat	35	700	77	1.07	82
Protein	15	300	75	0.42	32
TOTAL					264
				264/2000 =	13.2 ml/100 kcal

and people engaged in strenuous physical activity drink more than sedentary people. The amount of fluids consumed daily by an adult varies from 3¾ to 6½ cups (900 to 1500 ml), with an average intake of 38 oz (1100 ml) under normal circumstances. Intakes in excess of 3⅓ cups (800 ml) per hour exceed the rate at which water can be absorbed from the stomach. Alcoholic beverages, tea, and coffee are sources of water but also act as diuretics, causing an increase in the loss of water through the kidney as urine.

Food. So-called solid foods, which include all foods except beverages, are the second most important source of water; they can consist of from 0% to 96% water. Data on the water content of some representative foods presented in Figure 9-3 show that the majority of solid foods contain over 50% water. A 2000 kcal diet chosen from the four food groups provides 500 to 800 ml of water.

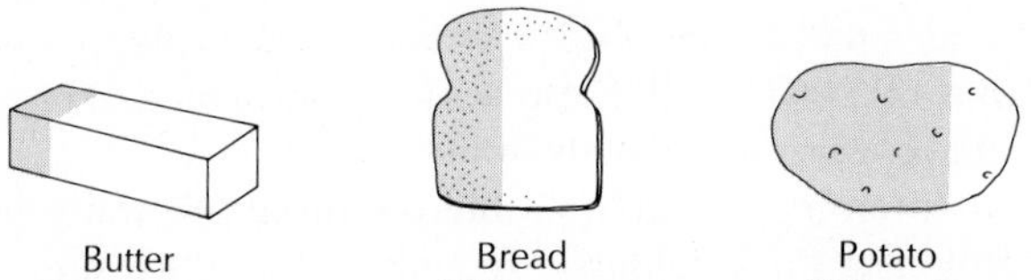

Metabolism. Water, in addition to carbon dioxide and energy, is an end product of the combustion of carbohydrate, fat, and protein. This water is referred to as the **water of metabolism.** A constant amount of water is released during the oxidation or burning of each of the three nutrients (Table 9-2). For an individual on a 2000-kcal diet, with 50% of kilocalories from carbohydrate, 35% from fat, and 15% from protein, the water of metabolism amounts to 264 ml/day (Table 9-3), or 13.2 ml/100 kcal.

water of metabolism
The water that results from the metabolism of carbohydrate, lipid, and protein

When either muscle or liver glycogen is used for energy, the additional water stored with it is also released. An athlete who relies on this energy source during intense physical activity may produce as much as 1 additional quart (liter) of water as a result of metabolizing 500 grams of glycogen.

Loss of Body Water

To counterbalance water intake and maintain fluid equilibrium, water is eliminated from the body in the urine, through the skin, through the lungs, and through the digestive juices and feces.

Urine. Once it has been absorbed throughout the gastrointestinal tract, water is taken up by the bloodstream, where it makes up 80% of blood volume. The bloodstream circulates throughout the body, acting as a solvent for nutrients and for waste products of metabolism. Some of these excesses and waste products are excreted in the urine, which itself is 97% water. Blood is filtered through the kidneys at a rate of 125 ml (½ cup) per minute, or up to 180 quarts/day. The kidneys reabsorb sufficient water to retain normal blood volumes, and excrete the rest. If fluid intake is high, urine volume is increased above the normal level of 1 to 2 liters (quarts), and the concentration of waste products in the urine is lower. Such urine has a low specific gravity. When fluid intake is low, a greater portion of the intake must be reabsorbed to maintain blood volume, and a much smaller amount will be left to act as a solvent in the urine for waste products. As a result, the concentration of the waste products in the urine will be high. Such urine will have a high specific gravity. Because the capacity of the kidneys to concentrate urine is limited, a minimum volume of urine is necessary to rid the body of its usual waste. This minimum is between 300 and 500 ml and depends on the **solute load.** Solute load is composed primarily of electrolytes such as sodium and potassium and urea, which must be excreted. If less than the minimum amount of fluid is available for urine formation, waste products of metabolism will be retained in the blood and in the tissue, where they may accumulate to levels that eventually interfere with cellular functions.

solute load
The combined amount of electrolytes and waste products of metabolism that needs to be excreted by the kidneys

Under some circumstances such as natural disasters and space flights, available fluid is extremely limited and must be conserved. In these situations, it is wise to limit the intake of foods that normally give rise to the metabolites that are excreted in the urine. Restricting protein to reduce urea and salt to reduce sodium to be excreted are the easiest, most effective methods of reducing the thirst and the necessary urine volume. An intake of sufficient carbohydrate (100 grams) to prevent ketosis will help reduce the solute load of ketones and electrolytes. All young infants, who initially have poorly developed kidney functions, are able to excrete only very small amounts of electrolytes. For this reason, they should not be given excessive salt, a high-protein intake, or too concentrated a formula, all of which overtax the kidneys.

During starvation or the ingestion of a high-protein/low-carbohydrate diet, excessive body water, potassium, and sodium are lost through the urine. This accounts for the rapid initial weight loss and weakness often reported by people on starvation-like reducing diets. The loss of water and weight peaks after about 4 days. By the ninth day, a new balance is usually established. Even as little as 60 grams of carbohydrate can prevent an undesirable change in body fluid volume and electrolytes by preventing the accumulation of ketones.

Skin. Loss of water throught the skin amounts to 350 to 700 ml (12 to 14 oz) each day. Water loss has been reported to be as high as 2.4 quarts (2500 ml)/hr; 2 cups (500 ml)/hr is not uncommon at high environmental temperatures and low humidity. If this water is not replaced, the body becomes **dehydrated.** When dehydration occurs total body water decreases, which causes a drop in blood volume and blood pressure. Infants lose a large amount of water by evaporation from the skin, which means that extra water should be provided when the temperature is high.

dehydration
Excessive loss of body water

Athletes lose appreciable amounts of water through the skin (up to 15 pounds in one afternoon for football players) as a result of strenuous physical activity. Those who are in good condition lose water but relatively little sodium; those who are not in good condition lose both and must therefore replace both. When water losses exceed 3 liters (quarts) per day, it is usually necessary to replace sodium as well

For further discussion of water and exercise, see Chapter 19

Table 9-4 ◆ Water balance in gastrointestinal tract

	Amount (ml)	
Sources		
Gastric secretions		8200
Saliva	1500	
Gastric juice	2500	
Bile	500	
Pancreatic juices	700	
Intestinal juices	3000	
Water intake		2000
TOTAL AVAILABLE		10,200
Uses		
Reabsorbed	10,000	
Fecal loss	200	
TOTAL USED		10,200
BALANCE		0

Symptoms of Dehydration
Thirst
Loss of appetite
Decreased blood volume
Decreased urination
Impaired physical performance
Nausea
Impaired temperature regulation
Muscle spasms
Increased pulse
Increased respiration
General debilitation

as water. This can be done by adding more table salt to the regular diet. Salt tablets are seldom if ever needed. If salt tablets are used, water is drawn into the gastrointestinal tract, where it causes bloating and cramping.

Lungs. Water, along with carbon dioxide, is constantly being lost through the lungs. The amount released this way is a little over 1 cup (300 ml) per day but increases at high altitudes because of increased respiration rates. If the atmosphere is unusually dry, the total amount of water lost through the lungs and skin may be as high as urinary losses.

Digestive juices and feces. During a 24-hour period, as much as 8 to 10 liters (quarts) of water (with 3700 ml, or 3.7 quarts, considered a minimum) may be secreted into the digestive tract as digestive juices (Table 9-4). These secretions include saliva, gastric juices, intestinal and pancreatic juices, and bile. Practically all of this is reabsorbed as it passes down the gastrointestinal tract, so that as little as 200 ml may be lost in the feces each day.

The volume of the digestive juices secreted is determined to a certain extent by the moisture content of the food. When food is dry, the amount of saliva increases to lubricate it and to aid in swallowing and the action of digestive enzymes. Secretion of bile is stimulated by the intake of large amounts of fat, and the volume of gastric, pancreatic, and intestinal juices may fluctuate in response to variations in the moisture content of food.

With diarrhea, there is a significant increase in the amount of water in the feces. Vomiting causes a similarly high loss of water. Either condition results in dehydration, a severe problem if the fluid and sodium are not replaced quickly.

In summary, it is important to note that fluid intake must be at least 2 liters (quarts) from food and beverages to compensate for water losses in the urine and feces and through the skin and lungs. Even under conditions of low solute load, minimal physical activity, and absence of sweating, the total water from food, drink, and metabolic water should be as least 1.5 liters (quarts) per day. Table 9-5 summarizes water balance within the body.

Requirements

The need for fluid in relation to body weight varies with age: the younger the person, the greater is the fluid requirement per unit of body weight. Fluid requirements under various conditions of age and environmental temperatures are shown in Table 9-6.

Table 9-5 ◇ Typical water balance in adult

	ml
Sources of Water	
Beverages	1100
Solid food	500-1000
Water of oxidation	300-400
TOTAL	1900-2500
Loss of Water	
Urine	900-1300
Insensible perspiration	500
Perspiration and evaporation from lungs	300-500
Feces	200
TOTAL	1900-2500

Table 9-6 ◇ Fluid requirement per kilogram of body weight

Subjects	ml/kg
Infants	110
10-year-old children	40
Young adult	40
Older adult	30
Elderly (>65 yr)	25
Adults (by environmental temperature)	
22.2° C (72° F)	22
37.8° C (100° F)	38

As a guide, it is suggested that adults consume 1000 ml (1 quart) of water for every 1000 kcal in the diet. This compensates for losses through the skin, respiration, and kidneys when 1000 kcal are metabolized. (For infants, 1500 ml, or 1.5 quarts, is suggested.) Usually about two thirds of this amount comes from beverages; the remainder comes from solid food. Because this intake is considerably less than the 4700 to 17,000 ml (4.7 to 17 quarts) of water that may be turned over in the body each day, it is obvious that the body must have extensive mechanisms for conserving water.

Regulation of Fluid Balance

Fluid balance is achieved in two ways: regulation of fluid intake through changes in thirst sensations and regulation of fluid loss through the kidneys.

When too much fluid is lost, the concentration of electrolytes, particularly sodium, in the extracellular fluid increases. This increase will cause water to be absorbed from the saliva, leaving a dry sensation in the mouth that stimulates thirst and then fluid intake. In addition, the hypothalamus in the brain responds to the higher sodium content of the blood in two ways: it stimulates the thirst sensation, and it also signals the pituitary gland to release the **antidiuretic hormone (ADH),** which influences the kidneys to reabsorb more water, restoring blood volume to a normal level. As water is reabsorbed, the concentration of waste in the urine decreases. Stimulation of thirst and secretion of ADH are triggered by changes in sodium concentration of as little as 1%.

antidiuretic hormone (ADH)
A hormone secreted by the pituitary gland that reduces the loss of fluid through the kidneys

An increase in blood sodium concentration or a decrease in blood volume triggers a series of hormonal changes to restore both to normal levels

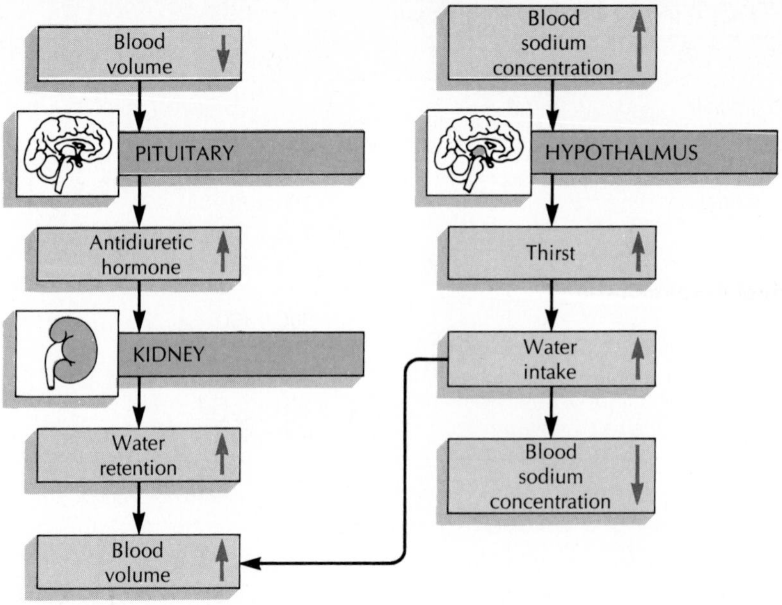

Disturbances in Water Metabolism

Because water is an essential part of all cells and the functioning of the cell depends on a certain concentration of nutrients, any abnormal loss or accumulation of fluid in cells can lead to problems. These problems may result from losses caused by diarrhea, nausea, or fever; abnormal retention of fluid; a defect in intestinal absorption; or an altered distribution of fluids within the body. When body fluids are reduced as much as 10%, symptoms of severe dehydration appear; a 20% reduction is fatal. An increase to levels 10% above normal results in edema. (For more discussion of edema, see Chapter 6).

When the environmental temperature is high, large amounts of water are lost through perspiration. This water loss is accompanied by an appreciable reduction in sodium. Similarly, nausea and vomiting leads to excessive loss of water, sodium, and potassium. The loss of water will stimulate the thirst center in the brain, leading to an increased consumption of water. If the resulting intake is very high and rapid and is not accompanied by an intake of enough sodium to replace that also lost, a condition known as **water intoxication** results. With this condition, the sodium concentration in the extracellular fluids becomes very low. Water then enters the cell (or potassium leaves the cell) to help equalize the concentration of electrolytes on the inside and outside. Overhydration of the cell causes muscle cramps, and a decrease in the extracellular fluid (as fluid enters the cell) causes a drop in blood pressure and a feeling of weakness. Employees who work for industries with high environmental temperatures, travelers in tropical areas who are unaccustomed to high temperatures, and people who engage in strenuous physical exercise, even in a temperate climate, may need *small* amounts of sodium when they drink to replace fluids. On the other hand, they should be careful not to use too much sodium.

water intoxication
The condition that results when the water content of a cell gets so high that the cell cannot function

Another form of water intoxication occurs when the intake of water is greater than the rate at which urine is excreted. This results in the cells taking up the extra water, again causing a dilution of cellular constituents in addition to the swelling of cells. When this form of water intoxication occurs in brain cells, the results include convulsions, coma, and sometimes death.

FLUORINE (Fl)

Because most people associate the element fluorine with the water supply, it seems appropriate to discuss it along with water rather than with other trace elements. The role of fluorine in controlling tooth decay has been recognized for some time. In addition, although there is evidence that growth and possibly reproduction are dependent on a supply of fluorine, there is lack of agreement on whether it is an essential nutrient.

Historical Background

Interest in the possible nutritional role of fluorine dates back to 1931. At that time it was shown that in some communities people had a remarkable freedom from tooth decay but also suffered from dental **fluorosis,** an undesirable brownish stain on the tooth surface. It was found that these same communities had a much higher than usual fluorine content in their water supplies; it was also discovered that people living in areas with slightly less fluorine had a reduced incidence of tooth decay but no fluorosis. By 1942, it had been established that water supplies containing 1 ppm (part per million) of fluorine were associated with a 50% to 60% reduction in tooth decay. Only when the fluorine content was above 2.5 ppm did dental fluorosis occur.

fluorosis
Chalky discoloration on the teeth; caused by excessive fluoride

In 1945, the Public Health Service recognized the possibility of adding fluorine to the water supply as a means of protecting the population against tooth decay. In a classic study, they added 1 ppm of fluorine to the water supply in Newburgh, a city on the Hudson River in New York, and used Kingston (across the river) as a control city that received no added fluorine. After 10 years of study, it was found that children under 10 years of age in Newburgh had a **DMF index** that was 60% to 65% lower than children of the same age in Kingston. Children 12 to 14 years of age, who had drunk fluoridated water since early childhood but not since birth, had a 48% reduction in their DMF index, whereas 16-year-olds had only a 40% reduction. Continued study of these communities showed that the advantages persisted and that there was no detectable adverse effect from the addition of fluorine to the water. Results of this and several other studies provided further support for the benefits from **fluoridation** of the water supply. Furthermore, records showing an increase in tooth decay in communities where the program was terminated confirmed that fluorine was responsible for the beneficial effect.

DMF index
The number of decayed, missing, and filled teeth (does not consider the extent of the decay or filling)

fluoridation
The addition of fluoride to a community water supply to bring total fluoride content to 1 ppm

By 1974 over 80 million people in over 4000 communities, including Chicago and New York City, were consuming water with added fluorine, and another 10 million people were drinking water in which the natural fluorine content was at a protective level. Currently, over 50% of the population in 32 of the 50 states (mostly in the central and eastern part of the country) is served by public water supplies with natural or controlled fluoridation.

In spite of evidence that there are no adverse effects from the addition of fluorine to the water supply to provide a total fluorine content of 1 ppm, and in spite of the endorsement of fluoridation by every medical and dental group in the United States, the United States Public Health Service, and many Asian and European countries, fluoridation remains a controversial issue.

Metabolism

Fluoride is absorbed readily from the stomach, although some fluoride continues to be taken up by the intestine. Of the 90% of fluoride that is absorbed by the body, half is excreted and half readily becomes an integral part of the tooth and bone structure. Regardless of the amount ingested, fluoride levels in the blood remain amazingly constant, reflecting the ability of the kidneys to control the levels in body tissues by excreting the excess in the urine. The amount of fluorine appearing in the tissues, including soft tissue, saliva, milk, and fetal blood, parallels the amount in the blood but at a slightly lower level.

Mode of Action

hydroxyapatite
A calcium phosphate complex found in tooth enamel

Where fluorine is available, some crystals of fluorapatite replace the crystals of **hydroxyapatite** normally deposited during tooth formation. Fluorapatite in tooth enamel is less soluble in acid and more resistant to the cavity-producing action of acids.

The enamel is still capable of taking up fluorine shortly after the teeth erupt. Fluorine available in the saliva is presumably absorbed on the tooth surface to add strength and rigidity. Larger, more nearly perfect fluorapatite crystals in bone have been observed as the fluorine concentration of human bone increases. As much as 5000 to 6000 ppm of fluorine in bone is physiologically safe.

Another benefit of fluorine intake includes greater stability of the skeleton to protect against the loss of calcium that occurs during menopause, when the body is immobilized, and (as recently observed) during space flights.

Sources

Fluorine Content of Some Representative Foods (mg/100 grams)

Mackerel	2.70
Tea	0.47
Coffee	0.25
Rice	0.07
Buckwheat	0.17
Soybeans	0.40-0.67
Spinach	0.02
Onions	0.05
Lettuce	0.01
Wine	6.3 mg/liter

From Gordenoff T, and Member W: Fluorine, World Review of Nutrition and Dietetics 2:213, 1962.

When water has 1 ppm fluoride, an adult usually ingests up to 1.5 mg of fluoride from water daily. Tea and solid foods provide another 0.25 mg of fluoride/day and fish products, especially mackerel and salmon, are considered good sources. The amount of fluorine in processed foods may be two to three times higher than that in fresh foods if fluoridated water has been used in preparation. Similarly, the fluoride content of vegetables reflects the fluoride content in water in areas where they are grown.

Fluoridation of the water supply has proved to be the most feasible way to provide protection against tooth decay. However, for people who either do not have access to a community water supply or who live in communities that have not introduced it, other methods of obtaining the benefits of fluorine are possible. These include using sodium fluoride tablets, which are effective if taken consistently throughout the growth period; adding fluorine at a level slightly higher than 1 ppm to school water supplies; injecting fluoride into the gum area before the time the teeth erupt; applying stannous fluoride to the surface of newly erupted teeth by a dentist; and using infant drops as a supplement for newborns being breast-fed in an area where the water is not fluoridated or where formula is not made with fluoridated water.

The recent dramatic reduction in tooth decay among people of all ages has been attributed to the almost universal use of fluoridated toothpastes. Although there is minimal benefit from the amount absorbed on the tooth surface, it appears that people swallow sufficient toothpaste that the amount ingested this way provides protection. If this evidence persists over time, the necessity of fluoridation of the water supplies may be greatly reduced.

Toxicity

Although there is some concern about the possibility of fluorine toxicity associated with fluoridation of the water supply, no evidence that this is a practical problem exists; the kidneys appear capable of excreting any excess. Based on the health records of 2 million people living in artificially fluoridated areas, the U.S. Public Health Service found no evidence of increased deposition of fluorine in soft tissues such as the kidneys or heart, no increase in mortality and morbidity rates, no growth depression or abnormalities, no increase in cancer or nephritis, and no increase in the births of mentally retarded children, all of which had been claimed by the antifluoridation forces. Claims that fluorine interferes with cell growth and protein synthesis have been discredited by studies showing that cellular reproduction continues in the presence of an amount of fluorine far in excess of the amount that is brought into the circulating fluids when fluorine is ingested.

Acute toxicity, which requires a daily intake of 2 to 10 grams, is rare. Chronic toxicity also occurs infrequently and is usually the result of prolonged use of water with a high natural fluorine content of 20 to 80 mg/day or with industrial contamination. Any danger from the consumption of artificially fluoridated water can be discounted; the continued use of this water and of processed foods with higher fluorine contents should have beneficial rather than detrimental effects.

ELECTROLYTES

The term **electrolyte** is applied to the positively and negatively charged ions that result when a chemical salt dissolves in water. Two of these, sodium and potassium, are major factors influencing the way water is distributed throughout the body. They also influence the contraction of muscles and the way in which impulses are carried in the nerves.

electrolyte
Any substance that splits into positively and negatively charged ions in solution

Because at least 20% of the population has sodium-sensitive hypertension (high blood pressure), reducing dietary sodium intake is recommended as a way of reducing the likelihood of developing the disease, which is one of the leading causes of death in many developed countries.

Electrolytes are often measured in milliequivalents (mEq) rather than weight (mg) because we are usually interested in knowing the comparable effect of an electrolyte on osmotic pressure rather than its concentration. Because 1 mEq of one element has the same effect as 1 mEq of another, by knowing the number of milliequivalents of one or more elements in one or more tissues, we can readily compare their effects. One milliequivalent of any element is the same as 1 mEq of hydrogen. To convert weight of an element to milliequivalents, divide the weight by the atomic weight of the element, which can be obtained in periodic tables of elements.

SODIUM (Na)

The major source of sodium in the diet is sodium chloride (NaCl), or common table salt. Discussion of requirements and functions often use the terms "salt" and "sodium" interchangeably, and as a result they are frequently confused (and confusing). Sodium is present naturally in many foods, as well as being added to foods during processing or cooking.

Confusion in discussing sodium and salt results not only from uncertainty about which one is being discussed but also what measure is being used: milligrams, grams, or milliequivalents. We have chosen to use "milligrams" consistently throughout this discussion since this is the way information is given in tables of food composition and on food labels. Laboratory reports often use milliequivalents. The boxed information on p. 242 will permit you to make the conversion between milligrams and milliequivalents and between sodium and salt.

Historically, salt has always played important roles, both as a seasoning and as a preservative. In fact, many of the major conquests of the world were motivated by a search for a salt supply to satisfy this need. In many countries the only source of salt is the evaporation of seawater, which is frequently carried out on a small scale in the home. In other areas, mines containing rock salt deposits are the major sources of supply. In spite of sodium's many functions, it was not until 1937 that its role as a dietary essential was established. Current interest in salt focuses on the relationship of salt intake to health, especially its role in **hypertension,** a condition in which **blood pressure** is abnormally high. This occurs when the intake of salt exceeds the kidneys capacity to excrete an excess. This causes blood

hypertension
A condition in which blood pressure is at an abnormally high level

blood pressure
The pressure or force exerted on the inner walls of arteries as the heart pumps blood throughout the body

Salt and Sodium Conversions

• Grams of sodium to milligrams	Multiply weight in grams by 1000
• Sodium into salt (NaCl) equivalent	Milligrams of sodium × 2.5 = milligrams of salt
• Salt into sodium	Milligrams of salt × .40 = milligrams of sodium
• Sodium in milligrams to sodium in milliequivalents (dietary prescriptions are often given as milliequivalents, or mEq)	Milligrams of sodium ÷ 23 (atomic weight of sodium) = milliequivalents of sodium
• Milliequivalents of sodium to milligrams of sodium	Milliequivalents of sodium × 23 = milligrams of sodium; milliequivalents of sodium × 58.5 = milligrams of table salt (NaCl)
• 1 tsp salt (5 grams or 5000 mg)	2000 milligrams of sodium

sodium levels to increase. This, in turn, results in an increase in blood volume to dilute the sodium. The increase in blood volume is reflected in increased blood pressure and increased work for the heart to pump more fluid.

Distribution

Sodium is a positively charged base-forming ion, or cation, present in the body primarily in the extracellular fluids: the intravascular fluids within the blood vessels, as well as the intercellular fluids surrounding the cells. About half of total body sodium is found in these fluids. Under normal conditions, as little as 10% of body sodium is present within the cell; but this is only because it is constantly pumped out of the cell to maintain the appropriate low level. The remaining sodium is found in the skeleton, tightly held or bound on the surface of bone. About half of this skeletal sodium acts as a reserve of exchangeable sodium, available to the extracellular fluids when dietary sodium is low or when losses from the body are high. Even when low intakes occur along with an increased need caused by losses, it takes a long period of sodium restriction to use up all the body reserves.

Absorption and Metabolism

Normally, 3000 to 7000 mg of sodium, or 7.5 to 18 grams of sodium chloride, is taken in daily. However, the amount varies greatly depending on the extent to which table salt, often called discretionary salt, is added during cooking and at the table.

A small portion of sodium is absorbed in the stomach, but most of it is absorbed rapidly from the small intestine. Absorbed sodium is carried through the bloodstream to the kidneys, where it is filtered out and returned to the bloodstream in amounts that maintain the blood levels within the narrow range required by the body. Any excess, which usually amounts to 90% to 99% of ingested sodium, is excreted in the urine. This regulation of sodium metabolism by the kidneys is controlled by **aldosterone,** a hormone secreted by the adrenal gland in response to blood sodium levels.

aldosterone
A hormone secreted by the adrenal gland; it acts on the kidneys to influence the amount of sodium that is reabsorbed

Normally, the amount of sodium in the urine parallels dietary intake, being high when intake is high and low when intake is low. When dietary intake is low or need is high, the secretion of aldosterone increases, stimulating the kidneys to resorb more sodium. Conversely, when blood sodium levels are high, the secretion of aldosterone diminishes and less sodium is retained. Some sodium is also deposited in bone, becoming a reservoir available in time of need.

Because there is a limit to the amount of sodium that can be excreted in a certain volume of urine, sodium in the blood and in extracellular fluid will rise if dietary intake exceeds the kidneys' ability to excrete it. When blood sodium rises, the thirst receptors in the hypothalamus of the brain react by stimulating the thirst sensation. This leads to greater fluid consumption, which in turn allows the kidneys to excrete more urine and sodium. Blood sodium levels drop, followed by a lessening of thirst.

Sodium is also lost from the body through perspiration. There is usually about 200 mg of sodium in a liter of perspiration. Normally, this loss per day is minimal (1000 mg), but under conditions such as a high environmental temperatures or fever, which cause excessive perspiration, the loss of sodium and water may be appreciable. Losses of 2000 to 2400 mg/day in the summer are not unusual in the tropics. If losses through the skin are great, aldosterone secretion increases, causing the kidneys to retain more sodium to help minimize the loss.

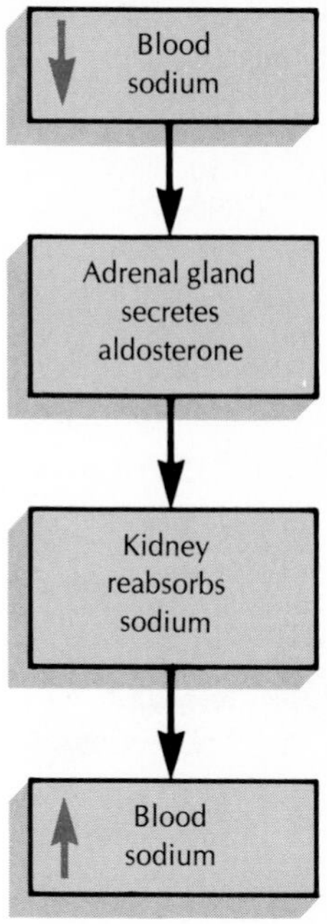

When blood sodium levels drop, the adrenal gland secretes aldosterone, which stimulates the kidneys to reabsorb more sodium to restore blood sodium levels

Functions

Sodium, as the predominant positively charged ion in the extracellular fluid, accounts for most of the osmotic pressure that keeps water from leaving the blood and going into the cell. This osmotic pressure balances a similar pressure caused by potassium within the cell, which acts to keep fluid in the cell. When the level of either sodium or potassium ions gets out of balance, water shifts in or out of cells to keep the concentration of sodium or potassium at the correct level. Normally the body is able to maintain the appropriate balance between sodium outside the cell and potassium inside the cell and is able to regulate water balance.

If, however, the amount of sodium within a cell rises, water enters the cell. The cell then has more than the usual amount of water, which causes it to swell. When cells swell, the tissue becomes waterlogged (edematous). Keeping low sodium levels in the cell is so important that cells constantly "pump out" any extra sodium that enters them. Water balance can also be upset when sodium is lost. Water then enters the cell to dilute intracellular potassium, to keep its concentration similar to that of sodium outside the cell, and the extracellular fluid decreases. These changes can then result in a drop in blood pressure.

Sodium, which is basic or alkaline in solution, accounts for 90% of the alkalinity of the extracellular fluids and helps to maintain body neutrality by counteracting the effects of acid-forming elements. Additional sodium can be released from the bone to offset the acid. One of the major causes of **alkalosis** (an excess of base-forming elements) is the ingestion of sodium-containing antacid preparations.

alkalosis
A condition in which the blood becomes too alkaline ($pH > 7$)

Sodium is essential for the absorption of glucose and in the transport of other nutrients across membranes, particularly the wall of the intestine.

Requirements

The dietary requirement for sodium has not yet been determined, but the usual intake far exceeds what is needed. The requirement is based on needs for growth, sodium losses in sweat and other secretions, and the amount of potassium in the diet.

Obligatory losses of sodium, which represent the minimum amount of sodium that has to be replaced, have been estimated to average about 115 mg/day. These include losses in the urine, stools, and sweat and nonsweat losses from the skin. The usual sodium intake of 3000 to 7000 mg therefore represents many times the minimum requirement. Because a diet that provides only 100 to 150 mg of sodium would be extremely unpalatable and practically impossible to achieve, insufficient intake is very unlikely. The estimated sodium allowances for adults (1100 to 3300

obligatory loss
The amount of water that must be lost from the body to get rid of wastes and to regulate body temperature

Safe and Adequate Daily Dietary Intakes of Sodium (mg)

0-1 yr	115-750
4-6 yr	450-1350
7-10 yr	600-1800
11-18 yr	900-2700
Adult	1100-3300

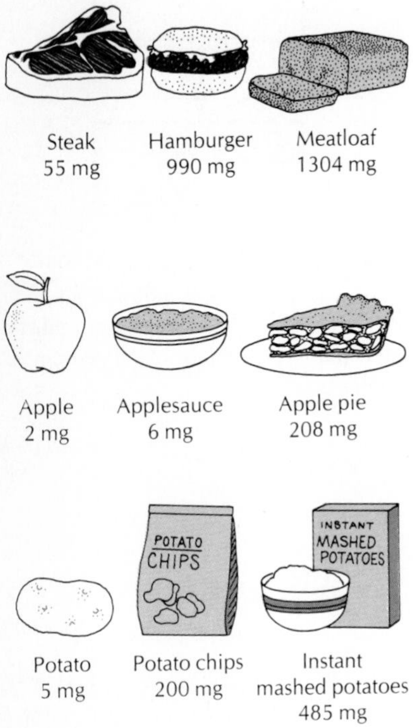

Sodium content of various forms of the same food

mg) represent over 10 times the 115-mg amount that maintains sodium balance. This allowance is equivalent to 3 to 8 grams (½ to 1½ teaspoons of salt) of sodium chloride (table salt). Canadian standards recommend an intake of 9 mg of sodium/kg of body weight/day, that is 1.6 grams sodium chloride.

Infants have a greater fecal loss of sodium and a modest need for growth. They have a higher need per unit of body weight than adults do.

Food Sources

Dietary sources of sodium fall into two main categores: naturally occurring salt and discretionary salt, that is, salt added during processing and preparation or at the table.

Sodium is present in food in widely varying amounts; in contrast to most minerals, more sodium is generally found in foods of animal origin than in those of plant origin. The sodium content of the commonly eaten foods is shown in Figure 9-4. The amount of salt in a person's diet is as much a function of the salt and other sodium-containing compounds added in processing as of the amount present in the food. For example raw potatoes have only 5 mg of sodium/100 grams, but the same potato as chips has 200 to 300 mg of sodium. Cured ham has 20 times as much sodium as raw pork does. Although fresh peas have less than 1 mg of sodium/100 grams, frozen peas have 85 mg of sodium and canned peas have 220 mg; the higher amounts result from the use of a salt solution in a specific gravity method of sizing and grading peas. (These amounts do not include any sodium added as table salt or salted butter.) In many countries monosodium glutamate, or MSG, is used as a flavor enhancer and contributes appreciable amounts of sodium to the diet. Because a large and growing proportion of food is commercially prepared and processed, there has been an increase in the use of salt by industry and a decrease in home use. Table 9-7 summarizes the functions of sodium-containing components in processed foods.

Salt is added to processed foods for many reasons besides the enhancement of flavor. In the manufacture of cheese, salt is used to control the growth of microorganisms (which in turn affects flavor and texture); in butter, salt acts as a flavoring agent and a preservative; in meat, it serves to control spoilage.

Sodium is also added in food processing as monosodium glutamate, as part of baking powder and several preservatives, and is used in many medicines. Altogether, however, these uses account for only 10% of total sodium intake.

In response to current health concerns, most food processors are seeking ways to reduce the sodium in food and at the same time retain a safe, palatable, and

Table 9-7 ◇ Functions of sodium-containing compounds in processed food products

Sodium-Containing Compounds	Functions
Baking powder	Leavening agent
Baking soda	Leavening agent; alkali
Monosodium glutamate	Flavor enhancer
Sodium benzoate	Preservative
Sodium caseinate	Thickener and binder
Sodium citrate	Buffer; used to control acidity in soft drinks and fruit drinks
Sodium nitrate	Curing agent in meat; provides color, prevents botulism (a food poisoning)
Sodium phosphate	Emulsifier, stabilizer, buffer
Sodium propionate	Mold inhibitor
Sodium saccharin	Artifical sweetener

acceptable product. Since 1986 information on the sodium content of foods has been a mandatory aspect of nutrient labeling. Many food processors who do not use nutrient labeling provide information on sodium voluntarily. The percentage contribution of various food groups to the total sodium intake is shown in Figure 9-5.

The discretionary use of added salt at the table varies greatly; however, the average use is 2000 mg/person/day (about 1 teaspoon), which usually accounts for almost half the daily sodium intake. There is evidence that salt preference is established very early in life but that it can be modified by stepwise reduction in salt intake over a period of time.

In some areas the sodium content of the water supply may be high enough—up to 250 mg/quart (or liter)—in one fifth of the sources to make it an important source of sodium, perhaps exceeding the amount of sodium provided by food. Most water supplies have less than 20 mg/quart (liter). However, many of the ion ex-

What Does the Label Say?	
Sodium free	<5 mg per serving
Very low sodium	<35 mg per serving
Low sodium	<140 mg per serving
Reduced sodium	Sodium reduced at least 75%
Unsalted	No salt
No salt added	No salt added to a product
Without added salt	When normally processed with salt
All foods that are so labeled will also list milligrams of sodium per serving on the label	

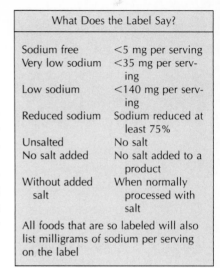

Food and Drug Administration Regulations on Sodium Labeling (1986)

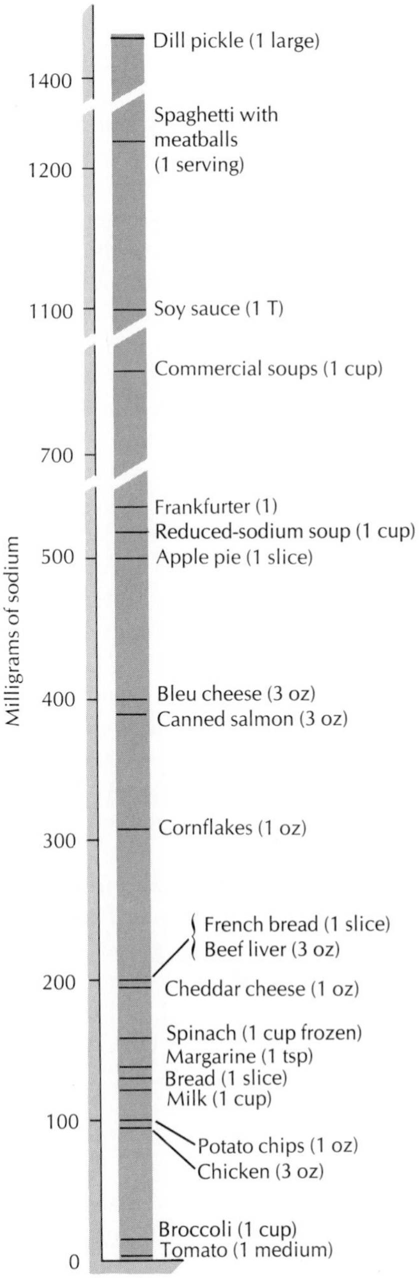

Figure 9-4 Sodium content of commonly eaten foods.

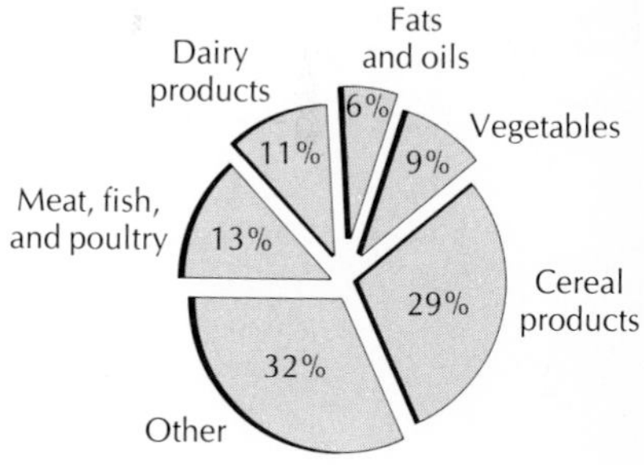

Figure 9-5 Contribution (by percent) of various food groups to sodium in the North American diet.

change units used as water softeners also produce water with a high sodium content (as much as 100 mg per liter). There is some evidence associating high sodium levels in water with incidence of atherosclerosis.

Intake

Because it is almost impossible to estimate the amount of salt added at the table or in home preparation of food, it is difficult to get a reasonable estimate of the amount consumed. The National Health and Nutrition Examination Survey (NHANES) estimated nondiscretionary intakes to be 2660 mg/day for men and 1840 mg/day for women; discretionary salt intake was estimated to be 2700 mg/day. In NHANES, "nondiscretionary" salt was defined as salt that the consumer has no choice in adding.

Restriction

Estimates of the number of people in the United States suffering from hypertension (elevated blood pressure) vary from one sixth to one fourth of the population, with as many as 75% of those in the 65- to 74-year-old age group having symptoms. Restriction of sodium intake results in lowering blood pressure to normal for only some people. It is generally conceded that the usual daily sodium intake of people in the United States is generous, and for some it would be desirable to restrict sodium to somewhat lower levels; however, there is no need to suggest therapeutic levels of 300 mg daily for the general population. As a result, the Dietary Guidelines for Americans urge the public to restrict or decrease their intake of sodium. In many cases, the adverse effects of an elevated sodium intake appear to be counteracted (at least somewhat) by a comparable increase in potassium and possibly calcium.

Mild restriction of sodium, with intake limited to 500 to 700 mg, can often be accomplished by limiting the use of salt at the table. It is unlikely, however, that this will correct serious problems such as hypertension and kidney disorders.

1 tsp salt = 2000 mg sodium

For a strict limitation of sodium to 300 mg, it is necessary to choose foods naturally low in sodium; eliminate all foods in which sodium is used in processing; and use sodium-free salt substitutes and low-salt milk, from which much of the sodium has been removed by a process using an exchange of ions. Spices and herbs except for celery and garlic salts, parsley flakes, and vegetable salts may be used because they contain virtually no sodium.

The long-standing use of low-sodium diets to treat toxemia, a major complication of late pregnancy, is no longer defensible because clinical studies all confirm that pregnant women need a moderate rather than a low salt intake. These needs (that is, an additional 70 mg of sodium daily) are the result of the expansion of blood volume, requirements of the fetus, and the need for sodium in the amniotic fluid.

There has been concern that infants with diets high in sodium are less able to excrete excess sodium and therefore develop a predisposition to hypertension. As a result, processors of baby foods have either eliminated all added salt from their products or have voluntarily restricted it to 0.25%. In addition, they advise parents to refrain from adding salt to make the food more acceptable to their adult tastes. Studies have shown that infants do not discriminate between salted and unsalted food. Infants fed human milk receive about 140 mg of sodium/day; this increases to about 1400 mg—day when the infant reaches 1 year of age.

When reducing discretionary salt in cooking, increase herbs and spices by 25%, double marinating time, or add 25% of spices in last 10 minutes of cooking.

Excess Sodium

Although it is obvious that sodium is an essential element, excessive amounts are not only unnecessary but also may be detrimental. In some people, dehydration is associated with increased blood sodium levels, known as **hypernatremia.** On the other hand, restriction of sodium intake results in lowering blood pressure to normal for only some people.

hypernatremia
Too much sodium in the blood

Toxicity

Doses of several grams of sodium per kilogram of body weight can be lethal for adults. Fortunately this amount is so unpalatable that it would not be taken voluntarily. Much lower intakes are toxic to infants whose immature kidneys have a limited ability to excrete sodium.

Deficiency

When body stores of sodium are depleted rapidly, symptoms of lethargy, nausea, and vomiting result. The person also becomes irritable, confused, weak, and sometimes hostile. Low body stores of sodium are also reflected by low levels in the blood, or **hyponatremia.** Water restriction will help increase the sodium concentration in body fluid. If the sodium loss continues, coma and ultimate death follow. However, a gradual change to a low-sodium diet results in few if any symptoms.

hyponatremia
Too little sodium in the blood

POTASSIUM (K)

Distribution

Potassium is a positively charged base-forming ion (or cation) with chemical properties similar to those of sodium. However, potassium is physiologically unlike sodium in that it is concentrated inside the cell rather than in the extracellular fluid. A sodium to potassium ratio of 1:10 is maintained within the cell, compared to a ratio of 28:1 in the extracellular fluids. Because most of the 250 grams of potassium normally present in the body is within the cells, blood potassium is a poor indicator of potassium status.

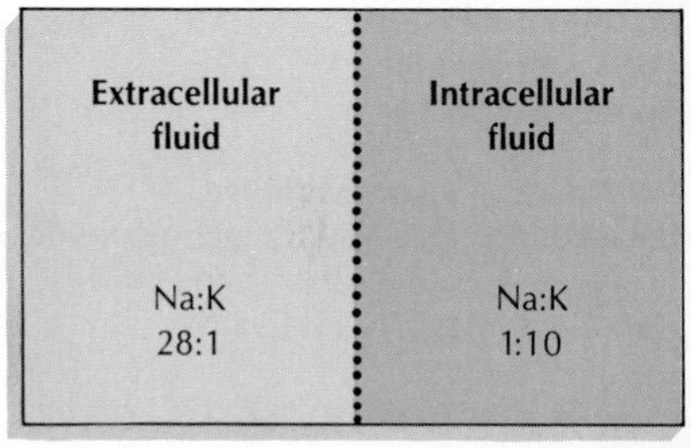

Sodium is constanly pumped out of the cell to maintain these different ratios

The amount of potassium in the blood reflects the nature of cellular metabolism rather than body reserves. Potassium levels rise in the blood when there is a breakdown of body tissue (catabolism) and also in acidosis, which occurs with diarrhea and indicates that potassium (a base-forming element) is leaving the cell to help establish a normal acid-base balance. Potassium levels decrease in the blood when the rate of protein synthesis or glycogen deposition within the cell increases and in alkalosis, which indicates that potassium is leaving the blood and entering the cell. If the level of potassium in the blood and therefore in the extracellular fluids increases above 0.5 gram/liter, muscular coordination is disturbed, and in severe cases cardiac arrest occurs. This is usually the result of failure of the kidneys to excrete potassium.

The kidney is less efficient in conserving or reabsorbing potassium than it is for many other body constituents. Normally, about 7% of blood potassium is lost in the urine after blood has filtered through the kidneys.

Potassium levels in the body are a constant percentage in lean body tissue. Because **potassium^{40}** is a constant percentage of total dietary potassium, it is assumed that the same ratio holds in the body. Therefore, by using a relatively simple technique known as a whole body counter to determine the amount of radioactive potassium (and from this, total potassium) in studies of body composition, it is possible to estimate the amount of lean body mass.

potassium^{40}
Naturally occurring stable isotope of potassium

Functions

Potassium is an integral part of the cell and is required for growth; for every pound gained, 1050 mg is required. Within the cell, potassium acts as a catalyst in many biological reactions, especially those involved in the release of energy and in glycogen and protein synthesis. Potassium is a major factor in maintaining osmotic pressure. As a base-forming element, it is important in the maintenance of acid-base balance; it also plays a role in the transmission of nerve impulses and in the release of insulin from the pancreas. Potassium acts along with magnesium as a muscle relaxant in opposition to calcium, which stimulates muscular contraction.

Although sodium is usually considered the dietary factor most related to blood pressure, it appears that the sodium/potassium ratio is more important than the absolute amount of sodium. Potassium intakes in a ratio of 1:1 to sodium intakes may protect against the adverse effects of high sodium.

Requirements

Estimated Safe and Adequate Daily Intakes of Potassium (mg)

0-1 yr	350-1275
1-6 yr	550-2325
6-10 yr	1000-3000
10-18 yr	1525-4575
Adult	1875-5625

Although potassium is a dietary essential, there is little information about minimal needs, which are estimated to be about 2000 mg/day for adults. Infants and children need from 15 to 65 mg/day for growth. Intake must be higher to cover losses in urine, feces, and perspiration. The usual intake of potassium in the North American diet is estimated at 2 to 6 grams/day, or 0.8 to 1.5 grams/1000 kcal. Intakes are highest among people eating large amounts of fruits and vegetables. Because potassium is found in a great many foods, especially meat, milk, and some fruits, its presence in the diet tends to parallel the diet's caloric value.

Food Sources

Naturally Occurring Potassium
Potassium sulfate
Potassium chloride
Potassium phosphate

Potassium as a Food Additive
Potassium alginate—thickener, emulsifier
Potassium iodate—dough conditioner
Potassium nitrate—preservative

The amount of potassium generally found in the North American diet is neither too much nor too little. The potassium content of some representative foods is shown in Figure 9-6. Potassium in food is very soluble, increasing the possibility that a considerable amount may leach (dissolve) into the cooking water. Potassium is also lost in whey when cheese is made. In addition to naturally occurring potassium in foods, potassium also occurs in food additives.

Deficiency

Potassium chloride can be used as a salt substitute for people who need to restrict sodium. Lithium chloride is also available as a salt substitute.

Potassium-deficiency symptoms seldom occur as a result of less than optimal dietary intakes. A potassium deficiency may occur in infants suffering from diarrhea, when food passes through the intestine so rapidly that absorption of potassium is decreased and the potassium not reabsorbed from digestive secretions is lost. Vomiting, including that induced by bulimics; diuretics, often used in treating hypertension; severe protein-kilocalorie malnutrition; and surgery may also lead to potassium

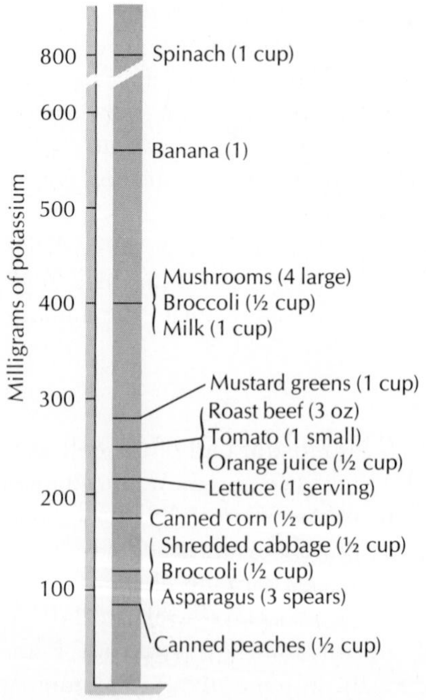

Figure 9-6 Potassium content of commonly eaten foods.

depletion. Overall muscle weakness, poor intestinal tone with abdominal bloating, heart abnormalities, and weakness of respiratory muscles are characteristic of the deficiency. Infants suffering from kwashiorkor respond to treatment only when potassium is given along with an increased protein intake.

When too much potassium is lost, it is best to replace it through dietary sources to minimize the possibility of an excess intake. Excessive intake can lead to excessively high blood levels (or **hyperkalemia**). High potassium intake is especially a problem with the elderly, who may have impaired kidney function and a resulting difficulty in excreting excess potassium. Both too much or too little potassium can lead to cardiac arrest.

hyperkalemia
Too much potassium in the blood

CHLORINE (Cl)

Chlorine, which makes up 0.15% of body weight (1900 mg/kg), is distributed throughout the body tissues as chloride but is found in highest concentration in the cerebrospinal fluid and in the gastric secretions. Muscle and nerve tissue are relatively low in chloride.

As a part of hydrochloric acid, chlorine is necessary to maintain the normal acidity of stomach contents, which is needed for the action of gastric enzymes. Chlorine is a negatively charged acid-forming element, or **anion;** along with the other acid-forming elements phosphorus and sulfur, it helps to maintain acid-base balance in the body fluids. Chloride ions are easily able to pass out of the red blood cell into the blood plasma to help the blood carry large amounts of carbon dioxide to the lungs. As carbon dioxide is taken up and released from the blood, chloride shifts in and out of the plasma to counteract any change in the acid-base balance that might otherwise occur. This transfer of chloride in and out of the red blood cell is called a **chloride shift.**

anion
A negatively charged ion

chloride shift
Transfer of chloride in and out of red blood cells to maintain acid-base balance in the blood

In other tissues, chloride occurs in the extracellular fluids rather than the intracellular fluid. Chlorine is necessary as the amounts of extracellular fluid, bone, and connective tissue increase during growth.

Chlorine is provided almost exclusively by sodium chloride (table salt); some water supplies may provide as much as 300 mg/liter (or quart), but the average is closer to 20 mg. When salt intake is restricted, the chlorine level drops, first in the urine and then in the tissue. Whenever there are excessive losses of sodium (such as those resulting from diarrhea, sweating, or vomiting), chloride is also lost. In vomiting, chloride losses may be excessive and should be replaced.

Human milk contains more chloride than sodium. Failure to include chloride in one commercial infant formula led to the death of several infants—stark evidence of the essential nature of the element in early life when milk is the sole source of food.

Chloride is excreted in the urine, but the kidneys are very efficient in reabsorbing it when the dietary intake is low.

Estimated Safe and Adequate Dietary Intakes of Chloride (mg)

0-1 yr	275-1200
1-6 yr	500-2100
6-10 yr	925-2775
10-18 yr	1400-4200
Adult	1700-5100

BY NOW YOU SHOULD KNOW

- Water is the most essential of all essential nutrients.
- Water is a constituent of every cell of the body. The greatest percentage of water is found in blood, muscle, and fat-free body mass.
- Water is distributed in blood, in cells, and between cells.
- We lose body water as we age.
- Water is obtained from beverages, food, and the end products of metabolism within the body.

- Water is eliminated from the body in urine, through the skin, through the lungs, and through digestive juices.
- There are many mechanisms by which the body maintains a fine water balance.
- Water serves as a solvent for nutrients and waste products, a catalyst for biological reactions, a lubricant, a temperature regulator, an essential factor for growth, and a source of minerals.
- For every 1000 kcal in the diet, 1000 ml or 1 quart of water is recommended.
- A shift in body water of as little as 3% can have a profound effect on performance and body function.
- The addition of fluorine to the water supply is considered a safe and effective way to reduce the incidence of tooth decay.
- For those who do not have a fluoridated water supply, topical application of fluorine or the use of fluoride supplements provides similar protection during tooth formation.
- Sodium and potassium are the electrolytes that influence body water distribution.
- Sodium and potassium are base-forming ions, whereas chloride is an acid-forming ion.
- Because the intake of sodium is many times the amount required by the body, over 90% is usually excreted.
- For people with a predisposition to hypertension, it is important to avoid high intakes of sodium.
- Sodium functions not only in fluid balance and acid-base balance, but also in transporting nutrients across cell membranes.
- This estimated safe and adequate daily dietary intake of sodium for adults is 1100 to 3300 mg per day.
- Processed foods and cereal products contribute the greatest percent of sodium to the North American diet.
- Sodium information is mandatory on food labels that reveal nutrition information.
- The Dietary Guidelines for Americans suggest avoiding too much sodium.
- Potassium, which functions primarily within the cell, is found in fruits and vegetables.
- Chlorine is a part of hydrochloric acid and functions to maintain the normal acidity of the stomach.

STUDY QUESTIONS

1. Name four functions of water in the body.
2. What foods would you choose if you were asked to increase your potassium intake?
3. How can a child who gets water from a home well be protected against tooth decay?
4. What happens when the need for sodium in the body increases?
5. What happens when the intake of sodium exceeds the ability of the kidneys to excrete the excess?
6. What is the major dietary source of chlorine in the diet?
7. What function do sodium and potassium have in common?
8. Name five foods high in sodium and five foods low in sodium.
9. What is dental fluorosis?
10. How does water regulate body temperature?
11. How much water is provided in a 2000 kcal diet?
12. A food recipe for Spanish green beans calls for 1 tablespoon of salt. The recipe will feed 50. How many milligrams of sodium per serving? (Use the salt and sodium conversions chart on p. 242; convert the milligrams to millequivalents.)
13. A patient is told to follow a low-sodium diet with a dietary prescription of 43 mEq per day. How many milligrams of sodium does that equal?
14. Why does either too little or too much potassium effect the heart?

Applying What You've Learned

1. **Keep a Record of the Fluids that You Take In During One Day**

   How does it compare to the recommended amount of 8 to 10 cups per day?

2. **Investigate if Your Local Water Supply is Fluoridated**

   Write or call your local water company. Ask if the water supply is flouridated. If so, to what level? Is it natural or controlled?

3. **Study the Nutrition Information on Your Favorite Breakfast Cereal**

   How many milligrams of sodium are in one serving? Now convert the milligrams of sodium to milligrams of salt, then from milligrams of salt to teaspoons of salt by using the conversions chart on p. 242. Are you suprised at the amount of sodium? Do this same exercise using your favorite packaged soup or snack food.

4. **Blood Pressure**

   Have your blood pressure taken at least once a year.

5. **Learn Your Family History of High Blood Pressure**

   Ask a member of your family for information on familial hypertension; who has it, what kind of medication they take, and whether they follow a low-sodium diet.

6. **Evaluate the Sodium Content of Your Diet**

   To get a clearer understanding of how much sodium is in your diet, complete the following statements with rarely, often, or daily.

   I eat cured or processed meats such as ham, bacon, sausage, frankfurters, and lunch meats
   I eat canned vegetables
   I eat commercially prepared meals, main dishes, or canned or dehydrated soups
   I eat cheese
   I eat salted nuts, popcorn, pretzels, corn chips, or potato chips
   I add salt to cooking water for vegetables, rice, or pasta
   I use the salt shaker

7. **Read the Label on All Foods that Bear Nutrition Information**

   Look for the sodium content per serving and start estimating your daily sodium intake from processed foods. If there is no nutrition information, refer to the list of ingredients to determine sources of sodium. If there are sodium-containing ingredients, check their function according to the chart on page 244. Remember, these ingredients are in decending order—those at the end of the list are present in very small amounts compared to those at the start.

SUGGESTED READINGS

Council on Scientific Affairs: Sodium in processed foods, Journal of the American Medical Association 248:784, 1983.

This article reviews the current regulations governing the sodium content of processed foods, anticipated regulations, and attempts to reduce the amount of sodium in the food supply and gives the amount of sodium in a variety of food products.

Richmond VL: Thirty years of fluoridation: a review, American Journal of Clinical Nutrition 41:129, 1985

This review explores the evidence of the effectiveness of water fluoridation; the problems and extent of misinformation about the program; the lack of evidence of toxicity or adverse effects at levels well above those used; and the economic, as well as health, benefits. It concludes that fluoridation is an appropriate action for the government to take to promote the health and welfare of society.

Water and electrolytes. In Recommended Dietary Allowances, ed. 9, Washington, D.C., 1980, National Academy of Sciences.

This book includes a comprehensive review of the considerations on which the provisional recommended dietary allowances for water and electrolytes were based. It also contains a nontechnical discussion of the physiology of water and electrolyte metabolism. It is a succinct and clearly written overview.

ADDITIONAL READINGS

Water

Anderson B: Thirst and brain control of water balance, American Scientist 59:408, 1971.

Anderson B, Leksell LG, and Rungren M: Regulation of water intake, Annual Review of Nutrition 2:73, 1982.

National Academy of Sciences: Drinking water and health, Washington, D.C., 1980, National Acedamy of Sciences.

Robinson JR: Water and life, World Review of Nutrition and Dietetics 12:172, 1970.

Walker JS and others: Water intake of normal children, Science 140:890, 1963.

Sodium

Altschul A, and Grommet JK: Sodium intake and sodium sensitivity, Nutrition Reviews 38:393, 1980.

Guyton AC, and others: Salt balance and long-term blood pressure control, Annual Review of Medicine 31:15, 1980.

Institute of Food Technology. Dietary Salt, Food Technology 1(85):49, 1980.

Joossens JV, and Geboers J: Dietary salt and risks to health; American Journal of Clinical Nutrition 45:1277, 1987.

Shank FR, and others: Perspective of Food and Drug Administration on dietary sodium, Journal of the American Dietetic Association 80:29, 1982.

Swales JD: Dietary salt and hypertension, Lancet 1:1177, 1980.

Weinberger MH: Sodium chloride and blood pressure, New England Journal of Medicine 317:1084, 1987.

Potassium

Freyly MJ: Sodium and potassium. In Present Knowledge of Nutrition, Washington, D.C., 1984, Nutrition Foundation.

Hodges RE, and Rebello T: Dietary changes and their possible effect on blood pressure, American Journal of Clinical Nutrition 41:1155, 1985.

Tobian L: Potassium and hypertension, Nutrition Reviews 46:273, 1988.

Fluorine

American Academy of Pediatrics: Fluoride as a nutrient, Pediatrics 49:456, 1972.

Dunning JM: Current status of fluoridation, New England Journal of Medicine 272:30, 84, 1965.

Evans CA, and Pickles T: Statewide antifluoridation initiatives: a new challenge to health workers, Public Health 68:59, 1978.

Korns RF: Relationship of water fluoridation to bone density in two New York towns, Public Health Reports 84:815, 1969.

Latham M, and Grech P: The effect of excessive fluoride intake, American Journal of Public Health 57:651, 1967.

Leverett DH: Fluorides and the changing prevalence of dental caries, Science 217:26, 1982.

Singer L, Ophaug RH, and Harland BF: Fluoride intake of young male adults in the United States, American Journal of Clinical Nutrition 33:328, 1980.

Smith EH: Fluoridation of water supply, Journal of the American Medical Association 230:1569, 1974.

Sognnaes RF: Fluoride protection of bones and teeth, Science 150:989, 1965.

FOCUS Water—A Precious and Diminishing Resource

Just as we tend to take for granted that the water we drink is a constant component of our diet, we also take for granted the quality and quantity of our public water supplies. Most of us are jarred into recognizing how dependent we are on water when our water source is temporarily taken away and we are unable to perform almost any of our daily tasks. Perhaps even more devastating is to have water available but contaminated so that it is no longer safe to use. Under those circumstances it is usually what we don't see that can hurt us.

The purity of the water depends on the *absence* of microorganisms and contaminants. Contaminants may take the form of pesticides and herbicides that have filtered into the water supply following their use in agriculture, microorganisms capable of causing illness or disease, or heavy metals such as lead and cadmium that have dissolved out of the pipes into the water or have been introduced in industrial or commercial effluent. Microorganisms are controlled by the addition of chlorine to almost all public water supplies, but the control of contaminants is much more difficult. It depends largely on the location of the water source and the storage area for the water supply in relation to drainage from contaminated soils or from industrial or sewage plants. We depend on our public health officials to monitor the quality of the water supply and to protect us from the potential danger of consuming impure water.

From a nutritional standpoint our health is influenced by the nature of the water supply. Soft water, which tends to come from sources well below the surface, has a relatively high concentration of sodium, averaging 20 mg/liter but as high as 100 mg/liter in some areas. The latter level is the maximum permissible if we are to protect people with a susceptibility to hypertension or kidney disease.

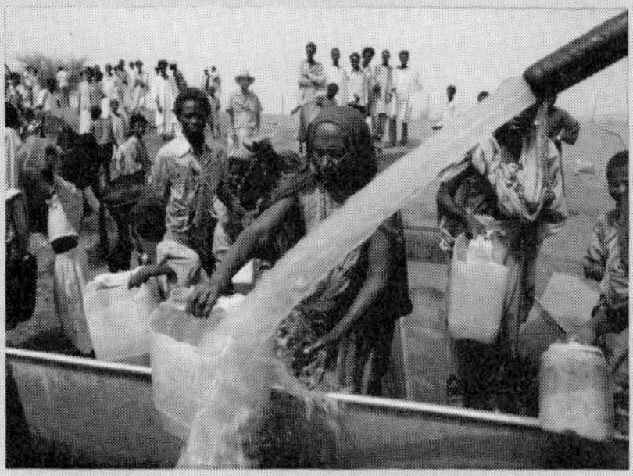

Hard water contains an appreciable amount of the elements magnesium and calcium, both of which are essential in normal nutrition. In tropical areas where the consumption of water may be substantial, hard water can make a significant contribution to the day's intake of these elements. Soft water, on the other hand, is a better solvent for the elements cadmium and lead. Although cadmium is probably needed in small amounts for some biological functions, large amounts are known to have detrimental effects. The cumulative effect of lead ingestion from the water supply is a concern in many areas. The presence of all these elements in the water supply complicates the process of renal dialysis used to prolong the lives of persons suffering from kidney failure.

Many water supplies have enough naturally occurring fluorine to provide additional strength to the tooth enamel and increase its resistance to tooth decay. Fluorine may be added in controlled amounts to provide comparable protection to those whose water supply has less than 1 ppm. Fluoridation, like chlorination, is feasible only in public water supplies and cannot be controlled in wells or private water supplies.

The amount of trace elements in water depends largely on the amount present in the terrain from which the water originated. There can be appreciable differences in the amounts from almost adjacent supplies, particularly if one originates from deep in the earth and the other from shallow sources.

In addition to concern about the quality of the water we consume, there are increasing and even more pressing reasons to be concerned about the quantity of our water supply. Many urban centers are faced with the realization that their water supplies are not infinite and that before permitting additional growth they have a responsibility to identify additional water resources. In other parts of the world population centers and agriculture are shifting as the water sources become depleted or recede. Modern technology is making it possible to desalinate (take the salt out of) some water sources to capitalize on the vast amount of salt water in the oceans. In other attempts to deal with the diminishing water reserves, agriculturalists are identifying plants that can flourish in brackish soils that have previously been unsuitable for cultivation.

The necessity of protecting our watersheds by preserving our forested areas is a high priority nationally. More recently, there has been considerable concern about the effect of "acid rain." The increased acidity of our lakes and streams, as well as of the soil, resulting from industrial waste that is carried great distances in the atmosphere, has had adverse effects on the growth of plants, fish, and other animals.

The importance of water to our survival cannot be overemphasized. Water is as vital for the survival of society on a long-term basis as it is for the survival of any one person on a short-term basis

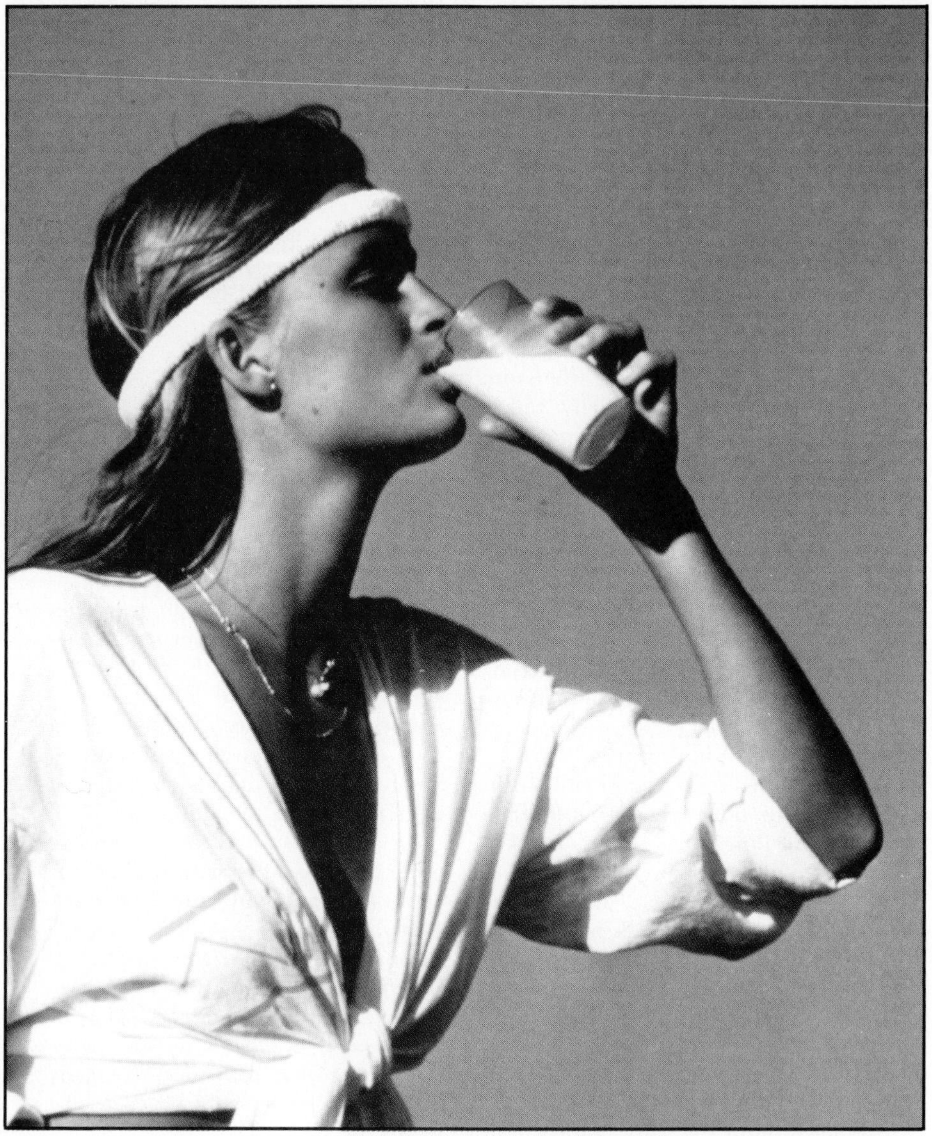

AWARENESS CHECK

Truth or Fiction?

- Calcium supplements will prevent osteoporosis.
- Most multiple vitamin supplements will provide 100% the U.S. RDA for calcium.
- Osteoporosis is a disease affecting only women.
- Dolomite is a dependable and safe source of calcium.
- Long-term alcohol consumption may lead to a magnesium deficiency.

Macronutrient Elements

CHAPTER 10

The four macronutrients—calcium, phosphorus, magnesium, and sulfur—that are discussed in this chapter perform many functions as mineral elements. These nutrients are influenced by each other with complex interrelationships in absorption, metabolism, and excretion. Their metabolism is controlled by many body hormones. Each, however, has one or more unique roles in metabolism and is found independent of the others in the food supply. Although phosphorus and sulfur are provided in adequate amounts in most diets, magnesium intakes appear marginal, and intakes of calcium are at less than recommended amounts for a large segment of the population. The consequences of a lack of calcium are most evident among postmenopausal women, who frequently suffer from osteoporosis. The best way to ensure an adequate intake of most macronutrients is to select a diet from a wide variety of foods.

Our knowledge of the importance of mineral elements goes back to the middle of the nineteenth century. Scientists of that time fed mice a mixture of carbohydrate, fat, protein, and water, which they thought were the only nutrients in food. They were baffled, however, when the animals died. They then attempted to find out the missing element from food that was obviously needed for growth. For a clue, they began looking at the very small amount of ash that was left over after a food was burned. When this was added to the diet the animals still died. By 1912 they learned that both vitamins and a mineral (ash) were essential for growth; since then, we have learned that the ash is composed of numerous mineral elements, many of which have a vital role in human nutrition. Research on the unique roles of these elements, as well as their relationship to others, is providing many of the previously missing links in our understanding of nutrition.

MINERAL ELEMENTS

Essential Mineral Elements

Before a mineral is considered essential, it must perform functions that are vital for life, growth, or reproduction. This means that there must be an improvement

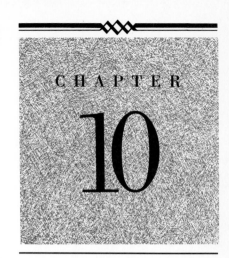

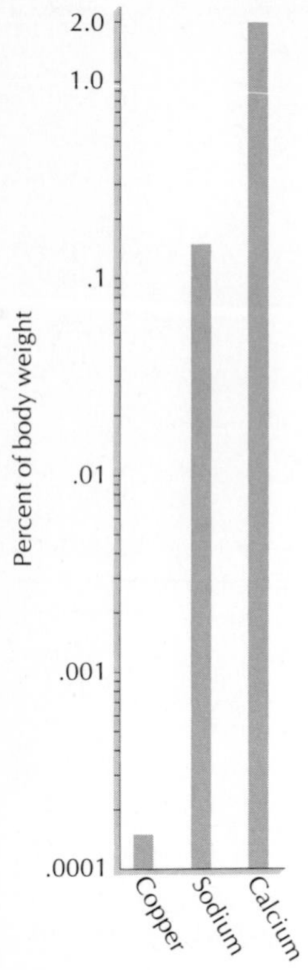

Relative amount of representative minerals in the body (log scale)

1 nanogram (ng) = 1 part per billion (ppb)

1 Microgram (μg) = 1 part per million (ppm)

in growth or health when the element is included in the diet in physiological amounts, compatible with normal body functioning. There must be evidence of a deficiency when the element is removed, some evidence that blood levels reflect low intake and are associated with impaired functions, and some indication that the element cannot be replaced by something else.

There are now 22 mineral elements considered essential, and tin is under review. Chromium and silicon, which only a few years ago were considered contaminants, are now considered essential. It is not only possible but probable that at least some of the 20 to 30 other elements now considered to be either contaminants or toxic substances will be found to be essential in small amounts. In general, an element is included in the list only when it has been established as essential by more than one independent investigator and in more than one animal species.

Much of the progress in our knowledge of mineral metabolism has been possible because of refinements in analytical techniques used to study minerals. These have made it possible to study the concentrations of minerals in quantities as low as 1 part per billion, or ppb, in biological tissue. (A ppb is also known as a *nanogram*.)

The body has several means of controlling the amount of essential mineral elements in the body. One of these is control over the amount that is absorbed. After absorption, the body can regulate the amount of mineral elements retained; this is done by the excretion of excess minerals in urine, bile, and feces. Some excess may also be lost through the skin in sweat. For some elements, a wide range of intakes can be tolerated. For others such as iron, copper, selenium, and zinc, the intake must be kept within a very narrow range to prevent complications from either a deficiency or an excess of the elements. If an element is needed in small amounts but toxic if we have too much, it is difficult to decide whether it is essential or not. This dilemma also creates concern about lack of control over the amount of trace elements readily available in supplements.

There appears to be no comparable mechanism for controlling the absorption and excretion of nonessential elements. Therefore, at the same time that nutritionists want food processing methods to ensure that essential elements are not removed from the food supply, they also want to be certain that excessively high amounts of other potentially toxic elements are not introduced.

Classification

organic
Having its origins in living material, either plant or animal

inorganic
Related to nonliving material, usually mineral in origin

macronutrient element
An element present in the body at more than 50 ppm

micronutrient element, or **trace element**
An element present in the body at less than 50 ppm

There are basically two types of substances: **organic** substances, all of which contain carbon and are part of living material, and **inorganic** substances with no carbon, and derived from nonliving material. Essential minerals, which are all inorganic substances, are often classified as either macronutrient or micronutrient elements (also known as *macroelements* or *microelements*). **Macronutrient** elements are those present in relatively high amounts (>50 ppm) in animal tissue; **micronutrient** elements, also called **trace elements,** are present at less than 50 ppm (0.005%) of body weight. It is important not to interpret the term "trace" to mean "unimportant." Even though some nutrients are needed in inconceivably small amounts, they are as important to body function as those needed in much higher amounts. For example, the consequences of a deficiency of iodine, representing 1 part per 80 million of body weight, may be more debilitating than a deficiency of calcium, which accounts for 2% (2 parts per hundred) of body weight.

Some of the elements listed in the Table 10-1 as essential for humans are also vital for plant growth. Other dietary essential elements, such as sodium and iodine, which are not, do occur in foods of plant origin. In contrast to protein and vitamins, mineral elements cannot be synthesized. The amount of a mineral element in an animal tissue reflects the amount present in the plants that the animal eats. This amount in turn is a function of the amount of the element present in the soil and the extent to which the plant concentrates it during growth.

Minerals are present in a higher concentration in foods of animal origin than in plants and are often in a form that is more readily absorbed. These foods may therefore be superior to foods of plant origin as sources of minerals. In grains, trace elements are concentrated in the outer layers and the germ, both of which are at least partially removed with extensive milling. Because **phytic acid** and fiber in the outer husk of grain tend to interfere with absorption of many minerals anyway, the difference between the amount of some minerals available from refined grain and the amount from whole-grain cereals is not as great as might be expected.

phytic acid
A phosphorous-containing organic acid found in plants; decreases mineral absorption

For a review of milling and processing grains see Chapter 4

Table 10-1 ◊ Classification of mineral elements

Classification	Elements*	Percent of Body Weight	Amount in Body	Suggested Daily Intake for Adults
Macronutrients (>0.005% body weight, or 50 ppm)				
Elements essential for human nutrition	Calcium	1.5-2.2	1.02 kg	800 mg‡
	Phosphorus	0.8-1.2	0.68 kg	800 mg‡
	Potassium	0.35	0.13 kg	1875-5625 mg
	Sulfur	0.25	0.20 kg	
	Sodium	0.15		1100-3300 mg
	Chlorine	0.15	0.14 kg	1200-5100 mg
	Magnesium (1950)	0.05	0.025 kg	350 mg‡
Micronutrients (<0.005% body weight)				
Elements essential for human nutrition	Iron (17th century)	0.004	4.5 grams	10-18 mg‡
	Zinc (1934)	0.002	1.9 grams	15 mg‡
	Selenium (1957)	0.0003	0.013 grams	.05-.20 mg
	Manganese (1931)	0.0002	0.016 grams	2.5-5.0 mg
	Copper (1928)	0.00015	0.125 grams	2-3 mg
	Iodine (1850)	0.00004	0.015 grams	.15 mg
	Molybdenum (1953)	0.0002		15-05 mg
	Cobalt (1935)	0.00003		.15-.5 mg
	Chromium (1959)	0.00003		.05-.2 mg
	Silicon (1972)			
	Vanadium (1971)	0.00045		
	Nickel (1971)	0.00023		
	Arsenic (1980)			
	Boron (1987)			
	Fluorine (1972)†			1.5-4.0 mg
Elements for which essentiality has not yet been established, although there is evidence of their participation in certain biological reactions	Barium			
	Tin (1970)†			
	Bromine			
	Strontium	0.0006		
	Cadmium	0.0006		
Elements found in the body that have not been assigned a metabolic role yet	Gold			
	Silver			
	Aluminum			
	Mercury			
	Bismuth			
	Gallium			
	Lead			
	Antimony			
	Lithium			
	+20 others			

*Dates in parenthesis identify year in which essentiality was established.
†Essentiality almost certain.
‡RDA established; For all others, figures represent intakes considered safe and adequate.

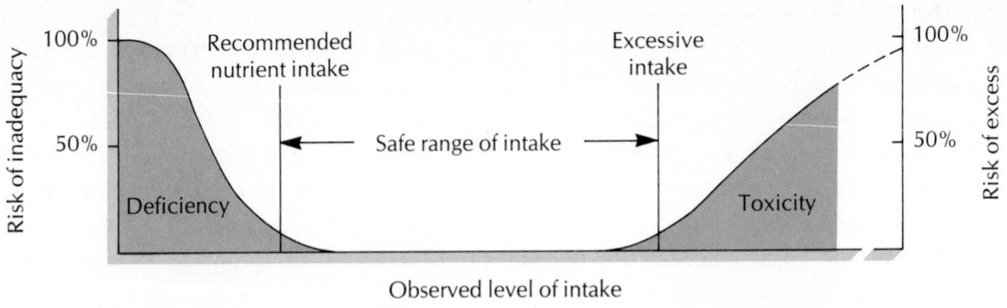

Figure 10-1 Concept of safe range of intakes. It is assumed that there is individual variability of both requirement for the nutrient and tolerance for high intakes of the nutrient. Safe range of intakes is associated with very low risk of either inadequacy or excess. The white area represents uncertainty about the point at which an intake becomes lethal.

Toxicity

As illustrated in Figure 10-1, lack of a trace element that is essential will result in deficiency symptoms and even death when the available amount is below a certain critical level. Above this level, it will permit marginal functioning until it reaches recommended levels, at which point it results in optimal functioning. At a somewhat higher level, there is a gradual decline in functioning until the nutrient has a negative rather than positive effect and eventually interferes with cell functioning. The amount of a nutrient needed to cause this **toxicity** varies from one person to another, just as the amount needed for optimal functioning varies. The range of intakes represented by the base in Figure 10-1 is considered safe and adequate.

toxicity
Quality of being poisonous, or toxic

Interactions

Mineral elements interact with one another in a variety of ways—both positive and negative. These interactions may occur during absorption, transport, metabolism, excretion, or storage. For example, selenium protects against mercury toxicity, or poisoning, and calcium protects against lead toxicity. On the other hand, high intakes of calcium interfere with iron absorption and too much iron with zinc absorption. Problems result when there is an imbalance in the intakes of the two nutrients that interact. Imbalances are unlikely to occur when food is selected from a variety of sources but may result from the indiscriminate use of mineral supplements.

Dietary Needs

The amount of minerals needed for adequate nutrition varies from a few micrograms (for elements such as cobalt) to 400 thousand times as much (for example, 800 mg of calcium). Regardless of the amount needed, insufficient intake results in some clearly identifiable changes such as low hemoglobin with an iron deficiency or abnormal heartbeat with a potassium deficiency. The Committee on Recommended Dietary Allowances has established standards for the macroelements calcium and phosphorus and for the microelements iron, zinc, and iodine. The board also suggests estimated safe and adequate daily dietary intakes for three electrolytes and six other elements for which there were enough data on which to make a recommendation.

General Functions

Because of the complex interrelationships that exist among the mineral elements, several general functions of minerals will be discussed here. Details of functions of individual minerals of special dietary significance are outlined later in the chapter.

Maintenance of Acid-Base Balance

Most of the many biological reactions within the cell can occur only when the pH, or acidity or alkalinity, of the cell is within a very narrow range. Anything that changes the pH of the cell environment may change the way cellular enzymes act. Inactivation of the enzymes results in cellular starvation and death.

Normal pH = 7.35-7.45

Among the many factors that can influence pH are the minerals available to the cell from the extracellular fluids. The minerals chlorine, sulfur, and phosphorus, which form acids when dissolved in water, are considered acid-forming. The acid-forming properties of a food depend on the presence of these elements rather than on organic acids such as citric acid, which gives the acid taste to fruits. Acid-forming elements predominate in foods containing protein such as meat, fish, poultry, eggs, and cereal products. These foods are called acid-forming foods.

Acid-Forming Elements	Base-Forming Elements
Chlorine	Sodium
Sulfur	Potassium
Phosphorus	Magnesium
	Calcium

Mineral elements that are basic, or alkaline, in solution are calcium, sodium, potassium, and magnesium. These elements tend to predominate in fruits, vegetables, and nuts; therefore even citrus fruits such as grapefruit, lemons, and oranges are base-forming.

Acid-Forming Foods	Base-Forming Foods	Neutral Foods
Meat	Fruits	Milk
Eggs	Vegetables	Sugar
Cereals	Nuts	Starch
		Fats and oils

Neither milk, which contains an internal balance of base-forming calcium and acid-forming phosphorus, nor pure carbohydrates and fats, which contain virtually no minerals, influence acid-base balance.

Most mixed diets contain a slight surplus of acid-forming mineral elements, but we all have ways of counteracting this. We can get rid of excess acid by excreting carbon dioxide through our lungs and slightly acid urine through our kidneys.

In addition, our blood contains *buffers*, or neutralizing substances, such as carbonates, phosphates, and proteins. These buffers react with either excess acid or excess base to prevent it from influencing the pH of the blood. If the buffers cannot neutralize excess base, our bodies can form carbonic acid from carbon dioxide and water, which are normally excreted. Carbonic acid then neutralizes excess alkali-forming (base-forming) elements and prevents **alkalosis,** a condition in which the blood becomes too alkaline. Similarly, excess acid may be neutralized by a base formed from NH_2, which results from the deamination of proteins, and water. This prevents **acidosis,** a condition in which the blood becomes too acidic. With these methods for coping with an excess of either base-forming or acid-forming elements, we seldom have a disturbance in acid-base balance caused by diet alone.

alkalosis
A condition in which the blood becomes too alkaline; pH > 7

acidosis
A condition in which the blood becomes too acid; pH < 7

Catalysts for Biological Reactions

Mineral elements are **catalysts** or **cofactors** for biological reactions with some, such as zinc, catalyzing as many as 100 different reactions. They are not part of initial compounds or end products but serve as the vital link between an enzyme and the substance on which it acts. They catalyze many of the separate steps involved in the metabolism of carbohydrate, fat, and protein (Figure 10-2).

catalyst
Substance that speeds up or facilitates a reaction that would occur at a much slower rate without the catalyst

cofactor
A substance that is essential for a given reaction to occur

The synthesis of hemoglobin depends on several mineral elements that are *not* a part of hemoglobin; similarly, although calcium is a catalyst for blood clotting, it is *not* part of the clot.

The absorption of nutrients from the gastrointestinal tract and the uptake of nutrients by the cell often depend on minerals. For example, calcium facilitates the absorption of vitamin B_{12}; magnesium and sodium do the same for carbohydrate. Several digestive enzymes (such as pancreatic lipase) are activated by minerals.

In addition to the carbon, hydrogen, oxygen, and nitrogen that are part of all vitamins, some vitamins contain minerals. For example, thiamin contains sulfur and vitamin B_{12} contains cobalt.

Components of Essential Body Compounds

Many of the hormones, enzymes, and other vital body compounds synthesized in the body contain minerals as essential parts of their structure. If a required mineral is absent, the body will be unable to produce adequate amounts of these essential substances.

Components of Essential Body Compounds

Iodine	Copper
Iron	Molybdenum
Chlorine	Zinc

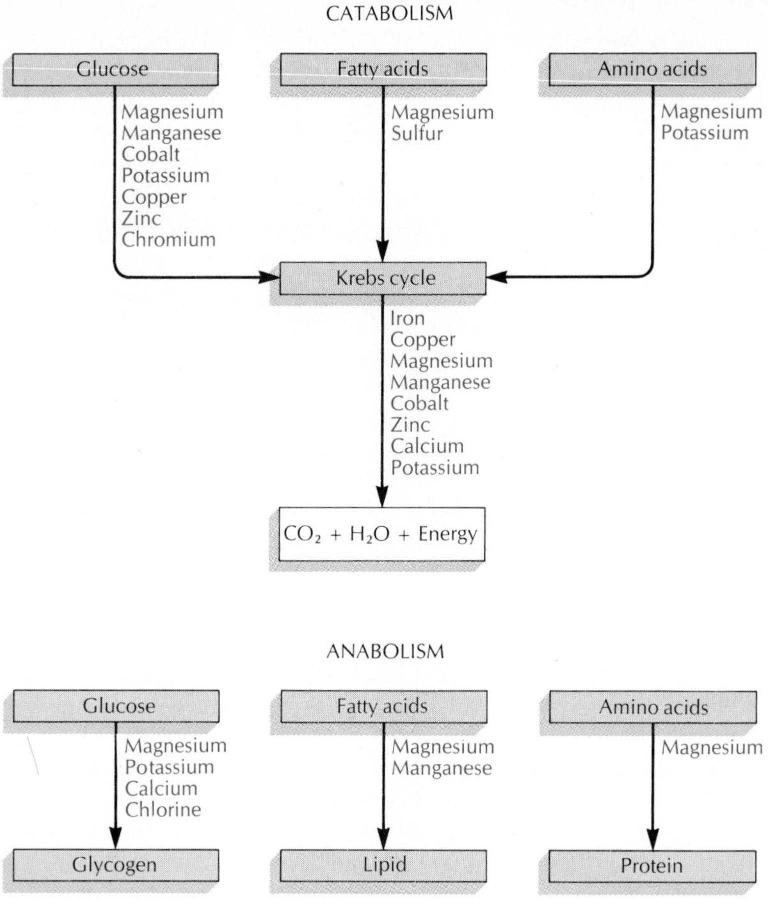

Figure 10-2 Role of minerals in metabolism. Minerals act primarily as catalysts to enzyme action. Some function as essential parts of enzymes.

For example, thyroxin, the hormone that controls energy metabolism, requires an adequate supply of iodine. Hemoglobin, which is essential for the transport of oxygen to the cells and carbon dioxide away from them, is an iron-containing compound. Chlorine is essential for the hydrochloric acid secreted into the stomach to provide acidity needed for gastric digestion.

metalloenzyme
An enzyme with a mineral element as an essential part of its structure

Mineral-containing enzymes are sometimes called **metalloenzymes** because, if the metal (that is, mineral) is not available, the enzyme will not be synthesized or will be ineffective. To point out only a few examples: both copper and iron are part of an enzyme involved in the release of energy; molybdenum is part of an enzyme needed to release liver stores of iron; and zinc is part of a protein-splitting enzyme that is secreted in the pancreatic juice. These enzymes cannot function if different minerals are substituted.

Transmission of Nerve Impulses

Minerals Essential for Transmission of Nerve Impulses
Potassium
Sodium
Calcium

Minerals play a vital role in conducting nerve impulses along nerve fibers. As a nerve impulse passes along a nerve fiber, the permeability of the membrane of each nerve cell changes, allowing potassium to leave the cell. At the same time, some sodium enters each cell but is quickly pumped out. This creates a temporary change in the electrical charge on the cell membrane. This charge in turn changes the permeability of the next segment of the fiber, which changes the electrical charge again. In this way, the message is passed down the fiber. The exchange of sodium and potassium ions across the cell membrane is therefore responsible for the tranmission of nerve impulses. Anything that changes the concentration of these ions in the fluids bathing nerve cells may interfere with their ability to transmit nerve impulses.

The transmission of a nerve impulse from one nerve cell to another is also dependent on the presence of the **neurotransmitter** acetylcholine (ACh) at the junction of the two fibers. The release of acetylcholine is regulated by calcium.

neurotransmitter
A chemical substance that is able to carry a message from one nerve fiber to the next

Regulation of Contractility of Muscles

The muscles of the body are constantly bathed in intercellular fluid. For muscles to function normally, the composition of this fluid must reflect a balance between elements such as calcium, which tend to stimulate muscular contraction, and elements such as sodium, potassium, and magnesium, which exert a relaxing effect. This balance is steadfastly maintained by the body under normal conditions; any disturbance is usually the result of a hormone shift rather than dietary changes.

Minerals Essential for Regulation of Muscle Contraction
Sodium
Potassium
Magnesium
Calcium

Growth of Body Tissue

Some mineral elements such as calcium and phosphorus occur in large concentrations in the bones and teeth and are the building materials for these tissues. An absence of these elements will result in stunted growth or in bones of inferior quality. Other minerals are indirectly involved in the growth process as catalysts to reactions that lead to the synthesis of body compounds or to the release of energy needed for growth.

Minerals Essential for Growth of Body Tissue
Calcium
Phosphorus
Magnesium
Iron

Maintenance of Water Balance

The role of mineral elements in maintaining the balance of fluids among the various fluid compartments of the body—the intracellular and extracellular with its three subcompartments (intravascular, intercellular, and transcellular)—is discussed in Chapter 9. Sodium as an extracellular ion is kept out of the cell by a sodium pump that works constantly to prevent it from attracting water into the cell.

Minerals Essential for Maintenance of Water Balance
Sodium
Potassium

CALCIUM (Ca)

Most people correctly associate calcium with bones, teeth, and milk. This association reflects the nutrition concept that is emphasized in basic health messages, which are often reinforced in the public press, as well as in increasingly complex discussions of diet and health. Indeed, this association suggests that the major functions of calcium are in bone and tooth formation and identifies milk as the major dietary source of calcium. Calcium is, however, only one of many nutrients necessary for effective bone and tooth formation. Calcium also regulates many vital biological functions. Most recently, interest in calcium has centered around its role in preventing **osteoporosis,** a bone disease in which the amount of bone is decreased but the composition remains normal.

osteoporosis
A bone disease in which the amount of bone is decreased but the composition remains normal; most often affects women after menopause

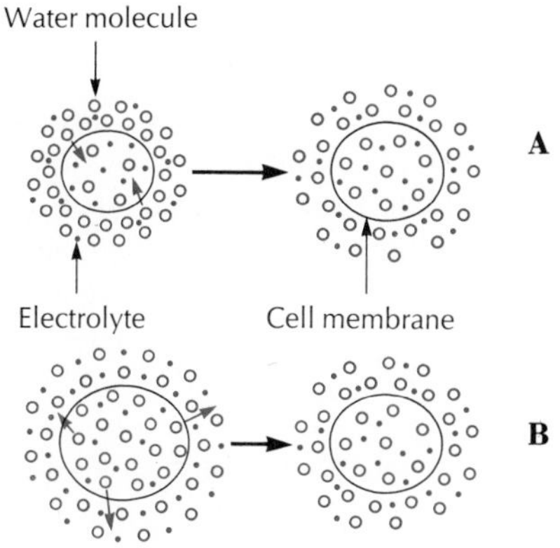

The process of osmosis—water passes in and out of the cell to maintain same concentration of electrolytes inside and outside. Cell size increases when water enters **(A)** and decreases as it leaves **(B).**

Distribution of calcium in the blood

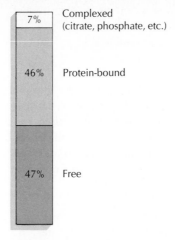

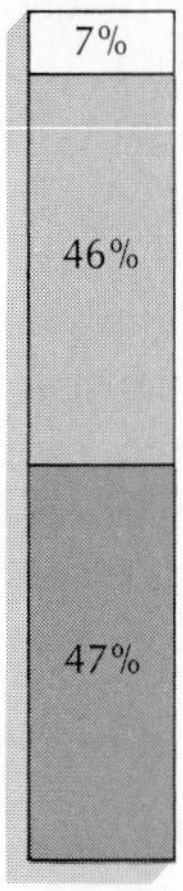

Distribution

Calcium makes up between 1.5% and 2% (850 to 1200 grams or 2 to 3 pounds) of the weight of the adult body. Of this, 99% is in the hard tissues: bones and teeth. The remaining 10 grams, or about 2 teaspoons, is widely distributed in the blood and soft tissues such as muscle, liver, and heart. In the blood, calcium levels are maintained within a very narrow range of 9 to 11 mg/dl, with about half loosely bound to protein and almost all the rest present as a free calcium ion. A very small amount (4 to 5 grams) is vital to the functioning of every body cell. Calcium in the blood and **soft tissues** is so important that it will be mobilized from reserves in the bones to maintain constant blood levels, which seldom vary more than 3% during a day.

soft tissues
Organs and tissues of the body that are not normally calcified—for example, the liver, kidneys, and muscle

Functions

Like most nutrients, calcium is essential for general functions, as part of an essential compound or as a regulatory substance.

Bone Formation

Early in fetal development a strong but flexible **matrix,** or pattern, for bone made of the protein collagen is formed; it has the same general shape as the mature bone but lacks strength and rigidity. The matrix, which accounts for about one third of the bone, remains rather flexible until after birth, possibly to make the birth process easier. It is composed of fibers of the protein **collagen** embedded in a gelatinous substance. Shortly after birth the matrix starts to gain strength and rigidity, primarily as a result of the growth of mineral crystals in the matrix in a process known as **calcification,** or **ossification.** During early growth, the calcification process proceeds rapidly so that by the time the child is ready to walk the bones are capable of supporting the weight of the body. Crystals in bone are composed of either calcium phosphate or a combination of calcium phosphate and calcium hydroxide called **hydroxyapatite.** Because calcium and phosphorus are the predominant mineral elements in these compounds, an adequate supply of both must be present in the fluids surrounding the bone matrix before they can start growing as crystals. The general structure of a long bone is shown in Figure 10-3. The bone shaft, which is the rigid part of the bone, contains calcium phosphate, magnesium, zinc, sodium, carbonate, and fluoride in addition to hydroxyapatite. This part of the bones is constantly being remodeled and reshaped throughout life as the weight of the body shifts, putting different stresses on the bones. At the end of the long bones is the epiphysis, which regulates bone growth. Under this is a more porous part

matrix
The form, or "mold," for the bone—make up of collagen and a carbohydrate-related material

collagen
The protein that forms the "mold" (matrix) for the bone

calcification (ossification)
The process by which calcium and phosphorus are deposited in the flexible bone matrix to give it strength and rigidity

hydroxyapatite
A compound made up of calcium and phosphate that is deposited into the bone matrix to give it strength and rigidity

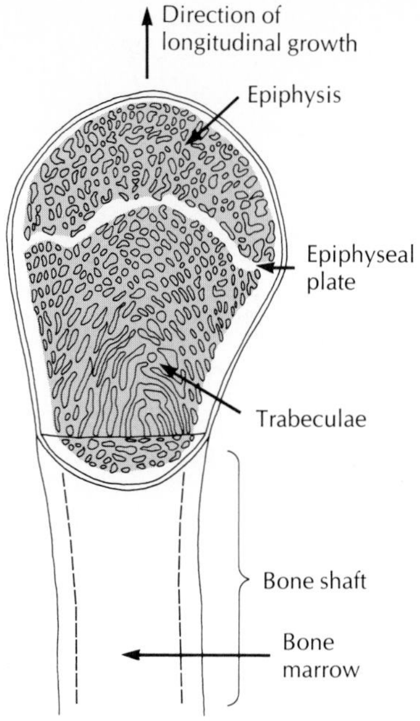

Figure 10-3 Diagrammatic representation of bone structure.

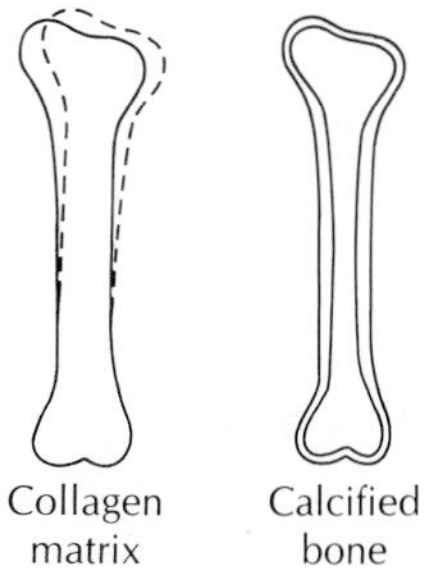

known as the **trabeculae,** which provides a readily available supply of calcium to help maintain levels in the blood. Trabecular bone also predominates in the vertebrae in the spine.

trabeculae
A portion of the ends of long bones that is porous to permit contact with the blood supply, so that calcium can be withdrawn to meet needs when the dietary intake is inadequate

Tooth Formation

Hydroxyapatite, the mineral compound found in bones, is the same one that forms **dentin** and **enamel,** which are the middle and outer layers of the tooth. However, the crystals in teeth are more dense and the water content lower. The protein in enamel is **keratin,** whereas that in dentin is collagen. In contrast to bones, teeth undergo microscopic changes once they have erupted into the oral cavity. The slow rate of exchange between the tooth calcium and that of the blood is confined almost entirely to the dentin layer, although there may be some calcium exchange between the tooth enamel and saliva.

Calcification of **deciduous teeth,** which make up the child's first set of teeth, begins by the twentieth week of fetal life but is completed shortly before they erupt. Permanent teeth begin to calcify when the child is between 3 months and 3 years old, whereas wisdom teeth, the last to erupt, may not begin to calcify until the child's eighth to tenth year. A full complement of adult teeth contains only about 1% of total calcium in hard tissues.

Because teeth have practically no ability to repair themselves once they have erupted, there is no need for calcium to maintain or repair teeth. A deficiency of calcium during the formative period for teeth may show up in an increased susceptibility to tooth decay. As with bone, the integrity of tooth structure involves many nutrients in addition to calcium.

dentin
The middle layer of the tooth; it is less calcified than the outer enamel layer

enamel
The very dense and highly calcified outer portion of the tooth; it is quite resistant to decay

keratin
A protein found in the skin, and nails, and tooth enamel

deciduous teeth
The first set of teeth, which are usually lost by ages 5 to 10

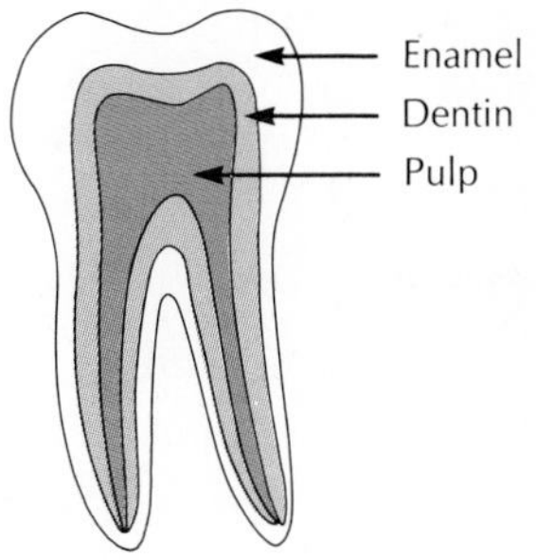

Structure of tooth

Growth

The observation that natives of Japan raised on a diet low in calcium are frequently shorter than Japanese people raised where the diet is adequate in calcium has led to the suggestion that calcium is necessary for normal growth. However, diets low in calcium are also low in protein; because protein is a specific growth factor and is also essential for the formation of the bone matrix, it is difficult to argue that a lack of calcium is a primary cause of growth failure. It may, however, be a contributing factor.

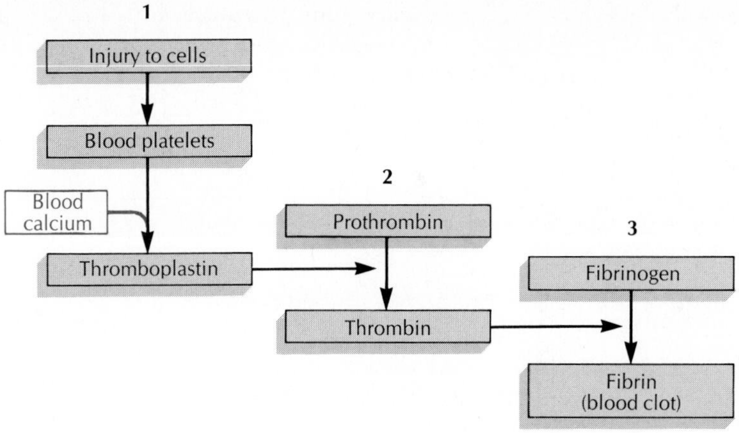

Figure 10-4 Schematic diagram of the role of calcium in blood clotting. Reaction begins when calcium triggers the release of thromboplastin from injured platelets.

Blood Clotting

The role of calcium in blood clotting is one of the best understood of its functions. Once cells have been injured, ionized calcium in the blood stimulates the release of a phospholipid, **thromboplastin,** from the injured blood platelets. Thromboplastin in turn catalyzes the conversion of **prothrombin,** a normal blood constituent, to thrombin. Thrombin then aids in changing **fibrinogen,** another normal component of the blood, to fibrin, which is the clot. A schematic representation of the blood-clotting mechanism (Figure 10-4) shows that calcium must be present as a catalyst in the first step to initiate the series of changes needed for the formation of the clot. Because blood calcium levels are maintained at a high enough level to aid in the blood-clotting process, no benefit is achieved from increasing dietary calcium before surgery.

thromboplastin
A protein released from the blood platelets at the time of injury to a blood vessel

prothrombin
A protein that is essential for the blood-clotting mechanism; a precursor of thrombin

fibrinogen
A protein that is a precursor of fibrin, which is essentially the clot in the blood

Catalyst or Cofactor for Biological Reactions

Calcium functions as a cofactor in many biological reactions. Among these reactions are the absorption of vitamin B_{12}; the action of the fat-splitting enzyme, pancreatic lipase; the secretion of insulin by the pancreas; the formation and breakdown of acetylcholine, the substance that is necessary for the transmission of an impulse from one nerve fiber to the next; and the contraction of myofibrils in muscle fiber. The level of calcium needed to catalyze these reactions will be maintained at the expense of skeletal calcium. Thus dietary calcium has little immediate effect on these reactions.

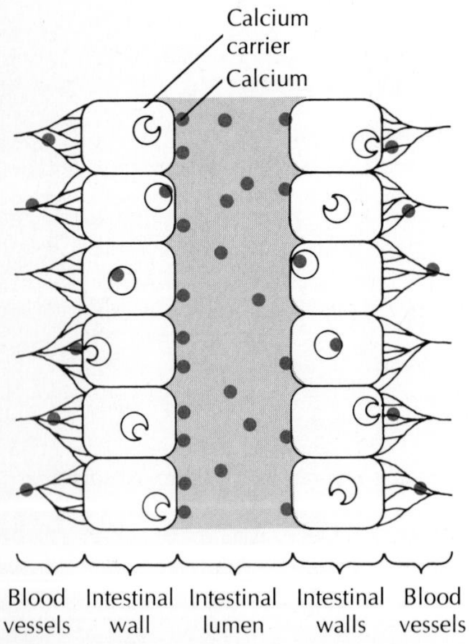

In active transport a calcium carrier shuttles calcium across the intestinal wall from lumen to the blood

Absorption

Adults are normally very inefficient in absorbing calcium. They absorb only 20% to 30% of the calcium in the typical American diet when the need is greatest but only 10% to 30% under most other conditions. The absorption of calcium is a complex process. It is influenced by the amount of dietary calcium available, the need for calcium, a person's age and sex, the use of certain drugs, and the presence of certain nutrients such as lactose, glucose, and vitamin D. The proportion of calcium absorbed varies inversely with the amount in the diet. For adults, who may absorb as little as 10%, an intake in excess of 1000 mg/day may be needed to maintain calcium balance. In growing children, however, up to 75% of dietary calcium can be absorbed. In general, women absorb less calcium than do men, and for both absorption declines with age.

Most absorption occurs in the upper three fourths of the small intestine, where the digestive mass is more acidic. Before being absorbed, calcium must be separated from any complex in which it may occur in food. Calcium is absorbed primarily by *active transport,* an energy-requiring process in which calcium attaches to a calcium-binding protein, enters the cells of the intestinal wall, and is transported across the cell and released through the membrane on the other side of the cell into the blood. Occasionally, calcium is absorbed by passive diffusion.

Factors Favoring Calcium Absorption

Factors Favoring Calcium Absorption
Adequate vitamin D
Acidity of digestive contents
Presence of lactose
Calcium/phosphate ratios of 1 : 1 to 1 : 2
Need for calcium

Vitamin D. The importance of the role of vitamin D in calcium absorption has been recognized since the early 1920s, but only recently have we discovered how it acts. We now know that vitamin D is changed to an active form which catalyzes the synthesis of a protein. This protein serves as a calcium carrier in the cells lining the intestinal wall. It is this carrier that takes calcium across the cells of the intestinal wall to the blood. This active form can result in a 10% to 30% increase in calcium absorption.

Acidity of digestive mass. Calcium is more soluble in acid and therefore is more readily absorbed from an acid medium than from an alkaline medium. Because calcium is absorbed primarily from the small intestine, anything that increases the acidity of the digestive mass before it enters the small intestine from the stomach prolongs the time before the acid is neutralized. Hydrochloric acid, normally secreted in the stomach, is responsible for the acidity of the contents of the digestive tract. The normal decline in hydrochloric acid in old age results in impaired calcium absorption.

Presence of sugars. It has been known for some time that the absorption of calcium in infants is improved from 15% to 50% in the presence of the disaccharide lactose. Fortunately, lactose is found along with calcium in milk. Attempts to explain lactose's effect on the basis of its slower rate of absorption, or changes in the growth of microorganisms in the lower gastrointestinal tract, or changes in the acidity of intestinal contents, have failed. A relatively high ratio of lactose to calcium is necessary to promote absorption. Other sugars such as ribose and fructose also enhance calcium absorption, but lactose is the most effective. More recently it has been shown that as little as 10 grams (1 tsp) of the monosaccharide glucose also enhances calcium absorption as much as 25%.

Calcium/phosphorus ratio. The relationship between calcium and phosphorus levels in the diet plays an important role in the absorption of both. A dietary ratio of calcium to phosphorus of from 1:1 to 1:2 promotes absorption. For infants, a calcium/phosphorus ratio of 1.3:1 is advised. Because of the low intake of milk and the high intake of phosphorus-rich foods, such as protein foods, carbonated beverages, and foods with phosphorus-containing additives, in the current North American diet, the calcium/phosphorus ratio is presently 1:1.6. Ratios below 1:2 and above 2:1 are not recommended, but the latter can be obtained only by misusing calcium supplements.

Protein. The favorable effect of protein in enhancing calcium absorption and reducing calcium losses in the urine has been attributed to both the phosphorus in protein and, specifically, to the amino acids arginine and lysine.

Need for calcium. The extent to which calcium is absorbed may be influenced by the body's need for calcium. During pregnancy, lactation, and adolescence, when the needs for calcium are greatest, absorption rates as high as 50% have been observed. In addition, when calcium intakes are low, the body adapts by absorbing more dietary calcium and excreting less.

Protein and Calcium Absorption

Studies on humans have shown that experimental diets with increased protein have little effect on calcium absorption but cause large increases in urinary losses of calcium. The resulting negative calcium balance was cause for concern because of the tendency of people in affluent countries to consume high amounts of protein and marginal amounts of calcium. Further studies showed that when comparably high amounts of protein from natural protein sources such as meat were consumed, the urinary excretion of calcium was reduced sufficiently to permit calcium balance. It is believed that the phosphorus present along with protein in the natural diets promoted calcium retention (there was a lack of phosphorus in the experimental diets). Therefore high-protein diets have no practical effect on calcium utilization.

Factors Depressing Calcium Absorption or Bone Formation

Factors Depressing Calcium Absorption
Oxalic acid
Phytic acid
Dietary fat
Emotional instability
Increased gastrointestinal motility
Lack of exercise
Dietary fiber
Caffeine
Drugs

Oxalic acid. Oxalic acid, which is found in some green leafy vegetables, such as spinach and kale, combines with calcium to form an insoluble complex, calcium oxalate. The calcium in calcium oxalate cannot be freed to be absorbed. In most food containing oxalic acid, sufficient calcium is present to tie up all the oxalic acid; thus, no surplus of oxalic acid is left to bind calcium from other foods eaten at the same time. For example, the oxalic acid of spinach binds the calcium in the spinach but does not interfere with the absorption of the calcium in milk at the same time. The fact that there was unbound oxalic acid in lower grades of cocoa led to questions about the use of chocolate milk for children. However, studies on college women showed that they could only tolerate 1 oz of cocoa—not enough to cause any depression in calcium absorption with either a low or high calcium intake. Comparable studies have not been done on children, but similar results would be expected. The studies indicate that there is no reason to discourage the use of chocolate milk on the basis of decreased calcium absorption.

Phytic acid. Another organic acid, phytic acid, binds calcium but is of little consequence in most diets. Phytic acid is found primarily on the outer husk of cereals. Only when calcium-rich foods are eaten with foods such as oatmeal or whole wheat pita bread, which are high in phytic acid, could this become a problem.

Presence of dietary fat. The effect of fat on calcium absorption is unclear. On the other hand, improved absorption results from the slower passage of food through the digestive tract—and as we have learned, foods that are high in fat move slowly. On the other hand, high-fat diets promote the formation of insoluble soaps of fatty acids and calcium; they can result in **steatorrhea** (fatty stools) and a reduction in calcium absorption.

steatorrhea
Condition in which feces contains abnormally high amount of fat; usually the result of incomplete digestion or absorption of fat

Emotional instability. The efficiency of calcium absorption can be influenced by the emotional stability of the individual. Emotional states such as stress, tension, anxiety, grief, or boredom can interfere with calcium absorption. In one study, a group of emotionally distressed young women required a higher intake of calcium to maintain calcium balance than a comparable group of happy, relaxed women. Another study of college men indicated a lower absorption and increased excretion of calcium under conditions of stress such as examinations.

Increased gastrointestinal motility. Anything that increases the rate of passage of food through the intestinal tract decreases calcium absorption by reducing the amount of time that the contents of the intestinal tract are in contact with the intestinal wall. Laxatives and foods high in bulk may have this effect.

Lack of exercise. People who do not engage in weight-bearing exercise, such as walking, and bedridden people who are essentially immobile lose as much as 0.5% of bone calcium in a month and have a reduced ability to replace it. This may be a cause of (or at least a complicating factor in) the decalcification of bone so often experienced by older people. Some evidence suggests that it is the lack of weight on the bones rather than immobility per se that causes negative calcium balance during bed rest. Similarly, swimmers may have less bone density than walkers or joggers. Astronauts have negative calcium balance because of either weightlessness or immobility.

Negative Calcium Balance
calcium output > calcium intake

Dietary fiber. Various types of dietary fiber depress the absorption of calcium and other minerals, either by decreasing the time needed to pass food through the digestive tract, by increasing the bulk of the food mass, or by diluting the intestinal contents or binding the mineral.

Caffeine. High intakes of caffeine affect calcium bioavailability by increasing the loss of calcium in the urine and the secretion and loss of calcium through the gastrointestinal tract.

Drugs. Some medications such as anticonvulsants; cortisone, and thyroxine reduce calcium absorption.

Metabolism

Once calcium has been absorbed through the wall of the intestine, it is transported in the blood and released to the fluids bathing the tissues of the body. From there, the cells take up whatever calcium is needed for their normal functioning and growth. As the blood is filtered through the kidneys, about 99% of the calcium (10 grams/day) is resorbed. The remaining 1% that is excreted in the urine usually amounts to 100 to 175 mg/day. Some calcium becomes a part of the digestive secretions in the stomach and intestine. Much of this calcium is resorbed, but the calcium lost in the feces amounts to about 130 mg, regardless of dietary intake.

Most of the absorbed calcium is used in the calcification of bones to give strength and rigidity. This process is facilitated by vitamin D.

The calcium in the blood is in equilibrium with bone calcium, about a third of which can be used to maintain blood calcium levels. The parathyroid gland has a major role in maintaining these levels, which do not fluctuate more than ±3% throughout the day. If blood calcium levels fall from the normal 10 mg/dl to below 7 mg/dl, the parathyroid gland secretes a hormone, **parathormone,** that has several functions. Within minutes, it stimulates the kidneys to resorb calcium that might normally be excreted in the urine. Within hours, it has acted on bone to cause some of the exchangeable bone calcium to be released by stimulating the metabolism of some of the carbohydrate of bone to citrate and lactate, in which the calcium is soluble. This in turn is released into the blood where it raises the calcium in the blood and the intercellular fluids to more normal levels. The parathormone also stimulates the absorption of calcium from the gastrointestinal tract; this occurs after several days and results from the formation of the active form of vitamin D—that leads to synthesis of a calcium-binding protein. When blood calcium levels return to normal, the secretion of the parathyroid gland also returns to normal.

parathormone
Hormone secreted by the parathyroid gland in response to low blood calcium; signals kidney to resorb calcium and the intestine to absorb more

Opposing the action of parathormone, is a second hormone **calcitonin.** This is a polypeptide formed in the thyroid gland. Calcitonin is secreted when blood calcium levels become elevated, acting to lower both calcium and phosphorus levels by inhibiting bone resorption. These two hormones are responsible for maintaining the level of calcium in the blood within the very narrow limits demanded by the body.

calcitonin
Hormone produced in the thyroid gland in response to normal or elevated blood calcium levels; signals bone to stop resorption and kidney to excrete calcium

The effect of the parathyroid hormone is integrated with the action of the active form of vitamin D, which also stimulates the absorption of calcium from the intestinal tract, increases the retention of calcium by the kidneys, and allows the parathormone to act to release bone calcium to maintain blood levels. An excess of vitamin D may lead to decalcification of bone and an increased absorption of calcium from the gastrointestinal tract; the result is hypercalcemia, or an excess of calcium in the blood.

The absorption and metabolism of calcium are summarized in Figure 10-5, and Figure 10-6 depicts the hormonal control of calcium metabolism.

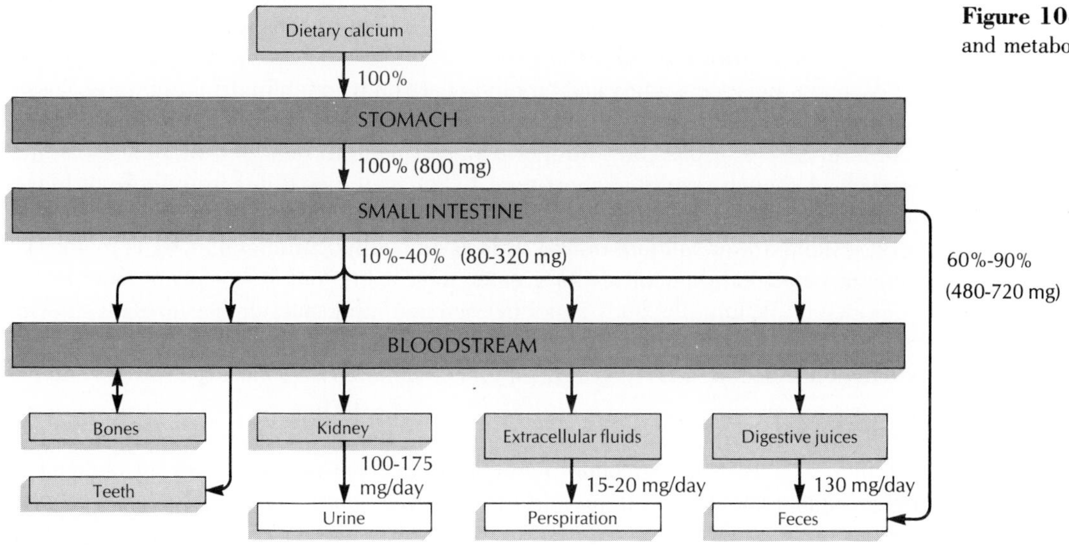

Figure 10-5 Summary of absorption and metabolism of calcium.

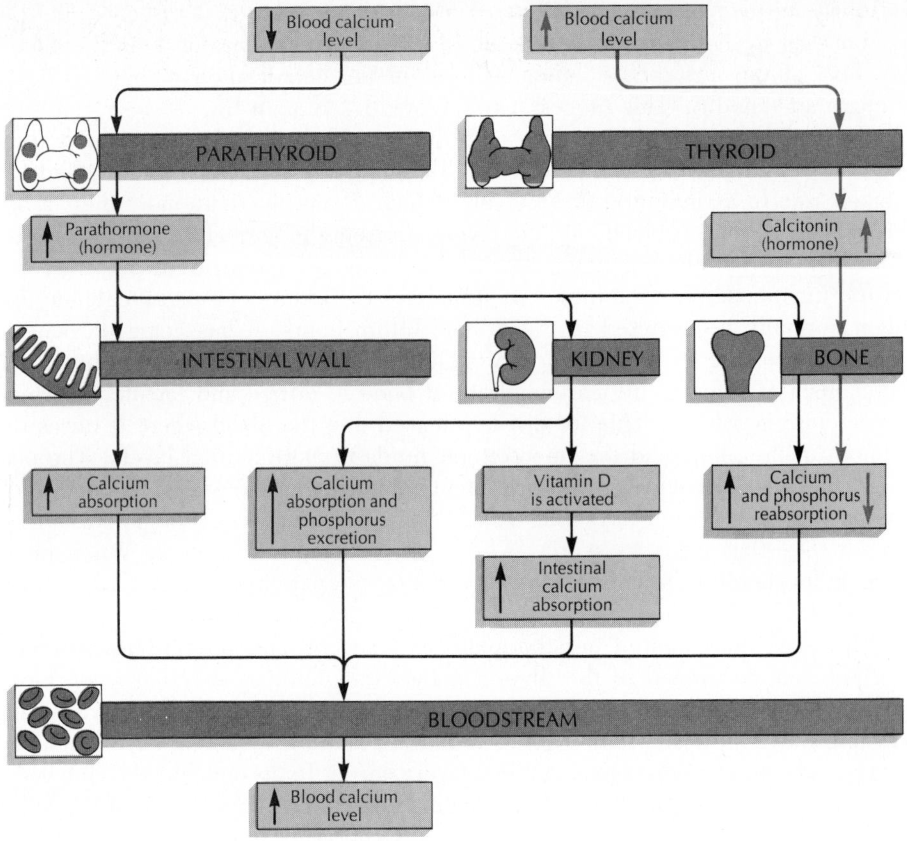

Figure 10-6 Summary of hormonal control of calcium metabolism.

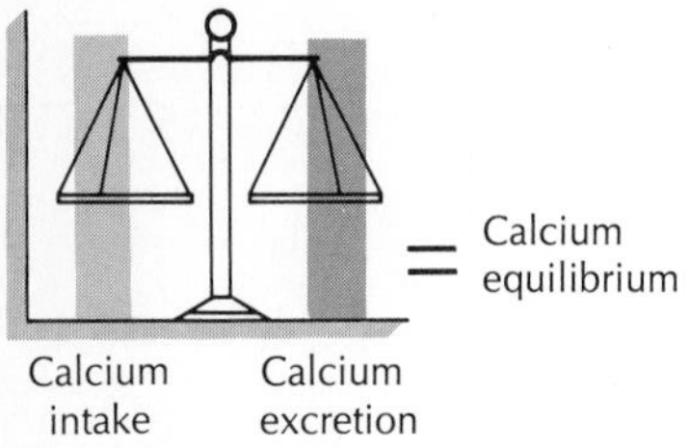

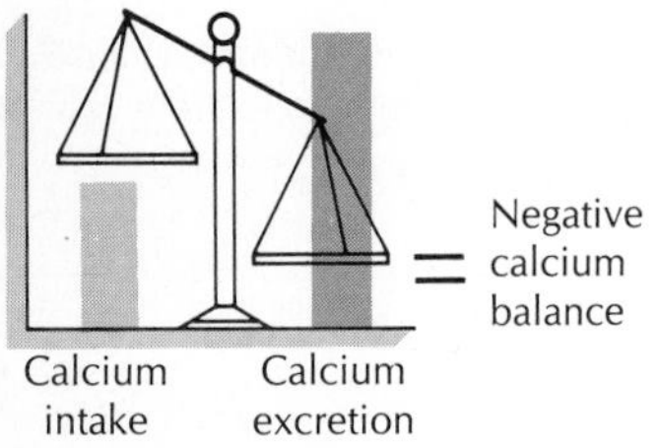

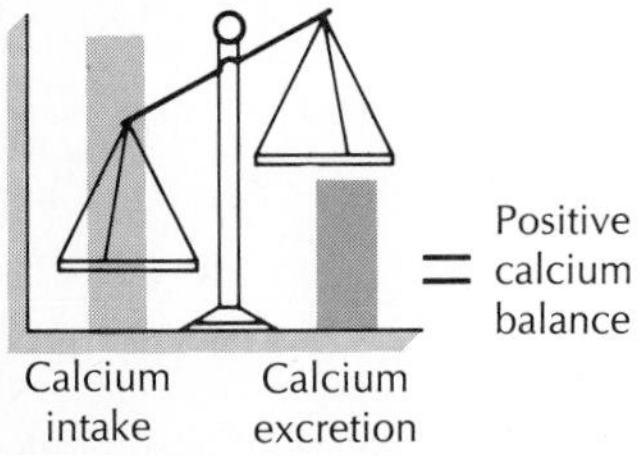

Requirements

Calcium Balance Studies

Estimates of calcium needs have been based on the results of calcium balance studies. These studies, which are quite difficult, require the collection and analysis of the intake of calcium in food and beverages, as well as analysis of urine and fecal excretion over a period of several weeks. Urinary calcium represents blood calcium that has not been reabsorbed by the kidneys; fecal calcium represents the endogenous calcium of digestive secretions plus any unabsorbed dietary calcium, known as **exogenous fecal calcium.**

exogenous fecal calcium
Calcium excreted in the feces that had its origin in the diet rather than being excreted into the intestine

Calcium balance studies must include data on calcium in drinking water, losses in perspiration and tears, and information on the history of calcium intake, phosphorus intake, and possible nitrogen-balance data all of which influence calcium balance. Although results of short-term balance studies differ from those of longer duration because of adaptation to changing intakes, balance studies are still used to set a standard for calcium intake. It is assumed that, when the body is in positive calcium balance, when intake is greater than excretion, it is storing calcium. In calcium equilibrium, the body is neither accumulating calcium nor losing it showing that calcium intake is adequate. In negative calcium balance, there is a net loss of calcium from the body that reflects decalcification of bone tissue.

Bone Quality

The lack of a measure for bone quality that is sensitive to short-term changes in dietary intake has made it impossible to use bone quality as an indicator of calcium needs.

For further discussion of assessing bone quality see "Assessment of Calcium Status"

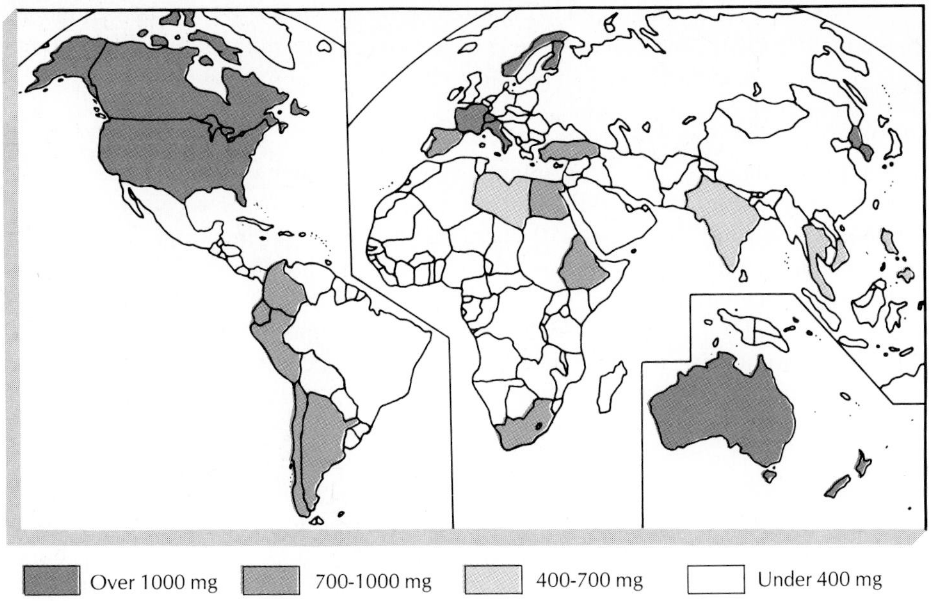

Figure 10-7 Amount of calcium available per person in food supply in different parts of the world.
Based on data from Calcium requirements, Report of Joint FAO/WHO Expert Committee, WHO Technical Report Series No. 230, Geneva, 1962.

Table 10-2 ◆ Comparison of recommended calcium intakes (mg)

	Age	Recommended Nutrient Intakes, Canada (1983)*	Recommended Daily Amounts, United Kingdom (1979)†	NRC Recommended Dietary Allowances (1980)‡	FAO/WHO Suggested Practical Allowances§
Children	7-12 mo	400	600	540	500-600
	1-10 yr	700	600-700	800	600-700
Males	16-19 yr	900	500-600	1200	500-600
	Adult	800	500	800	400-500
Females	16-19 yr	700	500-600	1200	500-600
	Adult	700	500	800	400-500
	Pregnancy	1200	1200	1200	1000-1200
	Lactation	1200	1200	1200	1000-1200

*Recommended nutrient intakes for Canadians, Dept. of National Health and Welfare, Ottawa, 1983.
†Department of Health and Social Security: Recommended daily amounts of food energy and nutrients for groups of people in the United Kingdom, Reports on Health and Social Subjects, No. 15, London, 1979, Her Majesty's Stationery Office.
‡Food and Nutrition Board: Recommended dietary allowances, ed. 9, Washington, D.C., 1980, National Academy of Sciences–National Research Council.
§Calcium requirements, Report of Joint FAO/WHO Expert Committee, WHO Technical Report Series No. 230, 1962.
158

Dietary Allowances

In spite of some disagreement about the best way to assess calcium needs, most countries have arrived at a set of dietary intake recommendations. The recommended allowances for the United States proposed in 1980 have been set at a level that the committee believes will meet the needs of essentially all healthy individuals.

Recommended Dietary Allowances for Calcium

1-10 yrs	800 mg
11-18 yrs	1200 mg
19+ yrs	800 mg

The Food and Agricultural Organization has released suggested practical calcium allowances that can be met more readily by a larger segment of the world's population. This includes people in a developing country who sometimes get very little calcium because of the limited amount in their country's food supply. The FAO group suggested that there is no evidence of any harmful effects from diets containing only 300 mg of calcium/day or more than 1000 mg of calcium/day, provided that vitamin D, which facilitates calcium absorption, is adequate. As seen in Figure 10-7 there is wide variation in the calcium available in the diets of various countries.

A comparison of American, Canadian, British, and FAO recommendations (listed in Table 10-2) shows that there is no general agreement regarding the optimal level of calcium intake, even for people living under similar conditions.

Infants

The calcium in the infant's skeleton is almost entirely replaced in the first year of life

It is assumed that the breast-fed infant, who receives about 50 mg of calcium/kg of body weight from breast milk and retains two thirds of it, receives adequate calcium. (Breast milk contains 210 mg of calcium in usual intake of 750 ml.) For the formula-fed infant, who retains less than half of the 65 mg of calcium/kg of body weight received from cow's milk formula, the intake is essentially the same. (Cow's milk contains 300 mg of calcium/750 ml.) If undiluted whole milk is fed, calcium absorption is greatly reduced because of the relatively high fat content of the milk. Vitamin D is essential for the body to use calcium at this age.

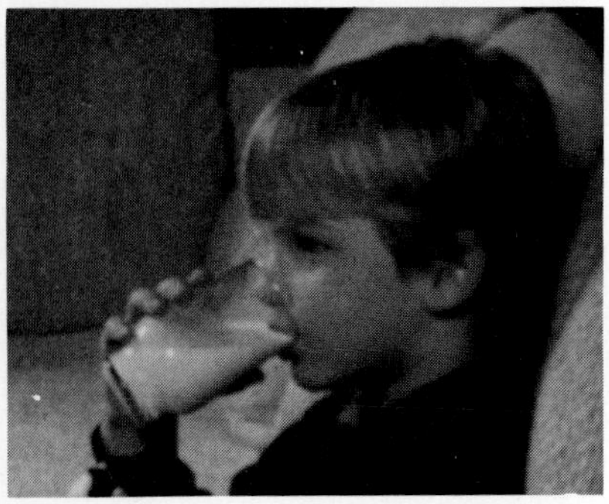

Milk products are the major source of calcium and vitamin D in a child's diet.

Children

Calcium needs are met by daily intakes of about 800 mg for children, 1 to 10 years of age, who may be able to absorb as much as 75% of the intake. The rapidly growing skeleton of an adolescent requires the retention of as much as 500 mg of calcium/day, calling for a daily intake of 1200 to 1500 mg. Except for variations in body weight, the need for calcium declines once peak bone mass is achieved, at least by age 30 and possibly earlier. Thus, children and adolescents need two to four times as much calcium to meet the needs for growth as adults need to maintain the mature skeleton.

Pregnancy

Although a child is born with relatively poorly calcified bones, the full-term fetus contains approximately 30 grams (1 ounce) of calcium, two thirds of which is deposited during the last 3 months of pregnancy. It is thought that calcium is stored in the mother's body early in pregnancy to be transferred to the fetus during the last 3 months at a rate of about 300 mg/day. Studies using stable isotopes of calcium show that up to 90% of the calcium in the fetal skeleton comes from the mother's diet; the rest is withdrawn from the reserves in her bones. To help meet this increased need pregnant women absorb more calcium and excrete less than nonpregnant women. Even so, to meet these additional needs, the expectant mother requires an additional 400 mg of calcium in her diet. The pregnant adolescent who needs 400 mg over the 1200 mg required for her growth must make a special effort to obtain this amount.

Lactation

A breast-fed baby receives calcium from the mother at a much faster rate than during fetal development. Calcium is provided from current maternal intake and from the stores that the mother accumulated during the sixth and seventh months of pregnancy, when the calcium retained far exceeded that needed by the fetus. Thus a lactating woman continues to need an additional 400 mg dietary calcium to prevent excessive depletion of her reserves of bone calcium. Over a 6-month lactation period, about 50 grams of calcium are secreted in human milk. To meet this demand, which amounts to just over 200 mg of calcium/day in 750 ml of milk, a maternal intake of 630 mg of calcium is required (assuming 30% efficiency of absorption). This calls for the use of large amounts of dairy products (a minimum of 1 quart of milk or its equivalent), as well as generous use of other calcium-rich foods. Few women maintain calcium balance during lactation; rather, they draw on the calcium reserves built up during pregnancy to provide some of the calcium that is transferred to breast milk. The ability of some women to maintain a successful calcium level in their breast milk on very low calcium intakes is unexplained.

Adults

There is considerable evidence that the greater the bone mass a person acquires in the first 20 to 30 years of life (the time during which peak bone mass is achieved), the greater the protection against the loss of bone mass in later years. Intakes of calcium during early adulthood have a marked influence on the total amount of bone accumulated. Based primarily on the results of calcium balance studies, the RDA for calcium has been set at 800 mg/day for all adults, assuming that 20% to 30% of dietary calcium is absorbed. There is some evidence that higher levels may provide additional benefits to adult women, who are particularly likely to lose bone with aging after they no longer have the protection against bone loss from estrogens secreted prior to menopause. As a result, based on the advice of a panel of experts, the National Institutes of Health recommends a daily intake of 1000 mg of calcium for premenopausal and **estrogen**-treated postmenopausal women and 1500 mg for postmenopausal women who are not on estrogen therapy. They believed that these intakes were necessary to maintain calcium balance or even to reduce the rate of bone loss, which is associated with an increase in bone fractures. These levels are considerably above the 530 to 630 mg average intake reported by adult women. To attain the recommended levels would require a substantial change in food intake patterns or the use of supplements or calcium-fortified foods. There is currently considerable research underway to provide more information on which to base dietary recommendations.

estrogen
Sex hormone, which is produced in lower amounts after menopause; may inhibit bone remodelling

There is little basis on which to suggest an increase in calcium intake with age for men. All evidence points to the need for men to maintain an adult intake of 800 mg/day throughout their later years to reduce the likelihood of demineralization of the skeleton.

Adequacy of Calcium in the North American Diet

Results of the Nationwide Food Consumption Study (1977-78) of 37,000 people found calcium intakes to be 979 mg/day for adult males and 679 mg/day for females. One third of the men and over half of the women had calcium intakes that fell below 70% of the RDA (Figure 10-8). A resurvey of adults in 1985 and 1986 showed no change. HANES II found similar intakes for women and slightly higher ones for men. The average reported intake for children under the age of 10, however,

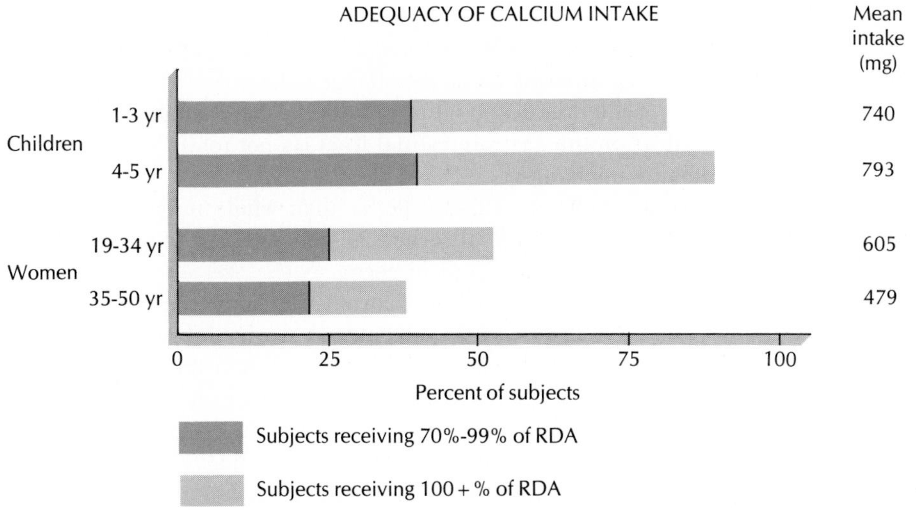

Figure 10-8 Adequacy of calcium intake in the North American diet. Based on data from the CSFII, USDA, 1986.

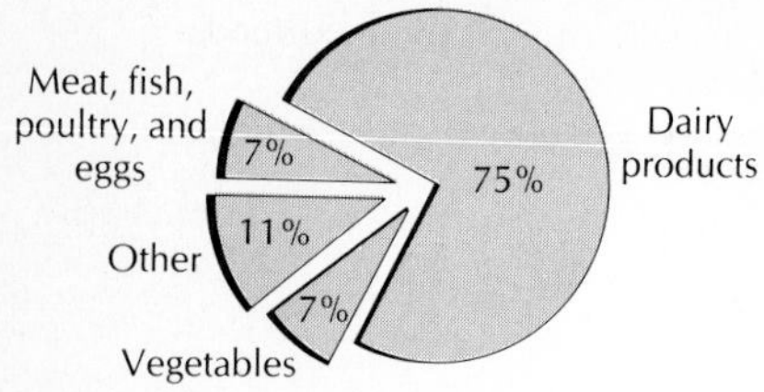

Figure 10-9 Contribution of various food groups to the calcium in the North American food supply.
USDA, 1985.

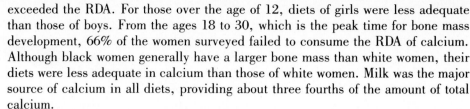

exceeded the RDA. For those over the age of 12, diets of girls were less adequate than those of boys. From the ages 18 to 30, which is the peak time for bone mass development, 66% of the women surveyed failed to consume the RDA of calcium. Although black women generally have a larger bone mass than white women, their diets were less adequate in calcium than those of white women. Milk was the major source of calcium in all diets, providing about three fourths of the amount of total calcium.

Food Sources

Calcium is present in significant amounts in a very limited number of foods. Figure 10-9 shows the contribution of various food groups to the total amount of calcium available in the North American diet. It is evident that milk and milk products are the most important dietary sources of calcium, with cereal products and fruits and vegetables each making a much smaller contribution. The calcium content of the foods consumed most frequently in the United States and some recommended sources of calcium are shown in Table 10-3. The amount of calcium available in the food supply has declined from a peak of 1.07 grams/person/day in 1945 to 0.88 gram in 1988.

Milk and dairy products are the most dependable sources of calcium because of the many forms in which they can be consumed, their availability in the food supply, and their relatively low cost. In addition, the calcium in milk is readily absorbed because all milk contains the sugar lactose and almost all milk is fortified with vitamin D, both of which facilitate absorption.

If dairy products were excluded from the diet, the bulk of other foods needed to supply comparable amounts of calcium would be so great that it would be difficult to use them as significant sources of calcium. The cost of comparable amounts of calcium from dairy and nondairy foods shows that nondairy foods are expensive calcium sources.

Sources of Calcium Providing the Calcium Equivalent of 1 Cup of Milk

- ¾ cup yogurt*, plain or flavored
- ⅞ cup yogurt*, fruited
- 1½ oz cheddar cheese
- 2 cups ice cream
- 2 cups cottage cheese
- ⅘ cup almonds
- 2½ oz sardines

*dried milk solids added

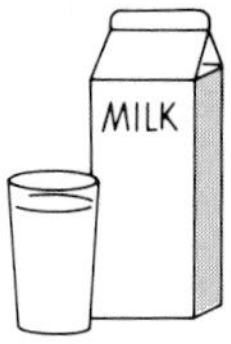

Foods of low water content such as sardines, almonds, and sesame seeds have an appreciable amount of calcium in 100-gram portions. However, their usefulness in most diets is limited if cost, as well as their high contribution to calories, is considered. (The latter is an especially important consideration for people on calorie-restricted diets.)

Many adults of black and Oriental ancestry lack the enzyme lactase, which is necessary for the digestion of lactose, the carbohydrate in milk. Lack of this enzyme causes digestive discomfort, which explains why these people cannot tolerate milk. Although milk cannot be promoted as a source of calcium for them, cheeses in which the carbohydrate lactose has been changed to lactic acid provide an acceptable alternative. Yogurt, a partially fermented milk, still contains some lactose but also has an enzyme that can bring about the change to lactic acid in the intestine. Sweet acidophilus milk, which is designed to provide the microorganisms thought to have a beneficial effect on the gastrointestinal tract, is not really useful because the carbohydrate remains unchanged.

Nonfat milk and buttermilk are slightly better than whole milk as sources of calcium. Calcium in chocolate milk is absorbed as well as that in unflavored milk in spite of the small amount of oxalic acid in cocoa.

Cheddar cheese is often more palatable than milk as a source of calcium for adults, even though it has a high caloric density and relatively high sodium content. Cottage cheese is a less dependable source of calcium. When rennin coagulation is used to prepare cottage cheese, more calcium is retained in the curd than when either acid coagulation or a combination of acid and rennin coagulation is used. All three methods are used commercially, but the consumer has no way of knowing which process is used. Cream cheese is a poor source of calcium because it is made from the fat portion of milk, which has practically no calcium.

Table 10-3 ◇ Calcium, phosphorus, and magnesium in average servings and per 100 kcal of most frequently used foods and recommeneded sources

Food	Amount	Kcal	Calcium			Phosphorus			Magnesium		
			Mg per Serving	Mg per 100 kcal	INQ*	Mg per Serving	Mg per 100 kcal	INQ	Mg per Serving	Mg per 100 kcal	INQ
Meat, Fish, Eggs, Poultry, Nuts											
Egg, fried	1 large	83	25	31	0.6	78	94	1.87	5	6	0.3
Beef roast	3 oz	318	11	4	0.1	202	63	1.1	22	7	0.4
Hamburger	3 oz	285	11	4	0.1	207	72	1.2	25	9	0.4
Chicken	3 oz	242	15	6	0.1	182	75	1.3	23	10	0.5
Tuna	3 oz	170	8	5	0.1	234	138	2.3	35	20	1.0
Peanut butter	2 T	178	18	10	0.2	114	64	1.1	59	33	1.7
Bacon	3 slices	89	12	13	0.2	188	211	3.5	21	24	1.2
Salmon, canned†	3 oz	120	167	133	2.7	243	200	4.2	81	134	1.6
Almonds†	1 oz (10)	165	75	45	1.0	147	90	1.8			
Pizza†	⅛ of a 12-in pie	145	86	59	1.2						
Tofu†	4 oz	114	102	90	2.2	145	120	2.5			
Cereal Products											
Cornflakes	1 cup	88	1	1	0.0	11	13	.21	4	5	0.2
Shredded wheat	1 biscuit	83	13	16	0.3	388	467	7.80	4	48	2.4
Saltines	4 crackers	43	2	5	0.1	9	21	.40	3	7	0.3
Rice	1 oz, dry	109	10	9	0.2	28	25	.40	8	7	0.4
White bread	1 slice	81	28	34	0.6	22	27	.50	5	6	0.3
Whole-wheat bread	1 slice	73	28	39	0.6	52	71	1.20	18	25	1.0
Dairy Products											
Whole milk†	8 oz	157	91	182	3.5	223	142	2.4	31	20	1.0
2% fat milk†	8 oz	121	297	254	4.2	240	198	3.3	34	28	1.4
Cheddar cheese†	1 oz	114	204	190	3.2	154	135	2.3	8	7	0.4
Cottage cheese‡	4 oz	103	75	73	1.5	340	330	7.1	6	6	0.1
Yogurt, plain†	8 oz	139	274	197	3.8	326	234	3.4	26	36	0.5
Ice cream†	8 oz	349	151	43	0.8	115	33	0.2	16	56	0.3
Nonfat milk†	8 oz	86	302	345	6.9	247	281	6.5	23	24	0.6
Fruits											
Apple	1 medium	81	10	12	0.2	14	17	0.3	11	14	0.7
Banana	1 medium	105	7	9	0.2	32	30	0.5	41	39	2.0
Orange juice, frozen	4 oz	56	11	19	0.3	19	34	0.6	12	22	1.1
Peach	1 medium	37	4	24	0.4	19	51	0.86	10	27	1.4
Vegetables											
Corn, canned	4 oz (½ cup)	84	5	5	0.1	71	72	1.2	19	20	1.0
Green beans	4 oz (½ cup)	52	39	75	1.2	32	61	1.0	19	37	1.8
Green peas	4 oz (½ cup)	88	19	22	0.4	84	95	1.6	19	22	1.1
Lettuce	¼ head	13	20	154	2.6	22	169	2.8	11	85	4.2
Tomato	1 medium	22	13	59	1.0	27	122	2.0	14	64	3.2
Potato, baked	1 medium	93	9	10	0.2	65	69	1.2	31	33	1.7
Broccoli†	3.5 oz, cooked	26	205	207	4.1	37	10	0.8	47	12	0.9
Turnip greens†	½ cup, cooked	15	99	15	2.0	21	3	0.4	16	2	0.3

*INQ = % U.S. RDA for nutrient/% Energy requirement (2000 kcal). (i.e. INQ (Ca) for fried eggs = ([25/1000] × 100)/([83/2000] × 100) = 2.5/4.15 = 0.6.)

†Recommended sources.

‡Variable source.

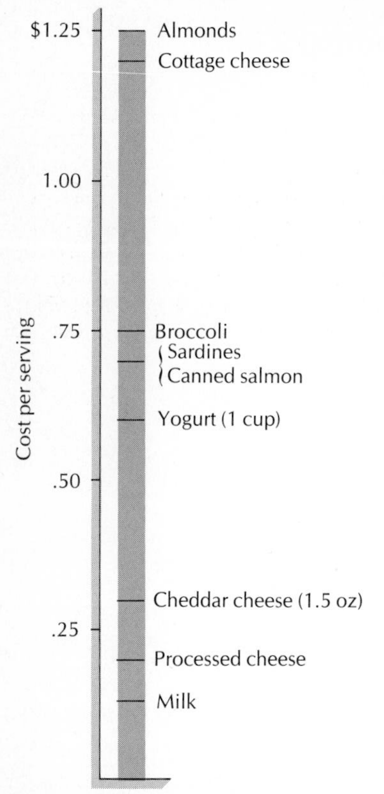

Relative cost per serving of various calcium sources, Northeast, U.S., 1988.

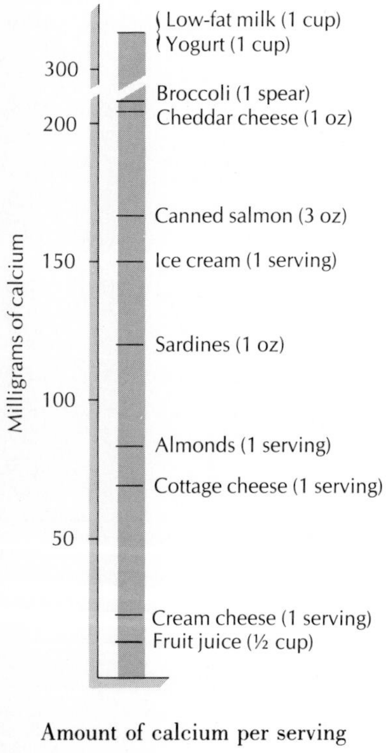

Amount of calcium per serving

Goat's milk contains slightly more calcium than cow's milk and is often substituted for it when an infant is allergic to cow's milk. Calcium-enriched soybean milk preparations in either powdered or liquid form are also satisfactory.

Broccoli and green leafy vegetables such as turnip greens, which do not contain oxalic acid, have appreciable amounts of available calcium but are not used often enough to be considered a consistent source. The calcium in vegetables is not as well utilized as that in milk because the bulk of the vegetables increases the rate of passage of food through the intestinal tract and therefore reduces the amount of time that calcium can be absorbed. In addition, a component of cellulose binds some calcium. Considerable calcium may be lost in the preparation of vegetables if thick skins are removed or if dark green leaves are discarded.

Soybeans, which contain 70 mg of calcium/oz (in mature seeds), become a significant calcium source when consumed in large amounts although the high fiber and phytate content reduces absorption.

Although bread has not traditionally been considered a source of calcium, the use of dried milk solids and calcium-containing mold inhibitors raises available calcium in some breads to the point that many adults can receive as much as one seventh of their daily requirement from them. The optional enrichment of flour with 500 to 1500 mg of calcium/pound also makes some bread with 20 to 60 mg of calcium/slice a significant source for the 10% of the population who eat three or more slices per day. Similarly, the calcium value of baked products (such as muffins, waffles, and cakes) made with milk or enriched flour should not be overlooked. Data from the Nationwide Food Consumption Study (1977-1978) show that in diets adequate in calcium, grain products provided 16% of the calcium.

Developing countries in tropical areas, where milk products are generally unavailable, rely on less traditional sources of calcium. There is, however, virtually no information on how well calcium from these sources is used. Since water consumption is high in the tropics, when its mineral content is also high (50 mg or more of minerals per quart, or liter), water may provide up to 200 mg of calcium/day. Other sources of calcium include small whole fish or fermented fish pastes; the mill powder used in grinding rice; soybean products such as tofu, saridele, and tempeh if calcium sulfate is used to coagulate the curd; the lime used in making tortillas in Mexico and by betel chewers; and a ground rock called *cal* that is used in porridges by the Peruvians. Even such foods as sweet potatoes, which are a dietary staple in the Papuan highlands of New Guinea, and aged eggs, which are packed in lime in China, may contribute to the limited total calcium consumed. In Malaya, pregnant women eat a small shellfish, rich in calcium, that is ground up whole. These represent only a few of the ways in which various populations acquire sufficient calcium although they consume practically no dairy products.

Table 10-4 ◆ Amount of calcium in various calcium supplements

Supplement	Percent Calcium	Milligrams in 1000-mg Tablet (1 gram)
Calcium carbonate	40	400
Calcium lactate	13	130
Calcium gluconate	9	90
Calcium citrate	18	180
Dibasic calcium phosphate	23	230
Bone meal*	28-33	280-330
Dolomite*	20	200
Tums	20	200

*Not recommended because of lead content of 6 ppm exceeding FDA limit of 5 ppm in food.

Because of the difficulty in getting adequate dietary calcium, many dietary supplements containing oyster shell or calcium salts, such as calcium carbonate, lactate, or gluconate, are being promoted. The percentage of calcium in the more common types of supplements is given in Table 10-4. Some antacids, such as Tums, contain up to 200 mg of calcium in the form of calcium carbonate. New products such as calcium gluconate must be dissolved in water; therefore the possible problem of poor solubility in the stomach is avoided. Some supplements, such as calcium citrate, are absorbed better on an empty stomach whereas others, such as calcium carbonate, are better absorbed if taken with food. Products such as bone meal and dolomite should be avoided because analyses have shown that they contain potentially dangerous levels of heavy metals such as lead.

In selecting a calcium supplement, read labels carefully; multivitamin-mineral pills seldom contain much calcium. A separate calcium supplement is usually necessary to obtain any appreciable amount; even then, several large pills of the supplement will be needed each day.

Those who sell special food-blending devices often promote the ingestion of pulverized eggshell as a feasible way to get an adequate calcium intake. An eggshell does contain 2 grams of calcium. However, because there are no data on the utilization of calcium from this source and there is danger of contamination with *Salmonella,* reliance on crushed eggshells is risky.

High Calcium Intake

In general, the body adapts to high intakes of calcium by decreasing the proportion that is taken up by vitamin D–facilitated absorption. However, since about 15% of ingested calcium is absorbed by passive diffusion a portion of high intakes is not affected by adaptation and continues to be absorbed.

Since it has been only in the past few years that people, especially women, have been using supplements and eating many foods fortified with calcium, we may not yet have had time to see the effects of very high intakes. Up to now, however, we have no evidence that high oral calcium intakes (more than 2 grams) alone have any effect on the level of calcium in the urine of normal subjects, and hence on kidney stone formation, or on the deposition of calcium in other soft tissues. Any abnormal deposition of calcium in soft tissues is more likely a result of low magnesium than of high calcium.

Animal studies have suggested that excessively high intakes of calcium have a depressing effect on the utilization of other nutrients, such as phosphorus, copper, iodine, zinc, magnesium, and iron, when these nutrients are present at minimum levels. The ratios of calcium to other minerals at which this depressing effect can occur are considerably beyond those possible on a normal diet; however, it is possible that imbalances could result from irrational supplementation.

Assessment of Calcium Status

Assessing calcium status is difficult because we do not yet have a feasible and sensitive method to make this assessment. Blood calcium levels are readily determined; however, blood levels rarely change because the parathyroid gland mobilizes bone calcium to maintain blood calcium and a drop in blood calcium is a more sensitive measure of parathyroid efficiency than of calcium status. Considerable work has been done to test x-ray measurements of bone density to reflect the degree of mineralization of the bones, but in general the x-rays are not sensitive to variation within the normal range of human calcium intake to be of any use in assessing calcium status. The problem is further complicated by the fact that from 10% to 40% of the bone must be demineralized before any change will be reflected in x-ray measurements. New techniques, known as single or dual photon, absorptiometry, and computed tomography show promise in the assessment of calcium status, with single photon useful only for cortical bone. Absorptiometry merely involves focusing a special light source on the wrist. Aside from changes in bone structure, there are no obvious symptoms of calcium deficiency.

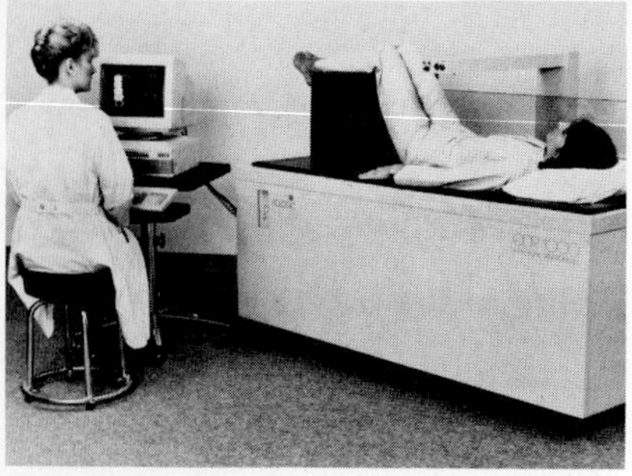

Bone density can now be measured with practically no radiation exposure using bone densitometer scan of lumbar region of spine.

Calcium-Related Health Problems

Osteoporosis

Osteoporosis is a condition found primarily among middle-aged and elderly women. In osteoporosis the mass, or amount, of bone in the skeleton has been diminished, but the remaining bone mass is of normal composition. Women with osteoporosis are usually shorter than they were when they were younger, are susceptible to bone fracture, and suffer from low backache. Estimates of the incidence of osteoporosis in people over 50 years of age range from 10% to as high as 50%. The fact that women lose their compact bone mass in the long bones once their estrogen levels drop at menopause, coupled with the fact that they do not acquire as much bone during adulthood, are major reasons why the incidence of this condition among women is 10 times that among men.

Bone fracture among osteoporotics (people with osteoporosis) may be caused by spontaneous fractures in which the break precedes the fall rather than being caused by it. Osteoporotic bone breaks as a result of loads that are 40% less than normal, and the healing period for fractures is considerably longer than average. Of the 6 million spontaneous fractures that are suffered annually, 80% occur in women, with nine out of ten fractures after age 60 resulting from osteoporosis.

Osteoporosis is now regarded as a condition of multiple origins. This has led to the proposal that it be referred to collectively as the osteoporosities. The concept of multiple causes may help to explain why high dietary calcium levels are not necessarily protective and low levels not necessarily associated with bone loss. The osteoporosities have been attributed to

- **A decrease in bone mass as the result of long-standing dietary inadequacy**
- **Poor absorption or utilization of calcium**
- **Irregularities of the action of the parathyroid gland in stimulating bone resorption**
- **A failure by the body to synthesize the collagen matrix of bone**
- **Immobility**
- **A loss of the stimulus for bone formation provided by the estrogens.**

In osteoporosis the rate of bone formation is normal but bone reabsorption occurs at an accelerated pace, leading to a decrease in bone mass. Bone reabsorption may occur to maintain normal blood levels of calcium when dietary intake is low or when dietary needs are abnormally high because of poor absorption. Other factors in the development of osteoporosis are heredity, age, level of physical activity, smoking, and certain medications.

A diet high in calcium (15.5 mg/kg of body weight), with 50 mg/day of sodium fluoride and with adequate vitamin D, has been shown to arrest the resorption of bone and has led to the observation that the best way to prevent osteoporosis is with an adequate calcium intake throughout life. Fluoride may protect against bone loss by stimulating bone formation and by producing a more stable bone mineral. The recent identification and synthesis of **DHCC,** which is the active form of vitamin D that increases calcium absorption, has raised hopes for its potential in preventing or treating osteoporosis. DHCC is now undergoing the clinical trials that are necessary to obtain FDA approval for general use.

DHCC (dihydroxycholecalciferol)
The active form of vitamin D formed by the addition of OH (hydroxylation) to dietary vitamin D first in the liver and then in the kidneys

More adequate intakes of calcium throughout adult life, either from food, supplements, or both, help maintain a larger bone mass to reduce the possibility of osteoporosis. Once the bone mass has diminished, however, supplements of calcium have no apparent effect in restoring the lost bone; they merely depress further loss.

Osteomalacia

osteomalacia
A condition in which the quality but not the quantity of bone is reduced

Osteomalacia is a condition in which the quality but not the quantity of bone is reduced. It is most likely to occur among women who live in areas of low sunshine (a nondietary source of vitamin D), those taking anticonvulsive drugs, which depress the absorption of calcium, or those who have depleted mineral reserves resulting from the demands of successive pregnancies and prolonged lactation. Most people with osteomalacia respond to vitamin D therapy. The differences in bone changes in osteoporosis and osteomalacia are shown in Figure 10-10. Although osteomalacia is also associated with low phosphorus levels, low blood calcium levels are the most frequent cause.

Hypercalcemia

Hypercalcemia, or too much calcium in the blood, occurs in infants as the result of high intakes of vitamin D. It has been observed when many different baby foods, supplemented with vitamin D, were included in an infant's diet. It is best corrected by reducing vitamin D intake rather than lowering the amount of calcium in the diet.

hypercalcemia
Too much calcium in the blood

Tetany and Calcium Rigor

When calcium in the blood (and therefore in the extracellular fluids) drops below a critical level, there is a change in the stimulation of nerve cells, resulting in increased excitability of the nerve and spasmodic and uncontrolled contraction of muscle tissue. This condition is known as **tetany.** Conversely, when calcium levels in the blood rise above normal, the muscle fibers contract; this is known as **calcium rigor.** Neither of these conditions is the result of abnormal dietary levels of calcium; rather, both indicate that the parathyroid gland (the primary source of control over calcium metabolism) is not functioning properly.

tetany
A condition in which the muscles are alternately relaxed and contracted because of low blood levels of calcium

calcium rigor
A condition in which the muscles are in a constant state of contraction because of high calcium levels in the blood

Blood Pressure

Recent research on the relationship of diet to blood pressure suggests that low calcium intake (<400 mg/day) are associated with increased blood pressure and hypertension. When calcium intake is increased, there is a marked decrease in the incidence of elevated blood pressure.

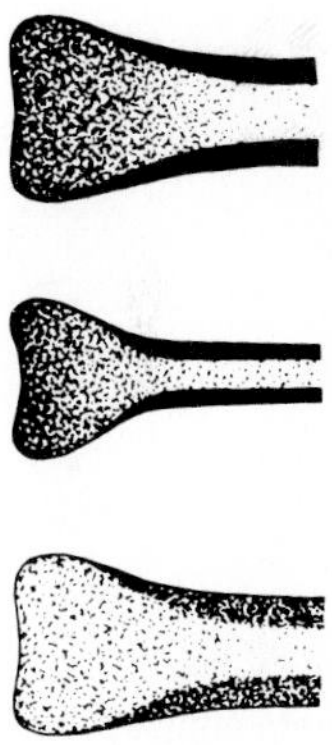

Figure 10-10 **A,** Normal bone. **B,** Osteoporosis, in which there is a reduced amount of bone of normal composition. **C,** Osteomalacia, in which the amount of bone is normal but the composition is abnormal.
USDA, 1985.

PHOSPHORUS (P)

Because phosphorus constitutes 22% of the mineral ash in the adult human body (or 1% of the body weight), it is classified as a *macroelement*. Its role as a major constituent of bones and teeth is recognized by even casual students of nutrition. The fact that it is often discussed in connection with calcium has further emphasized its role in the formation of hard tissues. As a result, however, its other equally vital roles are often overlooked.

Distribution

It is estimated that the adult body contains 1½ pounds of phosphorus. Of this, 85% to 90% is in the form of insoluble calcium phosphate (apatite) crystals in the bone. The remaining 10% of 15% is distributed throughout all living cells of the body, with about half of it in muscle.

Functions

Because it is impossible to describe all the biological reactions in which phosphorus plays a key role, the following have been chosen to illustrate the diversity of phosphorus functions.

Regulation of Energy Release

Phosphate, the form in which most phosphorus occurs in the body, is necessary for the controlled release of energy resulting from the oxidation of carbohydrate,

ADP + PO_4 (phosphate) + Energy = ATP

fat, and protein. Energy is stored when a third phosphate molecule is attached to ADP (adenosine diphosphate) to form ATP (adenosine triphosphate). As energy is needed, the ATP is changed back to ADP. The energy that held the phosphate to ADP is released to supply energy for many body reactions. If the cells were unable to convert energy into these high-energy bonds for storage, they would be incapable of regulating the rate at which the energy is available.

Absorption and Transportation of Nutrients

The combination with phosphorus (primarily in the form of phosphate) makes it possible for many nutrients to cross a cell membrane, be carried in the blood, or to become a large enough molecule that they do not "leak" out of a cell.

phosphorylation
The addition of phosphate (PO_4) to a substance, usually to aid in its transfer in and out of a cell

This process is known as **phosphorylation** and occurs in the processes of absorption from the intestine, release of nutrients from the bloodstream to the intercellular fluids, uptake into the cell, and uptake by the organelles of the cell. Fats, in the form of phospholipids (a combination of phosphate with the fat molecule) are part of the structure of the cell membrane.

Part of Essential Body Compounds

Some vitamins and enzymes can function only when they are phosphorylated—thiamin pyrophosphate, a vitamin B_1-containing enzyme, is an example. Phosphate is an essential part of the nucleic acids DNA and RNA. Both of these nucleic acids are essential for cell reproduction, playing roles in the replication of genes and in protein synthesis.

Calcification of Bones and Teeth

The calcification process starts when phosphate is deposited in the bone matrix. Use of the term "calcification" suggests that calcium is the major factor in this process. However, failure of bone calcification is often the result of an imbalance of calcium and phosphorus in the blood. When this occurs, the enzyme phosphatase increases to release phosphorus compounds into the blood to create the proper calcium/phosphorus ratio for bone growth.

Regulation of Acid/Base Balance

Because of their ability to combine with additional hydrogen ions, phosphates play an important role as buffers to prevent a change in the acidity of body fluids.

Absorption and Metabolism

phosphatase
An enzyme that catalyzes the release of a phosphate molecule from a compound

Phosphorus is released from food by intestinal enzymes known as **phosphatases** and is absorbed into the bloodstream with the help of vitamin D. The level of phosphorus in the blood is regulated by the parathyroid gland, which interacts with vitamin D to control the amount of phosphorus absorbed, the amount retained by the kidneys, and the amount released from and deposited in the bone. At the same time, the parathyroid gland is regulating calcium metabolism.

Requirements

The RDAs suggest a phosphorus intake at least equal to but no more than twice the calcium allowance indicated for the growth period. Most diets, however, provide much more phosphorus than calcium, and it is almost impossible to have a diet with a calcium/phosphorus ratio as high as 1:1. The ratio can be as low as 1:4 in diets with few dairy products and high protein content. There is, however, little likelihood that the phosphorus content of normal diets will be high enough to cause a problem.

Recommended phosphorous allowance = Recommended calcium allowance

For infants less than 6 months old, the recommended intake of phosphorus is 'wo-thirds that of calcium, the same ratio as is found in human milk.

Food Sources

Just as phosphorus is present in all cells of the body, it is present in practically all foods—especially protein-rich foods. Meat, fish, poultry, eggs, dairy products, and cereal products are the primary sources of phosphorus in the average diet. The amount of phosphorus in the most frequently eaten foods is given in Table 10-3.

The food supply provides 1500 to 1600 mg of phosphorus per person. Food consumption intake data show women consuming 1000 mg/day and men consuming 1500 mg/day in both the United States and Canada.

The phosphorus in carbonated soft drinks (up to 75 mg/12-oz bottle) and other phosphorus-containing substances in processed foods also contribute to phosphorus intakes, which in turn contribute to a low calcium/phosphorus ratio in the diet. The amount of phosphorus in our diets has changed little over the past 70 years in spite of the changes in our diet and food processing methods. The contribution of various food groups to the phosphorus in the North American food supply is shown in Figure 10-11. Most diets in the United States provide about 650 mg of phosphorus/1000 kcal.

Amount of Phosphorus in Soft Drinks
Colas—52 mg/12 oz
Club soda—none
Diet colas—39 mg/12 oz

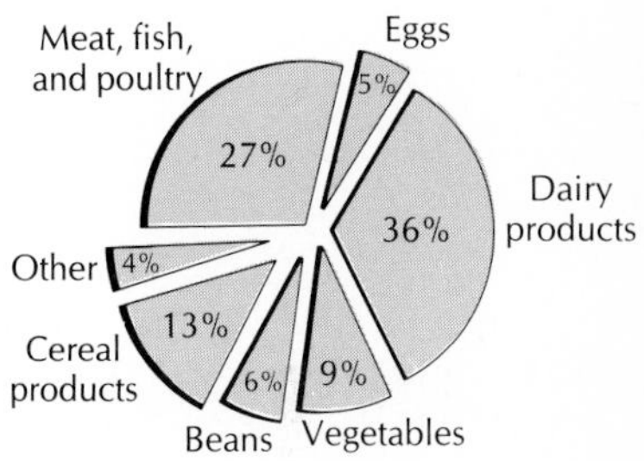

Figure 10-11 Contribution of various food groups to the phosphorus in the North American food supply.

Deficiency

Because of the distribution of phosphorus in both plant and animal food, there is practically no evidence of a deficiency in humans. Exceptions include people who consume large amounts of antacids, especially those made with aluminum hydroxide, which interferes with phosphorus absorption. Those who suffer excessive urinary losses associated with kidney dialysis may also have a phosphorus deficiency. Symptoms such as fatigue, loss of appetite, and demineralization of bone result.

Premature infants, because of their need for more phosphorus than is provided in human milk, are about the only other group known to show a phosphorus deficiency.

MAGNESIUM (Mg)

The presence of magnesium in living organisms was discovered in 1859. Even before that time it had long been used as a healing substance, an anesthetic, and an anticonvulsant. By 1926 magnesium had been identified as a dietary essential for mice and by 1932 as an essential for rats. Most of our information about its role in human nutrition was established after 1950. It is difficult to study the effect of magnesium deficiency in humans because of the sizable reserve of this nutrient in bone, some of which can be released to help meet the needs of the soft tissues. In addition, the kidneys have the ability to reabsorb magnesium when needed. Magnesium is now recognized as an essential element that occurs predominantly within the cell. It is involved in over 300 different enzyme reactions.

Distribution

The magnesium content of an infant's body at birth is approximately 0.5 gram; most of this was transferred to the fetus in the latter part of pregnancy. In the adult, the magnesium content of the body is a little less than 1 oz (30 grams), 60% of which is concentrated in bone. About a third of this magnesium is closely bound with phosphate; the remainder adheres to the bone surface, from which it is readily mobilized to maintain normal blood and tissue levels. In the blood, which contains a mere 1% of body magnesium, over half of the magnesium is free, one third is bound to the protein albumin, and the rest is part of a variety of other compounds. Magnesium occurs primarily in the red blood cells rather than in the serum. In a deficiency, the magnesium level in the red blood cells drops; in an excess, the serum level rises. The remaining body magnesium is evenly distributed between muscle and soft tissues. In the soft tissues magnesium, like potassium, is concentrated within the cell.

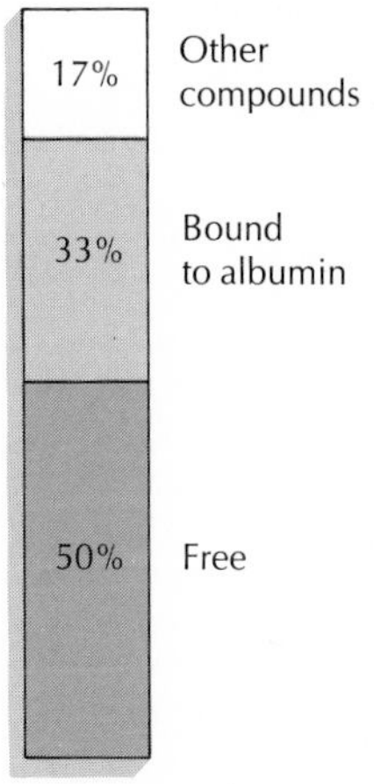

Blood magnesium

Absorption and Metabolism

Magnesium is absorbed primarily in the small intestine, probably with the help of a specific carrier. Approximately 35% to 40% of an average magnesium intake is absorbed; less is absorbed from diets with high intakes and more with low intakes. Absorption is reduced by the presence of calcium, alcohol, phosphate, phytates, and fat but is increased by dietary vitamin D and lactose. Cellulose has little effect. The absorption of magnesium is enhanced when parathyroid hormone is secreted, which results from a drop in serum magnesium.

Softened water has most of the calcium and magnesium of hard water removed.

Magnesium excretion is regulated through the kidneys. When magnesium intake is low, the kidney reabsorbs almost all magnesium so that practically none is lost. As a result, variation in dietary intake seldom affects magnesium blood levels. Urinary losses of magnesium do increase with the use of diuretics and the consumption of alcohol. Most of the magnesium that appears in the feces is unabsorbed dietary magnesium. The amount lost in perspiration is usually small, but at high temperatures it may amount to 15% of magnesium losses. The magnesium secreted in the pancreatic juice is normally almost all reabsorbed. There is considerable evidence that the metabolism of magnesium is controlled by the thyroid gland.

Functions

Within the cell, magnesium plays an important role as a catalyst to several hundred biological reactions, a major portion of which take place in the mitochondrion of the cell. Magnesium is necessary in all reactions involving the expenditure or release of energy; in almost all reactions involving carbohydrate, lipid, protein, and nucleic acid metabolism; and in those reactions related to the synthesis, degradation, and stability of the genetic material, DNA. To take care of these needs, the level of intracellular magnesium in the muscle tissue and liver is seven times that in the blood.

Although only 1% of magnesium occurs in extracellular fluids, it is necessary for the conduction of nerve impulses and for normal muscular contraction. In these reactions, magnesium and calcium play antagonistic roles; calcium stimulates and magnesium relaxes. The relaxing effect of magnesium is evident from the fact that with increasing levels of the element in the blood, there is an increasing anesthetic effect. At extremely high serum magnesium levels, coma and eventually heart failure result. These levels may be reached when there is kidney failure, in which the excretion of magnesium is depressed. The competitive nature of the calcium-magnesium interrelationship shows up again during absorption and excretion. When a large amount of one is being absorbed or excreted, there is usually a simultaneous reduction or increase in the amount of the other. Magnesium is necessary for the release of the parathyroid hormone and for its action in the bone, kidney, and intestine. It is also needed for the reactions involved in converting vitamin D to its active form.

Requirements

The Food and Nutrition Board recommends an intake of 300 mg of magnesium/day for women and 350 mg/day for men, or 5 mg/kg of body weight. These amounts are based on consideration of data from balance studies and usual dietary intakes. It is estimated that a typical North American diet provides 120 mg of magnesium/1000 kcal—a level that will barely provide the recommended intake. In one study, when intakes were increased to 10 mg/kg of body weight in an experimental situation, there was a period of high magnesium retention that later dropped, apparently after body stores were replenished.

Because information on magnesium requirements in pregnancy indicates an increased need, especially after the first child, an additional 150 mg of magnesium/

Table 10-5 ◆ Recommended Dietary Allowances for magnesium in the United States and Recommended Nutrient Intakes for magnesium in Canada (in mg/day)

Age	United States	Canada
1-3 yr	150	65
4-6 yr	200	90
7-10 yr	250	110
Boys, 10-12 yr	350	150
Girls, 10-12 yr	300	160
Men, 16-18 yr	400	240
Women, 16-18 yr	300	220
Men, 19-49 yr	350	240
Women, 19-49 yr	300	190
Men, 50-74 yr	350	210
Women, 50-74 yr	300	165

day is recommended for pregnant women. Similarly, for lactation, 150 mg/day above the needs of nonpregnant women seems adequate.

The recommendation of 50 to 70 mg of magnesium/day for infants is based on information that human milk provides approximately 40 mg/liter or quart.

Recomended Dietary Allowances for the United States and Recommended Nutrient Intakes for Canada are presented in Table 10-5.

Food Sources

The magnesium content of the most frequently used foods is shown in Table 10-3. When the magnesium content of food is related to caloric content, vegetables are the best source of magnesium, followed by legumes, seafood, nuts, cereals, and dairy products. Since magnesium is an essential structural element in chlorophyll, the green pigment in plants, green leafy vegetables are major contributors to dietary magnesium. Magnesium absorption is reduced with diets high in calcium, fat, or phytic acid, which is normally found in the outer husks of cereal grains such as rice or oats. Refining of flour or rice may remove 80% of the magnesium.

Although milk is a relatively poor source of magnesium, it appears to be adequate for the needs of either breast or bottle-fed infants.

Fresh water contains 1 to 16 ppm of magnesium. Soft water has considerably less magnesium than hard water, which may provide one fifth of daily magnesium intake. Some advertisements promote seawater because of its high magnesium content (1300 ppm); however, seawater has little relevance to human nutrition because it is totally unpalatable and never consumed because of its high salt content.

The contribution of various food groups to the daily 331-mg magnesium content of the food supply is shown in Figure 10-12.

Table 10-6 gives relevant dietary data on calcium, phosphorus, and magnesium.

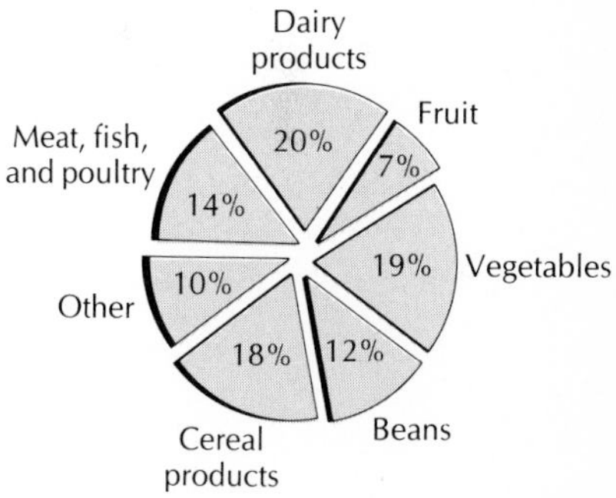

Figure 10-12 Contribution of various food groups to magnesium in the North American food supply.
USDA, 1985.

Deficiency

A magnesium deficiency is associated with starvation, persistent vomiting, the trauma of surgery, very high calcium intakes, or the rapid transit of food through the gastrointestinal tract, which reduces absorption time. It seldom shows up merely as the result of limited dietary intake because of the efficiency with which the kidneys resorb magnesium. Low serum magnesium levels are associated with ir-

Table 10-6 ◇ Calcium, phosphorus, and magnesium: relevant dietary/biological data

	Calcium	Phosphorus	Magnesium
U.S. RDA	1000 mg	1000 mg	400 mg
Amount available in food supply	920 mg	1510 mg	320 mg
Average adult intake			
NHANES II	979 mg	—	—
NFCS (% of RDA)	87	136	83
Major food sources (by percent)			
Milk and milk products	75	33	20
Fruits and vegetables	8	10	27
Cereal products	7	19	18
Meat, fish, poultry, and eggs	7	34	15
Percent of intake absorbed	20%-30%	50%-70%	30%-60%
Total amount in body (in grams)	860-1400	675	21-28
Distribution in body tissues (mg)			
Bones and teeth	850-1390	600	16
Blood	5-6	—	0.25
Soft tissues	4-5	30	9
Extracellular tissues	1	—	0.25
Indicators of nutritional status			
Blood levels			
Normal	8.5-11 mg/dl	3-4.5 mg/dl	1.6 mg/dl
Deficient	<7 mg/dl	<3 mg/dl	<1.5 mg/dl

ritability, nervousness, and convulsions as the result of stimulation of nerve impulses and increased muscular contraction.

A recognized form of magnesium deficiency is *low magnesium tetany*. This is diagnosed first as uncontrolled neuromuscular tremors that progress until convulsive seizures occur. These symptoms most often arise when a low dietary intake is superimposed on conditions that reduce the absorption and increase the excretion of magnesium. Both alcohol and diuretics increase the rate of magnesium excretion.

The undesirable calcification of soft tissues in magnesium deficiency may reflect the increase in calcium absorption that occurs when there is less magnesium to compete with calcium for absorption. At the same time, there is an increase in the amount of calcium mobilized from the bone. High calcium and low magnesium diets also lead to an increase in magnesium excretion, further evidence that the two elements compete with one another. Inadequate magnesium also results in **vasodilation** (an increase in the size of the blood vessels) and skin changes. Because the kidneys are so efficient in excreting magnesium in excess of needs, **hypermagnesemia,** or an excess of magnesium in the blood, will occur only when they are not functioning properly.

vasodilation
An increase in the size of blood vessels, usually evident in a flushing of the surface of the skin

hypermagnesemia
Too much magnesium in the blood

New methods of measuring magnesium in body fluids have demonstrated that magnesium depletion occurs more often than previously assumed.

Assessment of Reserves

Serum levels of magnesium do not provide a sensitive indication of the level in cells because about 33% of blood magnesium is bound to a protein and is not measurable with current analytical techniques. The levels of magnesium found in the red blood cells reflect only the amount of magnesium available as the cells were formed. Measurement of the amount excreted in the urine after a large oral dose is considered the most sensitive test for children. Retention of more than 40% of dietary magnesium indicates that the body needs to correct a deficiency.

SULFUR (S)

Sulfur, which represents 0.25% of body weight, is present in every cell of the body. It is concentrated in the cytoplasm of the cell. The highest concentrations of sulfur are found in the hair, skin, and nails, as evidenced by the characteristic odor of sulfur dioxide given off when these tissues are burned. The sulfur-containing amino acids, cystine, cysteine, and methionine, are characteristic of the protein keratin, found in high concentration in these tissues.

Sulfur in combination with hydrogen plays an important role in metabolism; it is involved in the formation of blood clots and in the transfer of energy. Sulfur is part of at least three vitamins (thiamin, pantothenic acid, and biotin) and is also part of lipoic acid (a vitamin-like substance). These are part of coenzymes, which are necessary to activate several enzymes. Compounds containing sulfur act as detoxifying substances by combining with toxic substances, converting them into harmless compounds that are excreted. Sulfur is necessary for collagen synthesis and the formation of many mucopolysaccharides.

Sulfur is available to the body primarily as the organic sulfur in the amino acids methionine and cysteine. Inorganic sulfur, or *sulfate,* can contribute to the pool of sulfur in the body, but its availability depends on the ratio of organic to inorganic sulfur. Any excess of inorganic sulfur is excreted in the urine.

Interest in sulfur in the food supply has been heightened by the realization that sulfiting agents, which have been used in salad bars to prevent the discoloration of ingredients, such as lettuce and mushrooms, caused severe reactions in many of the 10 million asthmatics in the United States. As a result in 1987, the Food and Drug Administration ruled that sulfites could not be used to preserve fresh fruits and vegetables and that its use in processed foods must be declared on the label. The amount used this way had little or no impact on the dietary intake of sulfur.

So far there is insufficient information on sulfur needs to make a dietary recommendation.

BY NOW YOU SHOULD KNOW

- Mineral elements perform two major functions: building body compounds and regulating body processes.
- Minerals are classified as macronutrient elements and micronutrient or trace elements.
- Minerals may interact with one another in either a positive or a negative way.
- Calcium is a component of bones and teeth. It regulates the action of many enzymes, controls the blood-clotting mechanisms, and is involved in the regulation of nerve impulses and the contraction of muscles.
- A variety of factors influence calcium absorption.
- Calcium is provided in relatively few foods; milk and milk products are the only dependable sources.
- Calcium deficiency in the diet results in a depletion of the body reserve of calcium in the bones. Several body hormones are able to protect against dietary deficiencies.
- Osteoporosis, which affects about 60% of postmenopausal women, is the major health problem resulting from an inadequate calcium intake. Women with osteoporosis are likely to suffer from spontaneous fractures, primarily of the hip.
- Phosphorus, which is found in all foods but particularly protein-rich foods, is essential for many functions, including absorption, transport, and metabolism of many nutrients. It also serves as a major component of bones and teeth.

- The typical North American diet provides adequate amounts of phosphorus but marginal amounts of magnesium and limited amounts of calcium.
- Magnesium helps to regulate enzymes that aid the metabolism of energy.
- The use of diuretics and alcohol consumption can increase the excretion of magnesium.
- Sulfur is part of all cells, but highest concentrations are in skin, hair, and nails.
- Sulfur is found in three amino acids: methionine, cystine, and cysteine.

STUDY QUESTIONS

1. Describe the role of calcium in forming a blood clot.
2. List the reasons why milk is such a good source of calcium.
3. How can an individual with milk or lactose intolerance obtain adequate calcium?
4. How can a postmenopausal woman plan a reasonable diet that includes as much as 800 mg of calcium/day but still supplies the required amounts of all the other nutrients?
5. How do the mineral elements discussed in this chapter participate in the maintenance of acid/base balance in the body? What other mechanisms does the body have to prevent a shift in pH in the body fluids?
6. What hormones are involved in regulating calcium metabolism?
7. What functions do phosphorus and magnesium have in common?
8. On the basis of nutrient density, what are the three best sources each for calcium, phosphorus, and magnesium?
9. Discuss the role of bone and of the kidneys in the absorption, metabolism, and excretion of calcium, phosphorus, and magnesium.

Applying What You've Learned

1. **Calculate Your Calcium intake**

   Write down everything you ate yesterday. How much milk or how many milk products did you consume? Using Table 10-3 on page 273, on Appendix F, calculate how many milligrams of calcium you had from these products. Compare your total to the RDA for calcium. If you were below the RDA, how would you add calcium-rich foods to your current diet?

2. **Assess Absorption of Your Calcium Intake**

   Considering all the food you ate yesterday, review the factors that favor and inhibit calcium absorption, which were relevant in your diet. Make concluding statements to describe your calcium intake and the factors that affect its absorption.

3. **Assess Fat Content of Calcium Sources**

   Often the best sources of calcium in the diet are also high in fat. Review again your sources of calcium, only this time circle those high in fat. For those foods you circled, list some low-fat substitutes that are high in calcium. (For example—whole milk could be replaced with low-fat milk, or ice cream with frozen yogurt or ice milk.)

4. **Plan a Menu**

   Plan one day of meals for a lactose-intolerant individual. Make sure the person receives at least 800 mg of calcium for the day.

5. **Examine Food Labels**

   Read the list of ingredients on several food labels. Do you find phosphorus used as an additive? List the foods and the sources of phosphorus.

6. **Calcium/Phosphorus Ratio**

   Calculate your calcium/phosphorus ratio for 1 day's food intake (Use Appendix F).

SUGGESTED READINGS

Allen LH: Calcium bioavailability and absorption: a review, American Journal of Clinical Nutrition 35:783, 1983.

A comprehensive and authoritative discussion of the factors that influence how much of the calcium in the food we eat is actually available to meet our metabolic needs. This article discusses not only the nature of the food itself but the form in which the nutrient is present.

Avioli LV: Calcium and osteoporosis, Annual Review of Nutrition 4:471, 1984.

This paper presents a comprehensive review of the dietary factors involved in osteoporosis. It offers convincing evidence about the merits of increased calcium intakes to protect against and treat the disease.

Wardlaw G: The effects of diet and life-style on bone mass in women, Journal of the American Dietetic Association 88:17, 1988.

This paper reviews the physiology of bone, the assessment of bone mineral, the definition and characteristics of osteoporosis, and the effect of life-style factors, diet, supplementation on bone mass. This is an excellent "state of the art" paper, but the student is warned that this is a rapidly developing field of inquiry in which the consensus is evolving rapidly.

ADDITIONAL READINGS

Minerals/general

Maugh TH: Trace elements: a growing appreciation of their effects in man, Science 181:253, 1973.

Mertz W: Mineral elements: new perspectives, Journal of the American Dietetic Association 77:258, 1980.

Mertz W: The essential trace elements, Science 213:1332, 1981.

Mills CF: Dietary interaction involving the trace elements, Annual Review of Nutrition 5:173, 1985.

Newberne PM: Disease states and tissue mineral elements in men, Federation Proceedings 40:2134, 1981.

Pennington J, Young B, Wilson DB, Johnson RD, and Vanderveen JE: Mineral content of foods and total diets: the selected minerals in foods survey, Journal of the American Dietetic Association 86:876, 1988.

Calcium

Allen LH, Barlett RS, and Block GD: Reduction of renal calcium reabsorption in man by consumption of dietary protein, Journal of Nutrition 109:1345, 1979.

Alvioli LV: Calcium and osteoporosis, Annual Review of Nutrition 4:471, 1974.

Bronner F: Intestinal calcium absorption; mechanisms and applications, Journal of Nutrition 117:1347, 1987.

Chinn HI: Effects of dietary factors on skeletal integrity in adults: calcium, phosphorus, vitamin D, and protein, Washington, D.C., 1981, Bureau of Foods, Food and Drug Administration, DHHS.

Heaney RP, Gallagher JC, Johnston CC, Neer R, Parfitt AM, Chir B, and Whedon GD: Calcium nutrition and bone health in the elderly, American Journal of Clinical Nutrition 36:986, 1982.

Heaney RP, Recker RR, and Saville PD: Calcium balance and calcium requirements in middle-aged women, American Journal of Clinical Nutrition 30:1603, 1977.

Hegsted DM: Calcium and osteoporosis, Journal of Nutrition 116:2316, 1986.

Holly J, McCarron D, Morris CD, and Parrot-Garcia M: Increasing calcium intake lowers blood pressure: the literature reviewed, Journal of the American Dietetic Association 85:182, 1985.

Irwin MI, and Kienholz EW: A conspectus of research on calcium requirements of man, Journal of Nutrition 103:1019, 1973.

Kerr RR: How important is dietary calcium in preventing osteoporosis? Science 233:519, 1986.

LSRO (Life Sciences Research Office): Effects of dietary factors on skeletal integrity in adults: calcium, phosphorus, vitamin D, and protein, Bethesda, MD, 1981, Federation of American Societies for Experimental Biology.

Nilas L, Christiansen C, and Rodbro P: Calcium supplementation and postmenopausal bone loss, British Medical Journal 289:1103, 1984.

Nordin BEC, and others: The problem of calcium requirements, American Journal of Clinical Nutrition 45:1295, 1987.

Pitkin RM: Calcium metabolism in pregnancy: a review, American Journal of Obstetrics and Gynecology 121:724, 1975.

Resnick LM: Dietary calcium and hypertension, Journal of Nutrition 117:1806, 1987.

Riggs BL, and Melton LJ: Involutional osteoporosis, New England Journal of Medicine 314:1676, 1986.

Riis B, Thonsend K, and Christiansen C: Does calcium supplementation prevent postmenopausal bone loss, New England Journal of Medicine 316:173, 1987.

Spencer H, and others: Calcium requirements in humans, Clinical Orthopaedics and Related Research 184:270, 1984.

Spencer H, Kramer L, and Osis D: Do protein and phosphorus cause calcium loss? Journal of Nutrition 118:666, 1988.

Wasserman RH: Intestinal absorption of calcium and phosphorus, Federation Proceedings 40:68, 1981.

Weinsier RL, and Norris D: Recent developments in the etiology and treatment of hypertension: dietary calcium, fat, and magnesium, American Journal of Clinical Nutrition 42:1331, 1985.

Phosphorus

LSRO (Life Sciences Research Office): Effects of dietary factors on skeletal integrity in adults: calcium, phosphorus, vitamin D and protein, Bethesda, MD, 1981, Federation of American Societies for Experimental Biology.

Zemel MB, and Linkswiler HM: Calcium metabolism in the young adult male as affected by level and form of phosphorus intake and level of phosphorus intake, Journal of Nutrition 111:315, 1981.

Magnesium

Abraham GE, and Lubran MM: Serum and red cell magnesium levels in patients with premenstrual tension, American Journal of Clinical Nutrition 34:2364, 1981.

Altura BM: Role of magnesium ions in regulation of muscle contraction, Federation Proceedings 40:2644, 1981.

Caddell JL: Magnesium in the nutrition of the child, Clinical Pediatrics 13:263, 1977.

Lakshmanan FL, Rao RB, Kim WW, and Kelsay JL: Magnesium intakes, balances and blood levels of adults consuming self-selected diets, American Journal of Clinical Nutrition 40:1380, 1984.

Levine BS, and Coburn CW: Magnesium, the mimic/antagonist of calcium, New England Journal of Medicine 310:1254, 1984.

Shils ME: Magnesium. In Present Knowledge of Nutrition, Washington, D.C., 1984, Nutrition Foundation.

Wester PO: Magnesium, American Journal of Clinical Nutrition 45:1305, 1987.

Sulfur

Expert Panel on Nutrition· Sulfites as food ingredients, Food Technology 40:47(June), 1986.

FOCUS Osteoporosis

Osteoporosis is fast becoming one of the major nutrition-related health problems in developed countries, largely because people are living longer and osteoporosis is a disease of the elderly. This problem affects primarily postmenopausal women, with less than 10% of the cases occurring in men. It is considered to be the result of the loss of bone mass, which occurs at an accelerated rate of about 2% to 3% per year once the level of estrogen production drops.

Symptoms of osteoporosis are the result of the decrease in bone mass, which is greater in the trabecular bone in the spine and hip than in the outside portion of the bone shaft of the long bones, known as the cortical bone. Hip fractures, many of which are spontaneous, resulting from a break in the bone at the head of the femur where it joins the hip socket, occur at a rate of 1.3 million per year. In addition to a great deal of pain there is an average financial cost of $18,000 per break. Of equal concern is the fact that many women experience a loss of height as a result of the compacting of the vertebrae, which occurs as the more porous, trabecular-like bone in the spine is lost. For most women the decrease in height may amount to 2 to 3 inches. It is accompanied by a stooped appearance characterized as a "dowager's hump." The resulting change in the body contour is accompanied by a crowding of the intestinal tract and the lungs, which interferes with normal functioning.

Some of the changes with osteoporosis are age-related and reflect the loss of bone calcium, which is associated with the decrease absorption of calcium resulting from the decline in the kidney's ability to convert vitamin D into a form that stimulates the absorption of calcium. The rest of the cases result from loss of bone and failure in bone remodeling that occur as the result of a decrease in estrogen production. Contrary to expectations, an increase in dietary calcium has little or no effect in slowing the loss of bone. The total bone mass that has accumulated by the time of menopause, however, determines the amount of available bone on which to draw.

As a result of the concern about osteoporosis, many older people are turning to the use of calcium supplements. The food industry is producing an array of products fortified with high levels of calcium in forms that are readily absorbed. While the use of one or two of these products may be reasonable, there is legitimate concern that if people switch to all of the available calcium-fortified products the calcium intake may reach a level that could have as yet unidentified health hazards. Since intakes above 2000 mg are seldom available from regular food products, we have practically no knowledge of the effect they may have, particularly on soft tissues. While there is general agreement that the goal of preventing a negative calcium balance is desirable, there is concern about the effect of a positive balance, particularly since there is little evidence that the extra calcium retained is contributing to an increase in bone mass.

In the absence of calcium-fortified foods, however, the only way to achieve high intakes from unfortified foods is to rely on dairy products. For a woman whose energy requirement is declining at the same time she needs to maintain or increase her calcium intake, dairy products of low calorie content such as lowfat or nonfat milk and cheese must be selected. This limits the variety of other foods she can choose, resulting in a less palatable diet and possibly one that will be deficient in other nutrients.

At this point the evidence that there is a need for an intake of calcium above the current recommendation of 800 mg is flimsy. Studies of women taking from 300 to 2000 mg/day over a 4-year period failed to provide evidence that there was any difference in bone loss related to calcium intake. The fact that the average calcium intake in women in the United States is slightly less than 75% of their RDA has provided the rationale for the current flurry of fortification and supplementation. Yet there is little or no recognition of the fact that the average requirement of calcium of 77% of the RDA is very little different than the average intake. Rather than promote higher intakes in the postmenopausal period, it is likely more beneficial to put more emphasis on encouraging women to consume the recommended intake during the period of bone formation (up to 30 years of age).

Research on the causes, prevention, and possible treatment of osteoporosis is commanding a great deal of attention. Until there is more convincing evidence of the best course of action, nutritionists suggest emphasis on the intake of adequate calcium during adolescence and early adulthood to permit maximum bone growth; maintenance of a good intake throughout adult years; and the use of estrogen replacement therapy, weight-bearing exercise, and enhanced vitamin D intake in the postmenopausal years.

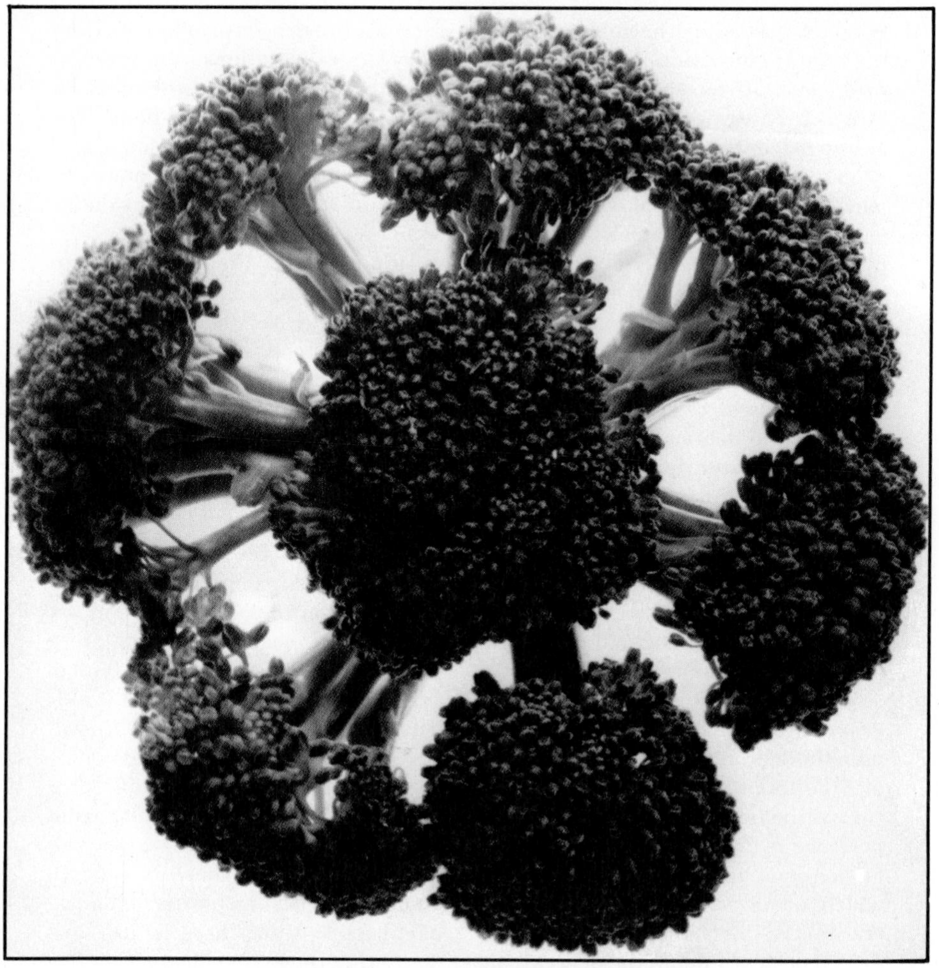

AWARENESS CHECK

Truth or Fiction?

- Supplements are the only good way to ensure an adequate intake of trace elements.
- Tea or coffee with a meal will inhibit iron absorption.
- Cooking in a cast iron skillet will increase the amount of dietary iron.
- It is simple for women to meet the RDA for iron from food alone.
- The processing of grain products reduces the zinc and selenium content of the food.

Micronutrient Elements

CHAPTER 11

Some trace elements such as iron and iodine have been known to be dietary essentials for many years. As more sensitive techniques for studying these elements have been developed, we have learned that zinc and ultratrace elements such as selenium, chromium, and molybdenum are needed in amounts as small as several parts per billion (ppb). Scientists are constantly attempting to establish the essentiality of other trace elements. At the same time they continue to learn more about the ways in which those that are known function and interact. Knowledge of the amounts of trace elements in food and some provisional estimates of human requirements have raised questions about the adequacy of these elements in the North American diet. These questions are of concern because an increasing portion of our diet consists of processed foods from which trace elements may have been unintentionally removed.

The discussions of iron and iodine in this chapter reflect the many years over which we have been accumulating information on their functions and sources. Discussions of zinc and selenium reflect a rapid accumulation of data in a relatively short period of time, whereas those of other trace elements are indicative of a growing but as yet incomplete store of knowledge.

IRON (Fe)

The element iron was first recognized as a constituent of body tissue in 1713. Since that time, we have learned that the total amount of iron in the body measures 1 teaspoon (3 to 5 grams), varying slightly with age, sex, size, nutritional status, general health, and size of iron stores. Virtually all iron exists in combination with protein and is responsible for the ability of every cell of the body to accept and release oxygen and carbon dioxide readily. Such reactions are essential to life.

Table 11-1 ◆ Distribution of iron throughout the body

		Approximate Amount (mg)	
	Total (%)	Men	Women
Functional			
Hemoglobin	60-75	2100	1750
Myoglobin	3	100	100
Tissue iron (enzymes)	5-15	350	300
Storage and Transport			
Storage iron (liver, spleen, and bone marrow)	0-30	1000	400
Transport iron (transferrin)	0.1	3	3
Serum ferritin	1	0.3	0.1
TOTAL		3553.3	2553.1

Distribution

hemoglobin
The iron-containing protein in the red blood cell that is responsible for its ability to carry oxygen to the cells and carbon dioxide away from the cells

myoglobin
The iron-containing compound in muscle that is responsible for providing oxygen to the cells

transferrin
The protein in the blood that is capable of transporting and picking up absorbed iron

ferritin
The form in which iron is stored in the liver and spleen; a small amount of ferritin that parallels the amount of storage iron also circulates in the blood (fer = iron)

hemosiderin
An insoluble iron complex in which iron is stored in the liver

Iron is concentrated in the blood, but some is present in every living cell, as shown in Table 11-1. Over two thirds of the iron in the body is functional iron, most of which is present in the **hemoglobin,** or iron-containing protein molecule of the red blood cell. A small portion of functional iron exists as part of **myoglobin,** an iron-containing protein similar to hemoglobin but found in muscle. The rest of functional iron is in the tissue enzymes, which are present in every living cell and are essential for cellular respiration, involving the exchange of oxygen and carbon dioxide.

In addition to hemoglobin iron, the blood contains a very small amount (about 4 mg) of iron that at any given time is being transported to the cells; it is tightly bound to the protein **transferrin.** This transport iron is turned over so rapidly that up to 10 times the 4-mg amount is exchanged each day. **Ferritin,** another iron-containing substance, is present in the blood serum in amounts paralleling storage iron.

The remaining one third of body iron is stored in the liver, spleen, and bone marrow. The amount of storage iron in the body is quite variable, generally being higher in men (approximately 1000 mg) than in women (approximately 400 mg). Iron is stored as the soluble iron complex ferritin, which is one-fifth iron, or **hemosiderin,** an insoluble iron-protein complex that is one-third iron.

Functions

Carrier of Oxygen and Carbon Dioxide

The major role of iron is to permit the transfer of oxygen and carbon dioxide from one tissue to another. Iron carries out this role primarily as a part of both hemoglobin in the blood and myoglobin in the muscle, but also as part of several tissue enzymes essential in cell respiration. The exchanges are involved primarily in the release of energy within the cell.

Blood Formation

erythrocyte
A mature red blood cell (erythro = red; cyte = cell)

erythropoietin
Hormone produced in the kidneys that stimulates the production of red blood cells in the bone marrow

erythropoiesis
Formation of red blood cells (poiesis = formation)

erythroblast
Earliest form of a red blood cell (blast = precursor cell)

Hemoglobin is an essential component of the mature red blood cells, or **erythrocytes,** formed in the bone marrow. When the number of red blood cells drops, the level of **erythropoietin,** a hormone produced in the kidneys, increases. Erythropoietin stimulates **erythropoiesis,** the production of more red blood cells.

Erythrocytes begin in the bone marrow as immature cells known as **erythroblasts,** each of which contains a nucleus. As these cells mature in the bone marrow, they synthesize heme, an iron-containing protein, from the amino acid glycine and iron (along with the help of vitamin B_6 and the mineral copper). The heme unites with a protein called globin, which is synthesized at the same time from other amino acids. Hemoglobin-containing immature red blood cells, known as **reticulocytes,** are thus formed and are released into the bloodstream, where they lose their nuclei to become erythrocytes capable of functioning as carriers of carbon dioxide and oxygen. (Figure 11-1.)

reticulocyte
An immature red blood cell

Because a red blood cell has no nucleus, it cannot produce the enzymes essential for its own survival. As a result, it lives only as long as the enzymes present at its maturity remain functional—usually about 4 months. As red blood cells die, they are removed from the blood by the cells of the liver, bone marrow, and spleen, which are part of the reticuloendothelial system. In the spleen, the iron and amino acids of the hemoglobin molecule are salvaged to be recycled. The iron is stored as hemosiderin and ferritin in the liver and spleen or is returned to the bone marrow, where it is incorporated into new hemoglobin molecules. In this way, iron is carefully conserved and reused. The amino acids are returned to the blood, where they are available for the synthesis of new protein. The remaining portion of the erythrocytes, mainly the cell structure, is excreted in the bile (Figure 11-2).

The adult male has 15 grams of hemoglobin/dl of blood, and the adult female has 13.6 grams/dl. The total hemoglobin content of the 5 liters (quarts) of blood in the adult male is 750 grams. Because the average life span of erythrocytes is

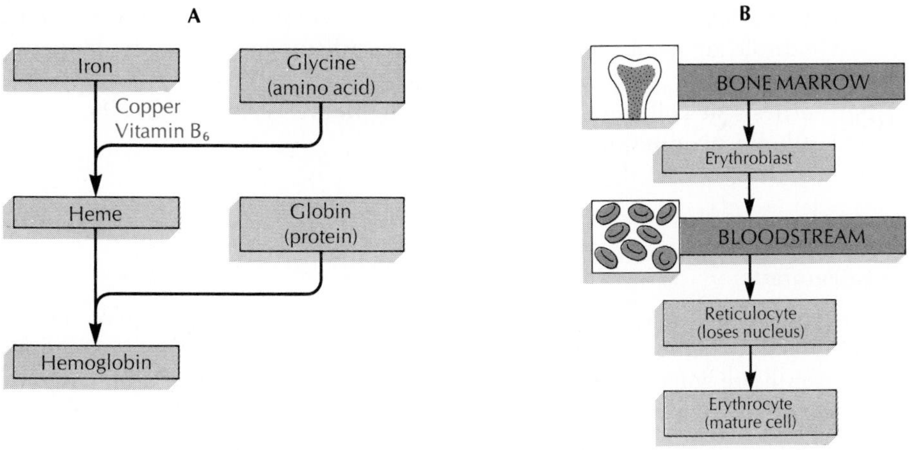

Figure 11-1 **A,** Hemoglobin synthesis. **B,** Red blood cell formation.

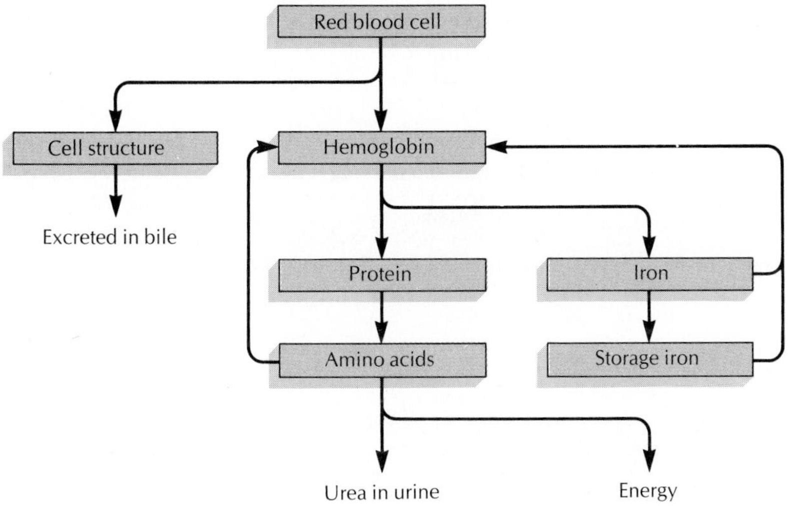

Figure 11-2 Process of destruction of red blood cells, in which iron is saved and recycled.

Blood volume = ~5 liters (50 dl)
Hemoglobin = 15 grams/dl
Total hemoglobin = 750 grams
Hemoglobin contains .034% iron
Total blood iron = 750 grams × 0.34
= 250 mgs
Life expectancy of blood cell = 120 days
Iron replaced daily = ~20 mg

only 120 days, 1/120 of these cells needs to be replaced every day. This is accomplished when 1/120 of the total amount of iron (20 mg) is released each day from old cells and is incorporated into the hemoglobin in the cells that replace them. Because it would be impossible to get this much iron a day from dietary sources, conserving iron is essential to survival.

Anti-infective Agent

Studies of the role of iron as an anti-infective agent suggest two conflicting roles. On the one hand, since iron is essential for the growth of microorganisms, potential harmful bacteria will be able to grow if it is available and will not thrive as well in iron-deficient people. On the other hand, if iron is not available, there is a decrease in the production of iron-containing enzymes and other immune substances needed to destroy infectious organisms. In this case, iron-deficient people are less able to fight infections. **Lactoferrin** in human milk is an iron-containing substance that is especially effective against *E. coli* organisms in the gastrointestinal tract of infants. In this case, lactoferrin binds iron so that it is not available for bacterial growth.

lactoferrin
Iron-containing protein found in human milk; serves as anti-infective agent for infants

Other Functions

Iron performs many other important functions including:

- **Catalyzing the conversion of beta-carotene (a vitamin A-like substance) to vitamin A (the active form).**
- **The synthesis of purines, which form an integral part of nucleic acid.**
- **Synthesis of carnitine, a vitamin-like substance needed to transport fatty acids.**
- **Synthesis of collagen, the structural protein surrounding cells.**
- **Antibody production.**
- **Detoxification of drugs in the liver.**

Requirements

The amounts of iron necessary each day to meet the body's need for maintenance of hemoglobin, to maintain adequate levels of storage iron, and to allow for a normal rate of growth are summarized in Table 11-2. These amounts are in addition to the 20 mg recycled each day. From the data, it is evident that adolescent girls and pregnant women have needs at least twice those of adult men. A discussion of the body's various needs for iron follows.

Replacing Losses of Body Iron

Although absorbed iron is conserved and there is no mechanism for excreting it, the relatively small loss each day must be replaced. Iron is present in every cell

Table 11-2 ◇ Summary of iron requirements (mg/day)

Age Group	Loss in Feces	Losses in Urine, Perspiration, and Desquamation	Needs for Menstruation	Needs for Growth	Needs for Pregnancy	Total Needs*
Adult men	0.7	0.2-0.5				0.9-1.2
Adult women	0.7	0.2-0.5	0.5-1.0			1.4-2.2
Pregnant women	0.7	0.2-0.5			1.0-2.0	1.9-3.2
Children	0.7	0.2-0.5		0.2		1.1-1.4
Adolescent girls	0.7	0.2-0.5	0.5-1.4	0.5-1.0		1.9-3.7

*Absorbed iron—dietary needs are 3 to 10 times this amount depending on the source of iron and the composition of the diet.

of the body. The amount lost in the urine, perspiration, and **desquamated** (or sloughed off) cells from the skin, hair, and nails varies from 0.2 to 0.5 mg/day. Losses in the feces (that is, loss of cells lining the intestinal tract) amount to 0.7 mg/day. Total losses range from 0.9 to 1.2 mg/day.

desquamated
Lost or removed from the surface

These small losses are the only ones that an adult man must replace. Women, however, must also replace the iron lost in menstruation. Although this amount varies greatly among women, it is fairly consistent from month to month in the same woman, amounting to 0.5 to 1 mg/day calculated over the month. When these needs are added to other adult needs, it becomes apparent that before menopause women must absorb from 1.4 to 2.2 mg of iron daily to replace losses—a need that is almost twice that of men.

Iron is Lost from the Body
In the hair and nails
In cells sloughed off from the skin and body surface
In cells lost from the mucosa or lining of the gastrointestinal tract
In bleeding

Growth

During growth, an increase in blood volume and tissue mass requires iron for both hemoglobin and myoglobin synthesis. An increase in body iron from 0.5 gram at birth to 5 grams in the adult (over a 20-year growth period) amounts to 225 mg/yr, or 0.6 mg/day. Others have estimated growth needs at 35 mg/kg of increase in body weight.

Replacing Losses from Blood Donation

The donation of 1 pint (0.5 liter) of blood represents a loss of 25 mg of iron that must be replaced. The blood volume and the cell number will return to normal quickly, but the resynthesis of hemoglobin is much slower.

Absorption

Iron occurs in food primarily in the oxidized form known as *ferric* iron which is iron with three positive charges, Fe^{+++}. Most iron that is used to enrich food products or in nutrient supplements and present in a few foods is reduced *ferrous* iron with two positive charges, Fe^{++}. In meat, about half the iron is part of the hemoglobin molecule and is known as **heme iron.** All other iron in food (either from myoglobin or plant sources) is referred to as **nonheme iron.**

heme iron
Iron provided in animal tissues as hemoglobin; about 50% of the iron in meat is heme iron

nonheme iron
Iron provided from plant foods and from the iron-containing components other than heme in animal tissues; for example, cereal, milk, eggs, and cheese.

Before iron can be absorbed, two conditions must exist. First, the iron must be separated from any organic material such as protein; second, in almost all cases, any ferric iron must be changed (chemically reduced) to ferrous iron. This change is accomplished in the presence of acid—either hydrochloric acid normally found in the stomach, or vitamin C (ascorbic acid), which is provided in many fruits and vegetables.

Ferric Iron (Fe^{+++})
Reduction (+H) ↓ ↑ Oxidation (−H)
Ferrous Iron (Fe^{++})

The absorption of iron occurs primarily in the upper part of the small intestine, usually the duodenum. Once nonheme iron has been released from food and reduced to ferrous iron (if it is not already in that form), it is combined with an amino acid. This combination, or **chelate,** is then readily taken into the muscosal cell of the small intestine. There, one of three things occurs, depending on the need for iron. First, if the body has an immediate need for iron, transferrin—a protein in the blood with the specific function of transporting iron—comes in contact with the mucosal cell. The iron that was taken in by the cell from the intestine will be carried across the cell and immediately released on the other side to combine with transferrin, which can bind two atoms of iron per molecule. This iron-transferrin complex in turn carries iron to any cells of the body needing it or to a storage site. This process can occur very quickly.

chelate
Substance, usually an organic acid such as one of the amino acids, that binds to a mineral element and influences the ease with which it is absorbed, utilized, or excreted

If transferrin is about 33% saturated with iron, it does not pick up any more. In that case, ferrous iron is released from the amino acid chelate and changed to ferric iron within the mucosal cell. In this form, it combines with another protein, apoferritin, to form ferritin. It stays in this combination until transferrin calls for more iron. The iron is then given up from ferritin, changed to ferrous iron while it is still in the cells lining the intestine, and released into the blood to transferrin.

If, however, there is no need for iron, the young mucosal cell still containing the stored iron migrates up the villi (projections on the intestinal wall). After 3 to 4 days, the cell (and its iron) will be lost and excreted in the feces. This mechanism, then, keeps the blood from picking up more iron than is needed.

The absorption of heme iron follows a slightly different path. The heme molecule is absorbed intact. Then, within the cell, the iron is split off by a special enzyme. From then on it is treated the same as other iron.

Factors Affecting Absorption

The amount of iron absorbed depends on a variety of factors; a discussion of these factors follows.

Body's need for iron. The body's need for iron is reflected in the amount of unbound transferrin in the blood and possibly in the amount of messenger or chelated iron in the mucosal cells of the intestinal wall. A rise in the **total iron-binding capacity,** or **TIBC,** of the blood, caused by an increase in unsaturated transferrin, indicates that iron has been removed from the blood to tissues or storage sites. More iron is then absorbed to keep transferrin about 15% saturated with iron. When the transferrin is up to one-third saturated with iron, less iron is absorbed; this indicates that the iron absorption mechanism responds to the body's need for iron.

total iron-binding capacity or **TIBC**
The ability of the blood to remove iron from cells lining the intestine; high TIBC, as a result of unsaturated transferrin capable of picking up more iron, indicates a need for iron.

A person with normal hemoglobin levels absorbs from 2% to 10% of dietary nonheme iron and 23% of heme iron. Iron-deficient individuals with low hemoglobin levels may absorb as much as one third of dietary iron from heme iron and one fifth of dietary iron from nonheme iron.

The need for iron is increased with exercise because of increased destruction of blood cells. There is also an increased synthesis of red blood cells when a person suffers from **hypoxia,** or loss of oxygen to the brain; this may occur among people living at high altitudes who need more hemoglobin to take oxygen to the brain than people at lower altitudes.

hypoxia
A condition in which there is too little oxygen reaching body cells, particularly brain cells

Form of iron. Although the body can absorb both reduced ferrous and oxidized ferric iron, the ferrous form is absorbed more readily. As a result, vitamin C, a reducing agent, is often included with iron supplements. In the diet of older people, the acids in citrus fruits can compensate for reduced hydrochloric acid in the stomach and can aid in changing ferric iron to ferrous iron.

Factors Favoring Iron Absorption
- Increased need
- Increased acidity
  - Vitamin C in diet
  - Hydrochloric acid in stomach
- Ferrous form of iron
- Dietary heme
- Smaller doses
- High altitudes

Factors Inhibiting Iron Absorption
- Dietary fiber
- Excessive coffee or tea intake
- Steatorrhea
- High calcium intakes
- High phosphorus intakes

Composition of the meal. When meat is eaten along with plant sources of iron, the absorption of iron from these sources increases from 2% or 3% to 8%, apparently because of the action of amino acids that are released during digestion to form soluble iron chelates. This is sometimes referred to as the "meat factor," or MPF (meat, poultry, and fish) factor. Up to 60 mg of vitamin C in the meal has a similar effect.

Dietary fiber. High fiber or cellulose depresses the utilization of iron, accounting for the poor absorption of 1% to 2% often noted from green leafy vegetables such as spinach. Similarly, the iron in whole-grain products is poorly absorbed.

Size of dose. The percentage of iron absorbed varies inversely with the size of the dose. Iron in smaller divided doses, given three or four times a day, is much better utilized than a single large dose.

Other factors. Phytic acid, an organic acid found in some whole-grain cereal products, combines with iron to form an insoluble iron complex that the body cannot absorb. In some cereals, phytic acid is bound to a protein and has no adverse effect on iron absorption; however, bran does.

The consumption of coffee or tea within 1 hour after a meal leads to a decrease in iron absorption of 40% and 85% respectively: this is attributed to somewhat bitter, iron-binding substances called *polyphenols*, such as **tannins** in tea.

tannin
A type of polyphenol; an astringent substance found in tea that binds iron

Steatorrhea, in which higher than normal amounts of fat appear in the feces, is associated with decreased iron absorption.

High intakes of calcium interfere with iron absorption. This is a growing concern with the increasing use of calcium supplements. Excessive phosphorus intake also inhibits iron absorption.

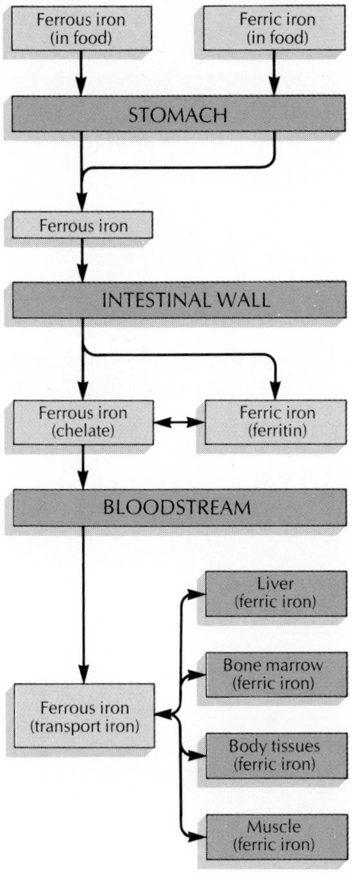

Interconversion of ferrous and ferric iron in the body

Transportation and Metabolism

Once iron has been absorbed, it is carried throughout the body bound to the protein carrier transferrin. It travels in the blood along with iron from the breakdown of body cells or from storage sites. From this it is released for use in the synthesis of respiratory enzymes or in the manufacture in the bone marrow of hemoglobin for red blood cells. Iron in excess of the immediate needs of cells and bone marrow will be deposited in the iron storage sites of the body. Of the approximately 1000 mg of iron stored in the adult male, 30% is in the liver, 30% is in the bone marrow, and the rest is in the spleen and muscles.

Individuals using calcium supplements should take them several hours after or before a meal to prevent interference with absorption of dietary iron. If both iron and calcium supplements are used, they should not be taken at the same time of day.

If dietary iron coupled with that obtained from the breakdown of red blood cells is not adequate to meet needs, iron will be obtained from reserves in the liver; it will be bound to transferrin in the blood and recirculated throughout the body. Only when the body's reserves of iron have been depleted will there be any evidence of iron deficiency symptoms. In infants, the liver stores of iron can last 3 to 6 months. A reserve of 1000 mg in an adult man lasts 1000 days; in an adult woman, it lasts over 500 days. The absorption and metabolism of iron are summarized in Figure 11-3.

Recommended Dietary Allowances

Adults

The National Research Council recommended that adult allowances for iron be based on the assumption that an adult man must obtain approximately 0.9 to 1.2 mg of iron daily to replace body losses in urine, feces, and perspiration and that an adult woman needs from 1.4 to 2.2 mg/day to cover additional losses in menstruation. Because an average of 10% of ingested iron is absorbed, it has been recommended that men obtain 10 mg/day and women 18 mg/day from dietary

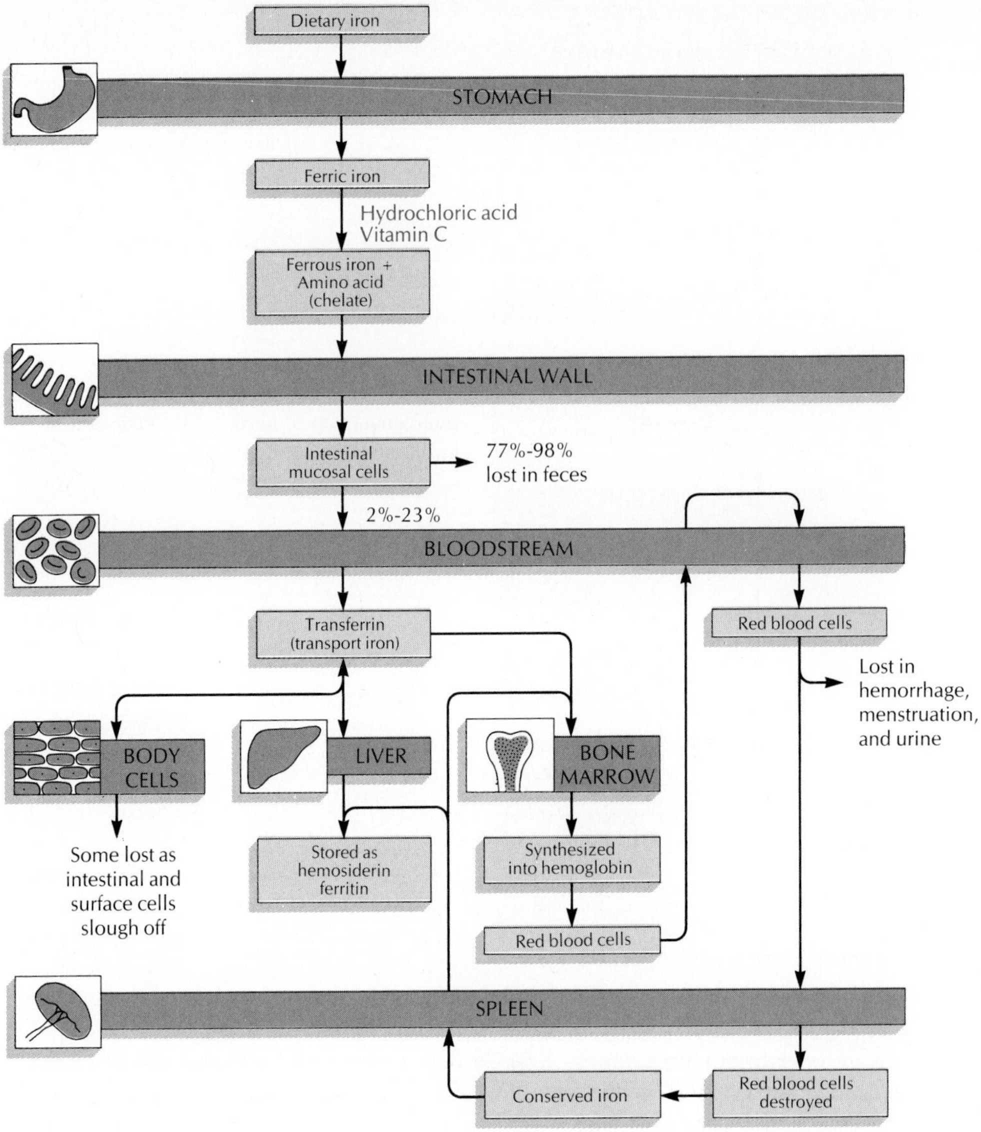

Figure 11-3 Schematic representation of absorption and metabolism of iron. Note how iron is conserved and recycled once it is absorbed.

Recommended Dietary Allowances for Iron (mg/day)

0-6 months	10
6 months-3 yr	15
4-10 yr	10
11-18 yr	18
Males	
19+	10
Females	
19-50	18
51+	10
Pregnancy	18*
Lactation	18*

*A supplement of 30 to 60 mg iron is recommended.

sources. For women, this amount actually represents a narrow margin of safety and may fail to meet the needs of those with high menstrual losses of iron—that is, as much as 32 mg/month.

There is general agreement among recommendations in various countries that men need 10 to 12 mg/day. There is little consensus for women, with recommendations ranging from 10 to 18 mg.

Pregnancy

During pregnancy, a total of 300 mg of iron is needed for the growth of the fetus, 70 mg for the placenta, and 500 mg for the synthesis of hemoglobin that is associated with a 50% increase in blood volume. Iron accumulates in the fetus at a rate of 0.5 mg/day in the first trimester but increases to 3 to 4 mg/day in the last two trimesters. Iron is stored in the fetus during the latter half of pregnancy, being transferred irreversibly to fetal blood even if the mother's hemoglobin level drops. Even with increased iron absorption and the saving of iron resulting from the absence of menstrual periods, it is almost impossible for a pregnant woman to obtain the required amount of iron from food alone, especially since the increase in calorie requirement during pregnancy is relatively small. As a result, the Food and Nutrition

Board recommends that pregnant women, in addition to obtaining 18 mg of iron/day from dietary sources, take a supplement providing about 30 mg of elemental iron (which is equivalent to 150 mg of ferrous sulfate). Because of the constipating effect of iron supplements, however, physicians have found that women have difficulty complying with this recommendation. Larger supplements should not be used.

Continued supplementation of a mother's diet for 2 to 3 months after delivery is encouraged to help ensure that iron reserves, usually depleted in pregnancy, are replenished. However, as blood volume drops, iron is recaptured from the extra hemoglobin synthesized during pregnancy.

In selecting an iron supplement, the amount of *elemental* iron provided is important not the amount of an iron salt (e.g., ferrous sulfate). The amount of elemental iron in various iron salts can be calculated from the following information

Iron Content (mg/100 mg) of Iron Salts in Supplements

Ferrous sulfate	20
Ferrous fumarate	33
Ferrous gluconate	12
Ferro-glycine sulfate	16

Lactation

Human milk, which contains about twice the amount of iron as cow's milk, is still a relatively poor source of iron. The amount of iron in breast milk is higher at the end than at the beginning of the nursing period but is not influenced by the amount in the maternal diet. Because only 0.5 to 1 mg of a woman's dietary iron is transferred to milk, the recommended intake during lactation is the same as for any nonpregnant adult woman.

Infants and Children

The reserve of iron in the liver of a full-term infant is sufficient to last from 3 to 6 months, during which time the infant doubles its birth weight. In addition, as infants shift from the uterine environment, where the oxygen pressure is low, to the extrauterine environment, which has higher oxygen pressure, the need for hemoglobin and heme iron to carry oxygen decreases—therefore a drop in hemoglobin from 18 grams at birth to 12 to 14 grams in the first 6 months of life is to be expected. In fact, it can't be prevented.

Because the reserve of iron in twins and premature infants is usually lower, it may be necessary to supplement these infants' diets with iron earlier than at 4 to 6 months recommended for fullterm infants. Since little iron is absorbed in early infancy, adding iron to infant formula or giving an iron supplement from birth does not prevent a drop in hemoglobin levels. It may, however, provide some protection against anemia after 4 months of age when dietary iron should be provided for the synthesis of hemoglobin and for newly formed cells. This need usually amounts to 1 mg of iron/kg of body weight/day. Hemoglobin values of 12 grams at 4 to 6 months of age are maintained throughout childhood before rising in late adolescence to adult levels.

The recommended children's dietary allowances for iron proposed by FAO/WHO vary, based on the proportion of the intake that is provided by animal foods. This reflects the increase in the absorption of dietary iron as the proportion of heme iron increases.

For children iron is needed for synthesis of new tissue and production of hemoglobin as blood increases. This requires from 0.35 to 0.70 mg/day over the 20-year growth period for boys and 0.30 to 0.45 mg/day over the 15-year growth period for girls. Assuming that 10% dietary iron is absorbed, a daily dietary intake of 3 to 7 mg is needed for growth needs over and above need for maintenance of body tissue.

Adequacy of Diet as It Relates to Iron

A diet adequate in most other nutrients will provide only 6 mg of iron/1000 kcal. This makes it difficult for an adult woman to obtain the recommended 18 mg of iron/day, especially if caloric intake is below 3000 kcal.

Data from NHANES II showing a mean iron intake of 10.6 mg/day for women between the ages of 18 and 50 and from the NFCS of 11.2 mg confirm that the recommended intake for women is very difficult to achieve. Failure to do so does not necessarily indicate iron deficiency; it merely suggests the increased possibility of a deficiency as intake falls below the recommended level. Only biochemical data on iron status can confirm iron deficiency.

Iron Content of Various Types of Liver (mg/3-oz serving)

Beef	5.3
Chicken	7.6
Calf	12.8
Lamb	16.1
Pork	27.2

Food Sources

The iron content of the most frequently eaten foods in the North American diet is given in Table 11-3. Liver is the only very rich source of iron, with the amount depending on the type of liver used. Since liver has never been a popular diet item in North America, most persons depend on a variety of moderately good alternative

Table 11-3 ◇ Amount of iron in average servings and per 100 kcal of foods most frequently reported in surveys and additional recommended sources

Food	Amount	Kcal	mg per Serving	mg/100 kcal	INQ*
Meat, Fish, Eggs, Poultry, Nuts					
Egg, fried	1 large	95	1.0	1.1	1.0
Beef roast	3 oz	315	2.0	0.6	1.1
Ground beef	3 oz	230	2.8	1.3	1.2
Chicken	3 oz	140	0.9	0.6	0.7
Tuna	3 oz	165	1.6	1.0	1.0
Peanut butter	2 T	190	0.6	0.3	0.3
Bacon, lean	3 slices	80	0.3	0.4	0.4
Liver, beef†	3 oz	185	5.3	2.8	3.2
Cereals					
Cornflakes	1 cup	110	1.8	1.6	1.5
Shredded wheat	1 biscuit	100	1.2	1.2	1.3
Saltines	4 crackers	50	0.5	1.0	1.0
Rice	1 oz, dry	109	0.9	0.8	0.9
White bread	1 slice	65	0.9	0.6	1.5
Whole-wheat bread	1 slice	70	1.0	0.7	1.6
Dairy Products					
Whole milk	8 oz	150	0.1	0.1	0.1
2% fat milk	8 oz	120	0.1	0.1	0.1
Cheddar cheese	1 oz	115	0.2	0.2	0.2
Fruits					
Apple	1 medium	80	0.2	0.2	0.3
Banana	1 medium	105	0.4	0.4	0.4
Orange juice, frozen	4 oz	55	0.2	0.4	0.4
Peach	1 medium	35	0.1	1.3	1.5
Raisins†	1 oz	80	0.6	0.7	0.8
Vegetables					
Corn, canned	4 oz-½ cup	82	0.8	1.0	0.9
Green beans	4 oz-½ cup	22	0.8	3.5	4.4
Green peas	4 oz-½ cup	62	1.2	1.9	2.1
Lettuce	¼ head	20	0.7	3.5	4.3
Tomatoes	1 medium	25	0.6	2.4	2.5
Potato, baked	1 medium	130	1.8	1.4	1.6

*INQ is the ratio of iron content to iron need divided by ratio of energy content in food to energy need. Based on U.S. RDA for iron (18 mg) and energy need of 200 kcal. INQ = % U.S. RDA iron/% Energy requirements. INQ > 2.0 = good source.

†Foods not in most frequently eaten group, but usually included in lists of recommended sources.

sources to meet their needs. Liver has recently fallen into disfavor because of its high cholesterol content.

From Figure 11-4, showing the contribution of various food groups to the iron in the North American food supply, it is clear that no one food group is responsible for a large share of the iron in the diet but that the meat, cereal, and vegetable groups make significant contributions.

Because of wide differences in iron absorption from various sources, knowledge of the iron content of foods does not always give a true picture of its availability. The extent to which iron from various sources is absorbed is illustrated in Table 11-4.

In eggs, iron is concentrated almost entirely in the yolk, from which only 2% is absorbed. In contrast, up to 30% of the iron in chicken is absorbed. Other animal sources fall between these extremes. Soy products often used as meat extenders have nonheme iron which is poorly absorbed.

Fruits and vegetables are fairly good sources of iron, but it is relatively poorly utilized. Vegetables provide three times as much iron in the North American diet as fruits. Fruits and fruit juices are rated as poor iron sources; potatoes and green stalks and leaves are good sources; and leguminous plants (peas and beans) are excellent sources. The pulp of fruits contains twice as much iron as the juice. Canned fruits and vegetables or acid foods cooked in an iron container will pick up additional iron, which is just as available as naturally occurring iron. This has led some people to propose a return to iron pots and pans for cooking.

Although raisins and other dried fruits are often recommended, they have no more iron in the dried form than they had in their original form. It should be remembered that dried fruit contributes many calories in addition to iron. For example, one-fourth cup of raisins, which provides 0.7 mg of iron, also provides 109 kcal. In addition, sticky raisins may contribute to dental problems.

Breads, either enriched or whole-grain, provide small amounts of iron per unit of weight, but because of the large amounts used by adolescent boys and families

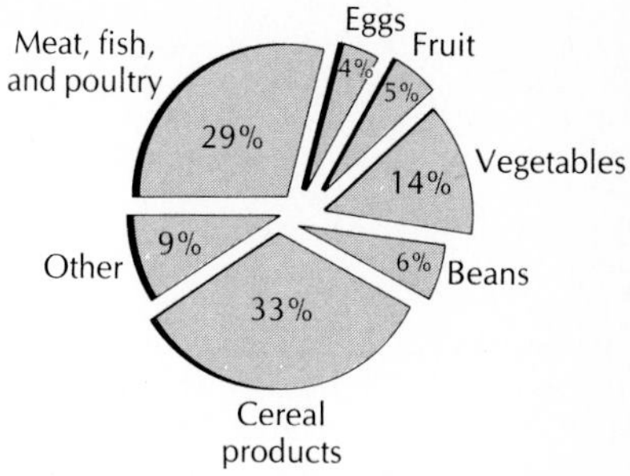

Figure 11-4 Contribution of various food groups to iron in the North American diet.

Table 11-4 ◆ Iron absorption from various plant and animal foods

Food	Amount of Iron in Food (mg)	Iron Absorption (Percentage of Intake)
Foods of Vegetable Origin		
Rice	2	0.3
Spinach	2	3.5
Black beans	3-4	3.6
Corn	2-4	2.5
Lettuce	1-17	7.8
Wheat	2-7	7.5
Soybeans	3-4	5.2
Foods of Animal Origin		
Egg yolk	1	2.0
Ferritin*	3	4.2
Veal liver	3	28.0
Fish muscle	1-2	11.0
Hemoglobin*	3-4	10.0
Veal muscle	3-4	22.0
Chicken		30.0

From Layrisse M, and Martinez-Torres C: Progress in Hematology 7:137, 1971; updated, personal communication, 1984.

*Iron-containing components of animal foods.

on restricted food budgets, they often make a significant contribution to daily iron intake even though less than 5% of the iron in them is absorbed. Enriched bread, macaroni, and corn grits contain slightly less iron than the whole-grain cereal from which they are derived. Infant cereals and some prepared dried cereals are enriched with amounts of iron to provide a full day's allowance in one serving. These levels are considered excessive.

Unbleached flour is refined flour that has not been treated to make it whiter. It is not necessarily enriched and does not have the trace elements of whole wheat.

The only food group characterized as a poor source of iron is the milk and milk products group. The small amount of iron in milk is well utilized but still makes an insignificant contribution to total intake.

Some food sources are relatively rich in iron but are less important because of the infrequency with which they are consumed. They include oysters (6.3 mg/3-oz serving), clams (6.1 mg/3-oz serving), and cocoa (1 mg/T).

Iron in the drinking water (present as ferric hydroxide) is a significant source only when iron values of water exceed 5 mg/liter. Typical amounts in the United States exceed 1 mg/liter (or quart).

Blackstrap molasses, a by-product of the sugar-refining process, contains about 2.5 mg of iron per tablespoon. Because of the bitter flavor of the product, however, it cannot be considered a significant dietary item.

Effect of Food Preparation

The major causes of loss of iron in the preparation of food are the discarding of iron-rich cooking water and the removal of vegetable peelings, with the loss of the iron concentrated near the skin. Any cooking method that minimizes the possibility of iron dissolving in the cooking water, such as using relatively large pieces of food, cooking foods with skins on, and simmering rather than boiling food, will increase the amount of iron available in the diet. Steamed vegetables have more iron than boiled vegetables, as do those cooked for a short time in a small amount of water; those cooked in their skins have more iron than peeled ones. The use of vegetable stock in soups or gravies also help minimize iron losses. The use of iron cooking pots increases the iron in food products by two-fold to six-fold. In fact, the switch away from iron cooking utensils may partially explain the increase in iron deficiency.

Trends in dietary sources of iron in the North American diet are shown in Figure 11-5. During the last 70 years, available iron in the diet has increased from 15 to 17.6 mg/person/day.

Figure 11-5 Trends in dietary sources of iron in the North American diet.
From Agricultural charts, Washington, D.C., 1978, U.S. Department of Agriculture; updated to 1984.

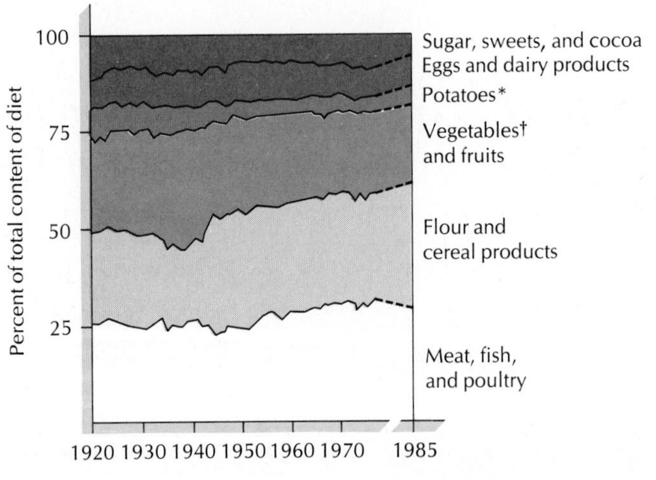

*Includes sweet potatoes.
†Includes dry beans, peas, nuts, and soya products.

Table 11-5 ◇ Permissible levels of iron enrichment in representative foods (1980)

Food	mg/kg
Bread, rolls, and buns	17.6-27.5
Flour	28.6-36.3
Corn grits, corn meal, and rice	28.6-57.2
Macaroni products	28.6-36.3

From Food and Drug Administration: Nutritional quality of foods: addition of nutrients, Federal Register 45(18):6314, 1980.

Iron Fortification or Enrichment

Ensuring an adequate intake of iron has depended on effective **fortification** or **enrichment** programs. These must be based on several considerations. First, the food to be fortified must be consumed in significant amounts by the general population. It should be produced in relatively few centers so that quality control can be maintained. The enrichment iron should be soluble and readily available to the body. Finally, the food should be of a type that remains stable and palatable over an extended period of time.

Sources of Dietary Iron
Foods (for naturally occurring iron)
Enriched foods
Fortified foods
Nutrient supplements

fortification
Addition of nutrient to food

enrichment
Addition of a nutrient to a food to replace that lost in processing

Bread and cereal meet this last criterion in developed countries. In developing countries, salt, sugar, and beverages may be effective carriers for iron fortification. Infant cereals and powdered milks are also acceptable carriers. However, foods that become discolored by the addition of iron salts are not candidates for fortification.

In the United States, certain foods such as bread, flour, macaroni, and corn grits have a **standard of identity** that permits them to be labeled "enriched" as long as the amount of iron added to the foods falls between certain specified limits; some examples are given in Table 11-5. For other foods, the added nutrients (which can be added in any safe amount) must be identified on the label. In 1975, the consumption per person of added iron in the United States was estimated at 8.3 mg/day.

standard of identity
Precise description of the ingredients or characteristics of a specific food

Although only 30 states have laws requiring the enrichment of flour, about 90% of the flour and breads sold in the United States is enriched with at least iron and three vitamins, thiamin, riboflavin, and niacin.

Supplementation

Supplementation with iron may be the only way to treat iron-deficient people. Any of over 30 different iron salts may be used in supplements, but ferrous sulfate is usually the least expensive and also seems to be the most effective. Unfortunately, many common gastrointestinal problems, ranging from nausea to constipation to diarrhea, are associated with iron supplementation. Vitamin C or folacin will enhance the effectiveness of a supplement. In addition, iron supplements are absorbed almost twice as completely when taken before rather than after a meal.

Evaluation of Iron Status

Although there are many indicators of iron status in the human body, only the four most commonly used will be discussed.

Tests of Iron Status (from Most Sensitive to Least Sensitive)
Serum ferritin
Red cell protoporphyrin
Transferrin saturation
MCV—Mean corpuscular volume
Hemoglobin/hematocrit

Serum Ferritin

The most sensitive indicator of iron stores is serum ferritin, an iron-protein complex that is present in normal serum in very small amounts (nanograms or ng/liter) with 1 μg/liter reflecting 10 mg of storage iron.

Protoporphyrin

protoporphyrin
A compound that is a precursor of the heme in hemoglobin; accumulates when there is inadequate iron to make heme

Protoporphyrin is a precursor of heme, the iron-containing portion of hemoglobin in red blood cells. An increase in protoporphyrin in the red blood cells indicates that heme synthesis has been depressed by lack of iron.

Transferrin Saturation

An increase in the amount of the unsaturated transport protein transferrin or the total iron-binding capacity (TIBC) occurs with a depletion of iron stores. Transferrin saturation of less than 16% indicates that iron reserves are inadequate to meet the needs for iron. An individual suffering from this is said to have a "latent iron deficiency."

Hemoglobin Content

Hemoglobin = 90 means that the hemoglobin level is 90% of the standard—usually 15 grams/dl for men and 13.6 grams/dl for women.

The use of hemoglobin content of the blood, a traditional indicator of the adequacy of iron status, has several limitations. First, there is lack of agreement on the level that is indicative of iron deficiency. For some people, a hemoglobin level of 12 grams/dl is adequate, whereas for others, this amount will result in a limited ability to exercise. Second, hemoglobin levels fluctuate over a 24-hour period, and a single determination may give erroneous information. Third, hemoglobin levels drop only after stores have been depleted; low hemoglobin values therefore represent an advanced stage of iron deficiency. Fourth, low hemoglobin values may be caused by a deficiency of other nutrients besides iron, such as protein or vitamin B_6. Finally, since depressed hemoglobin is a normal response to illness, it is hard to interpret hemoglobin levels in sick people. Values are sometimes reported as a percentage of the standard rather than as an actual amount (gm/dl).

Hemoglobin determinations are insensitive to the early stages of iron deficiency but are useful in assessing the severity of anemia. The relationship of various indicators to iron status is shown in Figure 11-6.

It is proposed that one or two sets of criteria be used to assess iron status: either the ferritin model or the *MCV*, or *mean corpuscular volume*, model. Both models include the measurement of erythrocyte protoporphyrin and transferrin saturation. In addition, the ferritin model includes the measure of serum ferritin, and the MCV model includes the mean corpuscular volume, which is the measure of the volume of blood cells. People with two out of three of these measures below the cutoff points indicated in Table 11-6 are described as having *impaired iron status*. Among this group, only those who also have hemoglobin values below an acceptable standard for age and sex should be considered to have *iron-deficiency anemia*. When these criteria are used, a relatively small number of people are considered to be anemic compared to when hemoglobin values alone are used. The

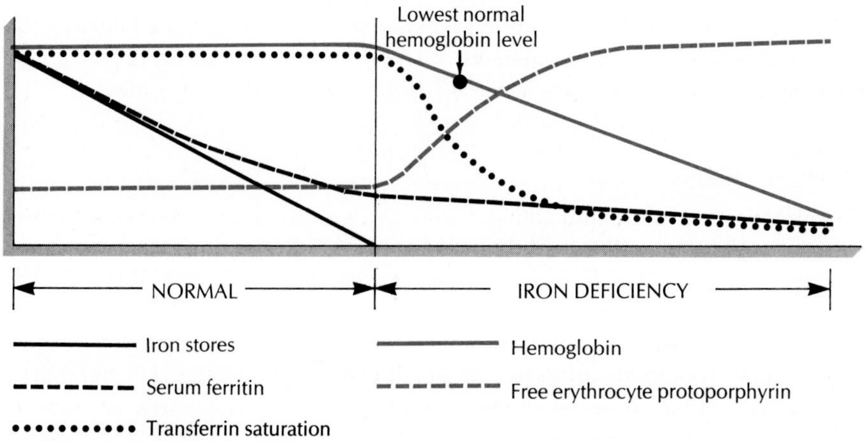

Figure 11-6 Relationship of various indicators of iron status to iron deficiency.

Table 11-6 ◆ Criteria for assessment of iron status—levels indicative of deficiency

Age (yr)	Hemoglobin gram/dl	Serum Ferritin (ng/ml)	Transferrin Saturation (%)	Erythrocyte Protoporphyrin (μg/dl RBC, or Red Blood Cells)	MCV
1-2	<9	—	<12	>80	<73
3-4	<10	<10	<14	>75	<75
5-10	<10	<10	<15	>70	<76
11-14	<12 (Male)	<10	<16	>70	<78
	<10 (Female)	<10	<10	>70	<78
15-74	<12 (Male)	<12	<16	>70	<80
	<10 (Female)	<12	<12	>70	<80

resulting incidence is much more in keeping with our best estimates of functional iron deficiency.

Deficiencies

Because the body is extremely efficient in conserving iron supplies, simple iron deficiencies occur only during the growth period, when intake fails to meet needs, after loss of blood, or when women have experienced frequent pregnancies in rapid succession. In iron deficiency, however, a gradual and well-defined sequence of changes ultimately results in anemia. In the first phase, there is a depletion of iron stores (a decrease in serum ferritin) and a compensatory increase in iron absorption represented by increased iron-binding capacity. These changes are followed by a stage in which iron stores are exhausted, transferrin saturation is reduced, the amount of the heme precursor protoporphyrin that is converted to heme decreases, and serum ferritin drops. In the third stage, anemia develops, characterized by low hemoglobin levels.

Evidence of these deficiencies may show up in decreased work capacity, altered behavior such as apathy and irritability, decreased secretion of hydrochloric acid, and altered susceptibility to infection.

Anemia

Nutritional Anemia

Nutritional anemia is caused by the absence of any dietary essential that is involved in hemoglobin formation or by poor absorption of these dietary essentials. Some anemias have been reported to be caused by a lack of either dietary iron or high-quality protein; by a lack of pyridoxine (vitamin B_6), which catalyzes the synthesis of the heme portion of the hemoglobin molecule; by a lack of vitamin C, which influences the rate of iron absorption and the release of iron from transferrin to the tissues; and by a lack of vitamin E, which affects the stability of the red blood cell membrane. Copper is not part of the hemoglobin molecule but aids in its synthesis by influencing the absorption of iron, its release from the liver, or its incorporation into a hemoglobin molecule.

Nutritional Anemia is Caused by Dietary Deficiencies of One or More of
Iron
Vitamin B_6
Protein
Vitamin C
Vitamin E
Copper

Nutritional anemia is usually characterized as both **hypochromic** and **microcytic.** Hypochromic suggests a lack of the pigment hemoglobin; microcytic indicates the presence of small red blood cells. Nutritional anemia is most common in adolescent girls because their growth demands, made more severe by menstrual losses, are difficult to supply from food alone. A cursory diagnosis of hemoglobin status can often be made by a visual examination of the mucous membranes, especially those on the underside of the eyelid or in the mouth where the blood

hypochromic microcytic anemia
An anemia characterized by small cells with too little hemoglobin, causing a lack of color (hypo = too little; -chrome = color; micro = small; -cyte = cell)

Table 11-7 ◆ Changes in measures of iron status indicative of developing iron deficiency

Measure of Iron Status	Normal	Iron Depletion	Iron-Deficient Erythropoiesis	Iron-Deficient Anemia
Iron stores (bone marrow, liver, spleen)	Adequate	Very low	0	0
Erythron iron (iron in red blood cells)	Normal	Normal	Slightly reduced	Less than half of normal
TIBC	330	360	390	410
Iron absorption	Normal	Increased	Increased	Increased
Plasma iron (μg/dl)	115-50	115	60	40
Transferrin saturation (%)	35	35	16	16
Red blood cell photoporphyrin (μg/dl in red blood cell)	30	30	100	100
Erythrocytes	Normal	Normal	Normal	Microcytic hypochromic
Hemoglobin (grams/dl)	12	12	12	<12

vessels are close to the epithelial surface. Pale membranes usually signify low hemoglobin values.

Nutritional anemia occurs frequently in young infants who continue to receive a diet consisting only of milk past the ages of 3 to 6 months. (Up until this time, fetal liver reserves are adequate. In fact, infants utilize little dietary iron during the first 3 to 4 months of life.) After this early stage, the use of an iron-fortified formula for bottle-fed babies and iron supplements for breast-fed babies are recommended. Meat, eggs, fruits, and vegetables in the amounts consumed by infants are incapable of meeting their iron need; enriched cereals must be used.

Pernicious anemia. Pernicious anemia is a form of nutritional anemia in which the number of red blood cells, not the hemoglobin level, is low. It is caused primarily by a failure in the absorption of vitamin B_{12} (cobalamin) rather than by a dietary lack of a nutrient. For a more detailed discussion of pernicious anemia, see discussion of vitamin B_{12} in Chapter 12.

Hemorrhagic Anemia

Hemorrhagic anemia is caused by an excessive loss of blood—a result of surgery, internal hemorrhaging, excessive menstrual losses, blood donations, or intestinal parasites. After a loss of blood, the blood volume is restored almost immediately and is followed by an increase in the number of red blood cells and finally by the restoration of hemoglobin levels.

Loss of blood represents a loss of 0.05 mg of iron/ml of blood or 25 mg/pint of blood. Even with the increased rate of iron absorption that occurs after blood loss, it takes at least 50 days following a blood donation to replace the iron lost. This period may be reduced to 35 days if iron supplements and vitamin C are given to the donor. For this reason, there is wisdom in limiting blood donations to from 2 to 3 liters a year, especially for women.

The various stages of iron deficiency and the biochemical changes associated with them are shown in Table 11-7.

Excess

At one time, there was general agreement that it was impossible to absorb too much iron. However, this theory was questioned when it was reported that the Bantu tribe in Africa suffered from **siderosis** (also known as **hemosiderosis**), in which their iron reserves were found to be up to 30 times the normal 1-gram reserve. The absorbed iron, as much as 200 mg/day, came from kettles that the Bantu used to ferment beer. A similar iron toxicity has been reported among infants and adults who take excessive iron supplements (that is, 3 to 10 grams of ferrous sulfate daily).

siderosis (hemosiderosis)
Condition in which there is an excessive amount of iron stored in the liver, usually because an individual does not have the ability to regulate the amount that was absorbed; this occurs in about 0.25% of the population

In siderosis the excess iron accumulates in the normal storage sites: the liver and spleen and in the mitochondria of all cells. Serum iron increases, and the bone marrow becomes **hyperplastic,** which means that it has too many cells. The failure of the body to regulate iron absorption occurs at very high levels of iron intake among the 0.25% of the population that has a genetic tendency toward iron overload. For these people, the transferrin of the blood is saturated to three times its normal level and is incapable of binding all the absorbed iron in this harmless complex. Any excess free iron stimulates the growth of pathogenic organisms in the blood, resulting in an increased susceptibility to infection.

hyperplastic
Producing too many cells

Hemochromatosis is another form of iron-storage disease that occurs in less than 0.1% of the population (about 22,000 people in the United States). These people have an inherited defect in the regulation of their iron absorption, which allows them to absorb unusually high amounts of iron and to store it in tissues that normally do not store iron. Opponents of an increased level of iron in enriched bread feel that it may intensify the problem of regulating iron uptake in people with hemochromatosis. Bread enrichment cannot, of course, increase the number of people with the disease because it is an inherited problem. However, since the findings from NHANES II data indicate that a very small proportion of the population (less than 2%) can be considered truly iron deficient based on biochemical data, there is little justification for increasing the levels of iron in enriched products.

hemochromatosis
Condition in which an individual absorbs unusually high amounts of iron; this occurs in less than 0.1% of the population

IODINE (I)

Distribution

The essential trace mineral element iodine is present in the body in a minute amount—about 0.00004% of body weight (15 to 23 mg), or less than a hundredth of the amount of iron in a healthy human adult. Over three fourths of this iodine is concentrated in a single tissue, the thyroid gland, which uses it in the synthesis of the hormone thyroxin. The remainder is in the other tissues, particularly the salivary, mammary, or gastric glands, and in the kidneys. In the circulation, iodine occurs either as free iodine or as protein-bound iodine (PBI).

The study of iodine focuses on the study of the thyroid gland. This gland consists of two lobes, or parts, located in the neck area on either side of the windpipe just below the voice box (Figure 11-7). It weighs about 25 grams (1 oz).

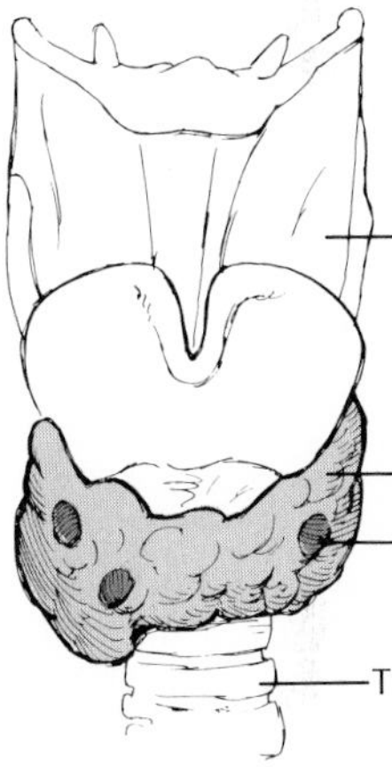

Figure 11-7 Diagrammatic representation of location of thyroid and parathyroid glands in neck area on either side of trachea (windpipe).

Absorption and Metabolism

The absorption and metabolism of iodine provide another example of the exquisite way in which the body controls the use of nutrients.

Iodine occurs in food either as the reduced iodide, as inorganic iodine, or bound to an organic component from which it must be freed. Free iodine is reduced to iodide and absorbed, primarily in the small intestine. Some may also be absorbed through the skin or inhaled as a contaminant from the combustion of fossil fuels.

Absorbed iodide appears immediately in the bloodstream, from which one third is absorbed by the thyroid gland, and the rest is taken up by the kidneys to be excreted in the urine, a protection against the accumulation of toxic levels. Small amounts are lost in perspiration and excreted in the feces. The excretion of iodine protects against the accumulation of toxic levels.

The iodide picked up, or "trapped," by the thyroid gland is oxidized to iodine, which unites with the amino acid tyrosine to be stored as part of the protein **thyroglobulin.** When the hypothalamus senses a drop in blood thyroxin levels, it releases to the blood a substance known as the thyroxin-releasing factor, TRF. TRF travels to the pituitary gland, which in turn triggers the release into the blood of a hormone called the thyroid-stimulating hormone (TSH). This hormone is carried to

thyroglobulin
Storage form of iodine in the thyroid gland

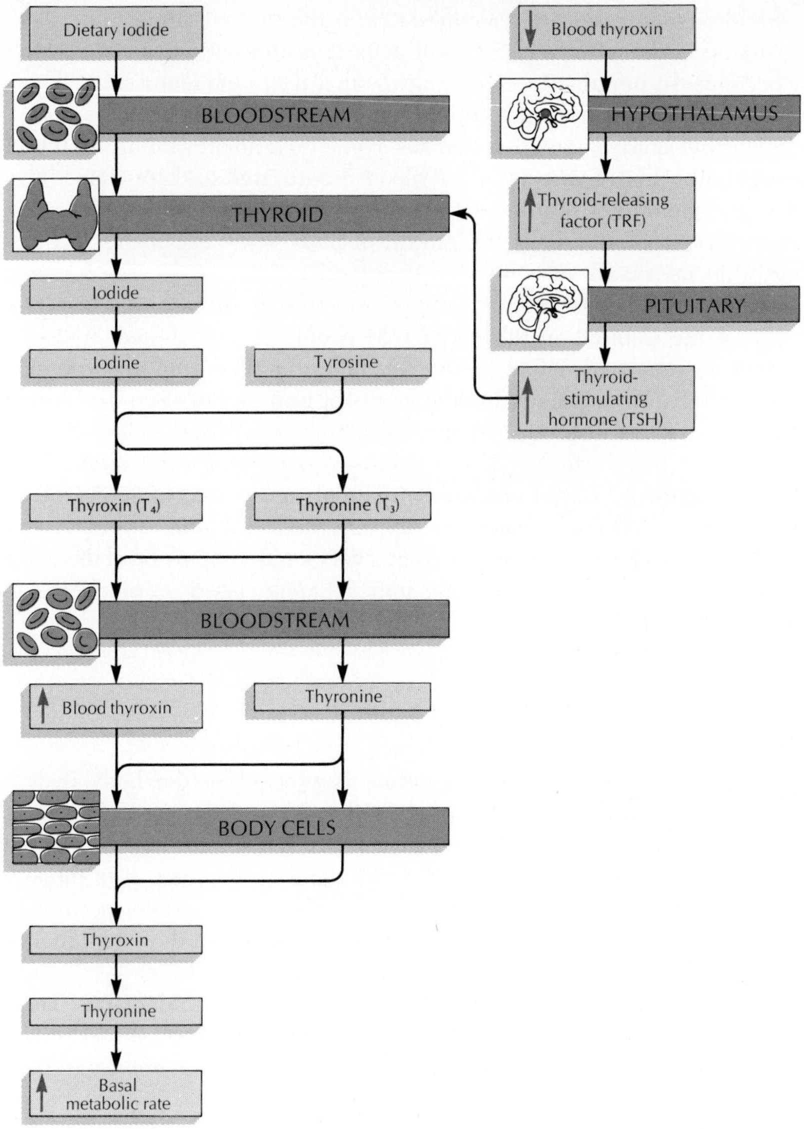

Figure 11-8 Summary of metabolism of iodine and synthesis and metabolism of thyroxin. As blood levels of thyroxin drop, a series of hormonal changes in the hypothalamus and pituitary cause the release of thyroid-stimulating hormone (TSH), which causes the thyroid to synthesize and release more thyroxin.

the thyroid gland, where it stimulates the production of an enzyme that acts on thyroglobulin to break away the iodine-containing tyrosine portions of thyroglobulin. These portions unite to form two forms, thyroxin, $\mathbf{T_4}$ with four molecules of iodine, or thyronine, $\mathbf{T_3}$ with three molecules. These hormones are then released into the blood in a ratio of 4:1 (T_4:T_3) to travel to each body cell, where they regulate cellular respiration. T_3 is considered the more active of the two hormones, and there is some evidence that once T_4 is within the cell, one iodine atom is removed to form T_3.

T_4
Thyroxin with 4 molecules of iodine

T_3
Thyronine with 3 molecules of iodine

T_4:T_3 in blood = 4:1

The salivary gland has the capacity to remove iodine from thyroxin, therefore inactivating it. The iodine is secreted in the saliva and can be reabsorbed in the gastrointestinal tract. This neatly orchestrated control over thyroxin synthesis and release is shown in Figure 11-8.

Functions

Regulator of Growth and Development (as Part of Thyroxin)

As part of the thyroid hormone, thyroxin, iodine plays a major role in regulating growth and development. Thyroxin can stimulate metabolism by as much as 30%, with the effects of a single dose persisting for 6 days or more. When the rate of metabolism increases, more oxygen is used, indicating that more energy is being released. Much of this energy appears as heat rather than as ATP.

Before the Food and Drug Administration ruled that thyroxin be available by prescription only, promoters of weight-reducing aids were selling thyroid extract on the theory that it aided in weight loss. Actually, it does; however, undesirable side effects, such as excessive stimulation of metabolism, make its use hazardous.

Other Roles

Although most of the attention regarding iodine has been focused on the role of thyroxin in energy metabolism, an increasing number of other roles is becoming apparent. The conversion of carotene, the precursor of vitamin A, to the active form of vitamin A; the synthesis of protein; and the absorption of carbohydrate from the intestine are examples of processes that are more efficient when thyroxin levels are normal. The synthesis of cholesterol is influenced by thyroxin, with above normal cholesterol levels occurring in hypothyroidism and below normal levels in hyperthyroidism. Additionally, thyroxin is essential for reproduction.

Requirements

The Food and Nutrition Board finds that an intake of 1 μg of iodine/kg of body weight is adequate for most adults. To ensure a margin of safety to provide for individual variations, a daily intake of 150 μg for both adult men and adult women is recommended. For pregnant and lactating women, the need is 25 μg and 50 μg higher, respectively. A wide range of intakes (between 50 and 1000 μg) is considered safe. Most North Americans consume at least 300 μg of iodine daily.

The needs of growing children for iodine, especially girls' needs, may exceed the suggested level of 1 μg/kg of body weight.

Recommended Dietary Allowances for Iodine (μg/day)

Adolescents and Adults, 11+ yr	150
Pregnancy	175
Lactation	200

Food Sources

Both food and water provide iodine in the human diet. The amount of iodine in water varies from one area to another and tends to parallel the iodine content of the soil. The iodine content of the soil is reflected in plants grown or animals raised in the area. An iodine content in water of less than 2 μg/liter, or 2 ppb, is associated with iodine-deficiency conditions; that of 2 to 15 μg is associated with an absence of iodine deficiency. In the United States, the iodine content of fresh water varies from 0.5 to 2 ppb, with the lowest levels in glacial rivers and lakes. Levels in seawater vary from 17 to 50 ppb.

The variation in iodine content of vegetables from various geographical areas is illustrated in the margin. Modern marketing practices, in which the food supply of any one community comes from widely varied geographical areas, have done much to ensure a uniform and adequate level of dietary iodine throughout the United States.

In general, the leaves of plants have higher iodine concentrations than the roots, with spinach leaves having 300 μg/serving. Different types of seafood such as lobster, shrimp, and oysters (with 15 to 150 μg/serving) are among the richest dietary sources of iodine. However, because of the relatively minor role they play in most diets, their contribution to dietary iodine is small. Saltwater fish provide 10 to 100 times as much iodine as do freshwater fish.

An FDA analysis of iodine in fresh whole milk showed a content ranging from 20 to 1320 μg/liter, or quart. The study also found that the iodine content of foods in a typical "market basket" diet—that is, foods readily available in grocery stores—ranged from 550 to 850 μg in a 3000-kcal diet. The average adult intakes were 180% of recommended dietary allowances for women and 350% for men. In addition to reflecting variations in the iodine content of the soil and water, these

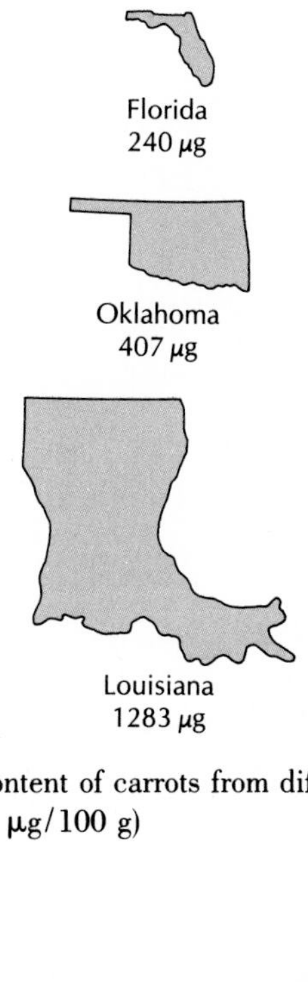

Iodine content of carrots from different areas (in μg/100 g)

values reflect the iodine contributed by the use of iodine-containing compounds in sanitizing processing equipment, especially dairy equipment; the use of iodate dough conditioners in bread making; and the use of iodine-containing coloring agents. The study did not, however, include the use of **iodized salt,** which at an average level of 4.5 grams/day contributes an additional 340 μg iodine. The findings of the FDA study suggest that it may no longer be necessary to promote the use of iodized salt for cooking and table use except in areas of the United States where the soil is known to be very low in iodine. About 55% of salt in the United States is iodized at a cost of ½¢ to 3¢/person/year. Federal labeling laws require that iodized salt bear the legend, "This salt contains added iodine, an essential nutrient"; noniodized salt must be labeled, "This product does not contain iodine, an essential nutrient." Iodized salt is used in only 20% of processed foods because of the technical and quality control problems associated with its use. Contrary to popular opinion, sea salt is not a good source of iodine because iodine **volatilizes** (converts to vapor) as the salt dries. Seaweed, which is a source of iodine, is a reasonable dietary source only for cultures accustomed to its use.

iodized salt
Salt to which potassium iodate has been added at a level of 1 part per 10,000. (as little as 1 part per 100,000 is used in some countries)

volatilize
Change from a solid to a gas

The contribution of various food groups to iodine in the North American food supply is shown in Figure 11-9.

Evaluation of Iodine Status

Comparison of the excretion of iodine in a single sample of urine related to the amount of excreted **creatinine** is used to evaluate iodine status. When little iodine is available, about 25 μg/gram of creatinine is excreted; when more iodine is available, at least 50 μg is excreted. Because neither dietary intake nor urinary excretion data correlate with evidence of a deficiency, factors other than reduced intake may cause a deficiency. The uptake of a **stable isotope** of iodine by people with a normally functioning thyroid is also useful in assessing iodine status.

New analytical techniques make it possible to measure T_3, T_4, and thyroid-stimulating hormone levels in the blood, all of which are indicative of iodine status. Another method is the assessment of protein-bound iodine (PBI) in the blood. This amount parallels both the level of thyroxin in the blood and the basal metabolic rate. PBI values of 4 to 8 μg/dl are normal; those >11 μg/dl indicate hyperthyroidism and those <3 μg/dl, hypothyroidism. Since basal metabolic rate reflects thyroxin levels, it is an indirect measure of iodine status.

creatinine
A nitrogen-containing substance, excreted in the urine; the amount excreted is directly proportional to lean body mass

stable isotope
A radioactive form of an element that does not deteriorate and can be used safely in the body to measure changes during metabolism

Tests for Iodine Adequacy
Urinary excretion
Uptake of labeled isotopes of iodine
T_4, T_3, and TSH blood levels
Protein-bound iodine test (PBI)
Basal metabolic rate (BMR)

Deficiencies

Goiter

Iodine deficiency is responsible for simple goiter, a condition characterized by swelling in the neck. This swelling is the result of the enlargement of the thyroid gland (Figure 11-10) as it attempts to compensate for the lack of iodine essential in the synthesis of thyroxin. Both cell number and cell size increase.

Simple goiter is a painless condition but has some undesirable effects on physical appearance. If the thyroid gland continues to grow, it exerts pressure on either side of the trachea, leading to difficulty in breathing. Appropriate iodine therapy will result in a slow reduction in the size of the enlarged thyroid gland. For more severe cases, treatment involves the surgical removal of part of the thyroid gland. This operation is complicated by the fact that the parathyroid gland, which is vital in the control of calcium metabolism, is embedded in the surface of the thyroid gland.

A deficiency of iodine is the primary but not the only cause of simple goiter. Certain foods contain substances called **goitrogens,** which increase susceptibility to goiter and account for about 4% of all goiters. Goitrogens act by blocking the absorption or utilization of iodine. Foods of the cabbage family, such as rutabagas, turnips, and cabbage, contain a heat-stable substance, pregoitrin, and a heat-labile

goitrogen
A substance that interferes with the absorption or utilization of iodine and therefore may cause iodine-deficient goiter

activator that converts the pregoitrin to goitrin, which interferes with iodine utilization. Goitrin is formed in raw foods but not in cooked foods. Peaches and almonds contain goitrogens, as do soybeans and cassava, which is a dietary staple in tropical countries. Ground nuts and peanuts contain a substance called arachidoside that also interferes with iodine utilization.

Sulfonamides, which are widely used antibiotics, reduce the conversion of iodide to iodine and are potentially goitrogenic, but at the levels used in treating infection they have little effect on thyroid activity. The vitamin-like substance para-aminobenzoic acid (PABA) has a similar goitrogenic effect. Both high calcium and high fat diets may also be goitrogenic.

Goiter may also be the result of defects in the enzymes necessary for the synthesis and release of thyroxin. Whatever the cause, the thyroid gland enlarges to compensate for the lack of iodine needed for its normal functioning.

Incidence. Goiter occurs primarily in areas where the soil is of glacial origin or where flooding or tropical rains have leached the iodine from the soil (Figure 11-11). It is almost nonexistent in areas where iodine-laden vapors from the sea

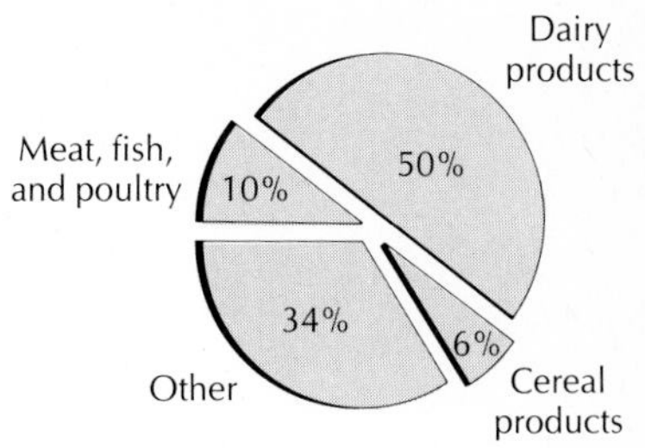

Figure 11-9 Contribution of various food groups to iodine in the North American food supply.

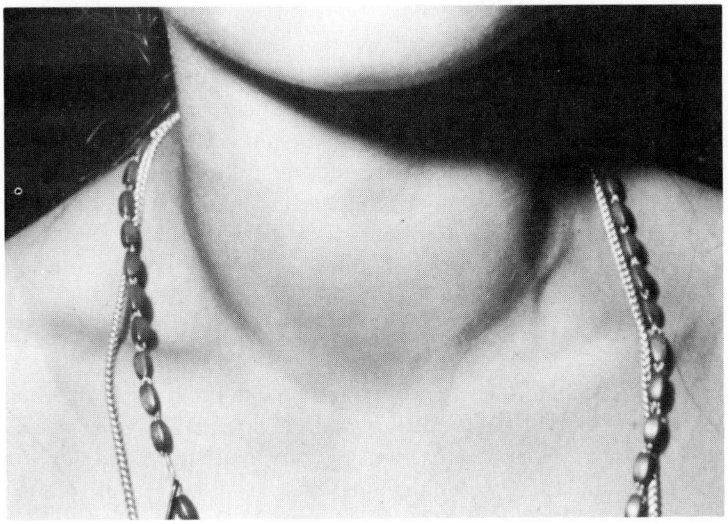

Figure 11-10 Swelling in the neck characteristic of goiter.
Photo from ICNND (International Committee on Nutritional and National Defense).

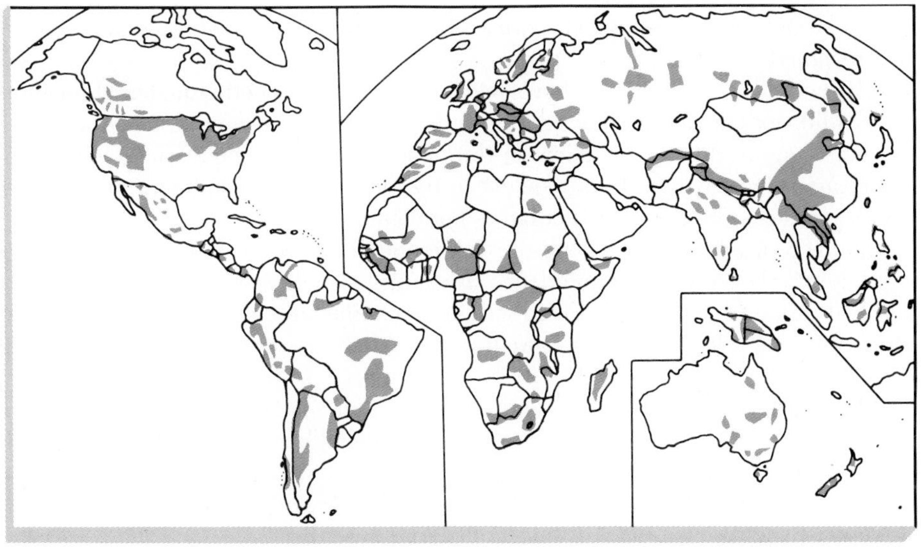

Figure 11-11 Goitrous areas of the world. Shaded areas indicate low iodine in the soil and water.

condense and deposit iodine on the soil. Coastal areas are relatively free of goiter. The contents of the soils and water supplies of goitrous areas show a very low concentration of iodine.

The incidence of goiter is about six times as high in females as in males. The most susceptible groups are adolescent girls and pregnant women. Practices such as limiting the use of iodized salt in an effort to control adolescent acne and restricting salt intake in pregnancy should be questioned because of the risk of goiter.

Of the estimated 200 million cases of simple goiter in the world today, the majority are caused by a dietary lack of iodine and tend to occur in definite geographical regions. In 1970, a nutritional status survey in 10 states revealed that in some areas as many as 7.2% of the population was afflicted—an incidence considered to be endemic. (A follow-up study, however, showed that many of the people with enlarged thyroids had intakes that met established standards and iodine excretions indicating that intake exceeded need. This indicates a prevalence of goiter unrelated to iodine deficiency.) Since 1970, there has been no evidence of an iodine deficiency in the United States.

Treatment. The treatement of goiter is a public health success story in the Western world. The use of iodine in treatment was recognized as early as 1820, and 30 years later a lack of iodine in the body was associated with low iodine levels in the soil and water. When it was shown that iodine was a normal constituent of the thyroid gland, there was a renewed interest in the use of iodine therapy in the treatment of goiter. Several investigations confirmed that endemic goiter (that is, goiter affecting many people in a particular region) could be controlled by raising dietary iodine intakes. Of many methods tried, only the iodization of salt has proven to be effective in reaching the majority of the population in developed countries. Most manufacturers absorb the small cost involved in iodizing salt. In developing countries intramuscular injections of "lipidoil," an iodine-containing poppy seed oil, every 2 to 4 years has proved successful.

Other Abnormalities

cretinism
The result of an iodine deficiency over several generations; victims are physically dwarfed and mentally retarded

Cretinism. This condition is encountered among children born to mothers who have had a limited iodine intake during adolescence and pregnancy and who live in areas where goiter is endemic. Because the mother's need for iodine takes precedence over that of the developing fetus, cretins suffer from an iodine deficiency during prenatal, as well as postnatal, development. These children, who suffer from hypothyroidism, are physically dwarfed and mentally retarded and have thick, dry, pasty skin and enlarged protruding abdomens. If treatment is started soon after birth, many of the symptoms of cretinism are reversible. However, if the condition persists beyond early childhood, permanent mental and physical retardation cannot be prevented.

myxedema
A condition caused by lack of thyroxin throughout the developmental period

Myxedema. Adults who have had symptoms of hypothyroidism throughout their childhood and adolescence suffer from **myxedema,** a condition characterized by coarse, sparse hair; dry, yellowish skin; poor tolerance to cold; and a low, husky voice. Myxedema results from a defect in the thyroid gland or the pituitary gland, which produces the thyroid-stimulating hormone.

Both cretinism and myxedema are still found in the world, but the use of iodized salt has greatly reduced the incidence in countries such as Switzerland, where the soil and water are extremely low in iodine. A similar program in the Andes mountains, which is a low-iodine area, would undoubtedly lower the incidence of iodine deficiency diseases.

Hyperthyroidism. Hyperthyroidism, in which the basal metabolic rate may be elevated as much as 100% above normal, is also known as Graves' disease or exophthalmic goiter. Persons suffering from overactivity of the thyroid gland experience nervousness, weight loss, increased appetite, intolerance to heat, tremors when the hand is outstretched, and protruding eyeballs.

ZINC (Zn)

Although zinc has been known to be a dietary essential in rats since 1934, it was not until 1961 that a zinc deficiency in humans was recognized. At that time, retarded growth and delayed sexual maturity were identified as symptoms clearly associated with a lack of dietary zinc. Other symptoms observed since then include delayed wound healing, loss of appetite, and decreased taste acuity, with a severe deficiency. These symptoms can be reversed by the addition of zinc to the diet. There are many other roles for zinc in human nutrition, but in only a few instances has the mechanism of action been clarified.

Zinc deficiency is most prevalent in Egypt and Iran, where it has been associated with a diet of unleavened whole-wheat flour (tanok) with little animal protein. The effect of this diet has been complicated by losses of zinc in sweat, resulting from high environmental temperatures. In Egypt, the deficiency has been further aggravated by hookworm and *Giardia* infestation and in Iran, by **geophagia,** which is the practice of eating a clay that apparently binds zinc. In Guatemala, zinc absorption is low because the diet consists largely of corn, tortillas, and black beans, from which the limited amount of zinc is poorly absorbed. In the United States, some cases of retarded growth have been attributed to a lack of dietary zinc, failure to absorb zinc, or use of the drug penicillamine.

geophagia
The practice of eating earth

In 1974, knowledge of the metabolic role of zinc, its importance in human nutrition, and food sources of the nutrient had advanced to the point that the Food and Nutrition Board felt confident in establishing a recommended dietary allowance. Realization of the possibility of a zinc deficiency in the human diet and the availability of techniques for detecting small amounts of zinc in tissues and food have resulted in much research on the role of zinc in nutrition. In 1988, several hundred papers pertaining to zinc were presented at a single scientific meeting.

Distribution

The human body contains from 2 to 2.5 grams of zinc, with three fourths of this amount concentrated in the skeleton from which it is removed only very slowly. A high concentration of zinc appears in the skin, hair, and testes, all of which seem particularly affected by a lack of zinc. In the blood, most of the zinc occurs in the red blood cells; a small amount is found in the white blood cells, platelets, and the blood serum. About a third of serum zinc is tightly bound to the protein macroglobulin, and the remainder is loosely bound to the protein albumin or to the amino acids histidine and cysteine. Blood serum levels of zinc fall during infections, pernicious anemia, hyperthyroidism, pregnancy, and the use of oral contraceptives.

Absorption and Metabolism

Zinc is absorbed primarily in the upper part of the small intestine, but little is understood about the mechanism. Absorption appears to be regulated in the cells in the intestinal wall, which respond to zinc levels in the plasma. It is likely that absorption is aided by a *ligand,* or binding substance, such as dietary histidine, citric acid, or one that is secreted in pancreatic juices. Zinc enters the mucosal cells (attached to the protein metallothien) lining the intestinal tract, where it is either stored until the mature cells are sloughed off, utilized in the metabolism of the absorbing cell, or released to pass through to the blood. In the blood, zinc is bound to a protein and carried to the liver; there it is stored until needed. In the average adult, one third to one half of the 10 to 15 mg provided daily in the diet is absorbed. Increased needs during pregnancy and lactation are reflected by up to a twofold increase in absorption.

Absorption is decreased as the stores of zinc increase or when the diet contains large amounts of whole grains in which either phytic acid or fiber may bind zinc as an insoluble complex. Oxalic acid in some vegetables has a similar effect. Typical diets usually do not contain enough fiber to depress zinc absorption. High levels of dietary calcium or copper also result in lowered absorption of zinc. Although this does not appear to be a problem with normal dietary intakes, the current trend toward high levels of calcium supplements is a concern.

In addition, nonheme iron interacts competitively with zinc and interferes with absorption when its ratio to zinc reaches 2:1 (because they compete for the common carrier, transferrin). This may be of concern if large iron supplements are taken during pregnancy. Except for the presence of a zinc-binding substance in human milk, there is no evidence of any dietary component that enhances zinc absorption.

It is unclear how zinc is distributed from the blood to the cells, but in humans zinc appears in the tissues within 15 minutes of intake. Tissues such as the liver, kidneys, lungs, pancreas, and testes release absorbed zinc rapidly, whereas the brain, muscle, and red blood cells turn it over slowly and hair and bone turn it over even more slowly.

Zinc is excreted in the feces, but again, the mechanism is unknown. Unabsorbed zinc, along with zinc from mucosal cells and that secreted in the pancreatic enzymes, is excreted in the feces. Fecal zinc varies in proportion to dietary zinc but always includes about 1.5 mg from pancreatic secretions. A small amount is lost in the urine (0.4 to 0.6 mg), in sweat (1 to 3 mg), and in semen (1 mg).

Functions

The functions of zinc fall into four main categories:

1. As part of metalloenzymes, at least 120 of which have been identified
2. In stabilization of membranes
3. In the protein-synthesizing structures in the cell
4. As a free ion within the cell where it functions as a cofactor in many reactions.

As a result, zinc affects many body functions.

Reproduction

Because zinc has its most profound influence on rapidly growing tissues, its effect on reproduction is significant. Offspring of zinc-deficient rats were either born with congenital malformations or serious defects in the central nervous system and brain. Figure 11-12 illustrates the difference in specific brain cells, the Purkinje cells, when zinc is adequate or deficient. Severely deficient animals are not able to reproduce.

In humans, the mother has transferred about 150 mg of zinc to the fetus by the time of birth. Maternal zinc deficiency is clearly associated with low-birth-weight infants and is suggested as a cause of central nervous system problems. Zinc-deficient men have shown retarded gonadal development. Impaired sexual maturity in both sexes is another result of zinc deficiency.

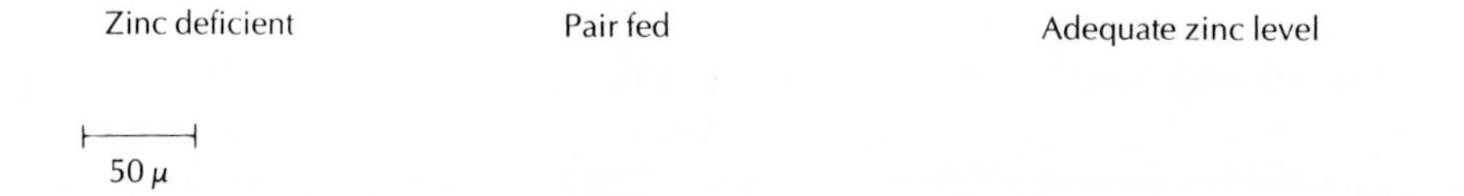

Figure 11-12 Specialized brain cells (Purkinje cells) from 21-day-old rats on a diet adequate in zinc and deficient in zinc, compared to pair-fed controls, which are given the same amount of diet with zinc as was eaten by the zinc-deficient rats.

Courtesy Gary Fosmire, Pennsylvania State University, and Christopher Dvergstein, University of North Dakota.

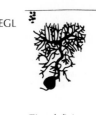

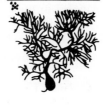

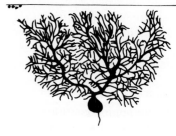

Skin Health

Zinc concentrates in wound tissue and plays a role in the incorporation of the amino acid methionine into the protein of the skin. In humans, zinc is most critical in the latter part of the healing process, when the epidermal (or surface) layers of the skin are healing. Supplementary zinc is effective in promoting healing only when people have low zinc intakes. There is no added advantage from high levels of zinc.

The role of oral zinc in the treatment of acne showed that a supplement of zinc sulfate in the diet resulted in a decrease of from 15% to 100% in acne scars, over a period of 4 weeks. Zinc is also successful in the treatment of an often fatal condition known as *acrodermatitis enteropathica,* which is believed to be caused by reduced absorption of zinc from a genetically caused failure to produce the zinc-binding protein. This condition usually appears within the first few months of life and is associated with the change from breast milk, which contains a zinc-binding protein that aids absorption, to formula, which contains unbound zinc. Skin rashes, diarrhea, and loss of hair are common symptoms in these infants.

Symptoms of zinc deficiency.
Photos courtesy Dr. Harold Sanstead, University of Texas Medical Branch, Galveston.

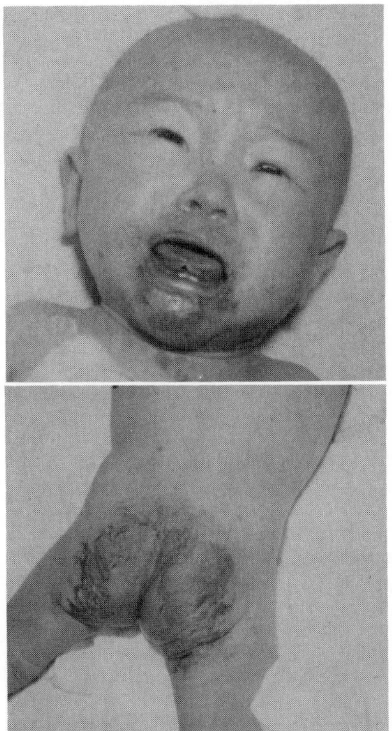

A, Infant with acrodermatitis on mouth, *top,* and on buttocks, *bottom,* as a result of zinc-deficient formula.

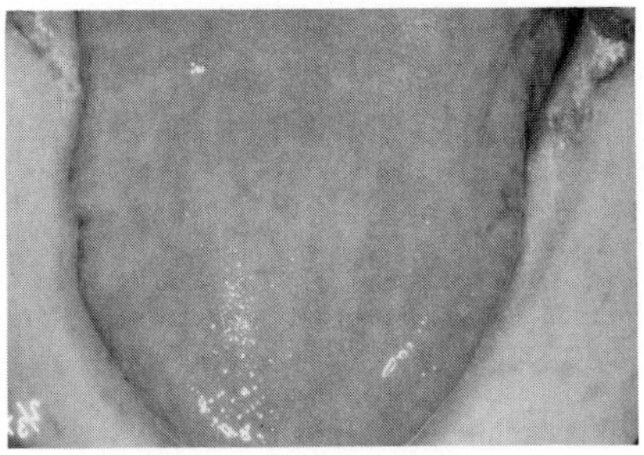

B, Smooth tongue (glossitis)–zinc deficiency as a result of giardiasis (parasitic infection).

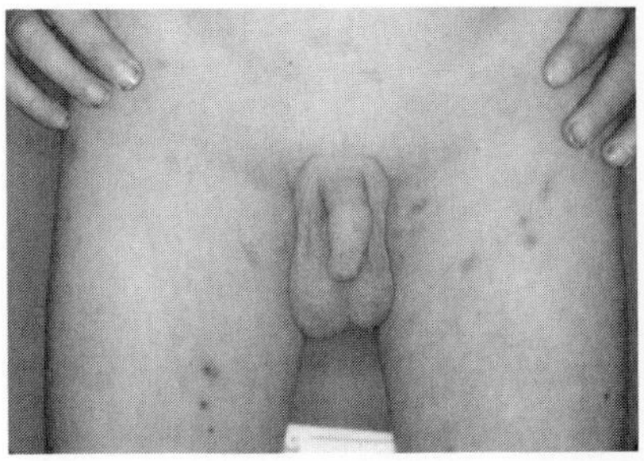

C, Delayed sexual development in late adolescence.

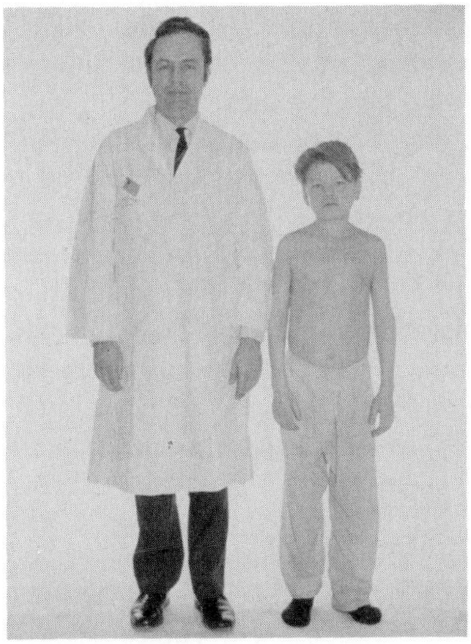

D, Short stature or delayed growth. On the left, a male of normal stature and development; on the right, a zinc-deficient adult male with impaired development.

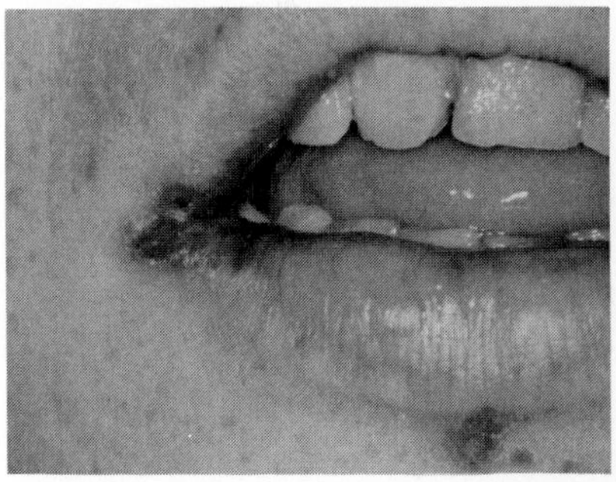

E, Bilateral oral lesions at corners of mouth.

hypogeusia
Loss of sense of taste

hyposmia
Loss of sense of smell

Taste

Low blood levels of zinc have been associated with **hypogeusia,** in which there is a loss of a sense of the taste. Hypogeusia is usually accompanied by **hyposmia,** or loss of the sense of smell. These abnormalities often occur under the stress of burns, bone fractures, and infections and may partially account for the poor appetite of hospitalized patients. Both conditions seem to characterize slight to moderate deficiencies, but only in severe zinc depression is hypogeusia clearly related.

When depressed appetite is caused by low dietary zinc, zinc sulfate (2 mg/kg of body weight/day) has been helpful in restoring taste and appetite, which may be critical in the recovery of the patient. Zinc sulfate (with 40 mg zinc/100 mg) has been used to counteract the anorexia experienced by cancer patients.

Growth

Growth in humans suffering from zinc deficiency is severely stunted, reflecting its role in protein synthesis. A diet high in animal protein, supplemented with zinc, results in a very rapid growth response.

Other Roles

As a part of many vital enzymes, zinc is involved in many other functions. It aids in the action of insulin and, hence, affects glucose tolerance. Zinc also helps mobilize vitamin A from its storage site in the liver and facilitates the synthesis of DNA and RNA necessary for cell reproduction. It is essential for the metabolism of alcohol, is necessary for many digestive enzymes, such as pancreatic lipase, and protects against exposure to heavy metals such as cadmium and lead.

Requirements

Recommended Dietary Allowances for Zinc (mg/day)

Children 1-10 yr	10 mg
All other 10+ yr	15 mg
Pregnant women	20 mg
Lactating women	25 mg

Isotope studies of body zinc show a daily turnover of 6 mg. Studies of adult men who consumed a liquid formula diet with less than 0.3 mg of zinc/day showed a daily loss of 2.6 mg of zinc in urine, feces, skin, semen, hair, and nails. After allowing for individual variations and 25% absorption, a dietary intake of 15 mg of zinc/day is suggested. For women, whose menstrual losses are negligible, 15 mg should be adequate unless the diet is devoid of animal foods. Canadian standards have been set considerably lower, at 8 mg for women and 9 mg for men. During growth spurts, needs are slightly higher for both boys and girls, who retain approximately 0.8 and 1.06 mg of zinc/day, respectively.

For pregnant women, an additional 1, 2, and 5 mg of zinc is recommended to ensure that 0.1, 0.4, and 0.75 mg are available in successive trimesters to meet the needs of the growing fetus and placenta. For lactation, an additional 10 mg is suggested to ensure that the mother can provide 1.6 mg of zinc, which is transferred to the milk each day. In setting these allowances, the Food and Nutrition Board assumed a diet with 25% zinc absorption.

colostrum
The first thin, yellow, watery secretion of the human breast following birth; earliest breast milk

Allowances for infants based on the zinc concentration of human milk, which drops from 20 mg/liter in **colostrum** (the earliest form of breast milk) to 2.6 mg/liter in the mature breast milk, are set at 3 to 5 mg/day for early infancy. Formula-fed infants require more because zinc in cow's milk is less available.

Food Sources

Only recently has it been recognized that the North American diet may not provide optimal amounts of zinc. The relatively frequent incidence of hypogeusia, delayed wound healing, and growth failure, which are all signs of zinc deficiency, support the notion that inadequate intakes may be more common than suspected and that a significant portion of the population may have marginal intakes. Recent analyses of the zinc content of typical diets in the United States show a mean content of 9.0 mg of zinc/day for women and 14.3 mg for men. Zinc available in the food supply is estimated at 12.5 mg per person, suggesting that careful dietary planning is necessary if RDAs are to be met.

The zinc content of the most commonly used foods and recommended zinc sources are shown in Table 11-8. From these data, it is evident that the best sources of zinc, seafood and meat, are expensive foods. Less expensive foods such as cereals and legumes contain significant amounts of zinc, but they also contain phytic acid and other substances that can appreciably interfere with intestinal absorption of zinc. In addition, up to 80% of the zinc in whole-grain cereals may be lost in milling. The availability of zinc from leavened whole-wheat bread is enhanced 30% to 50%, compared with the availability from unleavened bread; this

Table 11-8 ◇ Amount of zinc in average servings of most frequently used foods

Food	Amount	Kcal	Zinc per Serving (mg)	Zinc per 100 Kcal	INQ*
Meat, Fish, Eggs, Poultry, and Nuts					
Egg, fried	1 large	95	0.5	0.5	0.7
Roast beef	3 oz	315	5.3	1.7	2.0
Ground beef	3 oz	230	3.8	1.6	2.2
Chicken	3 oz	140	2.5	1.7	2.4
Tuna	3 oz	165	0.9	0.5	0.7
Peanut butter	2 T	190	1.0	0.5	0.6
Bacon	3 slices	110	0.6	0.6	0.7
Lunch meat	3 oz	190	1.8	0.9	1.3
Oysters†	½ cup	80	8.2	10.3	15.5
Pork†	3 oz	275	3.2	1.1	1.5
Cereals					
Cornflakes	1 cup	110	0.1	0.1	0.1
Shredded wheat	1 biscuit	100	0.8	0.8	1.0
Saltines	4 crackers	50	—	—	0
Rice, dry	1 oz	109	0.3	0.3	0.4
White bread	1 slice	65	0.2	0.3	0.4
Whole-wheat bread	1 slice	70	0.5	0.7	0.9
Beans, dried (cooked)†	1 cup	210	1.8	0.9	1.1
Dairy Products					
Whole milk	8 oz	150	0.9	0.6	0.8
2% fat milk	8 oz	120	0.9	0.7	1.0
Cheddar cheese	1 oz	115	0.9	0.7	1.0
Fruits					
Apple	1 medium	80	0.1	0.1	0.2
Banana	1 medium	105	0.2	0.2	0.3
Orange juice, frozen	4 oz	55	0.1	0.2	0.3
Peach	1 medium	35	0.1	0.3	0.4
Vegetables					
Corn, canned	4 oz (½ cup)	82	0.4	0.5	0.7
Green beans	4 oz (½ cup)	22	0.2	1.0	1.1
Green peas	4 oz (½ cup)	62	0.7	1.0	1.5
Lettuce	¼ head	20	0.4	2.0	2.6
Tomatoes	1 medium	25	0.2	0.8	1.0
Potato, baked	1 medium	130	0.4	0.3	0.4
Lima beans†	½ cup	95	1.7	1.7	2.4

*INQ = % US RDA zinc (15 mg)/% Energy requirement (2000 Kcal). INQ > 2.0 = good source.
†Sources of zinc usually included in recommended lists.

is apparently because of the release of bound zinc in phytates in the leavened bread. Fruits and vegetables are low in zinc.

The observation that people with low incomes may have less than optimal intakes was confirmed in an analysis of the diets of preadolescent girls, from low-income families, who were ingesting only 4.7 mg of zinc—considerably lower than the recommended 10 mg. Drinking water, with less than 0.1 mg of zinc/liter, is a negligible source.

Diagnosis of a Deficiency

Assessment of zinc status is difficult because neither serum nor plasma zinc levels reflect body stores, and the validity of measuring zinc-containing enzymes has not been established. Assessment is complicated by inflammations or low blood albumin levels. Neither red blood cell levels nor urinary zinc excretion are sensitive indicators.

The analysis of zinc in a sample of hair may be useful in detecting a severe deficiency or excess but is questionable for assessing a marginal deficiency. In hair analysis, care must be taken to prevent contamination from zinc in shampoos or other preparations used on the hair.

Taste acuity, as well as testing for levels of zinc in saliva, skin, fingernails, and white blood cells, are under investigation as possible diagnostic tools. So are measures of the uptake, retention, and turnover of stable isotopes of zinc. Until an acceptable test is available, it will be difficult to assess zinc status.

Toxicity

Although intakes of 2 grams or more of zinc sulfate cause acute gastrointestinal problems and vomiting, there have been few reports of toxicity from its ingestion even with doses up to 200 mg. However, we have had inadequate opportunity to assess the effect of these doses of zinc over months or years. For this reason, unsupervised supplementation of the diet with zinc is discouraged. The ingestion of excess zinc resulting from the storage of food and beverages in galvanized containers has resulted in fever, nausea, vomiting, and diarrhea. Moreover, toxicity has been associated with the inhalation of zinc chloride from industrial pollution. Among the metabolic effects of zinc toxicity are impaired immune function, a loss of as much as 50% of iron in the liver, followed by a loss of copper much later. Both of these losses may result in anemia. The possibility of an **atherogenic** effect (hardening of the arteries) from overuse of zinc was suggested by reports of a 25% decrease in HDL in healthy men taking a daily supplement of 440 mg zinc sulfate. This level also has an effect on copper metabolism and could aggravate a marginal copper deficiency by blocking copper absorption.

atherogenic
Causing atherosclerosis, or hardening of the arteries

Table 11-9 gives a summary of relevant biological data from iron, copper, and zinc.

SELENIUM (Se)

Scattered findings of selenium deficiencies in humans and animals were reported as far back as 1295 by Marco Polo, but it was not until 1957 that selenium was found to be an essential element. At that time, it was shown that selenium was effective in curing animal diseases that had previously been considered the result of vitamin E deficiency. Before 1957, selenium had been of interest only as a substance that was toxic to livestock.

The explanation for the presence of both selenium toxicity and deficiency in the United States lies in the variation of the selenium content in the soil. This variation, in turn, influences the amount of selenium in plants grown in the soil; the plants are then directly responsible for the selenium in the diet of animals.

Table 11-9 ◆ Relevant biological data on iron, copper, and zinc

	Iron	Copper	Zinc
U.S. RDA	18 mg	2 mg	15 mg
Amount available in food supply	17.6 mg		12.5 mg
Average daily intake			
NHANES II	13.1 mg		
NFCS	103% RDA		
FDA, 1982	18 mg	1.6 mg	12.7 mg
Major food sources			
Meat, fish, poultry	36%		
Cereal products	31%		
Fruits and vegetables	21%		
Milk and dairy products			
Total amount in body	2.5-3.5 grams	70-80 mg	2-2.5 grams
Distribution in body tissues			
Blood	60%-75%	15%	<1%
Liver, spleen, and bone	0%-30%	22-30	
Muscle	3%		
Skeleton	—	25%	75%
Skin	—	15%	1.5%
Brain		8%	
Indicators of normal nutritional status	Hemoglobin: 15.0 g/dl (men) 13.6 g/dl (women) Total iron-binding capacity: 30%-40% Serum ferritin: 10 ng/dl	Serum copper: 90 μg/dl	Red blood cell zinc: 10.2-13.4 μg/ml Serum zinc: 75-100 μg/dl Hair zinc: 180 μg/g Urinary excretion 230-600 μg/gram creatinine

Regions near the Great Lakes, along the Atlantic seaboard, and on the Northwest coast are generally deficient in selenium, while a belt of land stretching through the Midwest from Canada to Venezuela includes isolated areas with very high selenium contents.

Distribution

Selenium reserves of approximately 15 mg are believed to be concentrated in the liver. Plasma levels of 150 μg/liter, considered normal in the United States, are considerably above the 50 μg/liter found in adults in New Zealand where the soil is selenium deficient but there is no other evidence of a deficiency.

In choosing a multinutrient supplement, you should look for one containing selenium. About half of the supplements on the market contain selenium. Do *not* take separate selenium supplements without medical advice.

Functions

For years, there was a puzzle regarding the overlap between the functions of selenium and vitamin E. This was resolved when it was discovered that selenium was an essential part of the enzyme glutathione peroxidase, which inactivates the enzymes that cause the oxidation or rancidity in fats. Vitamin E, an antioxidant, was known to function similarly by competing with fat for available oxygen. Because of this similar function, there is an inverse relationship between vitamin E in the diet and the selenium requirement.

Other possible roles for selenium are associated with liver function, the release of energy to the cells, and the development of the structural protein of sperm cells. These roles are under study but are not yet confirmed.

Role in Human Nutrition

The selenium-containing enzyme glutathione peroxidase is necessary for the breakdown of peroxides, which are formed when fats are oxidized (become rancid). There is currently considerable speculation that selenium may play a protective role against cancer, primarily because of its antioxidant capacity. Studies in China, where selenium levels are very low, indicate that *Keshan disease,* in which the heart muscles of children and women of childbearing age undergo degeneration, can be cured by selenium supplements. In New Zealand, where the selenium content of the soil is low, there is evidence that the use of selenium alleviates discomfort in abdominal muscles following surgery.

Patients on intravenous feedings devoid of selenium have shown muscular discomfort, fingernail defects, and biochemical abnormalities in red blood cells that have responded to selenium.

Total Dietary Selenium

Because selenium in foods varies so much depending on the area in which each food is grown, it is difficult to estimate the amount present in typical diets. In New Zealand, where selenium is very low, intakes fall as low as 28 μg daily; in Venezuela, where selenium is high, the intake is over 200 μg daily. In the United States, it is estimated that the average daily selenium intake per person can be as low as 60 μg in areas with marginally low selenium in the soil or as high as 150 μg where soil is high in selenium. Water with less than 1 μg of selenium/liter is not a major contributor to the selenium intake.

Requirements

Several balance studies have helped us estimate selenium requirements. One study of women in New Zealand showed that 24 μg of selenium/day was enough to maintain balance. On the other hand, a study of adult men and women in the United States showed that men needed 80 μg daily and women, 57 μg. These higher values probably reflect the fact that body stores in the United States are higher than those in New Zealand, where the selenium content of the soil is much lower. In 1985, the RDA Committee thought there was enough evidence to propose an RDA for selenium. So far their recommendation of 1 μg/kg of body weight has not been accepted.

A pregnant woman, who transfers a total of 1.25 mg of selenium to her fetus, needs 14 μg/day during the last trimester. If 80% of the selenium is absorbed, her intake should be increased by 18 μg. During lactation, an additional 16 μg is recommended.

Those using selenium supplements, especially over 150 μg of selenium daily, should recognize the potential dangers associated with these higher intakes. In one reported case of selenium toxicity a subject took one 27.3-mg tablet daily for 77 days, which resulted in a loss of hair, nail changes, nausea, and vomiting. There is currently increasing evidence that selenium at moderate daily levels of 250 to 300 μg protects against cancer or heart disease, but the question is still under study.

Proposed (but as yet unpublished) Dietary Intakes for Selenium (μg/day)

Children	1-1.9 yr	20
	2-5.9 yr	25
	6-9.9 yr	35
Males	10-11.9 yr	45
	12-17.9 yr	60
	18-24.9 yr	75
	25-69.9 yr	80
	70+ yr	95
Females	10-14.9 yr	50
	15-17.9 yr	60
	18-49.9 yr	65
	50+ yr	70

Safe and adequate daily dietary intake for children, age 7 yr—50 to 200 μg

Table 11-10 ◇ Selenium content of total diet and of pork muscle in various parts of the country

	Dietary Intake (μg/day)	Content of Pork Muscle (μg/100 gram)
New York	46	125
Iowa	278	800
Nebraska	313	1140
South Dakota	521	1700

Food Sources

The selenium content of plant foods reflects the content of the soil in which they were grown. The soil content also influences the amount of selenium in the muscle, eggs, or milk of animals raised on crops grown in the soil. Data in Table 11-10 illustrate this. Although seafood has a high selenium content, its value as a dietary source is reduced because of the poor availability of its selenium. For example, selenium in tuna is only 50% available, possibly because it tends to bind to heavy metals such as mercury. Organ meats, muscle meats, cereals, and dairy products rank in descending order as good sources of selenium. The amount of selenium present in food tends to parallel the protein content of the food. Selenium is reduced by the milling process and is lost as vegetables are boiled.

OTHER MICRONUTRIENTS

In addition to the seven macronutrient elements discussed in the previous chapter and the micronutrient elements iron, iodine, zinc, and selenium discussed in this chapter, 11 other mineral elements, designated **ultratrace elements,** are present in the body in small and variable amounts and are essential in human metabolism. In the human body, these micronutrients are almost always bound to organic compounds rather than being free inorganic elements. They are: manganese, copper, molybdenum, chromium, nickel, vanadium, silicon, tin, arsenic, boron, and cobalt. Because of its close association with water, the trace element fluorine was discussed in Chapter 9.

ultratrace elements
Elements needed in amounts smaller than a trace element
- Manganese (Mn)
- Copper (Cu)
- Molybdenum (Mo)
- Chromium (Cr)
- Nickel (Ni)
- Vanadium (V)
- Silicon (Si)
- Tin (Sn)
- Arsenic (As)
- Boron (B)
- Cobalt (Co)

Nanogram (ng) = 1 part per billion (ppb)

Microgram (μg) = 1 part per million (ppm)

The use of the term trace element or the newer term ultratrace to describe this group of micronutrients is unfortunate because for some people it may imply a lack of nutritional importance. The term "trace" dates back to a time when analytical techniques were sensitive enough to detect the presence of elements but not sensitive enough to measure the minute amounts needed. The use of new analytical techniques has made it possible to detect amounts as low as 1 ppb (1 μg/kg) in natural material. Additionally, the use of isotopes has made it possible to study the metabolism of many of these elements. The concentrations at which trace elements are functional are often extremely small; for example, 1 part in 10 million is often all that is needed. Micronutrient deficiencies in the soil in various parts of the country influence the growth of both plants and animals in these areas.

Seven other micronutrients, whose essential nature has not yet been established on the basis of present criteria, may eventually be classified as essential.

Because some aspects of metabolism are common to many of these 11 microelements, they will be discussed as a group. A brief discussion of the unique aspects of each one follows the general discussion. The limited space allocated to these elements relative to those just discussed reflects only our limited knowledge of them, not their importance.

Relative body stores of minerals

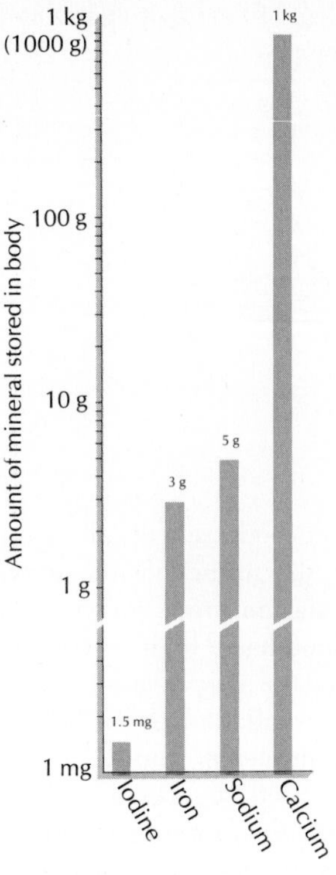

Roles in the Body

As mentioned before, the small amounts of micronutrients needed in the diet or stored in the body bear no relationship to their importance. A lack of one of these micronutrients can be just as serious as a lack of an element needed at levels hundreds of times higher. Some of these elements may be cofactors to biological reactions, acting as a link between the enzyme and its substrate; others are part of essential body compounds such as hormones and enzymes; others are involved in the growth of tissue. For some enzymes, nonessential elements can satisfactorily replace essential elements. It may well be that some trace elements are the most limiting factor in our diets, because many diets may be unable to provide even the minute amounts needed.

Incidence of Deficiencies

In the average diet, food comes from varied geographical sources, and the amount of micronutrient elements present in food varies with the nutrients in the soil on which they are grown. However, there is little evidence of naturally occurring dietary deficiencies. As a result, it has been difficult (but not impossible) to formulate experimental diets with an inadequate level of one micronutrient and adequate amounts of all others. Most of the evidence of the biological role of trace elements has come from animal studies. However, it has often been possible to demonstrate a similar function in human nutrition.

Interrelationships

One of the major difficulties in getting information on the functions of many mineral elements has been the extent to which the presence or absence of one element may influence the role of a second and therefore modify the requirement of the first.

The interactions among minerals may occur in the diet, during absorption in the intestine, at the sites of excretion in the kidneys or lungs, at uptake by cells, and at specific sites within the body cells. The interactions may be either **synergistic** (reciprocally helpful) or competitive.

synergistic
Working together to enhance the effect

As an example of this type of interrelationship, an increase in the molybdenum content of the diet without a simultaneous increase in copper or sulfur results in depressed growth and restricted hemoglobin production. The copper-molybdenum antagonism apparently works in both directions. Other examples include increased copper, which interferes with iron and zinc metabolism; high levels of manganese, which affect iron metabolism; and excess cobalt, which interferes with the synthesis of the iodine-containing hormone thyroxin.

Mineral Elements Interact Synergistically or in Competition with Each Other
In the diet
During absorption in the intestine
In the kidneys or lungs
At uptake by the individual cells
Within individual cells

Abnormally high levels of some elements can displace other elements that are essential parts of enzymes; this exchange makes the enzymes biologically inactive. These high levels may also interfere with the use of effective enzymes.

The ability of one element to replace another in a key compound and render it inactive is one of the hazards of using some of the mineral supplements on the commercial market. Too often, formulas for supplements are developed to give the producer a competitive advantage rather than to meet the nutritional needs of the individual. Unbalanced mineral supplements are potentially harmful; in fact, the FDA has suggested that calcium, iron, and iodine are the only mineral elements that can be justified as dietary supplements. In 1973, the FDA supported legislation to restrict the amounts of nutrients to be included in supplements, but its authority to do this was withdrawn. Therefore it is now possible for the public to buy almost any amount of most mineral elements on the open market without a prescription. The hazards of self-medication with mineral supplements are many but are insufficiently documented to support legislation that would lead to the control of their indiscriminate sale.

Because of the complexities of the interrelationships among trace mineral elements, it is necessary to assess the whole pattern of nutrient intake in studies of deficiency, toxicity, and requirements. Uncomplicated deficiencies of single micronutrient elements seldom occur under normal conditions.

Toxicity

Some trace mineral elements that are essential in small amounts may be toxic when present at higher levels. Most of the cases of toxicity from a trace mineral have been the result of exposure to an environment saturated with the element; minerals can enter the body through the respiratory tract and the skin, as well as the gastrointestinal tract. Manganese and selenium toxicities found among miners are believed to be caused by breathing air containing above-normal concentrations of the elements. Fluorine toxicity, which takes the form of dental fluorosis (mottled enamel), is the result of ingesting large quantities of water containing over 2.5 ppm of naturally occurring fluorine (see p. 239, Chapter 9).

Selenium poisoning in animals is common in areas where the selenium content of the soil is high. High urinary levels of selenium are found in humans in the same areas, although no definite evidence of selenium poisoning exists.

There are some trace elements, such as lead and cadmium (often referred to as "heavy metals"), for which no biological function has been established; they are also known to have toxic effects. For example, high levels of cadmium are associated with hypertension. On the other hand, some essential trace elements play a role in combating the toxic or damaging effects of high amounts of nonessential trace elements.

Deficiencies

Deficiencies of most trace mineral elements become evident only after prolonged dietary inadequacies and even then only when decreased absorption and other changes lead to increased need. Generally, the first evidence of inadequacy is a reduction of the enzymes for which the mineral is an essential part or a reduction in enzyme activity, which depends on a mineral cofactor. Because body stores will be drawn on to keep blood levels up in the event of a dietary deficiency, it is only when these body stores are depleted and intake is inadequate that blood levels drop.

Requirements

Until 1980, there had been no attempt to estimate human requirements for trace elements other than zinc, iron, and iodine. In the 1980 Recommended Dietary Allowances, however, the Food and Nutrition Board established standards for safe and adequate levels of several elements. In 1985, it was proposed that these should be called provisional recommended intakes.

The widespread presence of trace elements in foods, the minute amounts needed, the limited deficiency states that can be directly attributed to the lack of specific nutrients, and the interrelationships among trace elements have made the assessment of dietary needs difficult. Modification of the level of other nutrients, such as protein, in the diet may also influence the amount of a particular element needed.

Food Sources

The amounts of trace elements present in vegetable foods depend on the amounts present in the soil in which crops are grown and whether or not the elements are essential for plant growth. Because the elements must be in an inorganic form before they can be used by plants, those in "organic fertilizers" must be freed from the organic matter, usually by bacteria. In foods that come from animals, amounts of some elements reflect the diet of the animal, whereas amounts of the other elements—especially those essential for the particular species—may be controlled by the animal through the excretion of excesses. However, the ultimate source of trace elements in food is always the soil or the fertilizer used on it.

The possibility of a trace mineral deficiency is greatly reduced with modern marketing techniques that allow us to eat a diet from widely scattered areas rather than from a restricted geographic region. However, the increased use of highly refined, fabricated, or processed foods may result in a marginal intake of some trace elements. On the other hand, some elements may be introduced into foods through contamination during processing or from containers.

Milk is a relatively poor source of most micronutrient elements. In addition, it has been shown that the trace element content of human milk decreases as lactation progresses. Therefore it is suggested that other foods be added to an infant's diet after 4 or 5 months of age.

The following information is included as reference material for students, in the hope that it will provide answers to the various questions that may arise about trace elements.

Manganese (Mn)

Although no deficiency has been demonstrated in humans, manganese is considered an essential nutrient because of our knowledge of its many biochemical roles. In addition, it is essential for every animal species studied. Manganese is necessary for normal skeletal and connective tissue development. In addition, it acts as a catalyst or as part of the essential enzymes involved in the synthesis of fatty acids and cholesterol; in the formation of urea, in which nitrogen is excreted; in the

Table 11-11 ◇ Dietary sources of manganese

Rich Sources (>20 ppm)	Moderate Sources (1-5 ppm)	Poor Sources (<1 ppm)
Nuts	Green leafy vegetables	Animal tissues
Whole-grain cereals	Dried fruits	Poultry
Dried legumes	Fresh fruits	Dairy products
Tea	Nonleafy vegetables	Seafood

release of lipid from the liver; in the metabolism of carbohydrate; in the structure and function of the mitochondrion of the cell, which is essential for the release of energy; and in the synthesis of mucopolysaccharides. Both an excess and a deficiency of manganese adversely affect brain function.

Absorption and Metabolism

Manganese is absorbed in the body (in amounts of only 3% to 4%) in a way that is similar to that involved in iron absorption. A specific protein carrier, transmanganin, is available to transport manganese in the blood. Of the 10 to 20 mg of manganese stored in the body, most is concentrated in the pancreas, bone, liver, and kidneys. The amount of manganese in the body is controlled by the amount excreted in the bile. (Little is excreted in the urine.) Large intakes of calcium and iron depress manganese absorption. Newborn infants apparently lose manganese in the first few weeks of life but do not suffer any adverse consequences because of it.

Requirements and Food Sources

The provisional recommended intake of manganese has been estimated at 2.5 to 5 mg (35 to 70 μg/kg of body weight) for adults. Intakes less than 0.7 mg are considered inadequate. Therefore the 3.6 mg of manganese/day in a typical North American diet, obtained from plants, is considered sufficient.

Estimated Safe and Adequate Daily Dietary Intakes for Manganese (mg/day)

Children	1-3 yr	1.0-1.5
	4-6 yr	1.5-2.0
	7-10 yr	2.0-3.0
Adults	11 + yr	2.5-5.0

Whole-grain cereals and green vegetables are among the better sources of manganese, but the amount present depends on the part of the plant used as food and the geographical source. Tea is an extremely rich source, and in English diets it provides 2.3 mg of manganese. Relative amounts of manganese in common foods are given in Table 11-11.

Toxicity

Although the accumulation of excessive amounts of manganese is toxic, it is usually the result of inhalation of industrial contamination rather than high dietary intake. Weakness and psychological and motor difficulties are manifestations of high tissue levels of manganese. Manganese toxicity occurs more often with iron deficiency, and high levels of dietary protein protect against it.

Copper (Cu)

Copper was first recognized as a dietary essential in 1928, when it was shown that anemia could be prevented only if both copper and iron were available to the body. The first case of copper deficiency in a human was reported in 1966. Since that time, we have learned about many metabolic functions of copper but have had difficulty identifying them because of the interaction of copper with other trace elements such as zinc, molybdenum, and sulfur. A number of important copper-containing proteins and enzymes are known.

Functions

Copper has already been identified as an essential component of many enzymes. Copper plays a part in preventing anemia, either by (1) aiding in iron absorption, (2) stimulating the synthesis of the heme or globin fractions of the hemoglobin molecule, or (3) releasing stored iron from the ferritin in the liver. It now appears that, as part of the multifunctional enzyme ceruloplasmin, copper plays a role in the oxidation of ferrous to ferric iron.

Copper-Containing Enzymes are Involved in
Synthesis of hair pigment
Synthesis of elastin in the aorta
Synthesis of collagen

In addition to its role in preventing anemia, copper (1) is required for the synthesis of the phospholipids, which are essential in the formation of the *myelin* surrounding nerve fibers; (2) is part of the respiratory enzyme cytochrome oxidase, which is necessary for the release of energy in the cell; (3) maintains the activity (in conjunction with vitamin C) of enzymes involved in the synthesis of both elastin, a protein in the wall of the aorta, and collagen, which is part of connective tissue; and (4) is part of the enzyme tyrosinase, needed for the conversion of the amino acid tyrosine to melanin, which is the dark pigment of hair and skin. The absence of this enzyme is associated with *albinism*, a condition in which there is no color in the hair or eyes.

Absorption and Metabolism

Typical diets provide 1 mg or less of copper, about 25% to 40% of which is absorbed. Copper is taken up rapidly from the stomach and upper intestine, where the contents are still acid. Its absorption from the intestine is dependent on a copper-binding protein, metallothionein, that also functions in the absorption of cadmium and zinc. Absorption of copper decreases when intakes of vitamin C are high, which implicates high intakes of the vitamin in copper deficiency.

Absorbed copper appears in the bloodstream in as little time as 15 minutes after being consumed. Initially, it is loosely bound to albumin or to some amino acids to produce chelates, which are combinations of a trace element with another substance. These chelates appear to have the special function of aiding in the transport of copper across the membranes and into the cells. Transport copper represents only 7% of serum copper.

Copper is removed from the blood serum by the liver. From there, copper is either excreted into the bile; stored in a protein complex containing 2% copper; or used in the synthesis of **ceruloplasmin,** another protein-copper complex that is released back into the blood, where it accounts for 60% of serum copper. Serum copper values, however, are not necessarily a valid measure of copper status because plasma copper can be maintained at the expense of liver stores.

ceruloplasmin
A copper-containing protein synthesized in the liver; the major transport form of copper in the blood

The release of copper from the liver is controlled by the adrenal gland. Some serum copper enters the bone marrow, where it is used in the synthesis of eryth-

Table 11-12 ◇ Dietary sources of copper

Rich Sources (>8 ppm)	Moderate Sources (2-8 ppm)	Poor Sources (<2 ppm)
Liver	Leafy vegetables	Milk
Shellfish (especially oysters)	Eggs	Butter
Nuts	Muscle meat	Cheese
Cocoa	Fish	Sugar
Cherries	Poultry	Fresh fruits and vegetables
Mushrooms	Peas	
Whole-grain cereals	Beans	
Gelatin	Fresh fruit	
	Refined cereals	

From Pennington JT, and Calloway DH: Copper content of foods, Journal of the American Dietetic Association 63:143, 1973.

rocuprein, the form of copper within the red blood cells. Erythrocuprein is identical to hepatocuprein in the liver and cerebrocuprein in the nerve tissue. To reduce confusion, it has been suggested that all these compounds be referred to as either cytocuprein, which reflects their structure, or as **superoxide dismutase (SOD),** which reflects their function as enzymes in red blood cells. The activity of these enzymes may suggest a technique for assessing copper status.

superoxide dismutase (SOD)
A copper-containing enzyme found in red blood cells; also known as erythrocuprein, hepatocuprein, cytocuprein, or cerebrocuprein

Copper is excreted in both feces and urine. Fecal copper includes unabsorbed dietary copper, copper released in the bile, and copper lost through the intestinal wall. Urinary copper accounts for only 4% of copper loss.

The total copper content of the body is estimated at 75 to 150 mg, with half of this concentrated in the bones and muscles. The liver, which stores 10% of body copper, is the major site for storage. The newborn infant has liver stores that are 5 to 10 times those of an adult, but they drop to adult levels as early as 3 months of age.

Requirements

Assuming 40% absorption, a dietary intake of 2 mg of copper/day replaces losses in the urine, feces, and skin. This intake maintains copper balance in men, women, and the elderly. Because estimated intakes are often less, it is possible that people adapt to lower intakes. Intake in the United States for adults is 0.93 mg/day for women and 1.24 mg/day for men, about 50% below estimated needs. Infants have an exceptional need for copper: 0.05 to 0.1 mg/kg of body weight per day. Premature infants have an even higher need.

Estimated Safe and Adequate Daily Dietary Intakes for Copper (mg/day)

1-3 yr	1.0-1.5
4-6 yr	1.5-2.0
6+ yr	2.0-3.0

Pregnant women need approximately an extra 0.3 mg copper/day to transfer 20 mg to the developing fetus. During the first 6 months of breast feeding, the mother needs an additional 0.5 mg daily. After that, 0.3 mg/day is enough.

Food Sources

Copper is widely distributed in foods, with the amount reflecting the copper content of the soil. The copper content of representative foods is given in Table 11-12. The use of copper pipes in water systems may be a source of some ingested copper. The usual copper content of the diet is close to 1 mg. Human milk has 0.25 mg/liter, and cow's milk has 0.09 mg/liter, or quart.

Deficiency

Copper deficiency, although rare in humans, was found in 7- to 9-month-old infants on a milk diet who were hospitalized because of malnutrition associated with severe diarrhea. The deficiency was recognized by a drop in ceruloplasmin (the copper-carrying protein) levels and low blood copper levels. Because infants are born with stores of copper that normally last until foods other than milk are introduced at 3 to 6 months, the copper deficiency reported here may have been caused by failure to reabsorb the copper secreted in the bile.

The copper content of hair decreases with age but may not reflect nutritional status because of contamination.

An inherited condition known as Menkes' kinky hair syndrome, which is characterized by slow growth, degeneration of brain tissue, and peculiarly stubby white hair, is associated with low serum copper and ceruloplasmin levels. The condition results from defective copper absorption, when copper taken up by intestinal cells is not released into the bloodstream.

Toxicity

Copper is toxic to humans only when it exists as the unbound copper ion. In that form, it acts as an inhibitor to many enzyme systems. There is no evidence of copper toxicity as the result of environmental contamination. Intakes of copper salts at levels 10 times higher than are found in a normal diet lead to nausea and vomiting. Chronic copper toxicity occurs in the hereditary condition called Wilson's disease, in which there is an accumulation of copper in the liver, brain, kidneys, and cornea of the eyes (where it is identified visually by brown or green rings). Penicillamine, a penicillin derivative that promotes the excretion of copper, has been used to help reduce these stores to normal levels.

Molybdenum (Mo)

Molybdenum, which has long been recognized as essential for plant growth, is now considered an essential element in human nutrition. The 9 mg of molybdenum found in the body are concentrated in the liver, kidneys, adrenal glands, and blood cells.

Functions

Molybdenum is an essential cofactor in two enzymes, xanthine oxidase and aldehyde oxidase. The former is involved in the formation of uric acid from purines and also aids in mobilizing iron from the liver reserves; the latter is necessary for the oxidation of aldehydes. Molybdenum may help in the prevention of tooth decay by promoting the retention of fluoride. Molybdenum deficiencies in humans are unknown, but it is recognized as essential in early development.

Absorption

Molybdenum is readily absorbed (25% to 80%) and is excreted mainly in the urine. The amounts absorbed and excreted are influenced largely by the amount of sulfate in the diet, with high sulfate diets increasing urinary excretion.

Requirements

Estimated Safe and Adequate Daily Dietary Intakes for Molybdenum (mg/day)

Children	1-3 yr	0.05-0.10
	4-6 yr	0.06-0.15
	7+ yr	0.10-0.30
Adults	11+ yr	0.15-0.50

The estimated recommended molybdenum intake has been set between 0.15 and 0.5 mg/day for adults. Because the usual average daily intake is 0.2 mg and varies from 0.1 to 0.46 mg, there seems little likelihood of a deficiency, except among vegetarians and people who eat a diet composed largely of very refined foods. Supplementation during pregnancy may be desirable.

Estimated safe and adequate intakes for infants and children are extrapolated from adult values on the basis of smaller body weights.

Food Sources

Legumes such as peas and beans (3 to 5 ppm) and meat (2 to 5 ppm) are relatively rich sources of molybdenum. Whole-grain cereals (0.6 to 5 ppm) and fruits and vegetables (<1 ppm) are poor sources.

Toxicity

Evidence of molybdenum toxicity is rare. Symptoms include diarrhea, a depressed growth rate, and anemia, which is associated with failure of the red blood cell to mature.

Interrelationships

Most of the interest in molybdenum has centered around its metabolic interrelationships with copper and sulfate. Depressed growth and low hemoglobin production in animals on high levels of molybdenum are associated with high urinary losses of copper and can be overcome by the addition of copper. High intakes of molybdenum may interfere with removal of copper from the blood or synthesis of the ceruloplasmin needed to transport copper.

Chromium (Cr)

Chromium was first identified as an essential element in mammals in 1959 and was first associated with human dietary deficiency in 1966. It is now considered an essential element in human nutrition.

The average amount of chromium in a person's body in the United States is about 20% that of people in the Far East. Chromium is excreted primarily in the urine; unabsorbed chromium appears in the feces; absorbed chromium tends to accumulate in the skin, muscle, and fat. The amount of chromium in the hair is a relatively sensitive indicator of chromium nutriture, but the level indicative of deficiency is not known.

Functions

Although its biochemical role has not been clearly defined, chromium has been identified as part of the glucose-tolerance factor, which is required for optimal utilization of glucose. Chromium is believed to aid in the binding of insulin to the cell, which in turn allows glucose to be taken up by the cell.

Requirements

At the present time we have sufficient information to estimate requirements but not to establish recommended dietary allowances. The fetus obtains a generous supply of chromium from the mother; the amount in the body steadily declines throughout life.

Estimated Safe and Adequate Daily Dietary Intakes for Chromium (mg/day)

Children	1-3 yr	0.02-0.08
	4-6 yr	0.03-0.12
	7-10 yr	0.05-0.20
Adults	11+ yr	0.05-0.20

Food Sources

Chromium is found in foods of plant origin, in which its level varies with plant species, soil, and season. Vegetables provide from 30 to 55 ppm; whole grains and cereals, from 30 to 70 ppm; and fruits, 20 ppm. Meat products and cheese are also good sources. White sugar and raw sugar contain undetectable amounts of chromium, whereas brown sugar and commercial syrups have appreciable amounts. Typical North American diets contain from 50 to 100 μg/day (approximately 25 μg/1000 kcal), an amount sufficient to meet a suggested adequate intake for adults of 50 to 200 μg. Lower intakes have been associated with the use of refined sugars and cereals, which contain much smaller amounts of chromium than do products that are less refined. Only 1% to 2% of dietary chromium is absorbed.

Deficiency

Low intakes of chromium have been associated with a reduced tolerance to glucose and an increasing incidence of diabetes, both of which occur with increasing age. Many cases of mild glucose intolerance can be treated successfully with chromium.

Other symptoms of chromium deficiency include decreased glycogen reserves, retarded growth, disturbed amino acid metabolism, and increased aortic lesions. This last symptom is associated with elevated blood cholesterol levels. Chromium is absent from the aorta but not from other tissues of people with coronary heart disease.

Toxicity

Inhalation of chromium from industrial waste can be toxic, and the ingestion of excess chromium in drinking water has resulted in moderately acute toxicity. There is no evidence of toxicity from excessive dietary intakes. However, the effects of chromium are known to vary with the form available, and there are many uncertainties about the effects of excessive amounts and imbalances with other nutrients. Therefore the use of chromium supplements should be discouraged.

Nickel (Ni)

An understanding of the role of nickel in metabolism has led to its inclusion in the list of mineral elements considered essential. Nickel is present in all human tissues and is firmly associated with DNA and RNA. It is also found in human blood serum as a metalloprotein.

There is little likelihood of a nickel deficiency in the human diet, although a diet devoid of fruits and vegetables would provide only marginal amounts. Malabsorption might further reduce the nickel available.

There is an interaction between nickel and iron. With an iron-deficient diet, symptoms are intensified in the presence of nickel. When iron is adequate, nickel enhances iron utilization.

Requirements appear to be between 16 and 25 μg/1000 kcal. Nickel is found in cereal grains.

Vanadium (V)

The possibility that vanadium is an essential element for humans was considered only recently. There is increasing evidence that it should be classified as a dietary essential because it is part of human tissues. Only 1% of ingested vanadium is absorbed; about 60% of this is excreted in the urine, and the remainder is retained in the liver and bones.

Estimates of the vanadium content of the average North American diet indicate that it is about 10 times higher than the estimated requirement of 0.1 to 0.3 mg/day. An intake of 100 to 125 mg/day in humans may inhibit the synthesis of cholesterol by counteracting the stimulating effect of manganese. However, failure to demonstrate a significant effect in middle-aged men has discouraged its use for reducing blood cholesterol levels.

Studies on animals indicate that vanadium plays an essential role in growth, iron, glucose, and lipid metabolism, reproduction, and bone development. There is some evidence to indicate that vanadium may be exchanged for phosphorus in the apatite crystals of tooth enamel, thereby retarding tooth decay.

Silicon (Si)

Until recently, interest in silicon centered on silicosis, or silicon toxicity, as the result of the absorption of excessive amounts of the element. It is now evident that silicon plays a role in stimulating growth, initiating calcification of bone, and promoting the synthesis of connective tissue (collagen). Although most of the evidence on a metabolic role for silicon has come from research on rats and rabbits, there is general agreement that it is essential in human nutrition. The human requirement is unknown, and information on food sources is scanty. Unrefined cereals seem to be good sources and animal foods, poor sources. Beer has a high concentration of silicon.

Tin (Sn)

Because tin is not found in the tissues of the newborn, nor is it widespread in the animal kingdom, there is still some controversy as to whether it is an essential micronutrient. However, in 1970, a definite growth response was fairly well established with the presence of 1 ppm of tin. Symptoms of deficiency range from poor growth and loss of hair to dermatitis.

Since there is very little information on the tin content of food, it is not surprising to find estimates of intakes ranging from 3 to 17 mg/day. Needs are estimated at 3 to 6 mg/day. Stannous sulfate, the most commonly available form of tin, is absorbed poorly and is excreted in the feces. Although up to 114 ppm may be dissolved from unlacquered cans into some acid-containing juices, there seems to be no basis for concern about possible toxicity.

Arsenic (As)

Through the years arsenic has been negatively associated with its poisonous potency and more recently with the occurrence of some forms of cancer. Nevertheless as early as 1937 arsenic was shown to have therapeutic value, but evidence was not conclusive until 1976 that arsenic is an essential nutrient. In experimental animal studies, depressed growth and abnormal reproduction are two of the first signs of arsenic deficiency. For humans, specific biochemical functions of arsenic are still unknown but recent findings suggest one role may be in the metabolism of the essential amino acid methionine. The estimated dietary recommendation for humans of 6.25 to 12.5 μg/1000 kcal is based on animal studies. Fish and seafood are among the richest food sources of arsenic. The biological availability of arsenic may be influenced by other dietary factors with which it interacts, such as zinc and the amino acids arginine and methionine. Arsenic is known to be an antagonist of selenium and therefore protects against selenium toxicity.

Boron (B)

Boron is the most recent element to be added to the list of essential ultratrace elements. It was discovered in 1982 as a missing growth factor, which had a definite effect on bone growth, for chicks. When postmenopausal women had their usual intake of 0.25 mg boron supplemented with 3.0 mg, they showed reduced loss of calcium and other changes, suggesting that boron may be effective in preventing the loss of bone mineral related to osteoporosis. Boron is present in high concentration in foods of plant origin, suggesting that a greater dependence on these in the diet might provide some protection against osteoporosis. Prunes, dates, raisins, and peanuts provide about 0.5 mg boron/oz, and honey 0.2 mg, while wine contains 1.0 mg/4 oz serving. Soymeal is a rich, but not very practical, source. At least two antibiotics contain boron.

Cobalt (Co)

Functions

In human nutrition, the major (and only known) role of cobalt is as an essential part of vitamin B_{12}, or cobalamin, which is necessary to prevent pernicious anemia. Humans do not have the ability to synthesize this vitamin and must depend on animal sources to get it. Therefore cobalt itself is not a dietary essential for humans, but the cobalt-containing vitamin B_{12} is.

There is increasing evidence that cobalt may be essential in the functioning of several other essential enzymes. It is absorbed primarily from the jejunum (part of the upper intestine) by the same pathway as iron. About 85% of cobalt is excreted in the urine; a small amount is excreted in the feces and sweat.

Food Sources

The average daily North American diet contains about 300 mg of cobalt. The amount of cobalt in some representative foods is given in Table 11-13. In spite of the large amount of cobalt taken in, only the 0.04 μg required in vitamin B_{12} is needed. The cobalt content of plants reflects the amount of cobalt in the soil where they are grown.

Toxicity

High intakes of cobalt may have toxic effects, one of which is a goitrogenic effect after prolonged ingestion of cobaltous chloride. The enlarged thyroid gland returns

Table 11-13 ◇ Dietary sources of cobalt (micrograms per grams of dry weight)

Rich Sources (>5 ppm)	Moderate Sources (1.5-5 ppm)	Poor Sources (<0.05 ppm)
Liver	Lean beef	Cereal grains
Kidney	Lamb	Leguminous seeds
Oysters	Veal	Green leafy vegetables
Clams	Poultry	Yeast
	Saltwater fish	
	Milk	

to normal after the use of cobalt ceases. High intakes in animals have caused *polycythemia*, an increase in the number of red blood cells, and hyperplasia (an increase in the quantity) of bone marrow. These effects are believed to be the result of the production of erythropoietin, the hormone that stimulates red blood cell formation in the bone marrow.

Polycythemia is also seen in cobalt toxicity associated with beer drinking. (Cobalt is added to beer to control foaming.) A synergistic effect between cobalt and ethanol has been identified as the cause of cardiac problems in people who drink large quantities of beer. The vasodilation observed with high dosages of cobalt has led to its use in treating hypertension in humans.

BY NOW YOU SHOULD KNOW

- Iron, iodine, zinc, selenium, manganese, copper, molybdenum, chromium, nickel, vanadium, silicon, tin, boron, arsenic, and cobalt are all essential micronutrient elements.
- There are other mineral elements that may eventually be considered essential as we acquire more sensitive techniques to study them.
- Iron is an essential component of hemoglobin; its presence permits oxygen and carbon dioxide to be transferred from one tissue to another.
- Iron-deficiency anemia is one of the most prevalent nutritional deficiencies in the United States.
- Iron-deficiency anemia can result from eating an iron-poor diet for a long period of time, from depressed iron absorption, from blood loss, or from all three.
- Women during childbearing years have the highest RDA for iron.
- Iron in food comes in two forms: heme and nonheme iron. Heme is found in the flesh of animal foods and nonheme is found in other animal foods (such as eggs and milk products) and plants.
- Breads and cereals are usually enriched with iron.
- Iodine is an essential component of thyroxin, and therefore it plays a major role in regulating the basal metabolic rate.
- Iodine deficiency results in goiter. Iodization of salt has decreased the incidence of goiter.
- Zinc has many functions in the body.
- Food processing may decrease the amount of zinc and many of the other trace minerals in a food product.
- Some trace elements may be introduced during processing for functional purposes or as contaminants.
- A diet high in phytates reduces the availability of both iron and zinc.
- It is difficult to make precise estimates of the requirements for trace elements in the diet, because of the difficulty in assessing the amount in the diet due to the wide variation in the content of food from various parts of the United States.

- For some elements, such as selenium, there is evidence of toxicity from the consumption of excessive amounts.
- The study of trace elements is already complicated and is likely to become even more so as research, which is increasing at a phenomenal rate, reveals more of the complex interrelationships among these elements.

STUDY QUESTIONS

1. Why have we only recently learned about many of the trace elements?
2. Name five commonly eaten foods that contain zinc.
3. How would you determine if you had iron-deficiency anemia?
4. Why is salt iodized?
5. Trace the absorption and transportation of iron.
6. If the body has no mechanism to excrete iron, why does iron-deficiency anemia occur?
7. What is the role of hydrochloric acid in the absorption of iron?
8. Sequentially list the steps that occur when the oxygen-carrying capacity of the blood decreases.
9. A food label lists the content of iron in one serving of the food to be 15% of the U.S. RDA. How many milligrams of iron are in that food? (Use the U.S. RDA table in Appendix C.)

Applying What You've Learned

1. Assess Your Iron Intake

Record all the foods and beverages you consumed today. Use Appendix F to add up the milligrams of iron in your diet. Compare your total to your RDA. From the foods you listed, circle the foods that contributed iron to your diet. Now divide those foods into heme and nonheme food sources.

Study the meals that contained iron, answering the following:

Did the meals include a food rich in vitamin C (citrus fruits or vegetables)? How will this affect availability of the iron?

Was coffee or tea consumed during the meal or within the hour following? If so, what influence will this have on iron availability?

Were foods high in bran or phytates part of the meal? If so, what is the effect on iron absorption?

List several ways you could improve the iron quality of your diet.

2. Quick Checklist to Determine the Adequacy of Iron in Your Diet

Evaluate your iron intake by considering:

Do you include at least 3 oz of meat in your daily food intake?
Is your diet rich in both heme and nonheme food sources?
Do you include fruits and vegetables in your meals that have iron-rich foods?
Do you buy enriched grain products?
Do you cook acid foods such as tomato sauce in cast iron pans?
Do you use dairy products in place of meat as your source of protein? (Remember dairy products are a poor source of iron)

3. Determine Your Zinc Intake

Record everything you consumed today and use Table 11-8 to determine your zinc intake. Compare your intake to your RDA.

Make a pie graph showing the contribution of various food groups to the zinc content of your diet.

4. Check Your Dietary Practices

Go to your cupboard and read the label on your salt. Is it iodized?

5. **Determine If You Live in a Goitrous Area**

   Use Figure 11-11 to determine if you live in or close to a goitrous part of the United States.

6. **Determine the INQ of Your Breakfast Cereal**

   Read the nutrition information on your breakfast cereal. What is the %U.S. RDA of iron in a serving? Equate the % iron to milligrams of iron. (Use Appendix C to determine the U.S. RDA.) Determine the INQ for iron in this cereal. Is the INQ greater than 1? Is your cereal nutrient dense in iron?

7. **Evaluate Your Trace Element Intake**

   You have learned that trace elements are lost in food processing. Evaluate your trace element intake by comparing the number of foods you take in that are highly processed versus those that are eaten most closely to their natural state. List the foods that contribute the greatest amount of trace elements in your diet. Now list the foods that have lost trace elements due to processing.

SUGGESTED READINGS

Baer MT, and King JC: Tissue zinc levels and zinc excretion during experimental zinc depletion in young men, American Journal of Clinical Nutrition 39:556, 1984.

This article, presenting the results of 10-week balance study to assess the zinc requirements of young men, is an excellent example of the complexity of trying to assess the need for a trace element. It is especially recommended for the student who is interested in experimental nutrition.

Finch CA, and Huebers HH: Perspectives in iron metabolism, New England Journal of Medicine 306:1520, 1982.

This slightly technical article presents an update of iron metabolism that deals with body iron and iron balance, exchange, deficiency, and overload.

Herbert V: Recommended dietary intakes (RDI) of iron in humans, American Journal of Clinical Nutrition 45:678, 1987.

This paper presents the evidence on which recommended dietary allowances are proposed. It covers minimum requirements, sources, absorption, measurement of nutritional status, and toxicity.

International Nutritional Anemia Consultative Group: Iron deficiency in infancy and childhood, Washington, D.C., 1981, Nutrition Foundation, Inc.

International Nutritional Anemia Consultative Group: Iron deficiency in women, Washington, D.C., 1981, Nutrition Foundation, Inc.

These are two comprehensive reviews (in nontechnical language) of the important features of iron metabolism, changing iron needs during development, iron requirements, methods of preventing iron deficiency, and diagnosis and treatment of iron deficiency. They provide the practitioner with a complete understanding of the problem of iron deficiency and the effectiveness of various prevention and treatment approaches.

Melki IA, Bulus NM, and Abumdrad NA: Trace elements in Nutrition, Nutrition in Clinical Practice 2:230, 1987.

The authors present a concise, articulate review of the role of the trace elements of concern in total parenteral nutrition, with special reference to the application of our knowledge in clinical situations. They include a discussion of the assessment of nutritional status of the elements, the deficiency symptoms, and the effects, if any, of high levels of intake. The heavy metals, lead and cadmium, are included.

O'Dell BL: Bioavailability of trace elements, Nutrition Reviews 42:301, 1984.

This well-documented article presents current information on the various factors that influence the amount of a trace element that can be absorbed and utilized to perform essential body functions. It focuses particularly on interactions among nutrients and their effect on all aspects of metabolism.

ADDITIONAL READINGS

Greger JL: Mineral availability/new concepts, Nutrition Today 22:4, 1987.

Forbes RM, and Erdman W: Bioavailability of trace mineral elements, Annual Review of Nutrition 3:213, 1983.

Jacob RA, and others: Whole body surface loss of trace metals in normal males, American Journal of Clinical Nutrition 34:1379, 1981.

Mills CF: Dietary interaction involving the trace elements, Annual Review of Nutrition 5:173, 1985.

Iron

Beard, J: Iron fortification—rationale and effects, Nutrition Today 21:17, 1987.

Brittin HC, and Nossaman CE: Iron content of food cooked in iron utensils, Journal of the American Dietetic Association 86:897, 1986.

Cook JD, and Finch CA: Assessing iron status of a population, American Journal of Clinical Nutrition 32:2115, 1979.

Dallman PR, Yip R, and Johnson C: Prevalance and causes of anemia in the United States, 1976 to 1980, American Journal of Clinical Nutrition 39:437, 1984.

Finch CA, and Huebers H: Perspectives in iron metabolism, New England Journal of Medicine 306:1520, 1982.

Finch CA, and Cook JD: Iron deficiency, American Journal of Clinical Nutrition 39:471, 1984.

Hallberg L: Bioavailability of dietary iron in men, Annual Review of Nutrition 1:123, 1981.

Hallberg L, and others: Low bioavailability of carbonyl iron in man: studies on iron fortification of wheat flour, American Journal of Clinical Nutrition 43:59, 1986.

Hallberg L, Rosander L, and Skanberg A: Phytates and the inhibitory effect of bran on iron absorption in man, American Journal of Clinical Nutrition 45:988, 1987.

Helman AD: Vitamin and iron status in new Canadians, American Journal of Clinical Nutrition 45:785, 1987.

International Anemia Nutritional Consultative Group: Measurements of iron status, Washington, D.C., 1987, Nutrition Foundation, Inc.

Lynch SR, and others: Iron status of elderly Americans, American Journal of Clinical Nutrition 36:1032, 1982.

Meyers LD, and others: Prevalences of anemia and iron deficiency anemia in black and white women in the United States estimated by two methods, American Journal of Public Health 73:1042, 1983.

Monsen ER: Iron nutrition and absorption: dietary factors which impair iron bioavailability, Journal of the American Dietetics Association 88(7):786, 1988.

Monsen ER, and Balintfy JL: Calculating dietary iron availability: refinement and computerization, Journal of American Dietetic Association 80:307, 1982.

Review: Interaction of iron, copper, and zinc, Nutrition Reviews 45:167, 1987.

Simmer K, James C, and Thompson RPH: Are iron-folate supplements harmful? American Journal of Clinical Nutrition 45:122, 1987.

Simpson KM, Morris ER, and Cook JD: The inhibitory effect of bran on iron absorption in man, American Journal of Clinical Nutrition 34:1469, 1981.

Zinc

Apgar J: Zinc and reproduction, Annual Review of Nutrition 5:43, 1985.

Bales C, and others: The effect of age on plasma zinc uptake and taste acuity, American Journal of Clinical Nutrition 44:664, 1986.

Craig WJ, Balbach L, and Vyhmeister N: Zinc bioavailability and infant formulas, American Journal of Clinical Nutrition 39:981, 1984.

Fosmire GJ, Al-Ubaidi YY, and Sandstead HH: Some effects of postnatal zinc deficiency on developing rat brain, Pediatric Research 9:89, 1975.

Gordon PR, and others: Effect of acute zinc deprivation on plasma zinc and platelet aggregation in adult males, American Journal of Clinical Nutrition 35:113, 1982.

Hambidge KM, and others: Zinc nutritional status during pregnancy: a longitudinal study, American Journal of Clinical Nutrition 37:429, 1983.

Haynes D, and others: Long-term zinc deprivation in Rhesus monkeys: effects on adult female breeders before conception, American Journal of Clinical Nutrition 45:1492, 1987.

Kay RG: Zinc and copper in human nutrition, Journal of Human Nutrition 35:25, 1981.

Life Sciences Research Office: Assessment of the zinc nutritional status of the U.S. population based on data collected in HANES II, 1976-1980, Bethesda, MD, 1984, FASEB.

Mills CF: Dietary interactions involving the trace elements, Annual Review of Nutrition 5:173, 1985.

Oberleas D, and Harland BF: Phytate content of foods: effect on dietary zinc bioavailability, Journal of the American Dietetic Association 79:433, 1981.

Prasad AS: Discovery and importance of zinc in human nutrition, Federation Proceedings 43:2829, 1984.

Solomons, NW: Factors affecting bioavailability of zinc, Journal of the American Dietetic Association 80:115, 1982.

Swanson CA, Turnlund JR, and King JC: Effect of dietary zinc sources and pregnancy on zinc utilization in adult women fed controlled diets, Journal of Nutrition 113:2557, 1983.

Thompson P, and others: Zinc status and sexual development in adolescent girls, Journal of the American Dietetic Association 86:892, 1986.

Walravens PA, Krebs NF, and Hambidge KM: Linear growth of low-income preschool children receiving a zinc supplement, American Journal of Clinical Nutrition 38:195, 1983.

Iodine

Park YK, and others: Estimation of dietary iodine intake of Americans in recent years, Journal of the American Dietetic Association 76:17, 1981.

Sokoloff L: Kashin-Bek disease: current status, Nutrition Reviews 46:17, 1988.

Manganese

Freeland-Graves JH and others: Metabolic balance in young men consuming diets containing 5 levels of dietary manganese, Journal of Nutrition 118:776, 1988.

Freeland-Graves JH: Manganese: an essential nutrient for humans, Nutrition Today 23(5):15, 1988.

Copper

Danks DM: Copper deficiency in humans, Annual Review of Nutrition 8:235, 1988.

Finley EB, and Cerklewski FL: Influence of ascorbic acid supplementation on copper status in young adult men, American Journal of Clinical Nutrition 37:553, 1983.

Clinical cases: Essentiality of copper in humans, Nutrition Reviews 45:176, 1987.

Klevay LM, and others: Human requirement for copper. I. Healthy men fed conventional American diets, American Journal of Clinical Nutrition 33:45, 1980.

Mason KE: A conspectus of research on copper metabolism and requirements of man, Journal of Nutrition 109:1979, 1979.

Sandstead HH: Copper bioavailability and requirements, American Journal of Clinical Nutrition 35:809, 1982.

Molybdenum

Pennington JT, and Long JW: Molybdenum, nickel, cobalt, vanadium, and strontium in total diets, Journal of the American Dietetic Association 87:1644, 1987.

Rajagopaian KV: Molybdenum—an essential trace element in human nutrition, Annual Review of Nutrition 8:401, 1988.

Tsongas TA, and others: Molybdenum in the diet: an estimate of average daily intake in the United States, American Journal of Clinical Nutrition 33:1103, 1980.

Selenium

Baker SS, and others: Selenium deficiency with total parenteral nutrition: reversal of biochemical and functional abnormalities by selenium supplementation: a case report, American Journal of Clinical Nutrition 38:769, 1983.

Levander OA: Considerations on the assessment of selenium status, Federation Proceedings 44:2579, 1983.

Robinson M: Selenium, the New Zealand experience, American Journal of Clinical Nutrition 49:521, 1988.

Schubert A, Holden JM, and Wolfe WR: Selenium content of a core group of foods based on a critical evaluation of published analytical data, Journal of the American Dietetic Association 87:285, 1987.

Smith AM, Picciano MF, and Milner JA: Selenium intakes and status of human milk and formula-fed infants, American Journal of Clinical Nutrition 35:521, 1982.

Snook JT, and others: Selenium content of foods purchased or produced in Ohio, Journal of the American Dietetic Association 87:744, 1987.

Yang GQ, and others: Endemic selenium intoxication of humans in China, American Journal of Clinical Nutrition 37:872, 1983.

Young VR, Nahapelian A, and Jangerhorbani M: Selenium bioavailability with reference to human nutrition, American Journal of Clinical Nutrition 35:1076, 1982.

Chromium

Anderson R, and Kozlovsky A: Chromium intake, absorption, and excretion of subjects consuming self-selected diets, American Journal of Clinical Nutrition 41:1177, 1985.

Offenbacher EG, Spencer H, Dowling HJ, and Pi-Sunyer FX: Metabolic chromium balances in men, American Journal of Clinical Nutrition 44:77, 1986.

Offenbacher EG, and Pi-Sunyer FX: Chromium in human nutrition, Annual Review of Nutrition 8:543, 1988.

Sokoloff L: Is chromium essential for humans, Nutrition Reviews 46:17, 1988.

Silicon

Carlisle EM: The nutritional essentiality of silicon, Nutrition Reviews 40:193, 1982.

Cobalt

Underwood EJ: Cobalt. In Present knowledge of nutrition, Washington, D.C., 1984, The Nutrition Foundation, Inc.

Boron

Nielsen FM, Hunt CD, Mullen LM, and Hunt JR: Dietary boron affects mineral, estrogen, and testosterone metabolism in postmenopausal women. FASEB Journal 1:394, 1987.

Nielsen FM: Boron—an overlooked element of potential nutritional importance, Nutrition Today 23:4, 1988.

FOCUS Hair Analysis

Our growing understanding of the essential nature of many of the trace elements has brought with it a concern that people may not be getting enough of these elusive substances. Doubts about the adequacy of the diet to provide optimal amounts of trace elements have been raised in the popular and scientific presses alike. Some entrepreneurs have been quick to capitalize on this concern by marketing trace elements either individually or in multimineral supplements; others have offered to diagnose deficiency conditions. The Food and Drug Administration is restrained from doing anything about such situations even when they feel they are worthless or even potentially dangerous. For example, the sale of nutrient supplements cannot be regulated unless proof is offered that the supplements are toxic and a threat to health.

As a result, the public is subjected to one of the most dangerous health frauds: hair analysis, designed to lead to the use of unnecessary and risky supplementation. Hair analysis has some legitimate uses but is often thoroughly abused. We know that, in assessing nutritional status, it is often useful to analyze body tissues, most frequently blood or urine. The theory is that the amount of a nutrient in these tissues will in some way reflect the amount available in the body. In the case of hair analysis, we know that, for some nutrients, the amount in the hair reflects the amount that was available at the time the hair was growing. However, we have also learned that there are a great many things in the environment that can affect the amounts of trace elements found in the hair. Sometimes, these include substances in the natural environment, such as pollutants in the air. At other times, the man-made environment—for example, shampoos, hair conditioners, and permanent solutions—affect the amounts of trace elements that show up in an analysis.

What is dangerous about hair analysis? Actually, there is no danger in obtaining the hair sample. It usually only involves cutting off a relatively small piece of hair at the nape of the neck close to the scalp. The problems arise from the doubtful nature of much of the analysis, the way in which the results are presented, the recommendations that accompany them, and the high cost of the analysis.

Most hair analyses are provided by mail. The cost ranges from a relatively inexpensive \$15 to \$100 or \$150. The client merely cuts the sample of hair according to the instructions, which are sometimes very vague, sometimes very explicit. Seldom if ever is the subject asked to provide information on the condition of the hair—the use of shampoos, the hardness of the water in the area, or any special beauty treatments.

Whether or not the hair is actually analyzed is open to question. Almost certainly, however, there will be a report of an analysis. The report is usually an impressive-looking computer printout, providing figures on the amounts of nutrients in a fixed amount of hair and ratios of one element to another. The reports usually provide standards against which you can compare your analysis. The fact is that we do not have standards of any kind for more than one or two trace elements, let alone information on appropriate ratios of one element to another. However, this does not seem to bother those "in the business." They not only report values and fictitious standards but in most cases also make a diagnosis regarding a health concern, based on the presumed findings.

Some of the diagnoses are reassuring. Many, however, hint at an actual or impending health problem. The diagnosis may be as benign as susceptibility to colds or as anxiety-producing as borderline diabetes, predisposition to schizophrenia, or impending arthritis. The report usually continues to prescribe trace element supplements, usually in unrealistic and often unsafe high doses. A particular brand that can be ordered by mail, especially formulated to meet the subject's needs, is offered; it can be bought in monthly units but will be much less expensive if a 6-month supply is purchased at one time.

Often the subject, impressed by the uncanny insights in the diagnosis—"Sometimes you have trouble sleeping at night," "You occasionally have an overwhelming urge for a particular food," "Your fingers feel numb when you drive a car in the cold"—will urge family members or friends to get their hair analyzed also. And so the enterprise continues to thrive.

The supplement prescription often calls for a large number of individual elements to be taken in a prescribed sequence and at a certain time in relationship to the meal. All of this specificity helps to increase confidence in the validity of both the diagnosis and the prescription. The cost of the program is of special concern when the "victims" are elderly people living on fixed incomes, worried that their health will fail and that they will become dependent on family and friends. However, the central problem lies in the health hazards associated with the prescribed remedies.

At usual intakes the body is fairly efficient in maintaining appropriate levels of trace elements in the blood and other tissues, either by regulating the absorption of nutrients or their excretion through the kidneys. When too much of a nutrient is taken in, exceeding the usual physiological amount, these regulatory mechanisms break down. Either too much is absorbed, or too little excreted, or both. In these cases, the element may accumulate in some tissue of the body and reach a level that interferes with the actions of essential enzymes or other body reactions.

In addition to the problems connected with ingestion of high amounts of an element, there are other problems resulting from an imbalance of nutrients. We have considerable information on the complex interactions among trace elements and the extent to which the amount of one influences the effect of another. Sometimes, an imbalance causes one nutrient to accumulate at excessive levels; in other cases, it may cause excessive loss of the nutrient from the body. Whatever the outcome, it is obvious that there are inherent dangers in high or unbalanced intakes of trace elements.

In spite of all the concerns about its misuse, hair analysis has many advantages in assessing nutritional status. Hair is a tissue that is readily obtained; it is stable under conditions of storage; and because of low water content, the concentration of elements in hair is high enough to be more readily measured. Unfortunately, we have almost no standards against which to assess results of hair analysis when it is actually done, and the way this potentially useful tool is being exploited must be considered a health fraud. We have spent this much time discussing hair analysis to familiarize the reader with the nature of health frauds. There is a need to be skeptical about any kind of health cure or diagnosis that is offered through the mail or without the permission and supervision of a doctor or other medical personnel. Hair analysis may some day be a legitimate and useful diagnostic tool. Under present conditions, however, we can only recommend extreme caution, if not avoidance.

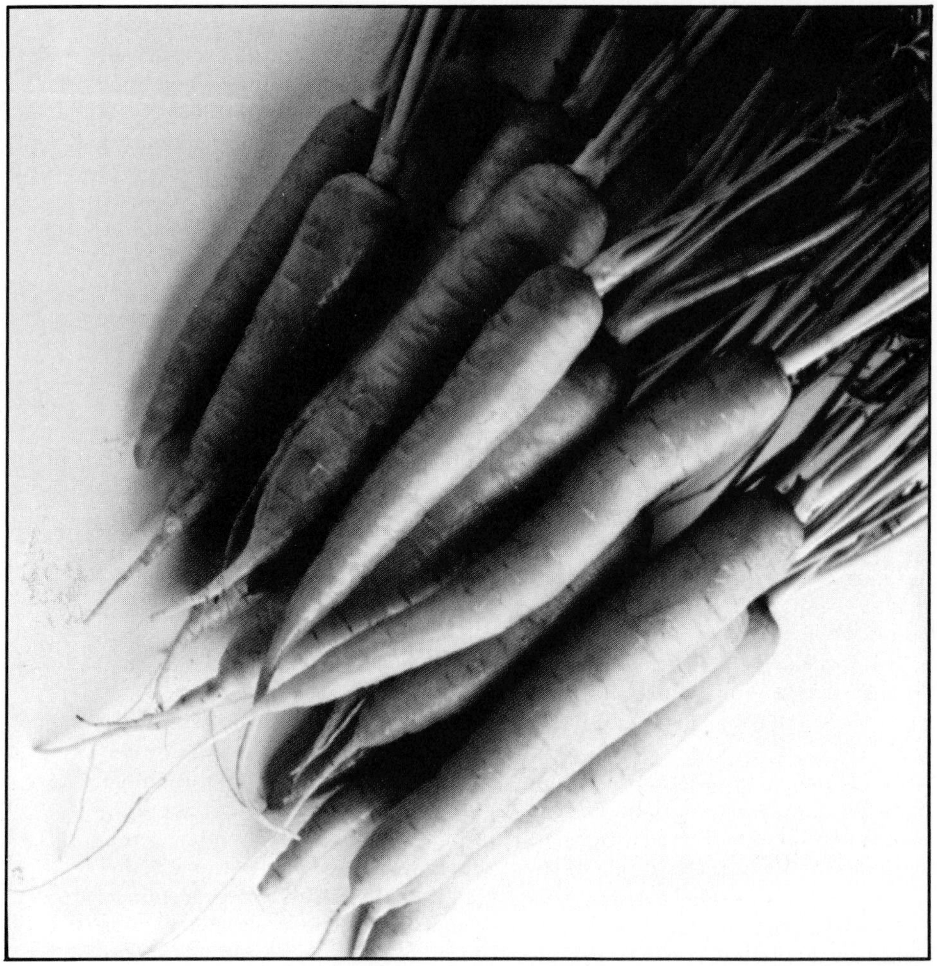

AWARENESS CHECK

Truth or Fiction?

- A person cannot meet the RDAs for vitamins from food alone.
- Eating carrots will improve your eyesight.
- Vitamin A prevents cancer.
- Megadoses of vitamins can be dangerous.
- Topical vitamin A promotes smooth and youthful skin.
- Nutrient supplements are regulated and controlled by the FDA.

Fat-Soluble Vitamins

CHAPTER 12

Although the last vitamin known to be essential in human nutrition was discovered in 1948, frequent and periodic claims are made about other substances with vitamin-like roles. None of these claims has been confirmed. We have, however, made great progress in determining the sources of known vitamins, the mechanisms by which they are absorbed, and their functions in the body. We also know that there are complex interactions among the vitamins and with other nutrients. Of the four fat-soluble vitamins to be discussed in this chapter, vitamins A and D have been studied most extensively. Both have beneficial effects in small amounts but may have detrimental effects in amounts that are too large. Vitamin A is most essential to vision and skin health, whereas vitamin D is essential for normal bone and tooth formation. The other two fat-soluble vitamins (E and K), equally as important but seldom deficient, have roles as antioxidants and as blood clotting factors. Any claims for miraculous uses of these or any vitamin should be viewed with a healthy bit of skepticism.

The first part of this chapter (pp. 339-345) presents an overview of both fat-soluble and water-soluble vitamins. These two groups will be discussed in this chapter through Chapter 14. The remainder of Chapter 12 discusses the four fat-soluble vitamins; Chapters 13 and 14 deal with the water-soluble vitamins.

OVERVIEW OF VITAMINS

Vitamins are nutrients that many people talk about, some people worry about, and other people rely on to solve a wide range of health problems. Although ample amounts of vitamins are provided by food, there is a growing industry devoted to their sale in pill or capsule form for those who fear they are not getting enough. This and the next two chapters are designed to provide perspectives on what vitamins are, what they can and cannot do, and what happens when we have too much or too little of any of them.

The discovery of vitamins provided the missing link in our knowledge about why some diets promoted growth and health and others did not. Because vitamins are present in food and needed in the body in such small amounts, it is easy to understand why they were overlooked as dietary essentials. The recommended daily adult intake of a vitamin varies greatly, but those needed in a small amount are just as important as those needed at a hundred or a thousand times that level.

vitamins
- Organic substances
- Needed in very small amounts
- Essential for health
- Must be provided in the diet because they cannot be synthesized in the body

organic
Having its origin in living material, either plant or animal; chemically speaking, it applies to any compound containing carbon

Vitamins are defined as **organic** substances, needed in very small amounts, that are essential for health and perform at least one specific metabolic function and which must be provided in the diet. Vitamins that are essential in the diet for one species of animal that *cannot* synthesize them may not be necessary vitamins for another species that *can* synthesize them. For instance, humans need vitamin C in the diet; rabbits do not. Plants can manufacture vitamins from the elements available to them in the soil.

The term "vitamine" was coined by Casimir Funk in 1912. He believed that disease might be caused by a lack of something in the diet and cured by adding it back. Since he thought this substance was necessary for life (vita), and contained nitrogen (amine), he proposed the term *vitamine.* Subsequent work showed that although there were many "vitamines," few were "amines." Thus the final *e* was dropped, giving us *vitamin.*

Shortly after Funk introduced his vitamin hypothesis, an unidentified substance in fat that was necessary for growth and reproduction in animals was reported. This substance was designated *fat-soluble A* to differentiate it from *water-soluble B,* which had been recognized earlier by Funk.

From this simple beginning, the list has grown to include four completely different and essential fat-soluble and nine water-soluble vitamins (Table 12-1). As our knowledge of each vitamin increased, names such as vitamin B_1, B_2, and B_6, B_c, and B_{12} which imply a common function, are being replaced by terms such as thiamin, riboflavin, pyridoxine, folacin, and cobalamin, which more adequately reflect their composition or structure. It will undoubtedly be some time, however, before the old terminology disappears.

Table 12-1 presents the discovery of vitamins in chronological order. Gaps in alphabetical and numerical names can be explained by the fact that scientists discovered some substances that they initially labeled as new vitamins, only to discover later that either they did not have vitamin activity or were identical to other factors. There is a slight possibility that other vitamins have yet to be discovered.

Although individual vitamins of the fat-soluble and water-soluble groups have unique functions, a few characteristics generally differentiate the two groups. These are summarized in Table 12-2.

Related Substances

precursor (provitamin)
Substance that is chemically related to a vitamin but must be changed by the body into the active form of the vitamin

antagonist (antivitamin)
Substance that is very similar to a vitamin but cannot take its place because of a very slight difference in chemical composition

Two groups of compounds chemically related to vitamins are of nutritional importance: vitamin **precursors (provitamins)** and **antagonists (antivitamins).**

Precursors, or provitamins, are substances that are chemically related to the biologically active form of the vitamin but cannot function as vitamins until the body converts them into the active form. This conversion takes place in different parts of the body, with varying degrees of efficiency.

Antagonists, also known as pseudovitamins or antivitamins, are usually chemically related to the biologically active "real" vitamin. The body does not discriminate between them and the useful form of the vitamin. Thus, not only do they fail to permit useful reactions, they cannot be replaced by the proper substance that would allow the reactions to proceed. Vitamin antagonists have been used to produce experimental vitamin deficiencies and medically to retard the undesirable growth of rapidly growing cells such as white blood cells in leukemia. They must, however, be used with caution because they also inhibit the growth of desirable cells.

Table 12-1 ◇ Discovery, isolation, synthesis, and nomenclature of vitamins essential for humans

	Discovery	Isolation	Synthesis	Other Names*
Water-Soluble Vitamins				
Thiamin (B_1)	1921	1926	1936	Aneurine Antineuritic factor Antiberiberi factor
Ascorbic acid (C)	1932	1932	1933	Antiscorbutic factor Cevitamic acid
Riboflavin (B_2)	1932	1933	1935	Yellow enzyme Vitamin G Lactoflavin Hepatoflavin Ovoflavin
Pantothenic acid (B_5)	1933	1938	1940	Pantotheine Pantothenol Antichromomotriclia factor
Pyridoxine (B_6)	1934	1938	1939	Pyridoxic acid Pyridoxal Pyridoxol Pyridoxamine
Biotin	1936	1942	1943	Anti–egg-white injury factor Bios II Vitamin H
Niacin (B_3)	1936	1936		Nicotinic acid Nicotinamide or niacinamide Pellagra-preventive factor
Folacin	1945	1945	1945	Adermine Folic acid Citrovorum factor Pteroylglutamic acid *Lactobacillus casei* factor Vitamin M Vitamin B_c Factor U
Cobalamin (B_{12})	1948	1948	1973	Antipernicious anemia factor Cyanocobalamin Hydroxycobalamin Erythrocyte maturation factor Animal protein factor (APF)
Fat-Soluble Vitamins				
Vitamin A	1915	1937	1946	Axerophthol Retinoic acid Retinal Retinol Dehydroretinol
Vitamin D	1918	1930	1936	Antirachitic factor Cholecalciferol Ergocalciferol Calcitriol Calcidiol
Vitamin E	1922	1936	1937	Tocopherol Antisterility factor
Vitamin K	1934	1939	1939	Phytylquinone Multiprenylmenaquinone Farnoquinone Antihemorrhagic factor Menadione (synthetic) Synkayvite (synthetic) Hykinone (synthetic)

*Terms appearing in the literature, many of which are no longer recognized as correct terminology.

Table 12-2 ◆ General properties of fat-soluble and water-soluble vitamins

Fat-Soluble Vitamins	Water-Soluble Vitamins
Soluble in fat and fat solvents (water-miscible derivatives available)	Soluble in water
Intake in excess of daily need stored in the body	Minimal storage of dietary excesses
Small amounts excreted in bile	Excreted in urine
Deficiency symptoms slow to develop	Deficiency symptoms often develop rapidly
Not absolutely necessary in diet every day	Must be supplied in diet every day
Have precursors or provitamins	Generally do not have precursors
Contain only the elements carbon, hydrogen, and oxygen	Contain the elements carbon, hydrogen, oxygen, and nitrogen and in some cases others, such as cobalt or sulfur
Absorbed into lymphatic system	Absorbed into blood through portal vein
Needed only by complex organisms	Needed by simple and complex organisms
Some are toxic at relatively low levels (6-10 times the RDA)	Toxic only at megadose levels (>10 times the RDA)

coenzyme
A substance, usually a vitamin, that must be present before certain enzymes can function

apoenzyme
An inactive protein portion of an enzyme; either a cofactor (a metallic ion) or a coenzyme (a vitamin) must be attached to it to form an active enzyme

holoenzyme
An active enzyme made up of a protein part (an apoenzyme), and either a cofactor (a mineral) or a coenzyme (a vitamin)

substrate
A substance on which an enzyme acts to change it in some way; for example, sucrose is a substrate for the enzyme sucrase because sucrase changes it to glucose and fructose

Functions

Despite a lot of knowledge about the chemical structure of vitamins, scientists still are unable to determine the exact biochemical role of many of them. It is known that some vitamins serve primarily as **coenzymes,** which aid in the action of enzymes. Some enzymes work alone to bring about required changes; others, however, require the help of coenzymes. Most of these coenzymes are vitamins that attach to a protein known as **apoenzyme**, to form an active enzyme known as a **holoenzyme**. The vitamin as a coenzyme is usually responsible for the attachment of the enzyme to the **substrate** on which it acts. The coenzyme can be compared to the last piece of a jigsaw puzzle to be fitted into place, making the picture complete.

Vitamins play a role at many stages in the metabolism of energy-yielding nutrients, as illustrated in Figure 12-1. If the vitamins are not available as coenzymes, the sequence of chemical changes cannot proceed. The product whose change is blocked accumulates in the tissues or blood, or metabolism proceeds in another direction. When an abnormal product accumulates, it is responsible for many of the symptoms associated with the lack of a specific vitamin.

Causes of Vitamin Deficiencies
Too little of vitamin in the diet
Poor absorption
Increased need

Deficiencies

There are several causes of vitamin deficiencies. The most common cause is the lack of the nutrient in the diet. Because needs differ, an amount adequate for one person may be insufficient for another. For example, some adults can function with 0.2 mg of thiamin daily, whereas others require as much as 0.8 mg. Because the person with high needs cannot be easily identified, the Food and Nutrition Board usually establishes the recommended dietary allowances to include a margin of safety over average needs to take care of the needs of most of the population. Unusually high losses from poor methods of harvesting, storage, or preparation of some foods reduce the actual content below the expected level and may result in a deficiency.

A second cause of a vitamin deficiency is failure of the body to absorb nutrients provided in food. For example, people whose secretion of bile is limited or absent

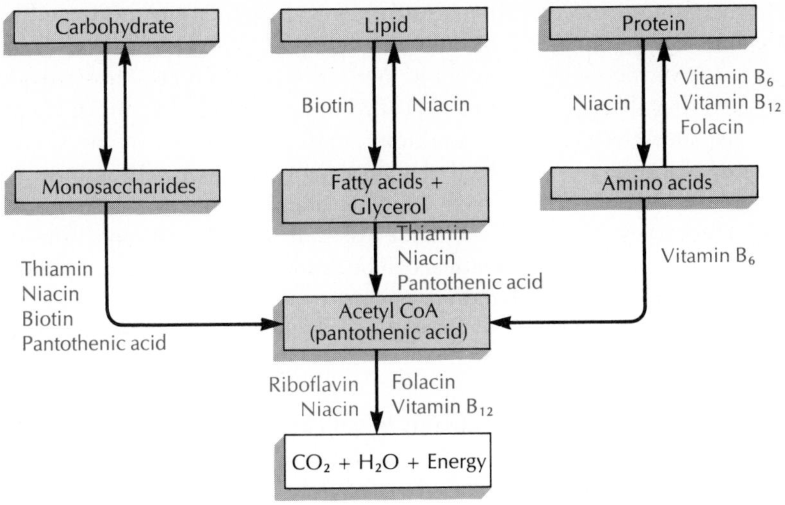

Figure 12-1 Examples of the reactions for which vitamins are essential in the metabolism of energy-yielding nutrients.

absorb lower amounts of the fat-soluble vitamins than those who have an adequate amount to aid in fat absorption. A lowered secretion of acid from gastric mucosa inhibits the absorption of cobalamin. A rapid passage of food through the gastrointestinal tract, which takes place with a high-fiber diet, reduces absorption of vitamins as well as minerals.

A third cause of vitamin deficiency is the increased need for a vitamin, leading to deficiency symptoms on an intake that would normally be adequate. For example, alcoholics experience an increased need for thiamin. People with tuberculosis and cigarette smokers need more vitamin C. There is even recent evidence suggesting that an infant can be conditioned to need abnormally high amounts of pyridoxine or vitamin C if the mother consumes large amounts during pregnancy.

Vitamins in Food

The contribution of a specific food to the vitamin content of the diet depends on several factors. First is the amount of the vitamin that is initially present in a food. Second is the amount that is lost or destroyed during harvesting (for plant foods), slaughtering (for animal foods), preparation, processing, and storage.

For plant foods, the vitamin content depends on the conditions under which the plant was grown. These include the rate at which the plant grew, the fertility of the soil, the particular type of plant, the availability of sunlight and moisture during critical growth periods, and the stage of maturity at harvest.

Once a plant is harvested, the loss of a vitamin depends on how the plant is stored and transported and how stable the vitamin is. In general, the higher the temperature, the longer the time of storage, and the more the exposure to air and sunshine during storage, the greater the losses. In preparation or processing, more nutrients will be lost when temperatures are high, cooking water is discarded, large surface areas are exposed to either air or water, acid or alkali is used in cooking, large amounts of air are incorporated during cooking, or the food is agitated. The vitamins that are most likely to be affected are those that are destroyed by heat and oxidation or are soluble in water. Actual losses can be reduced by (1) cooking at as low a temperature as feasible, (2) cooking in a minimum amount of water, (3) cooking just below the boiling point to reduce the amount of agitation of the food, (4) cutting the food in relatively small pieces (larger pieces take longer to cook, and smaller ones have more surface area exposed) to allow for fewer losses into the cooking water, (5) cutting with a sharp knife to avoid crushing the cells, (6) keeping the exposure to air to a minimum, and (7) using any cooking water in other dishes such as gravies and soups. Fat-soluble vitamins are not lost in cooking water but are much more susceptible to destruction from oxidation and rancidity than are water-soluble vitamins.

To preserve the vitamin content of food, it is generally best to store and prepare the food so that there is minimal exposure to heat, sunlight, air, acid, alkali, and oxygen because these are the conditions under which one or more vitamins are inactivated. In many cases, food that has been commercially grown, harvested, processed, or transported will have a higher vitamin content than food that is grown at home but harvested and stored under less than ideal conditions. However, fresh, home-produced fruits and vegetables can be (and often are) higher in vitamin content if they have been carefully handled.

Supplements

Giving the public information on the beneficial effects of an adequate intake of vitamins and the detrimental effects of an inadequate intake has had many positive effects. However, it sometimes has resulted in undue concern from people who are aware of their need for vitamins and are worried that their diets may be inadequate. Many of those who sell vitamin supplements have capitalized on this concern and have reinforced the public's doubts about obtaining sufficient amounts of vitamins from food. In addition, some supplements contain vitamins at levels well above any conceivable need. As a result, many people are buying and consuming vitamins far in excess of their daily requirements. (When a person's diet is low in a vitamin, supplements help; more often, however, the vitamins supplemented are ones that are already available in adequate dietary amounts.) Aside from the economic waste involved, little harm results from reasonably small excesses of most vitamins. However, as we will discuss later, excessive intakes of most of the fat-soluble vitamins and some water-soluble vitamins may have definite harmful effects.

Regulation

Attempts by the FDA in 1973 and 1976 to limit the nonprescription sale of vitamin supplements to those containing at least 50% but less than 150% of the U.S. RDA were overruled in 1978. Although the FDA believed there were no benefits from intakes above the U.S. RDA and that there was considerable cause for concern about indiscriminate and unsupervised uses of large amounts, opponents maintained that any such restrictions were an infringement on individual rights. Therefore, as of now, it is permissible to sell nutrient supplements alone or in combination at any level for adults, as long as no health claims are made on the label of the product or in its advertising. However, it is suggested that products designed for children and pregnant or breastfeeding women not contain over 150% of the U.S. RDA for any nutrient. Multinutrient preparations should contain a specified number of nutrients at or above a specified minimum level. This regulation is designed to encourage a more balanced composition of supplements and to preclude the omission of critical nutrients on the basis of price or complication of processing. Unfortunately, little is being done to enforce any of these regulations.

The FDA has proposed that disease-related health claims, such as "Product X contains fiber and prevents cancer," should not be permitted. Allowing nonspecific health claims, such as "Calcium builds bones," on generic statements is permissible.

Natural or Synthetic Vitamins

Because naturally occurring vitamins are biochemically identical to those produced synthetically in the laboratory, both are absorbed and utilized by the cell in exactly the same way. Therefore, vitamins from synthetic sources are just as useful as comparable amounts that occur naturally in foods. Advertisements for natural vitamins are often misleading because they usually promote products that are mostly synthetic, with an infinitesimal amount of a vitamin added from a natural source. For example, vitamin C with added acerola or rose hips; vitamin E mixed with beta-, gamma-, and delta-tocopherol; or B vitamins in a natural yeast base are primarily synthetic nutrients; however, ads for them imply a natural superiority.

Toxicity

Excessive intakes of water-soluble vitamins from natural food sources are excreted unchanged in the urine and present no problem of toxicity. However, **megadoses** in excess of 10 times the recommended dietary allowances may cause problems. (The doses are often described as unphysiological doses.) Problems may be the result of the formation of abnormal metabolites of the vitamin or of the interaction of one nutrient with another. Because the use of megadoses of nutrients without medical supervision is a very recent phenomenon, we have little information on the consequences. As the practice continues, we should learn more about any adverse consequences. In the case of some fat-soluble vitamins, we have known for some time about the adverse effects of megadoses. Until we know more about the effects of supplements we need to encourage people to choose the foods that will ensure an adequate nutrient intake. Contrary to many claims, it is quite possible to get all the vitamins that we need in food from the grocery store. Only when caloric intake is very limited is there a potential problem.

megadose
An amount of a vitamin at least 10 times the recommended intake

FAT-SOLUBLE VITAMINS

There are four fat-soluble vitamins, all of which are soluble in fat but otherwise have very little in common, either in terms of dietary sources or their roles in metabolism. Although the last fat-soluble vitamin was discovered in 1938, we still have much to learn about the biochemical roles of many of them. Each is concentrated in a specific body tissue such as the liver and each comes from a unique set of foods. A well-chosen diet can meet all known needs for fat-soluble vitamins. Because they are stored by the body, it is possible to have an intake of fat-soluble vitamins that is high enough to be toxic when supplements are used in addition to dietary sources.

VITAMIN A

Shortly after Funk introduced the term, the first "vitamine" was identified. It became known as *fat-soluble A*. Still referred to as vitamin A, it is now known to consist of several chemically related substances rather than one single active compound. The term **retinoids** is used for both synthetic and naturally occurring compounds similar to vitamin A and including its precursors, carotenes.

retinoids
All compounds, that are either natural or synthetic, similar to vitamin A (retinol) in chemical structure

In 1912, Osborne and Mendel reported that animals grew normally on diets containing milk fat but failed to grow when the milk fat was withdrawn. This growth failure was soon followed by an eye disease. About the same time, others observed that growth ceased in rats fed lard as a fat source; growth was restored when an ether extract of butter, cod liver oil, or egg yolk was used. Both groups concluded, correctly, that a fat-soluble substance was necessary for growth in animals.

Seven years later, dairy farmers reported better growth and improved fertility when cows were fed yellow corn rather than white corn. By 1928 carotene, one of the yellow pigments of plants, had been identified as a potent precursor of vitamin A. The term vitamin A is now used to refer to all forms of the vitamin that are sources of vitamin A.

Until 1967, the vitamin A activity of plant and animal tissue was always measured in International Units (IU) or United States Pharmacopeia (USP) units.

1 IU = 1 USP unit

retinol equivalent (RE)
A measure of vitamin A, used for requirements and amounts in the food supply; the sum of preformed vitamin A and the amount obtained by converting the precursor to the active form

In 1967, FAO/WHO recommended that **retinol equivalents (RE)** be used as measures of vitamin A and in 1974 the United States adopted **retinol equivalents** as the unit of measurement. Unfortunately tables of food composition and labels on food products continue to use either system, making it very difficult to relate intake to need.

Conversion of Information on Vitamin A into Retinol Equivalents (REs)

1 retinol equivalent (RE) = 3.3 IU retinol (animal foods)

or

$$= \frac{\text{IU of vitamin A precursor (plant foods)}}{10}$$

= 1 μg retinol

= 6 μg β-carotene

= 12 μg other carotenoids

Despite its early discovery, it was 1932 before scientists identified the chemical structure of vitamin A. In 1937 the vitamin was crystallized from halibut liver oil, with 2 to 36 million IU/gram. In 1946, it was synthesized. Synthetic vitamin A has about 1.2 million RE/gram at a cost of about 35¢ for a 3-year supply for an adult. It is used in the enrichment of many food products and in vitamin supplements. A water-miscible form is available for use in such nonfat products as dried milk solids. Over 700 tons of synthetic vitamin A were produced in the United States in 1984; much of it was used for food fortification and in supplements.

Vitamin A is a pale yellow substance that is soluble in fat or in fat solvents. In food, it attaches to a fatty acid. In the body, it functions in several chemical forms—retinol (an alcohol), retinal (an aldehyde), and retinoic acid (an acid). The relationship among these three forms is shown in Figure 12-2. Retinol and retinal can be reversibly oxidized and reduced. Once retinoic acid has been produced by oxidation, however, it cannot be reduced back to either of the other two forms.

The different chemical forms of vitamin A each perform specific functions. Retinoic acid, which has only limited functions and cannot be stored in the body, is sometimes referred to as a partial vitamin. A summary of the functions performed by each of the forms of vitamin A is given in Table 12-3.

preformed
The active form of the vitamin (retinol) provided in foods of animal origin

carotenoids
Substances chemically related to beta-carotene in chemical structure

With the exception of a small amount found in spinach, retinol, the **preformed** biologically active form of vitamin A, is found only in foods of animal origin. Many plants, however, are rich in a group of compounds called **carotenoids,** which are precursors (provitamins) of vitamin A. Ten of the over 50 known carotenoids have been identified in foods. Of these, only four (alpha-, beta-, and gamma-carotene and cryptoxanthin) are important in human and animal nutrition.

Beta-carotene is made up of two molecules of vitamin A; the others have one molecule of vitamin A and one molecule of a related, but metabolically inactive molecule with no vitamin A activity. Beta-carotene was produced synthetically in 1954. It is currently one of the few yellow pigments approved by the FDA for the

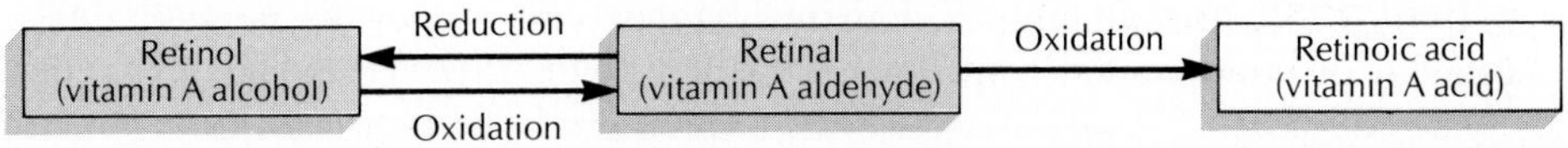

Figure 12-2 Relationship among biochemical forms of vitamin A.

Table 12-3 ◇ Effectiveness of various forms of vitamin A in various functions of the vitamin

Function	Retinol	Retinal	Retinoic Acid
Growth	+	+	+
Epithelial tissue	+	+	+
Bone	+	+	+
Vision	+	+	−
Reproduction	+	+	−

artificial coloring of food. It is used extensively in gelatin, margarine, soft drinks, cake mixes, and cereal products. Over 100 tons of beta-carotene were produced and used in the United States in 1983.

Functions

Although vitamin A was the first vitamin to be discovered and was chemically identified about 40 years ago, except for the part it plays in vision its roles are not well understood. Because vitamin A is required only by complex organisms, it has been difficult to study. However, it has been identified as essential for at least four distinct physiological functions: vision, growth, cell differentiation, and reproduction. It is also theorized that a common metabolic factor must exist in its effect on cartilage, bone, and **epithelium** (the surface cells of the body), but so far no one has been able to identify it biochemically. There are many clinical effects of vitamin A that seem to involve all human cells in one way or another, possibly through the vitamin's effect on DNA.

epithelium
The surface cells lining the outside of the body and all the external passages within the body

Vision

Vitamin A's action in the **retina** of the eye to allow vision in dim light is its only function that is clearly defined. The retinol that is provided in the blood is oxidized to retinaldehyde (retinal). This then combines with the protein opsin to form the pigment visual purple, or **rhodopsin,** located in the special cells known as rods in the retina of the eye. As light strikes the retina, the visual purple is bleached to visual yellow, and retinaldehyde is separated from opsin. With this action, a stimulus is transferred from the retina through the optic nerve fibers to the brain. During the process, some vitamin A is split off from the protein and changed to retinol. Most of this retinol is reconverted to retinaldehyde, which in turn recombines with opsin to regenerate rhodopsin. A small amount of retinol is lost in this process and must be replaced by the blood. The amount of retinol available in the blood determines the rate at which rhodopsin is regenerated and is available to act again as a receptor substance in the retina. Until this whole cycle has been completed, vision in dim light is not possible. It is slow when blood retinol levels are low and rapid when they are normal. The mechanism involved is shown in Figure 12-3.

retina
Inner layer of the wall at the back of the eye that contains the visual receptors

rhodopsin
A combination of the protein opsin and vitamin A in the retina of the eye; it is responsible for the ability of the eye to see in dim light

Two good examples of situations where vitamin A is needed are the inability of people to see upon entering dimly lit theaters from brightly lit streets and the blindness experienced by night drivers after meeting oncoming cars with bright headlights. In both examples, the bright light has caused excessive bleaching of rhodopsin, and vision in dim light will be possible only when a sufficient amount of visual purple has been reformed. This condition, known as night blindness, is due to a failure of a process known as **dark adaptation,** as illustrated in Figure 12-4. The speed with which the eye adapts after exposure to bright light is directly related to the amount of vitamin A available to reform rhodopsin. The "dark adaptation" test, which measures the speed of recovery of vision in dim light, is

dark adaptation
The ability of the eye to adapt to vision in dim light after being exposed to bright light

considered the most sensitive measure of vitamin A status. Unfortunately, it is a relatively complex and expensive test and is not very useful with children because it requires that subjects describe what they see.

Vitamin A is also part of other light-sensitive substances (opsins) in the cone cells of the retina. The cones are responsible for color vision in bright light. However, they are not as sensitive to changes in the available vitamin A as are the rods. In spite of the importance of vitamin A in visual processes, only 0.01% of the vitamin is found in the eye. Vitamin A supplementation does not improve normal vision but does improve poor vision caused by a vitamin A deficiency.

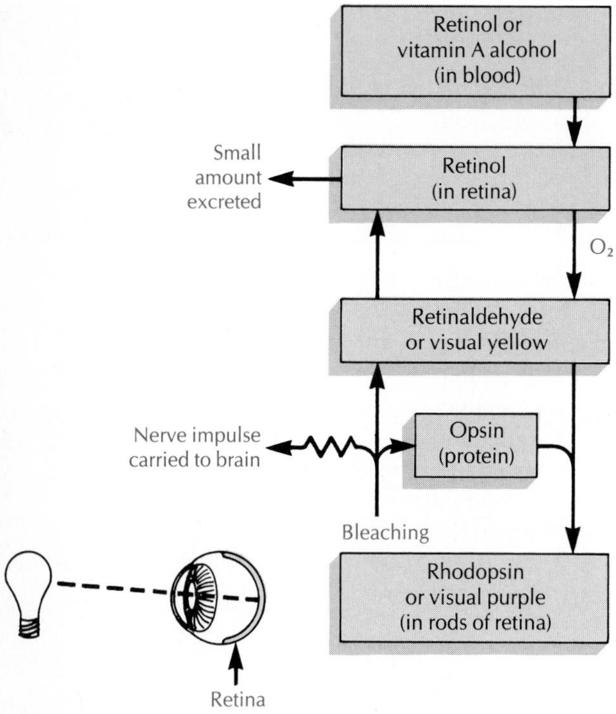

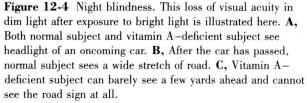

Figure 12-3 Role of vitamin A in dark adaptation. As light bleaches rhodopsin (visual purple) to retinaldehyde (visual yellow), a nerve impulse is generated and is carried by the optic nerve to the brain.

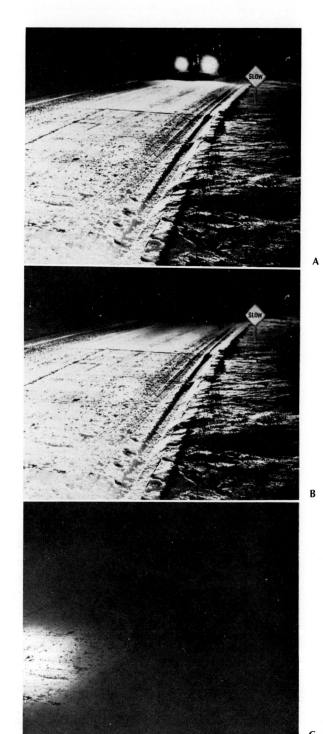

Figure 12-4 Night blindness. This loss of visual acuity in dim light after exposure to bright light is illustrated here. **A,** Both normal subject and vitamin A–deficient subject see headlight of an oncoming car. **B,** After the car has passed, normal subject sees a wide stretch of road. **C,** Vitamin A–deficient subject can barely see a few yards ahead and cannot see the road sign at all.

Courtesy The Upjohn Company, Kalamazoo, MI.

Growth

The role of vitamin A in promoting growth is best demonstrated when animals that are deprived of vitamin A cease to grow after their reserves of the vitamin have been depleted. This response is illustrated in Figure 12-5. Growth failure will occur before most other symptoms of vitamin A deficiency except night blindness.

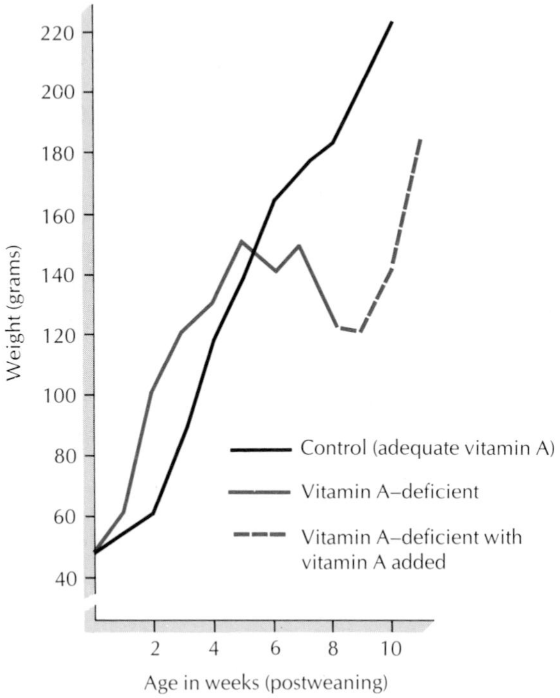

Figure 12-5 Growth response of rats to diets deficient or adequate in vitamin A. Note how the growth failure after vitamin A stores have been depleted is reversed by adding vitamin A to the diet.

Epithelial Cells

Epithelial cells are found not only in the outer protective layer of the skin, but also in the genitourinary and respiratory tracts. The formation of these epithelial cells, which normally secrete mucus, is dependent on vitamin A. Because epithelial cells are always being lost and replaced, the need for vitamin A in maintaining their health is continual.

When vitamin A is absent, dry and hardened *(keratinized)* cells develop. In addition to lacking the ability to form and secrete mucus, which keeps the linings of the body moist, keratinized cells lack **cilia.** These hairlike projections that prevent the accumulation of foreign material on the surface of the cells by constantly moving back and forth normally protect the body against infection. Figure 12-6 illustrates the difference between normal epithelial cells and those that are deficient in vitamin A. As a result, vitamin A has often been called an anti-infective vitamin. When the cells lining the trachea and the lungs become keratinized, deciliated, and deprived of their mucous secretions, microorganisms that would not penetrate a healthy epithelial layer are able to gain admission into the body, leading to an increased susceptibility to respiratory infections.

cilia
Hairlike projections on the cells lining the surface of the body

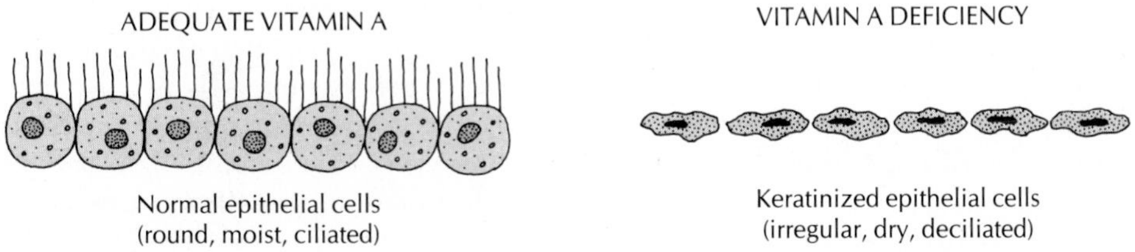

Figure 12-6 Changes in epithelial cells in a vitamin A deficiency.

Bone Development

It is well established that vitamin A is essential for normal bone growth. In a deficiency, bones fail to lengthen, are thick but weak, the **remodeling** process is poorly controlled, and the skull and spinal column do not continue to enlarge to make room for the growing nervous system. The function of vitamin A in bone growth may involve the conversion of immature cells to **osteoblasts,** which are responsible for an increase in the number of bone cells, and to **osteoclasts,** which are necessary for the breakdown of bone cells as bone is remodeled during growth. Retinoic acid can perform the function of vitamin A in the development of both bone and epithelial tissue.

remodeling
Reshaping of the bones that occurs as the bones adapt to bearing the changing weight of the body

osteoblasts
Cells that build bone

osteoclasts
Cells that destroy bone

osteo—bone
blasts—cells that build
clasts—cells that destroy

Reproduction

The promotion of animal fertility was one of the first functions discovered for vitamin A. Either retinol or retinal is necessary for normal reproduction in rats. In the absence of vitamin A, the male rat fails to produce sperm cells, and the female absorbs the fetus back into the body. The biochemical mechanism involved in normal reproduction is unknown; retinoic acid alone is not effective.

Other Functions

The production of proteins found in mucous secretions is altered when vitamin A is deficient. These mucous secretions are essential in keeping body linings moist and protecting the body against infection. The loss of appetite in a vitamin A deficiency may be caused by changes in the taste buds. Wound healing is also impaired as a result of changes in epithelial cells.

Vitamin A has a role in
Taste
Smell
Vision
Hearing

Absorption and Metabolism

From the time it is ingested until it is either used or excreted from the body, vitamin A changes its chemical form many times. Most of the preformed vitamin A in food combines with the fatty acid, palmitic acid, to form **retinyl palmitate.** Before it can be taken up by the intestinal cells, retinyl palmitate must be split by enzymes from either the pancreatic juice or mucosal cells to form free retinol. Bile is important for the uptake of retinol and is essential for carotenes. Once retinol is within the mucosal cell, it combines with a fatty acid (usually palmitic acid) and is incorporated into the small transport particles of fat called chylomicrons. These are then released into the lymphatic circulation, which eventually enters the regular blood system to be carried to the liver.

retinyl palmitate
An ester formed by the combination of retinol and the fatty acid palmitic acid

Because vitamin A is fat-soluble, factors that promote the absorption of fat enhance vitamin A absorption, and those that depress fat absorption depress vitamin A absorption. The absorption of vitamin A from foods is decreased in any condition in which the bile duct is obstructed. Vitamin E enhances the absorption of vitamin A and increases the amount of vitamin A stored in the liver.

The amount of retinoic acid in food is small. In the intestine, a small portion (less than 10%) of the retinol from food is oxidized first to retinal and then to retinoic acid, which is readily absorbed. In contrast to retinol, which is absorbed into the lymphatic system, retinoic acid attaches to the protein albumin, which increases its solubility in blood, and enters the general circulation through the portal vein.

The chylomicrons containing vitamin A are removed from the circulation by the liver after being slightly changed by the enzyme lipoprotein lipase. Vitamin A is deposited in the liver in lipid droplets for storage, most often in the form of retinyl palmitate and mainly in special fat cells. When vitamin A is needed, it is released as retinol. The retinol is then attached to a transport protein known as **retinol-binding protein (RBP),** which is synthesized in the liver. As this complex enters the blood plasma, it is attached to another protein, **prealbumin** (recently renamed **transthyretin),** which is also produced in the liver and present in the blood. In this form retinol is transported to the tissues, where it can be used for

retinol-binding protein (RBP)
A protein that serves as a carrier for vitamin A

transthyretin or **prealbumin**
A protein, which is produced in the liver and is present in the blood, that serves as a carrier for vitamin A

essential functions. Together, these two proteins—RBP and transthyretin—make retinol more soluble to facilitate its transport in the blood. They also make it part of a larger molecule to protect it from being filtered out and lost through the kidneys.

Once vitamin A is delivered to the cell, it is picked up by specific proteins within the cell known as CRBP (cellular retinol-binding protein) and CRABP (cellular retinoic acid-binding protein), which specifically bind retinol and retinoic acid. These proteins are distinctly different from the other vitamin A-binding proteins in the blood.

In addition to the intestine, both the kidneys and liver have enzymes capable of converting some absorbed retinol to retinoic acid. Retinoic acid from these sources is rapidly converted to a variety of metabolites that are excreted either through the kidneys in the urine or secreted by means of bile into the intestine.

The depressed utilization of vitamin A observed in protein deficiency can be explained by the need for proteins in vitamin A metabolism. Enzymes are needed at many stages, and transport proteins are needed to deliver vitamin A to the cells. In a protein deficiency, the synthesis of all these proteins is depressed. Thus protein appears to be necessary for the mobilization of vitamin A reserves from the liver. This may explain why low blood levels of vitamin A found in kwashiorkor increase when protein but no additional vitamin A is given.

Retinol

As a fat-soluble vitamin, vitamin A is absorbed in much the same way as lipid, being enhanced by the presence of bile and *vitamin E*. Preformed vitamin A from animal tissues is absorbed two to four times more efficiently than carotene from plant sources. As the amount of vitamin A in the diet increases, the proportion absorbed remains high, although the carotene absorption drops as the amount in the diet drops.

Carotene

After having been released from the plant cell during digestion, the four major plant precursors of vitamin A are absorbed intact in the presence of bile salts from the intestine. They are split in the intestinal wall to form retinol. This reaction is well regulated, so there is little possibility of producing too much vitamin A from carotene. The conversion of carotene to vitamin A, which involves splitting the carotene molecule into two parts, is not complete; some unchanged carotene is absorbed and enters the circulation. Blood carotene levels reflect dietary carotene, not the storage of vitamin A; therefore they have little significance as indicators of vitamin A status. Attempts to identify a function for carotene suggest that it may function to counteract the effect of oxidizing substances, which cause undesirable changes in various tissues.

For more details on the absorption, transport, and metabolism of vitamin A, and carotene see Appendix K

Unconverted carotene is stored in fat tissue and the adrenal glands rather than in the liver and may be responsible for a yellowish tinge to the skin when large amounts are stored. However, no toxic effects are associated with large doses of carotene.

The amount of vitamin A formed from precursors varies. Beta-carotene is made up of two vitamin A molecules, which can be split apart. The other precursors, however, yield only 1 molecule of vitamin A. Approximately one third of all the carotene in food is converted into vitamin A. Less than one fourth of the carotene in carrots and root vegetables and about half of the carotene in leafy vegetables is converted. Conversion occurs primarily in the intestinal wall, although some of it may take place in the liver and lungs. Vitamin A from carotene, after it is converted, is handled in the same way as the preformed vitamin. The absorption and metabolism of vitamin A and carotene are summarized in Figure 12-7.

The concentration of vitamin A in the human liver, which holds 90% of body stores, reflects long-term dietary intakes. It can range from 100 to 1000 IU/gram of liver tissue. A healthy person stores an estimated 500,000 IU in the liver, an

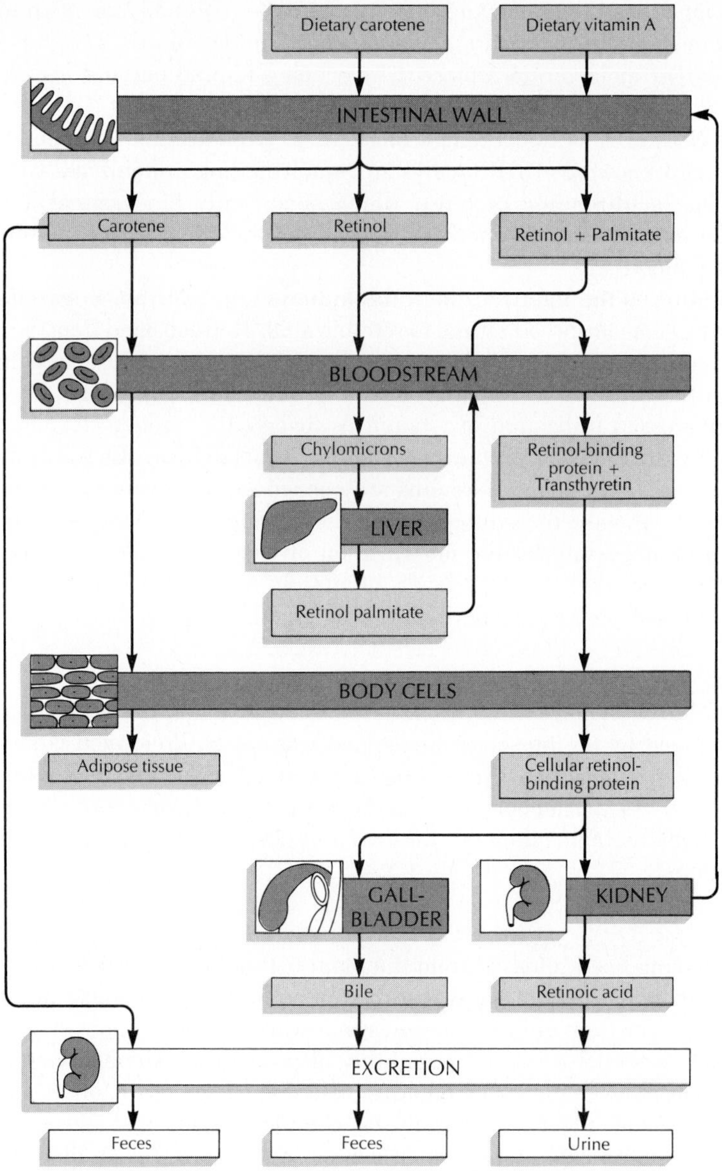

Figure 12-7 Summary of absorption, transport, and metabolism of vitamin A and carotene.

amount that may last several years. Autopsy data on the livers of Canadians, however, showed that 10% of those autopsied had no measurable reserves, and 20% had no more vitamin A than normally found at birth.

Recommended Allowances

Recomended Dietary Allowances of Vitamin A

		RE	IU
Children	1-3 yr	400	2000
	4-6 yr	500	2500
	7-10 yr	700	3300
Adult (14+ yr)			
Male		1000	5000
Female		800	4000
Pregnant		1000	5100
Lactating		1200	6000

The recommended allowances for vitamin A have been established assuming that half of the vitamin A value of a mixed diet comes from animal sources and half from vegetable sources. Studies on the amount of vitamin A required to maintain liver stores of at least 20 RE/gram of liver, to restore plasma vitamin A levels to normal, and to correct abnormalities in dark adaptation suggest that an intake of 10 μg of retinol/kg of body weight is sufficient for adults. This amount takes into consideration the 0.5% of body stores used each day and a variation of 20% in need among individuals. On this basis, 700 μg of retinol (700 RE) meets the needs of adult men, and 600 RE meets the needs of adult women. These amounts are slighly less than the 1980 recommended dietary allowances of 1000 RE and 800 RE for men and women, respectively. Because we have no information suggesting that older adults have higher or lower needs, the recommended intakes remain unchanged throughout life. During the last trimester of pregnancy, about 1.3 mg of retinol is transferred to the fetus. Except for women with low liver reserves, this can be provided without additional dietary vitamin A. For those women with low vitamin A reserves in the liver, an added intake of 200 RE of vitamin A daily is recommended. Because there is some danger that large doses (>20,000 RE/day) may cause birth defects, it is important for pregnant woment to avoid excessive intakes.

A mother produces milk with a vitamin A content of from 400 to 700 RE/liter, an amount that could use up to 50% of the mother's reserves during 6 months of breast feeding. To maintain maternal stores, it is recommended that an extra 400 RE of vitamin A/day be taken by the mother during lactation; this will provide 350 RE/day to the infant. For older children, daily intakes of 10 μg/kg of body weight are adequate.

Unless data on food composition are available in RE rather than IU, it is very difficult to assess the adequacy of dietary intake relative to the RDA, because tables do not give sufficient information to make the calculations.

Food Sources

The vitamin A value of food consists of the actual preformed vitamin A found only in foods of animal origin, as well as that from precursors that are found in foods of plant origin.

Table 12-4 shows the vitamin A value of the most frequently used foods and some recommended sources of vitamin A.

Liver, being the organ in the body in which vitamin A is stored, is the richest good food source. Pork liver has 12,000 RE/100 grams, whereas polar bear liver (the richest source and a toxic one) has 6000 RE/gram. Concentrates of fish liver oils, once widely used therapeutic sources of vitamin A, have been almost totally replaced by synthetic vitamin A in tablets and capsules.

Egg yolk, with 3300 IU of vitamin A or 1000 RE/100 grams (that is, 250 RE/egg) is a good source of vitamin A and is usually the first one introduced into an infant's diet. Because preformed vitamin A in animal foods is colorless, the deep yellow color in an egg yolk may reflect unconverted carotene rather than vitamin A activity. (Color also differs with the breed of hen.)

Vitamin A used to fortify foods is usually added as vitamin A palmitic, a combination of vitamin A and palmetic acid (a saturated fatty acid). The small amount used does not effect the P/S ratio of the diet.

The vitamin A value of butter shows a definite seasonal variation. In winter, butter averages 1900 IU or 570 RE/kg, whereas in summer, butter with more yellow coloring due to unconverted carotene has over 33,000 IU. Margarine is usually fortified with 30,000 IU/kg, usually as vitamin A palmitate.

In milk, vitamin A is present in the fat portion. Therefore vitamin A is absent in nonfat milk. However, most fresh fluid nonfat milk and dried nonfat milk solids are fortified with preformed vitamin A, with an average of 390 IU (130 RE) per cup. Aside from milk products, egg yolks, and liver, animal foods contain virtually no vitamin A.

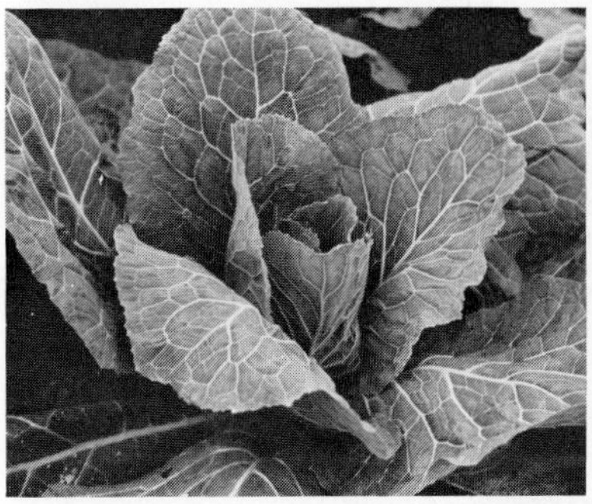

The amount of vitamin A in vegetables is directly proportional to the amount of carotene or chlorophyll in the food. Therefore, the deeper the color, the higher the vitamin A content.

Fruits and vegetables contain no preformed vitamin A, only precursors. Tables of food composition report IU of carotene. Vitamin A values (RE) for foods of plant origin, which are now included in some tables, depend on which particular carotene is present.

Generally, as can be seen from Table 12-4, the vitamin A value of fruits and vegetables is directly proportional to the color that comes from either the carotene or chlorophyll in the food. Therefore, the deeper the orange, yellow, or green colc of fruits and vegetables, the higher the vitamin A value. In addition, the vitamin A values of a food such as lettuce increase tenfold from the inner bleached leaves to the outer leaves, which are higher in the green pigment (chlorophyll) and yellow or orange pigment (carotenoids). Unfortunately, a high concentration of chlorophyll is often accompanied by an astringent bitter taste, as is found in very dark green endive leaves. Some potentially rich sources of vitamin A are therefore unpalatable. In some fruits such as mangos the carotene content increases with storage.

The pigments lycopene, found in watermelon and tomatoes, and xanthophyll, found in corn and egg yolk, do not have vitamin A value. Another yellow pigment in corn, cryptoxanthin, has a limited vitamin A potential of about 1 RE/gram. In countries where red palm oil (with 230 RE of vitamin A per gram) is used in cooking, its carotene content represents a major source of vitamin A activity.

Table 12-4 ◇ Vitamin A value of an average serving and per 100 kcal of foods most frequently reported in dietary survey and additional recommended sources

Food	Amount	Kcal	IU per Serving	IU per 100 Kcal	INQ*	Retinol Equivalent (RE)
Meat, Fish, Poultry, Eggs, Nuts						
Egg, fried	1 large	95	320	325	1.3	94
Beef, roast	3 oz	315	tr	tr		tr
Hamburger	3 oz	230	tr	tr		tr
Chicken	3 oz	140	20	14	0.5	5
Tuna	3 oz	165	70	42	0.2	20
Peanut butter	2 T	190	—	—	—	—
Bacon	3 slices	180	—	—	—	—
Beef liver†	3 oz	185	39,690	16,580	66	1,920
Cornflakes						
Cornflakes	1 oz.	110	—	—	—	—
Shredded wheat	1 biscuit	100	—	—	—	—
Saltines (10 grams)	4 crackers	50	—	—	—	—
Rice (cooked)	½ cup	109	—	—	—	—
White bread	1 slice	65	tr	tr	—	—
Whole-wheat bread	1 slice	70	tr	tr	—	—
Dairy Products						
Whole milk	8 oz	150	310	192	1.0	76
2% fat milk	8 oz	120	500	417	1.7	139
Cheddar cheese	1 oz	115	300	261	1.0	86
Fruits						
Apple	1 medium	80	70	88	.35	7
Banana	1 medium	105	90	86	.34	9
Orange juice, frozen	4 oz	55	95	173	.69	10
Peach	1 medium	35	470	1,343	5.40	47
Cantaloupe†	½ of a 5-in melon	45	8610	9,063	81.00	861
Vegetables						
Corn, canned	4 oz (½ cup)	83	255	310	1.2	26
Green beans	4 oz (½ cup)	22	235	1,208	4.2	24
Green peas	4 oz (½ cup)	62	655	1,129	4.5	65
Lettuce (100 grams)	¼ head	20	446	2,448	9.8	46
Tomatoes	1 medium	25	1,390	5,560	22.0	139
Potato, baked	1 medium	130	0	0	0	0
Broccoli†	½ cup	25	1,090	4,360	17	190
Spinach, cooked†	½ cup	20	7,370	10,425	146	737
Carrots†	½ cup	35	19,150	54,714	219	1,915

tr: trace; —: none.

*INQ based on U.S. RDA vitamin A = 5000 IU; energy need = 2000 kcal. INQ = % U.S. RDA (5000 IU)/% Energy requirement (2000 kcal). INQ ≥ 2.0 = nutrient-dense source.

†Recommended sources in addition to most frequently mentioned foods in dietary surveys.

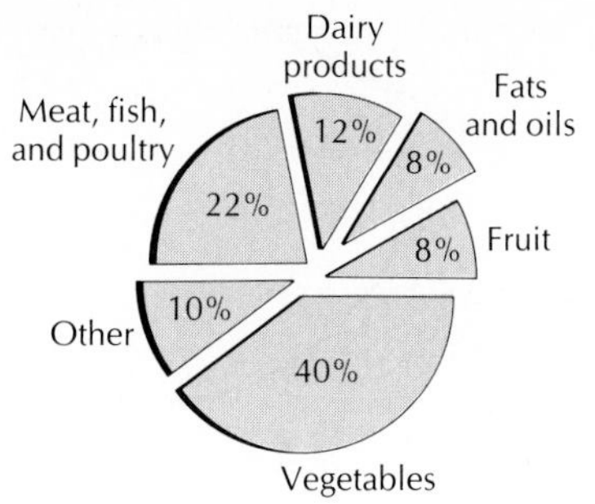

Figure 12-8 Contributions of various food groups to vitamin A in the North American food supply.
USDA, 1985.

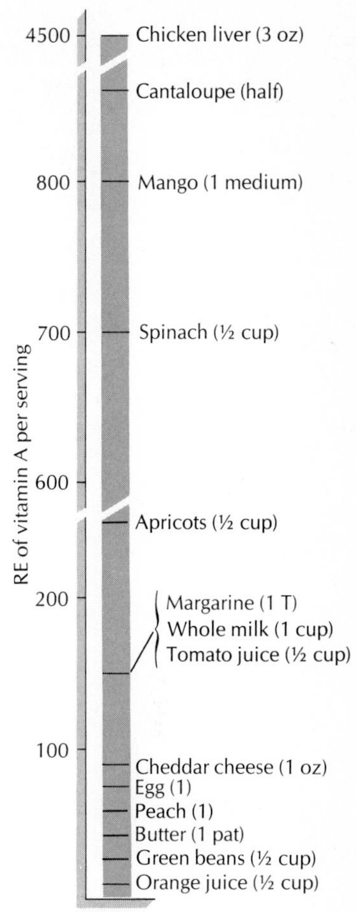

Figure 12-9 Relative amounts of vitamin A in various food sources.

Vitamin A is stable to heat and alkali but unstable to light, acids, and oxidation. Little vitamin A is lost under normal conditions of food preparation. Excessive temperatures in frying oils may cause the destruction of carotene, as will the oxidation that occurs in rancid fats. The small amount of green and yellow pigment that may appear in cooking water from fruits and vegetables represents an insignificant portion, if any, of the vitamin A that is actually present in the food. The drying of fruits in the sun and other forms of dehydration may lead to some loss of vitamin A.

The contributions of various food groups to the vitamin A content of the North American food supply are shown in Figure 12-8. The relative amounts of vitamin A in typical servings of various foods are shown in Figure 12-9.

In the United States, the average daily intake of vitamin A is 5400 IU, two thirds of which comes from vegetable sources. This can be compared to an average daily intake of 4300 IU in Britain, one third of which is from vegetables. In the tropics, the large amounts of palm oil used provide substantial amounts of vitamin A.

Deficiency

Deficiencies of vitamin A are found most often but not exclusively in preschool children. Deficiency symptoms show up after liver reserves of the vitamin have been depleted. These symptoms can also be the result of a deficiency of protein, needed to transport the vitamin, or zinc, needed to mobilize it from the liver. Symptoms may result from low dietary intakes, interference with absorption and storage, or interference with the conversion of carotene to vitamin A. Most symptoms of human vitamin A deficiency reflect the vitamin's role in maintaining the health of epithelial cells; they also usually involve the eyes.

Night Blindness

One of the earliest symptoms of vitamin A deficiency is **night blindness,** which is an inability to adjust to dim light following exposure to bright lights. Low vitamin A intakes cause liver reserves to drop, followed by a drop in blood levels and the amount of vitamin A available to the retina of the eye for formation of the visual pigment rhodopsin.

night blindness
An inability to adjust to vision in dim light

Changes in the Eye

The cornea of the eye is affected early with vitamin A deficiency. The tear gland fails to secrete tears, and there are distinct changes, including increased dryness, in the film covering the cornea. Other symptoms follow: keratinization, opacity, and sloughing of the epithelial cells of the cornea, which eventually rupture the cornea. Infection sets in, pus is released, and the eye hemorrhages. The symptoms occur in a condition known as *Bitot's spots* in its mildest form, as *xerosis conjunctiva* in moderately severe form, and as *xerophthalmia* in advanced states. Typical eye symptoms of severe vitamin A deficiency are shown in Figure 12-10.

xerophthalmia
A condition resulting from deficiency of vitamin A affecting the eye
(xero = dry; ophthalm = eye)

A

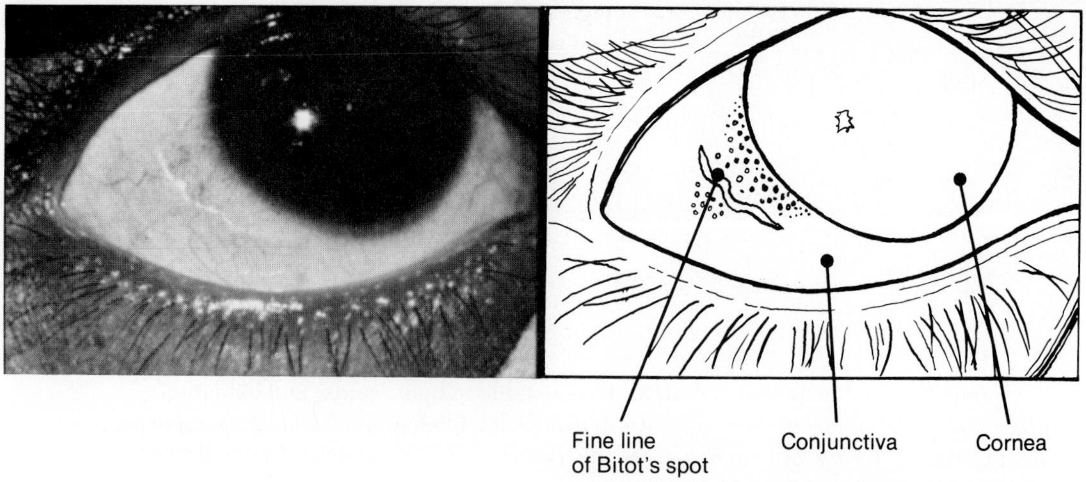

B

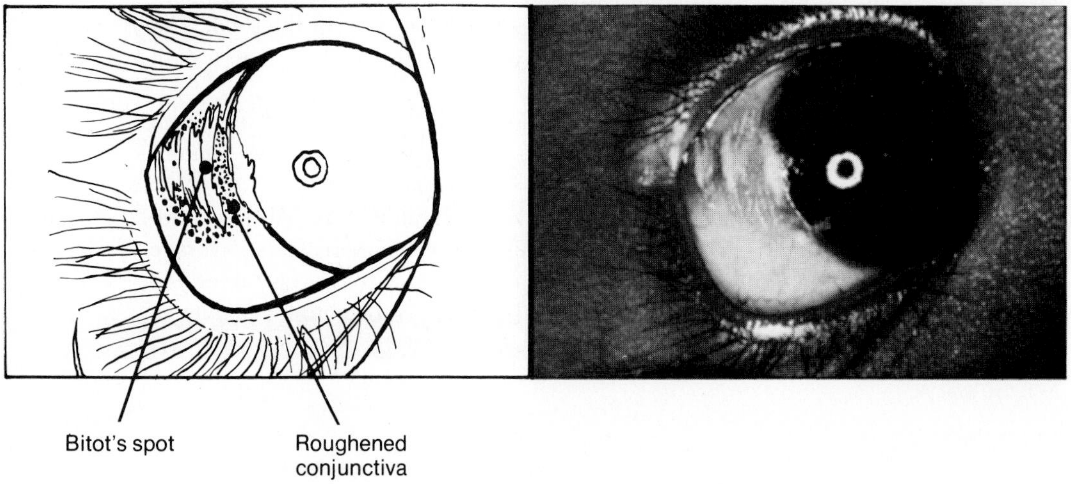

Figure 12-10 Development of eye symptoms of vitamin A deficiency. **A,** The first symptom of xerophthalmia is night blindness, followed by the occurrence of Bitot's spots on the conjunctiva. **B,** As the disease progresses the conjunctiva becomes dry and rough (conjunctiva xerosis).
Courtesy The Nutrition Foundation, Inc, NY, and American Foundation for Overseas Blind, Inc, NY.

Total blindness is a common outcome of vitamin A deficiency. This type of blindness frequently affects children; in fact, it is the leading cause of blindness in people under 21 years of age. It causes an estimated 250,000 cases of blindness a year in children in developing countries. Many children probably succumb to other forms of vitamin deficiency or infection before xerophthalmia develops. An infection (for example, measles) usually precedes xerophthalmia. The added stress of infection makes the child more susceptible to vitamin A deficiency and eventual blindness.

Epithelial Cells

folliculosis
A condition in which there is accumulation of hard material at the base of the hair follicle

Dry, rough skin, especially on the shoulders, may be an early sign of vitamin A deficiency. The condition known as **folliculosis,** in which there are small bumps near the base of the hair follicles that later become hard or keratinized, is used as an indication of possible vitamin A deficiency. This condition resembles permanent "goose bumps."

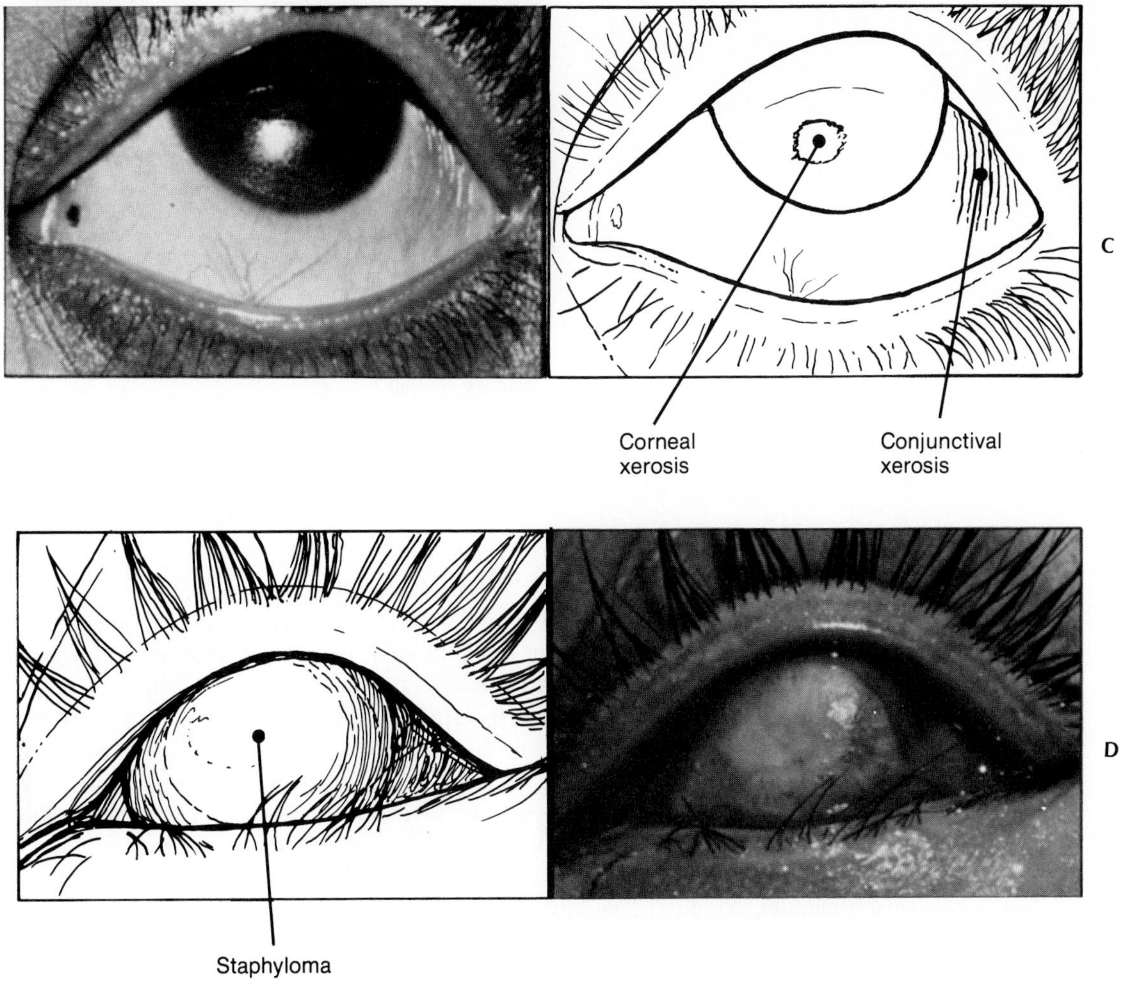

Figure 12-10, cont'd. C, Corneal dryness (corneal xerosis) may develop if the disease is not treated. **D,** If xerophthalmia is not treated, or is treated too late, it may result in damage or permanent blindness.

Other effects include changes in the gastrointestinal tract, with diarrhea linked to the changes in epithelial tissue; the absence of tooth enamel; and loss of both taste and smell, resulting in decreased appetite and food intake.

Dietary Intake

Data from the Nationwide Food Consumption Survey show that although the average intake of vitamin A was 134% of the RDA, only 50% of those evaluated had dietary intakes meeting the RDA, and 30% had intakes below 70% of the RDA. NHANES II data showed a mean intake of 98% of the RDA but a median intake of only 3300 IU. As shown in Figure 12-11, this pattern prevailed 10 years later in resurvey of women, children, and adult men.

Although there is little evidence of night blindness or other clinical signs of **hypovitaminosis** A (a condition in which the level of the vitamin in the blood is too low) about 5% of children ages 3 to 5 have serum vitamin A levels that are unacceptable. Beyond age 11, there are few low values.

hypovitaminosis
A condition in which the level of a vitamin in the blood is too low

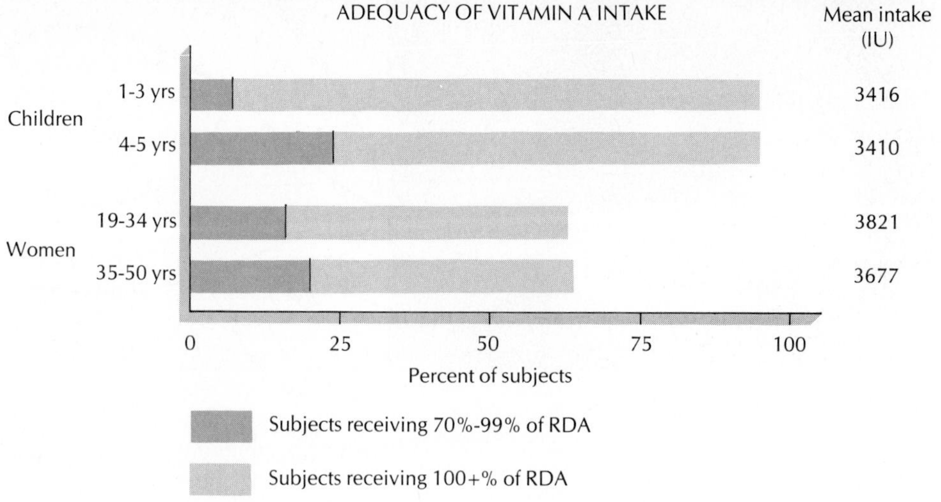

Figure 12-11 Adequacy of dietary intake of vitamin A as reported in USDA Continuing Survey of Individuals, 1985-1986.

Programs for the Prevention of Vitamin A Deficiency

Several countries in which vitamin A deficiency is rampant have programs to add vitamin A to a commercially processed staple food. In Central America, white cane sugar is the only such food that is universally consumed; in the Philippines, monosodium glutamate has been used. These supplementation programs have been very effective in reducing the incidence of vitamin A deficiency. Alternative programs to encourage the home production of vitamin A–rich fruits and vegetables or to promote the use of red palm oil in cooking have been considerably less successful.

In India, a program that provides each child under 5 years of age with a single dose of 100,000 IU (30,000 RE) of vitamin A in oil, dropped directly on the tongue every 6 months, has produced an impressive reduction in the incidence of vitamin A deficiency. Unfortunately, about 25% of the children are missed because it is difficult to administer such a massive program. An earlier use of vitamin A tablets in India was considerably less successful.

Evaluation of Vitamin A Status

The most sensitive indicator of vitamin A status is the measurement of vitamin A stores in the liver, but this is not feasible for the evaluation of populations. Because an inadequate protein intake or a possible zinc deficiency may prevent the release of vitamin A from the liver into the blood, plasma vitamin A levels are a poor indicator of vitamin A reserves. In addition, plasma vitamin values do not drop until liver reserves are depleted. Normal plasma levels for vitamin A are 20 to 50 μg/dl of blood. Any drop in plasma vitamin A levels below 10 μg/dl reflects a depletion of liver reserves. These reductions are associated with clinical symptoms such as follicular keratosis, which is a hardening of the base of the hair follicle; impaired dark adaptation; or severe acne.

Clinical Uses

Vitamin A and Acne

Like most vitamins, vitamin A has been used to treat a wide variety of conditions, including acne. Until recently, the use of high oral doses and topical applications of vitamin A (in the forms of retinol and retinal) to control acne had disappointing results. The topical use of retinoic acid, however, has proved considerably more successful, although it is very effective with some types of acne and totally ineffective with others. Oral doses of a naturally occurring form of retinoic acid have also had dramatic effects in several common forms of acne. However, retinoic acid should be used only under strict medical supervision; it should not be used by pregnant women or those likely to become pregnant because it may cause birth defects. Another synthetic analog of vitamin A with a significant effect on the health of aging skin is currently undergoing clinical tests. It may unfortunately have undesirable side effects.

Retinoids and Cancer

Studies on animals and humans have shown that several vitamin A–related substances (particularly carotenes) are associated with low rates of certain cancers. They appear to function in preventing the proliferation or progression of cancer rather than the initiation of the tumor. Epidemiological studies show that the dietary intake of carotenoids is inversely related to the development of lung cancer in later life. Their anticancer effect may be due to their ability to act as antioxidants. There is, however, no evidence that people on diets with recommended amounts of vitamin A or its precursors are at greater risk of cancer than those whose diets contain larger amounts. Several clinical trials to test the effectiveness of beta-carotene or other related carotenoids to control cancer growth are underway.

Toxicity

The possibility that too much vitamin A may be toxic has been recognized only recently. Symptoms have been reported after the consumption of polar bear liver, with 6000 RE of vitamin A per gram; after treatment of skin disorders in adolescents with vitamin A; and with high daily supplements for infants. The symptoms of vitamin A toxicity for adults are headaches, drowsiness, nausea, loss of hair, dry skin, and diarrhea; for infants, the symptoms are scaly dermatitis, weight loss, anorexia, and skeletal pain. Menstruation ceases in women, and rapid resorption of bone occurs in adults. The period between the initiation of high intakes and the onset of symptoms varies from 6 to 15 months. Some people show symptoms after long-term dosages of 16,000 RE/day, and others exhibit a reaction only at levels of 40,000 to 55,000 RE/day. (These amounts are readily available in over-the-counter supplements.) Infants have exhibited bulging of the head, hydrocephalus, hyperirritability, and increased intracranial pressure after dosages of 8000 RE/day for as little as 30 days.

Beta-Carotene (RE) in Fruits and Vegetables

Cantaloupe	500-900
Apricots	100-167
Cherries	50-83
Apple	33-57
Peach	27-83
Kale	635-985
Spinach	450-735
Carrots	400-815
Tomatoes	60-125
Asparagus	40-665
Broccoli	105-250

Range of values reflects degree of pigmentation.

Data Courtesy Dr. Paul LaChance, Rutgers University.

Recovery is rapid and complete after withdrawal of the vitamin, with symptoms frequently subsiding within 72 hours. Problems occur only from overuse of the preformed vitamin, not the precursor. Permanent effects of vitamin A toxicity are rare. There is some concern that long-standing daily intakes of 25,000 RE vitamin A by a pregnant woman may have harmful effects on her fetus. In animals, single injections of vitamin A in pregnant females have produced cleft palate in their young.

The FDA is concerned about the effects of toxicity but has been unsuccessful in attempts to impose a ceiling of 25,000 RE on the amount of preformed vitamin A that can be included in a nonprescription multivitamin preparation. The availability of inexpensive, high-potency vitamin A supplements is an ever-present danger because of the tendency of some people to oversupplement their diet.

On the other hand, carotene has never led to signs of toxicity, even at very large intakes, largely because the proportion absorbed decreases as intake increases. At the same time, much of the carotene that is absorbed does not get changed to vitamin A and ends up being stored in fat. When subcutaneous fat picks up carotene, it takes on a yellow color and the condition is called carotenodermia. This gives the body, particularly the soles of the feet and palms of the hands, a yellow and jaundiced look. Although completely harmless, this coloring is often distressing, especially when it occurs in young infants.

Women taking isotrenoid (Accutane) to cure acne should stop taking it several months before they expect to become pregnant because its use is associated with developmental defects in infants. Similarly, pregnant women should not take supplements with more than 5000 IU vitamin A.

VITAMIN D

rickets
A disease in which there are weaknesses and abnormalities in bone formation as the result of a vitamin D deficiency; infantile rickets is most common

antirachitic
Having the ability to combat rickets (anti = against or opposed; rachitic = having rickets)

Rickets, a condition characterized by defective bone formation in infants, has been prevented or cured by exposure to sunlight or by the regular ingestion of cod-liver oil. However, only in the last decade have we found out how these two seemingly unrelated cures work. The active substance responsible for curing rickets was originally known simply as vitamin D. Now, it is officially designated as cholecalciferol (vitamin D_3) if it comes from animal sources and as ergosterol (vitamin D_2) if it comes from sources such as yeast. Vitamin D had been known previously as the "sunshine vitamin," because sunshine is necessary to form vitamin D in the skin, and as the **antirachitic** factor, or rickets-preventive factor, because it prevents and cures rickets.

Because vitamin D can be produced in the body, it is considered by some scientists to be a hormone. However, when vitamin D is supplied by the diet, it is technically a vitamin. Regardless of whether the substance is considered a vitamin or a hormone, the nutritionist is concerned that adequate amounts be available for its role in promoting normal development of bones and teeth.

Discovery

In 1918, Mellanby presented evidence of a fat-soluble substance with antirachitic properties. Shortly afterward, the antirachitic properties of cod-liver oil, which had been used as a folk remedy since the early nineteenth century, were recognized. This fat-soluble substance, which was not destroyed by oxidation as was the vitamin A discovered earlier, was soon identified as vitamin D.

Provitamin D, or precursors ergosterol in plants and 7-dehydrocholesterol in the skin (which can be changed into vitamin D through irradiation by the short ultraviolet rays of the sun), were discovered in 1922. This antirachitic factor was isolated in crystalline form in 1930, and by 1937 its chemical structure has been determined. Most of the vitamin D used in supplements or in the fortification of food products has been obtained from irradiation of the precursors of vitamin D. It is now possible to synthesize two vitamin D derivatives that are even more effective than the naturally occurring vitamin in preventing several types of rickets.

Rickets

Rickets is a condition that has for centuries plagued infants in the temperate zone, that part of the world where the climate has marked seasons. It was so common in England that some writers referred to it as the "English disease" and believed it to be due to an environmental factor. The fact that rickets occurred very frequently among people living in the crowded, smoky, industrial sections of cities with poor sanitation suggested that it was caused by a bacteria. However, the children of the wealthy were even more prone to rickets than children of the poor. From time to time, it was suggested that sunshine helped prevent or cure rickets, but the relationship was not established until the late 1920s.

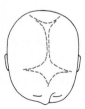

fontanel
The point at which the two hemispheres of the skull merge; the juncture is open at birth but should fuse before 1 year of age

Rickets is essentially a disease of defective bone formation. Deformities develop when poorly calcified bones are not strong enough to perform their functions; for example, bowing of the legs occurs when a child starts to walk before the bones are rigid enough to support the weight of the body (Figure 12-12). The ends of the long bones become enlarged, causing difficulties in movement. Knock knees result from the flattening that occurs in the poorly calcified ends of the bones. Deformities of the ribs result in a concave breast ("pigeon breast") that causes crowding in the chest cavity. Ribs also develop irregularly spaced areas of swelling that look like beads (this is also known as rachitic rosary). The **fontanel**, which is the opening on top of the skull in a very young infant, fails to close in early life. This allows rapid enlargement of the head, sometimes erroneously interpreted as a sign of health in the child. Teeth erupt later, are less well formed than normal, and decay earlier.

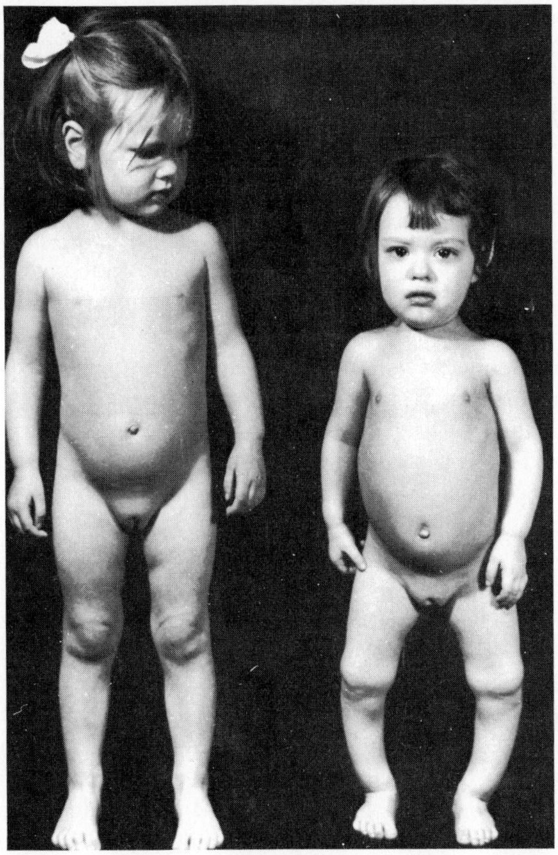

Figure 12-12 Typical case of rickets in a young girl *(right)* compared to a normal child *(left)*.
From Arneil GC: World Review of Nutrition and Dietetics 10:239, 1969.

Growth is generally retarded, but the severity of the disease as determined from other symptoms is frequently greater in children who have grown rapidly.

Rickets primarily affects children; the symptoms are reversed slowly if at all. Some symptoms produced during early childhood may remain throughout adulthood. Many of the cases of recurring rickets in the 1960s in both Great Britain and the United States were identified in children between the ages of 2 and 4; they showed a growth retardation and the typical bowed legs.

The term "adult rickets" is sometimes applied to the disease osteomalacia, in which there is a defect in bone formation but not necessarily because of vitamin D deficiency. Osteomalacia occurs most often in regions where customs prevent women from exposure to sunlight or where women bear and nurse children continuously throughout their childbearing years.

Although rickets was practically stamped out as a health problem in the Western world by the mid-1920s, there was a reappearance of the condition in the early 1960s. In Britain, over 500 cases of rickets were diagnosed; in addition, there were undoubtedly many people suffering from subclinical rickets. Most of those affected were immigrants whose dark skin pigmentation prevented the short rays of the sun from penetrating the skin. In the United States, there have been reports of rickets among children raised on strict vegetarian diets. Between 1974 and 1978, 24 cases of rickets were reported in Philadelphia; all were found in breast-fed infants who received no supplemental vitamin D.

Functions

Once the active form of vitamin D has been produced it is carried in the blood to the intestine, bones, and kidneys. It acts on all three tissues to stimulate a variety of reactions that increase the amount of calcium and phosphorus available for bone formation.

1. In the intestine, calcitriol (formed in the kidney from vitamin D) stimulates the synthesis of a calcium-binding protein and a phosphorus-binding protein. These two proteins increase the absorption of dietary calcium and phosphorus.
2. In the bone, calcitriol acts together with the parathyroid hormone to stimulate the release of calcium from the bone surface into the blood.
3. In the kidneys, calcitriol stimulates the reabsorption of calcium and phosphorus that might otherwise be lost as the blood is filtered through the kidneys.

When blood calcium has increased to normal levels, the parathyroid gland stops secreting the hormone that stimulates the production of calcitriol in the kidney. Without calcitriol, the intestine, bone, and kidneys can no longer effect the changes that increase blood calcium levels. A similar series of changes occurs with the level of blood phosphorus. These processes continue until normal levels of phosphorus are restored, after which the production of calcitriol is cut off.

Absorption and Metabolism

Dietary vitamin D is absorbed primarily in the upper part of the small intestine; both infants and adults absorb 80% of intake. The same factors that aid in or depress fat absorption also enhance or decrease the absorption of vitamin D.

Once absorbed, vitamin D is incorporated into small fat particles, or chylomicrons, and transported in the lymphatic system. From the lymphatic system, it is removed from the chylomicrons and transported in the blood plasma to the liver attached to a protein carrier called alpha-globulin$_2$, or DBP (vitamin D-binding protein).

irradiation
Process of treating with ultraviolet light (short wavelengths)

calcidiol
A metabolite of vitamin D, formed in the liver by adding a hydroxyl group to vitamin D, resulting in 25-hydroxycholecalciferol

calcitriol
A further metabolite and active form of vitamin D, formed when the kidney further hydroxylates calcidiol to produce 1,25-dihydroxycholecalciferol

Vitamin D that is formed from the **irradiation** of the precursor 7-dehydrocholesterol in the skin is bound to a transport protein and transferred to the liver. There, it is indistinguishable from the vitamin D provided in food.

Once vitamin D is removed by the liver, it is converted by a reaction called hydroxylation, which adds an OH group to form **calcidiol** (or 25-hydroxycholecalciferol). As soon as enough is produced, a feedback mechanism cuts off production. Calcidiol is then transported in the blood to the kidneys, attached to the same or a similar protein carrier that took its precursors to the liver. In the kidneys it is further hydroxylated (has another OH added) to form **calcitriol** (or 1,25-dihydroxycholecalciferol), which differs from the ingested or skin precursors only in the presence of two hydroxyl (OH) groups. It is calcitriol that is responsible for the vitamin activity. The regulation of vitamin D metabolism is another example of the sensitive way in which metabolism of several nutrients is interrelated.

Calcitriol (1,25-dihydroxycholecalciferol, or 1,25-DHCC) production is regulated indirectly by blood calcium levels. As blood calcium levels drop, the parathyroid gland, located on the surface of the thyroid in the neck area, is stimulated to secrete a dipeptide parathyroid hormone. This hormone travels to the kidneys, where it stimulates the enzyme responsible for converting calcidiol to calcitriol. When the level of calcium in the blood increases to a certain level, the thyroid gland secretes another substance, calcitonin, which causes a reduction in the production of 1,25-DHCC (the useful form) and diverts metabolism to another form—24-25-DHCC—that does not favor bone formation.

Similarly, low levels of phosphorus stimulate 1,25-DHCC production, and high levels stimulate 24,25-DHCC production. The substance 24,25-DHCC can be converted further to 1,24,25-trihydroxy vitamin D, with three hydroxyl groups. Neither of these substances functions as a vitamin.

A synthetic form of 1,25-DHCC is now being produced and tested for safety, after which the FDA will be able to release it for general use. It can be taken orally and eliminates the need for production of the active form in both the liver and the kidneys. If approved, this synthetic form will be useful for people with defective kidney or liver functions that prevent them from making the active form of the vitamin or for the elderly, whose kidney and liver function declines.

Excretion

Most vitamin D is excreted in the bile as part of bile acid. About 60% to 80% of an injected dose of vitamin D appears in the feces after being excreted in the bile into the gastrointestinal tract. The absorption and metabolism of vitamin D is summarized in Figure 12-13.

Requirements

Vitamin D is measured in International Units, which are defined in terms of a biological response to the feeding of this vitamin to a depleted animal. One International Unit (IU) of vitamin D weighs 0.25 μg; 1 μg contains 40 IU. Both IU and micrograms of cholecalciferol are used in expressing the vitamin D content of foods and vitamin D allowances.

40 IU of vitamin D = 1 μg of cholecalciferol

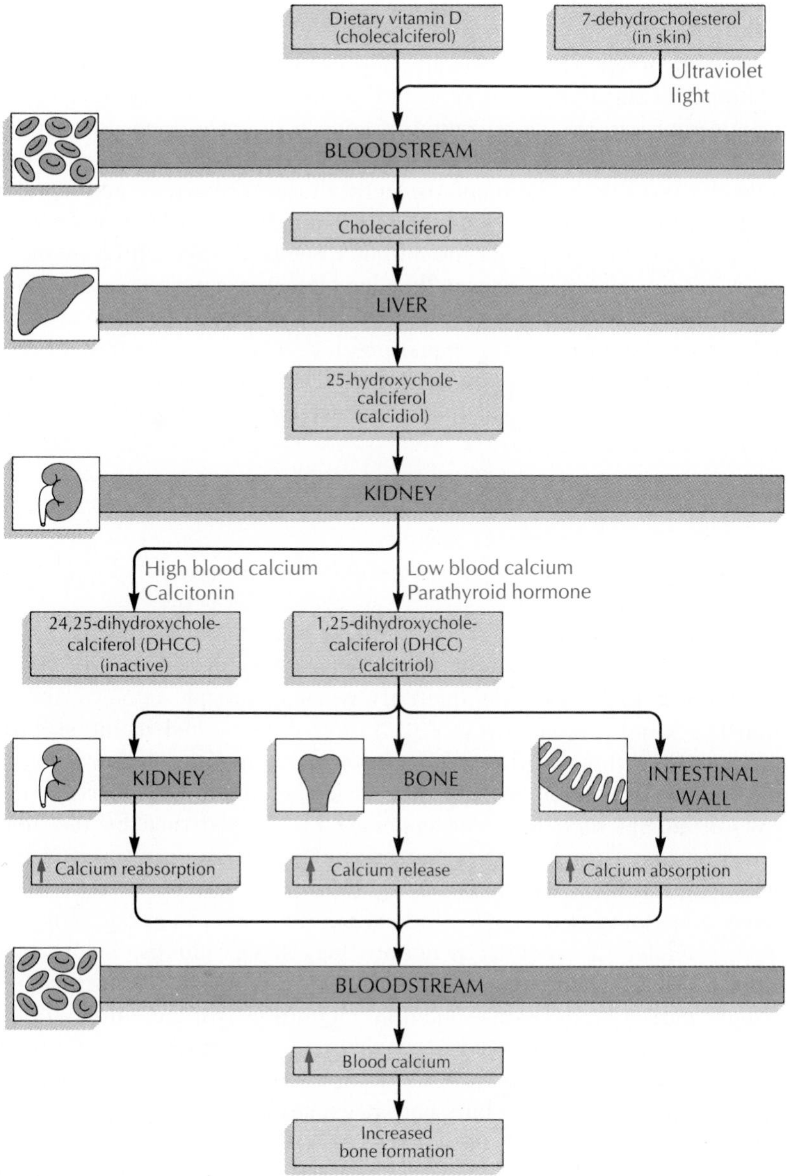

Figure 12-13 Summary of the absorption and metabolism of vitamin D.

Recommended Allowances for Vitamin D

Infants	10 μg	400 IU
Children (1-18 yr)	10 μg	400 IU
Adults		
19-22 yr	7.5 μg	300 IU
23 + yr	5 μg	200 IU
Pregnant women	+5 μg	+ 200 IU
Lactating women	+5 μg	+ 200 IU

There are two sources of vitamin D: food and the skin. It is therefore difficult to determine minimum vitamin D requirements. Indications are that 100 IU of vitamin D/day will protect against rickets and will promote growth when adequate amounts of calcium and phosphorus have been ingested. However, because daily intakes of 300 to 400 IU (7.5 to 10 μg) seem to promote better calcium absorption and some increase in growth, the RDA has been set at 10 μg (400 IU)/day for infants, children, adolescents, and pregnant and lactating women. Intakes above 20 μg (800 IU) appear to provide no greater protection against rickets than more conservative amounts.

If fortified milk or commercial infant formulas are used, it is not only unnecessary but also possibly undesirable to use supplements because the milk or formulas alone provide adequate amounts. Reports that breast milk contains a water-soluble form of vitamin D have been discredited, confirming that breast milk is low in vitamin D.

Because half of fetal calcium is deposited in the last 6 weeks of fetal life, premature infants have much lower calcium reserves than do full-term ones and need vitamin D to aid in the absorption of the high levels of calcium necessary to meet the demands of rapid growth. The apparent ineffectiveness of dosages of 400 IU of vitamin D in breast-fed premature infants may be a function of the low calcium content of breast milk rather than an indication of an abnormally high need for vitamin D.

During both pregnancy and lactation, a woman's blood level of calcitriol increases sharply. This increase is reflected in an enhanced absorption of calcium from the intestine and the mobilization of bone calcium to meet the needs of the developing fetus and young infant. Possibly the response is stimulated by the increase in the level of the hormone prolactin during pregnancy and lactation. An intake of 15 μg of vitamin D per day is recommended to meet this need.

It is more difficult to evaluate the minimal needs of older children and adults, who seldom develop rickets. Because they have greater exposure to ultraviolet light and to many food sources, their needs seem to be met. If occupational or clothing habits (such as those of miners or nuns) preclude exposure to sunlight, an intake of 400 IU of vitamin D per day is suggested. Deficiency symptoms develop only when exposure to sunlight is inadequate, dietary intake of vitamin D is restricted, or needs are relatively high.

Sources

Sources of Vitamin D
Irradiation of precursor in the skin
Foods (fortified milk, egg yolk)

Vitamin D is available to the body by two separate pathways: the skin and the diet.

The Skin

The precursor 7-dehydrocholesterol, when exposed to short (275 to 300 μm) ultraviolet rays from the sun or from mercury vapor sunlamps, is converted into the previtamin D_3, which over the next 2 to 3 days is converted in the skin into the active vitamin D_3 without further exposure to sunlight. The amount of vitamin D produced through irradiation of the precursor in the skin is influenced more by the amount of ultraviolet light to which a person is exposed than by the amount of precursor available. During the summer in a temperate zone, ultraviolet rays may reach far enough north for a maximum of 4 hours in the middle of the day, more than enough time to meet needs. In winter, this time may be reduced to less than an hour. Ultraviolet rays cannot penetrate fog, smog, clouds, smoke, ordinary window glass, window screening, clothing, or skin pigment. The presence of any or all of these barriers reduces the potential vitamin D available through radiation. The pigment in the skin, which acts as a protection against overproduction of vitamin D in dark-skinned persons when they live in the tropics, reduces benefits when they live in a more temperate zone because there is less sun and a smaller amount of irradiation.

The Diet

The diet is the primary source of vitamin D in the temperate zone. Foods of animal origin such as eggs, milk, butter, and fish-liver oils are the major sources of preformed vitamin D. However, food sources are characteristically unreliable because the amount of vitamin D present varies with the diet and breed of the animal. Most foods contain cholecalciferol, but some may contain 25-HCC, the metabolite of vitamin D formed in the liver. Even when all potential dietary sources are used, including egg yolk, butter, and milk, it is possible to obtain only about 125 IU of vitamin D a day. Therefore it is now customary to rely either on foods fortified with vitamin D or nutritional supplements when the need for vitamin D is high.

Milk, a carrier of the calcium and phosphorus needed for bone calcification, is the food most commonly fortified with vitamin D. Evaporated milk, irradiated to provide 400 IU per quart or liter of reconstituted milk, was the first food to be sold as an irradiated product. Now 95% of homogenized milk, practically all of nonfat milk, and much of the dried nonfat milk solids have added vitamin D. Most of the milk sold in North America is fortified with vitamin D at a level that will permit maximum utilization of calcium and phosphorus in the milk. The cost of fortifying 100 gallons (380 liters) of milk is estimated to be a mere 4¢.

Vitamin D is not added to buttermilk or acidophilus milk.

Although milk is the only product that has been endorsed for fortification, vitamin D is being added to many other products such as infant cereals, prepared breakfast cereals, milk flavorings, bread, and even some beverages. If a person consumed one serving of each of these products along with 1 quart (liter) of fortified milk a day, intake could easily reach 1000 IU daily. Assessing the amount of vitamin D in the diet is difficult without access to labels on the products. For example, in the United States, flour producers have the option of adding from 250 to 1000 IU of vitamin D per pound (0.45 kg) of flour. Although the United States does not allow the addition of vitamin D to margarine, England requires the addition of 1300 to 1600 IU/pound, and Germany, 135 IU/pound.

In temperate zones, pediatricians routinely introduce a supplementary source of vitamin D into infant diets. Cod-liver oil, used the early 1920s, has been completely replaced by water-soluble vitamin D preparations. (Water-soluble preparations also contain vitamin A and vitamin C.) Most drug companies had voluntarily reduced the recommended vitamin D dosage to provide only 400 IU/dose even before the FDA made that limit mandatory in 1965. Labels usually carry warnings against excessive use of vitamin D supplements.

In Europe, doctors have found that massive injections of 300,000 IU of vitamin D at intervals of 6 weeks to 3 months are effective in controlling rickets. Apparently, there are no adverse effects from such large doses.

Toxicity

With the demonstration over 60 years ago that cod-liver oil was effective in preventing rickets, the disease has ceased to be a cause of concern to public health authorities. Now the concern lies at the other end of the continuum: the problem of overuse of vitamin D. Early studies showed that no extra benefit was derived from levels above 400 IU/day and that levels of 1800 IU/day actually retarded linear growth. More recently, reports of infant **hypercalcemia**, in which practically all tissues of the body are adversely affected, have focused attention on the possibility that high levels of vitamin D are toxic.

hypercalcemia
Condition in which the calcium content of the blood is above normal levels

The level of vitamin D intake that brings on hypercalcemia ranges from a low of 10 μg/day in very sensitive infants, to 100 μg/day (for 4 months) in children, to 1000 μg/day in adults. Adults receiving 100,000 IU of vitamin D for periods of weeks or months will develop symptoms; most cases have involved intakes of 25,000 to 60,000 IU/day for 1 to 4 months. The withdrawal of all sources of vitamin D alleviates symptoms of appetite loss, nausea, weight loss, and failure to thrive associated with high blood-calcium levels.

Although the effect of hypervitaminosis D (excessive vitamin D) in human pregnancy has not been established, studies with pregnant rats showed that changes in the placenta and impaired maturation of osteoblasts (the bone-forming cells) resulted in defective bone formation. There is no evidence of toxicity from overexposure to the sun.

Interrelationship with Drugs

Increases in the incidence of rickets and osteomalacia, associated with anticonvulsant therapy in epilepsy and with the use of sedatives and tranquilizers have been attributed to the breakdown of vitamin D from active to inactive forms.

VITAMIN E

Among the fat-soluble vitamins, vitamin E is probably the most familiar and at the same time the one most frequently misused. It is estimated that 11 to 12 million adults in the United States are taking supplements of vitamin E in the hope that it will be a panacea for a variety of ailments ranging from infertility to heart disease to aging.

Vitamin E was recognized in 1922 by Evans and Bishop as a dietary factor in plants that was essential for normal reproduction in rats. It was not until 1933 that it was identified as a group of substances known as **tocopherols** and **tocotrienols** and established as a dietary essential for humans. Because of its role in preventing permanent sterility in male animals, vitamin E became known as the antisterility vitamin. The term has persisted in spite of the fact that it is now known that vitamin E has no unique role in human reproduction and that failure of reproduction in animals is only one of the results of a lack of vitamin E. The level of interest in vitamin E is evident from the fact that over the past 10 years there have been an average of over 650 scientific publications yearly dealing with it.

tocopherol
One of the compounds in food having vitamin E activity; d-alpha-tocopherol is the most biologically active.

tocotrienol
Another compound in food with vitamin E activity

Vitamin E is actually not a single compound but a mixture of at least eight naturally occurring tocopherols and tocotrienols, each of which makes a unique contribution to the vitamin E content in a food. Four different tocopherols have been identified: alpha, beta, gamma, and delta, all of which are oily yellow liquids. Of these, d-alpha-tocopherol is the most biologically active. RRR-alpha-tocopherol is a form with a specific chemical configuration, which is the current standard for measuring the vitamin E content of foods. The amount of vitamin E in the other forms is expressed in **tocopherol equivalents (TE),** so that values in tables of food composition represent the sum of the equivalents of RRR-alpha-tocopherol from all forms in the food. Chemically, these various forms differ from one another very slightly, but the difference is enough to mean that the biological value of the various forms is reduced to 10% to 50% of the value of tocopherol. Although much of the vitamin E used in supplements is naturally occurring alpha-tocopherol, concentrated from vegetable oils, the majority is vitamin E succinate or vitamin E acetate, both of which are more stable to light and oxidation and therefore do not lose their potency over time in pills or capsules. The synthetic form of vitamin E, which is usually labelled as All-rac-dl-α-tocopherylacetate, has about 50% of the biological activity of the naturally occurring alpha-tocopherol.

tocopherol equivalents (TE)
Units of measure for vitamin E in foods and for vitamin E requirements

1 mg tocopherol =
1 IU alpha-tocopherol =
1 tocopherol equivalent (TE).

Functions

Because deficiencies of vitamin E occur in humans only when there is a defect in fat absorption, such as that occurring in **cystic fibrosis** (also known as abetalipoproteinemia), or among premature infants, much of our knowledge of the functions of vitamin E has come from studies on animals.

It is generally agreed that the main function of vitamin E is as an **antioxidant,**

cystic fibrosis
A genetic disease in which the absorption of fat and fat-soluble nutrients is inhibited

antioxidant
Substance such as vitamin E or selenium that prevents the oxidation of another substance by taking up the oxygen itself

or substance that prevents oxidation. In this role it acts as a "scavenger," seeking out **free radicals** that either enter the body from the atmosphere (ozones and nitrogen dioxide) or are formed within the body through normal metabolic processes. Free radicals that cause the oxidation of polyunsaturated fats that are part of the structure of many cell membranes leave the membranes changed and weakened. By inactivating these oxidizing agents, vitamin E protects many tissues against destruction from oxidation of these components. (The change that occurs when lipid in the cell membrane is oxidized is similar to the change that occurs when a cooking fat becomes rancid on exposure to air.) The two tissues that are most susceptible to oxidation in a deficiency of vitamin E are the red blood cell membranes and the cells of the lungs. When lipid in the red cell membrane becomes oxidized, the membrane weakens and breaks and the cell loses its contents—this is the process of hemolysis. The lungs, which are exposed to more of the oxidizing substances from the environment than any other tissues, are particularly susceptible to oxidative changes. They are protected, however, when naturally occurring antioxidants such as vitamin E are available in the blood to help stabilize polyunsaturated fatty acids and phospholipids in the lung membranes.

free radicals
Very reactive molecules that seek other molecules with which to react

The antioxidant properties of vitamin E are also thought to explain its role in preventing the formation of **lipofuscin,** a pigment that forms in the uterus and may be a factor in the reabsorption of fetal tissue during miscarriage. Lipofuscin is considered characteristic of the aging process and shows up as brown spots under the skin.

lipofuscin
A colored substance formed from the breakdown of the cell wall during aging

Vitamin E also plays an important role in protecting vitamin A, vitamin C, and unsaturated fatty acids in the food against undesirable changes as the result of oxidation. The study of its role as an antioxidant is complicated by the fact that other substances, such as the mineral selenium, also function as biological antioxidants and perform some but not all of the roles of vitamin E.

Absorption and Metabolism

As a fat-soluble vitamin, vitamin E is absorbed best in the presence of fat and under the conditions that favor fat absorption. Most tocopherol is absorbed into the lymph, where it is incorporated into the chylomicrons. In the plasma, tocopherol circulates in association with the lipoproteins, primarily low-density lipoproteins (LDL), and undergoes rapid exchange with lipid membranes, especially red blood cell membranes. From 40% to 60% of dietary tocopherol is absorbed, but as the dose increases the proportion absorbed decreases. Vitamin E is stored primarily in the adipose tissues, muscle, and liver. Plasma levels of tocopherol normally range from 0.5 to 1.2 mg/dl but drop rapidly to half that level when vitamin E is withdrawn. Vitamin E stores are relatively abundant in normal people, and it usually takes several months for depletion to occur.

Recommended Allowances

It is well established from both human and animal studies that, as the dietary intake of polyunsaturated fatty acids goes up, so does the requirement for vitamin E, with the range of requirement apparently increasing by as much as tenfold. Although it has been difficult to devise a formula for relating vitamin E requirement to intake of polyunsaturated fatty acid (PUFA), an intake of 5 mg of vitamin E daily plus 0.5 mg/gram of PUFA in the diet has been proposed. However, there is no evidence of inadequacy with intakes considerably below those recommended on the basis of the formula; moreover, oils, which are the most common sources of PUFA, are also the best sources of vitamin E. Thus, such a formula is likely unnecessary. As a result, the recommended allowance for vitamin E for adults has been set at 10 mg TE/day for men and 8 mg TE/day for women. These amounts

Recommended Dietary Allowances for Vitamin E (TE/day)

Children (to 11 yr)	3-7
Adults	
Males (>11 yr)	10
Females (>11 yr)	8
Pregnancy	+2
Lactation	+3

will support a blood level of at least 0.5 mg/dl, which is considered adequate and which tends to increase with age. These recommended amounts are readily obtainable in the North American diet, in which the vitamin E/PUFA ratio of 0.6 mg of vitamin E/gram of PUFA is considered quite satisfactory.

For infants, whose stores at birth are limited, the recommended intake of vitamin E is based on the amount that is supplied in breast milk: approximately 2 mg/day. The breast-fed infant, however, has the advantage of the vitamin E content in **colostrum,** which is five times higher than the amount found in mature breast milk. The vitamin E content of human milk is four times that in cow's milk. Thus, during lactation, when the mother is transferring 2 mg/day to milk, an additional 3 mg of vitamin E is recommended on the assumption that 50% will be absorbed. All infant formula has added vitamin E to provide at least 5 mg/100 kcal, a level considerably above that provided in human milk. Recommended intakes for children range from 3 to 7 mg TE of vitamin E/day. For older children, the recommended amounts increase to reflect growth and increase in weight.

colostrum
Fluid secreted from breast of lactating women immediately after giving birth

Premature infants are born with very low levels of vitamin E in the blood, undoubtedly reflecting the fact that much of the vitamin E is transferred to the fetus during the latter part of pregnancy. To prevent hemolysis of the blood cells, it is usually necessary to supplement the diet of premature infants with up to 35 mg TE of vitamin E for the first 2 months of life.

During pregnancy, when the expectant mother's level of vitamin E increases in relation to her increase in blood lipid, an additional 2 mg TE is recommended.

Food Sources

The major source of vitamin E in the North American diet is vegetable oil, which accounts for about 60% of the estimated TE available. The vitamin E content of various oils ranges from 4 mg/100 grams of coconut oil, to 94 mg/100 grams of soybean oil (Figure 12-14). The use of a specific oil as a source of vitamin E in the United States is determined largely by relative price and availability because for most commercial purposes, corn, cottonseed, peanut, coconut, and soybean oils can be used interchangeably. (Current labeling laws require manufacturers to list on the label every oil that might have been used in a product. Because the mix of

Vitamin E content of margarine = 3 to 15 mg/100 grams

Table 12-5 ◆ Vitamin E content of 100 grams of some representative foods

Food	mg/100 g	mg/serving*	Food	mg/100 g	mg/serving*
Mayonnaise	50.0	8.0	Tomatoes, fresh	0.85	
Margarine (made with corn oil)	46.7	8.0	Green peas, frozen	0.65	
			Ground beef	0.63	
Yellow cornmeal	2.2	0.4	Pork chops, pan-fried	0.60	
Whole-wheat bread	2.0	0.6	Chicken breast	0.58	
			Cornflakes	0.43	0.12
Spinach	1.4	0.7	Banana	0.42	
Beef liver,	1.3		White bread	0.23	0.40
broiled	1.2		Carrots	0.21	
Egg	4.0	0.8	Orange juice, fresh	0.20	
Broccoli	1.0	0.1	Potato, baked	0.06	
Fillet of haddock, broiled	0.5	0.5	Peanuts	5.40	
Butter	2.5	0.1			

From Brunell RH, Keating J, Quaresimo A, and Parmin GK: Alpha-tocopherol content of foods, American Journal of Clinical Nutrition 17:1, 1965.
*Where serving size is not approximately 100 grams (3 to 4 oz).

oils varies from time to time, a food processor is forced to put a rather long list of oils on a label—even though only one or two may be present in the product at any one time.) Currently, about 75% of the oil used in the United States is soybean oil. However, the success of commercial production of alternate oils such as rapeseed oil, now known as Canola, and sunflower seed oils may cause a change in the relative amounts used commercially. Only when a product lists one oil can the consumer be sure which oil is actually present. In general, the amount of vitamin E in an oil increases in proportion to the amount of PUFA. Animal fats have practically no vitamin E.

Fruits and vegetables provide about 10% of the remaining vitamin E in the diet; the rest comes from all the other food groups, with each providing relatively small amounts. The amount of vitamin E in some representative foods is shown in Table 12-5. Wheat germ, which was the first dietary source identified, continues to be promoted as a rich dietary source.

Tocopherol is relatively stable at normal cooking temperatures but suffers considerable destruction at temperatures used for deep-fat frying. Foods stored at freezing temperatures lose an appreciable amount of their vitamin E content unless the temperatures are very low. Vitamin E is also destroyed by exposure to light and oxygen.

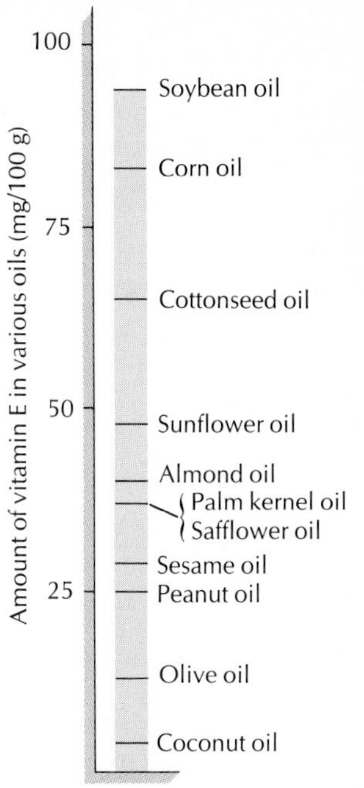

Figure 12-14 Relative amount of vitamin E in various oils.

Deficiencies

In Humans

In vitamin E deficiency in humans, in addition to a drop in blood tocopherol levels, the most common symptom observed is an increase in hemolysis of the red blood cells, which shows up also as vitamin E–induced anemia. These symptoms are also seen when the relative need for vitamin E is increased resulting from increased intake of PUFA.

In the only study of an induced vitamin E deficiency in humans, men receiving an intake of 4 mg of tocopherol/day for 30 months showed a steady drop in plasma vitamin E to half the normal values. After 30 months, plasma values reached a plateau as the reserves in adipose tissue were mobilized to maintain blood levels. The eventual drop in tocopherol blood levels to 1 mg/dl was accompanied by an increase in hemolysis of red blood cells. When lard (low in PUFA) was replaced with corn oil (high in PUFA), there was a further drop in serum tocopherol but no increase in the already high rate of red cell hemolysis.

In infants, the anemia that results from the breaking down of the red blood cells is exaggerated when large amounts of iron are given. Because premature infants and children with cystic fibrosis have difficulty absorbing lipid, it may be necessary to give them vitamin E by injection or by mouth in **water-miscible** form, a form of the vitamin that is more readily absorbed. Vitamin E–deficient infants are particularly sensitive to oxygen therapy, which is often used to help them through early critical periods; one undesirable result of oxygen is damage to the retina of the eye, which can cause permanent blindness. Vitamin E in doses up to 100 mg/day protects against the severity of this condition known as *retrolental fibroplasia (RLF)*, which is fairly common in newborns.

water-miscible
Able to be mixed in water; substances that are water-miscible can be dispersed in water but not dissolved

Infants and adults who suffer from cystic fibrosis, in which the ability to absorb fat and therefore fat-soluble vitamin E is impaired, have low blood levels of tocopherol. Most people with the disease respond to vitamin E supplementation of 50 to 400 mg/day.

In Animals

A lack of vitamin E in animals shows up in a variety of seemingly unrelated ways, with symptoms involving the muscles, nervous system, reproductive organs, vascular system, and glandular system. The severity of the symptoms increases as the amount and proportion of calories from unsaturated fat increases. At least some of the many claims made for uses of vitamin E in humans are made on the basis of these studies.

Nutritional muscular dystrophy, which is characterized by muscle weakness caused by fragmentation of the muscle fibers and the accumulation of fluid, is seen in vitamin E-deficient guinea pigs and rabbits. It apparently bears no relationship to human muscular dystrophy, which is a hereditary condition in which victims have normal plasma vitamin E values and symptoms that do not respond to vitamin E therapy.

Toxicity

Because vitamin E is a fat-soluble vitamin that can be stored in the body, there has been much concern over the possible consequences of large amounts that are being taken without adequate medical supervision. So far, we have only anecdotal evidence to suggest that there are problems associated with its use. Gastrointestinal distress has been reported when intakes of vitamin E reach the level of 300 to 600 mg. Some people experience nausea and diarrhea after taking vitamin E in excess, and there may be problems with blood clotting if vitamin D status is also marginal. Because we have no scientific evidence to support the use of high levels of this vitamin, it is unwise to use **unphysiological levels** of over 100 mg/day. Vitamin E does not appear to cause the toxicity problems of other fat-soluble vitamins, however.

unphysiological levels
Amounts that exceed those that are needed and which the body would be expected to handle

VITAMIN K

Vitamin K was first discovered in 1934 by a Danish scientist named Dam, who recognized it as the fat-soluble factor necessary for the coagulation of blood. Because the Danish word for the process is spelled *koagulation*, he designated the vitamin as vitamin K. "Vitamin K" now actually refers to several substances belonging to a chemical group known as the *quinones*. These include the naturally occurring phylloquinone in plant foods; menaquinone, which occurs in animal tissues and is synthesized by bacteria; and the synthetic substances menadione, Synkayvite, and Hykinone. These substances were formerly known as vitamins K_1, K_2, and K_3 (the synthetics), respectively. Menaquinone and the synthetic K vitamins have 70% and 20%, respectively, of the biological activity of the first. Phylloquinone occurs primarily in green leafy plants and was first isolated from alfalfa meal in 1939, which explains why alfalfa is such a popular "health" food. Menaquinone is synthesized by bacteria in the gastrointestinal tract; it has also been obtained as the result of bacterial synthesis from fish meal.

Quinones with Vitamin K Activity
K_1—phylloquinone—plants, animal tissue.
K_2—menaquinone—animals, bacteria
K_3—menadione—synthetic

In addition to naturally occurring vitamin K (phylloquinone and menaquinones) and synthetic menadione, all of which are fat soluble, there are two water-soluble forms, Hykinone and Synkayvite, and three water miscible forms: Mephyton, Konakion, and Mono-Kay. These latter forms are especially suitable for the treatment of vitamin K deficiencies when fat absorption is impaired. Table 12-6 attempts to clarify the interrelationships among these forms and tabulates the special properties of each.

The naturally occurring fat-soluble forms of the vitamin may be stored in the body, primarily in the liver. However, these stores of vitamin K are relatively small and are rapidly used up.

Vitamin K is stable to heat and oxidation but is destroyed by light, acid, alkali, oxidizing agents, and alcohol.

Table 12-6 ◆ Interrelationship and properties of compounds with vitamin K activity

Naturally Occurring (Fat-Soluble)	Synthetic		
	Fat-Soluble	Water-Soluble	Water-Miscible
Form			
Phylloquinone (green plants)	Menadione	Synkayvite Hykinone	Mephyton Konakion Mono-Kay
Menaquinone (bacterial synthesis)			
Mode of Administration			
Orally (except for infants) Intravenously Subcutaneously	Subcutaneously Intramuscularly		Orally Intramuscularly Subcutaneously Intravenously
Uses			
Orally to mother several days before delivery To counteract anticoagulants Gastrointestinal surgery	Obstructive jaundice Woman in labor Newborn		1 mg to newborn
Special Precautions			
No side effects	Small margin of safety Safe after first few weeks of life Large doses produce hemolytic anemia, hyperbilirubinemia, and kernicterus		Wide margin of safety

Functions

The major function of vitamin K is its use by the liver in the synthesis of various proteins needed for blood clotting. Among these are prothrombin (or factor II) and factors VII, IX, and X. Vitamin K appears to be necessary to catalyze the conversion of the precursor of prothrombin to prothrombin in the liver; it does this by helping to convert the glutamic acid of the protein to a new amino acid, gamma-carboxyglutamic acid. In turn, prothrombin in the blood catalyzes the conversion of fibrinogen, another factor involved in blood coagulation, into fibrin. Prothrombin levels in the blood determine the rate at which the blood will clot.

Blood-Clotting Essentials
Calcium
Vitamin K
Prothrombin
Fibrinogen
Fibrin

An anticoagulant called Dicumarol, which is chemically similar to vitamin K, stimulates the formation of vitamin K oxide in the liver. This substance then interferes with the role of vitamin K in stimulating the conversion of the prothrombin precursor to prothrombin. The widespread use of anticoagulant drugs in treating phlebitis and thrombosis has made the use of vitamin K therapy important in counteracting undesirable side effects such as hemorrhaging.

Other vitamin K–dependent proteins not involved in blood coagulation have been found in blood plasma, bone, and the kidneys. The function of the most abundant of these, **osteocalcin**, is unknown, but its calcium-binding properties and abundance in bone suggests that it may be involved in calcium metabolism, transport, and deposition.

osteocalcin
A protein found in bone that is dependent on vitamin K for synthesis

Absorption and Excretion

As is the case with other fat-soluble vitamins, the absorption of vitamin K is affected by the same factors as those that affect fat absorption. Absorption from the intestine into the lymphatic system requires bile and pancreatic secretions. From 40% to 70% of dietary vitamin K is absorbed. An obstruction of the bile duct, which limits the secretion of fat-emulsifying bile salts, reduces absorption, as does the use of mineral oil as a laxative.

Fat soluble forms of vitamin K are excreted as metabolites in both the bile and urine, whereas water-soluble forms are excreted rapidly, primarily in the urine. The amount stored is very small and its turnover very rapid.

Requirements

Estimated Safe and Adequate Daily Dietary Intake of Vitamin K (μg/day)

Infants	12
Children	15-60
Adolescents	50-100
Adults	70-140

The Food and Nutrition Board recognizes vitamin K as a dietary essential and has recommended safe and adequate intakes. Of special concern are needs in the first few days of life when the danger of hemorrhage is high. The relatively sterile intestinal tract of an infant does not contain the bacteria that synthesize vitamin K. Little vitamin K has been transferred from the mother to the infant during pregnancy unless vitamin K is given to the mother at the time of delivery. Furthermore, milk is low in vitamin K.

Therefore infants, who routinely receive only milk in the first few days of life, do not get an appreciable amount of the vitamin. Breast-fed infants are at an even greater disadvantage than bottle-fed infants because mother's milk is often not produced in significant amounts for several days. In addition, human breast milk, with 2 μg/liter, contains only one fourth the amount of vitamin K that cow's milk does. Also, there is little chance that vitamin K-synthesizing bacteria will develop in the lower intestine, where *Lactobacillus bifidus*, the predominant organism, does not promote synthesis.

As a result of all these factors, breast-fed infants have a prolonged blood-clotting time compared to bottle-fed infants. On the basis of these findings, both the American Academy of Pediatrics and the Food and Nutrition Board estimate that the newborn infant requires from 5 to 30 μg/day, assuming 10% absorption of orally administered vitamin K. This is often provided as a single intramuscular injection at the time of delivery. Estimated adult requirements of 1 μg/kg body weight/day assume that one half is contributed by food and one half is synthesized by intestinal bacteria. These estimates are considered generous, possibly double more recent calculations of need. No increase is recommended for pregnancy and lactation. Although, there is some evidence that needs in pregnancy may indeed increase.

Sources

For most people, adequate levels of vitamin K are provided both from green leafy vegetables and from the synthesis of the vitamin by intestinal bacteria. The North American diet provides from 300 to 500 μg of vitamin K per day. The concentration of vitamin K in foods is highest in dark green leafy vegetables (50 to 800 μg/100 grams) but is also found in fruits, tubers, seeds, eggs and dairy and meat products, with 1 to 50 μg/100 grams. The total dietary intake is estimated at 200 to 500 μg/day. Vitamin K usually occurs in association with chlorophyll in the chloroplasts of plants. Alfalfa is an especially rich source and on that basis (not its palatability) it is touted by health-food advocates. The average diet provides enough vitamin K so that there is no need for a supplement.

Although much of the synthesis occurs in the jejunum and ileum of the intestine and only a small portion of it may actually be absorbed, half of the vitamin K stores in the liver have been synthesized. The amount of vitamin K synthesized is reduced with the use of salicylic acid, an ingredient in most pain depressants of the aspirin type, certain antibiotics, and certain sulfonamides.

Deficiency

A prolonged blood coagulation time and a related increase in hemorrhage are the only known symptoms of a vitamin K deficiency. Prolonged prothrombin (clotting) time has been routinely used to assess a reduced vitamin K status, but it is now possible to measure prothrombin directly.

Because vitamin K can be easily synthesized and is provided in adequate amounts in practically all diets, any deficiency in adults is invariably caused by a failure in absorption. Recent studies have linked the bruising and increased blood clotting time observed in over 50% of a group of elderly people to a vitamin K deficiency. The deficiency was attributed to liver disease, poor absorption, and use of salicylates (aspirin).

In infants, however, the lack of bacteria to synthesize vitamin K, the infant's low stores of vitamin K at birth, and the small amount provided in milk characteristically lead to low prothrombin levels and a prolonged coagulation time. This occurs at a time when the risk of hemorrhage is high. In an attempt to reduce neonatal deaths due to hemorrhaging, vitamin K was routinely given either to the mother just prior to delivery or to the infant in the first few days of life. However, the uncontrolled use of menadione (over 5 mg), the synthetic form of vitamin K, resulted in an increase in a hemolytic type of anemia, an accumulation of bilirubin in the blood, and a condition known as **kernicterus**, in which bile pigment accumulates in the gray matter of the central nervous system. Kernicterus is characterized by mental retardation, jaundice, hemorrhaging, and a variety of neurological symptoms. Fortunately, intramuscular injections of 0.5% to 1 mg of naturally occurring phylloquinone at birth significantly reduced the incidence of hemorrhage (1 in 400 infants) with no undesirable side effects. Synthetic vitamin K cannot be given orally because it causes vomiting. The FDA does, however, permit the inclusion of vitamin K in prenatal supplements.

kernicterus
A condition characterized by mental retardation, jaundice, hemorrhaging, and neurological symptoms

Deficiencies show up in adults who take antibiotics for extended periods, who have difficulty absorbing fat, and/or who have a low dietary intake primarily because of limited use of dark green leafy vegetables.

BY NOW YOU SHOULD KNOW

- Vitamins are organic, needed in small amounts, perform at least one specific metabolic function, and must be provided in the diet.
- Vitamins are classified as either fat-soluble or water-soluble. Fat-soluble vitamins are soluble in fat, stored in the body, and needed in the diet every other day. Water-soluble vitamins are soluble in water, excreted in urine, and must be provided in the diet daily.
- People on a diet that provides a variety of nutrient-dense foods with adequate kilocalories should not need additional vitamin supplementation.
- Generally, vitamin deficiencies are caused by an inadequate diet, malabsorption, or an increased need.
- Vitamins A, D, E, and K occur in a limited number of foods. They are absorbed better in the presence of fat and under conditions that favor fat absorption.

- Vitamin A, also known as retinol, aids in improving vision in dim light, in maintaining the health of epithelial cells, and in bone remodeling.
- Vitamin D, also known as cholecalciferol, aids in the absorption of the changes that occur during the growth and remodeling of bone throughout life.
- Vitamin E, also known as alpha-tocopherol, functions as an antioxidant and therefore is able to protect the polyunsaturated fatty acids in the lipid portion of cell membranes from oxidation.
- Vegetable oils are rich in vitamin E.
- Vitamin K, found primarily in dark green, leafy vegetables and provided by bacterial synthesis in the gastrointestinal tract, is essential for normal clotting of the blood.
- Excessive intakes of vitamins A and D can lead to toxic symptoms, but these amounts will seldom be obtained from food alone without supplements to the diet.
- Fat-soluble vitamins are stable in heat, acid, and alkali conditions and are not soluble in water. As a result, losses during storage and food processing are relatively small.
- The North American diet provides ample amounts of all fat-soluble vitamins except vitamin D. Vitamin D should be supplemented for infants and children in the temperate zone, who may not get enough exposure to sunlight to synthesize the vitamin from the precursor in the skin.

STUDY QUESTIONS

1. Why are we reasonably confident that we have discovered all the essential vitamins?
2. In what ways do fat-soluble vitamins differ from water-soluble vitamins?
3. For what groups of people are each of the fat-soluble vitamins likely to be a problem?
4. How do the factors that affect the absorption of fat affect the utilization of vitamin A? vitamin K?
5. Why are vitamins D and K of special concern for infants?
6. Why might vitamin A intakes be higher in the summer than in the winter?
7. Explain how vitamin K is important in blood clotting.
8. Explain why milk is a good source of vitamin D.
9. Explain the relationship between the skin and vitamin D, the small intestine and vitamin K, and the liver and vitamin A.

Applying What You've Learned

1. **Interview Users of Vitamin Supplements**

   Do a survey of 10 young adults and five older adults to find out if they are taking vitamin supplements. Do they know what is in the supplements? Why are they taking supplements? Who advised them as to which supplement to buy? How much did they cost? Do they take them daily? What are your conclusions?

2. **Study the Different Supplements Available**

   Visit the vitamin section in a drug store, grocery store, or a health food store. Note the number of different supplements available. Choose one vitamin and gather information on the amount included in each supplement and on various costs at each of the stores.

3. Assess Vitamin A in Your Diet

List the best sources of vitamin A in your diet this week. Did you have sources of beta-carotene at least every other day?

4. Convert %U.S. RDA to IU, and Calculate INQ

Find nutrition information for a food product you have eaten or will soon eat. Locate the %U.S. RDA for vitamin A in Appendix C. Convert the %U.S. RDA to International Units (IU) of vitamin A. Then calculate the INQ to determine if this product is nutrient dense in vitamin A.

5. Evaluate the Vitamin Content in Your Diet

Many Americans have chosen to supplement their diets with vitamins and minerals, although in reality most of them do not need supplementation. If you take vitamins, now is a good time to evaluate your diet and assess your need. Record your meals for at least 3 days. Use Appendix F to total your vitamin and mineral intakes. Find your average intake. Compare this intake to your RDA. Unless you are taking in less than 67% of your RDA for any given nutrient, there is no dietary reason for you to take a supplement.

SUGGESTED READINGS

Bieri JG, Corash L, and Hubbard VS: Medical uses of vitamin E, New England Journal of Medicine 308:1063, 1983.

This review discusses the rationale for vitamin E therapy for medical conditions in which the vitamin may have a positive effect. It covers exposure to toxicants and environmental pollutants, malabsorption syndromes, blood disorders, cardiovascular disease, and prematurity. It also discusses the possibility of toxicity from high doses.

Deluca HF: New developments in the vitamin D endocrine system, Journal of the American Dietetic Association 80:231, 1982.

This review, written by one of the most productive researchers in the field of vitamin D, is a lucid account of the advances in vitamin D metabolism. It is authoritative and scientific but also practical in its approach.

Kolata G: Does Vitamin A prevent cancer? Science 223:1161, 1984.

This article is an overview of the proceedings of a conference sponsored by the National Cancer Institute, which explored evidence that some forms of vitamin A may have a protective effect in reducing the possibility of some forms of cancer. The article points to reasons both for and against the possibility that such a relationship will be confirmed.

Olson JA: Recommended Dietary Intakes (RDI) of vitamin A in humans, American Journal of Clinical Nutrition 45:704, 1987.

This paper discusses the rationale for the recommended dietary allowances as proposed by the 1985 Committee of the Food and Nutrition Board. Data on the vitamin A content of foods, body stores of the vitamin, its major functions, results of a deficiency, usual intakes, and evidence of nutritional status are included.

Olson JA: Recommended Dietary Intakes (RDI) of vitamin K in humans, American Journal of Clinical Nutrition 45:687, 1987.

The author provides the rationale for the proposed recommended dietary allowance for vitamin K in 1985. He discusses food and bacterial sources, its role in the nutrition of the newborn, its functions, and the effects of a deficiency, especially in newborns.

Vitamins

Levy AS, and Schucker RL: Patterns of nutrient intake among dietary supplement users: attitudinal and behavioral correlates, Journal of the American Dietetic Association 87:754, 1987.

Stewart ML, and others: Vitamin/mineral supplement use: a telephone survey of adults in the United States, Journal of the American Dietetic Association 85:1585, 1985.

Vitamin A

Bates CJ: Vitamin A in pregnancy and lactation, Proceedings of the Nutrition Society 42:65, 1983.

Bauernfeind JC: The safe use of vitamin A, International Vitamin A Consultative Group, Washington, D.C., 1980, The Nutrition Foundation, Inc.

Bauernfeind JC: Vitamin A deficiency: a staggering problem of health and sight, Nutrition Today 23:34, 1988.

Burton GW, and Ingold KU: B-carotene: an unusual type of lipid antioxidant, Science 224:569, 1984.

DeLuca LM, and others: Recent advances in the metabolism and function of vitamin A and their relationship to applied nutrition, International Vitamin A Consultative Group, Washington, D.C., 1979, The Nutrition Foundation, Inc.

Olson JA: Vitamin A. In Machlin, L, editor: The handbook of vitamins, New York, 1984, Marcel Dekker Inc.

Olson JA: Vitamins A and C—Proposed allowances, Nutrition Today 21:26, 1986.

Raica N, Jr, and others: Vitamin A concentration in human tissues collected from five areas in the United States, American Journal of Clinical Nutrition 25:291, 1972.

Ritenbaugh C: Carotenoids and cancer, Nutrition Today 22:14, 1987.

Rodriguez ME, and Irwin MI: A conspectus of research on vitamin A requirements in man, Journal of Nutrition 102:909, 1972.

Rosa RW, Wilk AL, and Kelsey FO: Teratogen update: Vitamin A congeners, Teratology 33:355, 1986.

Smith JE, and Goodman DS: Retinol-binding protein and the regulation of vitamin A transport, Federation Proceedings 38:2504, 1979.

Sommer A: Nutritional blindness, Oxford, 1982, Oxford University Press.

Sommer A, Tarwotjo I, and Katz J: Increased risk of xerophthalmia following diarrhea and respiratory disease, American Journal of Clinical Nutrition 45:977, 1987.

Sporn MB, Roberts AB, and Goodman DS, editors: The retinoids, New York, 1985, Academic Press.

Wolf G: Is dietary B-carotene an anticancer agent? Nutrition Reviews 40:257, 1982.

Ziegler RG, and others: Seasonal variations in intake of carotenoids and vegetables and fruits among white men in New Jersey, American Journal of Clinical Nutrition 45:107, 1987.

Zile MH, and Cullum ME: The function of vitamin A: current concepts, Proceedings of the Society for Experimental Biology and Medicine 172:139, 1983.

Vitamin D

Bronner F: Recent advances in vitamin D: clinical implications, American Journal of Clinical Nutrition 29:1253, 1976.

DeLuca HF: Some new concepts emanating from a study of metabolism and function of vitamin D, Nutrition Reviews 38:169, 1980.

Food and Nutrition Board: Hazards of the overuse of vitamin D, Nutrition Reviews 33:61, 1975.

Henry HL, and Norman AW: Vitamin D metabolism and biological action, Annual Review of Nutrition 4:493, 1984.

Rudolf M, Arulananthan K, and Greenstein RM: Unsuspected nutritional rickets, Pediatrics 66:72, 1980.

Webb AR, and Holick MF: The role of sunlight in the cutaneous production of vitamin D_3, Annual Review of Nutrition 8:375, 1988.

Vitamin E

Bieri JG: Vitamin E. In Present Knowledge of Nutrition, Washington, D.C., 1984, Nutrition Foundation.

Booth VH, and Bradford MP: Tocopherol content of fruits and vegetables, British Journal of Nutrition 17:575, 1963.

Bunnell RH, Keating J, Quaresimo A, and Parman GK: Alpha-tocopherol content of foods, American Journal of Clinical Nutrition 17:1, 1965.

Haeger K: Long-time treatment of intermittent claudication with vitamin E, American Journal of Clinical Nutrition 27:1179, 1974.

Hale W, and others: Vitamin E effect on symptoms and laboratory values in the elderly, Journal of the American Dietetic Association 86:625, 1986.

Horwitt MK: Vitamin E symposium: biochemistry, nutritional requirements, and clinical studies, American Journal of Clinical Nutrition 27:939, 1974.

Horwitt MK: Interpretations of requirements for thiamin, riboflavin, niacin-tryptophan and vitamin E plus comments on balance studies and vitamin B-6, American Journal of Clinical Nutrition 44:973, 1986.

Tappel AL: Will antioxidant nutrients slow aging processes? Geriatrics 23:97, 1968.

Wasserman RH, and Taylor AN: Metabolic roles of fat-soluble vitamin D, E, and K, Annual Review of Biochemistry 41:179, 1972.

Watson R, and Leonard T: Selenium and Vitamins A, E, and C: nutrients with cancer prevention properties, Journal of the American Dietetic Association 86:505, 1986.

Vitamin K

Ansell J, Kumar E, and Deykin RD: The spectrum of vitamin K deficiency, Journal of the American Medical Association 238:40, 1977.

Olson RE: The function and metabolism of vitamin K, Annual Review of Nutrition 4:281, 1984.

Vitamin K and prothrombin structure, Nutrition Reviews 32:279, 1974.

FOCUS Vitamin E—What Can We Expect It To Do?

Of all the nutrients that are taken as supplements to the diet, vitamin E is at the top of the list on almost every count—the number of people using it, the variety of conditions they are trying to cure, the amount of money they are spending on it (over $200 million/year), and the range of sources that give advice about it. Interest about vitamin E has also caught hold in the scientific community, which is publishing the results of research, at an unprecedented rate, that tries to determine the function of vitamin E and its possible relationship to many conditions. What *do* we know about what vitamin E can and cannot do? How much is in doubt? Because vitamin E has been proposed as a cure for almost every disease, including heartburn, heart attacks, sterility, menstrual disorders, skin diseases, angina, leg cramps, muscular dystrophy, and diabetes, it would be impossible to cover its relationship to all of them. In this section, at least we can get an idea of the magnitude of interest in vitamin E and maybe even some insights into what is myth and what contains at least a grain of truth. Is it a panacea for medical problems or merely a placebo?

Vitamin E as a supplement is promoted in three different forms. The most common is natural vitamin E, which is a concentrate obtained by extracting the vitamin from vegetable oils that are rich sources of it. Natural vitamin E is usually available as an oil in capsule form or in larger amounts to be taken by spoon; it is important to keep it cool and away from exposure to air so that it will not take up oxygen and lose its potency. A second type of supplemental vitamin E is in pill form in a range of potencies from 5 mg to 300 mg per tablet. This type is usually synthetic vitamin E; it is used by the human body in exactly the same way as the natural vitamin once it is absorbed, although a smaller proportion of the dose will usually be absorbed. Most synthetic vitamin E is labeled as all RAC alpha-tocopherol, meaning that it is a mixture of the eight different forms of vitamin E that are known to function as vitamin E. They may also have the words "acetate" or "succinate" added at the end of the name; that means that the vitamin is present combined with another compound to make it much less susceptible to being destroyed by exposure to oxygen. The third way in which vitamin E is marketed is in the form of wheat germ, wheat germ oil, or wheat germ concentrate. Why wheat germ? Wheat germ is the portion of the cereal grain that contains the oil. The germ of wheat has the highest concentration of vitamin E of any of the oils and was the first source discovered. As a result, it became one of the "super foods," promoted as a health food.

Some theorists are advancing the idea that vitamin E may be useful in delaying the aging process. This idea comes from the theory that one of the causes of aging is the change that occurs in cell membranes when the free radicals attack the unsaturated fatty acids that are part of the membrane structure. As the cell membrane is destroyed, some of the leftover parts accumulate as lipofuscin pigments, which are responsible for the brownish spots that appear under the skin quite often as people get older. The reasoning goes something like this: if we can keep the cell membrane from breaking down, we will not have the portions that accumulate to make lipofuscin; if lipofuscin in turn is responsible for aging, then aging will be retarded. However, evidence to support this theory is lacking. Vitamin E does have some effect on animals that have been subjected to toxic levels of oxidants.

There is also great interest in the relationship between vitamin E and heart disease. It began in the mid-forties, when relatively little was known about the cause of heart disease and even less about the role of nutrition in either preventing or curing it. With even the odds of gas rationing working against them, two doctors in Canada—brothers named Shute—were able to attract hundreds of people suffering from heart disease to make the trek to Ontario, where they received the "Shute treatment." This treatment reportedly consisted of a "shot" of vitamin E. Many people reported almost instant relief from their symptoms of angina, and the Shutes had a thriving business in the cure of heart disease. Their claims, which are very compelling, provided hope for a great many victims, income for the doctors, and material for several best-sellers on vitamin E and heart disease (they are still available in many book stores)—but not enough information to permit others to test their theories and procedures. More recently, efforts to show that vitamin E could lower blood cholesterol levels have led to conclusions that it does increase the desirable HDL cholesterol in women but not in men unless they have low values initially.

Studies on animals have shown that those animals that were fed diets deficient in vitamin E are more susceptible to the effects of environmental stresses, such as ozone, than are those fed doses many times the requirement. Animal studies have also shown that vitamin E protects against the free radicals that are apparently released when the body is exposed to various chemical toxicants such as selenium, mercury, lead, carbon tetrachloride, and benzene. This tells us that susceptibility is greater in vitamin E–deficient animals and that large doses provide protection, but it does not tell us whether the amount of vitamin E that *we* get in our diet is adequate or not. Before recommending that people take large doses, we need to establish that there is benefit in taking amounts beyond what we now ingest. Preliminary studies on humans suggest that the benefits, if indeed there are any, will not be as great as anticipated.

Claims that vitamin E provides a competitive advantage for athletes have not been supported by the research studies that have attempted to assess the claim.

The use of vitamin E in treating a condition called intermittent claudication, which is characterized by cramps in the calf muscles at night and extreme pain in walking, has met with considerable success and is an example of the legitimate use of a nutrient in dealing with a medical problem. There is also some reason to believe that vitamin E is helpful in a condition called fibrocystic breast disease, in which there are painful (but harmless) lumps in the breast. At one time, vitamin E was used to prevent hemolytic anemia in premature infants, who were getting high levels of PUFA in their formulas along with inadequate amounts of vitamin E. However, all commercial formulas now have enough added vitamin E to meet the needs of these infants.

The saga of vitamin E is far from over. We can't dismiss the possibility that some of the anecdotal reports of benefits may lead us to good, scientifically verifiable evidence of a role for vitamin E. It is reassuring that we have not yet found reason to worry about intakes several hundred times what we feel is necessary. Vitamin E is relatively inexpensive, so there is little reason to worry about excessive cost. However, it is still a good idea to use caution when claims are made about the effectiveness of vitamin E in curing a long and varied list of ailments. Suffering and even loss of life can result when faith in an untested cure increases the time before competent medical help is obtained. Also, vitamin E is important as a nutrient, but we have little reason to use it as a drug, that is, in amounts many times those that are provided in food. One study of elderly users of vitamin E supplements for 11 different disease states ranging from hypertension to diabetes, could identify only one biochemical measure and no difference in symptoms compared to nonusers over a 2-year period.

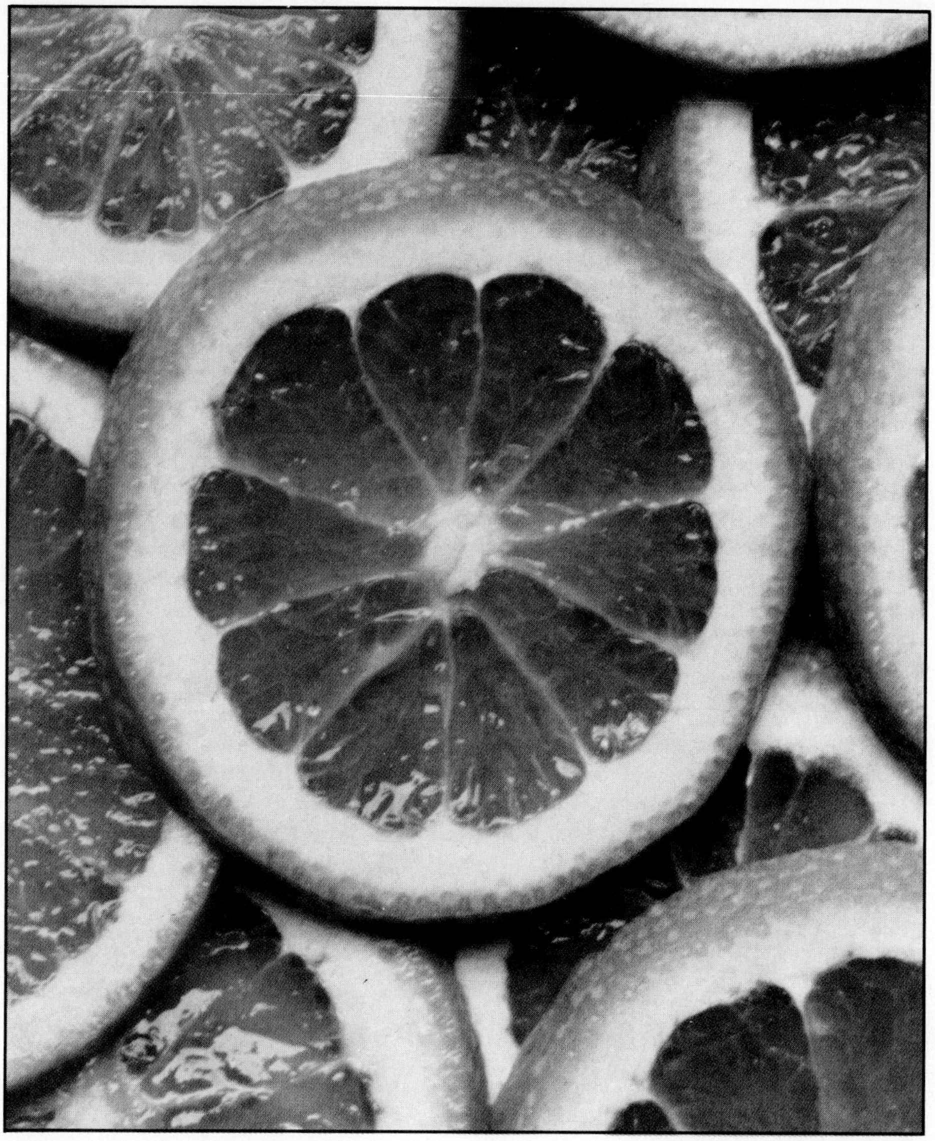

AWARENESS CHECK

Truth or Fiction?

- Vitamin C prevents and cures the common cold.
- Oranges and citrus fruits are the only dependable food sources of vitamin C.
- Megadoses of vitamin C are harmless.
- Megadoses of vitamin B_6 are harmless and should be taken to alleviate the symptoms of premenstrual syndrome.
- Cigarette smokers have an increased need for vitamin C.
- Cooking vegetables quickly in a small amount of water will help retain their folacin content.

Water-Soluble Vitamins: C, Folacin, B_{12}, and B_6

CHAPTER

13

The four nutrients discussed in this chapter are all classified as water-soluble vitamins. Aside from vitamin C, they are considered part of the B-complex vitamins, which serve as parts of coenzymes involved in many metabolic reactions. All function in blood formation, and each has at least one other unique function. The results of deficiencies are very specific for each, and the major food sources vary. There is every reason to believe that adequate amounts of each can be obtained from an appropriate choice of foods readily available in the food supply. Few people require supplements. If they do, however, the supplements should be taken at levels to correct inadequacies— not in large megadoses that can create nutrient imbalances and little-understood metabolic consequences.

The four water-soluble vitamins to be discussed in this chapter are vitamin C (ascorbic acid), vitamin B_6 (pyridoxine), folacin, and vitamin B_{12} (cobalamin). In contrast to the other water-soluble vitamins that will be discussed in Chapter 14, none of these four has a direct role in energy metabolism, and all are involved either directly or indirectly in blood formation.

VITAMIN C

Discovery

Perhaps the most talked about vitamin, and certainly the one most widely used as a supplement, is the one familiarly known as vitamin C (ascorbic acid), the *anti-scorbutic* (scurvy-preventive) dietary essential.

Other Names for Vitamin C
Ascorbic acid
Hexuronic acid
Cevitamic acid

The saga of the discovery of this vitamin is one of the longest and most interesting of all nutritional history. Descriptions of illnesses that were unmistakably scurvy were reported in a papyrus from 1500 BC found at Thebes and in the writings of Hippocrates in 400 BC. Scurvy was a major factor shaping the course of history, ravaging armies and navies and causing the death of many explorers and home-

"Legs became swollen and puffed up, while the sinews contracted and turned coal-black and, in some cases, all blotched with drops of purplish blood. Gums were so decayed that the flesh peeled off down to the roots of the teeth while the latter almost fell out. By February out of our group of 110 there were not ten left in good health. . . . Already eight were dead and over 50 more were given up for lost." *From the Journal of Jacques Cartier (1534)*

sour krout
Cabbage soup similar to sauerkraut

Cures Used in Lind's Scurvy Experiment

Oil of vitriol	Lemons
Vinegar	Oranges
Sea water	

steaders. It was known as early as the seventeenth century that scurvy could be controlled by eating certain foods, and since 1906 we have known that it is a vitamin-deficiency disease. The search for the responsible substance in the diet ended in 1932 with the isolation of the relatively simple white crystals of vitamin C from lemon juice, oranges, and cabbage.

It was in an effort to cure scurvy, which was sometimes called the "scourge of the navy," that the first carefully conceived nutrition experiment was conducted with humans. Seamen who embarked on long sea voyages did so knowing that a large number of the crew would die or be incapacitated by scurvy. This was true for Magellan, Vasco da Gama, and Cartier, whose vivid description of the disease, as it affected his men at Quebec in 1534, is classic. Some of Cartier's men were saved by drinking a brew of pine bark recommended by the Indians, and Captain Cook's crew was saved by his insistence that they eat a thick soup he called **"sour krout."**

In 1747 Lind, a British physician, suggested the theory that various "acidic principles" might have antiscorbutic properties. To test this he assigned sailors afflicted with scurvy into groups of two each to be fed the ship's basic diet, plus one of oil of vitriol (sulfuric acid) in water, vinegar, seawater, oranges, or lemons every day. The results of his experiment are now legendary. Both oranges and lemons had miraculous curative powers: the sailors assigned to this treatment were restored to active duty within 6 days, whereas those taking other treatments showed no improvement. Not only did Lind prove that scurvy could be cured, he also laid the foundation for the theory that lack of an essential food element could cause illness.

It was 50 years before the British navy recognized Lind's work by requiring that all ships leaving British ports carry sufficient lime juice for its crew throughout the whole voyage. This routine use of lime juice led to the term "limey" to refer to a British seaman, a term that now has extended to all British servicemen.

Although the British navy was the first to take steps to prevent scurvy, many other groups had suffered from the disease and some had found a cure. Crusaders of the Middle Ages believed that those who could survive the pain that attacked feet and legs and the changes that occurred in their gums would usually be cured by the warm temperatures of spring, a time coinciding with the availability of fresh fruit and vegetables. French and Spanish sailors did not succumb to scurvy because of the quantities of onions and leeks in their rations and sailors in the Mediterranean because they were seldom away long enough to use up their own reserves of vitamin C. When a potato crop failed, even rural European populations experienced scurvy outbreaks. One of the first tasks of Spaniards after they landed in California was to search for an herb or plant to cure scurvy. In 1846 Mormons making their way west to Utah were forced to winter in Nebraska, eating a diet of mush. Many succumbed to scurvy, as did troops during the Civil War. These are but a few examples of how the deficiency of a nutrient needed in amounts less than 2 tsp/yr shaped the history of the New World.

Infantile scurvy (Figure 13-1) was first reported in the late nineteenth century, at the time of the change from wet nurses to the use of preserved milk, and again when pasteurization of milk became mandatory. Infantile scurvy reappeared in the 1960s and 1970s, this time affecting infants fed home-prepared formula that had been subjected to prolonged heat treatment. Other scorbutic infants were born to mothers who had taken megadoses of vitamin C during pregnancy, conditioning these infants to need more vitamin C than is usually provided in milk or formula. Encouragement of breast feeding, the enrichment of infant formula, and the use of vitamin supplements are among the most effective methods of ensuring a vitamin C intake sufficient to prevent infantile scurvy.

Chemical Properties

Chemically, vitamin C is a simple compound of six carbon atoms, closely related to the monosaccharide, glucose. It is stable to acid but easily destroyed by oxidation, light, alkali, and heat, especially in the presence of iron or copper.

The synthetic form of the vitamin, first produced in 1933, is derived from the monosaccharides—glucose or galactose. Because the body cannot discriminate between natural and synthetic forms, they can be and are used interchangeably. Both function as a reducing agent, contributing electrons to other substances, and thus having the same effect as an antioxidant.

Vitamin C, usually present in food as reduced ascorbic acid, is susceptible to oxidation, causing it to change on exposure to air to **dehydroascorbic acid,** which has two fewer hydrogen atoms. It is transported to and enters the cell more easily in this oxidized form and is apparently reduced again within the cell before it can be used. Any further oxidation of dehydroascorbic acid is irreversible, having produced a biologically inactive form, diketogulonic acid, with no vitamin value. These changes are shown in Figure 13-2.

dehydroascorbic acid
An oxidized form of vitamin C that has lost two hydrogen atoms but still can function as the vitamin

Vitamin C occurs in two forms—D-ascorbic acid and L-ascorbic acid, the latter predominantly in food. Although they differ only in the way the atoms are arranged, L-ascorbic acid is well used by humans; D-ascorbic acid, on the other hand, can be used only in small doses. Because it is used extensively as a preservative in processing meat, D-ascorbic acid is identified as **erythrobic acid** on labels to avoid any implication that D-ascorbic acid is a vitamin.

erythrobic acid
Another name for the D form of vitamin C; it is used in meat processing to preserve the color of meat but cannot function as a vitamin in the same way as the L form found in most foods

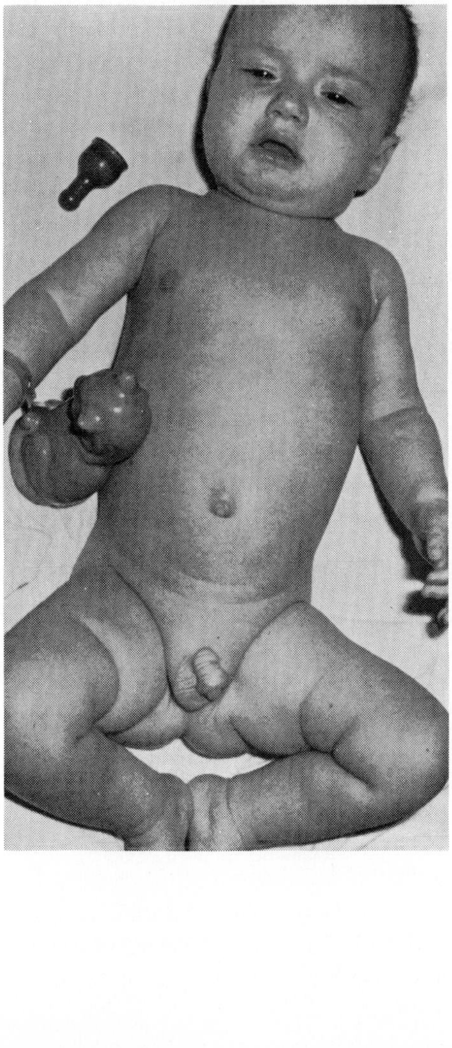

Figure 13-1 Infant with scurvy. Note frog position of legs and apprehension of infant in anticipation of handling tender limbs.
From Grewar D: Clinical Pediatrics (Philadelphia) 4:82, 1965.

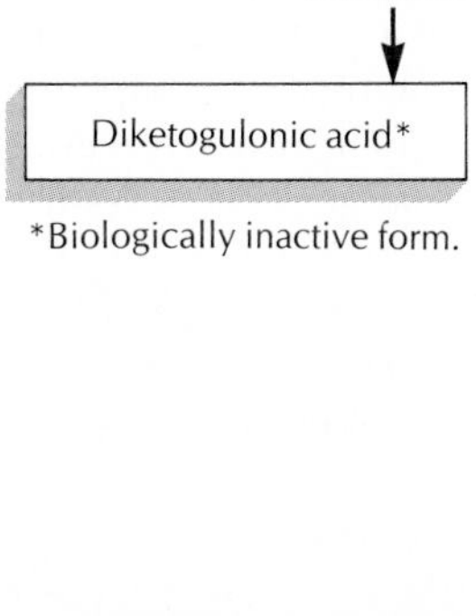

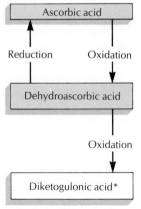

Figure 13-2 Relationship of various chemical forms of vitamin C.

Synthesis

Most animals can synthesize vitamin C from glucose, but a few, including human beings, lack the enzyme necessary to complete the conversion of glucose or galactose to vitamin C; thus they need to get it from food. Of the other animals needing a dietary source of vitamin C, the guinea pig and monkey have been used most extensively in research; fish, however, are proving increasingly useful. In plants, vitamin C accumulates during the ripening process, presumably synthesized in the plant cells from the natural glucose in fruit.

Functions

Functions of Vitamin C
Collagen formation
Dentin formation
Tyrosine metabolism
Synthesis of neurotransmitters
Utilization of iron, calcium, and folacin

Although vitamin C is a relatively simple compound that has been available in a purified form at reasonable cost for over 50 years, researchers have been unable to shed much light on its biochemical role. We do know, however, that it is essential for the health of both plant and animal cells. In contrast to most water-soluble vitamins, vitamin C has no clear-cut role as a coenzyme, nor is it part of any enzyme or body component. Vitamin C's more widely accepted roles include the following.

Collagen Formation

The most clearly identified function of vitamin C is the formation of collagen in connective tissue. Collagen is a protein component of all connective tissue, where it binds cells together in much the same way mortar binds bricks. In addition, it is a major component of skin, cartilage, teeth, and scar tissue, and it provides the structural framework of bone.

Vitamin C functions in collagen formation by promoting the change of the amino acids lysine and proline in strands of tropocollagen to hydroxylysine and hydroxyproline, necessary parts of collagen fibers. This process is called **hydroxylation.**

hydroxylation
A chemical process in which the OH group is added to a substance; in the formation of collagen, this must take place to make mature collagen fiber, which in turn makes strong connective tissue

This same process is involved in the formation of scar tissue. Some researchers suggest that it would be wise to increase vitamin C intake (up to 100 to 300 mg/day) both before and after an operation; others feel that is unnecessary as long as usual intake is adequate. Skin grafts for burned tissue heal more quickly when vitamin C is present.

Failure of collagen synthesis also causes small pinpoint hemorrhages, resulting from weakness in the membranes that line the capillaries and in the fibers that join the cells together under the surface of the skin. Blood then escapes into the enlarged intercellular spaces, accounting for the capillary bleeding associated with scurvy. These subcutaneous hemorrhages show up most often in areas subjected to mechanical stress, such as the gums, which often become soft and spongy and hemorrhage easily (Figure 13-3).

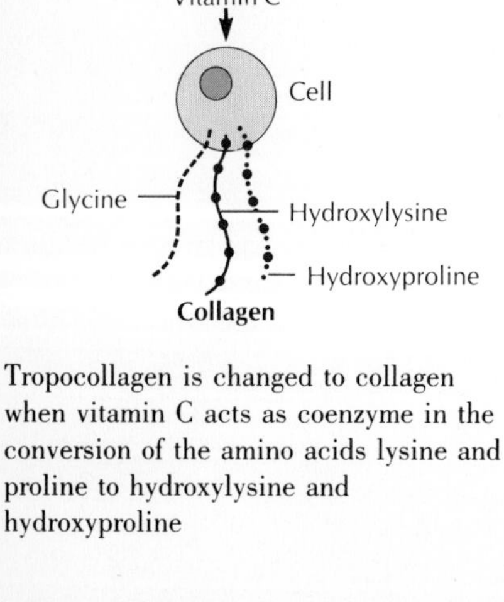

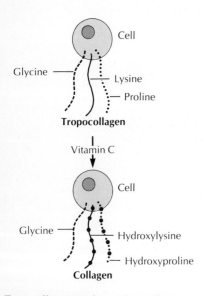

Tropocollagen is changed to collagen when vitamin C acts as coenzyme in the conversion of the amino acids lysine and proline to hydroxylysine and hydroxyproline

The bone matrix, which makes up one fifth of the weight of the bone shaft, is primarily collagen. If the matrix is defective, it is less capable of holding calcium and phosphorus during bone calcification, resulting in weakened or distorted bone structure. Sometimes bones are displaced when the supporting cartilage, which is also primarily collagen, is weakened as a result of a lack of vitamin C to maintain it.

Dentin Formation

The dentin layer of the tooth, derived from a group of cells known as odontoblasts, does not form normally when vitamin C is lacking. This, of course, produces a tooth with a structural weakness that is less able to resist mechanical injury or decay once it starts in the enamel layer.

Tyrosine Metabolism

Although it has been clearly demonstrated that vitamin C is necessary for hydroxylation of large amounts of the amino acid tyrosine, it does not appear necessary for the smaller amount present in most diets. Because tyrosine is a precursor of the hormone thyroxin and the neurotransmitter norepinephrine, vitamin C is indirectly involved in thyroid and adrenal function.

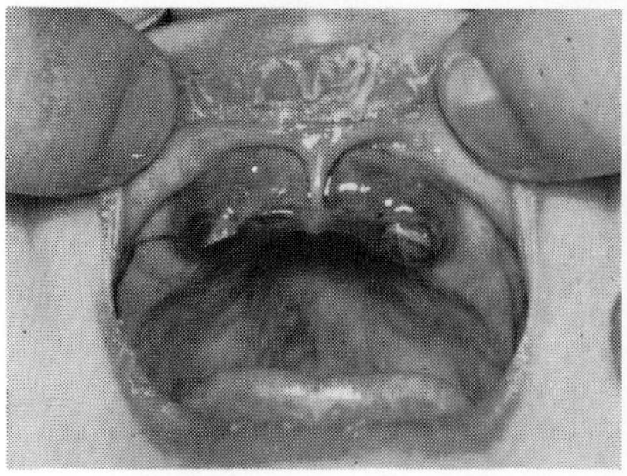

Figure 13-3 Gum hemorrhage in scorbutic infant. Note occurrence only where teeth have erupted; it does not occur in edentulous gum.
From Grewar D: Clinical Pediatrics (Philadelphia) 4:82, 1965.

Synthesis of Neurotransmitters

In the brain, two of the neurotransmitters needed to transfer nerve impulses from one cell to another can be produced only if adequate levels of vitamin C are available. Vitamin C is needed to convert tyrosine to the neurotransmitter *norepinephrine*, and the amino acid tryptophan to the precursor of the neurotransmitter *serotonin*.

Utilization of Iron, Calcium, and Folacin

Because vitamin C as a reducing agent keeps ferrous iron in the reduced form, it facilitates its absorption. It also aids in the transfer of iron from the blood into ferritin to be stored in the liver and activates some iron-containing enzymes. In diets with 25 to 75 mg of vitamin C present simultaneously with nonheme iron (iron from other than hemoglobin in animal foods), iron absorption increases as much as four times. Similarly, vitamin C aids calcium absorption by keeping it from forming an insoluble complex.

The conversion of the inactive form of the vitamin folacin to the active form is facilitated by vitamin C. Thus vitamin C may be indirectly involved in preventing the form of anemia in infancy caused by a folacin deficiency.

Other Functions

Many other functions have been attributed to vitamin C, including roles in alleviating allergic reactions, enhancing immune function, facilitating amino acid and drug metabolism, stimulating the formation of bile, and the release of some steroid hormones. Vitamin C is necessary for the synthesis of carnitine, which is required for the transport of fatty acids into the cells, the degradation of cholesterol to bile acids, and the detoxification of drugs in the liver.

Anecdotal testimony from convinced users shows that vitamin C is recommended for a staggering list of health problems. In most of these instances, if it has an effect at all it will be because of its biochemical role as a reducing agent rather than to correct a deficiency.

In assessing these roles for vitamin C it is important to differentiate between a nutritional or physiological role, relating to a function in normal metabolism, and a pharmacological or druglike role, involving **unphysiological** amounts many times more than normal. Intakes that have pharmacological effects for some people may be sufficiently high to produce undesirable or even toxic effects in others.

unphysiological intake
Intake that far exceeds needed or reasonable levels; such an intake could not be obtained from an unsupplemented diet

Whether vitamin C has a role in cancer control is highly speculative. As a reducing agent it could prevent the oxidation of harmless precursors to carcinogens, such as the conversion of nitrates to nitrites, the precursor of nitrosamines; it could promote the synthesis of mucopolysaccharides (ground substance), which inhibit the growth of cancerous cells; or it could provide protection against the stress of surgery, chemotherapy, or radiotherapy.

Evidence that vitamin C acts to detoxify histamine may explain its apparent effect in alleviating symptoms of many conditions, such as hay fever, frostbite, or poisoning. Vitamin C levels in the blood are lower among smokers. Although we have no biochemical explanation for this, it does suggest an increased need.

The presence of ascorbic acid sulfate in many tissues has suggested a role in the transfer of sulfate molecules necessary for the formation of many essential body compounds, such as mucopolysaccharide components of skin, nails, and mucous secretions.

Absorption and Metabolism

Vitamin C is absorbed by humans in the upper part of the intestine, either by simple diffusion or a **sodium-dependent active transport** mechanism, and is circulated in the blood.

sodium-dependent active transport
One mechanism by which nutrients are transported across a cell membrane; it requires energy and depends on an exchange of sodium from within the cell

Percent of absorption of vitamin C compared with intake; as intake increases, percent of absorption decreases

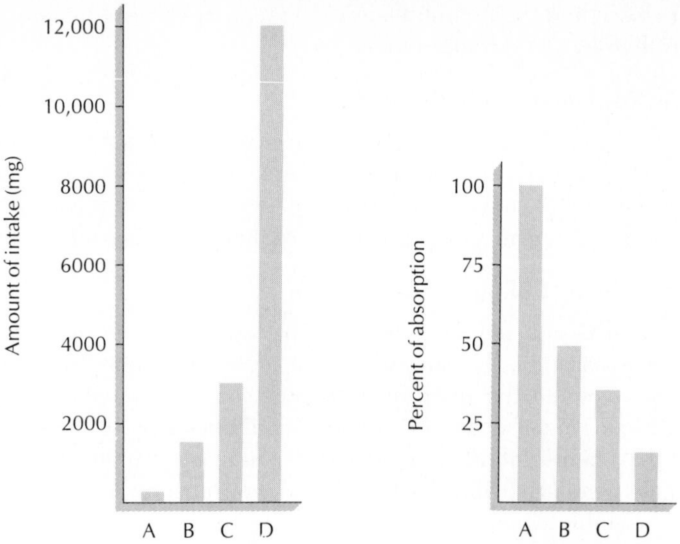

At low levels (30 to 60 mg) almost 100% of ingested vitamin C is absorbed, but as intakes increase, the absorption rate drops to 80% on intakes of 90 mg and further to 49%, 36%, and 16% on unphysiological intakes of 1.5, 3.0, and 12.0 grams, respectively. Any unabsorbed vitamin C would continue into the lower bowel, where it would have the same osmotic effect as other sugars, causing watery stools or diarrhea.

Organs Storing Some Vitamin C
Adrenal gland
Kidney
Lung
Liver
Blood
Muscle

Vitamin C in the serum reaches a maximum of about 1.2 mg/L on an intake of 100 mg/day and drops to 0.2 to 0.1 mg/L when the intake is less than 10 mg/day. Immediately after ingestion of larger amounts of vitamin C, the serum level of vitamin C is elevated until the excess is either picked up by the tissues or excreted in the urine. The highest concentration is found in the adrenal gland, with up to 50 times the concentration of serum levels. Other tissues, such as the kidneys, lung, and liver, have levels 3 to 10 times those of the blood. The amount in muscle is relatively small, but because of its mass, as much as 600 mg may be held in the muscles of a 70-kg person. Before it can be stored in the tissues, reduced ascorbic acid must be changed in the kidneys to the oxidized form, dehydroascorbic acid.

The total pool of vitamin C in the body reaches 1500 mg on an intake of 100 mg/day, sufficient to prevent the onset of scurvy for 90 days. There seems to be no benefit in maintaining stores at this maximum level. On a vitamin C-free diet, the pool declines at a rate of about 3% a day until it reaches 300 mg, when signs of scurvy begin to appear (Figure 13-4). After that the rate at which vitamin C stores are depleted declines noticeably.

Vitamin C is excreted primarily in the urine. As the vitamin passes through the kidneys, enough is reabsorbed to maintain a plasma level of 1.2 to 1.5 mg/dl and a body pool of 1.5 grams. Once that level is reached, little vitamin C is retained, and any excess is excreted in the urine.

Recommended Dietary Allowances for Vitamin C (mg/day)

Children	
1-10 yr	45
11-14 yr	50
Males (15+ yr)	60
Females (15+yr)	60
Pregnancy	+20
Lactation	+40

Requirements

There has been considerable controversy about the criteria for setting recommended allowances of vitamin C. Some nutritionists feel the recommended allowance should be 10 mg/day, the amount that will prevent scurvy. Others recommend 45 to 60 mg, amounts sufficiently high to permit tissue saturation and still not introduce any potential hazard.

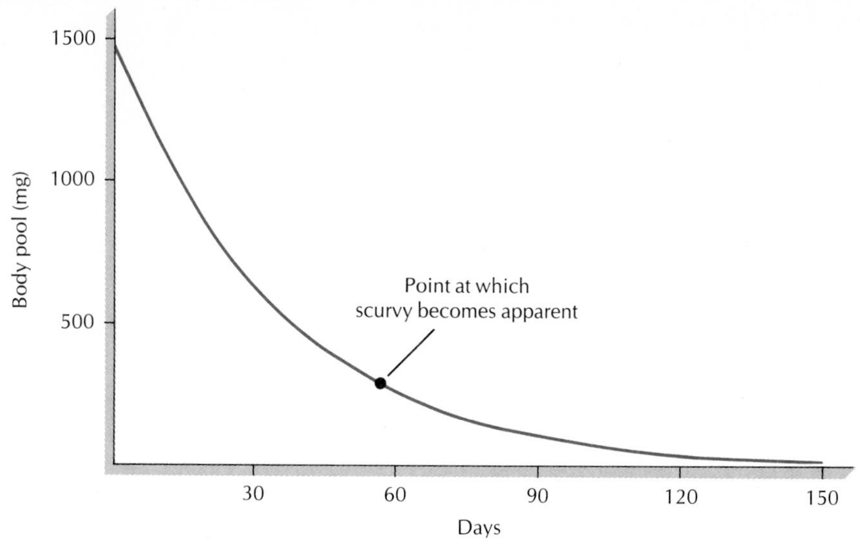

Figure 13-4 Depletion of vitamin C from body stores over time on a deficient diet.

Table 13-1 ◇ Comparison of dietary standards for vitamin C for selected age groups (in milligrams)

	US 1980	U.S.S.R.	Canada 1983	United Kingdom 1980	WHO/FAO	Sweden 1981
Children, 4-6 yr	45	50	25	20	20	45
Boys, 12-14 yr	60	70	40	25	20	50
Men	60	100	60	30	30	60
Women	60	70	45	30	30	60
Pregnant	80	100	65	60	50	80

On intakes moderately in excess of needs, vitamin C is excreted unchanged. At higher levels (500 mg), however, it is metabolized to oxalic acid. For most people urinary oxalic acid levels off at a harmless level less than 60 mg/day. For about 20% of the population, urinary oxalate levels continue to rise to a point where they contribute to the formation of kidney stones, which are made up largely of precipitated calcium oxalate.

Adults

Current standards reflect a philosophy that an intake leading to some degree of saturation of vitamin C reserves in the tissues is desirable. As a result, recommended levels, which vary from 30 to 100 mg/day in different countries, are many times the 10 mg/day known to prevent and cure clinically evident signs of scurvy. A comparison of U.S. standards with those of other nations (Table 13-1) is further evidence of lack of consensus.

Because an intake of 45 mg/day will permit storage of a reserve of 1500 mg of vitamin C to maintain optimal health, the RDA of 60 mg is generally considered a liberal allowance. The inclusion of the recommended four servings of fruits and vegetables in the diet each day will ensure even higher amounts.

Pregnancy

Recommendations for vitamin C intake for pregnant women include 20 mg above the needs of nonpregnant women. The developing fetus has plasma levels two to four times as high as maternal levels, and a high concentration is also found in the placenta, which has the ability to synthesize it.

Lactation

The vitamin C content of mother's milk usually varies from 4 to 8 mg/dl of milk. An intake of 100 mg/day by the mother should result in these levels in her milk.

Infants

Based on the amount of vitamin C found in mother's milk, a breast-fed infant receives 15 to 50 mg/day and has a plasma vitamin C level of 0.5 to 1.5 mg/dl. Because cow's milk provides only 4 to 6 mg/dl, which is less well-utilized and thus supports lower blood levels of vitamin C, it is recommended that bottle-fed infants receive a supplement of 35 mg, and premature infants receive double this dosage, beginning within the first 10 days of life. Most infant formula has enough vitamin C added to take care of the needs of the infant and to compensate for any losses during sterilization. No additional supplement is needed.

For children, the RDA increases only slightly from 45 mg/day for those 1 to 3 years of age to 50 mg/day for both boys and girls over 11 years of age and to 60 mg/day after age 15.

Food Sources

Vitamin C is found almost exclusively in foods of plant origin. Except for liver, no animal food is considered a significant source. The small amount in milk is usually destroyed by the heat of pasteurization. The amount present in a plant tissue depends on many factors.

Part and Type of Plant

The head of broccoli has more vitamin C than the stem, but in tests stems retained 82% during a 10-minute cooking period, whereas heads retained only 60%. In general, thin-stemmed vegetables contain more vitamin C than do thick-stemmed ones. Vegetables that wilt lose much more vitamin C than do those that do not wilt. Roots lose it slowly, but the loss is accelerated at higher temperatures.

Stage of Maturity

Because the vitamin accumulates in fruit throughout the maturing and ripening process, the longer it remains on the vine or tree up to peak maturity, the higher the vitamin C content. In contrast, immature seeds, such as peas and beans, contain some vitamin C but lose it all at maturity. However, sprouting of peas or beans results in a vegetable with an appreciable amount of vitamin C.

Conditions of Storage

To Help Retain Vitamin C as Food is Prepared for Use:
Harvest at the peak of maturity
Store in a cool, moist place
Limit exposure to air
Do not soak in water
Cook in a small amount of water
Leave food in large pieces if possible
Use microwave oven for cooking

Storing of vegetables at refrigerator temperatures in high humidity with a minimum of air movement will minimize vitamin C losses. The amount present in fresh vegetables bought in the temperate zone in the winter months depends on the storage conditions during harvesting, shipping, and display in stores before selling. Losses are minimized at low temperatures and minimum exposure to air.

Season of Year

The vitamin C content of vegetables such as broccoli fluctuates widely, undoubtedly reflecting weather, conditions of growing, harvesting, transporting, and storing, as well as the type of plant.

Method of Processing

Any method of food processing that involves the use of heat is likely to result in a reduced vitamin C content. If processing is done in the absence of air, losses will be much lower. When frozen and canned foods are picked at the peak of maturity and are processed immediately under optimal conditions, the resulting product may have a higher vitamin C value than the fresh product, for which the

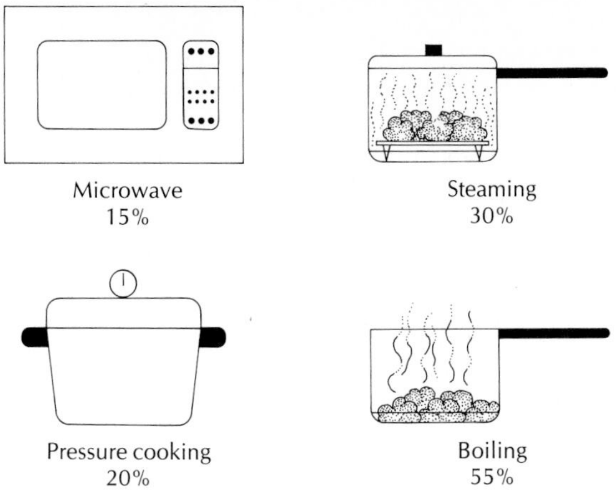

Loss of Vitamin C in cooking varies with the method of preparation (as illustrated with data on broccoli).

period between harvesting and consumption may be long and characterized by poor temperature and humidity control.

Blanching of vegetables before freezing is necessary to destroy certain enzymes that otherwise would catalyze the destruction of vitamin C.

Irradiation of potatoes results in no immediate decrease in vitamin C values, but a 50% loss occurs after 1 week. Freeze drying of fruit results in little or no loss.

Method of Preparation

Fortunately, many of the best sources of vitamin C are normally consumed raw. In cooked foods, most loss occurs in the early stages. For instance, broccoli heads when cooked lose 40% of their vitamin C value in the first 10 minutes by leaching or dissolving into the cooking water. Cabbage loses more by heat destruction than by leaching. The amount of water used has a greater effect on losses than does the total cooking time. Tests showed that losses of vitamin C in preparing broccoli by microwaving, pressure cooking, steaming, and boiling were 15%, 20%, 30% and 55%, respectively.

Adequacy of Food Supply and Diet

Figure 13-5 shows the contribution of various food groups to the vitamin C available in the American food supply. Fruits and vegetables provide 91%, and the remaining 9% comes from the relatively small amount in meat, fish, poultry, eggs, and dairy products. Although cereal products, such as grains, do not provide any vitamin C for the food supply, foods classified as cereal products are recently being enriched with ascorbic acid and therefore contribute up to 8% of daily intake. Vitamin C–enriched beverages, usually fruit drinks, contribute 6.5%

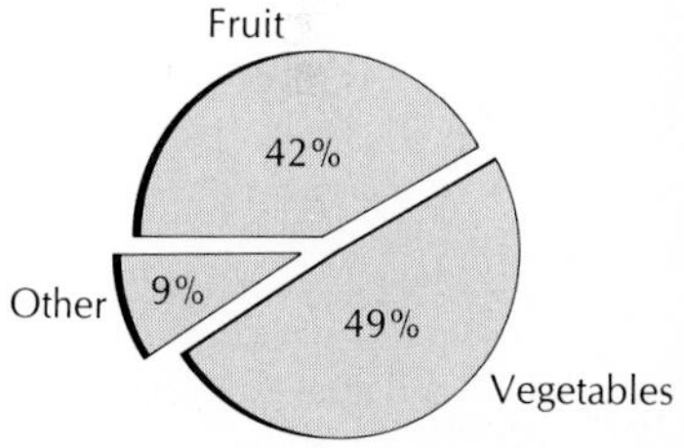

Figure 13-5 Contribution of various food groups to the vitamin C in the North American food supply.

Figure 13-6 shows the trends in per capita vitamin C available in the food supply, with a 25% increase in the last 20 years. The amount available in households and in individual diets has also increased appreciably, primarily as a result of the many ways it is used in processing food.

The adequacy of the dietary intake of vitamin C, as reported in the **CSFII,** is shown in Figure 13-7. The average intake in both NHANES and NFCS in 1977 to 1980 was 150% of the 1980 RDA, but about one in four participants had intakes less than 70% of the RDA. Persons with incomes below the poverty line and those who live in the South and rural areas receive less vitamin C than persons with incomes above the poverty line and who live in urban areas. In NFCS (1977-1978) persons who ate three meals each of the 3 days had intakes above those who ate only two meals a day. Similarly, the more snacks eaten, the higher the vitamin C

CSFII
Continuing Survey of Food Intake by Individuals, based on 6-day record

intake. Of the 3% of the participants in NHANES who had low serum vitamin C values, the majority consumed vitamin C–rich food infrequently, were cigarette smokers or were poor. Serum vitamin C levels decline with age. Men over 75 years old are 2 to 10 times more likely than women to have low serum values.

Tables of food composition continue to record only the reduced vitamin C content of fruits and vegetables, although the body utilizes both reduced and dehydroascorbic acid. The food composition tables in Appendix F are based on reduced

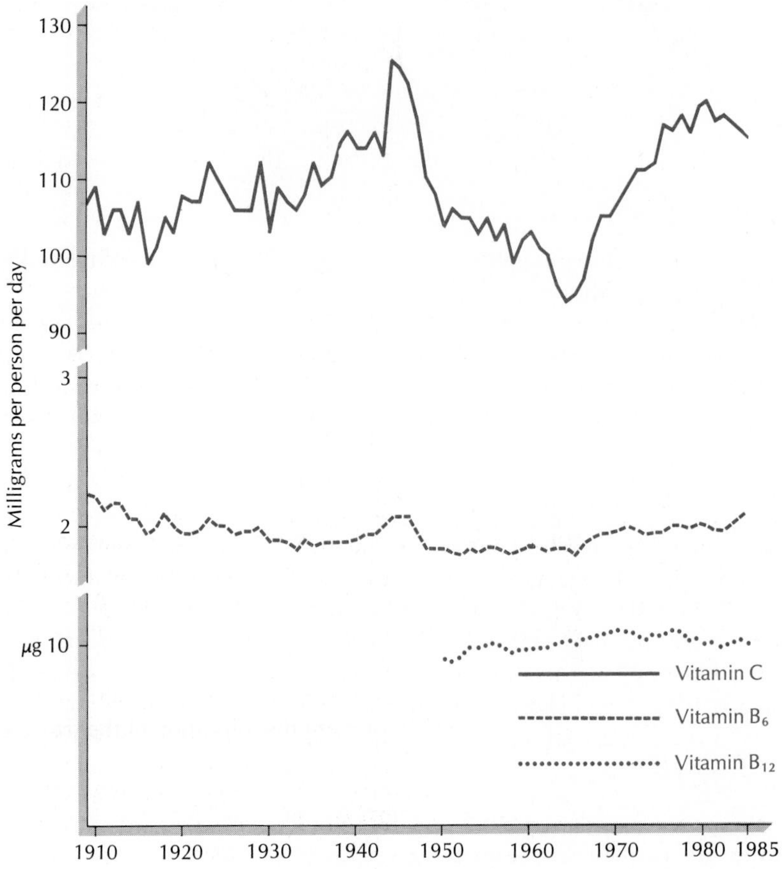

Figure 13-6 Trends in availability of vitamin C, vitamin B_6, and vitamin B_{12} in the North American food supply, 1910-1985.

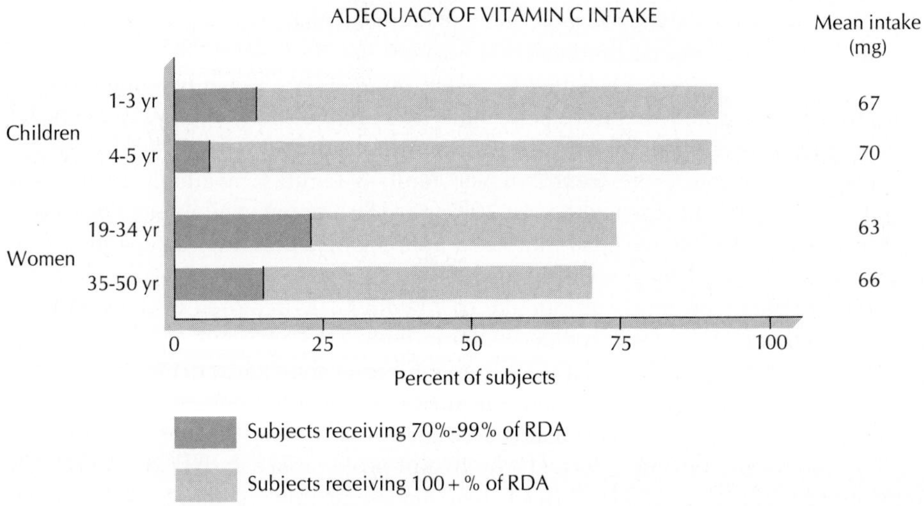

Figure 13-7 Adequacy of vitamin C intake in the United States, as reported in the CSFII(USDA) 1985-1986. In this figure and all subsequent figures with the same format, *subjects receiving 100% of RDA* also includes subjects receiving more than 100% of RDA; *subjects receiving 70% of RDA* refers to subjects receiving 70% to 99% of RDA. All others had intakes below 70% of RDA.

ascorbic acid, except for a few foods for which total values are provided. Table 13-2 gives reduced, dehydroascorbic, and total ascorbic acid values for some representative foods for which data are available, and Table 13-3 presents the vitamin C content of some more frequently eaten foods.

Aside from the more frequently used sources of vitamin C, such as citrus fruits and juices, broccoli, spinach, strawberries, and melon in season, there are several other rich sources. Parsley has a high content (175 mg/100 grams) but is consumed in such small quantities that it is not an important source. Many of the early concentrates of vitamin C, before synthetic vitamin C was readily available, were made from rose hips gathered mostly by Indians in northern Alberta. The acerola cherry, native to the tropics, is also an extremely rich source (1500 mg/100 grams), and although unpalatable alone, it is being used to fortify juices less rich in vitamin C, especially for infant feeding. Camucamu, a fruit native to South America, averages even more at 2000 mg/100 grams. Supplements labeled "with acerola," "with rose hips," or "natural vitamin C" usually have extremely small amounts, if any, from these sources, the rest is less expensive vitamin C.

In the processing of fruit juices, vitamin C is usually added at a level of about 30 mg per 4-oz serving to give them a better chance of competing with citrus juices. For persons who do not recognize the difference in vitamin C values of various juices, this is a commendable practice. Analyzed values vary considerably (they are usually higher) from those on labels to ensure that declared values are present after losses in processing and storage. In keeping with the policy of recommending the enrichment of food products only when there is evidence of a lack of the particular nutrient in a significant segment of the population, it is difficult to rationalize such a practice. However, in Canada the enrichment of apple juice with vitamin C has the approval of government agencies, because it conceivably puts a native product in a better competitive position with imported orange juice. The addition of vitamin C to dehydrated potatoes is a questionable practice because of the likelihood that vitamin C will be destroyed by heat and oxidation in preparation. The enrichment of milk or carbonated beverages with vitamin C, although practiced, has not been endorsed in the United States.

In processing of frozen fruits, such as peaches and apples, vitamin C is frequently added as a reducing agent to help prevent discoloration of the fruit. Vitamin C is used as a preservative in jams and jellies, a color stabilizer in fruit cocktail, a dough conditioner in white flour, an acidulant in frozen desserts, and in wine and beer to prevent darkening of color and deterioration of flavor. Although these amounts are usually small, they do contribute to vitamin C intake.

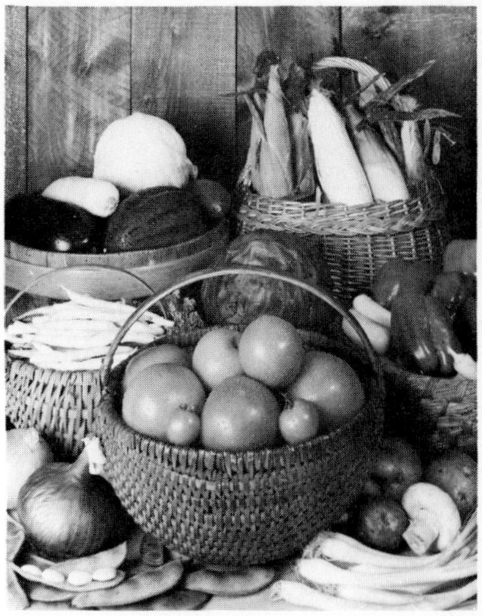

Almost everyone has learned that citrus fruits such as oranges and lemons are high in vitamin C. However, many vegetables also have a high vitamin C content

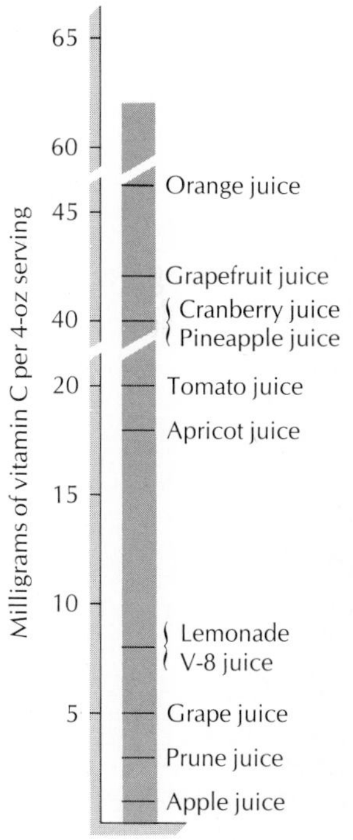

Amounts of vitamin C in various juices

Table 13-2 ◇ Reduced, dehydroascorbic, and total vitamin C (ascorbic acid) in 100 grams of some representative foods (in milligrams)

Food	Reduced Ascorbic Acid	Dehydroascorbic Acid	Total Ascorbic Acid
Asparagus	7.9	26.9	34.8
Broccoli	48.2	9.8	58.0
Brussels sprouts	60.9	4.4	65.3
Cabbage, raw	54.4	22.3	76.7
Cantaloupe	15.5	18.2	33.7
Green pepper	41.0	4.8	45.8
Strawberries	53.8	12.9	66.7
Sweet potatoes	18.8	8.1	26.9
Tomato juice	15.2	2.3	17.5

From Davey BL, Dodds ML, Fisher KH, Schuck C, and Shih DC: Utilization of ascorbic acid in fruits and vegetables. 1. Plan of study and ascorbic acid content of 24 foods, Journal of the American Dietetic Association 32:1064, 1956.

Table 13-3 ◇ Vitamin C, vitamin B_6, and folacin in average servings and per 100 kcal, and INQ of foods most frequently reported in nutrition surveys and additional recommended sources

			Vitamin C			Vitamin B_6			Folacin		
Food	Amount	Kcal	Per Serving (mg)	Per 100 Kcal (mg)	INQ*	Per Serving (mg)	Per 100 Kcal (mg)	INQ	Per Serving (μg)	Per 100 Kcal (μg)	INQ
Eggs, Beef, Poultry, Fish, Nuts											
Egg, fried	1 large	95				0.05	0.06	0.5	22	26	1.3
Beef roast	3 oz	315				0.47	0.15	1.3	3	1	0.04
Ground beef	3 oz	230				0.32	0.11	1.0	3	1	0.1
Chicken	3 oz	140				0.4	0.17	1.5			
Tuna	3 oz	165				0.42	0.25	2.2	3	8	0.4
Peanut butter	2 T	190				0.09	0.05	0.5	26	14	0.7
Bacon	3 slices	110				0.29	0.33	3.0			
Salmon, cured	3 oz	190				0.30	0.25	2.5			
Ham, cured	3 oz	205				0.20	0.08	0.8			
Brazil nuts	1 oz	185							1.1	1	0.03
Cereal Products											
Corn flakes	1 cup	110				0.54	0.06	5.6			
Shredded wheat	1 biscuit	100				0.07	0.08	0.8			
Saltines	4 crackers (10 grams)	50				0.001	0.002	0.02	13	14	0.7
Rice, dry	1 oz	109				0.03	0.03	0.3	2	4	0.2
Bread, white	1 slice	65				0.009	0.01	0.1	10	14	0.07
Bread, whole-wheat	1 slice	70				0.04	0.05	0.5	16	25	1.2
Dairy Products											
Milk, whole	8 oz	150	2	2	0.51	0.1	0.06	0.6	12	8	0.4
Milk, 2% fat	8 oz	120	2	2	0.66	0.12	0.1	0.9	12	10	0.5
Cheddar cheese	1 oz	115				0.02	0.02	0.2	5	4	0.2
Fruits											
Apple	1 medium	80	5	7	2.3	0.04	0.05	0.5	4	5	0.3
Banana	1 medium	105	12	12	3.9	0.63	0.6	5.5	23	22	1.1
Orange juice (frozen)	4 oz	55	49	96	32.0	0.04	0.07	0.7	55	92	4.6
Peach	1 medium	35	7	19	6.3	0.02	0.05	0.5	3	8	0.4
Grapefruit†	½ medium	45*	44	88	3.5						
Strawberries	½ cup	23*	42	160	7.0	0.04	0.16	1.6	13*	52	2.2
Cantaloupe	one half	94*	112	120	4.7	0.15	0.17	1.4	45*	49	2.3
Vegetables											
Corn, canned	4 oz (⅓ cup)	82	5	5	1.7	0.2	0.20	1.9	41	44	2.3
Beans, green	4 oz (⅓ cup)	22	5	10	3.2	0.07	0.14	1.2	22	83	4.2
Peas, green	4 oz (⅓ cup)	62	13	15	4.9	0.05	0.06	0.5	66	75	3.8
Lettuce	¼ head (100 grams)	20	6	46	15.4	0.04	0.31	2.8	13	100	5.0
Tomatoes	1 medium	25	23	105	34.9	0.1	0.46	4.1	53	212	10.8
Potato, baked	1 medium	130	20	22	7.2	0.22	0.24	2.2	56	65	3.3
Broccoli, frozen chopped†	½ cup	25*	53	212	70.4				86	374	18.7
Spinach, frozen†	½ cup	23*	20	87	27.5	0.28	1.22	12.2*	14	10	0.5

*INQ = % U.S. RDA for nutrient/% Energy requirement (2000 kcal) = (Amount of nutrient per serving/U.S. RDA for nutrient)/(kcal per serving/[kcal/serving/2000])
†Additional recommeneded sources not on list of most frequently used foods.

Evaluation of Nutritional Status

Although the biochemistry of vitamin C in the cell is less well understood than is that of other nutrients, the assessment of vitamin C status is more satisfactory. Since no single method is completely satisfactory, a more accurate assessment is possible by a combination of several methods.

The white blood cell, or leukocyte, level of vitamin C is the most sensitive test. When tissues are completely saturated, leukocyte values are between 27 and 30 mg/dl of blood. The fall in vitamin C in white blood cells parallels a decline in the saturation of the tissues and is indicative of the state of body reserves. Scurvy does not develop until tissues are less than 20% saturated.

When serum values fall below 0.4 mg/dl, they parallel white blood cell levels. When tissues are saturated, serum levels are close to 1 mg/dl of blood. The amount of a test dose excreted in the urine within a short period after intake has been the basis of a test for vitamin C status. It is assumed that when the intake has been adequate, the percentage of a test dose recovered in the urine will be high. When tissues are depleted, the proportion appearing in the urine decreases, showing that more has been retained in the body.

Deficiency

Scurvy, the most severe form of vitamin C deficiency, is relatively rare, especially in adults, now that its cause and cure are known. When it does develop, however, the early symptoms such as listlessness, fatigue, weakness, shortness of breath, muscle cramps, aching bones, joints, and muscles, and loss of appetite are relatively nonspecific. The skin becomes dry, feverish, and rough and is covered by reddish-blue spots. Hemorrhaging of the gums often leads to secondary infection.

A study of experimental scurvy in men found that clinical symptoms included enlargement, or hypertrophy, of the cornea, congestion of follicles or ducts, swollen joints, bleeding gums, muscular aches and pains, fatigue, and difficulty in breathing. **Petechiae,** or pinpoint hemorrhages under the skin resembling black and blue spots, developed when the vitamin C reserves fell below 300 mg. In this study, the first symptoms of petechial hemorrhages began to appear after 29 days on a deficient diet when urinary excretion had dropped to zero. By 90 days all subjects showed severe symptoms, with whole blood and plasma ascorbic acid almost depleted. Intakes from 6.5 to 130 mg of ascorbic acid/day were effective in reversing the symptoms of scurvy and repleting the body reserves.

petechiae
Small patches of bleeding just under the skin; they appear as intercellular substance weakens in a vitamin C deficiency

Infantile scurvy (Figure 13-1) is most likely to occur in the period of rapid growth between 5 and 24 months of age. Breast-fed infants never have scurvy, but infants who drink only cow's milk and whose diets are not varied by 6 months of age develop such symptoms as irritability, anorexia, growth failure, tenderness of hips, and anemia. The onset is extremely rapid, and unless treated promptly, the condition may quickly result in death. If the condition is treated, the recovery is equally dramatic.

Delayed or incomplete wound healing is a frequent sign of ascorbic acid deficiency, and anemia invariably occurs after 2 months of restricted intake.

Vitamin C and Smoking

The possibility that cigarette smokers have an increased need for vitamin C has been confirmed by an analysis of NHANES II data showing that six to nine times as many smokers as nonsmokers had low vitamin C serum values (less than 0.2 mg/dl). They absorb 10% less, have a decreased body pool, and have decreased levels in their leukocytes. Fewer than 1% of those who regularly used vitamin C supplements had similar low serum values. Those who used supplements regularly

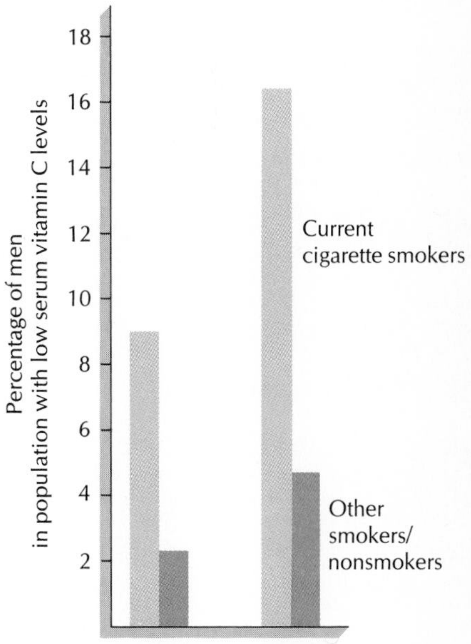

Relationships of smoking to serum levels of vitamin C

had more protection than those who used them irregularly. It appears that smokers may need up to twice as much vitamin C to maintain the body pool as do nonsmokers. Intakes above that, however, provide no additional protection.

Common Cold and Flu

The publication of a popular book by a distinguished chemist, Dr. Linus Pauling, promoting large (1 gram or more) doses of vitamin C in the prevention and cure of both the common cold and flu has led many people to follow this prescription. (He currently advocates 12-gram doses). Most of these people are interested only in positive benefits and have shown little concern for possible harmful effects of such large doses. Scientists, on the other hand, although they have somewhat conflicting test results, recommend a daily intake of 60 mg as adequate to meet adult needs, and well above the level necessary to prevent scurvy. They are not convinced that there are any benefits from the use of large amounts that would justify the use of supplements on a continuing basis.

double-blind study
A research design in which neither the investigator nor the participants know until all the data are collected whether a person was in the control or experimental groups

A **double-blind study** showed a 7% decrease in the number of days on which symptoms of any illness were recorded, and a 30% decline in the number of days subjects were confined to the house. The results did indicate that 1 gram of vitamin C reduced the severity of the symptoms. A concurrent study of children in Arizona showed a reduction in cold symptoms in children given 1 to 2 grams/day without an extra therapeutic amount at the time of illness.

Thus at this time there is reason to believe that the course of the common cold may be modified by vitamin C intake. However, there is still no precise information concerning what level will provide benefits and minimize the risk of side effects. The possibility that continued use of pharmacological doses of over 1 gram, which is many times the recommended intake, could lead to as yet unidentified metabolic changes, suggests the need for caution. If large doses are taken, they should be decreased gradually rather than abruptly to prevent any reactions to rapid withdrawal. The availability of synthetic vitamin C at very reasonable cost has made it easy for the public to obtain the vitamin at pharmacological levels of 2000 to 4000 mg.

Cancer

Evidence from population studies has suggested that people who consume more fruits and vegetables and who also have higher intakes of vitamin C and other nutrients as well, are less likely to develop some types of cancer. Most of the studies to confirm this have focused on the role of vitamin C as a reducing agent in inhibiting the conversion of naturally occurring nitrates in food to nitrites that are known carcinogens. Clinical studies on the use of ascorbic acid in the treatment of cancer patients have led to varying conclusions. The amounts used (>4 grams, more than 60 times the RDA) suggest that any effect is pharmacological and not related to its nutritional role.

Safety of High Doses

The extent to which the consistent use of very high doses of vitamin C impairs health is not clear at this time. The most frequently reported undesirable effects are an increase in urinary oxalate excretion (associated with increased risk of kidney stones), diarrhea resulting from the osmotic effect of unabsorbed ascorbic acid in the colon, excessive iron absorption in people with hemachromatosis, and vitamin C dependency. It is becoming increasingly clear, as more and more people are supplementing their diets with vitamin C pills, that the effects—both positive and

Table 13-4 ◆ Ascorbic acid (vitamin C)—relevant dietary biological data

U.S. RDA	60 mg	
Amount available in food supply	118 mg	
Average intake		
NHANES I	86.3 mg	
NHANES II	99 mg	
NFCS	147% RDA	
Major food sources		
Fruits and vegetables	91%	
Total amount in body	1000-4000 mg (average 1500 mg)	
Distribution in body tissues	Plasma: 1.2-1.4 mg/dl	
	Muscle: 600 mg (2 mg/gram)	
Indicators of nutritional status	*Normal*	*Deficient*
Serum or plasma levels	1.0-1.2 mg/dl	<0.2 mg/dl
Leukocyte levels	25-40 mg/dl	<3.0 mg/dl
Urinary ascorbic acid	60%-80% of intake	0.0 mg/dl

negative—are variable from one individual to another. Our concern relates to the as-yet-undiscovered metabolic effects of continued high-level supplementation. One fifth of the population reportedly takes over 300 mg/day.

A summary of relevant biological data for vitamin C is presented in Table 13-4.

FOLACIN

Discovery

Folacin, the second-to-last vitamin to be discovered, was found during the search for the factor in liver responsible for its effectiveness in curing **pernicious anemia.** Pernicious anemia is a fatal condition characterized by large red blood cells and degeneration of nervous tissue. Although folacin does not have the antipernicious anemia properties attributed to it in 1945, it is a dietary essential for human beings and for many animals and microorganisms, but not for rats, dogs, or rabbits. It has been isolated from spinach, yeast, and liver; occurs in a wide variety of foods; and functions in many biological reactions.

pernicious anemia
Blood disease characterized by very large, immature red blood cells with normal amounts of hemoglobin; it is caused by a genetic defect and is manifest in the inability to absorb vitamin B_{12}. For more discussion, see p. 404

The many names by which folacin has been known reflect the many paths by which it was identified. As early as 1930 the Wills factor in yeast and crude liver extracts was found to cure an anemia characterized by very large red blood cells. Soon after, a growth factor for monkeys was named vitamin M and one for chicks vitamin Bc. Factor U and the *Lactobacillus casei* factor were found to be essential for the growth of microorganisms. As the chemical nature of each of these substances became known, it became evident that the effectiveness of all of them resulted from **pteroylglutamic acid (PGA).** Because this substance could be extracted from green leafy vegetables such as spinach, it was designated as **folic acid** (folio = leaf). Folic acid is now used interchangeably with the official term, **folacin.** Because many substances give rise to folacin, the use of the term has been restricted to pteroylmonoglutamate, the form from which the active coenzymes are directly derived. The term **"folate"** is applied to the broader group of substances that give rise to folacin.

PGA
Pteroyl glutamic acid

folacin or **folic acid**
Designates the biologically active form of the vitamin with one glutamic acid molecule; also known as pteroyl monoglutamate

folate
All forms of the vitamin from which folacin can be formed; most common forms have three or seven glutamic acid molecules

Substances with folacin activity are synthesized by plants, in animal tissues, and by microorganisms in the human intestinal tract. By 1945 scientists knew the chemical structure of pteroylglutamic acid and had succeeded in isolating and synthesizing it inexpensively.

Chemical Composition

Folacin is a complex substance made up of the combination of the chemical compounds pterin and para-amino-benzoic acid together known as pteroic acid. To this is attached one molecule of glutamic acid, a nonessential amino acid. This vitamin occurs in food, however, with from one to seven (but primarily with one, three, or seven) glutamic acid molecules attached.[8]

Functions

megaloblastic anemia

A form of anemia characterized by large *(mega)* cells *(blast),* in which the cells continue to grow because they fail to mature and lose their nuclei

Shortly after the discovery of folacin in 1945 it was learned that the vitamin cures **megaloblastic** (or macrocytic) **anemia** by stimulating the regeneration of both red blood cells and hemoglobin. However, because it was ineffective in relieving the neurological symptoms of pernicious anemia, folacin was not the true antipernicious anemia factor. It does, however, play several essential roles in metabolism, especially in rapidly dividing cells such as red blood cells, white blood cells (leukocytes), or cells of the intestinal wall.

Folacin functions in all biological reactions involving the transfer of single-carbon units, such as methyl (CH_3) groups, from one substance to another. Examples of this function are the formation of the amino acids methionine and serine, the formation of vitamin-like choline from its precursor ethanolamine, and the synthesis of the amino acid histidine. The conversion of the vitamin niacin to N-methylnicotinamide, the form in which it is excreted, depends on the addition of a methyl (single-carbon) unit obtained from folacin.

The synthesis of the purines and the pyrimidines, all essential parts of the nucleic acids DNA and RNA, depends on folic acid coenzymes. Because of this role in nucleic acid synthesis and an equally important one in amino acid metabolism, folacin is especially important during growth and the regeneration of red blood cells and of those lining the gastrointestinal tract where rapid cell division is occurring. The formation of each new cell requires the synthesis of DNA to carry its genetic information. Because nucleic acids control protein synthesis, folacin exerts an indirect effect on the synthesis of enzymes and other essential proteins.

The metabolism of the essential amino acid phenylalanine to tyrosine also requires folacin, as does the formation of the porphyrin group of hemoglobin before iron is added, and the metabolism of long-chain fatty acids in the brain.

Absorption and Metabolism

Before the folacin in food can be absorbed, the extra glutamic acid molecules must be split off, leaving the monoglutamate, PGA. This usually occurs in the cells in the intestinal wall involving specific enzymes and vitamin B_{12}. Once absorbed into the portal blood, the folacin is carried to cells, where it functions as a coenzyme in many biological reactions or is stored in the liver.

Folacin is absorbed in the upper part of the intestine by both active transport and diffusion. From 50% to 90% of dietary folate is absorbed, depending on the form of the vitamin and the composition of the meal. Folates with from three to seven glutamic acid molecules are absorbed equally well. Absorbed folacin, which has one glutamic acid molecule, is removed rapidly from the blood into the tissues, which apparently have a protein that actively binds folacin. Within the cell, folacin may recombine with additional glutamic acid molecules to form large polyglutamate molecules that can leave the cell only with difficulty; this may be a way of preventing the loss of folates. Therefore little folacin is excreted. The liver is the major storage site, with reserves of 7 to 15 mg, largely in the form of methyl folate, that are sufficient to last 4 to 5 months. Amounts stored in other parts of the body may double or triple this body pool of folate. The release of folate from methyl folate requires the presence of vitamin B_{12}. Thus, even if folate stores are adequate, there may be a relative deficiency if it is trapped because of a lack of vitamin B_{12}.

Folacin, or PGA with one unit of glutamic acid, is changed (reduced) in the presence of ascorbic acid and the niacin-containing coenzyme NADPH to a substance known as tetrahydrofolic acid. This compound is relatively unstable; it reacts quickly with a single carbon unit, which can be obtained from many sources, to form one of several biologically active substances. This conversion of folacin to its biologically active forms must occur before the vitamin can perform its role. Anything that blocks the addition of the single carbon units prevents folacin from functioning as a vitamin. Minor changes in the structure of these active forms lead to the formation of the coenzymes responsible for many of the roles played by folacin. (See Figure 13-8.)

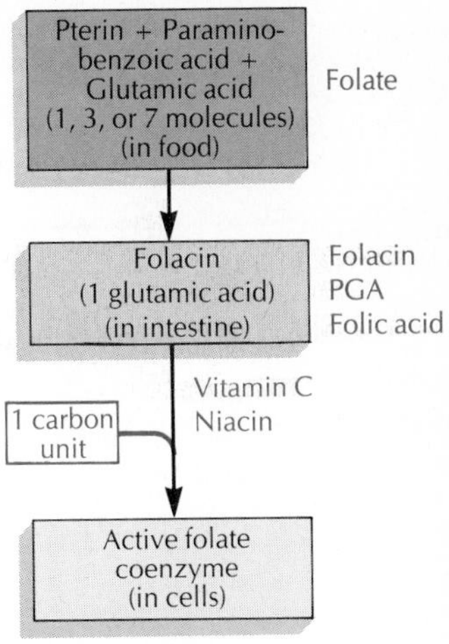

Figure 13-8 Relationship of various chemical forms of folacin.

Requirements

The need for folacin has not been clearly established. It is believed that approximately 3 μg/kg of body weight will meet the needs of most adults. One depletion/repletion study showed that 200 to 250 μg of dietary folate/day met requirements of normal adults and that 300 μg/day allows some storage. The Food and Nutrition Board, assuming a low 25% to 50% absorption and allowing a wide margin of safety for differences in availability from various food sources, has set the recommended dietary allowances for adult men and women at 400 μg/day.

As seen from Table 13-5, recommended intakes vary considerably from one country to another, for example, from 165 to 400 μg for adult women. Recent data suggest that intakes about half the current adult RDA of 400 μg will result in significant liver stores and no evidence of a deficiency. In correcting a deficiency, folacin will stimulate normal red cell production and normal bone marrow tissue but will not immediately cause an increase in serum folate levels or any storage of the vitamin.

The minimum requirement may also be influenced by body size and metabolic rate. It increases with an increased consumption of alcohol, which interferes with absorption, and with any condition that leads to a significant increase in the metabolism of single-carbon units associated with rapid cell growth, such as pregnancy, hyperthyroidism, and hemolytic anemia, and with the use of many drugs. The amount of folacin in food needed to provide the RDA level is variable because of uncertainty about how much is destroyed in cooking and processing and the extent to which it is absorbed, which varies greatly with the source. Synthetic folacin is much more completely utilized, with 100 μg protecting against folate deficiency.

Studies on infants have shown that stores at birth are small but that 3.6 μg/kg of body weight is adequate to meet their needs. The RDA for children has been based on a need of 3.3 μg/kg of body weight for children between 1 and 10 years of age, to reflect the role of folacin in cell division and growth. These recommendations, however, are based on limited data.

Recommended Dietary Allowances for Folacin (μg/day)

Children	
1-3 yr	100
4-6 yr	200
7-10 yr	300
Adults	400
Pregnancy	+400
Lactation	+100

Table 13-5 ◆ Comparison of dietary standards for folacin in different countries (μg/day)

	Great Britain	Canada	FAO/WHO	United States
Children, 5-8 yr	200	125	—	300
Girls, 12-14 yr	300	160	400	400
Women, 18-34 yr	300	165	400	400
Boys, 12-14 yr	300	160	400	400
Men, 18-34 yr	300	210	400	400
Pregnant women	500	305	800	800
Lactating women	400	305	600	500

Supplements for pregnancy are usually available by prescription in order to include the recommended additional 400 μg folacin. Over the counter products may have no more than 400 μg.

During pregnancy, when folacin needs are markedly increased to meet the needs of the rapidly growing fetus, the recommended intake is 800 μg/day. Since it is almost impossible to obtain this much from food alone, the use of a supplement in pregnancy is almost essential. However, because high folate levels depress zinc absorption, supplementation should be kept at a level close to the requirement.

There is evidence that folate plays a role in decreasing the incidence of "small-for-date" babies. Of even greater importance is the mounting evidence that adequate folate during pregnancy provides protection against neural tube defects, a severely handicapping problem in newborns.

During lactation, 100 μg daily in addition to 3 μg/kg of body weight, for a total of about 500 μg, will allow the secretion of milk with a minimum folacin content of 2 to 5 μg/dl, assuming that 50% of dietary folacin is absorbed. Human milk has about twice as much folate as cow's milk.

Food Sources

Data on the folacin content of food are now available on a sufficient number of foods to allow us to estimate the folacin content of diets. A comparison of data from food composition tables and analytical values shows very close agreement. Most diets provide from 200 to 240 μg, which maintains normal red cell folate levels for over 90% of the population.

Data on the folacin content of foods most frequently reported in dietary surveys are shown in Table 13-3. Wheat germ, with 178 μg/100 grams, is one of the most concentrated sources, followed by liver, kidney, yeast, and mushrooms. However, because those foods play a relatively insignificant role in most diets, fruits and vegetables make a much more important contribution to dietary intake. Oranges and orange juice, with 17 to 43 μg/100 grams or 25 to 55 μg per serving, are dependable sources in which the acidity helps protect the folacin from destruction.

Asparagus, broccoli, lima beans, and spinach rank highest as vegetable sources of folacin; lemons, bananas, strawberries, and cantaloupes are rich fruit sources. Milk contains relatively little folacin.

Figure 13-9 shows the contribution of various food groups to the total folacin available per person per day (280 μg) in the North American food supply.

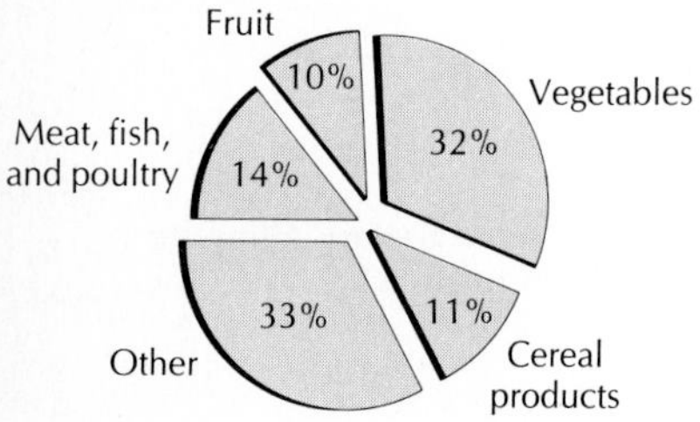

Figure 13-9 Contribution of various food groups to the folacin in the North American food supply, 1987.

Although 75% of the folacin in a mixed North American diet is present as polyglutamate, 35% of the folacin in orange juice, 53% in soybeans, and 60% in milk occurs as monoglutamate, which can be absorbed without the release of the extra glutamic acid molecules. The form of the folacin also influences its availability, stability, and nutritional value; that with more glutamic acid molecules attached is slightly less available. Folates, unlike many other nutrients, are present in practically all foods, but because they are very likely to be destroyed by heat, ultraviolet light, or oxidation, the actual amount in food or diets as consumed is often difficult to determine.

Losses of folate in processing and cooking may range as high as 50% to 90%, and even 100% when high temperatures and large volumes of water are used. In strained baby foods, losses are high in fruits and vegetables but minimal in meats.

Deficiency

Approximately 10% of the North American population has low folate stores. Deficiency may result from inadequate intake, impaired absorption due to degeneration of intestinal lining, excessive demands, or increased losses. It tends to show up in such tissues as the intestinal lining or red blood cells with a high rate of cell division.

pregnancy-induced hypertension A condition that occurs late in pregnancy; symptoms include high blood pressure, proteinuria, and edema. For further discussion, see Chapter 15

A deficiency of the vitamin has been implicated in **pregnancy-induced hypertension** with 20% of pregnant women found to be deficient. Whether caused by deficient intakes or lowered absorption, folacin deficiency has been associated with fetal damage and severe depletion of maternal reserves. In lactating women blood folate levels drop constantly, reflecting the stress imposed by maintaining folate content of breast milk at approximately 25 μg/day.

Oral contraceptives and drugs such as antitumor agents and anticonvulsants interfere with folate utilization, resulting in increased needs. About 50% of all persons admitted to hospitals in low-income communities and 20% to 30% in other communities show evidence of folate deficiency. It tends to occur more frequently among the elderly, the lonely, and the poor, all of whom have limited variety in their diets. An incidence of 50% is reported among alcoholics (in whom absorption is impaired) and chronic invalids. Low folacin levels among alcoholics are attributed to poor diet, malabsorption, liver damage, poor storage, excessive losses, and possibly a direct effect of alcohol on folacin metabolism.

People Subject to Folate Deficiency
Pregnant women
Elderly people
Alcoholics
People taking a variety of drugs, including oral contraceptives

In an experimental deficiency study, it took adults about 5 months to develop symptoms of megaloblastic anemia, the final step in a long series of changes. Infants with low reserves and higher needs for growth developed symptoms in 8 weeks. Inadequate folacin levels may reduce the production of leukocytes and thus the ability of the body to fight infection.

Many believe that as the relationship between folacin deficiency and biochemical disorders is clarified, it is very possible that folacin deficiency will be recognized as the most prevalent of all vitamin deficiencies. Almost all symptoms can be attributed to a failure to metabolize single-carbon units.

Clinical Uses

Folacin is effective in treating nutritional megaloblastic anemia caused by folate deficiency, megaloblastic anemia of pregnancy and infancy, and some other anemias that fail to respond to vitamin B_{12}, which is also essential in protecting against a special form of megaloblastic anemia, known as pernicious anemia. Although folacin does correct the large red blood cells and glossitis (a condition characterized by a smooth, inflamed surface on the tongue) associated with pernicious anemia, it not only fails to alleviate the degeneration of nervous tissue but also accentuates the changes. Therefore, in addition to failing to provide a complete cure for pernicious anemia, the use of folacin may be potentially dangerous, possibly allowing irreversible nervous system symptoms to progress undetected. Because folacin eliminates the most effective means of diagnosing the disease, the FDA has set a limit of 0.4 mg (400 μg) of folacin as the permissible amount in nonprescription vitamin supplements. This would be sufficient to protect against a folacin deficiency without curing megaloblastic symptoms used to detect pernicious anemia.

A folacin antagonist, such as aminopterin, which interferes with the formation of the active coenzyme necessary for the production of leukocytes, has been effective in treating leukemia, a fatal condition characterized by overproduction of white blood cells. Unfortunately, such treatment also inhibits the growth of other cells; therefore, it can be used only intermittently and provides only temporary relief.

Evaluation of Nutritional Status

The most common result of human folacin deficiency is megaloblastic anemia, in which abnormally large red blood cells known as macrocytes or megaloblasts are present in increasing numbers. These develop when the newly formed immature red blood cells (reticulocytes) fail to mature and to lose their nuclei, which would prevent further growth. These are easily identified by microscopic examination. Under these conditions the number of red blood cells decreases, but the cell increases in size as the amount of hemoglobin continues to increase.

Determination of folate levels in blood serum provides a sensitive indicator of folate status long before clinical symptoms of deficiency develop. Normal values drop in about 1 week on diets very low in folacin. In contrast, red cell folate levels, which drop after 15 to 20 weeks of deficient intake, provide a better guide to folate stores. Low values indicate a severe deficiency and are associated with changes in the bone marrow and depressed DNA synthesis. The urinary excretion of formiminoglutamic acid (FIGLU), a metabolite of the amino acid histidine, is increased in people deficient in folate. The test to assess this level is known as a histidine load test because a large dose of histidine is usually given to increase the sensitivity to a folacin deficiency.

Toxicity

There appear to be no toxic reactions to folacin; up to 15 mg may be taken daily for 1 month with no adverse effects. Larger amounts (100 times the RDA) may interfere with the action of drugs such as anticonvulsants, may promote the growth of certain cancers, and may interfere with zinc absorption. There is, however, no reason to ingest amounts in excess of the RDA.

COBALAMIN (VITAMIN B_{12})

Discovery

Until 1926 pernicious anemia was a fatal disease of unknown origin with no known cure. In 1926 Minot and Murphy determined that the condition could be cured if the patient was fed large amounts of raw liver—at least ⅔ pound (0.3 kg) each day. In 1934, together with Whipple, they were awarded the Nobel Prize in medicine for their discovery of this treatment for pernicious anemia.

extrinsic
From outside the body

intrinsic
From within the body

Also in 1926 Castle noted that pernicious anemia patients had a low gastric secretion. He postulated that the antipernicious anemia substance was formed by the combination of an **extrinsic** factor in food, especially liver, and an **intrinsic** factor in the normal gastric secretion. Both extrinsic and intrinsic factors were considered necessary for the prevention or cure of the disease. Castle's theory was held during succeeding years while scientists attempted to isolate and identify the active substance in food. This search led to the discovery of vitamin B_{12}, now recognized as Castle's extrinsic factor.

Attempts to identify this essential component of liver were hampered by the fact that no animal other than humans had exhibited a need for the substance. Thus all evaluations of new liver concentrates had to be made on human subjects suffering from pernicious anemia. Medical investigators were able to isolate progressively more concentrated extracts of liver with antipernicious anemia potency, but the progress was discouragingly slow. With each advance, however, pernicious anemia patients benefited. Only with the discovery that the microorganism *Lactobacillus lactis* also needed the antipernicious anemia factor for growth could more extensive experimental work be attempted to make possible the final isolation of vitamin B_{12}, now also known as cobalamin.

Clinical tests showing that an injected dose of the liver extract was much more effective than the same amount ingested began to cast doubt on Castle's theory that intrinsic and extrinsic factors combined to form an antipernicious anemia substance. They eventually led to the conclusion that Castle's extrinsic factor in food was itself the antipernicious anemia factor and that the intrinsic factor secreted by the gastric mucosa was necessary for absorption. Favorable results with the use of large amounts of liver resulted from the fact that when such large amounts of vitamin B_{12} are available, a small portion is absorbed by diffusion, which does not require the intrinsic factor. This small amount was adequate to prevent the disease.

Chemical Composition

In 1948, 2 years after folacin was discovered and determined *not* to be the antipernicious anemia factor, small red crystals with high antipernicious anemia potency were isolated from liver extracts. These were designated as vitamin B_{12}, which was found to contain the mineral cobalt as about 4% of its weight. The cobalt was present in the center of a large, complex molecule known as a corrinoid, which resembles hemoglobin or chlorophyll. With this discovery vitamin B_{12} was named cobalamin. One form of the vitamin, cyanocobalamin, was found to have a cyanide group closely bound in the molecule along with cobalt. This stable form obtained from bacterial synthesis is used in vitamin supplements. Other forms of the vitamin, hydroxycobalamin or methylcobalamin, are found in dairy products. In meat and in body tissues much of the vitamin B_{12} occurs as a coenzyme in which the hydroxyl or cyanide part of the molecule is replaced by a compound called adenosine. Because all these still contain cobalt, they all have vitamin B_{12} activity.

In 1973, 25 years after it had been discovered, vitamin B_{12} was synthesized. Before this, concentrates of vitamin B_{12} to be used in the treatment of pernicious anemia and in supplements were obtained from the growth of microorganisms and fungi.

Once vitamin B_{12} was isolated, chemically identified, and synthesized, it was much easier to study its role in biological reactions. In contrast to other vitamins, a deficiency of this vitamin results primarily from a defect in the mechanism by which it is absorbed rather than a dietary deficit.

Functions

Vitamin B_{12} is involved in DNA synthesis and thus in cell replication. It is necessary for normal growth, for maintenance of healthy nervous tissue, and for normal blood formation. The exact biochemical role of the vitamin in maintaining all these functions has not been determined.

The functional form of the vitamin is a coenzyme that is generally referred to as a "cobamide coenzyme." The conversion of the vitamin to this active form involves many nutrients, including niacin, riboflavin, and manganese—still another example of the interdependence of nutrients.

In the bone marrow where erythroblasts, the forerunners of red blood cells, are formed, vitamin B_{12} coenzymes provide the methyl groups for the synthesis of DNA. If DNA is not produced, the cells cannot divide; instead, they continue to produce RNA and to synthesize protein, increasing in size. These large red blood cells or macrocytes, which are characteristic of the blood of pernicious anemia patients, differ from the smaller mature erythrocytes (red blood cells) formed when cobalamin is available. The role of vitamin B_{12} in nucleic acid synthesis is important in all body cells, but its effect is more pronounced in erythrocytes, which develop very rapidly at a rate of at least 200 million per minute.

The way in which cobalamin affects the nervous system is not clear. The nervous system damage in vitamin B_{12} deficiency has also been attributed to damaged myelin, the sheath of lipoprotein surrounding nerve fibers. It is now thought that lack of one of the two vitamin B_{12}-dependent enzymes needed for fatty acid synthesis may be responsible for changes in metabolism that lead to the synthesis of "funny fatty acids." These are associated with demyelinization or destruction of myelin needed for normal nerve function. It eventually leads to degeneration of nerves in parts of the spinal column.

Whereas folacin aids in the transfer of single-carbon units from one substance to another, vitamin B_{12} is necessary for the synthesis of these units, which in turn are vital in the formation of many essential body compounds.

Vitamin B_{12} is necessary for the synthesis of the amino acid methionine from homocysteine, which appears in the urine when there is an inadequate intake of the vitamin. In addition, it facilitates the formation of the folate coenzymes needed for nucleic acid synthesis.

Vitamin B_{12} is also essential for the release of folacin from the methyl folate reserves in the liver and in human blood serum so that it can be used as a coenzyme.

Thus a vitamin B_{12} deficiency may cause a relative folacin deficiency by failing to free it from the storage form in which it is unable to make a useful active coenzyme. Such folate is considered to be trapped.

The animal protein factor known to stimulate growth in animals is identical with vitamin B_{12}. By promoting the retention of nitrogen and raising the biological value of the protein of the diet, it leads to more rapid growth per unit of food. The beneficial effects of the antibiotics aureomycin and penicillin in stimulating growth in animals is now attributed to the fact that these antibiotics inhibit the growth of organisms that destroy vitamin B_{12}. Their use, then, essentially increases the vitamin B_{12} available. The usefulness of vitamin B_{12} as a growth factor for children has been investigated. Although results are inconclusive, they suggest that it is effective only in underweight children, and only if the general nature of the diet improves.

Some patients with neuropsychiatric problems of memory loss, weakness, personality and mood changes have shown biochemical evidence of vitamin B_{12} deficiency without the usual megaloblastic anemia. Vitamin B_{12} also appears essential for the synthesis of the protein osteocalcin, needed for the formation of new bone cells.

Absorption and Metabolism

intrinsic factor
A heat-labile mucoprotein secreted from specific cells in the wall of the stomach as a normal part of gastric juice necessary for the absorption of vitamin B_{12}

The absorption of vitamin B_{12} is governed by the **intrinsic factor,** a heat-labile mucoprotein secreted from specific cells (known as parietal cells) in the wall of the stomach as a normal part of gastric juice. As food passes through the digestive tract, the acid of the gastric juice and proteases in the pancreatic juice cause the release of vitamin B_{12} from the protein complex in which it occurs in many foods. The intrinsic factor, which is different for each species, then binds itself to vitamin B_{12} and helps attach the vitamin to a receptor in the cells lining the upper portion of the intestine. This reaction is catalyzed by the mineral calcium. Vitamin B_{12} is released from the intrinsic factor to the absorbing cells in the intestinal wall by the action of intestinal enzymes, which also are different in each species. A failure in any of these stages means that dietary vitamin B_{12} will not be absorbed. For instance, one third of people over 60 no longer secrete gastric acid; they cannot absorb vitamin B_{12} from food because they are unable to split it from the protein complex. In addition, about 1% of those in this age group secrete less intrinsic factor and are therefore less able to reabsorb the vitamin B_{12} secreted in bile.

The percentage of the intake that is absorbed decreases as the actual amount in the diet increases. Efficiency of absorption is 56% at intakes of 1 μg and 28% at intakes of up to 5 μg but declines progressively at higher intakes. When amounts of crystalline B_{12} in excess of 10 μg are taken, absorption drops to 1%, casting doubt on the value of such a large oral intake. Normal subjects usually absorb 30% of the test dose and excrete most of it in the urine. People with pernicious anemia absorb and excrete only 2% of the test dose.

If an individual's gastric juice lacks the intrinsic factor necessary for absorption of vitamin B_{12}, no food source is absorbed. However, if amounts approximately a thousand times greater than the normal dosage are given in oral doses of liver extract or large supplements, sufficient amounts may pass through the intestinal wall by diffusion. Since the intrinsic factor in a hog's stomach is similar to that in a human's, it has been possible to use a concentrate of hog's stomach to facilitate human absorption of vitamin B_{12} from either food or pills. It is most effective, however, to inject vitamin B_{12} intramuscularly to bypass the defective absorptive mechanism.

The efficiency of absorption appears to diminish with increased age; with a pyridoxine deficiency, resulting in a decreased synthesis of intrinsic factor; with an iron inadequacy; and in hypothyroidism. Efficiency of absorption increases during pregnancy and when an intrinsic factor concentrate is fed along with vitamin B_{12}.

Malabsorption occurs in gastritis and with the use of some anticonvulsants and antibiotics, but the effect is usually not of concern.

Once vitamin B_{12} is absorbed, it passes into the bloodstream where it is bound again to a transport protein known as transcobalamin, the form in which it circulates to various tissues. The combination of a small molecule such as vitamin B_{12} with a larger protein molecule prevents the former from being lost in the urine as it passes through the kidneys. When sufficient transport protein is produced, the body is able to hold on tenaciously to the absorbed protein-bound vitamin and loses little of it.

About 2% of vitamin B_{12} stores are excreted in the bile each day, and much of this is reabsorbed along with dietary sources of the vitamin. Analogs of vitamin B_{12} are also excreted in the bile but are not reabsorbed. Daily loss of vitamin B_{12} is estimated to be between 1 and 2.6 μg. Vitamin B_{12} excess is stored in the liver, primarily in the form of a protein-bound B_{12} enzyme. The liver is able to store up to 2500 μg—enough vitamin B_{12} to last 6 years. Some is also found in muscle, skin, and bone, but bone marrow or red blood cells have none. The amount in the liver increases with age, more than doubling between 20 and 60 years of age. Appreciably higher values found in the United States as compared to Great Britain reflect higher dietary intakes in the United States.

There is considerable evidence that in humans, the amount of serum vitamin B_{12} is a sensitive indicator of body stores of the vitamin.

Requirements

The need for cobalamin in humans is extremely small and has been difficult to determine. Studies with labeled doses of the vitamin show a need for only 0.6 to 1.0 μg/day. Even this may decrease when intake is low, since the body then conserves vitamin B_{12} by excreting less in the bile. There is a turnover of 0.1% to 0.2% of body stores each day, regardless of how small the stores are. Vitamin B_{12} injected at levels as low as 0.1 μg/day will maintain normal DNA synthesis and other biochemial functions. However, because it is desirable to obtain vitamin B_{12} from food, a 3 μg/day intake is suggested, assuming at least 50% absorption.

Recommended Dietary Allowances for Cobalamin (Vitamin B_{12}) (μg/day)

Children	
1-3 yr	2.0
4-6yr	2.5
7+ yr	3.0
Adults	3.0
Pregnancy	+1.0
Lactation	+1.0

Breast-fed infants who receive from 0.2 to 0.8 μg/day from breast milk have an adequate vitamin B_{12} status and no evidence of a deficiency, even when mothers' stores are marginal. An intake of 0.15 μg/100 kcal is recommended for formula-fed infants, with amounts for children increasing in relation to calorie and protein intake up to 2 μg/day at age 10 years.

During the last half of pregnancy, a fetus draws approximately 0.3 μg/day of vitamin B_{12} from the mother, leading to the recommendation that pregnant women receive 4.0 μg/day. A similar amount will take care of the 0.3 μg/day that is transferred to milk during lactation.

The intakes recommended by FAO/WHO and Canada are the same as the RDA in the United States. The British do not include vitamin B_{12} in their recommendations.

Food Sources

All vitamin B_{12} found in food has been synthesized by microorganisms. Except for a minute amount produced by bacteria in the nodules on roots of legumes or present as contamination in unwashed root vegetables, no vitamin B_{12} is provided by fruits, vegetables, and grains. Thus, because plants cannot synthesize it, vitamin B_{12} is found only in foods of animal origin. Animals absorb the vitamin after it has been synthesized by bacteria in their rumen from the plant foods they eat, if enough cobalt is available. Any excess is stored in their tissues. Microorganisms in the gastrointestinal tract of humans can also synthesize the vitamin, but the site of synthesis is too far down in the colon to permit absorption. Thus humans must depend on animal foods for vitamin B_{12}.

Vitamin B_{12} is found only in food of animal origin

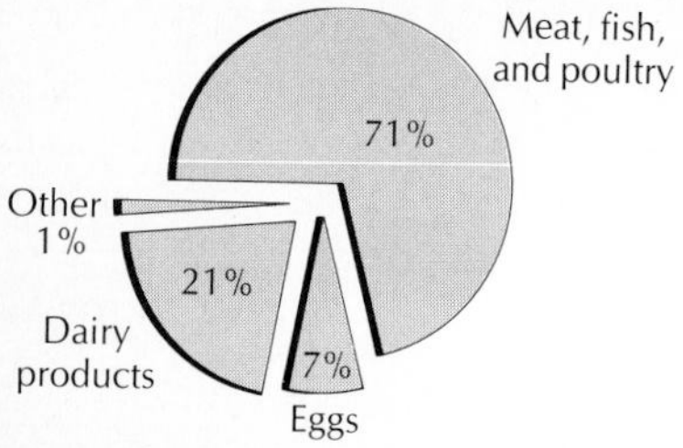

Figure 13-10 Contribution of various food groups to the vitamin B_{12} in the North American food supply, 1987.

The "average" North American diet provides 3 to 5 μg/day. True vegetarians (vegans) may have intakes as low as 1 μg/day and "meat eaters" as much as 100 μg/day. The contribution of various food groups to the vitamin B_{12} content of the diet is shown in Figure 13-10, and the adequacy of vitamin B_{12} intake in the United States is shown in Figure 13-11.

The best sources of vitamin B_{12} are animal foods—liver (containing about 1 ppm), kidney, and muscle (meat), where it occurs in a protein complex (Table 13-6). The practice of some manufacturers of adding it to cereals is hard to rationalize, especially because these cereal products are invariably eaten with milk, a source of the vitamin.

Over half the vitamin B_{12} in food is in the form of a coenzyme that is very unstable and is destroyed by processing and methods of food preparation. Otherwise, little of the remaining B_{12} is lost, except when very high temperatures are used.

Cyanocobalamin is stable to acid and oxidation but is destroyed by alkali. About 70% is normally retained in cooking.

Deficiency

Because of body stores of vitamin B_{12}, deficiencies develop slowly even on a diet devoid of the vitamin or in persons who have had their stomach removed. Children of vegans become vitamin B_{12}–deficient in 2 to 3 years, because they have no stores on which to draw. However, it takes many years for a "new" adult vegetarian to become deficient in vitamin B_{12}. Virtually no evidence is found of a deficiency state from a lack of dietary source of the nutrient, except among *strict* vegetarians.

Pernicious anemia, the major problem from an inadequate amount of the nutrient, results from several conditions—a lack of the intrinsic factor secreted by the glands of the stomach, from partial or complete removal of the stomach, a lack of the protein in the blood that binds absorbed cobalamin, or a lack of the substance that releases it from the mucosal cells to the blood. Atrophy or degeneration of the mucosal cells lining the stomach is an additional cause of a deficiency. This may result from genetic factors, alcoholism, iron deficiency, or dysfunction of the thyroid gland. Intestinal infestation with a tapeworm that avidly absorbs any available vitamin also produces a deficiency.

Diagnosis of vitamin B_{12} deficiency can be made on the basis of blood levels of the vitamin, which are determined microbiologically. Normal serum levels of 100 to 1000 μg/ml fall below 100 μg/ml in persons with pernicious anemia. Detection of changes in the nature of red blood cells from small nonnucleated cells to larger nucleated ones confirms the diagnosis.

Pernicious anemia can now be readily controlled by injections of cobalamin.

Figure 13-11 Adequacy of vitamin B_{12} intake in the United States.
Based on data from NFCS and CSFII, 1985-1986.

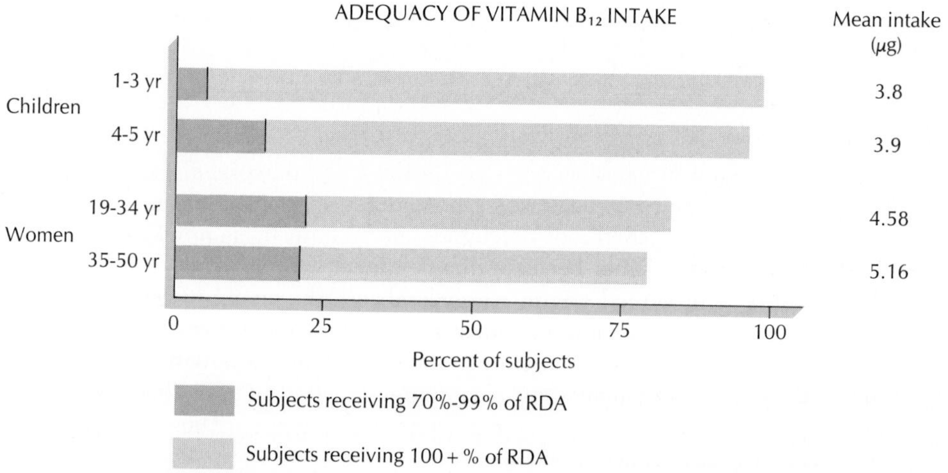

Table 13-6 ◇ Cobalamin (vitamin B_{12}) content in average servings and per 100 kcal of most frequently used foods,* and additional recommended sources

Food	Amount	Kcal	Per Serving (μg)	Per 100 Kcal (μg)	INQ†
Eggs, Beef, Poultry, Fish, and Nuts					
Egg, fried	1 large	95	0.57	0.61	3.8
Beef roast	3 oz	315	1.54	0.49	3.3
Ground beef	3 oz	230	1.52	0.66	4.4
Chicken	3 oz	140	0.3	0.21	1.4
Tuna	3 oz	165	2.2	1.3	8.9
Peanut butter	2 T	190	—	—	—
Bacon	3 slices	110	0.83	0.75	5.0
Oysters‡	3 oz	80	16.2	20.3	135.0
Ham‡	3 oz	229	0.72	0.31	2.0
Liver‡	3 oz	85	87.00	100.00	>700.00
Dairy Products					
Milk, whole	8 oz	150	0.86	0.57	3.8
Milk, 2% fat	8 oz	120	0.91	0.76	5.1
Cheddar cheese	1 oz	115	0.25	0.22	1.4

*Foods of vegetable origin provide no vitamin B_{12}; therefore they are not included in this table.
†INQ = %U.S. RDA for nutrient/% Energy requirement (2000 kcal).
‡Recommended sources.

About 1000 μg given twice in the first week, followed by 250 μg every 3 weeks, is usually enough to permanently protect against recurrence of the condition. The most crucial aspect of pernicious anemia therapy is early diagnosis, so that treatment can be begun before nerve degeneration has become irreversible. In contrast to the pernicious anemia victim before 1925, who was forced to eat large amounts of liver daily, today's patient can be treated relatively simply and inexpensively.

Clinical Uses of Vitamin B_{12}

Although vitamin B_{12} has been promoted for use in a wide range of conditions, from night blindness, psoriasis, and warts to menopausal problems and general malaise, there is no clinical evidence that these problems result from a lack of the vitamin or that they can be prevented or cured through its use. Fortunately, there is no reason to believe that the levels being given, usually by injection, have any harmful or detrimental effects, other than economic waste. It is possible, however, that if the widespread use of vitamin B_{12} therapy continues, we will begin to see evidence of adverse effects.

Practically all vitamin B_{12} produced commercially by bacterial fermentation is cyanocobalamin, a heat-stable form that is readily changed to the active form when given either orally or by injection.

Currently the only legitimate use for vitamin B_{12} therapy is when evidence is present of a metabolic defect in absorption.

PYRIDOXINE (VITAMIN B_6)

Pyridoxine, or vitamin B_6, is unique among the B-complex vitamins in that it functions primarily in protein metabolism. A deficiency of the vitamin was first identified in 1951 among infants of middle-class families who developed neuromotor seizures as the result of the use of an overprocessed infant formula.

The terms "vitamin B_6" and "pyridoxine" are used to denote at least three, related substances—pyridoxol, pyridoxal, and pyridoxamine—all of which func-

Vitamin B_6
Pyridoxine (or pyridoxol)
Pyridoxal
Pyridoxamine
Phosphorylated derivatives
  Pyridoxol phosphate
  Pyridoxal phosphate
  Pyridoxamine phosphate

tion as vitamins for all animals. Pyridoxine was first identified in 1934 as a substance capable of curing a characteristic dermatitis in rats that did not respond to any of the three factors then known in the B complex. This was followed by its isolation in 1938 and the identification of its structure and its synthesis in 1939.

Aside from reports of convulsive seizures in infants with inadequate pyridoxine intakes, we have no evidence of deficiency disease associated with vitamin B_6. However, there is considerable evidence of undesirable biochemical changes with diets containing suboptimal amounts of the vitamin.

Functions

Vitamin B_6 in the form of pyridoxal phosphate (PLP) functions as a coenzyme for many biological reactions. Zinc or magnesium are cofactors in the formation of this active coenzyme in both the liver and red blood cells.

Neurotransmitters Made from the Decarboxylation of Amino Acids
Serotonin from tryptophan
Norepinephrin from tyrosine
Histamine from histidine

Pyridoxine is essential for the process of *transamination*, in which the characteristic amino (NH_2) group from the one amino acid is transferred to another substance and *deamination*, which involves the removal of the amino group from amino acids, so that protein over and above needs for growth can be used as a source of energy. *Decarboxylation*, or the removal of the carboxyl (COOH) group from certain amino acids, a necessary step in the synthesis of the vital body regulators—*serotonin* from tryptophan, *norepinephrine* from tyrosine, and *histamine* from histidine—is also dependent on PLP.

Some of the reactions for which vitamin B_6 is an essential coenzyme are listed in Table 13-7.

Vitamin B_6 is involved in several biochemical steps in the conversion of the amino acid tryptophan to the vitamin niacin. In one, an intermediary product, kynurenine, is changed to xanthurenic acid and then to niacin. In the tryptophan load test, if no xanthurenic acid appears in urine after an intake of 2 grams of tryptophan, it is assumed that the pyridoxine intake is adequate. The appearance of xanthurenic acid indicates a deficiency of vitamin B_6.

Vitamin B_6 is also essential in the production of one of the precursors of nucleic acids and in the synthesis of heme, the iron-containing portion of the hemoglobin molecule.

The role of pyridoxine in the functioning of the central nervous system, especially in infants, is the focus of much research. In mild pyridoxine deficiency, *electroencephalogram* readings change, and in severe deficiency convulsive seizures take place. The development of the brain and its ability to transmit nerve impulses can be permanently impaired if pyridoxine is absent or low during the critical periods of brain growth in the first few months of life. In addition, the role of pyridoxine in the synthesis of serotonin, a brain neurotransmitter, will influence behavior.

The interrelationship between pyridoxine and hormones is evident in many

Table 13-7 ◆ Examples of biochemical changes for which pyridoxine (vitamin B_6) is an essential coenzyme

Function	Reaction
Protein metabolism	Conversion of tryptophan to niacin; methionine to taurine; and glutamic acid to GABA (gamma amino butyric acid)
	Formation of cross-linkages in elastin formation
	Synthesis of messenger RNA; heme, a part of hemoglobin; and antibodies to fight infection
Carbohydrate metabolism	Release of glycogen from liver and muscle as glycogen phosphate
Lipid metabolism	Conversion of linoleic acid to arachidonic acid
	Synthesis and turnover of cholesterol

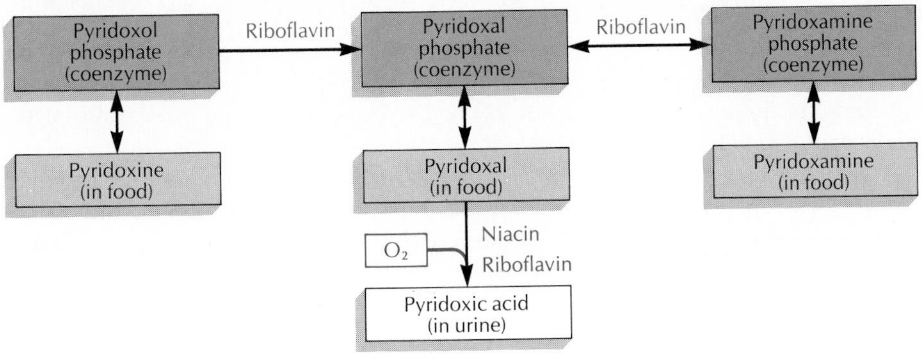

Figure 13-12 The relationship of various chemical forms of vitamin B_6.

ways. A large amount of thyroxin results in depressed levels of the enzymes dependent on pyridoxine, and a deficiency of vitamin B_6 results in decreased levels of insulin and growth hormone.

Absorption and Metabolism

Although vitamin B_6 is absorbed by passive diffusion in the jejunum, the phosphorylated coenzyme is absorbed very slowly. Vitamin B_6 is active as pyridoxal phosphate (PLP), which can be formed from any one of the three forms found in food—pyridoxine, pyridoxal, and pyridoxamine—that circulate in the blood attached to the protein albumin. The ways in which these substances can form pyridoxal phosphate are shown in Figure 13-12. Note that the vitamin riboflavin is necessary for the conversion to occur. Pyridoxal phosphate is the coenzyme form in which vitamin B_6 functions in performing many of its roles, and is the form found in muscles and red blood cells.

Although pyridoxine is a water-soluble vitamin, there is considerable storage in the body. Half of the pyridoxine found in the body is in muscle tissue. Excess vitamin B_6 is oxidized to pyridoxic acid, which is a metabolically inert substance, and is excreted in the urine. Pyridoxal, pyridoxamine, and pyridoxol phosphate also appear in the urine and have been measured in attempts to assess vitamin B_6 status. Some pyridoxine is excreted in the feces, but it arises primarily from synthesis by intestinal microorganisms and does not indicate loss of dietary pyridoxine.

Requirements

Because pyridoxine is necessary for practically all aspects of protein metabolism, the requirement for the vitamin varies directly with the protein content of the diet. Since the North American diet contains more than the recommended amount of protein, the requirement for vitamin B_6 is set proportionately high.

Not until 1968 did the Food and Nutrition Board believe adequate data existed on which to base recommendations for the vitamin B_6 intake. The current recommended intakes of 2.0 and 2.2 mg/day for women and men, respectively, are based on a requirement of 0.02 mg of vitamin B_6 per gram of dietary protein and average protein intakes of 100 and 110 grams, respectively.

Pregnant women transfer enough pyridoxine to the fetus to maintain a level of the vitamin in fetal blood three times that in the maternal blood; thus an additional intake of 0.6 mg/day is recommended.

The amount of vitamin B_6 in human milk is directly related to the amount in the mother's diet; an increase will be reflected in the milk within 4 hours. Because the recommended dietary intake of 2.5 mg/day may not ensure enough in the milk to provide at least 0.5 mg/L needed by the breast-fed infant, supplements of up to 5.0 mg/day may be recommended. Infants suffering from a pyridoxine deficiency have a wide variety of symptoms, including hyperexcitability, rigidity of the body, and a high, piercing cry.

Recommended Dietary Allowances for Vitamin B_6 (mg/day)

Children	
1-3 yr	0.9
4-6 yr	1.3
7-10 yr	1.6
11-14 yr	1.8
15-18 yr	2.0
Males 19+ yr	2.2
Females 19+ yr	2.0
Pregnancy	+0.6
Lactation	+0.5

Recommended intake of vitamin B_6 = 0.02 mg/gram of protein eaten for both men and women

The recommended intake for infants is based on the 0.015 mg/gram of protein in both human milk and cow's milk. Daily intakes of 0.5 mg allow for adequate metabolism of protein and permit normal development of the central nervous system. For the older infant and child, from 0.9 to 1.6 mg/day are suggested, and for the adolescent, from 1.8 to 2 mg/day.

Older persons may have increased needs for the vitamin. This is reflected in a lower blood plasma level of the enzyme transaminase, less pyridoxal kinase in the brain, and more xanthurenic acid excreted in the urine after a tryptophan load test. About one fourth of a test group of persons who were over 60 years old showed signs of a subclinical deficiency of vitamin B_6.

Food Sources

Estimates of the amount of vitamin B_6 available vary from 1.6 mg/day in the diet of individuals to 2.0 mg per person per day in the food supply. A biochemical analysis of representative diets showed intakes of 1.2 mg/day for adults. The amount in foods tends to parallel the protein content.

Vitamin B_6 is found widely distributed. In plants it occurs as pyridoxine, the alcohol form (formerly known as pyridoxol) bound to protein. Pyridoxamine and pyridoxal, the most prevalent forms in animal foods, are more easily absorbed.

Among the richest food sources are white meats (chicken and fish), liver, whole-grain cereals, and egg yolks. Aside from bananas, avocados, and potatoes, there are few good fruit and vegetable sources. Citrus fruit, milk, and cheese are poor sources. Figure 13-13 shows the sources of pyridoxine in the food supply.

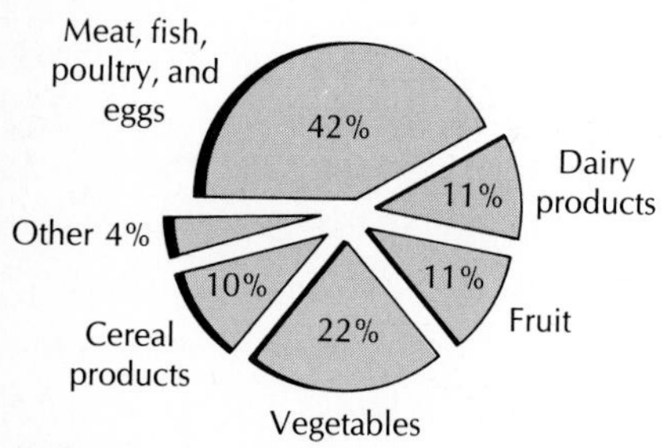

Figure 13-13 Contribution of various food groups to the vitamin B_6 in the North American food supply. Nutrient content of U.S. Food Supply.
USDA Human Nutrition Information Services HNIS 299-20, Washington, DC, 1987.

The pyridoxine content of the foods most frequently used is shown in Table 13-3. The adequacy of vitamin B_6 intake in the United States is shown in Figure 13-14. When the standard 0.02 mg B_6 per gram dietary protein is used, the assessed adequacy of diets increases appreciably.

Vitamin B_6 is relatively stable to heat and acid but is destroyed by oxidation and ultraviolet light. Pyridoxal is labile to alkali.

Freezing of vegetables causes a 15% to 70% reduction of the amount present, milling of cereals leads to losses as high as 50% to 90% of the original values and processing of meat and fish to losses of 40 to 60%. At present, the addition of vitamin B_6 to enriched bread and cereals is not mandatory. However, it is added to many cereals. The added nutrient must be declared on the label.

Studies on the bioavailability or the extent to which vitamin B_6 is absorbed from various foods show that 70% of the content in the typical North American diet is absorbed. Comparable values for milk and orange juice are 80% and 42%, respectively.

Figure 13-14 Adequacy of vitamin B_6 intake in the United States, as reported in CSFII, 1985-1986.
NFCS, Report No 85-4.

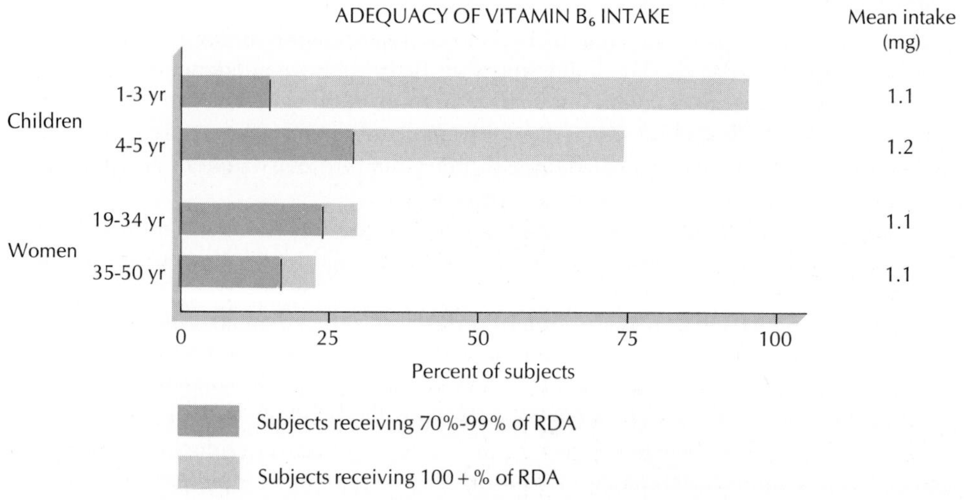

Table 13-8 ◇ Factors that may lead to pyridoxine (vitamin B_6) deficiency or dependency

Inadequate dietary intake
Impaired delivery of vitamin (intake adequate)
Defective intestinal absorption
Defective cellular and intracellular transport
Impaired oxidation of pyridoxine
Impaired phosphorylation to form active coenzyme
Excessive loss of vitamin
Through kidneys
Through oxidation
Inactivation by drugs
Relative deficiency (primary intake inadequate relative to demand)
Increased metabolic activity (pregnancy, fever, etc.)
Increased protein intake
Metabolic defects that alter use

Some naturally occurring vitamin B_6 antagonists in foods, such as mushrooms, have no effect on needs for the vitamin. There are, however, more than 40 drugs, in addition to oral contraceptives, that affect the use of vitamin B_6 and that could result in decreased availability and poor vitamin B_6 nutriture.

Evaluation of Vitamin B_6 Status

Although no specific nutritional deficiency disease can be attributed to a lack of vitamin B_6, certain biochemical changes do occur when intake is low or the needs of the individual are above normal. Many factors may be responsible for a deficiency of pyridoxine; these are enumerated in Table 13-8.

Vitamin B_6 status can be assessed by a variety of biochemical tests based on the functions of the vitamin. The details are beyond the scope of this text but include pyridoxal phosphate in the blood, the excretion of xanthurenic acid in the urine when a test dose of tryptophan is fed, the excretion of pyridoxic acid in the urine, and the measurement of vitamin B_6–dependent enzymes (particularly glutamic oxaloacetate transaminase [SGOT]) in the blood. Of these the amount of pyridoxal phosphate (PLP) in the blood is probably the most sensitive.

Clinical Uses of Vitamin B_6

The use of oral contraceptives leads to metabolic changes similar to those of a vitamin B_6 deficiency. These include elevated urinary levels of products of tryptophan metabolism in women taking estrogen-containing pills, and depression attributed to a failure to convert tryptophan to serotonin, a neurotransmitter substance in the brain. Both of these conditions can be corrected with daily supplements of 10 mg of vitamin B_6.

Both isoniazid (isonicotinic acid hydrazide), which is chemically related to pyridoxine and is used in the treatment of tuberculosis, and penicillamine, which is used in treating Wilson's disease, cystinuria, and rheumatoid arthritis, may increase the requirement for vitamin B_6.

Other conditions in which vitamin B_6 has been used with some, but variable, success are carpal tunnel syndrome, which causes paralysis of the fingers; nausea of pregnancy; premenstrual syndrome (PMS); and anemia. In each of these situations it is essential that the use of the vitamin be based on a medical diagnosis and prescription, which should not exceed 50 mg/day.

Deficiency

Vitamin B_6 deficiencies in both animals and humans result in a large number of abnormalities in amino acid and protein metabolism, with such clinical signs as poor growth, convulsions, anemia, decreased antibody formation, and skin lesions.

Infants on a formula providing less than 0.1 mg of vitamin B_6/day showed signs of hyperirritability and convulsions, which disappeared when the vitamin was added.

microcytic hypochromic anemia
(Micro = small; cyte = cell; hypo = too little; chrome = color)
Anemia characterized by small cells and too little hemoglobin

In adults the only symptom attributed to lack of pyridoxine is **microcytic hypochromic anemia.** Other less specific symptoms, such as weakness, nervousness, irritability, insomnia, and difficulty in walking, have been associated with inadequate intakes. When the vitamin antagonist deoxypyridoxine is fed, skin changes occur (glossitis, cheilosis, and stomatitis) that are different from those resulting from a riboflavin or niacin deficiency (see Chapter 14).

In a pyridoxine deficiency a decrease in the amount of urinary citrate, which aids in the solubility of oxalates, may account for the formation of urinary calculi (kidney stones). On the other hand, the lack of the transaminases necessary to convert oxalic acid to the nonessential amino acid glycine may be responsible. However, when both magnesium and pyridoxine levels are low, urinary calculi are not formed.

Table 13-9 ◇ Relevant biological and dietary data for vitamin B_6, folacin, and vitamin B_{12}

	Vitamin B_6	Folacin	Vitamin B_{12}
U.S. RDA	2.2 mg	400 μg	3 μg
Amount available in food supply	1.97 mg	280 μg	8.7 μg
Average dietary intake			
NHANES II	N/A	N/A	N/A
NFCS	75% RDA	N/A	174% RDA
CSFII	1.07 μg	175 μg	345 μg
Major food sources			
Meat, fish, poultry	42%	14%	79%
Fruit and vegetables	21%	42%	0
Cereal	15%	11%	0
Milk and dairy products	11%	33%	21%
Total amount in body	25 mg	5-10 mg	2-5 mg
Distribution in body tissues			
Muscles	50%		
Blood			
Bones and teeth			
Extracellular fluids			
Liver		50%	50%-90%
Indications of nutritional status			
Normal values			
Urine	> 20 μg vitamin B_6 1 g creatinine > 25 xanthurenic acid/24 hr urine excretion	5-20 mg FIGLU	12 mg methylmalonic acid/24 hr
Serum	> 5 ng PLP/ml	> 67 ng/ml of folate > 200 ng/ml of red cell folate	> 100 pg/ml

People with sensitivity to monosodium glutamate have a higher requirement of vitamin B_6 to maintain normal enzyme levels.

Toxicity

The first reported vitamin B_6 toxicity, in 1983, resulted from the use of 2 to 6 grams over a 2-month period. This resulted in severe loss of neuromotor coordination, which was reversed when vitamin B_6 was withdrawn. Earlier, adults on intakes of 200 mg/day for 1 month showed signs of vitamin B_6 dependency. Thus, although vitamin B_6 has been considered nontoxic, now that it is readily available and used for self-medication, it is very likely that further evidence of toxicity will appear.

Summaries of relevant biological data for vitamin B_6, folacin, and vitamin B_{12} are presented in Table 13-9.

BY NOW YOU SHOULD KNOW

- Vitamins C, folacin, B_{12}, and B_6 are water-soluble vitamins that function in blood formation.
- Vitamin C, ascorbic acid, has long been known as the antiscorbutic vitamin found primarily in fruits and vegetables.
- Ten milligrams of vitamin C per day will prevent scurvy; larger amounts (60 mg) are recommended to maintain a reserve of the vitamin.
- Large doses of vitamin C (from 250 to 12000 mg/day) have been promoted to cure a variety of conditions, such as the common cold, cancer, and allergies. However, there is still little if any evidence that this is effective, and there is considerable concern about the results of taking such large doses.
- Because vitamin C is destroyed by heat, oxidation, and alkali, it is important to store and prepare vitamin C–rich foods so that losses are minimized.
- Life-style factors such as smoking, drinking alcohol, and stress can influence the needs for several water-soluble vitamins.
- Folacin and vitamin B_{12} are both involved in growth and blood formation.
- High intakes of folacin will mask a vitamin B_{12} deficiency.
- Vitamin B_{12} is needed for synthesis of DNA, and folacin is required for synthesis of part of the DNA molecule.
- Vitamin B_{12} is found only in foods of animal origin. Therefore, individuals who choose not to eat animal products must find alternative sources of B_{12}.
- Because DNA is essential for cell replication, which must occur in growth, a deficiency of either folacin or vitamin B_{12} can result in poor growth and particularly in failure of normal blood formation.
- In contrast to other water-soluble vitamins, vitamin B_6, or pyridoxine, is required for almost all aspects of protein metabolism.
- Although B_6 has been considered nontoxic, reports since 1983 from clinical uses and popular self-medication indicated B_6 may be toxic. Furthermore, the level at which pyridoxine becomes toxic varies from one individual to another.

STUDY QUESTIONS

1. Under what circumstances or in what groups of people would you expect deficiencies of each of the water-soluble vitamins discussed to show up?
2. What parts have inadequate intakes of vitamin C played in the history of North America? Of the world?
3. Why are the requirements of vitamin B_6 related to protein intake?
4. List the three most important food sources of each of these water-soluble vitamins in the North American diet.

5. Explain the function of intrinsic factor in the absorption of vitamin B_{12}.
6. Explain why vitamin preparations can only have 400 μg of folacin per tablet.

Applying What You've Learned

1. **Keep a Record of Everything You Have Eaten Today**

   Which foods in your diet made the best contribution to each of the four water-soluble vitamins discussed in the chapter?

2. **Plan Adjustments in the Water-Soluble Vitamins You Ingest**

   If your intake was low in any one vitamin, how would you adjust your diet to make it adequate?

3. **Find a Food Label that has Nutrition Information**

   Locate the %U.S. RDA for vitamin C in Appendix C, and convert the U.S. RDA to milligrams of vitamin C per serving. Now determine the INQ, to determine if this product is nutrient dense in vitamin C.

4. **Analyze the Methods of Preparation to Retain Water-Soluble Vitamins**

   Because these water-soluble vitamins are so easily destroyed, it is important to consider the way in which the foods are handled and the possible destruction of the vitamins. For all the fruits and vegetables you buy, answer the following questions, summarize the nutrient losses, and make recommendations of ways you could improve your food handling to preserve the nutrients.
   - Form of purchase—canned, frozen, or fresh
   - Condition of home storage—on counter, refrigerator, cut up before storage, or stored whole
   - Home processing—chopping, blanching
   - Method of cooking—eating raw, washing, steaming, frying, cooking in water, stir frying, microwaving

SUGGESTED READINGS

Herbert V: Recommended dietary intakes (RDI) of vitamin B_{12} in humans, American Journal of Clinical Nutrition 45:671, 1987.

The evidence on which the recommended dietary allowances are based, the dietary sources, the evaluation of nutritional status, and the consequences of a deficiency are discussed. This article presents the information usually presented to support the RDA.

Herbert V: Recommended dietary intakes (RDI) of folate in humans, American Journal of Clinical Nutrition 45:661, 1987.

The author discusses the basis on which the RDI for folate has been proposed. The article covers the basis for the recommendations for all the affected age and sex groups in the United States.

Life Sciences Research Offices: A review of folate intake, methodology, and status, Bethesda, MD, Nov. 1981, Federation of American Societies for Experimental Biology. Life Sciences Research Offices: Assessment of the folate nutritional status of the U.S. population based on data collected in the Second National Health and Nutrition Examination Survey, 1976-1980, Bethesda, MD, Oct. 1984, Federation of American Societies for Experimental Biology.

These two reviews, which were prepared at the request of the Food and Drug Administration, include up-to-date discussions of our knowledge of folates in food, evidence of low folate status in the population, attempts to enhance folacin in the diet, and standards for assessing status. Together, these reviews represent the most complete discussion of folacin available.

Olson JA, and Hodges RE. Recommended dietary intakes (RDI) of vitamin C in humans, American Journal of Clinical Nutrition 45:693, 1987.

The authors present evidence for the recommendations of the 1985 Committee on Recommended Dietary Allowances for 1985. Data on its source, functions in the body, distribution in body tissues, results of deficiency, absorption, and metabolism are presented.

ADDITIONAL READINGS

Vitamin C

Buzina KS, and others: Vitamin C status and physical working capacity in adolescents, Bibliotheca Nutritio et Dieta 27:107, 1984.

Hodges RE, and others: Experimental scurvy in man, American Journal of Clinical Nutrition 22:535, 1969.

Kallner AB, Hartmann D, and Hornig DH: On the requirement of ascorbic acid in man: steady-state turnover and body pool of ascorbic acid in man, American Journal of Clinical Nutrition 34:1347, 1981.

Olson JA: Vitamins A and C—proposed allowances, Nutrition Today 21:26, 1986.

Sauberlich HE: Ascorbic acid. In Olson RE, and others, editors: Present knowledge of nutrition, ed. 5, Washington, D.C., 1984, Nutrition Foundation, Inc.

Szent-Gyorgyi A: Lost in the twentieth century, Annual Review of Biochemistry 32:1, 1963.

Folacin

Babu S, and Srikanita SG: Availability of folates from some foods, American Journal of Clinical Nutrition 29:276, 1976.

Folic acid: biochemistry and physiology in relation to the human nutrition requirement, Washington, D.C., 1977, National Academy of Sciences.

Rodriguez MS: A conspectus of research on folacin requirements of man, Journal of Nutrition 108:1983, 1978.

Rosenberg IH, Bowman BB, Cooper BA, Halsted CH, and Lindenbaum J: Folate nutrition in the elderly, American Journal of Clinical Nutrition 36:1060, 1982.

Sauberlich HE, and others: Folate requirement and metabolism in nonpregnant women, American Journal of Clinical Nutrition 46:1016, 1987.

Cobalamin (Vitamin B_{12})

Albert MJ, Mathan VI, and Baker SJ: Vitamin B_{12} synthesis by human small intestinal bacteria, Nature 283:781, 1980.

Beck WS: Cobalamin and the nervous system, New England Journal of Medicine 318:1752, 1988.

Carmel R, and others: Cobalamin and osteoblast—specific proteins, New England Journal of Medicine 319:70, 1988.

Halstead CH: The small intestine in vitamin B_{12} and folate deficiency, Nutrition Reviews 33:33, 1975.

McLaren DJ: The luxus vitamins, A and B_{12}, American Journal of Clinical Nutrition 34:1611, 1981.

Pyridoxine (Vitamin B_6)

Henderson LM: Vitamin B_6. In Present knowledge of nutrition, ed. 5, Washington, D.C., 1984, The Nutrition Foundation, Inc.

Gregory, JF, and Kirk JR: The bioavailability of vitamin B_6 in foods, Nutrition Reviews 39:1, 1981.

Guthrie HA, and Crocetti AF: Implications of a protein-based standard for vitamin B_6, Nutrition Reports International 28:133, 1983.

Leklem JE: Vitamin B_6 requirements and oral contraceptive use—a concern? Journal of Nutrition 116:476, 1986.

Leklem JE: Vitamin B_6: of reservoirs, receptors, and requirements, Nutrition Today 23:16, 1988.

Reynold RD, and Leklem JE, editors: Vitamin B_6 in human nutrition, Philadelphia, 1985, Alan R. Liss Inc.

Schuster K, Bailey LB, and Mahan CS: The effect of maternal pyridoxine supplementation on the vitamin B_6 status of mothers and infants and on pregnancy outcome, Journal of Nutrition 114:977, 1984.

Shultz TD, and Leklem JE: Vitamin B_6 status and bioavailability in women, American Journal of Clinical Nutrition 46:647, 1987.

West KD, and Kirksey A: Influence of vitamin B_6 intake on the content of the vitamin in human milk, American Journal of Clinical Nutrition 29:961, 1976.

FOCUS Nutrient Supplementation—More Hazard Than Help?

A mere 30 years ago, nutritionists could not have envisioned a day when they would be more concerned about the consequences of overuse of nutrients than of the health hazards of undernutrition. Yet that is exactly where they find themselves today. In their enthusiasm for informing people of the importance of nutrients in health, they have created a paradox of dismaying proportions. Although many people are concerned about the most appropriate choice of food, many have also lost confidence in the ability of the food supply to provide them with an adequate nutrition. Not surprisingly, there have been entrepreneurs more than ready to capitalize on these fears. The result is a multibillion dollar business generally referred to as the "health food industry." Annual sales of 1.8 billion dollars in vitamins alone, either as single nutrients or in multinutrient supplements, is evidence of the extent of the "vitamin mania."

Why are nutritionists so concerned about the situation? The reasons are many. First, because megadoses of vitamins have been available, marketed, and used for such a relatively short period, we have not had an opportunity to learn about their effects in amounts many times that generally regarded as adequate to meet the needs of healthy people. There is little doubt that intakes at or even slightly below the "physiological" intake are adequate for normal body function. It is when they are consistently taken at much higher levels that we begin to feel uneasy, not only because of what we do know, but also because of what we do not know. Our main concern is that the majority of people taking vitamin supplements are making their selection based on their own intuition or on some skillfully prepared advertising copy or strategically placed articles in the popular press—they have not sought a competent professional opinion.

Many supplement users are turning to vitamins because they fear illness rather than because they are ill. When people turn to vitamins as either a protection or a cure-all, they subject themselves to a risk of even more severe illness. If their problem is one that would respond to immediate and more conventional medical treatment, by delaying this they are increasing their chances of a more severe problem.

In most cases the vitamin is promoted on the basis of anecdotal evidence that neither has been subjected to nor withstood rigorous testing. Frequently people who start using vitamin supplements become very health conscious and take multiple steps to improve their health. This makes it impossible to attribute any benefits to a single change, whether it is vitamins, exercise, improved diet, or reduced use of tobacco or alcohol.

Studies on the use of vitamin supplements in relation to need for the vitamin have repeatedly shown that many are taking the nutrients that are already present in ample amounts in their diets and are failing to take those present at marginal levels. In addition to being an economic waste, this use of supplements may create an imbalance among the nutrients, which can make the situation worse rather than better.

Although the vitamin supplementation industry thrives only in relatively affluent societies, within these societies it is often those least able to pay who are enticed into investing their resources in the hope that vitamins will provide the health protection they seek. The elderly are frequent targets for door-to-door salespeople who prey on their fears that they will become ill and unable to look after themselves. To them any product that promises to help maintain their health and independence has tremendous appeal. Similarly, mothers who feel that the health of their children is of utmost importance are all too willing to accept the assurance of good nutrition that they feel supplements provide. Many of these supplements are sold in tasty, chewable, candylike pills that encourage the child to take more than one a day or other prescribed amount. Toxicity from overuse of vitamin D is but one example of the potential hazards from self-directed supplementation.

In addition to the many vitamins of known usefulness, many with no nutritional role are promoted from time to time for roles they cannot fulfill. Vitamin B_{17}, so named after the World War II bomber that attacked its target in much the same way that vitamin B_{17} was expected to attack health problems, is an example of a nonnutrient substance.

Because many of the true vitamins have not been used for any appreciable length of time at "megadose levels," we have little information on the potential hazards of their use. For some vitamins, the effects may not show up for several years, making it difficult to feel confident that they are safe and harmless until we have had experience with them over a much longer period. Reports of neurological problems resulting from use of excessive amounts of vitamin B_6 over long periods are an example of the kinds of problems to be anticipated if high-level supplementation is continued unsupervised. Diarrhea from the use of vitamin C is another unexpected problem that was recognized only when a sufficient number of people had taken large amounts for long periods so that there were enough reports to associate the changes with the supplementation.

When irrationally balanced formulas are used, the user, who may be told that 10 mg of vitamin B_1 provides many times the requirement, may be lulled into complacency on reading that the same product contains 10 mg of vitamin C, for which it will provide only one sixth the allowance. Similarly, a long list of ingredients, with the implication that they are essential nutrients, can be very misleading to the consumer, who may buy a product based on the number of nutrients it provides. It does not matter to them that some are rutin or hesperidin or some other nonnutrient item.

Another deceptive practice is the listing of ingredients by their less familiar names. This gives the seller a competitive edge over other companies, who may choose to list the more familiar name. Listing a protein by all its component amino acids rather

Statement on Vitamin and Mineral Supplements The American Institute of Nutrition, The American Society for Clinical Nutrition, The American Dietetic Association, and National Council Against Health Fraud—1987

The Committee has considered the issue of the health aspects of vitamin and mineral supplements. The following statement, drafted by the Committee, was approved by the Councils of the American Institute of Nutrition and the American Society for Clinical Nutrition.

Statement

Healthy children and adults should obtain adequate nutrient intakes from dietary sources. Meeting nutrient needs by choosing a variety of foods in moderation, rather than by supplementation, reduces the potential risk for both nutrient deficiencies and nutrient excesses. Individual recommendations regarding supplements and diets should come from physicians and registered dietitians.

Supplement usage may be indicated in some circumstances including the following:

- Women with excessive menstrual bleeding may need to take iron supplements.
- Women who are pregnant or breastfeeding need more of certain nutrients, especially iron, folic acid, and calcium.
- People with very low calorie intakes frequently consume diets that do not meet their needs for all nutrients.
- Some vegetarians may not be receiving adequate calcium, iron, zinc, and vitamin B-12.
- Newborns are given, under the direction of a physician, a single dose of vitamin K to prevent abnormal bleeding.
- Certain disorders or diseases and some medications may interfere with nutrient intake, digestion, absorption, metabolism, or excretion and thus change requirements.

Nutrients are potentially toxic when ingested in sufficiently large amounts. Safe intake levels vary widely from nutrient to nutrient and may vary with the age and health of the individual. In addition, high dosage vitamin and mineral supplements can interfere with the normal metabolism of other nutrients and with the therapeutic effects of certain drugs. The Recommended Dietary Allowances represent the best currently available assessment of safe and adequate intakes and serve as the basis for the U.S. Daily Allowances shown on many product labels. There are no demonstrated benefits of self supplementation beyond these allowances.

than as a single item can provide an impressive array of mysterious ingredients. Furthermore, when amounts are recorded in milligrams, the amounts look quite impressive.

The cost of vitamins will determine which ones are included. The public is being trained to believe that "natural" is desirable, with the implication that synthetic is bad. Because of many production difficulties, except for vitamin E, only a very small portion of those sold are in any way "natural." Our cells cannot tell whether a vitamin came from the chemistry lab (synthetic) or from a food source (natural). If you need a vitamin supplement, the least expensive should be equally as good as the most expensive; chances are they were all bought from the same supplier.

However, to decide if we do need a supplement, we should first determine by an assessment of our usual dietary practices (longer than 2 days) whether we are truly not getting enough of the nutrient from our food. It is the rare person who needs a supplement of more than 50% of the recommended amount. Anyone who needs more than 100% would have to be suffering from some condition that causes a high need. This we cannot diagnose ourselves.

The bottom line on vitamin supplementation is that if you feel better taking one, choose a low level (50% or less of the RDA) of a balanced supplement. They are often hard to find because the more a supplement provides the better the market. You can divide a higher-dose supplement if necessary. Avoid putting together a collection of many single pills at high levels, which could lead to excessive cost and potential danger. The hazards of excessive and unbalanced mineral supplementation are just as great as those of vitamin excesses and imbalances.

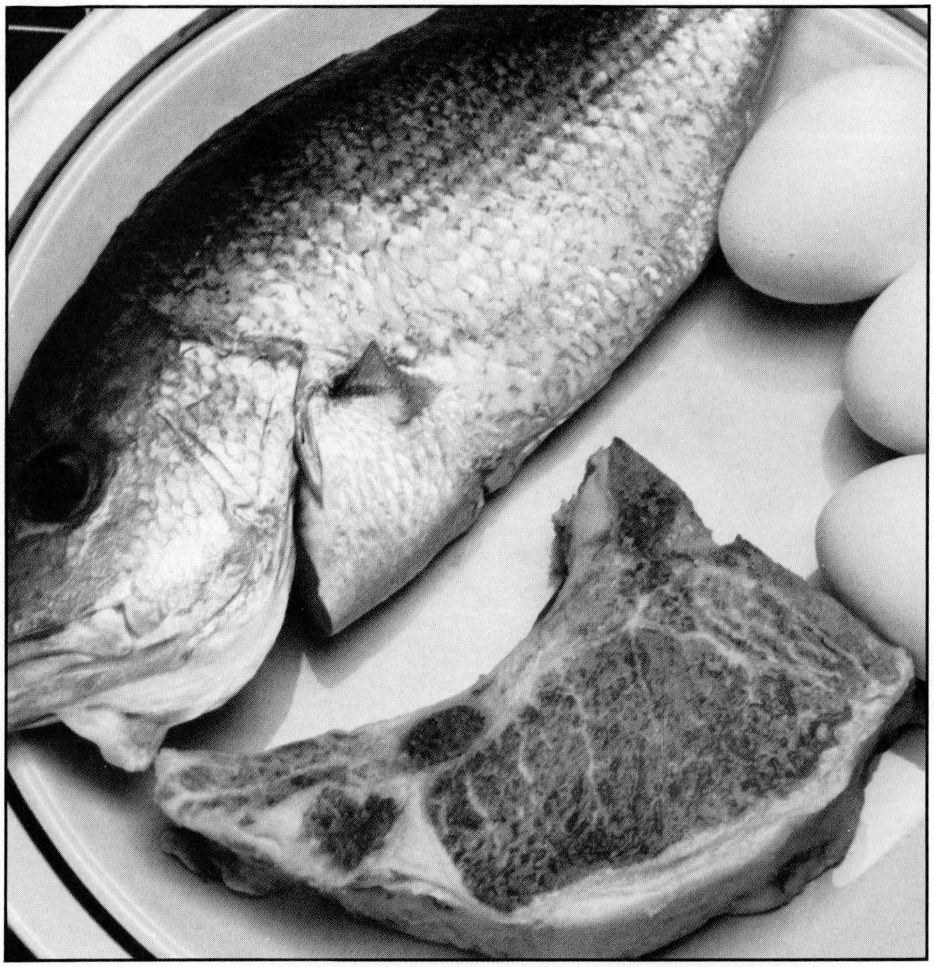

AWARENESS CHECK

Truth or Fiction?

- Thiamin, riboflavin, and niacin are nutrients used to enrich grain and cereal products.
- Body builders who eat raw egg whites may be setting themselves up for a biotin deficiency.
- Milk is one of the best food sources of riboflavin.
- It is almost impossible to meet dietary needs of pantothenic acid in our food supply.
- Milk is stored in opaque containers because its nutrients are readily destroyed by ultraviolet light.

Other Water-Soluble Vitamins

CHAPTER 14

Many people tend to equate vitamins with energy, an idea that has been fostered by the popular press. In the case of the vitamins discussed in this chapter, this concept is understandable; although vitamins do not provide energy, they are essential parts of many of the coenzymes that aid body cells in releasing the energy stored in carbohydrate, lipid, and protein. Three of the water-soluble vitamins—thiamin, riboflavin, and niacin—were discovered as cures for severe deficiency diseases. However, these diseases have practically been eliminated in the Western world, partly because of a program of enrichment of cereal products. Marginal deficiencies are still found, and in developing countries, where refined cereals are replacing whole-grain cereals, severe deficiencies still occur. Other vitamins and vitamin-like substances are also discussed in this chapter.

The vitamins to be discussed in this chapter are thiamin, riboflavin, niacin, pantothenic acid, and biotin. Almost all of these vitamins have a primary role in energy metabolism. Six additional vitamin-like substances are also covered.

THIAMIN

Discovery

Thiamin, also familiarly called vitamin B_1, is widely known for its role in preventing the deficiency disease **beriberi**. Although it had been described by the Chinese as early as 2600 BC, the disease was virtually unknown until the middle of the nineteenth century. The word "beriberi" means "I can't, I can't" and probably refers to the sufferer's inability to achieve neuromotor coordination. With the increasing use of more highly refined cereals, beriberi became a major health problem, especially in countries where cereals such as rice provided as much as 80% of the calories in the diet. Although many theories were advanced, a lack of an unknown substance in rice bran extract, which seemed almost magical in curing the disease, appeared to be the cause of beriberi.

beriberi
A vitamin B_1-deficiency disease that appeared when people began eating highly milled rice and other cereal grains instead of whole grain products

As early as 1855, Takaki had cured beriberi in the Japanese navy by using meat and milk to supplement the regular ship's diets. About the turn of the century, physicians in the Philippines and Indonesia recognized that the rice bran extract known as tikitiki contained something that cured both paralytic **polyneuritis** in chicks and beriberi in humans, especially infants. By the mid-twenties, scientists were able to produce 5 grams (1 teaspoon) of thiamin crystals from almost a ton of bran. Another 10 years elapsed before these crystals were chemically identified and synthesized in 1936. Immediately upon this discovery, both Swiss and American firms began the production of thiamin, which now exceeds an annual rate of 300 tons.

polyneuritis
Inflammation of the nerves
(poly- = many; neuro = nerves; -itis = inflammation)

Despite knowledge about the food sources of thiamin and the availability of synthetic thiamin at reasonable prices, beriberi still occurs in many parts of the world. In the Philippines, beriberi causes 75 infant deaths per 100,000 births and is the fourth leading cause of death in that country. In addition, an estimated 1.5 million people suffer from some less severe form of the disease. This incidence of beriberi is due to the fact that the small rice mills, which produce 95% of the rice, do not enrich it and are producing a highly polished rice that is very low in thiamin. The practice of repeatedly washing the milled rice causes a further loss of thiamin. After milling, washing, and cooking losses are considered, the Filipino diet provides less than the 0.27 mg of thiamin/1000 kcal that is required to protect against beriberi.

Infantile beriberi occurs most frequently in infants 2 to 5 months of age. Onset is frighteningly rapid, and unless treated within a matter of hours, the condition often results in death. The baby develops such symptoms as **cyanosis,** that is, too much carbon dioxide in the blood, causing a bluish color; **tachycardia,** a very fast heartbeat; and a change from a loud piercing cry to a thin, weak, almost inaudible one, sometimes accompanied by vomiting and convulsions. Once thiamin is taken, symptoms are dramatically relieved within a matter of hours. Beriberi occurs more often in breast-fed than bottle-fed infants because the lactating mother's dietary intake of thiamin is often too low to produce milk with enough thiamin to protect her infant. This situation is complicated by the transfer to mother's milk of pyruvic aldehyde, a toxic product of carbohydrate metabolism that accumulates in thiamin deficiency.

cyanosis
Too much carbon dioxide in the blood

tachycardia
Very rapid heartbeat (*bradycardia* is a very slow heart rate)

In adults, beriberi takes two distinct forms. In wet (edematous) beriberi, the victim suffers from swelling of the limbs, usually starting at the feet and progressing upward throughout the body, causing difficulty in walking. The accumulation of fluid in heart muscle leads to eventual heart failure and death. In dry (wasting) beriberi, a gradual loss of body tissue occurs; the victim becomes thin and emaciated. In both forms, symptoms include numbness in the legs, irritability, vague uneasiness, disorderly thinking, and nausea, all suggesting an involvement of the nervous system.

In the United States, alcoholics are almost the only group in which beriberi ever occurs.

Chemical Properties

Thiamin, which is usually available as the more stable and biologically active thiamin hydrochloride, is a white crystalline substance, soluble in water and easily destroyed by heat or oxidation (especially in the presence of alkali such as baking soda). The term "thiamin" indicates that it is a sulfur-containing and nitrogen-containing substance. Thiamin has also been known as "the antineuritis factor," a term indicative of its role in preventing symptoms involving inflammation of the nerves.

Thiamin
thio- = sulfur; amine = nitrogen-containing

Antineuritic
Substance that protects against condition affecting nerves
(anti = against; neur = nerves; itis = inflammation)

Functions

Vitamin B_1 is a part of the coenzyme thiamin pyrophosphate (TPP) made up of thiamin with two molecules of phosphate attached. It was previously known as *cocarboxylase* and is required in the metabolism of carbohydrate. The accumulation of the intermediary products of metabolism when the necessary thiamin-containing enzyme is absent is believed to cause typical symptoms.

TPP (thiamin pyrophosphate) = Thiamin + Two phosphates

There are three stages in the metabolism of carbohydrate during which the absence of thiamin as part of a coenzyme leads to a slowing or complete blocking of chemical changes. First, as part of TPP, thiamin is necessary for the decarboxylation (removal of carbon dioxide) of pyruvic acid as it is prepared to enter the Krebs cycle. When thiamin is lacking, pyruvic acid tends to accumulate.

A second and similar role for TPP in oxidative decarboxylation occurs at the stage in the metabolic cycle when another intermediary product of both fat and carbohydrate metabolism, α-ketoglutaric acid, is decarboxylated.

A third enzymatic role of thiamin is in activating *transketolase*, an enzyme necessary for the metabolism of glucose in all except skeletal cells. Even though this pathway involves less than 10% of all glucose, it is vital; it is the only way that the body can produce either ribose, which is the sugar needed for the synthesis of RNA (essential in cell reproduction), or an intermediary product that is needed for the synthesis of fatty acids.

Attempts to explain the neurological symptoms associated with thiamin deficiency have led us to investigate thiamin triphosphate in the nerve cell membrane, where it apparently acts in the transmission of high-frequency impulses at the nerve synapse. It does this either through the production or release of the neurotransmitter substance acetylcholine or through the formation of complexes with other neurotransmitters. Thiamin also plays a role in the conversion of the amino acid tryptophan to the vitamin niacin.

Absorption and Metabolism

Most of the absorption of thiamin occurs in the duodenum of the small intestine, reaching maximum absorption at intakes of 2.5 to 5 mg/day. Thiamin in small amounts is absorbed by active transport, a process requiring energy and sodium; larger amounts are absorbed by passive diffusion. Although thiamin is synthesized in the lower gastrointestinal tract, it is too far down to be absorbed.

Because the coenzyme TPP is too large a molecule to pass in and out of the cell, it is produced in the cell as needed. Thus the thiamin existing in either animal or plant foods as TPP must be split off before being absorbed by humans. This thiamin is then rejoined to phosphates as needed in individual cells to produce TPP.

The adult body contains 30 to 70 mg of thiamin, about 80% of which is TPP. Half of body thiamin is found in muscle. Although the body has no storage site for the vitamin, normal levels in heart muscle, brain, liver, kidneys, and skeletal muscle double after thiamin therapy and rapidly drop to half these values in all but the brain during thiamin depletion.

Recommended Dietary Allowances for Thiamin (mg/day)

Children	
1-3 yr	0.7
4-6 yr	0.9
7-10 yr	1.2
Males	
11-18 yr	1.4
19-22 yr	1.5
23-50 yr	1.4
50+ yr	1.2
Females	
11-22 yr	1.1
23+ yr	1.0
Pregnancy	+0.4
Lactation	+0.5

Requirements

Efforts to determine the minimal needs and optimal intakes of thiamin for humans have involved studies of the relationship between dietary intake and urinary excretion. These studies are based on the assumption that thiamin in excess of needs is excreted. An intake that leads to a small (but not zero) excretion is believed to represent minimal needs. Larger excretions indicate intakes above needs.

Because thiamin is part of the coenzyme needed in at least three places in the metabolism of carbohydrate, recommended intakes for all age groups assume a relationship between caloric intake and thiamin need. The current RDAs for the

United States are based on a level of 0.5 mg of thiamin/1000 kcal, while Canadian standards are 0.4 mg/1000 kcal. These figures represent optimal intakes, which for the most part are above minimum requirements. There are no benefits from intakes in excess of these levels; excesses are excreted. There is no indication of toxicity from thiamin use, although intakes of 10 to 20 times the recommended amount, which are often included in supplements, may have as yet unknown effects.

Studies of older people show that their need for thiamin is relatively high; they excrete less at all levels of intake, react more rapidly to moderate depletion, and respond more slowly to the addition of thiamin to the diet.

The need for thiamin increases with an increased consumption of alcohol, because the vitamin is necessary for the metabolism of acetaldehyde, an intermediary product in alcohol metabolism. At the same time, a degeneration in the intestinal wall of alcoholics results in decreased absorption of the vitamin.

The need for thiamin is inversely related to the amount of fat in the diet. Thus, fat has frequently been referred to as a "thiamin sparer." Since only one of the reactions for which thiamin is needed is involved in the metabolism of fatty acids, when fat calories replace carbohydrate calories, less thiamin will be required. When beriberi occurs, it is almost invariably in people on a high-carbohydrate (more than 80% of kilocalories) diet.

The need for thiamin increases when some sulfonamides and other antibiotics are given. Although several theories have been suggested to explain this effect, there is no clear-cut evidence to support any of them.

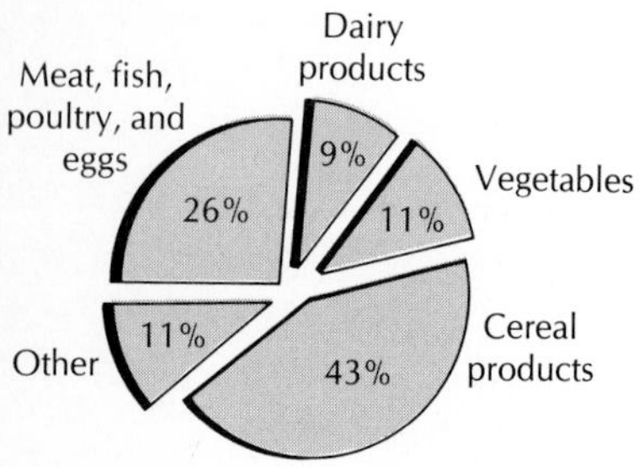

Figure 14-1 Contribution of various food groups to thiamin in the North American food supply.
USDA, National Food Review (Winter) 1987.

Food Sources

As shown in Figure 14-1, cereal products, most of which are enriched with thiamin, provide almost half of the thiamin available in the North American food supply; meat, fish, and poultry, about one fourth; and dairy products and vegetables, about one tenth each. Our food supply provides about 2.2 mg/day, which is higher than the amount that was available at the beginning of the century (Figure 14-2), largely due to added thiamin.

The richest sources of thiamin are pork products. For the segment of the population that eats pork frequently, it presents a dependable source. Those who do not use pork can obtain adequate amounts from other sources. The thiamin content of the most frequently used foods is shown in Table 14-1.

Peas and other legumes are good sources of thiamin. As can be noted from a comparison of fresh and dried peas, the amount of thiamin increases with increasing maturity of the seed. The amount of thiamin actually obtained from dried legumes will be reduced if they are soaked for a long time in water that is then discarded or if baking soda is used to hasten the cooking time by softening the cellulose. The use of minute amounts of baking soda (1/16 teaspoon/cup of beans) is satisfactory; shorter cooking time reduces thiamin losses sufficiently to compensate for the increased losses resulting from the addition of the alkaline baking soda.

Effect of Baking Soda (or Alkali) in Cooking
Softens the cellulose in food
Reduces cooking time
Destroys vitamin C
Destroys thiamin
Intensifies green color

It is important to assess the balance of negative and positive effects of using alkali in cooking.

Whole-grain cereals have 94% of their thiamin content in the outer husks and in the germ, both of which are removed in the milling of cereals. Enriched or whole-wheat bread may at first appear to be an insignificant source of thiamin. However, so much grain is consumed (about ½ pound/person/day), especially by low-income families, that the use of these products provides enough thiamin to ensure an adequate intake in diets that would otherwise be marginal. The use of enriched bread in the United States, the result of mandatory enrichment laws in 35 states, has been credited with decreasing the incidence of beriberi among alcoholics, many of whom eat much bread and bread products (which are cheap sources of calories). Ninety percent of the bread and flour marketed in the United States is now enriched.

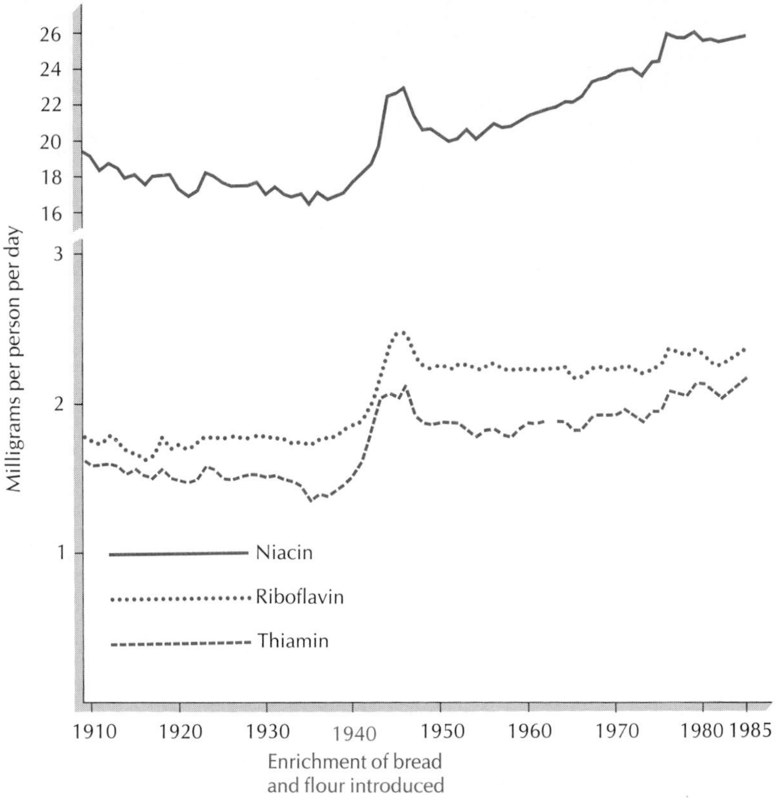

Figure 14-2 Trends in the thiamin, riboflavin, and niacin available in the North American food supply, 1910-1985.

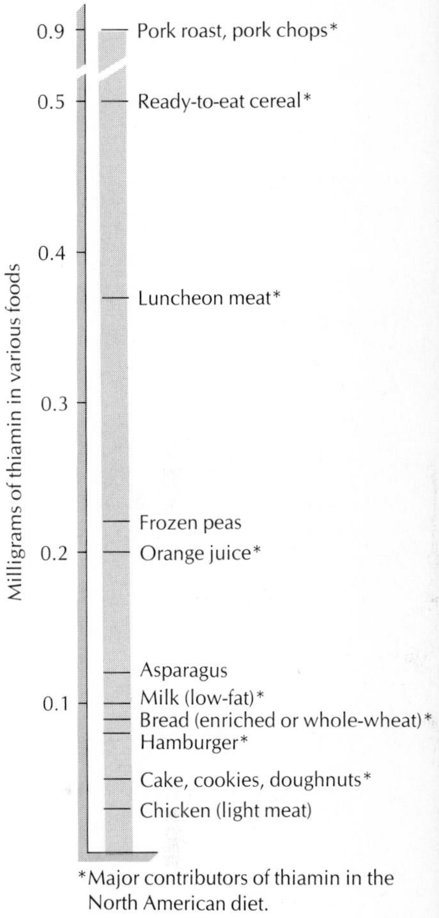

Amount of thiamin per serving in various foods

Despite being promoted in health food stores, dried brewer's yeast and wheat germ, both rich in thiamin, assume little importance in the North American diet because of the infrequency of their use. Live yeast cells, found in compressed yeast cakes, are high in thiamin; because they also require thiamin, however, they deprive the body of thiamin and may actually cause a thiamin deficiency. Cooking kills the yeast cells; problems therefore occur only when live yeast is eaten, which was once commonly done as a supposed cure for acne and other skin conditions.

The enrichment of other cereal products such as rice, macaroni, corn grits, and flour assumes practical importance depending on the extent to which each of these items is a dietary staple. The level of thiamin added is regulated by **standards of identity** for enriched foods shipped in interstate trade.

Certain freshwater fish, a few saltwater fish, and some shellfish such as clams, shrimp, and mussels, as well as bracken ferns and tea contain a thiamin-splitting enzyme, **thiaminase.** Fortunately, this enzyme is heat labile (that is, it is destroyed by cooking). Therefore only when raw fish is regularly consumed is the presence of this enzyme a concern. Tea, however, also contains a heat-stable thiaminase that can have an appreciable effect on the availability of thiamin when tea is consumed in large amounts (8 or more cups/day).

standards of identity
Federal regulation that specifies the types and amounts of ingredients (including nutrients) in a food product labeled in a specific way

thiaminase
An enzyme that splits or destroys thiamin

Dietary Adequacy

The adequacy of thiamin intake in the North American diet is shown in Figure 14-3.

Participants in the NFCS (1977 to 1978) had average intakes of over 110% of the RDA, with 54% having intakes greater than 100% and 83% having intakes over 70%. Results of both HANES I and II showed that the intake was at least 0.4 mg/1000 kcal for all economic, age, sex, and racial groups and averaged 0.6 mg/1000 kcal.

Table 14-1 ◇ Thiamin, riboflavin, and niacin contents in average servings and per 100 kcal of foods most frequently reported in surveys and recommended sources.

Food	Amount	Kcal	Thiamin Per Serving (mg)	Thiamin Per 100 Kcal (mg)	Thiamin INQ*	Riboflavin Per Serving (mg)	Riboflavin Per 100 Kcal (mg)	Riboflavin INQ	Niacin Per Serving (mg)	Niacin Per 100 Kcal (mg)	Niacin INQ
Meat, Fish, Eggs, Poultry, Nuts											
Egg, fried	1 large	95	0.03	0.03	0.4	0.14	0.15	1.6	tr	tr	—
Beef, roast	3 oz	315	0.07	0.02	0.3	0.19	0.06	0.7	4.0	1.2	1.3
Ground beef	3 oz	230	0.04	0.02	0.3	0.09	0.04	0.3	4.4	1.9	1.8
Chicken	3 oz	140	0.06	0.04	0.6	0.10	0.07	0.8	11.8	8.4	8.4
Tuna	3 oz	165	0.04	0.02	0.3	0.09	0.05	0.7	10.1	6.1	6.3
Peanut butter	2 T	190	0.04	0.02	0.3	0.04	0.02	0.2	—	—	—
Bacon	3 slices	110	0.13	0.13	1.7	0.05	0.04	0.6	1.4	1.2	1.2
Ham	3 oz	205	0.51	0.12	3.4†	0.19	0.09	1.1	3.8	1.8	1.9
Beef liver	3 oz	185	0.18	0.09	1.3†	3.52	1.90	23	12.3	6.6	6.8
Cereal Products											
Cornflakes	1 cup	110	0.37	0.34	4.1	0.43	0.39	4.2	5.0	4.5	4.2
Shredded wheat	1 biscuit	100	0.07	0.08	1.1	0.08	0.10	0.8	1.5	1.5	1.4
Saltines	4 crackers	50	0.06	0.12	1.3	0.05	0.12	1.4	0.6	1.2	0.5
Rice	1 oz, dry	109	0.11	0.10	1.3	0.01	0.009	0.1	0.9	0.8	1.1
White bread, enriched	1 slice	65	0.12	0.18	2.6	0.08	0.12	1.5	0.9	1.3	0.6
Whole-wheat bread	1 slice	70	0.10	0.14	1.6	0.06	0.09	1.1	1.1	1.5	1.4
Dairy Products											
Whole milk	8 oz	150	0.10	0.06	0.8	0.38	0.24	2.8	0.21	0.14	0.14
2% fat milk	8 oz	120	0.10	0.08	1.0	0.41	0.34	4.0	0.21	0.17	0.16
Cheddar cheese	1 oz	115	0.01	0.01	0.1	0.11	0.10	1.1	0.02	0.02	0.10
Cottage cheese, low-fat (2%)	4 oz	102	0.05	0.05	0.6	0.42	0.20	2.4	0.30	0.30	0.30
Fruits											
Apple	1 medium	80	0.02	0.05	0.5	0.02	0.03	0.3	0.11	0.13	0.4
Banana	1 medium	105	0.06	0.06	0.8	0.11	0.07	1.2	0.62	0.60	0.6
Orange juice, frozen	4 oz	56	0.11	0.20	2.6	0.01	0.02	0.2	0.06	1.1	0.4
Peach	1 medium	37	0.02	0.05	0.3	0.05	0.14	1.6	0.5	2.3	3.0
Vegetables											
Corn, canned	½ cup	82	0.04	0.05	0.6	0.07	0.08	1.0	1.2	1.5	1.3
Green beans	½ cup	22	0.04	0.18	2.6	0.06	0.27	3.5	0.4	1.8	2.0
Green peas	½ cup	88	0.26	0.3	3.9	0.08	0.09	1.1	0.7	0.8	0.8
Lettuce	¼ head	20	0.06	0.30	4.0	0.04	0.20	2.4	0.3	1.5	1.5
Tomatoes	1 medium	25	0.07	0.27	4.6	0.06	0.24	3.5	0.7	2.8	3.5
Potato, baked	1 medium	93	0.10	0.11	1.4	0.04	0.04	0.5	0.8	0.9	4.0
Asparagus	½ cup	22	0.18	0.60	12.0†	0.11	0.50	7.1†	0.9	4.1	4.5†
Broccoli	½ cup	22	0.13	0.59	8.6	0.16	0.50	5.2†	0.5	2.2	2.0

—; none: *tr*; trace.
*INQ = %U.S. RDA Nutrient/% Energy requirement (2000 kcal). INQ ≥ 2.0 = good source.
†Recommended source.

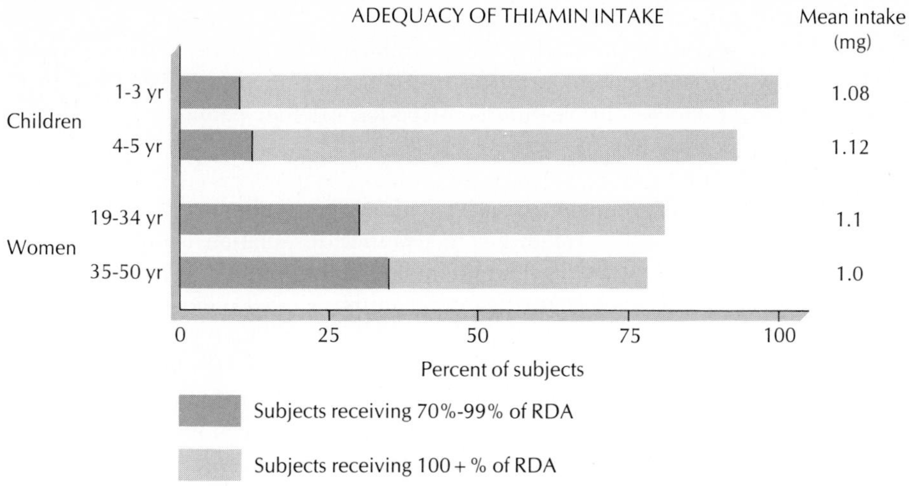

Figure 14-3 Adequacy of thiamin intake in the United States.
As reported in 1977-1978 NCFS and CSFII, 1985-1986.

Evaluation of Nutritional Status

The most sensitive test available for the determination of thiamin status measures the effect of thiamin pyrophosphate on the activity of red blood cell transketolase, an enzyme that can function only if TPP is present as a coenzyme. Values from this test reflect a decrease in dietary intake before any other signs of thiamin inadequacy are detectable.

The urinary excretion test measures the amount of thiamin excreted in the urine following a test, or "load," dose (that is, a dose several times the requirement). People with low levels of saturation in the tissues will retain more thiamin and excrete less than will people whose intake has been more adequate. Because so many other factors influence excretion, load tests are not considered reliable.

Deficiency Symptoms

Thiamin deficiency may result from a low dietary intake when the diet is very low in calories or limited in variety. Deficiency of this nutrient may also result from failure of absorption, which is usually caused by some abnormality in the gastrointestinal tract, possibly as a result of a folacin deficiency; the inability of tissues to accumulate adequate stores of the vitamin; failure to utilize available thiamin; or an increased requirement, such as occurs in a diet high in carbohydrate or alcohol, both of which need thiamin to be metabolized. There is no clear-cut indication of the relationship between clinical symptoms and biochemical changes that occur in a thiamin deficiency.

Because thiamin deficiency in humans usually occurs along with deficiencies of other B-complex vitamins, it is difficult to attribute symptoms specifically to a lack of thiamin. However, the following symptoms are more specific to a lack of thiamin.

Loss of Appetite

Loss of appetite, or **anorexia,** caused by thiamin deficiency has been clearly demonstrated in animals and frequently in humans. Anorexia accompanied by vomiting was the first sign of deficiency in a group of normal men when thiamin deficiency was induced. Even at intakes of 0.2 mg/1000 kcal, which did not cause any other symptoms, loss of appetite, nausea, and constipation occurred. Although increased intake of thiamin will restore a depressed appetite, it will not stimulate the appetite beyond a normal level.

anorexia
Loss of appetite due to physiological cause (anorexia nervosa usually has psychological cause)

Decreased Muscle Tone

The loss of *tonus* (tone) in the wall of the gastrointestinal tract results in decreased gastric motility, a distended colon, and constipation. Thiamin has been used with varying degrees of success in treating constipation in older people.

Depression

For description of beriberi, see p. 418

Mental depression and confusion have sometimes been alleviated by the use of thiamin. This has led to the somewhat misleading designation of thiamin as the "morale vitamin." People with low thiamin intakes show pronounced mood changes, vague feelings of uneasiness, fear, disorderly thinking, and other signs of mental depression. Mental changes associated with inadequate thiamin respond readily to thiamin supplements. This is well illustrated in a study of 10 older women who were limited to 0.33 mg of thiamin/day. They all showed irritability, complained of fatigue and headaches, and voluntarily restricted their social engagements. Urinary excretion of thiamin dropped progressively. Symptoms were alleviated when the women were given 1.4 mg of thiamin for only 1 day. Similar good results were obtained for men. In beriberi, the most acute symptom is the mental confusion that precedes coma.

Neurological Changes

Nystagmus (involuntary rapid eye movement), also known as Wernicke's syndrome, is a result of changes in the central nervous system that are quickly reversed by thiamin. Levels of thiamin in the brain can be reduced by 50% without any noticeable clinical signs. Further reduction to 30% of normal leads to slow and unsteady gait, and at 20%, severe disturbances of posture and equilibrium occur. Peripheral neuritis, in which the nerves that control the extremities fail to function properly, shows up in a variety of ways in human beings, with the legs usually affected first.

Neuromuscular coordination is affected in people on low thiamin intake, resulting in decreased mechanical efficiency and work output. Motor speed and eye-hand coordination that had deteriorated on a low thiamin intake were quickly restored with thiamin supplementation.

Clinical Uses

Thiamin has been used in the medical treatment of a wide variety of conditions besides beriberi. One survey of the literature showed that it had been tried therapeutically in 230 different conditions for neuritis, neuralgia, pains of various origins, diseases of the central nervous system, or cardiovascular symptoms. The results were generally inconclusive. Because we have no evidence of adverse effects from intakes up to 100 mg, the use of vitamin B_1 is probably safe although of unknown or questionable effectiveness.

RIBOFLAVIN

Riboflavin, which has also been known as vitamin B_2, vitamin G, and "the yellow enzyme," was recognized as a vitamin in 1917. At that time, it became clear that vitamin B retained some growth-promoting properties even after its antiberiberi properties (thiamin) had been destroyed by heat. To differentiate the heat-labile component of vitamin B from this heat-stable fraction, the two components were named vitamin B_1 and vitamin B_2, respectively. Riboflavin is now known to be essential for growth and tissue repair in all animals, from microorganisms to humans. So far, we have not identified any deficiency disease associated with it, although there are general symptoms.

Riboflavin
ribo- = ribose, a sugar; flavin = yellow fluorescence

At the same time that riboflavin was being identified, reports announced the isolation of four substances necessary for growth: hepatoflavin, lactoflavin, ovoflavin, and verdoflavin. Investigators, isolating factors from liver, milk, eggs, and grass, respectively, agreed that these were flavin compounds—substances that produce an intense yellow-green fluorescence in water. These substances had been concentrated from natural foods in 1925 and were isolated in 1932, at which time it became evident that the active factor was the same in all of them and was composed of a protein plus a pigment, or flavin. With the synthesis of riboflavin in 1935, it soon became clear that the five-carbon sugar ribose was common to all the flavin compounds, which were then designated "riboflavine." Shortly afterward, the final "e" was dropped in all countries except Britain.

Sources of Riboflavin
Liver *(hepato)*—hepatoflavin
Milk *(lacto)*—lactoflavin
Egg *(ovo)*—ovoflavin
Green vegetables *(verdo)*—verdoflavin

Chemical Properties

Riboflavin is a relatively stable vitamin; it is resistant to the effects of acid, heat, and oxidation. It is unstable in the presence of alkali and light. Because it is slightly soluble in water, some losses occur when small pieces of riboflavin-containing food are cooked in large amounts of water for long periods. However, the major loss of riboflavin (up to 70% in 4 hours) is caused by the action of sunlight on milk, which is ordinarily a significant source of riboflavin in the Western diet. The almost universal use of opaque wax-lined cardboard or plastic milk containers has essentially eliminated the problem.

Functions

At a biochemical level, riboflavin as a part of several coenzymes contributes to their capacity to accept and transfer hydrogen atoms, or positive charges. These reactions are essential for the release of energy from glucose, fatty acids, and amino acids within the cell mitochondrion. The two coenzymes, flavin mononucleotide (also known as FMN, or riboflavin mononucleotide) and flavin adenine dinucleotide (or FAD), are attached to a variety of proteins and are known as flavoproteins. Riboflavin is necessary before the amino acid tryptophan can be converted into the active form of the vitamin niacin. Riboflavin also aids in the conversion of both vitamin B_6 and folacin to their coenzymes and in their storage in the body. Because these coenzymes are needed for DNA synthesis, riboflavin has an indirect effect on cell division and therefore on growth.

Riboflavin-Containing Coenzymes
FAD (flavin adenine dinucleotide)
FMN (flavin mononucleotide)

Among the other biochemical roles of riboflavin are the production of hormones in the adrenal cortex, the formation of red blood cells in bone marrow, the synthesis of glycogen (glycogenesis), and fatty acid catabolism. Some substances chemically related to riboflavin can replace riboflavin completely, whereas other substances act as riboflavin antagonists.

Absorption

The absorption of riboflavin occurs primarily in the upper portion of the gastrointestinal tract, which regulates the amount taken up. Within the intestinal cells, riboflavin is *phosphorylated*, or linked with a phosphate molecule, to form FMN. Once absorbed, both riboflavin and FMN are transported and attached to albumin in the blood. FMN is readily released from the blood to the tissues, principally the liver, where it is converted into another coenzyme (FAD) by the addition of adenosine triphosphate. Tissue storage is in the form of FMN and FAD rather than as free riboflavin. With higher intakes, the amount in the liver will not increase beyond a certain level. Similarly, in a deficiency, liver reserves do not drop below 50% of saturation levels. The thyroid hormone appears to stimulate the absorption and storage of riboflavin and the synthesis of FMN and FAD.

Riboflavin is excreted primarily in the urine after the kidneys have allowed the reabsorption of enough of the vitamin to maintain tissue saturation. Riboflavin excreted in the feces is either unabsorbed dietary riboflavin or some of the riboflavin secreted in the bile, which is not reabsorbed. A small amount of this riboflavin is broken down by intestinal microorganisms into different end products. Relatively little riboflavin is stored in the body, although the liver and kidneys contain higher concentrations than do other tissues such as muscle.

More riboflavin is absorbed when it is taken with meals (70%) than when taken alone (15%). Older people absorb more riboflavin than do younger ones.

Recommended Dietary Allowances for Riboflavin (mg/day)

For all ages	0.6 mg/1000 kcal
Children	
1-3 yr	0.8
4-6 yr	1.0
7-10 yr	1.4
Males	
11-14 yr	1.6
15-22 yr	1.7
23-50 yr	1.6
51+ yr	1.4
Females	
11-22 yr	1.3
22+ yr	1.2
Pregnancy	+0.3
Lactation	+0.5

Requirements

Throughout various editions of the *Recommended Dietary Allowances*, riboflavin requirements have been based on caloric intake, protein allowances, or metabolic body size (weight in kg$^{3/4}$). Results do not differ significantly. When standards are related to energy allowances, 0.6 mg of riboflavin/1000 kcal with a minimum of 1.2 mg daily is recommended to ensure tissue saturation with the vitamin. This estimate was based on data from studies of excretion in relation to intake. During pregnancy and lactation, an additional 0.3 mg and 0.5 mg, respectively, are recommended daily, assuming 70% utilization. These amounts are just slightly higher than the amounts the FAO/WHO committee considers a practical goal. There are no known problems with high intakes of riboflavin, and there are some indications that riboflavin needs increase with age and possibly in exercising women.

Food Sources

Riboflavin is widely distributed in both animal and vegetable foods. The amounts present in various foods are given in Table 14-1. Figure 14-4 shows the relative contributions of the major food groups to the riboflavin available in the food supply. Daily intakes of riboflavin per person average 2.43 mg. Protein-rich foods contribute about one third of the amount of riboflavin in the North American diet; this amount is seldom affected by the usual methods of food preparation. The adequacy of the riboflavin intake in the North American diet is shown in Figure 14-5.

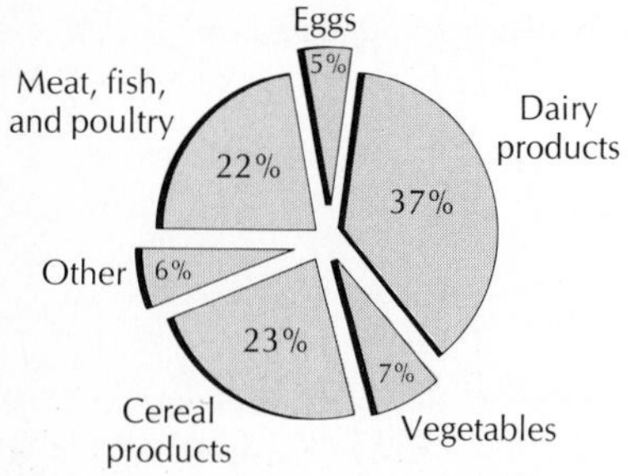

Figure 14-4 Contribution of various foods groups to riboflavin in the North American diet.
USDA, National Food Review (Winter) 1987.

About 60% to 90% of the vitamin in fruits and vegetables is retained in cooking. On the other hand, the milling of cereal causes up to 60% loss of riboflavin. Because of its intense yellow color, riboflavin is often not used in fortifying cereals such as rice; it is always added, however, to flour and bread to enrich them at a higher level than that found in whole-wheat products. Originally, the high standards were the result of errors in determining the amount of riboflavin present in whole wheat, but the standards have been retained as a way to prevent any deficiency.

Lactoflavin in milk makes a significant contribution to the amount of riboflavin in the diet, with 1 quart (about 1 liter) providing all the intake recommended for

Figure 14-5 Adequacy of riboflavin intake in the United States.
Based on data from the 1977-1978 NCFS and CSFII 1985-1986.

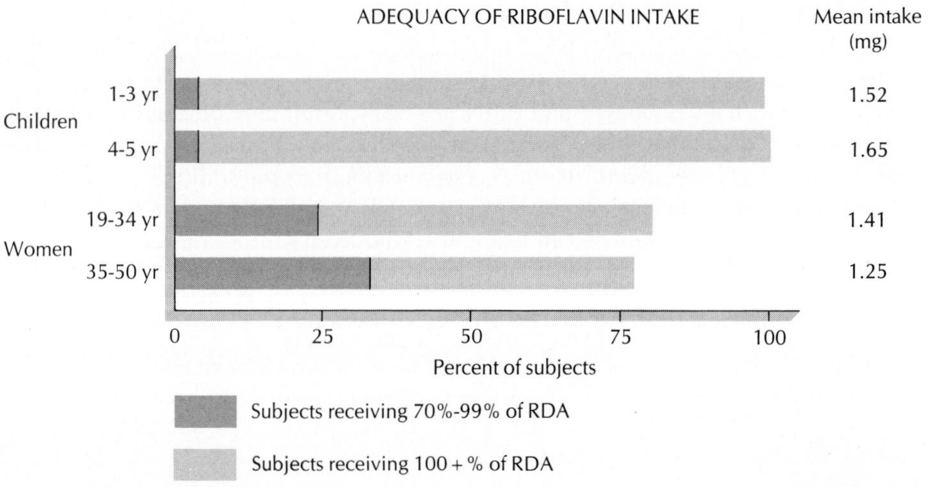

people of all ages and 2 cups providing a sufficient amount to meet minimal needs. Cheese retains about one fourth of the amount of riboflavin in the milk from which it was made. Liver and kidney are high in riboflavin, but other meats are only fair sources.

Although riboflavin in the human body is synthesized by bacteria in the gastrointestinal tract, there is little evidence that a significant amount is absorbed.

Evaluation of Nutritional Status

The measurement of the activation of the enzyme erythrocyte glutathione reductase, to which riboflavin is closely bound in red blood cells, is used as a functional indicator of riboflavin status. Neither urinary riboflavin excretion nor red cell riboflavin are considered sensitive enough to be good indicators.

Data from the 1977 NFCS showed that 66% of the people surveyed had over 100% of the RDA for riboflavin; only 12% had intakes less than 70%. The mean intakes of all ages and sex groups exceeded the RDA by 31%. Results of the NFCS' continuing survey (CSFII) in 1985 to 1986 yielded similar results (Fig. 14-5).

In an experimentally induced severe riboflavin deficiency (less than 0.07 mg of riboflavin for 39 to 56 days), six adult males showed measurable personality changes, including hypochondriasis, depression, and hysteria, as well as reduced hand-grip strength.

Deficiency

Riboflavin deficiency appears to be more common than previously suspected. In one study of 431 high school students, 16% of the girls and 6% of the boys had glutathione reductase activity coefficients that indicated inadequate riboflavin intakes. These were eliminated by a riboflavin supplement of 0.5 mg/day for 1 week. Other studies showed deficiencies in 11% of a group of children and in 26% of a group of girls, 13 to 19 years old, of lower socioeconomic status. These deficiencies were all associated with milk intakes of less than 1 cup/day.

The many manifestations of lack of riboflavin can be assessed clinically. In humans, an early form of **ariboflavinosis** (lack of riboflavin) is a condition known as **cheilosis** in which cracks appear at the corners of the mouth and the lips become inflamed. In a condition called **glossitis,** the tongue becomes smooth and takes on a characteristic purplish-red color. Intakes must be low for several months before these symptoms show up.

ariboflavinosis
A lack of riboflavin

cheilosis
A condition characterized by cracking at the corners of the lips

glossitis
Condition characterized by a purplish tongue with a very smooth surface

As is true in a deficiency of any vitamin, growth retardation occurs with a lack of riboflavin. Certain congenital malformations such as cleft lip and cataracts and skeletal deformities, which are associated with a deficiency at a crucial stage in development have been clearly demonstrated in riboflavin-deficient animals. The relationship is much more difficult to establish in human pregnancy. The loss of hair seen in riboflavin-deficient animals does not appear in human beings. Clinically, riboflavin deficiency seldom occurs in isolation, but rather in conjunction with other water-soluble vitamin deficiencies.

Toxicity

No reports of riboflavin toxicity have appeared in other animals or human beings. Individuals have a maximum absorptive capacity of about 20 mg/day.

NIACIN (NICOTINIC ACID)

Niacin, formerly known as nicotinic acid and on occasion as vitamin B_3, was originally obtained from the oxidation of nicotine in 1867. By 1912, it had been associated with the antiberiberi substance in rice polishings and had been isolated in crystalline form. However, not until 1937 was it recognized as the pellagra-preventive factor (that is, a vitamin capable of curing the disease pellagra in humans and blacktongue in dogs). Nicotinamide, which is chemically related to niacin, also has vitamin activity. The term niacin is now used to include nicotinic acid, nicotinamide, and other related compounds.

Discovery

pellagra
A condition characterized by a rough skin and caused by a lack of the vitamin niacin or the nutrients needed to convert tryptophan to niacin
(pellagragenic = causing pellagra)

The disease known as **pellagra** in Italy and "mal del sol" or "mal de la rosa" in Spain was first described in the eigtheenth century. It occurred mainly among the poor, who used corn (maize) produced in the New World as their dietary staple. Although the disease could be cured by changing the diet, only in 1917 was it associated with the absence of a dietary factor.

The association of pellagra with diets monotonously high in highly refined maize led to the theory that the disease was caused by a mold or a toxic or infectious substance in spoiled corn. Later, a lack of nitrogen was implicated; in addition, the absence in corn diets of the essential amino acids lysine or tryptophan, in conjunction with the high content of another essential amino acid, leucine, suggested that an amino acid imbalance was the cause. The skin symptoms of pellagra were aggravated by exposure to sunlight, leading to the belief that the disease was the result of "sun poisoning" (mal del sol). Because pellagra-causing corn diets, in which molasses and salt pork were often the only other foods, were consumed by people on limited incomes often living in crowded and unsanitary surroundings, theories suggesting that the disease had an infectious or parasitic origin received support. In addition, the fact that several members of the same family often developed pellagra seemed reason to look for hereditary factors.

Progress was made in controlling the disease in 1917, when Goldberger, a physician working with the United States Public Health Service, confirmed his theory of the cause of pellagra by producing it through dietary restriction. He conducted classic experiments with a group of prisoners who were promised a reprieve if they would switch from the prison diet to one typical of the villages in which pellagra was prevalent. Because this diet was the most familiar one to many of them anyway, they were willing subjects. After about 5 months, however, these men began to develop the classic symptoms of pellagra: dermatitis, diarrhea, and depression. Those eating the regular prison fare remained healthy. These results fairly well refuted the theory that pellagra was an infectious condition and established the theory that a dietary factor was involved. It took researchers an additional 20 years to identify the nutritional factor.

endemic
Restricted to a certain geographic locale—often used to refer to a nutrient deficiency

Pellagra, first reported in the state of New York in 1875, is the only vitamin deficiency disease that has ever been considered **endemic** to the United States and a major public health problem. Its incidence was fairly well confined to small cotton-mill towns in southern states where the diet was predominantly one of corn, molasses, and salt pork. In 1918, an estimated 10,000 deaths from pellagra and another 100,000 cases of the disease were reported, primarily in cotton-growing areas. At that time, a dietary deficiency was suspected but the lacking nutrient had not yet been identified; therefore the most effective means of controlling the disease was to encourage the increased use of meat and milk products by promoting home production of food.

Efforts to isolate the dietary factor responsible for preventing or curing pellagra were complicated by the fact that many other deficiencies produced similar skin symptoms. Not until 1937 did Elvehjem, at the University of Wisconsin, show that nicotinic acid was effective in curing blacktongue, a condition in dogs similar to human pellagra. The use of nicotinic acid in treating human pellagra brought dramatic results, and the number of pellagra victims in southern hospitals and mental institutions dropped sharply. Several recent reports have indicated that niacin deficiency is still prevalent in some areas, usually associated with alcoholism

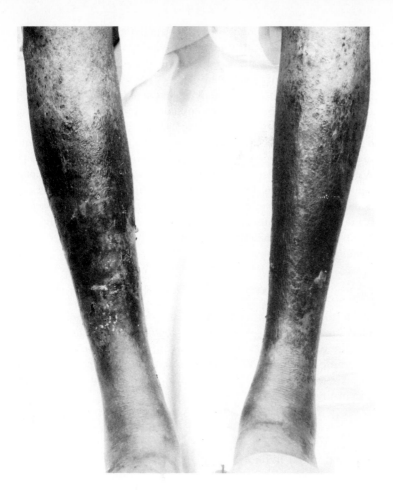

Figure 14-6 Severe dermatitis of the legs in a patient suffering from pellagra. Courtesy Dr. JL Spivak, Johns Hopkins University School of Medicine, 1982.

or an infection of the pancreas. The skin changes associated with a diet inadequate in niacin and protein are depicted in Figure 14-6, the photograph of a patient hospitalized with pellagra.

Pellagra is still found in corn-eating countries such as Romania, Yugoslavia, and some parts of Egypt and in sorghum-eating areas in India. It is not found in Central America, where corn provides 80% of the calories but where alkalis (usually soda lime) used in corn preparation liberate the niacin bound to a protein, making it available for absorption.

The pellagragenic (pellagra-causing) nature of a diet of sorghum has been attributed to the high content of the amino acid leucine. The condition can be corrected by the addition of isoleucine, suggesting that the leucine/isoleucine balance may be an important factor.

Tryptophan/Niacin Relationship

A chemical analysis of foods such as milk that are effective in curing or preventing pellagra shows that they may have a low niacin content. Moreover, diets low in niacin are not always pellagragenic. This apparent discrepancy was explained in 1945 with the discovery that the amino acid tryptophan was also effective in curing pellagra. The role of tryptophan as a precursor of niacin has since been well established through the use of radioactive isotopes, which proved that tryptophan was converted to niacin in the cells. Under most circumstances, 60 mg of tryptophan will yield 1 mg of niacin or one niacin equivalent (NE). Because protein is approximately 1% tryptophan, 60 grams of protein will provide 600 mg of tryptophan,

60 mg tryptophan = 1 mg niacin = 1 niacin equivalent (NE)

Protein is approximately 1% tryptophan

60 grams protein provides 600 mg tryptophan

600 mg tryptophan can be converted to 10 NE

or 10 niacin equivalents. Although current food composition tables record only the preformed niacin content and *not* niacin equivalent values for foods, the sum of the preformed niacin and the niacin equivalent of the tryptophan more accurately reflects the pellagra-preventive value of food.

Dietary requirements are expressed as niacin equivalents, representing preformed niacin plus that obtained from tryptophan. Therefore, a comparison of dietary intake of niacin, based on calculations from tables of food composition with recommended intakes, underestimates the values of the diet in meeting requirements.

The conversion of tryptophan to niacin requires at least three other vitamins—thiamin, pyridoxine, and riboflavin. (Biotin may also be needed.) Because vitamin B_6 (pyridoxine) is involved in the formation of niacin, it has not been surprising to find symptoms of pellagra appearing when a vitamin B_6 antagonist called isonicotinic acid hydrazide (INH, or isoniazid) is used in the treatment of tuberculosis. The conversion of tryptophan to niacin may be more efficient during pregnancy than at any other time.

Chemical Properties

Niacin is stable to heat, light, acid, alkali, and oxidation; in other words, little of the nutrient is lost in normal procedures of food processing and preparation. Although either the acid or the amide form (nicotinamide) of niacin can be used by humans, the amide is preferred for therapeutic doses. A large amount of the acid form acts as a vasodilator, sometimes leading to flushed skin and uncomfortable tingling and burning sensations.

Functions

Niacin-Containing Coenzymes
NAD (nicotinamide adenine dinucleotide)
NADP (nicotinamide adenine dinucleotide phosphate)

Niacin is required by all living cells. Like thiamin and riboflavin, it plays a vital role in the release of energy from all three energy-forming nutrients—carbohydrate, fat, protein, as well as alcohol—and is involved in the synthesis of protein, fat, and the pentoses needed for nucleic acid (DNA) formation. It is part of the coenzymes nicotinamide adenine dinucleotide (NAD), which is involved primarily in catabolic reactions, and nicotinamide adenine dinucleotide phosphate (NADP), which functions in synthetic reactions. Both can accept or release hydrogen atoms readily. Because of this, these coenzymes are effective in assisting a group of enzymes, known as dehydrogenases, in removing hydrogen in many biological reactions. No other biochemical role for niacin has been established yet, but its central role as a part of these coenzymes means that it aids the body in utilizing carbohydrate, fat, protein, and alcohol and in synthesizing fat.

Absorption and Metabolism

Niacin is readily absorbed from the stomach and small intestine. It is converted into the coenzymes in the blood, kidney, liver, and brain and is stored to a limited extent as the coenzymes NAD and NADP. Any excess niacin is excreted in the urine as a methyl derivative. Approximately two thirds of the niacin metabolized by adults may come from tryptophan.

Requirements

$$\text{Niacin equivalent (NE)} = \text{mg of preformed niacin} + \frac{\text{mg of tryptophan}}{60}$$

In establishing an RDA for niacin, a niacin equivalent has been defined as 1 mg of niacin or 60 mg of tryptophan.

Because niacin is crucial in the release of energy from nutrients, it is not surprising to find that the RDA for niacin is based on caloric intake. The minimum amount of niacin needed to prevent pellagra has been established at 4.4 niacin equivalents (NE) per 1000 kcal. A 50% margin of safety to take into account individual variations has been added, resulting in recommended allowances of 6.6 NE/1000 kcal. Regardless of caloric intake, a daily minimum intake of 13 NE is suggested. Recommendations of the FAO and WHO are essentially the same. The British have set their standard about 80% higher, at 11.3 NE/1000 kcal.

On the basis of the amount of niacin and tryptophan in human milk, the recommended intake for infants has been set at 8 NE/1000 kcal. The lack of any firm data on niacin requirements for children from infancy through adolescence has led to the recommendation that an estimated 6.6 mg/1000 kcal and a minimum of 8 NE/day will take care of growth needs.

Although pregnant women are more efficient in converting tryptophan to niacin during the second and third trimesters, an increase of 2 NE of niacin over normal needs is indicated. During breast feeding, when human milk contains about 0.15 mg of preformed niacin and 22 mg of tryptophan/dl (or per 70 kcal), the maternal diet should provide 5 NE more than what is needed under normal circumstances. This will provide the breast-fed infant with 3.5 NE/day, of which two thirds comes from tryptophan. Bottle-fed infants almost always have a higher intake.

Most North American diets are adequate in protein and as a result supply sufficient niacin. Animal protein contains 1.4% tryptophan, and vegetable protein, 1%. Therefore, a diet with 60 grams of protein provides a minimum of 600 mg tryptophan, which can yield 10 mg of niacin. Any tryptophan needed for the synthesis of body protein will not be available for niacin formation; however, whenever 60 mg of tryptophan is available, enough will be used to produce 1 mg of niacin.

Most diets contain 500 to 1000 mg of tryptophan to provide 8 to 14 mg of niacin. An additional 8 to 17 mg of preformed niacin in the diet makes a total of 16 to 33 mg of niacin altogether, an amount sufficient for practically all adult needs. Only when the diet is low in protein and relatively high in a tryptophan-poor cereal (such as corn) is a deficiency likely to occur. Gelatin is one protein that is completely devoid to tryptophan. In general, the niacin equivalent of North American diets is considered to be 50% above the preformed niacin content.

Recommended Dietary Allowances for Niacin (mg NE/day)

Infants	8.0 NE/1000 kcal
Children and adults	6.6 NE/1000 kcal
Children	
1-3 yr	9
4-6 yr	11
7-10 yr	16
Males	
11-18 yr	18
19-22 yr	19
23-50 yr	18
51+ yr	16
Females	
11-14 yr	15
15-22 yr	14
23+ yr	13
Pregnancy	+2
Lactation	+5

Food Sources

The amount of niacin in the most frequently used foods is shown in Table 14-1. Liver, meat, poultry, peanut butter, and legumes are the richest sources. Milk and eggs, although low in preformed niacin, contain high amounts of tryptophan and as such have a high niacin equivalent. Figure 14-7 shows the relative contribution of different food groups to niacin in the food supply. These values are based on niacin content and not niacin equivalents. The vitamin is present in plants as nicotinic acid and in animal foods as nicotinamide.

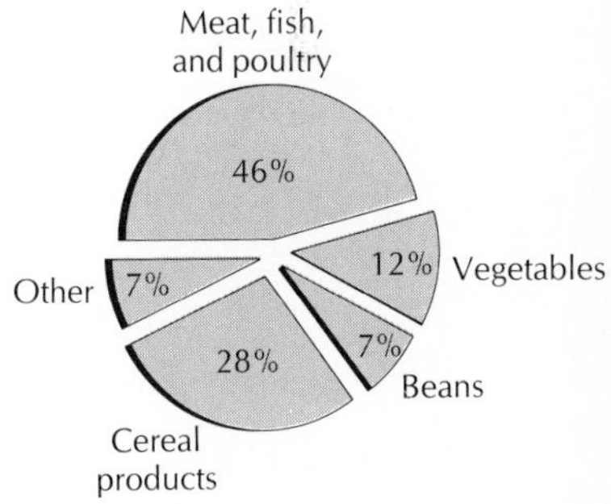

Figure 14-7 Contribution of various food groups to the niacin in the North American food supply, 1987.

Much of the niacin in cereals such as rice and corn occurs as niacinogen, a peptide of at least 17 amino acids. For this reason, the niacin in these foods has low biological value and contributes little to the niacin requirement unless the food is prepared with alkali, as in the preparation of corn tortillas. In wheat bran, niacin occurs as niacytin, which is usually not available at all and is excreted in the urine.

As much as 90% of the niacin in cereals is in the outer husk and is removed in the milling process. The addition of niacin in enriched cereal products has done much to compensate for this loss at a very low cost.

Dietary Adequacy

The adequacy of the niacin intake in the North American diet as reported in CSFII is shown in Figure 14-8. It is similar to data from the NRCS (1977-1978), which showed that two thirds of the 38,000 subjects surveyed had intakes of preformed niacin in excess of 100% of the RDA; 91% had intakes over 70% of the RDA. There were no differences that could be attributed to age, sex, race, income, region,

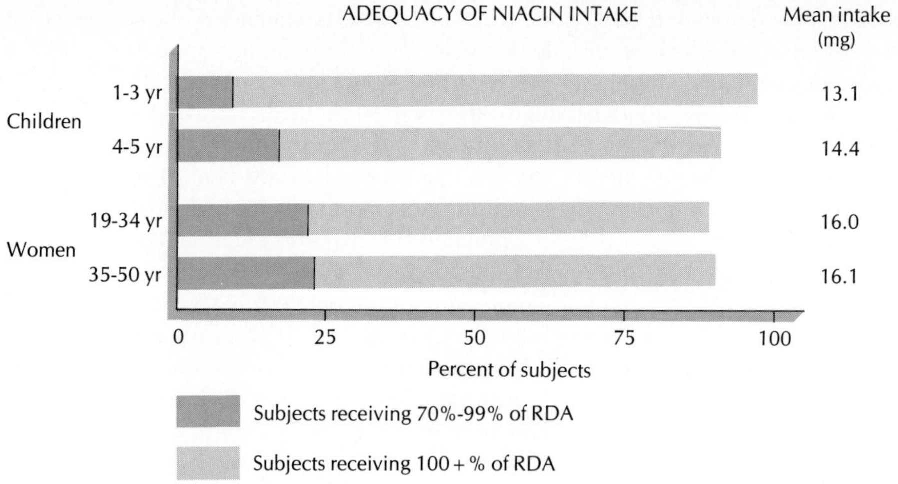

Figure 14-8 Adequacy of niacin intake in the United States.
Based on data from the 1977-1978 NFCS and CSFII 1985-1986.

or degree of urbanization. Because over 90% of the population had more than recommended amounts of protein, which serves as a source of tryptophan for the synthesis of additional niacin, there is little reason for concern about the adequacy of niacin in the North American diet. Mean intakes at all ages were over 100% of the RDA but fell below that level when calorie intakes were less than 70% of recommended levels, which occurred in about one third of the group. Similar data from the 20,000 people examined in two NHANES studies (1971 to 1974 and 1977 to 1979) show both mean and median intakes of preformed niacin in excess of their standard: 6.6 mg/1000 kcal.

Evaluation of Nutritional Status

Because little niacin is stored when the dietary intake is adequate, a large percentage of a test dose is excreted. If dietary intake has been low, less of the test dose is excreted, indicating that the body needs to retain more. Methyl nicotinamide appears in the urine at the time clinical signs of pellagra develop.

Deficiency

Four Ds of Pellagra
Dermatitis
Diarrhea
Depression
Death

Pellagra affects the skin, gastrointestinal tract, and central nervous system. The symptoms, sometimes called the four Ds of pellagra, are dermatitis, diarrhea, depression, and eventually death. The dermatitis of pellagra is often complicated by symptoms of other B-vitamin deficiencies. However, when a niacin deficiency occurs, there is a characteristic skin inflammation that appears almost exclusively on areas of the skin exposed to sunlight and in a symmetrical pattern on both sides of the body. A clearly marked line differentiates afflicted from healthy skin areas.

As the mucous linings of the gastrointestinal tract become affected, the patient suffers from diarrhea and other signs of infection. The irritability, headaches, and sleeplessness of early stages are soon followed by more severe mental symptoms such as loss of memory, hallucinations, delusions of persecution, and finally a severe depression that almost inevitably is followed by death.

Megavitamin Therapy

Large doses of niacin have been used in attempts to reduce blood cholesterol levels, which is a known risk factor in coronary heart disease, and to treat schizophrenia.

Under strict medical supervision, doses of 1 to 2 grams of niacin (not nicotinamide) three times a day may result in lowered blood cholesterol levels and may be beneficial in protecting against recurrent nonfatal heart attacks.

Table 14-2 ◇ Relevant biological and dietary data for thiamin, riboflavin, and niacin

	Thiamin	Riboflavin	Niacin
U.S. RDA	1.5 mg	1.7 mg	20 mg
Amount available in daily food supply	2.2 mg	2.4 mg	27 mg
Average intake			
NHANES II	1.30 mg	1.90 mg	16.7 mg
NFCS CSFII, women and children	113% RDA	132% RDA	124% RDA
Major food sources			
Grain products	43%	23%	28%
Meat, fish, poultry	26%	22%	46%
Fruits and vegetables	16%	—	16%
Dairy products	9%	37%	—
Total amount in body	30-70 mg		
Distribution in body tissues			
Heart	2.3 μg/g		
Brain, liver, kidneys	1 μg/g	25 μg (liver) 16 μg (kidney)	
Muscle	50%	2-3 μg/g	
Indicators of normal nutritional status			
Normal urinary excretion/gram of creatinine	>0.06 mg	>.08 mg	>1.6 mg of N-methyl nicotinamide
Enzyme (stimulation)	<15% transketolase	<1.2% glutathione reductase	

Blanks indicate not applicable or no information available.

In treating psychiatric problems, not only niacin but also other vitamins have been used in extremely large amounts, in what is known as **orthomolecular therapy.** The use of large doses of niacin (4 to 5 grams/day) in the treatment of schizophrenia is controversial. At the moment, the bulk of the evidence seems to question its value, and little scientific evidence supports its effectiveness.

orthomolecular therapy Treatment of disease with very large doses of vitamins

The use of nicotinic acid, the acid form, in single oral doses of 50 mg or more leads to severe flushing of the skin in a time period of from a few minutes to half an hour, with symptoms persisting up to 1½ hours. Some people report that the symptoms are merely inconvenient, whereas others are unable to continue the use of high doses. In addition to the flushing reaction of the skin, other symptoms such as gastrointestinal distress, unusual nervousness, recurring ulcers, increased uric acid excretion, and glucose intolerance are frequently reported. Intakes of as high as 3 to 9 grams of the nicotinamide form have none of these adverse effects, however.

Relevant biological data for thiamin, riboflavin, and niacin are included in Table 14-2.

PANTOTHENIC ACID

Discovery

Pantothenic acid, identified first as vitamin B_5, was so named to designate its widespread occurrence in foods (*pantos* means "everywhere"). Similarly, in its central role as a part of coenzyme A, its role in the metabolism of carbohydrate, fat, and protein has been recognized. Additionally, it functions in the synthesis of many hormones, neurotransmitters, and other essential body compounds. A second pantothenic acid coenzyme—acyl carrier protein (ACP)—has recently been identified.

Before it was finally isolated in 1939 and chemically identified in 1940, pantothenate had been known to be a growth factor in yeast and to be effective in the cure or prevention of dermatitis in chicks and the graying of hair in rats. A yellow, viscous oil, pantothenic acid has never been crystallized, although its synthetic calcium salt (calcium pantothenate) has been available in crystalline form for some time. It is in the form of calcium pantothenate that pantothenic acid is incorporated into most nutrition supplements. It is important to note that the amount of calcium in calcium pantothenate is so small that its presence in a supplement makes no contribution to calcium needs. The alcohol form of pantothenic acid, pantothenol, is used in cosmetics.

Chemical Properties

Pantothenic acid is a water-soluble vitamin that is stable in moist heat in neutral solution but is relatively unstable in dry heat, acid, or alkali. There is little loss in cooking at normal temperatures.

Chemically, pantothenic acid is a relatively simple compound containing the nonessential amino acid alanine and pantoic acid. Before pantothenic acid participates in biological reactions, it adds in succession a sulfur-containing compound, phosphate, and adenosine to form coenzyme A (also called CoA). Coenzyme A is the form in which most pantothenic acid is found in animal tissues and in which it plays a central role in most biological reactions. The activation of CoA involves the addition of acetate to form acetyl-coenzyme A, or acetyl-CoA. The acetate molecules, which come directly from the metabolism of either carbohydrate or fat and indirectly from protein, are readily accepted by and released from the CoA molecule.

The relationship between pantothenic acid and activated CoA is shown in Figure 14-9.

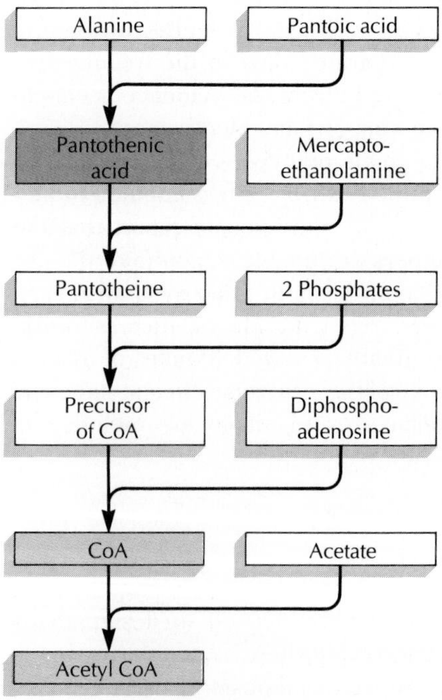

Figure 14-9 Relationship between pantothenic acid and CoA.

Because CoA appears within the cell but not in the blood, it must be synthesized within the cell and can pass out through the cell membrane only with difficulty, if at all. In red blood cells, CoA exists bound to a protein. It appears in highest concentration in the liver, adrenal glands, kidneys, brain, and heart, all of which are tissues with high metabolic activity.

Functions

As part of CoA, pantothenic acid participates in the release of energy from all three major energy-yielding nutrients—carbohydrate, fat and protein. Products formed during the metabolism of each of these nutrients eventually react with CoA in the Krebs cycle before their energy can be released. In addition, CoA—and therefore pantothenic acid—is necessary for the synthesis of fat. Besides functioning in the transfer of acetate groups to the Krebs cycle, CoA is involved as a source or acceptor of acetate groups, as in the formation of acetylcholine, which is needed in the transmission of nerve impulses.

CoA is also essential for the formation of porphyrin (a part of the hemoglobin molecule), for the stimulation of antibody responses, and for the synthesis of cholesterol and some of the hormones produced by the adrenal glands. In essence, because of its central role in energy metabolism, CoA can be considered vital to all energy-requiring processes within the body. It is indeed fortunate that pantothenic acid is present in almost all foods.

Requirements

It is well established that human beings, as well as practically all other animals and microorganisms, need pantothenic acid. The amount needed has not been estimated with any certainty. A 3000-kcal diet will usually provide form 13 to 19 mg of total pantothenic acid. Of this amount, from 2 to 7 mg/day is excreted in the urine and 1 to 2 mg in the feces, suggesting that from 4 to 10 mg is retained. The wide range of intakes, blood values, and urinary excretion levels that appear in people who have no evidence of deficiency makes it difficult to determine a minimum requirement. The estimated safe and adequate daily intake is 4 to 7 mg. Even during periods of stress, when needs may be relatively high, most diets will provide adequate amounts of pantothenic acid.

Estimated Safe and Adequate Daily Dietary Intakes of Pantothenic Acid (mg/day)

Infants	2-3
Children and adolescents	3-7
Adults	4-7

Food Sources

Pantothenic acid is a component of all living matter. Although organ meats, most fish, and whole-grain cereals are the richest sources, all food groups make a contribution. The richest sources found so far are royal jelly (from queen bees) and fish ovaries prior to spawning—doubtful items in the diet but great for health food promotors!

Of 507 foods analyzed for pantothenic acid content, 47% had over 5 ppm, a level that should provide an overall dietary intake of 5 to 10 mg daily.

Foods processed in dry heat are relatively poor sources. In canning, up to one third of pantothenic acid is lost from animal foods and three fourths from vegetable foods. About 50% is lost in the refining of wheat. Human milk contains 2 mg of pantothenic acid/dl, slightly more than half the amount found in cow's milk.

Deficiency

The wide variety of reactions for which pantothenic acid is necessary is paralleled by an equally wide variety of deficiency symptoms in many tissues. Low intakes may slow down many metabolic processes, resulting in many subclinical symptoms. The symptoms probably reflect the impaired health of cells in many tissues. Lowered resistance to infection is well documented, and higher intakes seem to improve the ability to withstand stress.

Pantothenic acid neither prevents nor cures the graying of hair in human beings, despite any claims to the contrary by promoters of food supplements.

Clinical Uses

Pantothenic acid in the form of its calcium salt has been used successfully in treating paralysis of the gastrointestinal tract after surgery, which causes the accumulation of gas and severe abdominal pain. It appears to stimulate gastrointestinal motility; however, high levels (from 10 to 20 grams) cause diarrhea.

BIOTIN

Discovery

Recognition of biotin as a dietary essential occurred in 1924, when it was identified as "bios II," one of three factors necessary for the growth of microorganisms. Between then and 1943, when it was synthesized, scientists tried to learn the nature of bios II and two other substances that they had named vitamin H and coenzyme R. As soon as the chemical nature of the sulfur-containing bios II was determined, it became clear (as it often does in the study of nutrients) that all three were the same substance. Identified as biotin, it is now considered as essential water-soluble vitamin.

Symptoms of biotin deficiency occur in human beings and some animals only after the ingestion of a diet that is low in biotin and includes many raw egg whites. Raw egg white has a carbohydrate-containing protein, avidin, that binds biotin in a complex too big to be absorbed and unaffected by digestive enzymes. Thirty percent of the dietary calories must come from raw egg white (about 2 dozen) to induce a biotin deficiency; thus it is obvious that the ingestion of an occasional raw egg white is no cause for concern. Cooking denatures, or changes, avidin so that it no longer has the ability to bind biotin.

Chemical Properties

Although biotin has been isolated in at least eight active forms from food, d-biotin is the most active. Other forms are biocytin, a combination of biotin and the essential amino acid lysine; biotin sulfone, a potent antagonist; and biotinal, which forms the active oxybiotin. In animal tissues, the protein-bound biotin is fat soluble, whereas the free biotin found in plants and excreted in the urine is water soluble. Biotin is stable in heat but unstable in alkali and oxidation; some is lost in cooking water.

Functions

At least four enzymes, primarily carboxylases, involved in the transfer of carbon dioxide, are dependent on biotin. Since carboxylation is common in nature, biotin plays a part in many reactions including the synthesis and oxidation of fatty acids and glucose. Other functions of biotin include roles in the metabolism of at least three amino acids; the synthesis of nicotinic acid, purines, and prostaglandins and the digestive enzyme pancreatic amylase; and antibody formation.

Requirements

In 1980, for the first time, the revision of the RDA included recommendations on dietary intakes of biotin. These were based on studies of usual biotin intakes and on fecal and urinary excretions of the nutrient. Although there is evidence that intestinal synthesis of biotin makes some contribution to the body's supply, it is not clear how much of that biotin is absorbed. There is no evidence of a biotin deficiency in the U.S. population, which consumes an average of 30 to 45 μg/day via self-selected diets. Blood levels are high but urinary excretion is below normal. Therefore, intakes in this range are apparently adequate. It is assumed that about half of the dietary intake of biotin is absorbed.

Infants consuming human milk with 4 μg of biotin/1000 kcal or formulas with 15 μg/1000 kcal have shown no evidence of a deficiency. Intakes of 3 to 12 μg of biotin daily, considerably less than the current RDA, are apparently adequate to meet the needs of very young infants.

Estimated Safe and Adequate Daily Dietary Intakes of Biotin (μg/day)

Infants	35-50
Children	65-120
Adolescents and adults	100-200

Food Sources

Biotin is present in almost all foods. Most of it occurs bound to protein, from which it is readily released. The richest food sources for biotin have been found to be liver, kidney, peanut butter, egg yolk, and yeast. Because these foods are often eliminated in low-cholesterol diets, there is concern that, as such diets are used more frequently, we may see an increase in diets low in biotin. Some vegetables such as cauliflower, nuts, and legumes are good sources but all other meats, fruits, diary products, and cereals are considered poor sources. Human milk has 0.10 times the amount of biotin of cow's milk.

Biotin in the diet is supplemented by biotin that is synthesized by bacteria in the intestinal tract; this synthesis is stimulated by a sucrose-containing diet. Antibiotics, including sulfonamides and oxytetracycline, are known to reduce the number of biotin-synthesizing organisms. There is no reason to include biotin in a multivitamin supplement; in particular, there is no evidence that large supplements of biotin relieve feelings of stress or enhance physical performance.

Sources of Biotin
Food
Synthesis within the intestinal tract

A B

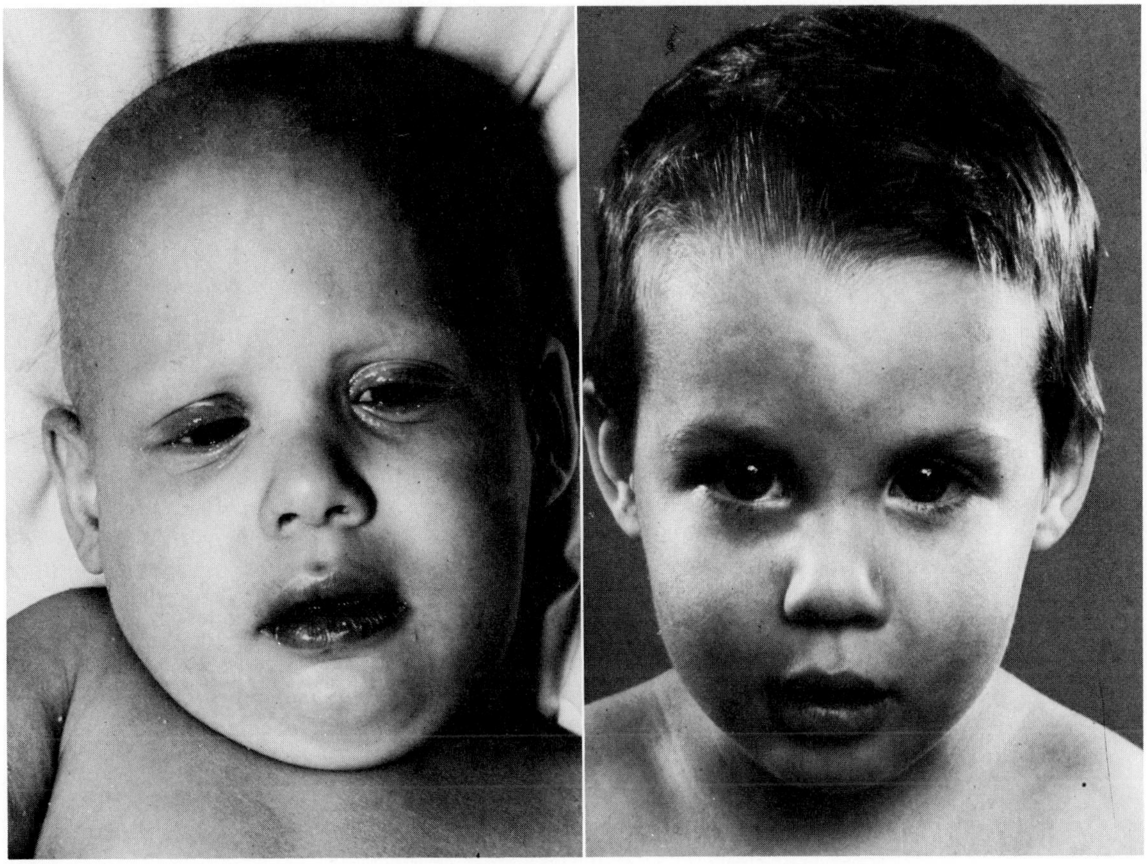

Figure 14-10 A, Infant with biotin deficiency. **B,** Same child after three months of treatment.
From Thoene J, Baker H, Yochino M, and Sweeetman L: Medical Intelligence 304:817, 1981.

TPN (total parenteral nutrition)
Process by which all nutrients, in specially formulated solutions, are provided through the veins rather than by mouth

Biotin Content of Foods (μg/100 grams)

Chicken liver	170-210
Peanut butter	38
Eggs	20-25
Oatmeal	15-30
Wheat germ	22-38
Poultry	10-11
Vegetables	2-4

Deficiency

Biotin deficiency can result from inherited carboxylase deficiency, prolonged use of **TPN**, or a diet very high in avidin from raw egg whites. In a study in which four human subjects became biotin deficient on a diet lacking in biotin and high in avidin, the symptoms observed were similar to those of a thiamin deficiency and included dermatitis, loss of appetite, nausea, mental depression, and glossitis, as well as many other symptoms. Both infants and adults receiving total parenteral nutrition have shown similar symptoms that are alleviated when biotin is added. A life-threatening metabolic defect that results in a failure to synthesize several carboxylase enzymes can be relieved by the use of larger amounts (10 mg) of biotin.

Although a natural biotin deficiency in human adults is not known, two types of dermatitis that occur in infants may be caused by a lack of biotin. Infants with these types of dermatitis respond rather dramatically to large doses (5 to 10 mg) of biotin given orally or by injection. Similar conditions in adults are not responsive. Neonatal biotin deficiency occurs in the first weeks of life; the juvenile form occurs after 2 to 3 months. A baby with a typical case of biotin deficiency is shown in Figure 14-10, both before and after treatment. Clinical problems related to biotin may be more common than previously recognized.

OTHER VITAMIN-LIKE SUBSTANCES

With the sustained and growing interest in nutrition among all segments of the population, it is not surprising that many claims have been made for vitamin-like substances. As a result, there is a lot of confusion about whether certain components of food are essential, helpful, harmless, or harmful. The six substances discussed in the following pages are among the many vitamin-like substances that come and go in popularity. They are part of a group that has some properties of vitamins but fails to meet all the criteria to be classed as vitamins. Some are present in larger amounts than vitamins. Some can be synthesized in sufficient amounts to meet needs for most people. It has been impossible to determine any essential biological role for some of them, even though they appear in the diet and in body tissues.

It is possible that, in the future, some of these vitamin-like substances will be established definitely as vitamins, whereas others will definitely be dropped from that classification.

Myoinositol

Myoinositol—also known as muscle sugar, inositol, and mesoinositol—is one of a group of six-carbon compounds closely related in chemical composition to the monosaccharide glucose. It was first recognized in 1928 as a growth-promoting factor for yeast and as a cure for alopecia, or loss of hair, in mice.

Myoinositol is present in practically all plant and animal tissues in concentrations higher than those normally associated with vitamins. In animal cells, it occurs primarily as a phospholipid that is sometimes referred to as lipositol. In grains, it is present as the more complex water-soluble compound phytic acid (inositol hexaphosphate), which is the organic acid found in husks of grains that binds calcium, zinc, and iron and decreases their absorption. In soybeans, myoinositol is in a free form. Apparently, sharks and certain other fish store carbohydrate as inositol rather than as glycogen.

Fruits, meat, milk, nuts, vegetables, and whole-grain cereals are the best food sources of myoinositol. Phytic acid is a major source.

The biological significance of myoinositol in human nutrition is unknown, although it is widely distributed throughout the body, especially in heart, brain, and skeletal muscle. Although it has been found essential for the growth of liver and bone marrow cells and helps to prevent fatty livers, a specific role for this substance has not been clearly established.

People apparently consume about 1 gram of myoinositol in food each day. In addition, we are able to use glucose within individual cells to synthesize enough myoinositol to meet our needs. The amount excreted in the urine is small and variable, ranging from 8 to 144 mg/day, although diabetics excrete much more.

Choline

Choline was identified in 1937 as a dietary factor that prevented the accumulation of fat in the liver of dogs. Since then, we have learned that choline is effective because of the presence of three methyl (CH_3) groups. As a methyl donor, choline transfers these groups to other biological compounds in a wide variety of biological reactions. Choline can be readily synthesized from the nonessential amino acid serine, provided another source of the methyl groups is available and vitamin B_6 is available to catalyze the reaction. The methyl groups are provided by another amino acid, methionine. They can be synthesized in the presence of adequate folacin or cobalamin. It appears that humans are not solely dependent on a dietary source of either choline or its direct precursor.

Even though choline is part of the chemical acetylcholine that is needed to send messages from one nerve cell to another, there is no evidence that choline will reverse or prevent memory loss in healthy people.

Choline occurs as a constituent of the phospholipid **lecithin** (phospatidyl choline), which facilitates the transportation of lipid in the blood. In bile it acts as an emulsifier. It is part of the cell membrane and is especially important in nerve cell membranes as part of a phospholipid called sphingomyelin. It does not catalyze any reactions or act as part of a coenzyme. Choline does, however, react with acetyl CoA to form acetylcholine, which is responsible for transmitting nerve impulses from one nerve ending to the next. It is also essential for normal lung development in the last trimester of pregnancy.

lecithin
A phospholipid that contains choline; it is found in eggs

For more on lecithin, see Chapter 5.

Choline is widely distributed in food, with eggs, liver, peanuts and fish as major sources. It is present in relatively large amounts in all foods that contain fat. Fruits and vegetables contain virtually no choline. The average North American diet provides from 500 to 900 mg/day. Most people's need for dietary choline is either small or nonexistent.

Choline Content of Foods (grams/100 grams)

Egg yolk	1.7
Beef liver	0.6
Soybeans	0.2
Fish	0.2
Cereal	0.1

Choline is not associated with any specific deficiency disease in most people. It does, however, exert a protective action against cirrhosis of the liver among alcoholics and is being used to stimulate the synthesis of the neurotransmitter acetylcholine. Reports of its effectiveness in lowering blood pressure and blood cholesterol have not been verified. Intakes of up to 5 grams choline chloride or 15 grams lecithin can safely be used. Dietary choline is not essential for the adult, but it may be for the young infant.

Coenzyme Q (Ubiquinone)

Coenzyme Q is a lipidlike substance that is somewhat similar in its chemical makeup to both vitamins K and E. It belongs to a group of compounds known as ubiquinones. The forms that appear to be biologically important have long carbon side chains containing anywhere from 30 to 50 carbon atoms.

Coenzyme Q is found in practically all living cells and appears to be concentrated in the mitochondria. There, it functions in the respiratory chain, in which energy is released from energy-yielding nutrients as the high-energy compound adenosine triphosphate. Coenzyme Q is easily, and reversibly, oxidized and reduced. Without this substance, incomplete release of energy would be anticipated.

It is probable that ubiquinones can be synthesized readily, with niacin, folacin, vitamin B_{12}, pyridoxine, and pantothenic acid all playing roles in their synthesis.

Coenzyme Q-type compounds are found in soybeans, vegetable oils, and a great variety of animal tissues.

Lipoic Acid

Lipoic acid, which has been isolated from liver and yeast, is essential for the growth of several microorganisms, although it has not yet been shown that people or other mammals require a dietary source. Lipoic acid does participate in biochemical reactions, but the amounts needed to meet these needs are probably synthesized in the body.

Lipoic acid is now identified in five distinct forms. One form, which is bound to protein, has also been called factor 11. Other forms include factor 11A, the pyruvic oxidation factor, thioctic acid, and protogen. Lipoic acid (the official name) and thioctic acid, which indicates the sulfur *(thio-)* found in the molecule, are the names most frequently used at this time. Fat-soluble lipoic acid can be reversibly oxidized to the water-soluble β-lipoic acid.

Lipoic acid is essential, along with a thiamin-containing coenzyme, for the reactions in carbohydrate metabolism that convert pyruvic acid to acetyl-CoA. In plant cells, lipoic acid may be necessary for some of the reactions of photosynthesis, the process by which plants synthesize carbohydrate.

Carnitine

Carnitine is an essential substance that is needed to transport long-chain fatty acids into the cell mitochondrion where they are metabolized to provide energy. Normally, carnitine is synthesized in the liver and kidneys from the essential amino acids lysine and methionine in reactions that require iron. In the absence of carnitine, triglycerides accumulate in the blood. Some people are unable to synthesize carnitine; as a result, several reports of carnitine deficiency have been made since a human deficiency was first recognized in 1973. Carnitine's role in the metabolism of fatty acids makes it essential for survival and development in young infants.

Meat (especially dark red meat) and dairy products are the major sources of carnitine in the North American diet, with most diets providing about 100 mg (with ranges of from 2 to 300 mg). Vegetarians have very low intakes. Carnitine is considered a dietary essential for bottle-fed infants but is provided in adequate amounts in breast milk.

After finding that D-L carnitine supplements are not only useless but also cause changes in heart and skeletal muscle, the FDA has ruled that D-carnitine may not be used. L-Carnitine, which is a useful form, is more expensive. It is the only supplement form of carnitine that should be used, and then only under strict medical supervision.

Taurine

Taurine is unique as an amino acid because it occurs free, not as part of a peptide, and because it has a somewhat different chemical structure than most amino acids. It accounts for 10% of the sulfur in the body and plays a major role in cardiovascular and central nervous system regulation. As a component of bile acids, it maintains membrane stability. It is widely distributed in the tissues of mammals and is present in especially high concentrations in heart, brain, and muscle. An absence of taurine leads to specific deficiency symptoms. The fact that human milk contains a relatively high amount suggests that it may have a function in the developmental process, particularly central nervous system growth. Taurine is present in large amounts (30 to 70 mg) in meat and fish, but almost absent in fruit, vegetables, and grains.

BY NOW YOU SHOULD KNOW

- Thiamin, riboflavin, niacin, pantothenic acid, and biotin are essential parts of the coenzymes necessary for the cell to release energy from carbohydrate, lipid, protein, and alcohol.
- The RDAs for thiamin, riboflavin, and niacin are based on caloric intake.
- The classical thiamin deficiency is known as beriberi. The classical niacin deficiency is known as pellagra.
- Although the severe deficiency diseases beriberi and pellagra are seldom found any more, many people do suffer from marginal deficiencies that may show up as symptoms when they experience physical and emotional stress.
- These B vitamins can be obtained in adequate amounts in the North American diet, particularly in cereals, meat, and milk.
- Thiamin, riboflavin, and niacin are added to cereal and grain products.
- Sixty milligrams of the essential amino acid tryptophan can be converted to 1 mg of niacin.
- Other substances such as myoinositol, carnitine, and taurine are essential for body functioning, but are needed in larger amounts than vitamins.
- Many other substances are being promoted as having vitamin-like properties.
- Some of these other substances have no effect, others have some physiological effects but are not essential, and others are useful at low levels but may have druglike effects at high levels. Still others are fraudulently represented; fortunately, most of these are harmless.

STUDY QUESTIONS

1. Under what circumstances or in what groups of people would you expect deficiencies of each of the water-soluble vitamins to show up?
2. Which of the water-soluble vitamins are sensitive to heat, light, alkali, acid, and oxidation?
3. What parts have inadequate intakes of the water-soluble vitamins played in the nutrition history of this country? of the world?
4. Why are the requirements of some vitamins related to energy intake and others to protein intake?
5. List the three most important food sources of each of the water-soluble vitamins in the North American diet.
6. Plan meals for a lactose-intolerant adult female, making sure to meet the RDA for riboflavin.

Applying What You've Learned

1. **Evaluate the Contribution of Water-Soluble Vitamins to Your Diet**

   Use the diet records you completed in previous chapters to see which foods made the best contributions to each of the water-soluble vitamins in your diet.

2. **Plan Adjustments in the Vitamins You Ingest**

   If your intake was low for any one vitamin, how would you adjust your diet to make it more adequate?

3. **Calculate Your Average Caloric Intake for Several Days**

   Determine your thiamin (0.5 mg/1000 kcal), riboflavin (0.6 mg/1000 kcal), and niacin (6.6 NE/1000 kcal) need based on those calories. Is this need greater than, less than, or about equal to your RDA for these vitamins?

4. **Read the List of Ingredients on Cereal Box and Bread Labels**

   Do you find the products enriched with thiamin, riboflavin, and niacin? In what form are they added?

5. **Storage and Preparation of Food**

   List the precautions you take in the storage and preparation of food to minimize the losses of thiamin, riboflavin, niacin, and pantothenic acid.

6. **Select Three Multivitamin Supplements**

   Compare the amount of the water-soluble vitamin provided in each. Did the price reflect the difference in potency?

SUGGESTED READING

Machlin LJ: Handbook of vitamins, New York, 1985, Marcel Dekker Inc.

This book pulls together in one volume a summary of the most recent information about 13 vitamins, as well as several other substances that behave in a vitamin-like way in the body. Each chapter is authored by the foremost authority on a particular nutrient. Much of the material is too technical for casual reading; however, the book provides perhaps the best source available for answers to questions ranging from need and function of vitamins to source and availability of nutrients in the diet.

ADDITIONAL READINGS

Thiamin

Dong MH, and others: Thiamin, riboflavin, and vitamin B_6 contents of selected foods as served, Journal of the American Dietetic Association 76:156, 1980.

Hilker DM, and Somogi JC: Antithiamins of plant origin: their chemical nature and mode of action, Annals of the New York Academy of Sciences 378:137, 1982.

Tandhaichitir V, and Wood B: Thiamin. In Present Knowledge of Nutrition, ed. 5, Washington, D.C., 1984, Nutrition Foundation, Inc.

Riboflavin

Belko AZ, Obarzanek E, Kalkwarf HJ, Rotter MA, Bogusz S, Miller D, Haas JD, and Roe DA: Effects of exercise on riboflavin requirements of young women, American Journal of Clinical Nutrition 37:509, 1983.

Lopez R, Schwartz JV, and Cooperman JM: Riboflavin deficiency in an adolescent population in New York City, American Journal of Clinical Nutrition 33:1283, 1980.

Roe D, Kalkwarf H, and Stevens J: Effect of fiber supplements on the apparent absorption of pharmacological doses of riboflavin, Journal of the American Dietetic Association 88:211, 1988.

Rivlin RS: Riboflavin. In Present Knowledge of Nutrition, ed. 5, Washington, D.C., 1984, Nutrition Foundation, Inc.

Niacin

Carte EGA, and Carpenter EJ: The bioavailability for humans of bound niacin from wheat bran, American Journal of Clinical Nutrition 36:855, 1982.

Horwitt MK, Harper AE, and Henderson LM: Niacin-tryptophan relationships for evaluating niacin equivalents, American Journal of Clinical Nutrition 34:423, 1981.

Rao BSN, and Gopolan C: Niacin. In Present Knowledge of Nutrition, ed. 5, Washington, D.C., 1984, Nutrition Foundation, Inc.

Pantothenic Acid

Fry PC, Fox HM, and Tao HG: Metabolic response to a pantothenic-deficient diet in humans, 22:339, 1976.

Olson RE: Pantothenic acid. In Present knowledge of nutrition, ed. 5, Washington, D.C., 1984, Nutrition Foundation, Inc.

Song WO, Chan GM, Wyse BW, and Hansen RG: Effects of pantothenic acid status on the content of the vitamins in human milk, American Journal of Clinical Nutrition 40:317, 1984.

Biotin

Marshall M: The nutritional importance of biotin, Nutrition Today 22:26, 1987.

McCormick DB, and Olson RE: Biotin. In Present knowledge of nutrition, Washington, D.C., 1984, Nutrition Foundation, Inc.

Other Nutrient Factors

Borum PR: Carnitine—Who needs it? Nutrition Today 21(6):4, 1986.

Borum PR: Carnitine, Annual Review of Nutrition 3:233, 1983.

Carroll JE, Carter AL, and Perlman S: Carnitine deficiency revisited, Journal of Nutrition 117:1501, 1987.

Chesney RW: Taurine: is it required for infants? Journal of Nutrition 118:6, 1988.

Feller AG, and Rudman D: Role of carnitine in human nutrition, Journal of Nutrition 118:541, 1988.

Jarvis WT: Food faddism, cultism and quackery, Annual Review of Nutrition 3:35, 1983.

McMahon K: Choline, an essential nutrient? Nutrition Today 22:18, 1987.

Picone TA: Taurine update: metabolism and function, Nutrition Today 22:16, 1987.

Zeisel SH: Dietary choline, Annual Review of Nutrition 1:95, 1981.

FOCUS Nutrients and Nonnutrients—A Nutrition Puzzle

Because of the increasing concern over nutrition questions and the eternal hope of some people that they can find a panacea for health problems, claims and counterclaims are being made for substances that are reported to be nutrients. As might be expected, this can sometimes lead to great confusion for the public. Because the list is constantly changing, it is impossible to guess which nutrients are likely to be popular next year—let alone 10 years from now.

The nutrients that have been selected for this Focus section are the bioflavonoids, laetrile, pangamic acid, spirulina, and caffeine and its related compounds. They are examples of the types of nutrients that appear and reappear in the popular literature; however, their popularity has persisted a little longer than many others. In general, it is best to be skeptical about substances that are advertised to the public before they are presented in the scientific literature and for which exaggerated claims are made.

The bioflavonoids, hesperidin and rutin, were first suggested as dietary factors in 1936, when it was found that substances in extracts of both red pepper and lemon increased the antiscorbutic (anti-scurvy) effect of vitamin C. For awhile these substances, of which hesperidin and rutin were the most common, were designated as vitamin P. They were also believed to reduce capillary bleeding. However, we now know that they do not enhance the utilization of synthetic vitamin C, although it is agreed that in large doses they may have some pharmacological effects. In fact, we know of no clinical usefulness for these compounds, which have been advocated at various times in the treatment of a wide range of unrelated conditions. There is also no evidence of a dietary need for bioflavonoids; certainly, their inclusion in nutritional supplements is not justified. Several bioflavonoids are being investigated as possible low-calorie sweetening agents, however.

Laetrile, also known as vitamin B_{17}, is a cyanide-containing, potentially toxic substance. It was first promoted in 1952 and belongs to a group of chemicals called the amygdalin group. Laetrile is derived from the pits of apricots, peaches, and bitter almonds and from apple seeds. It has been widely promoted as a substance that prevents and cures cancer. Because there is absolutely no evidence of laetrile's effectiveness, the FDA has prohibited its promotion as a cancer-curing drug. Laetrile's promoters have tried to circumvent this restriction by offering it for sale as a food under such names as "bitter food tablets" or "Seventeen" and by not making claims for its role in cancer therapy. Despite arguments that patients should have freedom of choice in treatment, the sale of laetrile has been legalized in only 16 states, and it still cannot be sold through interstate trade or in Canada. Those promoting laetrile claim either that the substance seeks out cancer cells and releases hydrocyanic acid, which in turn kills the cells, or that cancer is caused by a deficiency of vitamin B_{17}. Currently, there is no scientific evidence that laetrile is either a vitamin or a cancer cure or that it plays any positive role in known metabolic functions.

Pangamic acid was introduced to the public as vitamin B_{15} in 1978. Its promoters claim that it is helpful in alleviating such diverse problems as indigestion, alcoholism, hepatitis, heart disease, and schizophrenia. Although pangamic acid was patented in 1949, there is no scientific evidence that it has any physiological functions or that a lack of it results in adverse effects.

Pangamic acid is being marketed in the United States under a wide range of names and in a great variety

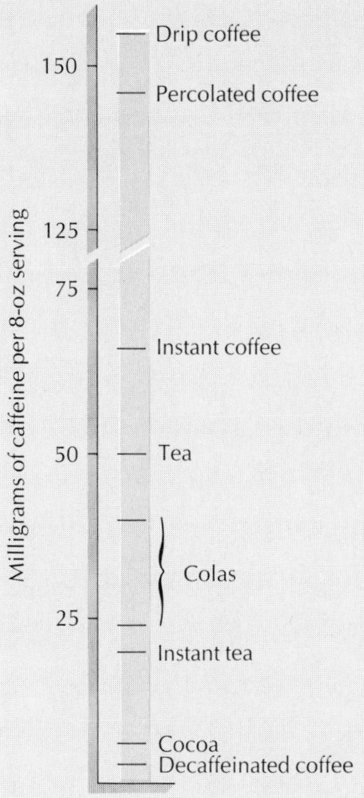

Caffeine content of various beverages

of forms. Although the majority of products that contain pangamic acid also contain calcium gluconate and a derivative of the amino acid glycine, the FDA has ruled that they are unidentifiable substances. The Canadian government has concluded that there is no proof that pangamic acid has any therapeutic benefit. Therefore its sale in Canada has also been prohibited.

In the absence of anything but anecdotal evidence, pangamic acid is considered nutritionally worthless and deceptively labeled as a vitamin.

In 1981, a new entry in the field of "miracle nutrients" was spirulina. It is now being promoted as a rich protein source. Derived from microorganisms, it is indeed mostly protein and provides a reasonable balance of amino acids. However, the few milligrams that constitute one dose are hardly significant, especially at a price of \$3.20 for 20 grams of protein—an amount provided in one serving of meat or three eggs. Spirulina is not really necessary because protein can be gotten from foods at a fraction of the cost, and with palatability and other nutrients as a bonus.

Caffeine, a methylxanthine, is a component of tea, coffee, and cocoa—common dietary items. It has been alleged to play a role in cancer, cardiovascular disease, and birth defects. It has no nutritional significance. However, caffeine does have physiological significance and is considered one of the most widely used drugs. With 80% of the adult population consuming caffeine, it is very appropriate to discuss it as a dietary component. The caffeine content of common beverages ranges from 6 to 85 mg/serving. The mean consumption in the United States is estimated at 2.6 mg of caffeine/kg of body weight, or 150 to 200 mg/day. About 60% comes from coffee, 30% from tea, and 10% from cola beverages, chocolate, and medications. Canadian authorities estimate an intake of 450 mg/day.

In addition to its well-known role as a central nervous system stimulant, caffeine acts as a diuretic, increasing urine production; relaxes smooth muscles; and stimulates the heart muscle and gastric acid secretion. It also increases oxygen consumption and free fatty acid and glucose levels in plasma. Caffeine apparently also has a depressing effect on iron absorption. It is absorbed completely and quickly and is distributed in the water component of various tissues; it is excreted in the form of xanthines and uric acid 3 to 6 hours after ingestion. Intakes of 65 to 130 mg of caffeine have beneficial effects on motor and mental performance, whereas intakes of 400 mg cause insomnia and poor performance.

Two caffeine-related compounds are theophylline and theobromine. Theophylline is found in tea and is also a central nervous system stimulant; theobromine is found in cocoa. Neither has any nutritional merit.

At this time, there is no conclusive evidence confirming a relationship between health and caffeine consumption. Pregnant women are advised to use it in moderation, however.

PART II

Applied Nutrition

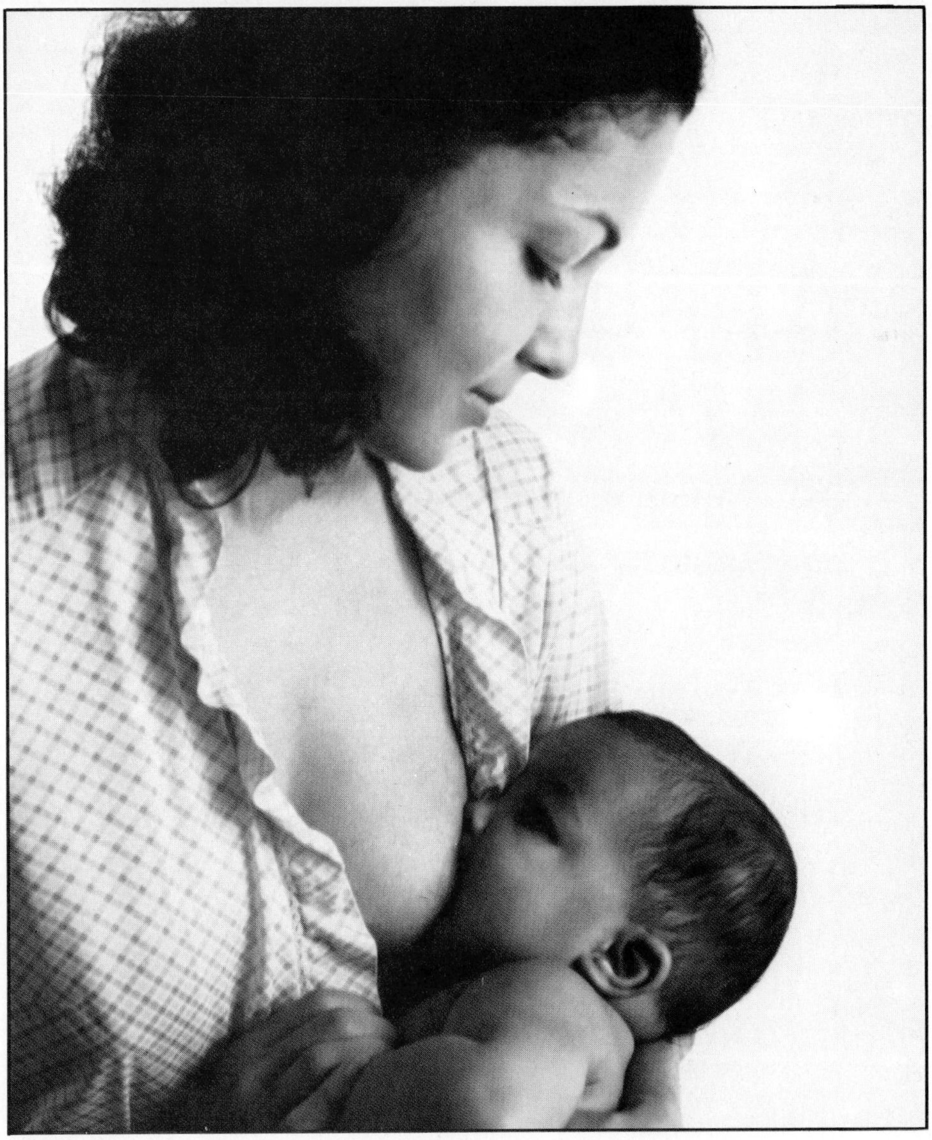

AWARENESS CHECK

Truth or Fiction?

- Nutritional needs of the pregnant teen are higher than those of a woman in her 20s or 30s.
- Because the risk of degenerative diseases is greater among the obese it is recommended that pregnant women restrict weight gain.
- During pregnancy, a woman should restrict her intake of sodium.
- The zinc status of the pregnant woman can be adversely affected by excessive supplementation of iron and folate.
- A woman needs more calories when breast feeding than during pregnancy.
- Almost all drugs taken by a mother during lactation appear to some extent in her milk.

Nutrition in Pregnancy and Lactation

CHAPTER 15

Adequate nutrition before and during pregnancy has greater potential for long-term health impact than it does at any other time. Infants who are well nourished in the womb have an enhanced chance of entering life in good physical and mental health. The effect of undernutrition during reproduction will vary depending on the nutrient involved, the length of time it is lacking, and the stage of gestation at which it occurs. The intake of substances such as caffeine, nicotine, alcohol, and many drugs; the presence of intrauterine infections; the age of the mother; and the physical and emotional stress to which she is exposed may all modify the nutritional status of both mother and child.

Although pregnancy is a normal, physiological event, from a nutritional standpoint, it is a vulnerable period. The nutrient demands of the **embryo** or **fetus** developing in the **uterus** must be met in addition to those for maintenance of the adult woman. This calls for quality nutrition both before and during pregnancy.

The importance of adequate nutrition for the fetus cannot be emphasized enough. The future health of the developing child depends to a large extent on the nutritional foundation established in prenatal life. It is difficult, however, to identify the precise effects of nutrition on reproduction. Maternal health is complex, being influenced by various genetic, social, and economic factors and by infections and environmental conditions, many of which affect fetal development. In addition, prepregnancy nutrition is as important as nutrition during pregnancy; both influence fetal growth and therefore the size and health of the infant at birth.

Fortunately, the needs of the pregnant woman are not the sum of the needs of the growing fetus added to those of a mature woman. The pregnant woman experiences a series of physiological adaptations that result in improved utilization of nutrients, either through increased absorption, decreased excretion, or alterations in metabolism. In addition, a woman who has been well nourished before conception

embryo
The term used to describe the developing fetus from the second to eighth week of gestation, when most of the cell differentiation takes place

fetus
A developing human from 2 months after conception to birth

uterus
The female organ in which the fertilized ovum becomes embedded and in which it continues to grow throughout gestation

Nutrient Needs
Mother + Baby
$1 + 1 \neq 2$

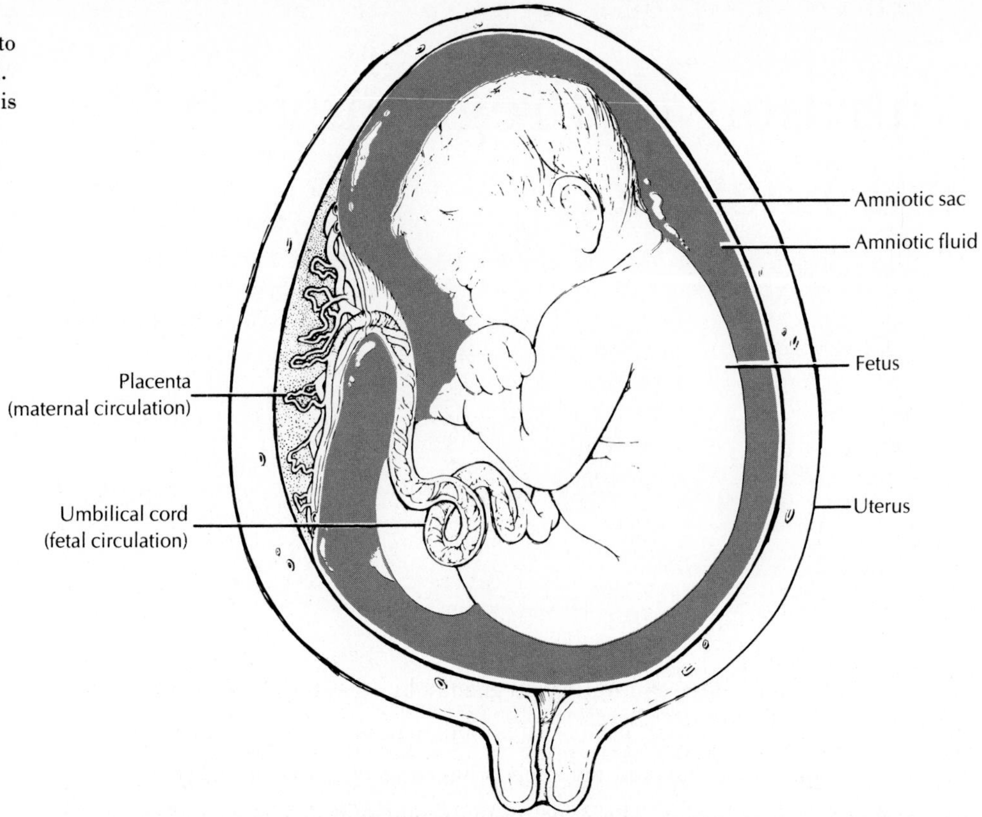

Figure 15-1 Diagrammatic representation of fetus in relationship to placenta through which it is nourished. Blood supply to placenta from mother is result of increase in blood vessels in uterine wall.

begins her pregnancy with reserves of several nutrients so that the needs of the growing fetus can be met without jeopardizing her health. As a result, the healthy woman whose diet was adequate before pregnancy is usually able to bear a full-term, viable infant without extensive modification of her diet. It is recommended, however, that the mother's diet provide sufficient nutrients so that maternal stores will not be depleted and the mother will be able to produce enough milk to adequately nourish her child after birth. For the pregnant teenager, nutritional needs are considerably higher.

The developing fetus is totally dependent on the mother for all nourishment. This nourishment is obtained primarily from the mother's blood, which comes in close contact with the fetal circulation in the **placenta** so that nutrients can be transferred (Figure 15-1) through the **umbilical cord** to the fetus. Besides regulating the transfer of nutrients, the placenta acts as an endocrine gland with responsibility for the synthesis of at least 10 different hormones that control the metabolism of the fetus and sometimes that of the mother. During the latter part of **gestation** (pregnancy), some nutrients are available to the fetus through the **amniotic fluid,** the liquid in which the baby lives during fetal development.

Nutrients are provided either from the mother's diet, from her stores of nutrients (primarily in the bones and liver), or from synthesis in the placenta. Because the placenta controls the transfer of nutrients, hormones, and other substances (such as drugs) to the fetus, the development of the placenta itself is crucial to the health of the fetus. The placentas of poorly nourished mothers contain fewer and smaller cells than those of well-nourished mothers. This reduces their ability to synthesize substances needed by the fetus, to aid in the flow of needed nutrients, and to inhibit the passage of potentially harmful substances. Once nutrients have crossed the placenta to the fetus, many are changed so that they are trapped in the fetus and cannot be transferred back to the mother. For example, vitamin B_6 becomes attached

placenta
Tissue embedded in the wall of the uterus; in the placenta, maternal and fetal circulations come in close enough contact with one another that nutrients from the mother and waste from the fetus can be exchanged

umbilical cord
A narrow tube through which blood flows from the placenta to the fetus

gestation
The period from conception to delivery; pregnancy

amniotic fluid
The liquid that fills the amniotic sac within the uterus, in which the baby lives during fetal development

to phosphate to make pyridoxal phosphate—a molecule too big to leave the fetal circulation.

Intrauterine nutrition is especially important in the development of the infant's central nervous system and kidneys, which mature rapidly in the latter part of pregnancy. Nutritional deficits before birth can often be partially, but never wholly, reversed by adequate nutrition after birth.

intrauterine nutrition
Provision of nutrients to fetus before birth (intra = within; uter = uterus)

BIRTH SIZE

In the United States, up to 15% of all infants (over a quarter of a million) are **low-birth-weight (LBW) babies,** weighing less than 5.5 pounds (2500 grams). More than two thirds of these babies are **premature**—that is, they are born after less than 37 weeks of gestation. The rest suffer from **intrauterine growth retardation (IUGR);** they are born after 40 weeks of gestation but are small because of malnutrition during uterine growth. LBW babies also have an increased susceptibility to infection, immature kidneys, difficulty regulating body temperature, and problems in both carbohydrate and protein metabolism. As a result, these infants have twice the risk of infants over 5.5 pounds of being hospitalized in the first year of life and 30 times the possibility of dying in the **neonatal** period, which is considered the first 28 days of life.

low-birth-weight (LBW) babies
Infants weighing less than 5.5 pounds (2500 grams)

premature babies
Infants born after less than 37 weeks of gestation

intrauterine growth retardation (IUGR)
Depressed growth of the fetus caused by poor nutrition during fetal growth; caused by congenital malformation, intrauterine infection, small or inefficient placenta, maternal smoking, alcoholism, drug addiction, or severe malnutrition

neonatal
First 28 days of life (neo = near; natal = birth)

These risks are high among babies born to adolescent mothers, who have high nutritional requirements for their own growth. Furthermore, many teenage pregnancies involve girls of low socioeconomic status who are frequently undernourished themselves and are therefore less capable of providing adequate nutrients to promote intrauterine growth. As a result, the half million children born each year to mothers under 18 years of age are more likely to suffer from deficits in physical, social, and psychological development than are babies born to more physically mature mothers. One fourth of these teenage mothers become pregnant again within 1 year and one third within 2 years. Regardless of age, the outcome of teenage pregnancy is influenced by the girl's physiological maturity. The closer the age of **menarche,** or the onset of menstrual periods, to the age of conception, the greater the nutritional demands on the mother and the greater the risks, including low-birth-weight infants and developmental abnormalities. These infants are often victims of child abuse and neglect.

menarche
Time of physiological maturity in girls; characterized by onset of menstruation

Intrauterine growth retardation, which results in babies who are **small for gestational age (SGA),** is most likely to occur in the offspring of women who are of low socioeconomic status; have poor nutritional status; are shorter and weigh less than their better-nourished counterparts at the time of conception; experience hypertension, viral infections, or other diseases; or use drugs extensively before or during pregnancy. The infants of these women may be undernourished because of poor nutritional status of the mother, or poor circulation to the fetus, resulting in a reduced supply of oxygen and nutrients; inhibition of the transfer of nutrients because of reduced size of placenta; or hormonal changes. The sequence of changes leading to fetal growth retardation is shown in Figure 15-2.

small for gestational age (SGA)
Full-term infants who weigh less than 5.5 pounds

Prematurity as a cause of low birth weight is more often a problem with multiple births or when mothers gain too little (less than 16 pounds, or 7 kg) or too much (more than 30 pounds, or 14 kg) weight during pregnancy, smoke excessively (over 11 cigarettes a day), or consume alcohol in excess (1 to 3 oz 100-proof alcohol/day). Because much of the development and maturation of the kidneys and lungs occurs in the latter part of pregnancy, the chances of defects in these tissues increase significantly among premature babies.

To reduce chances of having a low-birth-weight infant, pregnant women should:
- Gain between 16 and 30 pounds
- Smoke no more than 11 cigarettes/day—preferably none
- Limit alcohol consumption to 1 to 3 drinks/day (1 drink = ½ oz 200-proof or 1 oz 100-proof alcohol)

The malnourished pregnant woman is prevented in many natural ways from carrying a potentially undernourished child to term. Only an estimated 60% of conceptions survive the critical first 4 weeks of gestation. Of these, another 10% fail to survive to 20 weeks. Intrauterine deaths that occur from 20 weeks of gestation

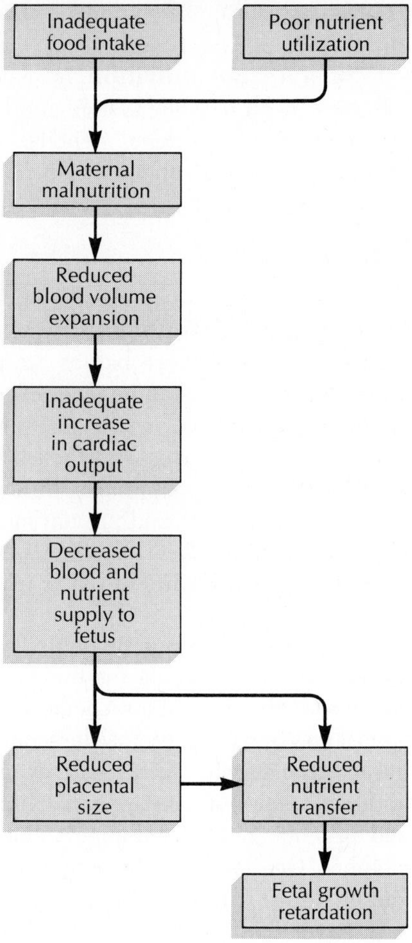

Figure 15-2 Relationship between maternal and fetal malnutrition.
From Rosso P: American Journal of Clinical Nutrition 34:744, 1981.

to term reduce to 50% the proportion of conceptions that result in viable births. In addition, approximately 1% of the newborns suffer from perinatal handicaps necessitating special care. In the United States, the mortality rate in the first 2 years of life is approximately 25 per 100 live births but is highest among blacks and low-income women. Infant mortality ranges from 8 per 1000 live births in Sweden to over 200 in many developing countries. There is general agreement that many infant deaths result from undernutrition and malnutrition before and during pregnancy and are therefore preventable.

PHYSIOLOGICAL ADJUSTMENTS

primipara
A woman having her first child (primus = first; parita = child bearing)

multipara
A woman who has had more than one child

During pregnancy, many physiological, biochemical, and hormonal changes occur that influence the need for nutrients and the efficiency with which the body uses them. Beginning with the third month of pregnancy, total blood plasma volume is known to increase about 33% above normal levels; it may reach up to 50% above normal in **primiparas** (women having their first baby) and even higher in **multiparas** (women who have already had at least one baby). These increases provide more blood to circulate through the placenta to carry nutrients to the fetus and to carry metabolic waste, such as carbon dioxide and nitrogenous end product, away from the fetus to the maternal kidneys. At the same time, the increase in the rate at which blood filters through the kidneys increases the ability of the mother to excrete waste products that could impair fetal development. Any loss of needed nutrients is prevented by an increase in the ability of the kidneys to reabsorb nutrients from the filtered blood. To aid in the circulation of this larger amount of blood, the capacity of the heart to pump fluid is also increased by one third. In addition to the increase in fluid within the circulatory system, intercellular water between the cells increases total fluid still further. The total increase in body water may therefore be as much as 20%.

This **hemodilution**, which occurs as blood volume increases almost twice as much as hemoglobin or albumin, results in decreased hemoglobin and plasma protein concentration, as well as a lowered per unit volume concentration of red blood cells and many nutrients. These observations in pregnant women are often erroneously interpreted as evidence of a deficiency. This means that we must use different standards in assessing the nutritional status of pregnant women. Frequently the total amount of a constituent in the blood may actually increase although the per volume value will have dropped. Blood lipids, cholesterol, phospholipids, and free fatty acids increase in concentration and total amount.

hemodilution
The dilution of the concentration of components in the blood, caused by an increase in blood volume during pregnancy.

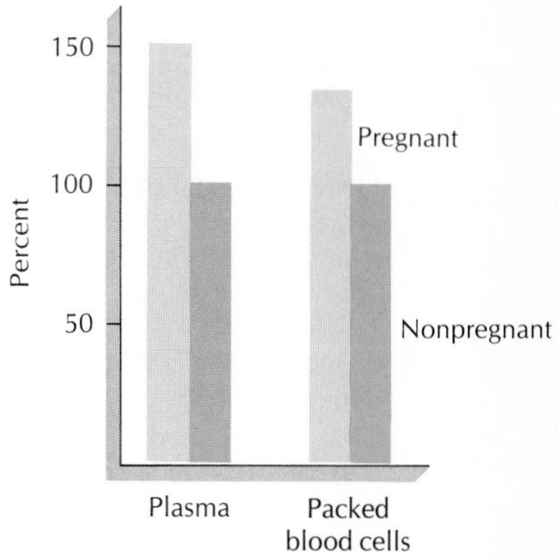

Increase in plasma and packed blood cells during pregnancy

The decrease in gastric motility and intestinal tone that is common in pregnancy is advantageous insofar as it slows the passage of food through the gastrointestinal tract and enhances the absorption of nutrients. On the other hand, it may result in nausea and constipation, the latter causing considerable discomfort in the latter part of gestation.

The increase in basal metabolic rate reflects the energy costs of the increased work of the kidneys and heart. The decrease in the secretion of hydrochloric acid during pregnancy reduces gastric acidity and depresses calcium and iron absorption. However, these effects are counterbalanced by other factors that lead to an increased absorption of calcium and iron in the last trimester of pregnancy.

In addition to the increased secretion of hormones that prepare the pregnant woman's body to permit the fetus to develop, there are other changes that have nutritional implications. These include the increased secretion of (1) aldosterone (the salt-conserving hormone) by the adrenal gland; (2) the growth hormone by the pituitary gland; (3) thyroxin, which regulates metabolism by the thyroid; and (4) the parathyroid hormone, which controls calcium, phosphorus, and magnesium metabolism by the parathyroid gland. Another nutritional implication is the increased uptake of iodine by the thyroid gland. Increases in the hormones progesterone and estrogen from both maternal and placental sources ensure a normal course of pregnancy.

PHYSIOLOGICAL STAGES OF PREGNANCY

From a physiological standpoint, pregnancy can be divided into three main phases, each with unique nutritional considerations: implantation, organogenesis, and growth.

Implantation

The first 2 weeks of gestation is a period of **implantation,** during which the fertilized ovum becomes embedded in the wall of the uterus. At this time, the embryo is nourished through the outer layers of the fertilized egg from secretions, known as **uterine milk,** of the uterine glands. About one third of conceptions fail to survive this period.

implantation
The process in which the fertilized ovum embeds itself in the wall of the uterus and begins to grow, receiving its nutrients from the uterine milk

uterine milk
A substance obtained from the walls of the uterus that nourishes the growing embryo before the placenta is fully developed

Organogenesis

The next 6 weeks are known as the period of **organogenesis,** or embryogenesis. During this time, the developing fetal tissue, known as the embryo, begins to differentiate into functional units that later become organs, such as heart, lungs, and liver. Skeletal development also begins during this time. Nourishment is obtained from the blood and degenerating cells in the space between the embryo and the wall of the uterus. The presence of specific nutrients is crucial for the continued growth of a normal fetus, with different tissues requiring different nutrients at various times.

organogenesis
The process in which the fertilized cell divides and differentiates into the beginnings of the human organs and tissues

critical period
The time in cell differentiation during which a particular tissue is especially sensitive to the presence or lack of a particular nutrient

Evidence from animal studies links the absence of certain nutrients during specific **critical periods** of organogenesis with specific congenital abnormalities in newborns. For example, riboflavin deficiency has been associated with poor skeletal formation, pyridoxine and manganese deficiencies with neuromotor problems, vitamin B_{12} deficiency with hydrocephalus and vitamin A, niacin, and folacin deficiencies with cleft palate. Comparable effects in humans are hard to confirm but are probable if deficiencies continue for long periods of time.

The stage in pregnancy at which a deficiency occurs influences the way in which it shows up. If the inadequacy occurs in very early stages, the result may be a spontaneous abortion; at other stages during differentiation, a deficiency may cause a variety of **congenital** abnormalities; after differentiation is complete, deficiencies may have virtually no effect on the developing fetus, except on tissue growth.

congenital
Existing at or dating from birth

Sequence of Developmental Changes During Pregnancy

Week 4	Brain development begins
Week 5	Heart function Liver function
Week 8	Skeleton mineralization begins
Month 3	Kidney function
Month 4	Lungs form
Month 5	Fetus kicks and turns
Month 6	Fetus swallows
Month 7	Fetal nervous system controls breathing
Month 8	Subcutaneous fat accumulates
Month 9	Lungs function

During organogenesis, the possibility of a nutritional inadequacy with its potential hazards to the fetus is high because this critical period occurs at an early stage in pregnancy—before a woman may know she is pregnant or have sought medical and nutritional advice. In addition, many women experience nausea during early pregnancy, which depresses appetite and food intake and often reduces the nutrients available for absorption to a critically low level. Under such conditions, the expectant mother who has had good dietary habits before conception has an advantage over her less well-fed counterpart, who may have entered pregnancy with minimal nutrient reserves.

At the end of the organogenesis period, the fetus weighs only 1 oz and is a little over an inch long; however, it has many of the features of a newborn. The outer layers of the embryo have already developed into the nervous system and are beginning to form the skin. The middle layers are forming muscles and internal organs, including a beating heart; from the center of the embryo, the glands and linings of the digestive and respiratory systems are taking on functional characteristics.

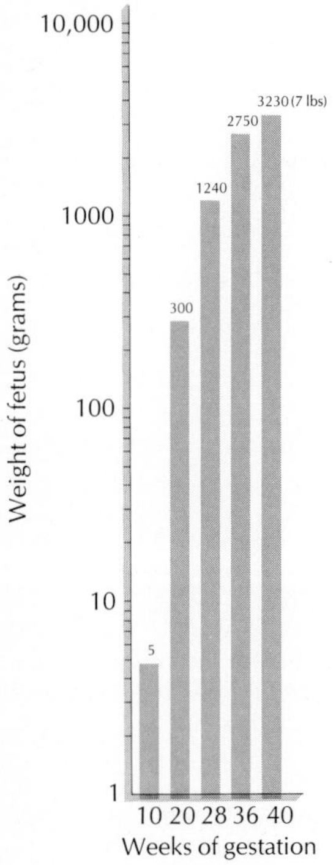

Weight of fetus at various stages in gestation

Growth

The remaining 7 months of pregnancy are known as the growth period. During this time, the differentiated tissues are nourished through the placenta and continue to grow until they reach a functional size capable of supporting life outside the womb. Some nutrients are available in the amniotic fluid that the infant swallows in the latter part of pregnancy. The need for nutrients at this time is high both in quantity and in quality. A deficiency will usually result only in prematurity or a smaller infant, rather than in the serious congenital problems as caused by a nutrient deficiency during organogenesis.

Growth occurs in three phases. During the first, known as **hyperplasia,** there is a rapid increase in the number of cells. This cell replication requires folacin and vitamin B_{12}, both of which play a role in the synthesis of the nucleic acids (DNA and RNA) that must be produced each time a cell divides. In the next phase, cell proliferation continues along with **hypertrophy,** or cell growth, which calls for the availability of amino acids and vitamin B_6, both of which are essential for protein synthesis. In the final phase, cells divide more slowly, and growth is primarily the result of hypertrophy. The age at which a particular tissue reaches mature size, when much less hyperplasia occurs, varies from the first year of life for the brain to several years for the liver. A reduced number of cells caused by inadequate diet at a later time does not necessarily result in impaired function because many tissues can function on fewer cells. In addition, if tissue growth is depressed during a period of undernutrition, it can be stimulated again when an adequate diet is available.

hyperplasia
Increase in cell number

hypertrophy
Increase in cell size

The Placenta

Early in the growth stage, the placenta develops and begins to play its role of providing nourishment for the fetus. The placenta, which weighs from 325 to 1000 grams (2.2 pounds) at birth, is the tissue through which the nutrients and oxygen needed for fetal growth are transferred from the maternal blood to the fetus and through which fetal waste is excreted. No direct circulatory connection exists between the fetus and the mother—that is, blood does not flow from one to the other. However, in the placenta the two independent circulatory systems come in close enough contact with one another for nutrients to pass from one to the other. In the placenta, approximately 13 square meters of contact exist between the two circulations. For some nutrients such as folacin, iron, vitamin C, and vitamin B_{12}, the placenta allows the passage of sufficient amounts to meet the demands of the growing fetus even at the expense of maternal reserves. For other nutrients such as thiamin, riboflavin, vitamin B_6, and vitamin D, it allows the maternal and fetal tissue to compete for the nutrients. The fat-soluble vitamins A and E are present in lower amounts in fetal blood than in maternal blood. The placenta becomes the regulator of fetal nutrition, the success of which depends not only on the nutrients available in the mother's blood but also on the way in which the placenta governs their transfer. In addition to promoting the active transfer of nutrients and permitting the diffusion of others, the placenta can synthesize some body compounds. Nutritional failure may be as much the result of an inadequate supply of blood to the placenta as of a low level of nutrients in maternal blood.

1 kg (1000 grams) = 2.2 pounds

Nutrients Given to Fetus at Expense of Mother
Folacin
Iron
Vitamin C
Vitamin B_{12}

Nutrients for which Mother and Fetus Compete
Thiamin
Riboflavin
Vitamin B_6
Vitamin D

Nutrients for which Mother Has Priority over Fetus
Vitamin A
Vitamin E

Rate

As is evident from Figure 15-3, the rate of fetal growth is very slow in the first 2 months of pregnancy. Even at a gestational age of 25 weeks, the growth increase is only 6 grams (0.2 oz)/day. By 34 weeks, the increase is estimated at 40 grams (1.4 oz)/day and by term has dropped again to 13 grams (0.4 oz)/day. Fetal weights at various ages of gestation and comparable increase in maternal weight are shown in Table 15-1. During the first **trimester** (3 months), growth is almost entirely in maternal tissue; during the second trimester, gain is in both fetal and maternal tissue; and in the third trimester, it is primarily in fetal tissue. Gain during the latter two periods is 350 to 450 grams (¾ to 1 pound)/week.

trimester
Term applied to each of the successive 3-month periods during the 9 months of gestation

The relatively slow development of the human fetus means that nutritional deficiencies must prevail over a long period of time if they are to have a measurable

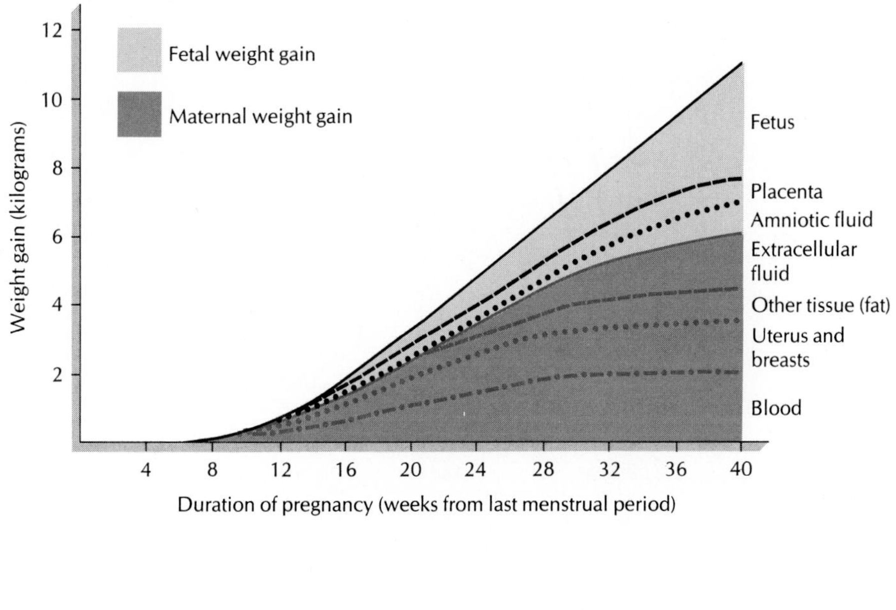

Figure 15-3 Pattern and components of weight gain throughout pregnancy.
From Pitkin RM: Clinical Obstetrics and Gynecology 19:489, 1975.

effect on fetal development. In contrast, many animals used in nutrition investigations develop at a very rapid rate, produce litters of larger size relative to maternal size, and therefore are much more susceptible to short-term dietary deviations. Comparisons of rates of development and the relationship of litter size to maternal weight for different mammals are shown in Figure 15-4. You can see from this figure that mice produce a litter weighing 30% of maternal weight in 3 weeks, whereas human mothers take 9 months to develop infants representing 5% of the mother's weight.

Table 15-1 ◇ Fetal weight and maternal weight gains at different ages in gestation

Age (weeks)	Total Fetal Weight (grams [pounds])	Maternal Gain including Fetus (grams [pounds])
First Trimester		
10	5 (0.01)	650 (1.4)
12	30	
Second Trimester		
20	300 (0.7)	4000 (8.8)
24	900	
Third Trimester		
28	1240	
30	1484 (3.3)	8500 (18.7)
32	1750	
34	2278	
36	2750	
38	3052	
40	3230 (7.1)	12,500 (27.5)
42	3310	

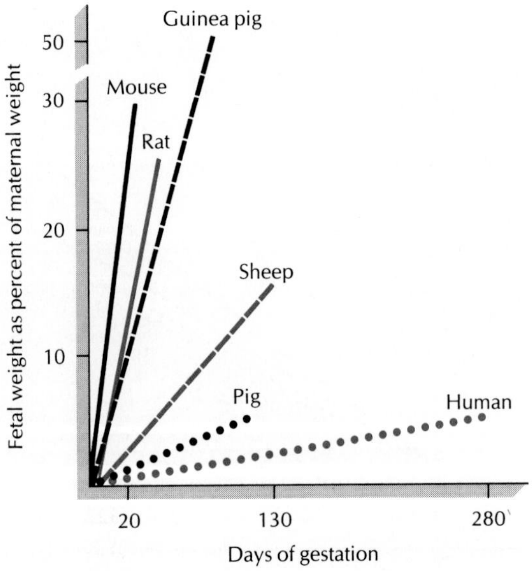

Figure 15-4 Products of conception of six mammalian species as a percentage of maternal weight.

NUTRITIVE NEEDS

The recommended increase over the normal nutrient need of a woman to meet the demands of pregnancy varies from one nutrient to another, as shown in Table 15-2. This table includes recommended base needs for adult women; needs for adolescents are even greater. The increase in energy needs is usually smaller than that for other nutrients, which becomes very evident when additional needs for pregnancy and lactation are expressed as nutrients per 1000 kcal (nutrient density) or percentage increase. For some nutrients such as iron and vitamin A, the recommended maternal intake allows the fetus to accumulate sufficient amounts to store reserves that last through the early stages of infancy. For others such as vitamin D, vitamin C, and calcium, virtually no storage occurs in the infant's body prior to birth; therefore the mother needs to provide only enough for fetal growth. Increases to meet the nutritional stresses of pregnancy depend on many factors such as the metabolic adjustments to meet increased demands and the nutrient reserves of the mother. The Recommended Dietary Allowances vary from 15% above normal for energy and niacin to 100% for folacin and vitamin D to more than 200% for iron.

Nutrients Stored in Fetus
Vitamin A
Iron

Nutrients Not Stored in Fetus
Vitamin C
Vitamin D
Calcium

Energy

During pregnancy, caloric needs are influenced by several factors. The growth of the fetus, although very slow at first, calls for some additional energy. As the fetus matures, it needs energy for growth and for some physical activity, which amounts to 125 kcal/day by the end of pregnancy. The growth of the placenta, the normal increase in maternal body size (including fat reserves of 4 to 5 pounds, the uterus, and mammary tissue), the additional work of carrying the growing fetus, and the

Energy Needs during Pregnancy
Fetus
 Growth
 Activity
Mother
 Increased basal metabolism
 Fat stores
 Growth of uterus and mammary tissue
 Increased blood volume
 Change in activity

Table 15-2 ◇ Recommended Dietary Allowances to meet needs of pregnancy and lactation; percentage increase over those of non-pregnant woman

	Adult Woman (25-49)	Pregnant Woman (Third Trimester)	Lactating Mother*	Percent of Increase in Need Over Nonpregnant Woman	
				Pregnancy	Lactation
Energy (kcal)	2000	2300	2500	15	25
Protein (grams)	44	74	64	70	45
Vitamin A (RE)	800	1000	1200	25	33
Vitamin D (μg)	5	10	10	100	100
Vitamin E (TE, mg)	8	10	11	25	35
Vitamin C (mg)	60	80	100	33	66
Thiamin (mg)	1.1	1.5	1.6	36	45
Riboflavin (mg)	1.3	1.6	1.8	23	38
Niacin (NE, mg)	14	16	18	14	29
Vitamin B_6 (mg)	2	2.6	2.5	30	25
Folacin (μg)	400	800	500	100	25
Vitamin B_{12} (μg)	3	4	4	33	33
Calcium (mg)	800	1200	1200	50	50
Phosphorus (mg)	800	1200	1200	50	50
Iron (mg)	18	18+	18	†	†
Zinc (mg)	15	20	25	33	66
Iodine (μg)	150	175	200	16	33
Selenium (μg)‡	55	73	71	32	29

*During first 6 months of lactation.
†The increased iron requirement for pregnancy and lactation cannot be met by the usual American diet or from body stores; thus, a supplement of 30 to 60 mg elemental iron is recommended.
‡Proposed 1985.

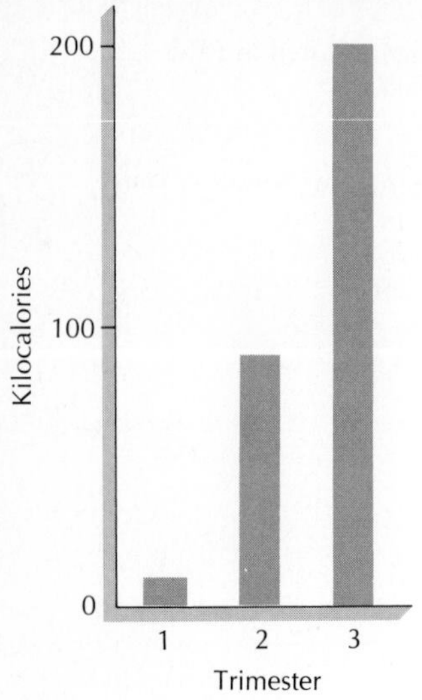

Additional daily energy needs for fetal growth

steady but slow rise in basal metabolism all contribute to additional energy needs. On the other hand, any decrease in activity of the mother depresses the caloric requirement.

Increases in caloric needs for fetal growth are not distributed evenly throughout gestation. They are very small (10 kcal/day) in the first trimester. In the second trimester an additional 90 kcal is needed, and in the final trimester about 200 kcal/day is needed, primarily for the growth of the fetus and placenta.

The growth of the fetus and maternal tissue and their maintenance (which is the amount for increased heart and respiration rate) call for an estimated net energy cost of 27,000 kcal over the 9 months of pregnancy. If it is assumed that 4.4 pounds (2 kg) of maternal body fat are added during pregnancy, total energy costs of pregnancy are increased by 18,000 kcal for a total of approximately 55,000 kcal. This amounts to 300 kcal/day, distributed over the last two trimesters. For mothers who greatly reduce their activity, no additional energy may be needed.

Table 15-3, which shows the components of maternal weight gain, makes it evident that a normal pregnancy calls for considerable weight gain over and above that represented by the size of the fetus. If the net gain in maternal weight is less than the combined weight of the fetus, placenta, and amniotic fluid (5 kg or 11 pounds), we must assume that the growth of the fetus has caused a depletion of the mother's tissue reserves. Failure in the development of the breast and some fat reserves during pregnancy may preclude a normal and successful lactation period.

Fat that accumulates throughout pregnancy, but especially the first 30 weeks, acts as an energy reserve for a time when food intake may be inadequate. Thus, it prevents the catabolism of the mother's tissue later in pregnancy. An increase in ketones in the urine in late pregnancy suggests that fat reserves are being used to provide for the high energy needs of the rapidly growing fetus and to spare protein for tissue growth. Fat stored during pregnancy also is used to meet needs for lactation.

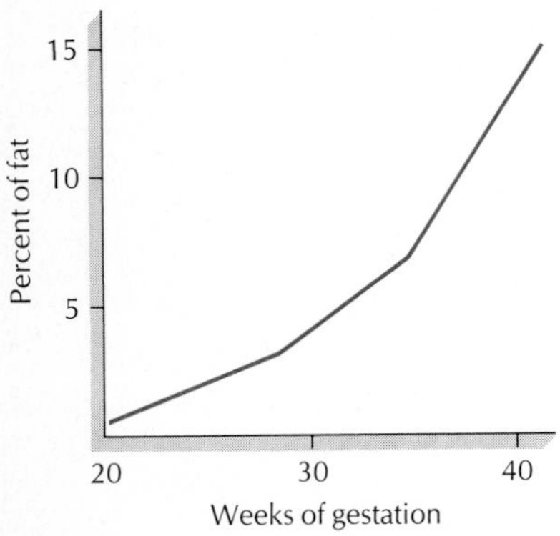

Change in fat content of fetus throughout pregnancy

In the first trimester, the fetus accumulates no fat other than that which is part of the essential lipids in its cell walls and nervous system. At 20 weeks, the fetus contains only 0.5% fat, but this rises steadily to 3.5% at 28 weeks, 7.5% at 34 weeks, and 16% at the end of pregnancy. Fat is synthesized by the fetus from glucose, which crosses the placental barrier readily. The only fatty acid to be transferred from the mother to the child is the essential fatty acid, linoleic acid.

Maternal weight gain. Recommendations about weight gain for pregnant women have changed markedly in the last 5 decades. Unrestricted maternal weight gain, encouraged on the theory that the mother was "eating for two," was widely accepted in the early part of the century. However, difficulties of pregnancy and labor with increased risk to the mother, and the birth of large babies who suffered

Table 15-3 ◊ Components of maternal weight gain in pregnancy

Tissue	Weight (grams)		Weight (pounds)		
Fetus	3150		7		(Range, 5-10 pounds)
Placenta	675		1.5		
Amniotic fluid	900		2		
Subtotal		4725		10.5	Relatively constant
Mother					
Uterus	900		2		
Breasts	450		1		
Increase in blood volume	1350		3		
Tissue fluids	1350		3		
Fat	2000		4.4		
Subtotal		6100		13.4	
TOTAL		10,825		23.9	

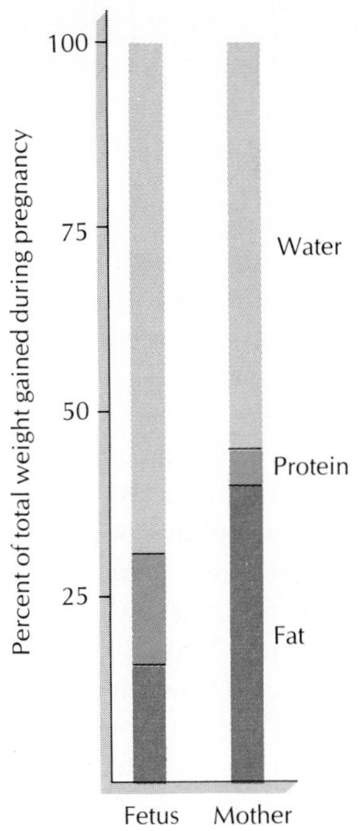

Distribution of total weight gained during pregnancy

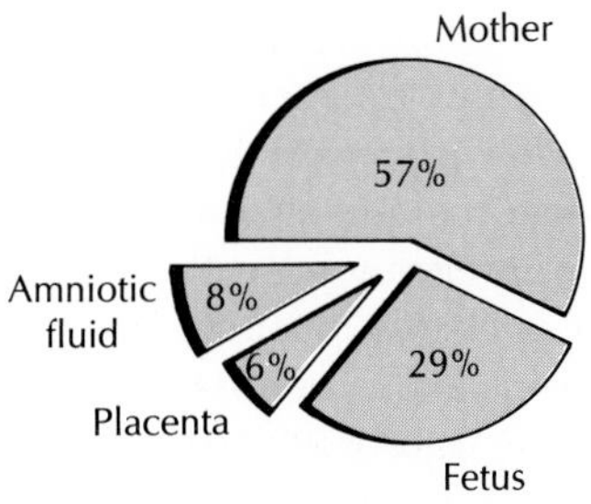

Composition of weight gain of mother and fetus during entire pregnancy

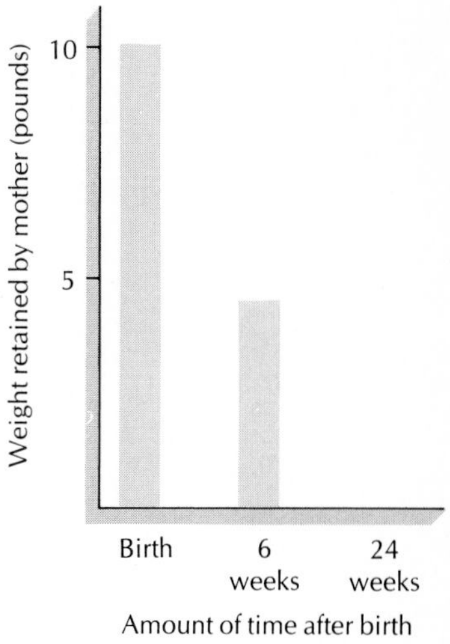

Retention (after delivery) of weight gained during pregnancy

many complications in early life were all recognized as consequences of this regimen.

The next recommendation, popular in the 1940s and 1950s that calories be restricted enough to limit weight gain to 10 to 15 pounds (4 to 6 kg) resulted in equally undesirable consequences. Current recommendations of a weight gain of 22 to 27 pounds are based on a more complete understanding of the physiology of pregnancy.

Both pattern of weight gain and total weight gain are important. In general, a gain of 2 to 4 pounds (1 to 2 kg) in the first trimester followed by a steady increase of approximately 400 grams/week to 10 pounds at 20 weeks, 19 pounds at 30 weeks, and 27 pounds at term is the normal pattern. Mothers who fail to gain weight in the second trimester are very likely to have premature deliveries with increased risk to the health of the baby.

Many women restrict their weight gain, fearing that part of it may be permanently retained after pregnancy. Studies show that about 10 pounds (4 kg) gained during pregnancy usually remain immediately after birth and only 4 or 5 pounds (2 kg) remain at 6 weeks postpartum (after birth). Most of the gained weight is usually lost in 6 to 8 months.

Some obstetricians maintain that a woman who is obese at the onset of pregnancy can successfully reduce her own body size without jeopardizing the health of her infant or herself if the quality of the diet is carefully maintained. Most of them suggest that any major adjustments in the mother's weight should be made under normal circumstances rather than during pregnancy. If weight gain is to be controlled, however, the only effective way to do it is through caloric restriction rather than restriction of salt or water intake.

One study found that gains of 30 pounds for women underweight at conception, 20 pounds for women of normal weight, and 16 pounds for overweight women were associated with the lowest perinatal mortality.

The Committee on Maternal Nutrition of the Food and Nutrition Board has concluded that a gain of 20 to 25 pounds (9 to 11 kg) minimizes the risks of pregnancy and is most desirable for the health of both mother and baby. Women who eat to the point of satisfying their appetites gain 22 to 27 pounds (10 to 12.5

Risk Factors for Toxemia
- Inadequate diet
- First pregnancy at < 20 or > 35 years of age
- Multiple gestation
- History of high blood pressure, kidney disease, or inadequate medical care
- Sudden weight gain
- Inadequate weight gain

kg). After a careful evaluation of all relevant data, the committee suggested a maximum of an additional 250 kcal daily after the first trimester of pregnancy, although the RDAs remains at an extra 300 kcal.

Protein

Recommendations for protein intakes during pregnancy consider (1) estimates of the theoretical amounts of protein deposited in the fetus, placenta, and maternal tissues, which amount to 3.3 grams/day; (2) data on nitrogen balance during pregnancy suggesting a retention that is twice the estimated amounts; (3) evidence that women with intakes throughout pregnancy that are higher than estimated needs have more successful pregnancies; and (4) evidence that there is increased risk associated with low protein intakes. Recommended dietary allowances (RDAs) for a pregnant woman include an additional 30 grams or a total of 76 grams of protein daily throughout pregnancy. In the United States, most nonpregnant women have intakes in excess of this amount. FAO, on the other hand, has suggested a daily increase of 3 grams above normal needs in the first trimester and 14 and 24 grams, respectively, in the next two trimesters. Amino acids are transferred from the mother to the fetus to be used in the synthesis of the fetus's protein. Up to 20 weeks into pregnancy, all amino acids must be provided to the fetus. After that, the fetal liver is able to synthesize some of the nonessential amino acids itself. Because the fetus cannot oxidize amino acids as a source of energy, they seem to be used exclusively for protein synthesis. Total weight gain during pregnancy includes 1 kg of protein, half of which is in fetal tissue.

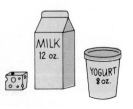

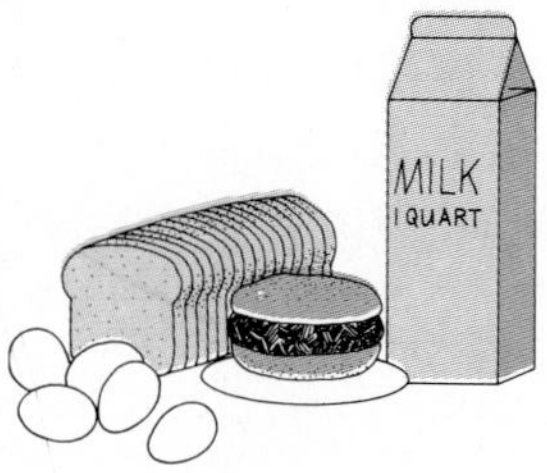

Amount of various food sources that provide 30 grams of protein each

After the development of the uterus, placenta, and mammary glands early in pregnancy, little if any protein is stored in maternal tissues. When dietary protein is restricted, it is definitely the amount in storage in the mother's body that is reduced rather than the amount transferred to the fetus. Reserves of energy in fat help make protein available during rapid fetal growth. Protein intake of the mother influences the extent to which the birth length of the infant approaches its genetic potential.

Severe protein restriction during fetal life is associated with a decrease in the number of cells in tissue at the time of birth. This is particularly serious in the brain, which is relatively well developed during prenatal life and may be irreversibly stunted by deficiency. Other tissues that reach less of their mature size in prenatal life are not as affected. Protein and caloric deficiencies during gestation may result in poor utilization of food by offspring after birth.

In addition to the amino acids that are transferred to the fetus, large protein molecules such as antibodies also cross the placenta. They give the infant immunity to any antigens (foreign substances) to which the mother has been exposed.

Minerals

Calcium

Although the infant's bones are poorly calcified at the time of birth, teeth begin to calcify at 5 months of gestation. Thus, an appreciable amount of calcium is involved in fetal development. This amounts to approximately 7 mg/day for the first trimester, increases to 110 mg/day in the second trimester, and jumps to 350 mg/day in the last trimester. As a result, the mother provides approximately 30 grams of calcium to the newborn infant. About 80% of this transfer occurs in the third trimester. Although the pregnant woman initially has more than 2 pounds (1000 grams) of stored calcium to draw on, she becomes even more efficient as the pregnancy progresses, absorbing twice as much calcium as under normal conditions.

Foods providing 400 mg of calcium (40% U.S. RDA = 400 mg)

It is estimated that 9 grams of fetal calcium comes from the mother's bones. Ideally, there should be extra calcium stored in the mother's bones during pregnancy to help meet demands for calcium during lactation. To prevent the mother from getting **osteomalacia** (loss of bone quality), her diet should contain reasonable calcium, no excess of phytic acid, and adequate vitamin D.

osteomalacia
Loss of bone quality; see Chapter 10 for further discussion

Iron

Infants are born with high hemoglobin levels of 18 to 22 grams/dl of blood and with a supply of iron stored in the liver to last from 3 to 6 months. To achieve these levels, the mother must transfer about 300 mg of iron to the fetus during gestation. Beyond needs for fetal growth, iron is also required for the placenta; for the formation of hemoglobin as a result of the increase in maternal blood volume; and to replace maternal iron losses in skin, hair, and sweat. These needs total over 1100 mg and represent almost twice the total iron reserves of the adult female. However, a saving of 100 to 200 mg results from the absence of menstrual losses. Most of the iron in the mother's extra hemoglobin will be returned to her iron pools when blood volume returns to normal after delivery. To provide the net need of 800 mg to meet the needs of pregnancy, 1 to 1.5 mg/day can be absorbed from the diet, and maternal stores can provide up to 300 mg. Unfortunately, however, many young women have practically no reserves at the beginning of pregnancy.

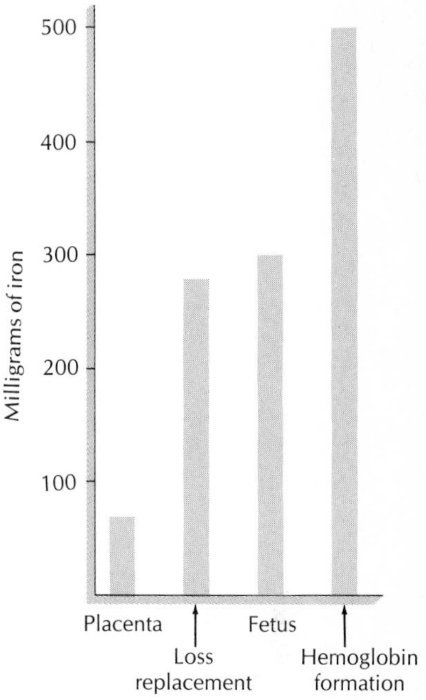

Distribution of iron needs in a pregnant woman

Iron absorption increases from 10% to 30% of dietary intake in the second half of pregnancy because of an increase in protein transferrin, which increases the body's capacity to absorb iron. The Food and Nutrition Board, however, suggests that the recommended dietary allowance of 18 mg for nonpregnant women should be supplemented with 18 mg of elemental iron (obtained from 30 to 60 mg of ferrous sulfate) for pregnant women to maintain maternal reserves and to meet the needs of the fetus. Others question the use of iron supplements because of the constipation they frequently cause. They argue that, with an increase of 50% in blood volume, a drop in hemoglobin concentration from 14 to 10 mg/dl actually represents an increase in the amount of hemoglobin available for carrying oxygen and that a woman with this level of hemoglobin should not be considered iron deficient.

The best method of combating iron deficiency during gestation is to ensure that a woman enters pregnancy with a store of at least 300 mg of iron. The injection of a single large dose of iron at the beginning of pregnancy is an effective way to build iron stores and protect against depletion of these reserves. This practice may be justified because many women fail to take an iron supplement regularly during pregnancy. One study showed that women whose hemoglobin levels stayed below 12 grams/dl had not been taking supplements, even though the level given (130 mg) was not high enough to cause side effects.

Sodium

During pregnancy, the increase in extracellular fluids calls for an 80% increase in body sodium. As a result, obstetricians are recognizing an increased need for sodium and are no longer advising a restriction of sodium intake, which had been a long-standing practice. Sodium is apparently so important that if its intake is restricted, the expectant mother experiences a series of hormonal and biochemical changes that help conserve sodium.

In another example of fine homeostatic control, when blood sodium levels first drop, the kidneys produce more of the hormone renin, which sets up a series of reactions with the final result being that the pregnant woman retains the sodium she obviously needs. If the system fails or is overtaxed, the result is a sodium deficiency with increased risk of eclampsia, prematurity, and low-birth-weight infants. Because the usual sodium intake in the United States is high, pregnant women are advised to continue their usual intake and not to increase or decrease it.

See Chapter 9 for a description of this mechanism for conserving sodium

Because they lead to a loss of sodium, the use of **diuretics** during pregnancy should be discouraged. The use of salt substitutes should also be discouraged because of limited information on their effect on pregnant women.

diuretics
Substances that stimulate the kidneys to excrete more fluid

Iodine

Intakes of iodine that prevent goiter under normal circumstances frequently prove inadequate during pregnancy, leading to goiter in the expectant mother, especially if she is an adolescent. A relative iodine deficiency may result in part from the increased urinary losses of iodine. When the mother has goiter, the chances that the child will develop goiter are increased 10 times. In addition, the incidence of cretinism, the most severe form of iodine deficiency, increases. In Western countries, the use of iodine-containing dough conditioners, colorings, and sterilizing materials in food processing is increasing, making the likelihood of an iodine lack therefore very slight.

Other Elements

Little work has been done to determine quantitative needs for other mineral elements during pregnancy. It does seem reasonable to expect that the ability of a woman to adapt to pregnancy with enhanced absorption and decreased excretion will take care of some but not necessarily all of the additional needs for mineral elements.

Low levels of zinc, magnesium, and manganese have all been associated with defects in the developing animal fetus. Excessively high levels also have adverse effects. Although levels of minerals used in experimental studies far exceed those found in usual diets, these findings warn us about the dangers of excessive supplementation.

Fat-Soluble Vitamins

Although it is fairly well established that pregnant animals have a series of adaptive mechanisms to cope with increased demands for minerals during pregnancy, there is no evidence that they have a similar system for adapting to vitamin needs. In general, fat-soluble vitamins are present at higher levels in maternal blood than in fetal blood. With the exception of vitamin D, the transfer of fat-soluble vitamins to the fetus is limited.

Vitamin A

Aside from the fact that animals on vitamin A–deficient diets have trouble conceiving and bearing young, little is known about the need for vitamin A during pregnancy. Congenital abnormalities result from a daily intake of vitamin A as low as 5000 RE throughout the first trimester. An infant is born with a reserve of vitamin A in the liver that can be provided by a small increase in the mother's intake to 1000 RE per day, assuming two thirds of this is preformed vitamin A.

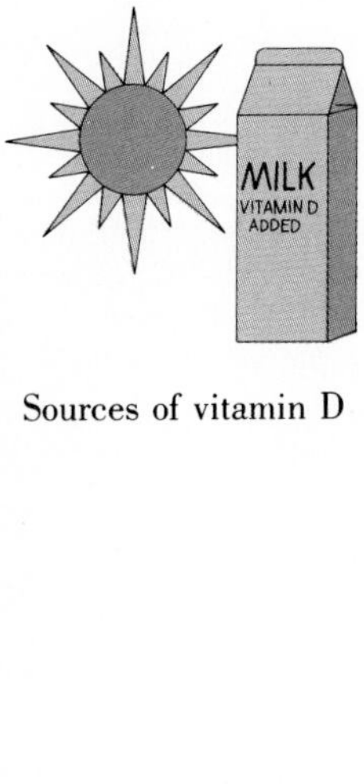

Sources of vitamin D

Vitamin D

The need for vitamin D is set at 10 μg (400 IU) per day. Vitamin D enhances maternal calcium absorption. Its active forms, calcidiol and calcitriol, both cross the placenta with ease and play an important role in calcium metabolism in the fetus. Since all milk, except buttermilk, is fortified with 400 IU of vitamin D/quart, there is no need for an additional source of the vitamin for those who meet their calcium needs with milk. In fact, too much vitamin D should be avoided.

Vitamin E

The role of vitamin E in promoting normal reproduction and reducing the number of spontaneous abortions and stillbirths in animals has led to many studies to try to find a similar role in humans. So far, no unique role for the tocopherols in human reproduction has been found, and in spite of some evidence that they may be beneficial to women who have had repeated spontaneous abortions or failure to conceive, it has not been shown that a vitamin E deficiency is responsible for pregnancy failure. Nevertheless, an increased intake of 2 mg/day is recommended. As with nonpregnant women, this requirement appears to be adequately met by a balanced diet, with little likelihood of a deficiency unless the diet contains abnormally high amounts of polyunsaturated fatty acids (PUFA). Because little vitamin E crosses the placenta, the human infant has low tissue concentrations that persist for at least 6 years.

Vitamin K

Vitamin K, which is necessary for normal coagulation of the blood, plays a role in preventing **neonatal hemorrhaging.** It became routine practice to give oral menadione (a synthetic form of vitamin K) to the mother in the last several weeks of pregnancy or even to inject it during labor to stimulate prothrombin synthesis. As a result of complications, however, the inclusion of menadione in over-the-counter supplements for pregnancy is prohibited. Similar and safe protection is afforded by giving the natural form of the vitamin either by injection or by mouth to the infant or mother.

neonatal hemorrhaging
Bleeding soon after the time of birth

Water-Soluble Vitamins

Because little of the water-soluble vitamins is stored, the pregnant woman must rely on a daily intake that is high enough to meet the added requirements of pregnancy. In general, maternal blood levels for water-soluble vitamins tend to fall; fetal blood levels tend to exceed those of the mother by 50% to 100%.

Thiamin

Although the relationship between thiamin needs and caloric intake is believed to remain the same during pregnancy, an increase of 0.4 mg of thiamin is recommended. The normal urinary excretion of thiamin drops, indicating that more is being retained and used by the tissues. In some cases, thiamin helps relieve the nausea of pregnancy.

Riboflavin

The increase in maternal body size and the growth of the fetus and accessory tissues call for an increase in riboflavin, which is present in higher amounts in fetal blood than in maternal blood. Animal studies have shown that a lack of riboflavin interferes with cartilage formation, resulting in skeletal malformations such as shortening of the long bones and a fusion of the ribs.

Vitamin B_6

Women under normal stress of pregnancy have an altered tryptophan metabolism and altered cell growth. Vitamin B_6 goes to the fetus to maintain a level in fetal blood that is much higher than that in maternal blood. Levels of pyridoxine that are about one third of the normal amount have been found in **toxemia** of pregnancy. Women who used oral contraceptives prior to conception often enter pregnancy with very low tissue levels of pyridoxine. There is no evidence that these low levels affect the outcome of pregnancy, but they do reduce the amount of pyridoxine in breast milk. The RDA for pregnant women has been increased by only 0.6 mg above what is recommended for nonpregnant women.

toxemia
Severe complication of pregnancy that threatens the life of both the mother and child; toxemia literally means *blood poisoning,* but this is neither a cause nor a symptom of toxemia

Pyridoxine has been used experimentally to help control the nausea of pregnancy. The results, although encouraging for some women, have been inconclusive, and no satisfactory theory explains this phenomenon.

Folacin

The recommended intake of folacin is based on its role in promoting normal fetal growth and preventing **macrocytic anemia** of pregnancy. Macrocytic (large cell) anemia, which frequently occurs in pregnancy, may be caused by a relatively inadequate intake of dietary folate. There are indications that iron deficiency puts additional stress on folate metabolism and may convert a subclinical folate deficiency

macrocytic anemia
An anemia characterized by very large red blood cells, which form when folate is lacking

into a megaloblastic anemia. Because folacin is needed for the synthesis of the essential components of DNA and RNA and because these components increase rapidly during growth, it is logical that folacin intake should increase. In addition, folacin is required for the development of red blood cells, which must increase as the mother's blood volume increases. As a result, the RDA for folacin is twice that for nonpregnant women. Once the folate (folacin) is transferred to the fetus, it is changed to a form that cannot be returned to the mother, therefore ensuring that the fetus will not subsequently be shortchanged to meet maternal needs. Although women can get the RDA of folacin in a carefully planned diet, a supplement of 200 to 400 μg will ensure a sufficient intake. This intake is especially important for high-risk women such as those who have had many pregnancies, have suffered from chronic hemolytic anemia, or are using anticonvulsant drugs. This added amount is available only by prescription or in supplements designed for use in pregnancy.

There is a notable decrease in folacin absorption and an increase in urinary excretion during pregnancy, which may contribute to the depletion of maternal reserves. Folacin deficiency is a major cause for concern in pregnancy—and pregnancy is the major cause of folacin deficiency.

The importance of folacin in promoting a normal pregnancy is emphasized by the fact that the use of a folacin antagonist, aminopterin, induces the resorption of fetuses in animals. Its use in humans does not lead to resorption or abortion of a fetus but does result in the birth of a child with congenital malformations such as hare lip, cleft palate, or hydrocephalus.

Complications of pregnancy such as abruptio placentae (premature detachment of the placenta), hemorrhage, and fetal malformation, which have been identified as results of folacin deficiency, cannot be alleviated or prevented by supplementation after the onset of the problem.

Vitamin B_{12}

The infant has priority over the mother in obtaining vitamin B_{12}, as evidenced by the levels in fetal blood, which are twice those in maternal blood even when maternal levels are depleted. Low maternal levels are associated with prematurity and occur more often in smokers than nonsmokers.

The capacity of the pregnant woman to absorb vitamin B_{12} is increased in pregnancy, but a large amount is transferred to the fetus. The recommended daily intake of vitamin B_{12} to maintain constant serum levels is 4 μg. If this amount is

Table 15-4 ◇ Comparison of dietary standards for pregnancy

	FAO	United States	United Kingdom	Canada
Energy (kcal)	2485	2300	2400	+500
Protein (gram)	38	74	60	68
Calcium (gram)	1-1.2	1.2	1.2	1.2
Iron (mg)	14-28	45	15	20
Vitamin A (μg RE)	1000	1000	750	900
Vitamin D (μg)	10	10	10	5
Thiamin (mg)	0.9	1.5	1	0.4/1000 kcal
Riboflavin (mg)	1.4	1.6	1.6	0.5/1000 kcal
Pyridoxine (mg)		2.6		0.015 mg/g of protein
Folacin (μg)		800		470
Vitamin B_{12} (μg)	4	4		3.0
Vitamin C (mg)		80	60	65
Zinc (mg)		20		10

not supplied, as is often the case with vegetarian mothers, the serum vitamin B_{12} levels drop but return to normal without supplementation after pregnancy.

Vitamin C

The recommended allowance for vitamin C is increased by 20 mg during pregnancy. Vitamin C does pass the placental barrier freely, and serum values of a fetus have been established as being two to four times those of the mother. There is some evidence that the placenta can synthesize vitamin C, which could account for higher levels in fetal tissues. Low maternal intakes of vitamin C are associated with the premature rupture of fetal membranes and increased neonatal death rates.

A comparison of the recommended dietary intakes during pregnancy as suggested for different countries as shown in Table 15-4, makes it clear that, for some nutrients, such as calcium and riboflavin, there is fairly close agreement. For others the differences are up to threefold, indicating that more data are needed.

Water

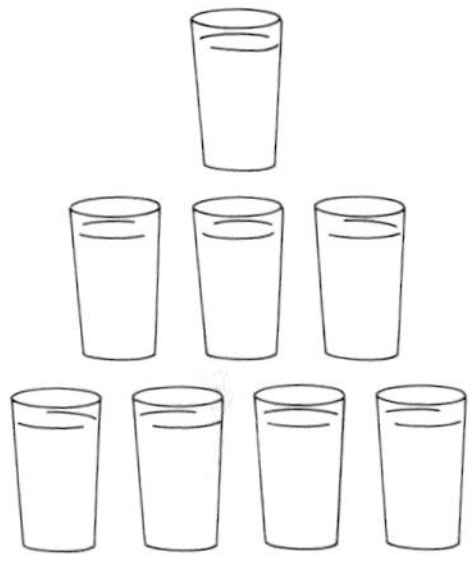

While we tend to rely on our sense of thirst to guide us to consume sufficient water, we need to encourage the pregnant woman to pay particular attention to her practices. It is recommended that she have at least 8 cups/day to assure that her water intake is sufficient to facilitate digestion and absorption of nutrients, the elimination of metabolic waste through the kidneys, and lubrication of fecal material in the colon. The pregnant woman should choose fluids that contribute to overall nutrient needs and restrict or avoid the use of alcohol, caffeine, and artificially sweetened beverages. The use of fluoridated water may contribute to bone and tooth development of the fetus.

ROLE OF NUTRITIONAL SUPPLEMENTS

Recommended dietary intakes during pregnancy call for increases over normal needs, ranging from 15% for niacin to 100% for folacin. At the same time, it is suggested that energy needs be increased by only 300 kcal—from 12% to 15% above normal for most women. Therefore, to meet added needs for pregnancy and not exceed caloric needs, it is absolutely essential to have foods of high nutrient density.

Supplements Recommended During Pregnancy
Iron
Folacin
Vitamin D (in temperate zone)
Vitamin B_6 (if oral contraceptives used prior to conception)

The selection of an adequate diet for pregnancy is relatively easy if we are concerned with an isolated day or two, but the pregnant woman must maintain a high level of nutritive intake for the normal gestation period of 280 days. To do this, she must constantly be aware of her food choices. Taking this responsibility may result in extra pressure during a period that, for some women, is already characterized by some degree of emotional stress. To allow women a little more freedom in the selection of foods and an occasional indulgence in a favorite low-nutrient food, it is reasonable to suggest the use of a supplement that provides a balanced formula at protective levels—possibly 50% of the day's recommended allowance, which is less than that found in many products. Excessive amounts of iron or folacin should be avoided because of possible adverse effects on zinc status.

The FDA ruled in 1977 that nutritional supplements labeled specifically for pregnant women should provide between 50% and 200% of the U.S. RDA for 10 vitamins and 5 minerals for which evidence of need had been established. This emphasizes the need to rely on a preformulated product rather than self-prescribed supplements of individual nutrients, which at worst might create a severe imbalance and at best might fail to include the most needed nutrients. Table 15-5 provides the permissible compositional ranges for dietary supplementation of vitamins and minerals for pregnancy and lactation.

Table 15-5 ◇ Permissible compositional ranges for dietary supplements of vitamins and minerals for pregnancy and lactation*

	Pregnant or Lactating Women		
	Lower Limit	U.S. RDA	Upper Limit
Vitamins			
Mandatory			
Vitamin A (IU)	5000	8000	8000
Vitamin D (IU)	400	400	400
Vitamin E (IU)	30	30	60
Vitamin C (mg)	60	60	120
Folacin§ (mg)	0.4	0.8	0.8
Thiamin (mg)	1.50	1.70	3.00
Riboflavin (mg)	1.7	2.0	3.4
Niacin (mg)	20.0	20.0	40.0
Vitamin B_6 (mg)	2.00	2.50	4.00
Vitamin B_{12} (μg)	6.0	8.0	12.0
Optional			
Biotin (mg)			
Pantothenic acid (mg)	0.300	0.300	0.600
	10.0	10.0	20.0
Minerals			
Mandatory			
Calcium (gram)	0.125	1.300	2.000
Iodine (μg)			
Iron (mg)	150	150	300
Magnesium (mg)	18	18	60
	100	450	800
Optional			
Phosphorus (gram)	0.125	1.300	2.000
Copper (mg)	1.0	2.0	4.0
Zinc (mg)	7.5	15.0	30.0

From Federal Register 4(203):46172, Oct. 19, 1976.
*There are no limits on supplements for other groups unless a health claim is made.

Iron supplements are recommended when hemoglobin levels drop below 10.5 grams/dl, indicating both depletion of iron reserves and hemodilution. Ferrous sulfate or ferrous gluconate are most frequently recommended. Since calcium or magnesium, in supplements, may interfere with the absorption of iron, iron is absorbed better if taken alone at bedtime or before a meal that also includes vitamin C. Supplements should have an iron/zinc ratio less than 3 to prevent iron from interfering with zinc absorption.

One additional reason for caution in the use of high-level nutritional supplementation during pregnancy is that infants may become conditioned to high intakes during fetal life. This can carry over as an increased need in the postnatal period and has explained, for example, the increase in infantile scurvy in developed countries. Vitamin B_6 dependency has also been noted, and the toxic effects of too much of the fat-soluble vitamins A and D have been well documented.

It is possible for some pregnant women to adapt to such a wide range of nutrient intakes during the stress of pregnancy that nutritional supplementation is not needed. This is especially true if they enter pregnancy in good nutritional health and do not suffer from nausea of pregnancy. However, supplements of iron, folacin, and (for long-term users of oral contraceptives) vitamin B_6 are usually suggested.

DIETARY MODIFICATIONS IN PREGNANCY

The selection of a diet to meet the needs of pregnancy requires careful choices of foods but is not particularly complicated. For the pregnant woman whose diet has conformed to the "Basic Four" food pattern, it is merely a matter of emphasizing the more nutrient-dense foods within each of the four food groups. (Nutrient-dense foods are those that give reasonable amounts of nutrients per calorie consumed.) Women who have not followed such a pattern before becoming pregnant must develop a new set of food choices. Because these women may enter pregnancy with depleted nutrient stores, it is even more important that a diet adequate in all nutrients be started as early as possible. Mothers who have had problems in previous pregnancies—miscarriages, premature deliveries, or low-birth-weight infants—should pay particular attention to their diets.

It must be emphasized that nutrition is only one of many factors that will determine the health of the baby. However, it is also one of the few factors over which the mother herself has complete control. Most women are concerned enough about the health of their offspring to have high motivation to "eat right." Pregnancy is perhaps the most effective time to attempt nutrition education. The ways in which the nutritive needs of pregnancy are met will vary depending on the preferred food habits or likes and dislikes of each woman. Canada's food guide for pregnancy, in the box below, provides a dietary plan on which to build a nutritionally adequate diet, applicable in most western countries.

Besides modifying the normal diet pattern to accommodate different quantitative needs for nutrients during pregnancy, other modifications may be indicated. From the fifth to the fourteenth week of pregnancy, 75% of women experience nausea due to hormonal changes; when appetite is disturbed, the consumption of smaller

Canada's Food Guide for Pregnancy

Food Group	Number of Servings Daily
Milk and milk products	3–4
Breads and cereals	8–10
Fruits and vegetables	6–10
Meat, fish, poultry, and alternates	2

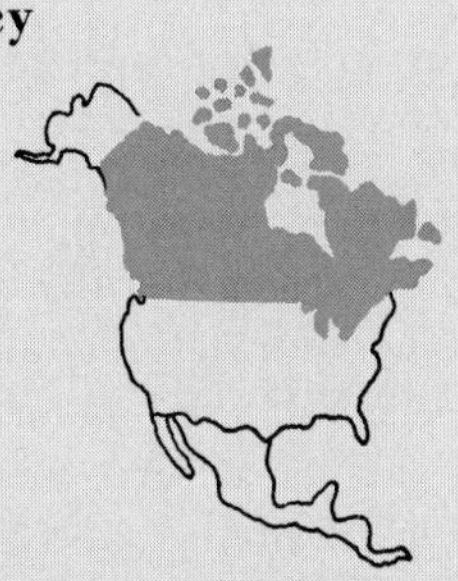

Notes

- This food guide provides 2200 to 2400 kcal. It meets the needs of the average, healthy Canadian woman in the second or third trimester of pregnancy.
- When choosing "extra" foods, such as cakes, cookies, or desserts, select those with nutritional value.
- Sodium (salt) should not be restricted. Moderate amounts may be used at the table and in cooking.
- 2 to 3 Tbsp. of fats and oils (for example: butter, margarine, salad oils) are recommended daily to improve the absorption of fat-soluble vitamins.
- Adequate fluid intake, 6 to 8 glasses including water, is important each day. Reduce alcohol intake. Use caffeine sources (coffee, tea, chocolate, and soft drinks) in moderation.
- The need for vitamin-mineral supplementation is individual. Before taking any supplement, discuss this with a dietitian/nutritionist, public health nurse, or doctor.
- Ask your doctor for a referral to a dietitian/nutritionist if you are underweight, a chronic dieter, very active, a teen, overweight, having twins or triplets.

Adapted from Nutrition for Pregnancy, British Columbia Ministry of Health Preventive Services, 1986.

and more frequent meals has been helpful to many women. This same pattern of consumption is also useful in the latter part of pregnancy when discomfort is experienced after large meals because of crowding by the fetus in the abdominal cavity.

In contrast, between the fourth and seventh months, many women experience an insatiable appetite. Eating a small meal just before hunger sensations usually become most severe has been a useful method of controlling total intake. Intake must be maintained at a level that results in a steady gain of 400 grams/week in the second and third trimesters. A diet relatively high in bulk and fluid may be helpful in maintaining normal gastric motility at a time when there is a tendency toward constipation.

The selection of a diet for pregnancy is complicated for many women who experience strong food dislikes and cravings. They often crave foods they do not ordinarily like or develop strong distastes for foods they previously liked. In some cases, the aroma or sight (even in ads) of a particular food evokes a strong reaction. Many times, the dislikes are for foods that have no nutritional consequences; however, should the dislike be for a food such as milk, which is the most reliable and frequently used source of calcium, nutritional consequences are of great concern. Similarly, most cravings such as those for pickles or fresh strawberries have few nutritional implications; however, if the craving is for calorie-dense foods such as chocolate cake and ice cream, there may be a problem of these foods crowding out more nutritious choices.

pica
Practice of eating nonfood items such as clay or coal; sometimes used to refer to unusual cravings for foods, such as often occur during pregnancy

Pica, or the consumption of nonfood items such as laundry starch, library paste, ice cubes, or clay, seems to occur more often in pregnancy than at other times. No one has come up with a physiological or psychological basis for these nonfood cravings, but they are well recognized and seem to occur most frequently among people with an iron deficiency. There is no evidence that the substances consumed contribute iron, however.

EFFECT OF NUTRITION ON PREGNANCY

The nutritional status of the mother at the time of conception is considered as important to the outcome of pregnancy as is the diet during pregnancy. Status at conception generally reflects long-standing food habits that change in relatively few women during pregnancy, in spite of the motivation prevailing at this time. Because of the influence of many nonnutritional factors such as maternal age, number of pregnancies, birth interval, and life-style factors such as use of alcohol, cigarettes, drugs, caffeine, and herbal teas, it is difficult to pinpoint specific dietary effects.

For more on Burke's study see Chapter 1.

The impact of the nutrition of the mother on the course of pregnancy and on the condition of the infant at birth has been the subject of many investigations, not all of which have led to the same conclusions. A now classic study by Burke points most conclusively to a relationship between maternal diet and the infant's well-being. The chance of a child with a high level of health being born to a mother with a good or excellent diet is much better than when the maternal diet is rated as poor or very poor. Studying Canadian women, Ebbs and his coworkers found a similar relationship; mothers on good diets experienced few complications during pregnancy and gave birth to infants with a greater chance of surviving the neonatal period. Somewhat later, however, investigators at Vanderbilt University (McGanity and others, 1969) failed to demonstrate a relationship between quality of maternal diet and the course and outcome of pregnancy; they believed that complications of pregnancy led to suboptimal intakes, rather than the converse. Although they found a relationship between diet and the course of pregnancy only at dietary intakes of less than 1500 kcal and 50 grams of protein, they emphasized that these findings should not be interpreted to mean that good nutritional practices should not be encouraged. None of the subjects in their study had notably suboptimal diets; therefore they may have entered pregnancy with good enough nutritional status to provide a buffer against the stress of pregnancy.

In 1959 in an English study, Thomson was unable to demonstrate any relationship between diet and the duration of gestation, birth weight of the infant, fetal malformation, perinatal death, or failure of lactation. This led to the conclusion that abnormalities of reproduction were not caused by dietary deficiencies. However, these data cannot be interpreted to mean that it is never possible for dietary inadequacies to cause abnormalities of pregnancy. A later review of 4300 obstetrical cases showed that incidence of prematurity, necessity for cesarean section, and perinatal deaths increased as the ratings for maternal health and physique dropped.

Since pregnant women consuming less than 1800 kcal/day are unable to maintain a positive nitrogen balance, the fetus can continue to grow and accumulate protein only at the expense of maternal tissue.

A widely publicized study in New York City (Susser, 1981) assessed the effect of dietary supplementation for high-risk women on the birth weight of their infants. The study failed to demonstrate a beneficial effect from a supplementary beverage providing 6 grams of protein and 322 kcal. There was actually a decline in birth weight when the supplement provided 40 grams of protein and 470 kcal; this latter group, however, had more premature infants and more neonatal deaths, possibly related to the higher incidence of intrauterine infection in the supplemented group. Supplemented mothers gained more than unsupplemented mothers. The diet did overcome the adverse effects of smoking on pregnancy outcome.

In contrast to these findings, an analysis of the results of using diet supplements with pregnant women at the Montreal Diet Dispensary (Higgins, 1976) showed that mothers who received food supplements of milk, orange juice, and eggs along with dietary counseling gave birth to slightly larger babies. However, supplements were less effective with mothers who had a previous problem with low-birth-weight infants. Similarly, an evaluation of the impact of the federally funded **WIC** program showed that providing vouchers for food supplements of iron-fortified cereal, milk, cheese, eggs, and fruit to women who had had low-birth-weight infants or had failed to carry a fetus to term resulted in decreased incidence of low birth weights. The earlier during pregnancy that the supplementation was available, the greater the benefits. Those who had been in the program for 7 to 9 months gave birth to infants weighing half a pound more than those who had not participated. The $1.2 billion invested in the program in 1984 was considered cost-effective because of savings resulting from hospitalizing a lower number of low-birth-weight infants.

WIC (Women, Infants, and Children) A federally funded program to provide nutrition counseling and supplemental food to pregnant women and to children who are considered at nutritional risk

The effect of diet preceding pregnancy can be illustrated from data on babies born during a period of wartime starvation in two countries: the Netherlands and Russia. In the Netherlands study, babies born during a hunger period had been conceived before that period by mothers whose previous diets had been good. Although these babies were shorter and 10% lighter than babies born to mothers whose diets were adequate throughout pregnancy, there were fewer stillbirths, premature infants, and congenital malformations compared to babies conceived during the hunger period. This indicates the protective effect that a good diet before pregnancy can exert during the course of pregnancy. In contrast, mothers whose babies were born during the siege of Leningrad and whose diets had been poor preceding pregnancy experienced a stillbirth rate double the normal rate, a 41% incidence of prematurity among live births, and a 31% incidence of neonatal deaths among low-birth-weight infants. A reduced rate of conception also occurred.

Many other studies have suggested that the better the state of the mother's nutrition before or at the time of conception, the greater the chance of normal pregnancy leading to the birth of a healthy child.

Nutrition-Related Concerns in Pregnancy
Pregnancy-induced hypertension
Exercise
Drug use
Aspartame
Nausea
Edema
Cigarette Smoking
Vegetarianism
Mothers over 35 years of age
Alcohol *(see Focus section)*
Caffeine *(see Focus section)*

NUTRITION-RELATED CONCERNS IN PREGNANCY

Pregnancy-induced hypertension (PIH). This condition occurs most frequently among women who are underweight at the time of conception, who fail to gain adequately in the early part of pregnancy, or who have a large and unexpected gain in the latter part of pregnancy. This condition is characterized by elevated blood pressure and is frequently accompanied by proteinuria, generalized edema, headache, and blurred vision. The treatment of PIH is quite different than that for nonpregnancy-related hypertension. Restriction of energy intake (weight gain) or salt intake and the use of diuretics all have adverse consequences such as reduced fetal weight and health complications during labor and delivery. Treatment involves bed rest. Women with PIH, also known as preeclampsia, who fail to correct the problem are at great risk of developing **eclampsia.** This is an advanced stage of PIH in which convulsive seizures in the mother place both the mother and infant at great risk.

eclampsia
The final and more severe stage of toxemia; it usually occurs toward the end of pregnancy, is characterized by convulsive seizures, and calls for induced delivery to reduce the risk to both mother and baby

Exercise. Many pregnant women continue to engage in active exercise programs throughout their pregnancy. In addition to having higher energy needs than in the nonpregnant state, they are more susceptible to hypoglycemia and to loss of fluids during exercise. They are therefore advised to avoid exercising on an empty stomach and to drink fluids both before and during exercise. They do have less constipation and fewer varicose veins. Strenuous exercise should be avoided since it causes the blood flow to be diverted to the exercising muscle causing as much as a 25% decrease in blood (and hence oxygen) reaching the uterus. There is also some danger of fetal damage when the mother's body temperature rises during exercise and causes an increase in fetal temperature—especially during the first trimester or when fetal heart rate increases or decreases following maternal exercise. Strenuous, but not moderate, exercise has also been associated with low-birth-weight infants in a few studies. On the other hand women in good physical condition have normal or improved birth outcomes.

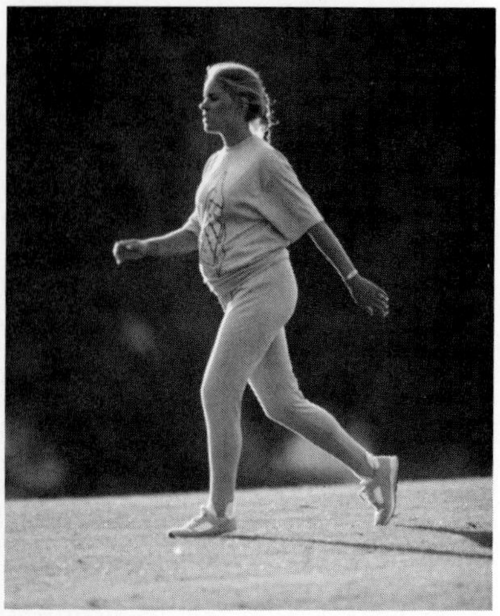

Recommendations for Exercise During Pregnancy
- "Moderate" exercise is acceptable
- Keep pulse rate below 140 beats/minute
- Limit "workouts" to 15 minutes or less, 3 times weekly
- If any pregnancy-related health problem is present, do not exercise
- Recommended activities are swimming, walking, and bicycling on a stationary cycle

Drug use. Although there is limited information on the adverse effects of either prescription or over-the counter drugs on the developing fetus, they often affect the intake, absorption, and metabolism of nutrients and, hence, the nutritional status of the mother. While the therapeutic benefit from the use of a drug must be weighed against any possible risks to the fetus or mother, no drugs should be taken during pregnancy without adequate medical supervision. Similarly the use of herbal teas should be avoided since many have components that could have adverse effects on fetal development.

Aspartame. Although evidence suggests that the use of aspartame does not pose a problem to pregnant women, its use should be restricted to the levels below the accepted daily intake (ADI) of 50 mg/kg of body weight. The use of aspartame-sweetened beverages in place of those that provide energy and other nutrients may have nutritional consequences.

Nausea. Severe nausea during the early stages of pregnancy has nutritional implications for the mother who enters pregnancy with low nutrient stores. Whether it is the result of psychological or, more likely, physiological factors, it can sometimes be alleviated by smaller, more frequent meals, eating dry crackers before rising in the morning, and avoiding foods that have offensive taste or odor to the pregnant woman. Severe and continued nausea **(hyperemesis)** calls for hospitalization to control dehydration, electrolyte imbalances, or excessive weight loss.

hyperemesis
Severe and continuing nausea

Edema. Some edema, primarily in the extremities, occurs in the majority of pregnancies, especially in the third trimester. Since the cause is more hormonal than diet-related neither diet modifications or salt restriction is beneficial.

Cigarette smoking. Cigarette smoking has been shown to decrease infant birth weight and increase the risks of perinatal morbidity and mortality. The effects may be the result of toxicity of carbon monoxide, nicotine, or other constituents of tobacco, reduced blood flow to the uterus, or reduced maternal food intake.

Vegetarianism. Well-planned vegetarian diets consisting of a variety of plant foods along with milk and eggs are quite adequate to meet the nutrient needs of the pregnant woman. Less well-planned vegetarian diets may pose risks of less than adequate intakes of available iron, zinc, calcium, or vitamin B_{12} and of poor

Factors That May Impose Nutrition Risks on the Outcome of Pregnancy

- Undernutrition (that is, inadequate energy or nutrient intakes)
- Failure to gain adequate weight according to the recommended pattern
- Underweight or overweight prior to conception
- Multiple gestation
- Adolescent pregnancy
- Maternal age over 35 years
- Close birth intervals
- Restrictive diets (that is, fad diets or vegan eating styles)
- Pathological hyperemesis
- Poor reproductive history
- Low socioeconomic status
- Existence of chronic systemic diseases/infection (diabetes, hypertension, renal disease, inborn errors of metabolism, allergies, anemia, chronic liver or bowel disease)
- Food cravings/aversions, pica
- Smoking
- Substance abuse (for example, alcohol, vitamins, or other drugs)

From Dept. of Health and Welfare, Canada, 1987.

quality protein. "New vegetarians" who avoid only some meats or animal foods are at minimum risk of dietary inadequacies.

Age. Women who enter pregnancy over 35 years of age have nutritional needs reflecting their longer medical history, the probable long-time use of oral contraceptives, and the possibility of a longer history of poor eating habits, which could be reflected in lower nutrient stores. Careful nutrition evaluation may reduce the risk of any nutrient-related poor pregnancy outcomes.

These and other risk factors involved in pregnancy are outlined in the box above.

LACTATION

Early Feeding Decisions

At or before the time of birth, the mother must make a major decision: how to feed the infant for the first 3 to 6 months of life. For the majority of mothers, it is a choice between breast feeding or bottle feeding with a modified cow's milk formula. For a few whose infants are allergic to cow's milk, the option will be between breast feeding and bottle feeding with goat's milk or a soy-based formula. In spite of the well-documented nutritional, psychological, physiological, and social advantages of breast feeding, in 1988 only slightly over 60% of the mothers of newborns had chosen breast feeding at time of discharge from the hospital. Although a decision to breast feed may be changed at any time, a decision to bottle feed can seldom be changed after the first few days of life. The Surgeon General's 1990 Objectives for the United States calls for having 75% of infants breast-fed at the time of hospital discharge and 35% breast-fed at 6 months of age.

For many mothers, this decision is an emotional one, possibly influenced by the opinions of husbands, mothers, doctors, peers, and friends. Interestingly, most women make this decision very early—many times in early adolescence, well before conception, and seldom later than early pregnancy. For those who do not have a total commitment to their decision, the attitudes of nurses, doctors, and other medical personnel and the practices in the hospital (such as rooming-in and provision for immediate physical contact with the baby) may be critical in either reinforcing or reversing an earlier decision.

The decision to either breast-feed or bottle-feed an infant is one with far-reaching consequences for both the mother and the child. The advantages of breast feeding will be discussed in greater detail in Chapter 16. A very strong consideration for breast feeding is that it represents a satisfying emotional experience for the mother. Once the decision has been made, the likelihood of success depends on not only on the health and nutritional status of the mother but also on the mother's attitude toward breast feeding, her understanding of the process occurring during the **lactation period,** and the support and encouragement she receives from medical personnel and the family. Fortunately, those who choose bottle feeding have available to them many satisfactory and carefully formulated products that are well suited to the needs of most infants.

lactation period
Period in a woman's life when her mammary glands produce milk to feed her young infant

colostrum
The first fluid secreted by the human breast to nourish the infant

The first fluid secreted by the human breast, **colostrum,** is thin, yellowish, and watery and bears little physical resemblance to milk. However, it has its own unique nutritional composition (Table 16-5) and provides many immune substances to help combat infections. The flow of colostrum may not begin for 2 to 4 days after birth—a delay that is often erroneously interpreted as a failure of lactation. In the interval, the baby may be fed a glucose solution but only after it has been allowed to attempt to nurse, which may provide the stimulation necessary to initiate lactation.

Nutritional Needs

The nutritive demands for the mother during lactation far exceed those during pregnancy, although after birth the mother may cease to feel the responsibility of "eating for two." In 4 months, a normally developing infant doubles the birth weight accumulated in 9 months of pregnancy. This is evidence of the high demand that the breast-fed infant makes on the mother. Milk secreted in 1 month represents more kilocalories than the net energy cost during the whole pregnancy. Fortunately, some energy and many nutrients stored during pregnancy are available to support milk production. The recommended intakes for specific nutrients to permit the synthesis and secretion of enough good-quality milk (which provides the sole source of nourishment for the infant) are summarized in Table 15-2. Most of these recommended intakes are based on our knowledge of the amount of milk produced, its nutritional content, and the extent to which the mother has reserves that she can use to meet at least part of the requirement.

These recommendations for dietary intakes during lactation are based on even less data on quantitative needs than are recommendations for intakes during pregnancy. However, it is fairly well established that the recommended intakes will support the average daily production of 750 ml of milk. It is entirely possible that satisfactory lactation can be maintained on somewhat lower levels of intake, but we also know that many women produce much more than 750 ml of milk; some studies have reported as much as 1000 to 1200 ml daily.

foremilk
Milk secreted at the beginning of one nursing period

hindmilk
Milk secreted at the end of one nursing period

Analyses of human milk have shown considerable variation in composition, not only among women but also in the same woman over time. The amount of some nutrients varies not only from day to day but from one time of day to another. In addition, the milk secreted first in any one nursing, known as **foremilk,** frequently differs nutritionally from that secreted at the end of that nursing period, known as **hindmilk.** For some nutrients, the composition remains constant. The fact that many mothers, especially in developing countries, can maintain a prolonged and satisfactory lactation period on diets well below currently accepted standards is baffling; it suggests that we need to reappraise the ability of lactating women to adapt to limited intakes.

In general, the total energy, protein, fat, and carbohydrate content of mother's milk is relatively constant. If energy or protein is lacking, there will be a reduction in milk volume rather than in milk quality. At very low protein intakes the proportion of casein may be reduced. The availability of more protein or more energy will not enhance the amount of protein in the milk nor increase the volume of milk beyond what is needed for the infant.

Although the total amount of fat in breast milk is not influenced by the mother's diet, the composition of the milk fat reflects the composition of the mother's diet. The content of the polyunsaturated fatty acids parallels that in the mother's diet; medium-chain fatty acids predominate when carbohydrate is the major energy source, and longer-chain fatty acids predominate when fat is a major energy source.

For some nutrients such as calcium and iron, the mother whose diet has been adequate before and during pregnancy has stores that can be used to maintain the quality of the milk if her postpartum intake fails to provide enough of the nutrients. The quality of the milk is relatively independent of the mother's intake for these nutrients, as long as reserves last. For vitamin A, however, the content in human milk reflects the diet of the mother, even though there may be reserves in the liver.

Amounts of both thiamin and vitamin B_6 in human milk reflect almost immediately the amounts in the mother's diet. A mother may produce milk with marginal or even inadequate amounts of both vitamins. Women who have used oral contraceptives for more than 30 months prior to conception have difficulty producing milk with sufficient vitamin B_6 without the use of a supplement of 2.5 to 5 mg/day. For most other water-soluble vitamins, low dietary intakes will result in the secretion of less milk rather than milk of an inferior quality. Except for folacin, vitamin B_{12}, and vitamin B_6, the amounts of vitamins in milk do not continue to increase with higher intakes. Although relatively little is transferred, the amount of fat-soluble vitamin D in breast milk reflects the mother's intake and exposure to sunlight; vitamins A and E reflect maternal intake alone.

Nutritional Needs of Lactating Woman Relative to Pregnant Woman

- Increased
  - Energy
  - Vitamin A
  - Thiamin
  - Riboflavin
  - Niacin
  - Vitamin E
  - Zinc
  - Iodine
- Decreased
  - Protein
  - Folacin
  - Vitamin B_6
- Unchanged
  - Calcium
  - Iron
  - Magnesium
  - Phosphorus
  - Vitamin D

Because trace elements cannot be synthesized, any that appear in breast milk must be provided by the mother. There is as much as a 15-fold difference in the amount of trace elements in milk from different mothers. There is little reason to believe that it is possible to transfer excessive amounts of trace elements to human milk. Iodine, which is needed to prevent goiter, is transferred efficiently and in adequate amounts, but fluorine, which is effective in enhancing resistance to tooth decay, is not.

Sodium appears in human milk in response to the mother's intake. In fact, some mothers have stopped breast feeding because they thought their milk was "too salty."

The energy required for lactation will be proportional to the amount of milk produced. The average 750 ml (25 oz) of milk secreted each day, with 67 kcal/100 ml, will contain 502 kcal. Because the mother is about 90% efficient in synthesizing this milk, approximately 550 kcal are required each day for milk production. It is assumed that about 200 kcal can be obtained from the fat stored during pregnancy. Therefore an additional intake of 350 kcal over normal needs should permit adequate daily lactation. In addition to the energy cost of milk production, the mother may need more calories because of her increased activity in caring for a small child. The recommended energy intake (REI) is 500 kcal over normal needs. Since the recommended increase in calorie needs for lactation is considerably smaller than the increase suggested for many minerals and vitamins (Table 15-2) this means that the extra energy must come from foods of high nutrient density—nonfat milk, eggs, fruit, vegetables, and enriched or whole-grain cereals. The amoung of extra energy needed for lactation is almost twice the extra energy needed for pregnancy, so it is appropriate for the nursing mother to add more food to her diet. The extra 20 grams of protein needed are readily available in the usual North American diet. The increases suggested can be met by the equivalent of an additional meal of approximately 500 kcal of protective foods each day, but again a moderate level of supplementation may be indicated.

Riboflavin

Milk is one of the most dependable sources of riboflavin in the adult diet, and human milk provides this vitamin for the infant. The mean content of riboflavin in milk is 0.04 mg/dl, which reflects dietary intake. This amount requires that 0.34 mg of riboflavin be transferred to human milk each day. Because only 70% of additional riboflavin is utilized in milk production, the nursing mother should increase her daily intake to 0.5 mg above normal. Four glasses of milk per day should be adequate.

Vitamin C

The amount of vitamin C in human milk is higher than that in cow's milk. Because of losses during heat processing, cow's milk cannot meet the vitamin C needs of the infant after the first 2 weeks. The recommended 100 mg of vitamin C for the mother is easily obtained from two servings of citrus fruit or juice.

Vitamin B_6

The amount of vitamin B_6 in human milk responds very rapidly to changes in the mother's intake. Only 4% of a maternal intake is transferred to breast milk, which results in milk with a level of vitamin B_6 barely adequate to prevent convulsive seizures in the infant. Maternal intakes of 2.5 to 5 mg, difficult to achieve from dietary sources alone, result in milk with a vitamin B_6 content that is considered optimal for normal infant growth. Long-term users of oral contraceptives have a special need for such a supplement if they are to provide the 35 μg of vitamin B_6/100 kcal in breast milk that the Academy of Pediatrics recommends for infants.

Folacin

The high incidence of folacin-deficient megaloblastic anemia in lactating women suggests that lactation drains maternal reserves. This problem is complicated by the fact that folacin deficiency is the most prevalant nutritional problem during pregnancy, with the result that many women enter lactation with practically no reserves.

Vitamin B_{12}

The ingestion of vitamin B_{12} is reflected in an increase in the vitamin in human milk from 1 to 6 days later.

Vitamin A

Although most infants have a fair reserve of vitamin A stored in their liver at the time of birth, human milk provides both vitamin A and related carotenoids. An intake of 6000 IU (1200 RE) of vitamin A, easily achieved by the mother's regular use of green and yellow vegetables, allows production of milk with 70 RE or IU/dl, which is sufficient to meet the needs of the infant.

Vitamin D

Vitamin D is needed to protect the infant against rickets. Because relatively little fat-soluble vitamin D is transferred to the mother's milk (1 IU/dl), breast-fed infants must receive protection through exposure to sunlight and from a dietary supplement. A daily intake of 400 IU of vitamin D, the amount in 1 quart of fortified milk, is considered adequate for lactating women.

Vitamin K

Although the amount of vitamin K in breast milk is not sufficient to provide for the needs of the infant, it can be increased by the addition of vitamin K to the mother's diet. However, vitamin K given to the mother is not transferred to her milk until the fourth day postpartum, which is too late to give the infant protection against postnatal hemorrhages during the critical first few days of life. Therefore breast-fed infants are given a supplement of natural vitamin K either orally or by injection immediately after birth.

Contaminants

The extent to which drugs, pesticides, herbicides, and other contaminants are transferred to mother's milk and their effects on the infant are poorly understood. When DDT (which can be stored in body fat) was more generally used, there was considerable concern that it might reach dangerously high levels in a mother's milk during her first lactation.

Oral contraceptives lead to lowered milk production, and sedatives lead to a decrease in the strength of the infant's sucking reflex. In fact, because it appears that almost all drugs taken by the mother appear to some extent in her milk (with variable and largely unknown effects), the safest advice is for the mother to avoid the use of all drugs during lactation. Certainly they should be taken only on the advice of a physician. Alcohol is found in human milk in relation to the amount used by the mother. The small amount associated with an occasional moderate drink has a minimal sedative effect on the infant and is probably relatively harmless. More frequent use of alcohol, however, should be avoided.

Contaminants That May be Found in Breast Milk
Drugs
Herbicides and pesticides
Alcohol
Heavy metals

Dietary Supplements

In view of the very high levels of nutritional intake needed for normal lactation it is probably a sound practice to recommend the mother's continued use of her prenatal supplement. However, supplements providing therapeutic levels of some nutrients and insignificant amounts of others cannot be endorsed. In addition, we should not minimize the importance of a varied and balanced diet to provide new mothers with dietary fiber, good quality protein, and trace elements that cannot be found in most supplements.

Stimulation

Many techniques have been suggested to stimulate lactation. The milk flow of lactation can be initiated only after the infant has begun to suck at the breast; vigorous sucking stimulates both the anterior and posterior pituitary glands (Figure 15-5). The former gland produces the hormone **prolactin,** which stimulates milk production. The latter releases the hormone **oxytocin,** which stimulates the "let-down" reflex whereby the smooth muscles surrounding the **alveoli** of the nipples contract to allow the release of milk. As the result of pain, emotions, or embarrassment, the let-down reflex may sometimes be inhibited; the action of oxytocin counteracts this. Oxytocin also acts on the walls of the uterus after birth, causing strong contractions that help it return to its normal size. The effect of these hormones is shown in Table 15-6.

Almost every culture has its own medicinal or food **galactagogues,** which are substances believed to stimulate lactation. These include garlic, cottonseed, candy, large quantities of milk, and sometimes small quantities of beer or ale. Whether or not they are effective is uncertain.

The relationship between the mother's fluid intake and volume of milk secreted has not been established. Even when fluid intake is low, the volume secreted remains constant. A decreased intake of fluids limits milk production only when total intake is less than the volume of milk produced. Drinking water beyond the level of natural thirst decreases milk secretion because of its action on pituitary hormones, which regulate milk production. Although high intakes do not stimulate milk production,

prolactin
A hormone produced in the anterior pituitary gland; it stimulates the production of milk in response to emptying of the breast at a feeding

oxytocin
A hormone produced in the posterior pituitary gland; it stimulates the release of milk from the breast in response to sucking by the infant

alveoli
Part of the ductal system of the breast into which milk is secreted and from which it is "let down"

galactagogue
Medicine, food, or treatment used to stimulate the flow of milk in lactation

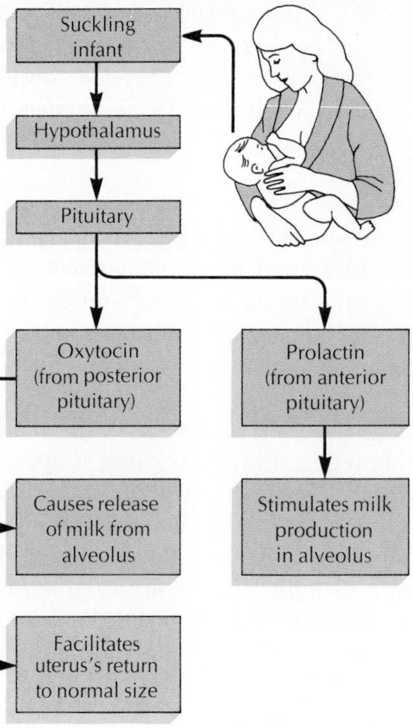

Figure 15-5 Suckling by infant initiates hormonal changes that lead to milk production and the let-down reflex, which releases milk.

Table 15-6 ◇ Hormonal control of lactation

Hormone	Source	Function
Estrogen	Ovary	Stimulates breast development during pregnancy
Progesterone	Placenta	Stimulates milk production
Prolactin	Anterior pituitary gland	Stimulates milk production
Oxytocin	Posterior pituitary gland	Let-down reflex

liberal fluid intake is suggested for general maintenance of good health in the mother.

Food Avoidance

There are widespread beliefs, not based on any sound data, that lead many lactating women to avoid certain foods. One study reported that 59% of lactating women avoid cabbage, beans, garlic, and onions; 52%, chocolate; 21%, alcohol; and 18%, carbonated beverages on the grounds that these foods produce gas or colic in their infants. Because there are no nutritional disadvantages and some advantages to limiting intakes of many of these foods, there is little concern when they are excluded from the diet. Another study showed that the use of milk by mothers of sensitive infants also produced colic.

Success and Duration

Many attempts have been made to predict the success of lactation. Some evidence suggests that the output of milk is directly proportional to the mother's metabolic size (body weight in $kg^{3/4}$)and that a strong positive correlation exists between the rise in temperature of mammary skin caused by nursing and milk supply. Other studies have shown that the course of lactation is established by the end of the first week, at which time the daily output should reach 500 ml. There is little doubt that a positive attitude on the part of the mother and the support that she receives from family and friends are determining factors in the success of breast feeding. Although a great many undernourished women do succeed in breast feeding satisfactorily, those who were severely malnourished in childhood may have impaired development of secondary sex characteristics, resulting in inadequate mammary tissue.

The length of the breast-feeding period varies depending on a great many factors, both social and physiological. Mothers in higher socioeconomic and educational groups breast-feed their infants more frequently and for longer periods; however, currently only one infant in five is breast-fed for 6 months in the United States.

Some mothers terminate lactation when the amount of milk produced declines to the point that extensive supplementary feeding is required, no longer making it feasible to breast-feed.

In many cultures, breast feeding continues for 2 to 3 years, with milk as the only, although nutritionally inadequate, source of food for a year or more. In other cultures, breast milk may be supplemented with other foods as early as 3 or 4 weeks. This early supplementation may lead to less vigorous sucking, which in turn results in a reduction in milk output and usually early weaning. Mothers of these infants experience an earlier return to a regular pattern of ovulation, with subsequent pregnancies occurring sooner.

Breast feeding has merit as a contraceptive method because when sucking is strong for a prolonged period, both ovulation and the return of a regular menstrual cycle are delayed. At least half of the first postpartum menstrual cycles do not involve the production of an ovum (egg). The risk of pregnancy during **amenorrhea** (absence of menstruation) caused by lactation is initially 5% but increases with each cycle. The use of artificial methods of contraception influences the course of lactation, with oral contraceptives inhibiting lactation. Nutrition plays a role in human fertility in several ways. The undernourished woman has a delayed menarche, longer adolescent sterility, irregular menstrual cycle, longer amenorrhea during lactation, and an earlier menopause.

amenorrhea
Absence of menstruation

• • •

This chapter has dealt with decisions and conditions that influence the health of a developing child from conception through the neonatal period. The next chapter will concentrate on the nutritional choices that are important throughout the whole period of early infancy—a time when these choices are made entirely by the mother or caretaker.

BY NOW YOU SHOULD KNOW

- The health of the infant is determined by the nutritional status of the mother before, as well as during, pregnancy.
- The nutritional needs of the pregnant woman are greater than her normal needs but less than the needs of the mother and fetus combined.
- Low-birth-weight infants are at greater risk of illness within the first year of their lives than are infants that weigh over 5.5 pounds at birth.
- Physiological adaptations such as decreased gastric motility and increased intestinal absorption occur to make the mother more efficient in using the nutrients in her diet.

- Growth of the fetus in the first 3 months of pregnancy amounts to a weight of only about 1 oz. However, it is during this period, when cells differentiate, that the quality of the mother's diet and the reserves that she brings to pregnancy are major determinants of fetal development.
- Because the increase in requirement for calories during pregnancy is proportionately less than the increase in requirement for other nutrients, the mother must choose foods carefully from among nutrient-dense sources.
- The need during pregnancy for all nutrients except iron and folacin can be readily met from the diet. Women are advised to use a supplement to ensure an adequate intake of these two nutrients and possibly to balance amounts of other vitamins and minerals.
- Weight gain during pregnancy should be between 22 and 27 pounds.
- Use of alcohol and caffeine should be kept to a minimum during pregnancy.
- Over 60% of women now choose to breast-feed their infants because of the nutritional, immunological, and psychological benefits.
- The Surgeon General's 1990 Objectives for the United States calls for 75% of infants breast-fed at the time of hospital discharge and 35% at 6 months of age.
- Needs of lactating women are higher for most nutrients than they are for pregnant women. However, needs for protein and folacin are less during lactation than during pregnancy.
- Because of the nutritional demands on the lactating woman, she is encouraged to continue taking a prenatal vitamin/mineral supplement.

STUDY QUESTIONS

1. Define the following terms: placenta, amniotic fluid, intrauterine growth retardation, uterine milk, implantation, organogenesis, fetus, pregnancy-induced hypertension, eclampsia, macrocytic anemia, colostrum, and lactation.
2. What are the particular nutritional needs of each trimester of pregnancy and of lactation?
3. How does the fertilized ovum develop into a viable infant?
4. How do the amount and pattern of weight gain influence the outcome of pregnancy?
5. List the reasons why a woman should not gain too little or too much weight during pregnancy.
6. Describe the way in which the fetus receives nourishment during gestation.
7. If a pregnant women is complaining of constipation, what dietary recommendations would you propose to her?
8. What are the precautions a pregnant woman should take to guard against osteomalacia?

Applying What You've Learned

1. **Assess Dietary Adjustments**

   Talk with at least two pregnant women about the dietary adjustments they have made during pregnancy and the reasons for these changes. Ask them about any distinct changes in their likes and dislikes of particular foods.

2. **Modify Your Diet for Pregnancy and Lactation**

   Whether you are male or female keep a record of what you eat for 1 day. Using the Canada's Food Guide for Pregnancy found on p. 467 modify your food intake to meet the needs of a pregnant woman in her first, second, and third trimester of pregnancy. What foods would you change to get the needed nutrients while keeping within the gradual increase of calories? Finally, modify food intake to meet nutritional needs for lactation.

3. **Vegetarian Menu**

   Plan three vegetarian meals and two snacks for a lactating woman.

4. **Assess Your Diet**

   List the foods or beverages in your present diet that would be recommended for pregnant women. List the foods that would not be recommended for pregnant women.

5. **Personal Interviews**

   Talk with your mother, grandmother, or aunt about her experiences during pregnancy, such as diet, exercise, food cravings, prenatal vitamins, morning sickness, and beliefs.

SUGGESTED READINGS

Council on Scientific Affairs, American Medical Association: Fetal effects of maternal alcohol use, Journal of the American Medical Association 249:2517, 1983.

This article is the report of an eight-member committee that reviewed the literature on fetal alcohol syndrome and other consequences of alcohol use during pregnancy. It presents a thoughtful, well-articulated summary of our current knowledge of the subject. It also points to the importance of an effective education campaign among young women to help eliminate overuse of alcohol as one entirely preventable cause of mental retardation.

Kennedy ET, Gerschoff S, Reed R, and others: Evaluation of the effect of the WIC supplemental feeding on birth weight, Journal of the American Dietetic Association 80:220, 1982.

This paper demonstrates the importance of dietary intervention early in pregnancy for women who may be at nutritional risk. It is based on an evaluation of a federally funded program that provides food supplements or vouchers for food to women throughout the course of pregnancy and to any high-risk children up to 4 years of age.

King JM: Dietary risk patterns during pregnancy. In Weininger J, and Briggs G, editors: Nutrition update, vol. 1, New York, 1983, John Wiley & Sons.

This article focuses on the three dietary patterns—insufficient food intake, poor food selection, and poor food distribution throughout the day—that lead to nutritional problems in pregnancy, primarily problems of energy imbalance and iron-deficiency anemia. It explains the links between these dietary patterns and clinical problems, and it presents four principles for guiding pregnant women in food selection.

Nichols BL, and Nichols VN: Nutrition in pregnancy and lactation, Nutrition Abstracts and Reviews 53:259, April, 1983.

This article, written by researchers at the USDA Children's Research Center, presents a straightforward and well-documented summary of the "state of the art" of nutrition in pregnancy and lactation. Dealing with each nutrient individually, it documents the current research and is a valuable tool for the student who wants more detail from an authoritative source.

Worthington-Roberts, B: Nutritional support of successful reproduction: an update, Journal of Nutrition Education 19:1, 1987.

This well-documented, comprehensive review of the influence of a host of environmental and nutritional factors on the outcome of pregnancy covers the role of early nutritional experiences, general prenatal nutrition, weight gain, energy requirements, protein controversies, vitamins and minerals, alcohol, and caffeine. A highly recommended reading, it discusses some of the rationale behind the more recent theories and the evidence to support them.

ADDITIONAL READINGS

Pregnancy

American Council on Science and Health: Alcohol use during pregnancy, Nutrition Today, p. 29, Feb., 1982.

Bailey LB, Mahan CD, and D'Imperio D: Folacin and iron status in low-income pregnant adolescents and mature women, American Journal of Clinical Nutrition 33:1997, 1980.

Beagle WS: Fetal alcohol syndrome: a review, Journal of the American Dietetic Association 79:274, 1981.

Belizan J, and Villar J: The relationship between calcium intake and edema, proteinuria, and hypertension gestosis: an hypothesis, American Journal of Clinical Nutrition 33:2202, 1980.

Brown JE, and Toma RB: Taste changes during pregnancy, American Journal of Clinical Nutrition 35:716, 1981.

Burke BS, Stevenson SS, Worchester J, and Stuart HC: Nutrition studies during pregnancy. V. Relation of maternal nutrition to condition of infant at birth: study of siblings, Journal of Nutrition 38:453, 1949.

Council on Scientific Affairs, American Medical Association: Fetal effects of maternal alcohol use, Journal of the American Medical Association 249:2517, 1983.

Dwyer J: Vegetarian diets in pregnancy and lactation: Recent studies of North Americans, Journal of the Canadian Dietetic Association 44:26, 1983.

Ebbs JF, Tisdall FF, and Scott WA: Influence of prenatal diet on mother and child, Journal of Nutrition 22:515, 1941.

Higgins AC: Nutritional status and the outcome of pregnancy, Journal of the Canadian Dietetic Association 37:17, 1976.

Hingson R, and others: Effects of maternal drinking and marijuana use on fetal growth and development, Pediatrics 70:539, 1982.

Huber, AM, Wallins LL, and DeRusso P: Folate nutriture in pregnancy, Journal of the American Dietetics Association 88:791, 1988.

Kennedy ET, Gerschoff S, Reed R, and others: Evaluation of the effect of the WIC supplemental feeding on birth weight, Journal of the American Dietetic Association 80:220, 1982.

King JC, Stein T, and Doyle M: Effect of vegetarianism on the zinc status of pregnant women, American Journal of Clinical Nutrition 34:1049, 1981.

Kurrpa K, and others: Coffee consumption during pregnancy and selected congenital malformations: a nationwide case-control study, American Journal of Public Health 73:1397, 1983.

Leader A, Wonk K, and Keitel M: Maternal nutrition in pregnancy. I. A review, Canadian Medical Association Journal 125:545, 1981.

McGanity WJ, and others: Pregnancy in the adolescent, American Journal of Obstetrics and Gynecology 101:773, 1969.

Mitchell M, and Lerner E: Factors that influence the outcome of pregnancy in middle-class women, Journal of the American Dietetic Association 87:711, 1987.

Naeye RL: Maternal blood pressure and the outcome of pregnancy, American Journal of Obstetrics and Gynecology 14:780, 1981.

Param RR: A new hypothesis on the etiology of essential hypertension and preeclampsia, Medical Hypothesis 18:193, 1985.

Pike RL, and Smicklas HA: A reappraisal of sodium restriction during pregnancy, International Journal of Gynaecology and Obstetrics 1:1, 1972.

Rossett HL, Weiner L, and Edelin KC: Treatment experience with pregnant problem drinkers, Journal of the American Medical Association 247:1429, 1982.

Rush, David, and others: The National WIC evaluation: evaluation of the special supplemental food program for women, infants, and children, American Journal of Clinical Nutrition 48:389, 1988.

Sandstead HH, Bodwell CE, Weaver F, and others: Maternal nutrition and fetal outcome, American Journal of Clinical Nutrition 35: 697, 1981.

Stearns G: Nutrition status of mother prior to conception, Journal of the American Medical Association 168:1655, 1958.

Susser M: Prenatal nutrition, birthweight, and psychological development: an overview of experiments, quasi-experiments and natural experiments in the past decade (review), American Journal of Clinical Nutrition 34: 784, 1981.

Taffel SM, and Keppel KG: Advice about weight gain during pregnancy and actual weight gain, American Journal of Public Health 76:1396, 1986.

van Bereest ECH, Schaafsma G, and de Waard H: Oral calcium and blood pressure, American Journal of Clinical Nutrition 44:883, 1986.

Widdowson EM: Fetal and neonatal nutrition, Nutrition Today 22(5):14, 1987.

Lactation

Adequacy of lactation in well-nourished mothers, Nutrition Reviews 40:136, May, 1982.

Brown RE: Breast-feeding and family planning: a review of the relationships between breastfeeding and family planning, American Journal of clinical nutrition 35:162, 1982.

Butte NG, Garza C, Stuff JE, Smith EO, and Nichols BL: Effect of maternal diet and body composition on lactational performance, American Journal of Clinical Nutrition 39: 296, 1984.

Byrne J, Thomas MR, and Chan GM: Calcium intake and bone density of lactating women in their child-bearing years, Journal of the American Dietetic Association 87:883, 1987.

Chan GM, Roberts CC, Folard D, and Jackson R: Growth and bone mineralization of normal breast-fed infants and the effects of lactation on maternal bone mineral status, American Journal of Clinical Nutrition 36:438, 1982.

Chan GM, Ronald N, Slater P, Hollis J, and Thomas MR: Decreased bone mineral status in lactating adolescent mothers, Journal of Pediatrics 101:767, 1982.

Greer FR, and Garn SM: Loss of bone mineral content in lactating adolescents, Journal of Pediatrics 101:718, 1982.

Hollas BW, Roos BA, Draper HH, and Lambert PW: Vitamin D and its metabolites in human and bovine milk, Journal of Nutrition 11:1240, 1981.

Jelliffe DB, and Jelliffe EFP: The volume and composition of human milk in poorly nourished communities. A review, American Journal of Clinical Nutrition 31:492, 1982.

Kirksey A, Ernest J, Roepke J, and Tsai T-L: Influence of mineral intake and use of oral contraceptives before pregnancy on the mineral content of human colostrum and more mature milk, American Journal of Clinical Nutrition 32:30, 1979.

Kramer M: Do breastfeeding and delayed introduction of solid foods protect against subsequent obesity? Journal of Pediatrics 98 (6):883, 1981.

Lactation, maternal nutrition and fertility, Nutrition Reviews 40:268, 1982.

Lunn PG, Austin S, Prentice AM, and Whitehead RG: Effect of improved nutrition on plasma prolactin concentration and postpartum infertility in lactating women, American Journal of Clinical Nutrition 39:228, 1984.

Miranda R, Saravita NG, Ackerman R, Murphy N, Berman S, and McMuray DW: Effect of maternal nutritional status on immunological substances in human colostrum and milk, American Journal of Clinical Nutrition 37: 632, 1983.

Rogan WJ, Bagniewska A, Damstra T: Pollutants in breast milk, New England Journal of Medicine 302:1450, 1980.

Sampsom DA, and Jansen GR: Protein and energy nutrition during lactation, Annual Review of Nutrition 4:43:1986.

Sneed SM, Zare C, and Thomas MR: The effects of ascorbic acid, vitamin B_6, vitamin B_{12}, and folic acid supplementation on the breast milk and maternal status of low socioeconomic lactating women, American Journal of Clinical Nutrition 34(7):1338, 1981.

The vitamin D activity of milk, Nutrition Reviews 40(1):27, 1982.

FOCUS Pregnancy—The Alcohol/Caffeine Dilemma

Up until 1973, pregnant women enjoyed the occasional alcoholic beverage and their morning cup of coffee without any concern about possible adverse effects on the children they were carrying. At that time, the publication of a research report describing fetal alcohol syndrome (FAS) caused pregnant women to think twice about the consequences of what had been considered safe drinking practices. A similar concern about the safety of caffeine-containing beverages arose as a result of a report to the FDA, which concerned the effects of caffeine among soft drink users.

Infants born with FAS (Figure 15-6) have characteristic facial malformations. They are usually below the third percentile in height, weight, and head circumference and suffer from retarded mental and motor development. The symptoms as described in the 1973 study were distressingly similar to those that had been recognized 5 years earlier in children of alcoholics but were now being seen in children of moderate drinkers, that is, those drinking 1 to 2 oz of alcohol or even less per day.

Further study led the Surgeon General to issue an advisory in 1981 that each pregnant woman should be told about the risk of alcohol consumption, counseled to avoid drinking alcoholic beverages, and urged to become aware of alcohol in food and drugs. Almost simultaneously, the Bureau of Alcohol, Tobacco, and Firearms asked the liquor industry to fund an educational campaign to increase awareness of the hazards of excessive use of alcohol during pregnancy. The bureau's concern was the result of findings that infants of mothers who used as little as 1 oz of alcohol/day were smaller than other infants and that there were more spontaneous abortions associated with the use of 1 oz/day. Infants of mothers who were heavy drinkers (3 oz/day) frequently exhibited FAS.

There was little controversy about the risks of heavy drinking, but there were considerable differences of opinion about the dangers of moderate drinking and about what constituted moderate drinking. To try to answer these questions and to separate the effects of other behaviors such as smoking or poor eating habits have been the goals of at least six major surveys and two major studies. Survey results based on the responses of at least 65,000 women showed a positive correlation between maternal alcohol consumption and the risk of fetal abnormality. Depending on the population group, the incidence of abnormality ranged from 1 in 300 to 1 in 2000 live births and affected 30% to 40% of infants of alcoholic mothers. Stillbirths were found to be twice as prevalent in women who had at least three drinks a day, and spontaneous abortions occurred in these same women three times as often as they did in those who had one drink or less per day. Few children are able to overcome the deficits in growth associated with maternal heavy drinking, but many do show some improvement in IQ. Malformations, however, will undoubtedly be life-long. Results of studies of 462 children showed a clear relationship between maternal alcohol use and impaired infant development after adjusting for the effects of nicotine and caffeine. The smallest quantity of alcohol associated with FAS was 2.5 oz/day

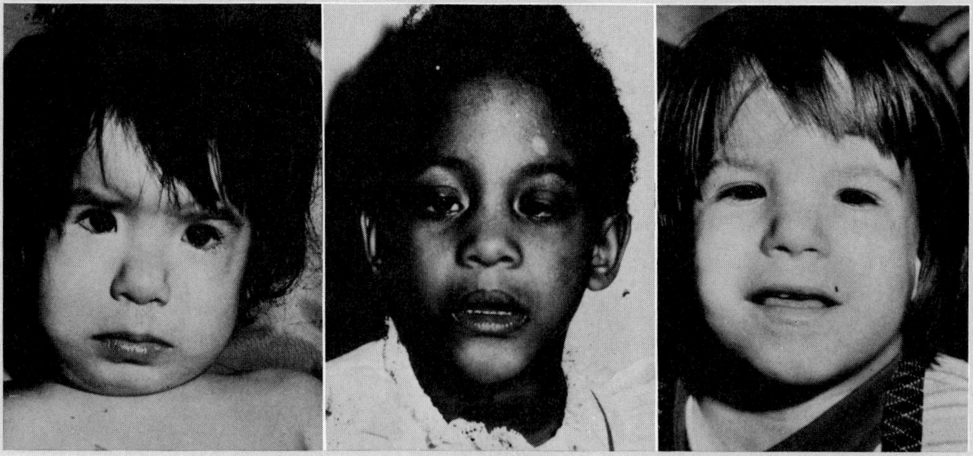

Figure 15-6 Children with fetal alcohol syndrome (FAS) from three different racial backgrounds: *(left)* American Indian, *(center)* black, and *(right)* white. All are mentally retarded.
From Streissguth A, and others: Science 109:353, 1980. Copyright 1980 American Association for the Advancement of Science.

throughout pregnancy, and the shortest period of drinking that resulted in FAS was the first 8 days of pregnancy. Mothers who had been drinkers before conception placed their children at greater risk than did those who drank only during pregnancy.

Although there are no data from humans, results of animal studies indicate that binge drinking at critical times in fetal development can also have tragic consequences. Until we have more information on the critical level above which there is significant risk, women of childbearing age should be advised that the only safe choice during pregnancy is abstinence. They should also be aware that the teratogen (or substance responsible for fetal abnormalities) is alcohol and that beer and wine can have effects that are just as serious as those of hard liquor. On the other hand, with minimal risk associated with the use of 1 oz/day, it would be unfortunate if women attributed all their infants' birth defects, growth retardation, or hyperactivity to use of alcohol during pregnancy.

We know that alcohol passes rapidly from the mother to the fetus. The fetus then retains it longer, presumably lacking sufficient alcohol dehydrogenase to start using, or metabolizing, it. The alcohol is excreted into the amniotic fluid, from which it is removed very slowly.

FAS is a completely preventable condition; young women should be sensitized to it before they are likely to conceive. The social cost of the resulting mental retardation makes it imperative to conduct an extensive educational campaign in high school, through physicians' offices, and in outlets where alcohol is sold. On the other hand, the American Council on Science and Health feels that a recommendation of complete abstinence without consideration of other risk factors (such as smoking) is unrealistic and unnecessary and places an undue burden of guilt on the pregnant woman. They believe that 1 oz of absolute alcohol (two 12-oz glasses of beer, two 4-oz glasses of wine, or two mixed drinks) is a safe upper limit. However, they do caution against binge drinking.

The evidence for any effects of caffeine on the developing fetus is much less convincing. Evidence is based almost entirely on studies of rats, mice, and rabbits, in which it was shown that intakes of caffeine as low as 80 mg/kg of body weight caused some irreversible defects in developing fetuses. At intakes as low as 6 mg/kg, less serious and more reversible defects were noted. The most frequently observed problems involved bone malformation, problems in the development of fingers and toes, and cleft palate. Because we know so little about the relative metabolism of caffeine across species, there are many unanswered questions about whether it is possible to extrapolate from animal studies to human studies.

If indeed the effects of caffeine are comparable, it would require the consumption of 25 to 35 cups of regular coffee with the highest caffeine content, 75 to 100 cups of tea, over 50 12-oz cola drinks, or an inconceivable amount of decaffeinated coffee to provide 80 mg of caffeine/kg of body weight for a woman weighing 110 to 132 pounds (50 to 60 kg). Even if there are detectable effects in some women at 6 mg/kg, it is unlikely that there will be problems with moderate consumption of coffee or cola drinks. Certainly a pregnant woman is placing neither herself nor her fetus at any significant risk if she restricts her daily intake to 4 to 6 cups of coffee. Similarly, moderate use of cola drinks leads to no significant risk. A Finnish study of 466 pairs of mothers of infants with and without deformities could find no difference in the incidence of deformity between mothers who had at least 4 cups of coffee and those who drank less. (There are 100 mg of caffeine in a cup of Finnish coffee, compared to 80 to 155 mg in a cup of coffee in the United States.)

Until we have definitive studies on humans, the possibility of an association of birth defects with the excessive use of coffee or cola drinks should not be ruled out. In the meantime, the FDA urges pregnant women to be prudent in their use of caffeine and, if given a choice, to avoid it.

As is true regarding the use of almost any food, moderate or prudent use of either alcohol or caffeine in pregnancy is wise. Because the possibility of minimal risk does exist, however, abstinence from alcohol and the limited use of small amounts of caffeine should reduce the risk to almost zero.

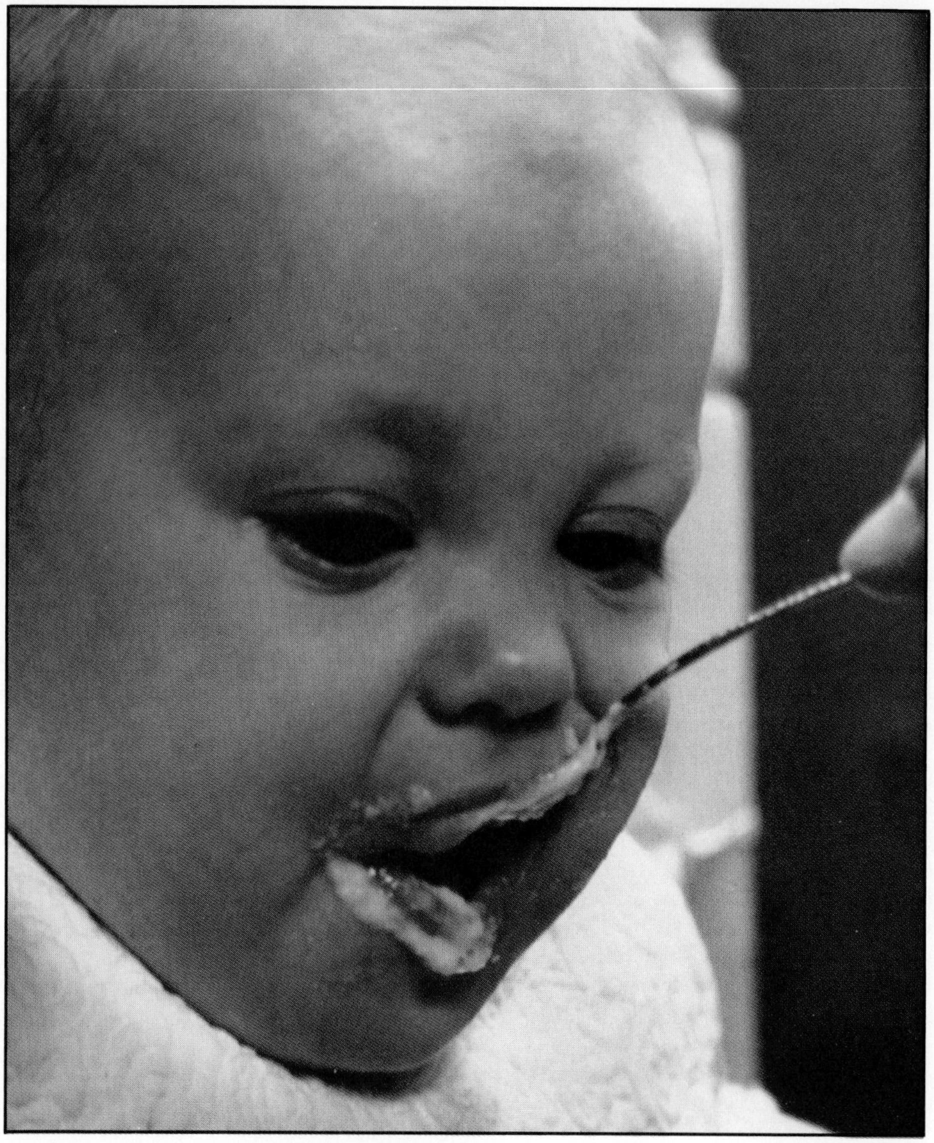

AWARENESS CHECK

Truth or Fiction?

- Breast feeding is always the best method of infant feeding.
- Solid foods should be introduced in the third month of life.
- Putting a baby to bed with a bottle of milk is a recommended pacifier that will keep the child from crying.
- Breast feeding can be an expensive form of infant feeding because of the actual food dollar spent on the foods needed to meet the increased calorie and nutrient needs of the mother.
- Whole milk or cow's milk is not recommended during the first 6 months of life.
- By 6 months of age milk alone cannot provide all the calories needed by the infant.

Infant Nutrition

CHAPTER 16

Although we cannot overemphasize the importance of the mother's nutrition during gestation in helping to ensure the health of her infant at birth, the infant's nutrition during the first year of life is also critically important. Most of the mother's time with her infant in the first 3 months is spent feeding the baby. Similarly, most of her concerns are about feeding, and most of her satisfactions come from seeing the child accept food, thrive, and grow. As nutritionists have learned more about the effect of early nutrition on later development and have discovered more sensitive ways of assessing the immediate consequences of different feeding patterns, recommendations have been modified. Although we know that the infant is amazingly resilient and will thrive on many different feeding regimens, we continue to look for the method that will increase the chances of optimal health throughout life.

Nutrition in an infant's first year has long-term consequences affecting health throughout life, largely because it is during this period that growth, development, and maturation occur more rapidly than at any other time. The adequately nourished infant is more likely to achieve normal physical and mental development. An infant who is inadequately nourished in one or more nutrients may suffer from stunted growth and a range of biochemical changes that adversely affect development.

The impact of any nutritional deficiency on an infant's health depends on when the deficit occurs and how long it lasts. Many problems can be prevented if the inadequacy is corrected within a critical period, but if it is delayed too long, the consequences will be more or less permanent. The critical periods and critical nutrients vary from one body tissue to another; for example, most brain growth, for which both protein and cholesterol are essential, occurs in the first 2 years and most tooth development, requiring calcium, phosphorus, and vitamins A, D, and C, occurs in the first 6 years of life. Therefore it is during such critical periods that we must be most concerned about the nutrients uniquely needed by a particular tissue.

Success of Nutrition in Infancy Depends On

- Choice of breast feeding or bottle feeding
- Timing of introduction of solid foods
- Monitoring of growth, morbidity, and nutritional status

Phases of Infant Feeding
Breast or bottle feeding
Transitional feeding
Modified adult diet

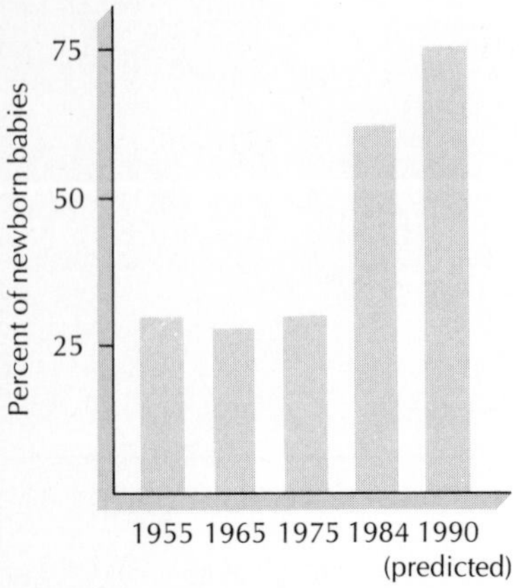

Changes in the incidence of breast feeding, 1955-1990 (predicted)

The success of early nutrition depends on the choice of early feeding methods, correct use of nutrient supplements, the pattern and timing of introduction of solid food, and careful monitoring of growth, morbidity, and nutritional status. Each of these choices is determined by a complex of social, environmental, economic, and behavioral variables, as well as nutritional considerations. Because there are many gaps in our knowledge about optimal nutritional practices, pediatricians and nutritionists have sometimes made seemingly contradictory recommendations. The more we learn, however, the closer the agreement on appropriate infant feeding practices. In the meantime, fortunately, healthy infants seem to thrive on quite diverse feeding practices. The long-term consequences of these may yet prove important, even though the differences are subtle and hard to identify in the short term.

Infant feeding practices should be considered in three overlapping phases: the nursing period, when breast milk or an appropriate formula is the sole source of nutrients; a transitional period, when specially prepared foods are introduced; and a modified adult period, when the majority of nutrients come from food available from the family table. One criterion, but not the only, of dietary adequacy is growth. It is expected that a full term infant will double its birth weight in 4 to 6 months and triple it in 1 year.

Percentage of Mothers Breast-feeding in 1983

College graduates	78%
Incomes over $25,000	71%
Incomes under $10,000	44%
Over age 35	60%
Under age 20	41%
Black	32%

Breast Feeding is Higher Among
College-educated women
More affluent women
Nonsmokers
Mothers who were breast-fed themselves

BREAST FEEDING

The one aspect of infant feeding on which there is almost complete agreement is that breast feeding is superior for practically all infants. In spite of this, and because reasonable alternatives are available, it is important that women not be coerced into breast-feeding. They should not be made to feel guilty if they choose not to breast-feed.

Breast feeding in the United States was an almost universal practice at the turn of the century, but by 1971 only 25% of mothers were breast-feeding. By 1976 more mothers were breast-feeding at the time of discharge from the hospital; by 1984 the percentage had risen to 62%, with a projection that by 1990 over 75% of mothers would use this method, a level already reached in the western United States.

Studies show that the women more likely to breast-feed are older and more educated and are from higher socioeconomic groups. They are also more likely to be concerned about environmental influences on health, to feel "natural is best," and to be nonsmokers. Other studies have shown that women report feeding their children in the way in which they themselves were fed. Current data show 27% of infants in the United States, compared to 12% in 1965, are breast-fed until 6 months of age. Thus it appears that more women are choosing to breast-feed and are also using this method of feeding for a longer period compared to 20 years ago.

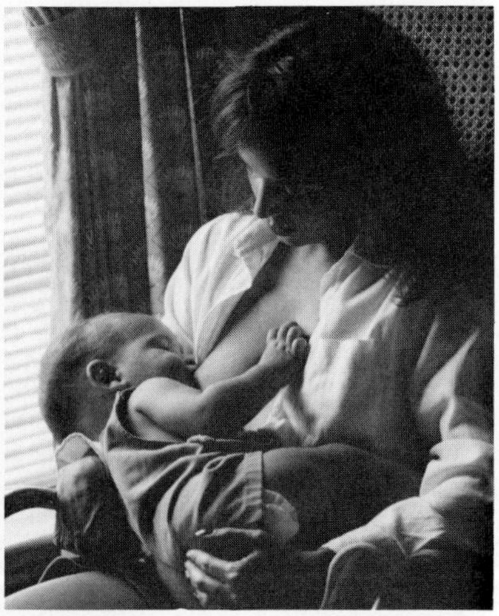

Many nutritionists advocate breast feeding not only for its nutritional benefits but also because of its roles in protecting against infection and promoting mother-infant bonding.

The pattern of feeding established by the better-educated group is frequently followed several years later by less-educated mothers and those of lower socioeconomic status. Current trends toward breast feeding are being reinforced by the recommendation from pediatricians that breast milk, or modified cow's milk formula, if breast feeding is impossible, be the *sole* source of nutrition for the first 4 to 6 months of life and the major source for 1 year.

The decision to breast-feed is influenced by consideration of the health benefits for the baby, the fact that it fosters a close relationship between mother and baby, and the belief that it is the "natural" thing to do. One study showed that over half the mothers chose their feeding method before pregnancy, 86% by the end of the first trimester, and all by the last trimester. This points to the wisdom of directing education programs to girls early in their schooling rather than waiting for them to receive information from a physician, which may have little influence on the choice.

Although many factors are involved, the lower incidence of breast feeding in developed countries compared to developing countries has been attributed to the large number of women who are working outside the home, the availability of acceptable substitute methods, and the lack of medical guidance and support. However, each mother usually makes the decision after considering the relative merits of breast versus bottle feeding, since either should be successful in a Western culture. In developing countries the situation is quite different. There suitable alternatives are too costly for most families, the water supply is often a source of contamination, refrigeration is unavailable, and knowledge of **aseptic** techniques for handling the formula is limited. If the child is to survive the neonatal period, breast feeding is almost essential. Failure to breast-feed results in the loss of one of a country's best natural resources—breast milk. However, when breast feeding is absolutely impossible, formula feeding, properly used, will be a life-saving alternative.

aseptic
Sterile; free from contamination

The following sections explore the relative advantages and disadvantages of breast feeding.

Considerations Favoring Breast Feeding

Nutritional Factors

In general it is believed that the nutrient composition of the milk of each species is best suited to the growth needs of its offspring, and when possible it should be used. If this is not possible, the milk of another species should be modified to approximate the composition of the maternal milk.

Factors Influencing Early Feeding Decisions
Nutritional
Immunological
Psychological
Economical
Physiological

The difference in nutritive composition of human and cow's milk is well documented; some aspects are presented in Figure 16-1 and Table 16-1. This shows that breast milk contains more of some nutrients and less of others, whereas for

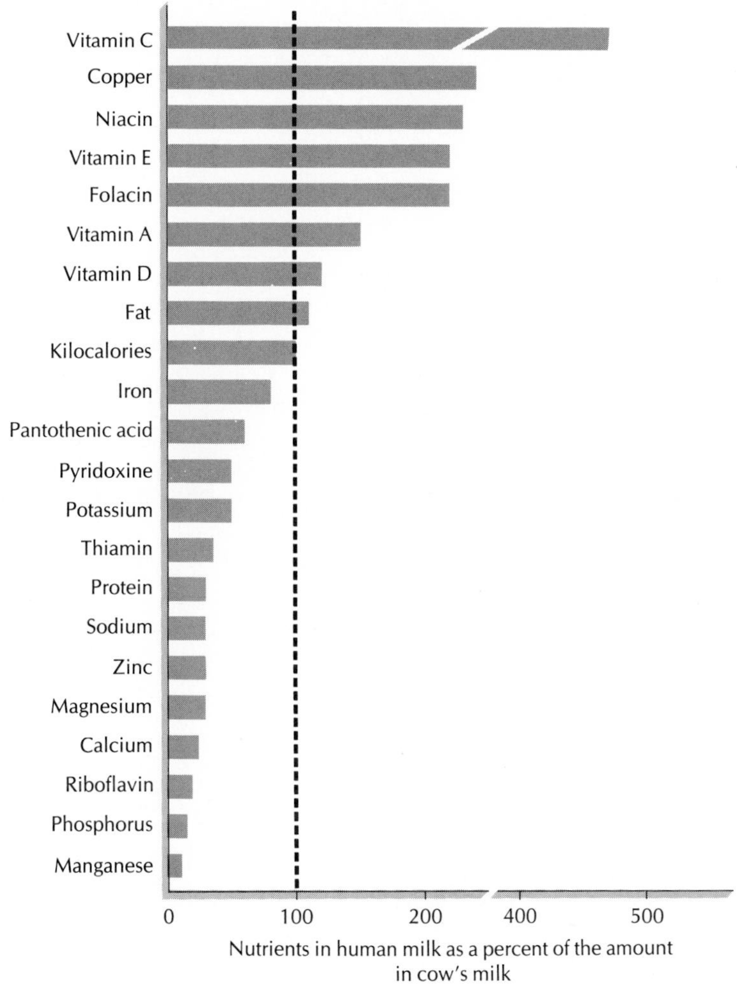

Figure 16-1 Differences in composition of human breast milk and cow's milk. Vertical dotted line represents the amounts in cow's milk, always considered 100% for each nutrient; solid bars represent the amounts in human milk relative to cow's milk; solid line represents the amounts in formula.

Based on data from Lonnerdal B: Composition of human milk, normative data. In Handbook of Nutrition, Evanston, Ill., 1985, American Academy of Pediatrics.

Recommendations for Early Feeding of Infants

Breast feeding completely for 4 to 6 months

Introduction of solid foods by 6 months

Transition to table foods when child shows readiness

some the composition is very similar. In addition, some nutrients are available in the form best suited to the digestive capacities of the offspring. The lower concentration of some nutrients in breast milk such as calcium and protein, is believed to reflect the differing growth needs between the human infant and the calf. The latter doubles its birth weight in 2 months, whereas the human infant takes 4 months.

Energy. The caloric value of human milk and cow's milk is similar (20 kcal/oz), as is the total fat content of 3.2% to 3.5%. The lower protein content of human milk is compensated by a higher amount of lactose. Fat provides 51%, protein 7%, and carbohydrate 42% of the calories in human milk, compared to 45%, 21%, and 34% in cow's milk.

Newborn infants, whose primary energy source during gestation has been glucose, use up their stores of liver glycogen as a glucose source within 24 hours after birth. They then turn to glucose and fatty acids from the diet and from body fat

Table 16-1 ◇ Composition of colostrum, immature (transitional) and mature human milk, and cow's milk per deciliter of milk

	Human Milk					
Nutrient	Colostrum (1-5 days)	Transitional (Immature) (6-10 days)	Mature	Mature Cow's Milk*	Ratio Human : Cow's	Typical Formula
Energy (kcal)	58	74	72	69	1.0	70
Fat (g)	2.9	3.6	3.9	3.7	1.0	3.9
Lactose (gram)	5.3	6.6	7.2	4.8	1.5	
Protein (gram)	2.7	1.6	0.9	3.3	0.3	1.4
Casein (gram)	1.2	0.7	0.3	2.8	0.1	
Lactalbumin (gram)		0.8	0.3	0.4	0.8	
Calcium (mg)	31	34	30	125	0.25	51.0
Phosphorus (mg)	14	17	15	96	0.16	39.0
Zinc (mg)	0.4		0.16	0.37	0.3	0.5
Iron (mg)	0.09	0.04	0.03	0.04	0.8	1.2
Vitamins						
A (IU)	296	283	240	303	0.8	300
Carotene (IU)	186	63	45	63	0.7	
D (IU)			5	4	1.2	60
E (mg)	0.8	1.32	0.2	0.06	3.3	2.0
C (mg)	4.4	5.4	4.3	0.9	4.7	9.0
K (μg)			2.3			5.5
Folacin (μg)	0.05	0.02	0.52	0.23	2.2	10
Niacin (mg)	0.075	0.15	0.20	0.085	2.0	1.0
Pantothenic acid (mg)	0.183	0.288	0.18	0.30	.6	0.45
Pyridoxine (mg)			0.02	0.048	0.5	0.04
Riboflavin (mg)	0.029	0.033	0.035	0.16	0.2	0.1
Thiamin (mg)	0.015	0.006	0.014	0.042	0.4	0.05
Carnitine (mg)	1.1	1.6	1	2.1	0.5	
Sodium (mg)	21		15	49	0.3	23
Potassium (mg)	150		53	152	0.3	80
Chloride (mg)	115		42			50
Magnesium (mg)			4	13	0.3	4.1
Copper (μg)			24	10	2.4	60
Iodine (μg)			11	500	0.50	1000
Manganese (μg)			0.3	2.5	0.12	10
Selenium (μg)	4.1		2			

Adapted form Lonnerdal B: Composition of human milk. In Handbook of nutrition, Evanston, Ill, 1985, American Academy of Pediatrics.

Blanks indicate data not available.

**Mature cow's milk* is cow's milk of normal composition, produced after 2 weeks of lactation.

stores. Free fatty acids are released from triglycerides by a lipase present in human milk. They are the preferred source of energy for the infant heart throughout the suckling period. The switch to fatty acids calls for a source of carnitine to transport fatty acids. Newborns do not have a fully developed ability to synthesize carnitine. Therefore, they must obtain it from breast milk, from cow's milk-based formula, or from those soy-based formulas to which carnitine has been added. Bottle-fed infants whose formula does not contain carnitine often have an impaired ability to use fatty acids and to regulate body heat and as a result have elevated blood lipids.

Carbohydrate. The disaccharide lactose, present at a higher level in human milk, has several advantages over other carbohydrates: it facilitates the absorption of calcium and magnesium and favors amino acid absorption and nitrogen retention. Lactose is also critical as the only source of the monosaccharide galactose. Galactose is essential to the formation of **myelin,** which is in turn essential to normal nerve function.

myelin
Protective sheath that surrounds nerve fibers and protects their ability to transmit nerve messages

Although the low solubility of lactose makes it impractical for use in formula prepared at home, it is the carbohydrate added to all milk-based commercially prepared formulas. In soy-based formulas, sucrose, the added carbohydrate, not only does not provide galactose, but promotes the growth of bacteria that often cause gastrointestinal distress. Human milk contains a salivary-like amylase, which accounts for the breast-fed infant's ability to digest starch.

Protein. Human milk, in which the protein is predominantly lactalbumin, contains only one third as much protein as cow's milk, in which most of the protein is in the form of casein. The lactalbumin in human milk **whey** differs from the casein in cow's milk **curd.** It not only has an amino acid pattern that more nearly approaches that of body proteins, but it also provides more of the essential amino acids than does casein. Casein forms a hard curd when acted on by the enzyme rennin in the stomach, whereas lactalbumin forms a soft, flocculent curd that is more rapidly digested and absorbed by the infant.

Benefits of Human Milk Protein
More lactalbumin
Less casein
Higher cysteine/methionine ratio
Less phenylalanine
More taurine
More peptidase

whey
The fluid portion remaining when protein in milk precipitates out

Human milk protein has a higher ratio of the amino acid cysteine to methionine. This is important because the liver of the human infant lacks the enzyme necessary to convert methionine to cysteine, which is used as a sulfur-containing amino acid.

curd
The solid portion that forms when proteins in milk are precipitated

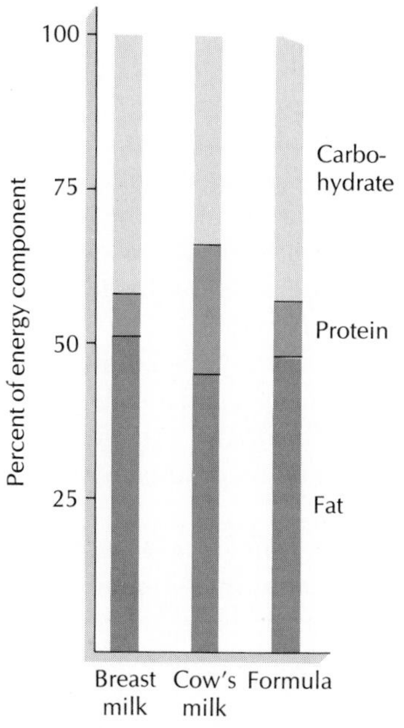

Comparison of energy components in different types of milk for infants

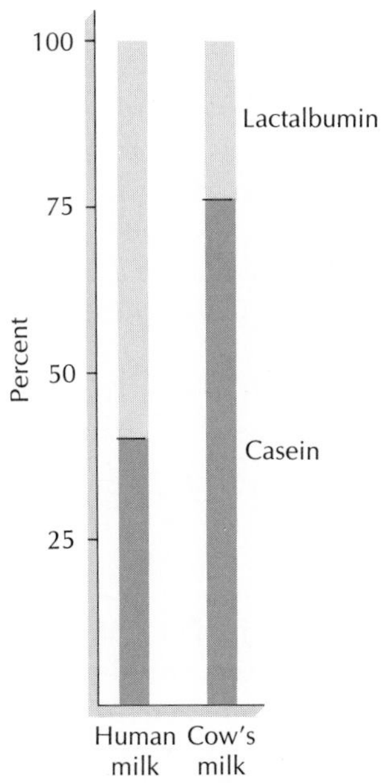

Comparison of amounts of types of protein in human milk and cow's milk

It also has a lower proportion of the amino acid phenylalanine, which is especially important for those infants with PKU, who can use only a small amount of this essential amino acid. In addition, 15% to 25% of its nitrogen, compared to 6% in cow's milk, is nonprotein nitrogen; the nutritional significance of this is unclear.

Taurine, the sulfur-containing amino acid, has recently been identified as a possible dietary essential for the development of the central nervous system in infants. It is present in adequate amounts in human milk of mothers fed an omnivorous diet but levels are low in cow's milk and the milk of vegans. Most infant formula based on either cow's milk or soy protein have taurine added (45 mg/liter).

The presence of a protein-splitting enzyme in breast milk reduces proteins to the less complex peptone stage, on which digestive enzymes act more effectively. These enzymes in cow's milk are destroyed by the heat of pasteurization.

Benefits of Human Milk Lipids
- Fewer saturated fatty acids
- More medium-chain fatty acids
- Fewer short-chain fatty acids
- More lipase
- Increased digestibility
- Palmitic acid on carbon 2 of glycerol molecule
- More linoleic acid
- Higher polyunsaturated/saturated fat ratio
- More fat in hindmilk
- Contains more cholesterol

Lipid. The fat in human milk, almost all of which is triglyceride, differs in several respects from that in cow's milk. Fatty acids in human milk are less saturated, are of medium-chain (10 to 14 carbons) formation, and are utilized more effectively than are the short-chain (8-12 carbons), more saturated fatty acids in cow's milk. About 95% of human milk fat, compared to 61% of butterfat, is digested. This results partly from a fat-splitting enzyme (lipase) in human milk.

Palmitic acid, when present in human milk, is present in the number 2 (middle) carbon position of the triglyceride, whereas in other milks it is attached in the number 1 or 3 position. Since human milk contains an enzyme that splits off the fatty acids in position 1 and 3, before the monoglyceride with the fatty acid attached in position number 2 is absorbed, there is little free palmitic acid available in the intestine of the breast-fed infant. This is desirable, since the free palmitic acid that will be released from cow's milk tends to interfere with calcium absorption.

The total lipid in human milk varies form 2% to 10%; it is uncertain if it is influenced by maternal diet. The fatty acid pattern of human milk, however, has changed as the dietary intake of fat in many Western countries has shifted from saturated animal fats to more unsaturated vegetable oils. Currently a higher proportion of the unsaturated fatty acids, linoleic and linolenic acid, contribute to an increasing P/S ratio in human milk. Human milk, in which linoleic acid accounts for 14% of the fat, protects the infant against a deficiency of essential fatty acid. The possibility of a deficiency of vitamin E, which is needed to prevent the oxidation of linoleic acid, is small. The intake of hydrogenated fats has been reflected in a higher amount of "trans" fatty acids in human milk. So far, it is unclear if the newborn can metabolize these as well as the naturally occurring "cis" forms.

The cholesterol content of human milk bears no relationship to maternal diet but is many times higher in mothers with hypercholesterolemia. The cholesterol content of human milk is important because very young infants are unable to synthesize cholesterol but need it for the formation of myelin as the nervous system develops. A little later, a dietary source of cholesterol is important so that the infant learns early in life to adjust the synthesis of cholesterol in the liver to complement that already provided in the diet to prevent its overproduction.

The increase in the fat content of human milk from the beginning of a feeding (foremilk) to the end (hindmilk) is believed to increase its satiety value and to make it easier for the breast-fed infant to regulate caloric intake and weight gain. Obviously, it is impossible for the fat content of cow's milk or formula to vary throughout the feeding.

Vitamins. In general, the vitamin content of human milk reflects maternal intakes and nutritional status. When the mother's supply of vitamins, either from body stores or from her diet, is low, the amount in milk is low and responds to dietary supplementation. When her supplies are high, the vitamin level in milk is high and, after reaching a plateau, is less likely to respond to supplementation.

Both vitamin A and vitamin D in breast milk are influenced by the mother's intake except when very large quantities are taken in. Mothers on strict vegetarian diets may have critically low vitamin D levels and may produce a milk that is incapable of preventing rickets in infants. A maternal intake of up to 100 mg vitamin C/day is reflected in milk. The content of riboflavin, pyridoxine, and vitamin B_{12} in human milk parallels the amount in the mother's diet. In contrast the folacin content remains stable regardless of maternal intake, unless the mother's diet has been very poor. Little is known about vitamin E in breast milk.

The amount of the heat-labile vitamins, thiamin, and vitamin C naturally occurring in human milk is almost completely available to the infant, whereas the higher amount originally in cow's milk may be substantially reduced as the result of the heat used in the pasteurization of milk and sterilization of the formula. The absorption of folacin is enhanced by a factor in human milk.

Minerals. Unlike vitamins, mineral content of human milk is minimally influenced by the mother's stores and immediate intake. This has been established for calcium, magnesium, phosphorus, iron, copper, zinc, sodium, potassium, and chloride. The manganese and selenium content is influenced by maternal intake. The calcium content of human milk, one fourth that of cow's milk, is well suited to the needs of the growing infant and contributes to a favorable calcium/phosphorus ratio of 2:1. Similarly, the low sodium content of human milk is advantageous to the infant, whose kidneys have difficulty handling excess sodium. Sodium content of breast milk declines from 640 mg/L in colostrum to 180 mg/L in milk at 3 months, but is influenced by mother's diet.

Benefits of Human Milk Minerals
Less calcium
Less sodium
Higher calcium/phosphorus ratio
Iron more available
Higher copper/zinc ratio

The phosphorous content of human milk is appreciably lower than that of cow's milk, providing only one sixth as much per liter or per 100 kcal, and one third as much per gram of protein. The low ratio of calcium to phosphorus in cow's milk may be a contributing factor in hypocalcemic tetany in formula-fed infants.

Trace elements. With advances in knowledge of the role of trace elements in nutrition, interest has increased in using breast milk as a standard to estimate the needs for infants and to provide a basis for formulating human milk substitutes. This is especially important, because certain processes used to modify cow's milk to more closely resemble human milk may result in the the removal of some of the trace elements. The use of distilled water by mothers concerned about environmental pollution may further reduce the amounts of these elements available to the bottle-fed child.

The iron content of human milk is quite low (0.4 mg/L) but has a much higher bioavailability (50%) than any other dietary source of iron. This higher availability of iron is attributed to the lactoferrin content of human milk. Because of this and the fact that most infants are born with a 3 to 6 month reserve of iron, breast-fed infants who have not had any significant blood loss, who are adequately nourished, and who do not have a higher than average rate of growth, do not need another source of iron until 4 to 6 months of age. Iron from fortified formula is less well absorbed. There is some evidence, however, that even before anemia is evident, iron deficient infants may show some behavioral changes associated with iron deficiency such as tension, decreased responsiveness to stimuli, and lethargy. Calculations that the infant needs to absorb 200 mg (0.55 mg/day) of iron over the first year of life further supports the notion that it is possible that human milk might be inadequate.

Human milk also contains a substance that enhances the absorption of zinc. Of recent interest is the observation that the high copper/zinc ratio (1:5) in breast milk compared to cow's milk (1:15) is associated with decreased cholesterol synthesis. There is no evidence of a copper deficiency in exclusively breast-fed infants.

For some elements, such as selenium, for which both a deficiency and an excess may be undesirable, the content in breast milk seems to be controlled within relatively narrow limits. Data from the analysis of human milk suggest that for such elements a certain minimum amount must be present in all breast milk. The upper limit may be up to 5 times the minimum for copper, 7 times for iron, and 17 times for zinc. Until more complete information is available, it will be impossible to judge whether formulas are indeed satisfactory substitutes for human milk in regard to trace elements.

Immunological Factors

immunity
Ability to resist or combat infection

Colostrum, the breast secretion that precedes the secretion of mature milk, differs from milk in appearance and nutritional properties. This watery, yellowish fluid contributes **immunity** to the infant through its effect in the gastrointestinal tract as well as after it is absorbed. Between the fifth and tenth day after birth, colostrum undergoes changes in chemical and physical composition, until by the tenth day it has usually assumed the characteristics of mature milk.

Immune Properties in Human Milk
- Lysozymes digest bacterial wall
- Peroxidases weaken bacterial cell wall
- Macrophages engulf and digest bacteria
- Macrophages synthesize complement, a protein
- Lactoferrin ties up iron needed by bacteria
- *Lactobacillus bifidus factor* discourages growth of infective bacteria
- Immunoglobulins combat infective organisms

After much work to identify the substances responsible for the anti-infective properties of human milk, nutritionists now believe that these are a group of substances called "colostrum particles," which are stable in the acid medium of the stomach and resistant to the digestive enzymes. Among these, lysozymes attack and digest the cell wall of bacteria after the bacteria have been inactivated by peroxides and vitamin C. Both human milk and the saliva of infants contain peroxides; vitamin C is present in colostrum. An enzyme, lactoperoxidase, acts by killing the *Streptococcus* organism.

The macrophages, which are large cells that are not absorbed, contribute to immunity in two ways. (1) They engulf and digest bacteria. (2) These cells also synthesize complement, a protein involved in establishing immunity to infectious organisms. These bacteria and viruses are responsible for such diseases as poliomyelitis, influenza, and diphtheria.

Lactoferrin, an iron-containing protein found in both colostrum and mature milk, inhibits the growth of *Staphylococcus* organisms and *E. coli* by tying up the iron they need for growth. If extra iron is added to the diet, the lactoferrin becomes saturated, and any additional iron is free to support the growth of infectious microorganisms. Thus infants whose diets are supplemented with iron could have increased susceptibility to infection.

A nitrogen-containing carbohydrate in human milk is known as *Lactobacillus bifidus factor*. It creates conditions in the gastrointestinal tract that encourage the growth of the microorganism *Lactobacillus bifidus*. By producing acetic or lactic acid from lactose, this microorganism depresses the growth of pathogenic or disease-producing organisms, thus decreasing the infant's susceptibility to infection. It also competes with undesirable *E. coli* and thus inhibits its growth. The factor in human milk is lactulose, a derivative of lactose known to occur in large amounts in breast milk and in higher amounts in heat-treated than in untreated cow's milk. The growth of *L. bifidus* is enhanced on a high-lactose, low-protein diet. The lactose/protein ratio is 7:1 in human milk, compared to 4:1 in cow's milk.

immunoglobulins
Antibodies that are not absorbed but are effective against viruses and bacteria in the gastrointestinal tract

A group of proteins in human milk called **immunoglobulins** also plays a major role in defending against infections. One of these, IgA, which is present in the highest concentration in the first few days of life, consists of many antibodies against viruses, bacteria, and other pathogens. It acts primarily in the stomach, and it is especially effective against those pathogens to which the mother is exposed, such as poliovirus, streptococcus, and pneumococcus. Immunoglobulins resist digestive enzymes and are stable at the high acidity (low pH) of the stomach. After 3 to 6 weeks this IgA is replaced by a related immunoglobin, secretory IgA, which appears in internal secretions and then in blood.

Some of the fatty acids and monoglycerides in human milk are able to penetrate the membranes of viruses and bacteria to destroy them. All of these factors contribute to what is called "passive immunity" in infants, meaning that, when children are breast fed, they have the protection they need without the use of any medicines or vaccines.

Psychological Factors

The psychological advantages of breast feeding have been freely discussed, but continue to be difficult to document. Certainly there are many emotional and psychological considerations in the decision to breast-feed or bottle-feed.

Women who are allowed close physical contact with their infants in the delivery room immediately following birth are more likely to breast-feed, and to do so more successfully, than mothers who are initially separated from their infants for 8 hours or more.

There is general agreement that the infant derives a sense of security and belonging in the early mother-child relationship or bonding from the warmth of the mother's body and from the comfort of being held rather than from the feeding process per se. A classic study with monkeys showed that those fed by a surrogate mother were as well adjusted as those fed by the real mother. Research with dogs and ducks has identified a critical period during the first few days of life when imprinting, or learning, which is remarkably resistant to modification, occurs. It may be that the impact of the mother's presence on the child in this critical period will be found to have implications for later development. So far psychologists have been unable to identify consistent differences in personality between bottle-fed and breast-fed infants. Breast feeding does, however, increase the mother's feeling of competence in dealing with her child. Some believe that the greater psychological advantages accrue to the mother, who feels that she is involved in a unique relationship with the child and is fulfilling her true maternal role for which there is no substitute.

Fertility Factors

Breast feeding has long been recognized as an important, although far from foolproof, factor in birth control. It appears that as long as a child is sucking vigorously at the breast the mother is very unlikely to return to a normal ovulation cycle. This probably results from the fact that prolactin, which stimulates milk production, also represses the synthesis of ovarian hormones. In developing countries, the interval between births decreases with the earlier introduction of solid foods to stimulate infant growth. In general, mothers whose infants are solely breast fed and who nurse at least every 6 hours do not begin to ovulate until 12 months after delivery. On the other hand, mothers of bottle-fed infants begin to ovulate and menstruate regularly by 6 months. The introduction of solid foods leads to a reduction in the strength of the nursing reflex and an earlier return to a normal ovulation cycle.

Breast feeding may prolong the period before conception can occur, but it does not provide total protection against becoming pregnant.

Other Factors

Scientists are constantly identifying new and different ways in which breast milk protects the young infant during the critical first months of life. The arguments favoring breast feeding are so compelling that in 1984 the Surgeon General set a goal of having 75% of all babies breast fed on discharge from the hospital by 1990 and 35% at 6 months.

The growth rate of breast-fed infants exceeds that of bottle-fed infants for the first 4 to 5 months of life. This may result from the protein-synthesizing properties of nucleotides in breast milk. After this period, bottle-fed infants experience a more rapid growth rate, but no differences between the two groups can be detected at 2 years of age.

Although the risk of breast cancer is lower among women who have had and breast-fed a child before they are 20 years of age and who later breast-fed more children, there is also evidence that cancer-producing viruses may be transmitted to the milk by mothers who have a family history of breast cancer. Formation of blood clots is also less common among women who breast-feed.

The list of other advantages of breast feeding is growing. The most relevant ones are listed in Table 16-2.

Contraindications to Breast Feeding

Since up to 50% of mothers choose alternate methods, it is obvious that either they see some advantages to alternatives or some objections or disadvantages to breast

Table 16-2 ◇ Additional advantages of breast feeding

Advantage	Explanation(s)
Infant's jaw is more fully developed and teeth are less crowded	Infant must work harder to extract milk from the breast than from the bottle
Less danger of contamination; no danger of incorrect formula	No need to mix formula or prepare bottle
Reduced likelihood of allergic reactions	Human milk proteins do not cause allergies
Reported lower rate of sudden infant death or cot death	Infant not sensitive to human milk protein, therefore there is less possibility of aspiration following regurgitation; or higher vitamin E in human milk may protect membranes in the lungs
No hypocalcemic tetany	Higher calcium/phosphorus ratio in human milk
Reduced renal solute load	Less urea and sodium to excrete
Less colic	Fats and proteins in human milk are more easily digested and less likely to create gastric and intestinal distress
Contains prostaglandins synthesized from fatty acids	Prostaglandins act to regulate many body processes
Provides epidermal growth factor (EGF)	Promotes growth of cells lining gastrointestinal tract and other rapidly growing tissues
Mother's uterus returns to normal size more quickly	Secretion of oxytocin during nursing stimulates uterine contractions
More rapid maturation of gastrointestinal tract	Many hormones and growth factors in human milk may be involved.

feeding. Among the latter are the mother's perception that she is failing to secrete adequate milk, the constant fatigue reported by many mothers, the lack of freedom to return to work or to a social life, the possibility of breast infection, and the mother's desire to quickly restore her figure to normal.

Contraindications to Breast Feeding
Cancer
Tuberculosis
Ingestion of DDT or PCBs
Transfer of drugs
Psychological breakdown

Some mothers abandon breast feeding early because they fail to understand that lactation may be delayed until 3 to 5 days after birth, that the physical appearance of colostrum is different from milk, and that their milk has not "turned to water." They may also have been unaware that there may be some physical discomfort from the engorgement of the breasts when milk first "comes in." The desire of mothers, for either economic or psychological reasons, to leave the hospital as soon as possible after delivery can mean that if lactation is not established shortly after birth, the mother will give up her plans in the interests of taking the infant home on a functioning bottle-feeding routine.

Contaminants

The possibility that unwanted substances will pass into the milk is a deterrent to some. The transfer of pregnanediol, a metabolite of the hormone progesterone, through the mother's milk can result in **hyperbilirubinemia** in some infants. The transmission of as little as 20% of any drugs taken by the mother, or any environmental contaminants, such as **PCBs**, to the infant, can present problems. Concern has subsided over high levels of DDT, PCBs, and other environmental contaminants in human milk as control over their use becomes more rigid.

hyperbilirubinemia
Presence of bile pigments in the blood

PCB (polychlorinated biphenyl)
A toxic industrial chemical that can accumulate in food (fish) through contaminated water

Drugs. Among the many drugs and other chemicals that should not be used by a nursing mother are the commonly used nicotine, caffeine, and amphetamines. The former causes shock, vomiting, rapid heartbeat, and diarrhea in the infant, while the latter two cause irritability and poor sleeping patterns. Some others suppress lactation. Tranquilizers are of particular concern, because they cause a child to suck less vigorously; this in turn can lead to a depressed secretion of milk. The presence of anticoagulants in human milk can increase the possibility of neonatal hemorrhaging.

Illness of Mother

Chronic or acute illness on the part of the mother may preclude breast feeding. Depending on the type and severity of the disease and its contagious nature, it may or may not be advisable for mothers with tuberculosis to breast-feed. Mothers who suffer from short-term infections such as mastitis may either be able to continue breast feeding during the duration of the infection and its treatment or may maintain lactation during this interval by pumping the breasts regularly until nursing can be resumed.

Economic Factors

Based on a USDA report outlining the extra food required by the nursing mother to provide the recommended 500 kcal, 0.4 grams of calcium, and 20 grams of high-quality protein over and above that suggested for non-pregnant, nonlactating women, the cost may be higher or lower than the cost of the formula needed by the infant—depending on whether a "liberal" or "thrifty" food plan is followed. On a liberal plan the addition of a quart of milk, 6 oz of orange juice, 2 slices of whole-wheat bread, 1 T of butter, and an egg provides the added nutrients at a cost of 82¢ per day ($5.74 per week) in 1988. On a low-cost food budget the USDA report considered the use of 3 oz of nonfat milk solids, 2 oz of cooking oil, 1 oz of enriched cornmeal, ⅓ pound of turnip greens, and a nutrient supplement every other day at a total cost of 45¢ per day ($3.15 per week). By comparison, as shown in Table 16-3, the cost of formula can range from $2.46 a week for a formula of evaporated milk and sugar to $15.75 a week for ready-to-use formula in individual 8-oz cans. The cost of equipment, such as bottles and sterilizers, has not been included. With inflation of food costs, absolute amounts will increase, but relative cost should not change appreciably.

Social Factors

For many mothers, the freedom and flexibility for professional and social life that bottle feeding affords are overriding considerations in the choice of feeding method. In fact, even among mothers who have had a satisfying breast-feeding experience, the loss of freedom and restriction of their social life are considered the prime disadvantages. Most mothers find, however, that an occasional bottle can be substituted with no problems for the child. The mother may experience some physical discomfort from the engorgement of the breasts when the infant does not remove

Table 16-3 ◇ Relative costs (in dollars) per week of breast feeding and bottle feeding (based on 750 ml/day)

Breast-feeding mother's food and supplement over nonlactating mother's	
Thrifty food plan	$ 3.15
Liberal food plan	5.74
Bottle feeding	
Whole fluid milk and sugar	2.85
Evaporated milk and sugar	2.46
Concentrated liquid formula (13 oz)	7.00
Powdered formula (1-pound can)	8.84
Ready-to-use formula	
Large can (32 oz)	10.65
Serving-size bottle (8 oz)	15.75

the milk on schedule, but pumping the breast is an easy solution to this dilemma. With more women in the work force, employers are taking many steps to meet the needs of lactating women. Among these are flex-time work schedules, on-site day-care centers, and the availability of nursing rooms where mothers can nurse their babies or express and refrigerate their milk. As a result, many mothers are able to successfully combine a career and social life with breast feeding.

BOTTLE FEEDING

Modified cow's milk formula. The availability of safe and satisfactory formula in which cow's milk has been modified to provide a suitable substitute for human milk leads many mothers to choose bottle feeding or a combination of breast feeding and bottle feeding. Whether the formula is prepared in the home or commercially, cow's milk must be modified to resemble human milk in nutrient composition and physical properties.

Modifications of Cow's Milk Needed
Dilute protein and calcium concentrations
Add carbohydrate
Decrease sodium
Replace butterfat with corn oil to increase linoleic acid

Dilution of cow's milk to provide a concentration of protein similar to that of human milk also causes a reduction in curd tension and leads to the formation of a softer, more flocculent curd that can be more readily digested by the infant's enzymes. Other methods of modifying the character of the curd used in place of, or in addition to, dilution include the use of pancreatic enzymes, heat treatment, the addition of an acid, such as citric acid, or acid-producing microorganisms, or the addition of alkali. One method seems to have a little advantage over another. The dilution of milk has the advantage of creating a calcium concentration more nearly approximating human milk and the disadvantage of reducing the caloric concentration to 20 kcal/oz. The addition of a soluble and readily usable carbohydrate, such as dextromaltose or sucrose, to soy-based formula and home-prepared formulas raises the caloric value to that of human milk. It fails, however, to provide the benefits of lactose, which is suitable for use only in commercially prepared milk-based products because of problems of getting it into solution. Most formulas provide 20 kcal/oz, so that infants consuming 25 oz (750 ml) receive about 500 kcal daily. If infants continue on formula after 6 months, it is probably desirable to limit its use to 1 quart (liter) per day to encourage the baby to consume other foods to provide a nutritionally balanced diet.

Reducing the amount of sodium in cow's milk or commercial formula to a level comparable with human milk is necessary to decrease the work for the infant's immature kidneys, which must excrete this electrolyte in the urine. Reduction of sodium is especially important when the baby is losing fluid as a result of excessive heat or diarrhea. This is accomplished by removing much of the sodium from cow's milk by dialysis. The possibility that essential trace elements may be removed at the same time must not be overlooked.

The linoleic content of human milk is simulated by replacing the butterfat (short-chain saturated fatty acid) with corn oil (long-chain unsaturated fatty acid). This fat is tolerated better by the infant and provides more adequate levels of linoleic acid. Substitution of butterfat with coconut oil, which has saturated fatty acids, has no advantages. Too high a level of PUFA, such as linoleic acid, however, increases the need for vitamin E. The use of medium-chain triglycerides improves fat absorption but results in decreased absorption of vitamins A and E.

Since most commercial preparations are based on nonfat dried milk, with vegetable oil added to provide the fat necessary to increase the caloric density, they contain almost no cholesterol. Nutritionists now believe that some dietary cholesterol should be provided, since it is needed for the synthesis of myelin, which surrounds nerve fibers and is essential for the normal functioning of the central nervous system. In addition, infants need to develop the ability to regulate cholesterol synthesis early in life. The fact that human milk does contain cholesterol suggests that is desirable in early life. But the presence of an inhibitor of cholesterol synthesis in the liver suggests that human milk provides enough.

The safety of bottle feeding has increased with greater awareness of the importance of aseptic techniques in the preparation of infant formulas. Sterilization of feeding equipment and formula has reduced disease caused by pathogenic organisms. Before it was recognized that microorganisms were the cause of disease, the hazards of bottle feeding were so great that infant mortality and morbidity rates were very high. In many parts of the world there is still significantly higher mortality and morbidity among bottle-fed infants than among breast-fed infants, but among infants born to middle-class parents in technologically developed countries, there is generally no significant difference. The increasing use of preprepared sterilized formulas in disposable bottles offers advantages of convenience and safety to those who can afford them.

The quality of infant formula is regulated by the FDA, which requires that each batch of formula be tested to assure that it meets minimal nutrient standards throughout the period of its shelf life and does not contain any contaminants such as heavy metals, pesticides, or carcinogens.

Whole cow's milk. Although at one time there was considerable support for the use of whole homogenized unmodified cow's milk in infant feeding, it is no longer considered appropriate for infants in the first 6 months of life because of the distribution of calories from carbohydrate, protein, and lipid. In addition, pasteurized cow's milk contains no vitamin C and very little iron. It is now evident that unmodified whole milk can cause stomach bleeding in infants up to 1 year of age and may be a factor in allergies in young infants, especially those whose parents have a history of allergies. The high sodium and protein content of whole milk causes an increased renal solute load that taxes the kidneys' ability to excrete the excess. For all these reasons, whole milk should not be used in the first 6 months or until solid foods are providing at least 200 kcal/day.

Whole Cow's Milk May Cause
Low vitamin C intakes
Gastric bleeding
Increased renal solute load
Allergies
High sodium and phosphorus intakes

Nonfat or skim milk. For some time nonfat milk was used in infant feeding on the theory that it would restrict weight gain and the tendency toward obesity and would eliminate any intake of cholesterol.

It is now evident that nonfat milk (less than 0.5% fat) feeding is undesirable in the first 2 years of life, primarily because of its low caloric density 11 kcal/oz (35 kcal/dl) compared to 21 kcal/oz (67 kcal/dl) in human milk. Although infants fed nonfat milk can increase their intake of milk and solids somewhat to gain some weight, they cannot increase their energy intake to 90 kcal/kg of body weight, the level necessary to prevent a significant loss of body fat. This is reflected in decreased skinfold thickness.

Nonfat Milk Feeding Not Recommended Because of
Low energy content
Lack of cholesterol
Lack of vitamin A, unless fortified
Lack of linoleic acid
High protein/energy ratio
High sodium
Low zinc and copper

If infants do take enough fat-free milk to meet their caloric requirements, the amount of protein and sodium ingested is too great. In addition, the lack of linoleic acid, an essential fatty acid, results in dermatitis and growth retardation. The lack of dietary cholesterol is also considered undesirable, since it is questionable whether infants are able to synthesize the amount needed for myelin formation. If the nonfat milk is fortified with vitamin A, there is little likelihood of a deficiency, unless lack of fat prevents its absorption. Since skim milk is not fortified with iron or copper, as are infant formulas, its use increases the chance of the infant developing anemia. In summary, the use of nonfat milk is considered inappropriate in infant feeding. The use of milk with 2% fat has many but not all of the same disadvantages.

A comparison of some of the characteristics of milks used in infant feeding is given in Table 16-4.

Mixed feedings (partial breast feeding). Because it is almost impossible for any mother to be present at every feeding, an occasional bottle feeding in place of breast feeding is not only acceptable but recommended. The feeding may be either breast milk that has been expressed (pumped or drawn out by hand) and frozen for later use or a commercially prepared formula. An infant accustomed to a bottle and nipple is less likely to reject them when it is either convenient or necessary to use a bottle later.

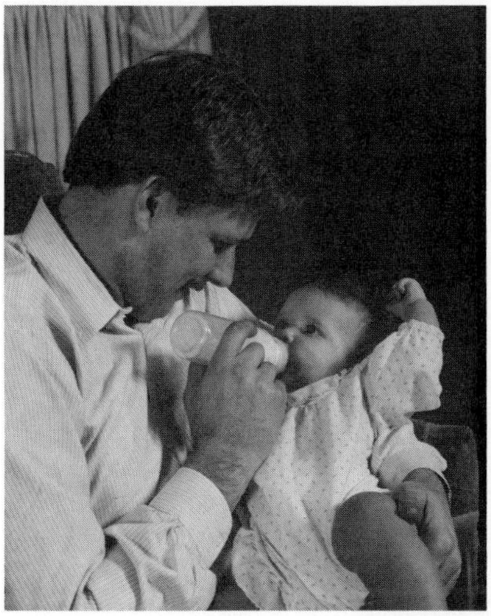

An infant accustomed to a bottle and nipple is less likely to reject them when it is either convenient or necessary to use a bottle.

Table 16-4 ◇ Comparison of caloric distribution and other nutritional factors in milk and formula

	Breast Milk	Formula	Whole Cow's Milk	2% Cow's Milk	Nonfat Cow's Milk
Energy (kcal/fl oz)	21	20	20	18	11
Carbohydrate (% calories)	42	41	30	41	57
Protein (% calories)	7	9-11	22	28	40
Fat (% calories)	51	48	35-55	31	3
Lipid (%)	3.7	3.6	3.6	2.0	0.1
P/S ratio	0.4-0.8	2-4.5	0.4	0.4	—
Cholesterol (mg/L)	140-200	20-40	110	80	30
Iron (mg/L)	0.8	12	Trace	Trace	Trace
Relative renal solute load* (mOsm/166 kcal)	22	33	76	100	142

Developed from USDA Nutritive Composition of Foods, Handbook 8-1, 1976.
*Amount of waste products of metabolism, primarily urea, to be excreted in the urine for 166 kcal.

Temperature of milk. Cold formula is well tolerated by 50% of young infants and 75% of older infants and gives as good a growth response as that which has been warmed to body temperature. On the other hand, feeding ice-cold milk lowers the temperature of stomach contents for at least an hour and delays digestion by decreasing the activity of proteolytic (protein-splitting) enzymes.

Nursing-bottle syndrome. The practice of offering infants a bottle at bedtime and allowing them to fall asleep with the bottle in the mouth causes **nursing-bottle syndrome.** This results in a high rate of tooth decay caused by the retention of the sugar-containing fluid, either milk, formula, or fruit juice, close to the teeth, where acid is formed from the sugar. For this reason fruit juices should be fed by cup, and infants should not be allowed to keep a nipple in the mouth for a long time.

nursing-bottle syndrome
The high incidence of tooth decay in infants who are allowed to fall asleep with a bottle in their mouth, which causes the fluid to be held close to the surface of the teeth; either milk or fruit juice contains enough fermentable carbohydrate to feed the bacteria in the mouth until they are capable of causing decay.

Cost. The relative costs of various feeding methods also influence a mother's choice (Table 16-3).

ADEQUACY OF MILK DIET

Recommendations for supplements to milk feedings for infants are shown in Table 16-5. At 3 to 6 months, when fetal iron reserves are depleted milk cannot provide sufficient iron to maintain hemoglobin levels. At that time an iron supplement or the use of iron-fortified formula is recommended.

Ascorbic acid intake is limited for infants on home-prepared formula. These infants should receive a supplementary source by the tenth day of life. Orange juice was recommended until it was discovered that the oil of the orange rind extracted with the juice caused allergic reactions. Now a synthetic source of vitamin C, usually as drops, is recommended for the first few months of life, after which the child can be given a fruit juice high in vitamin C. Some infants born to mothers who have an extremely high vitamin C intake during pregnancy have been reported to have a conditioned need for the vitamin that is higher than that in breast milk or formula.

The amount of vitamin D in either human or cow's milk is to some extent a function of the diet of the mother or cow, but even under ideal conditions it is not a dependable source. Thus, unless a child is regularly exposed to sunlight, it is necessary to provide a daily supplement of 400 IU of vitamin D, preferably by 5 days of age. Cod-liver oil, once a popular source, has been replaced by water-miscible preparations; this avoids the danger of lipoid pneumonia from the aspiration of the oily particles of cod-liver oil into the lungs. If a bottle-fed infant is given a

Table 16-5 ◆ Recommended supplementation of infant diets

Type of Feeding	Iron	Vitamin D	Fluorine	Vitamin C
Breast feeding	7 mg $FeSO_4$*	400 IU	0.25 mg	—
Iron-fortified formulas	—	—	0.25 mg†	—
Modified cow's milk	7 mg $FeSO_4$	400 IU	0.25 mg	20 mg
Evaporated milk formula	7 mg $FeSO_4$	—	0.25 mg†	20 mg

*After 3 to 6 months, Ferrous Sulfate.
†If fluoride content of water is <0.3 ppm.

prepared formula or a formula made with evaporated or homogenized milk, which is normally fortified with vitamin D, no supplementation is necessary, and because of toxicity from diets high in vitamin D, supplementation is probably undesirable. Reports of a water-soluble form of vitamin D in breast milk have proved false; thus is seems clear that breast-fed infants do need an extra amount of vitamin D.

Except for infants fed a formula with fluoridated water, a fluorine supplement of 0.25 mg/day in the first year is necessary to develop resistance to tooth decay. Because of the possible hazards from excessive ingestion of fluorine, such supplements are available only by prescription.

The small amount of iron in human milk is well utilized, with up to 50% absorbed. This results partially from the vitamin C, vitamin E, and copper content of human milk, all of which aid in iron absorption. Although human milk alone could provide the infant's needs for iron, it is recommended that a ferrous sulfate supplement be given, beginning at the age of 4 months. After the child is weaned, an iron-fortified formula is recommended. For bottle-fed infants the use of iron-fortified formula is recommended throughout the first year of life to prevent a drop in hemoglobin levels below 11 grams/dl of blood. Infants do not have the ability to absorb iron before it is needed. Once they need it, they are able to regulate absorption sufficiently well to prevent the uptake of excess iron, which could lead to iron overload when it is fed before it is needed.

NUTRITIVE NEEDS OF INFANTS

Precise information on the nutritive needs of infants is available for only a few nutrients, but levels of intake that appear to support growth in healthy infants are used in setting the RDAs (Table 16-6).

Supplements for Infants
Vitamin D
Fluorine
Iron
Vitamin C (?)

Energy. An intake of 54 kcal/pound or 115 kcal/kg of body weight (range 95 to 145 kcal/kg) has been considered adequate to meet the needs for the first 6 months but recent studies showed a drop to 71 kcal/kg/day by the fourth month. Because the body surface area of infants per unit of body weight is twice as great as that of adults, the insensible heat loss from the surface is also twice as great. Of the energy intake, 50% is used for basal energy, 25% for activity, and 25% for needs for growth of 5 to 7 grams/day.

By 6 months, energy needs have decreased to 43 kcal/pound (95 kcal/kg). A very placid infant may need as few as 32 kcal/pound, whereas a fretful infant may need as many as 60 kcal/pound.

Use of Energy Intake for Growth

1 month	25%-30%
2-11 months	7%
1 year	1%

An excessive intake of calories, leading to a rapid gain in weight, is as undesirable in infants as in adults, supporting the concept that maximal growth is not synonymous with optimal growth. However, attempts to show a relationship between weight in early life and obesity in childhood, adolescence, and adulthood have been far from conclusive.

One theory suggests that the number of adipose, or fat, cells is determined early in life and is proportionately larger in overfed infants, who have a greater need for more cells to store fat. As a result, these infants find the regulation of

Table 16-6 ◇ Proposed recommended dietary intakes (RDI, 1985) and recommended dietary allowances (RDAs, 1980) for infants

	RDI for Age (Months)			RDAs for Age (Months)	
Nutrient	0-3	3-6	6-12	0-5.9	6-12*
Kilocalories	wt (kg) × 115	wt (kg) × 105	1300	—	—
Protein (gram)	10	15	19	wt (kg) × 2.2	wt (kg) × 2.0
Calcium (mg)	225	440	600	360	540
Magnesium (mg)	30	40	50	50	70
Iron (mg)	—	7	9	10	15
Iodine (μg)	30	40	50	40	—
Zinc (mg)	—	3	5	3	—
Selenium (μg)	13	13	13	10-40	20-60
Vitamin A (μg RE)	375-420	375-420	375-420	420	400
Vitamin D (μg)	7.5	10	10	10	—
Vitamin E (mg α TE)	2	3	4	3	—
Vitamin C (mg)	25-35	25-35	25-35	35	35
Folacin (μg)	16	24	32	30	45
Niacin (mg NE)	4	5	6	6	8
Riboflavin (mg)	0.25	0.4	0.6		
Thiamin (mg)	0.2	0.4	0.5	0.3	—
Pyridoxine (mg)	0.15	0.3	0.4	0.3	0.6
Vitamin B_{12} (μg)	0.3	0.4	0.5	0.5	1.5
Provisional Allowances					
Chromium (μg)	—	10-20	15-30	10-40	20-60
Molybdenum (mg)	0.02-0.04	0.02-0.04	0.03-0.06	0.03-0.06	0.04-0.08
Manganese (mg)	—	0.4-0.6	0.6-1.0	0.5-0.7	0.7-1.0
Copper (mg)	—	0.4-0.6	0.6-0.7	0.5-0.7	0.7-1.0
Fluoride (mg)	—	0.25-0.50	0.25-0.75	0.1-0.5	0.2-1.0

*Only where different from RDI.

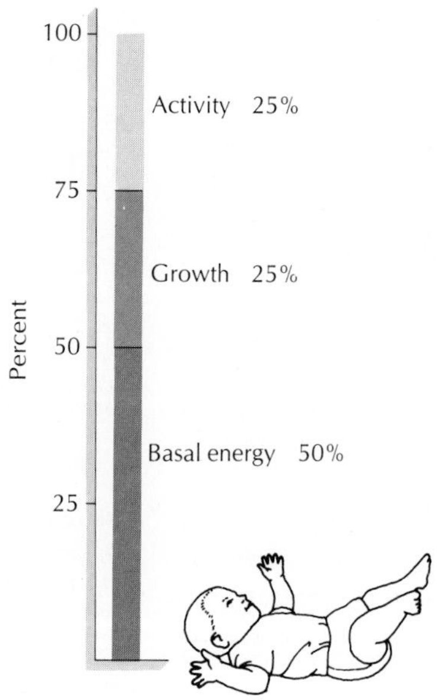

Use of energy by young infant

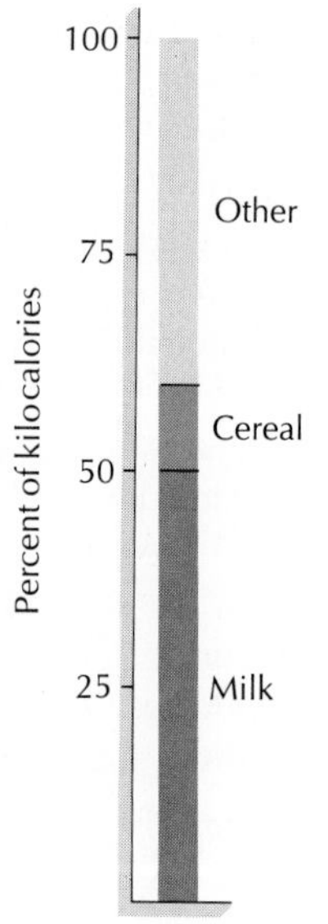

Sources of calories at 9 months of age

weight in later life more difficult because of a tendency for adipose cells to remain large and filled with lipid. This theory is now questioned, because although fat cells do proliferate in the first year of life in response to a need to store fat, they can increase in number and size whenever they are needed. There is little relationship between weight status at 1 year and 4 years to weight status in adulthood.

For a newborn infant, either breast milk or formula provides all the needed calories. Although it is recommended that milk be the sole source of energy up to the age of 6 months, in practice, the feeding patterns used by most mothers show that by that age 70% of the energy comes from milk and 10% from fruit, with cereal, meat, eggs, and vegetables each providing 5%.

Protein. The need for protein during the period of rapid skeletal and muscle growth of early infancy is relatively high. An intake of 2.2 grams of high-biological-value protein per kilogram of body weight permits nitrogen retention of about 45%, sufficient for normal growth as long as energy intake is adequate. At 3 weeks, from 60% to 75% of dietary protein is used for growth and the rest for maintenance. By 4 months of age, the proportions are 45% and 55%. By 5 months, the protein needs have dropped to 2 grams/kg. If protein of a lower biological value is used, the amount needed increases proportionately. Only proteins, such as milk, meat, and eggs, with a biological value (BV) of at least 70% to 85%, with almost half of the amino acids as essential amino acids, should be used for infants. A protein intake providing from 6.5% to 8% of the total dietary calories is capable of meeting the protein requirement. There is no evidence of advantages from protein intakes above these levels.

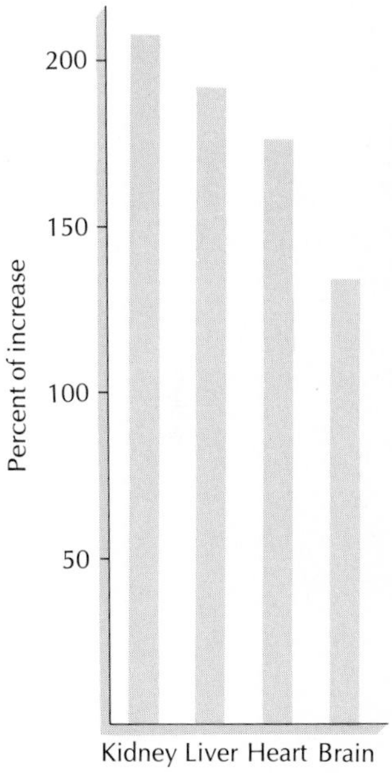

Increase in organ size during first 12 months of life

Protein in excess of the body's need for growth and repair of tissue must be deaminated in the liver so that the nonamine portion of the amino acids can be used as a source of energy, and the amino portion is excreted as urea. Since the infant has a limited capacity to concentrate waste metabolites, such as urea, in the urine, the excretion of more wastes requires a larger volume of water. If the necessary water is not available, urea will accumulate, and ironically, the infant will suffer from protein edema. In addition, the need for the liver to produce the enzymes (deaminases) necessary to remove the amino group may lead to an undesirable hypertrophy, or increase in size, of the liver. Also the higher rate of infection in infants fed cow's milk may occur because mechanisms normally related to the formation of antibodies to protect against infection are diverted to take care of excess milk protein. Protein intakes should not exceed 6 grams/kg body weight.

Infants receiving whole unmodified cow's milk, which has twice the protein of human milk, suffer from a hypochromic microcytic anemia. This is caused by gastric bleeding that leads to large blood losses in the feces, apparently the result of an allergy to the cow's milk protein.

Infants' amino acid requirements are proportionately higher than those of adults. In addition, histidine is essential for infants at a level surpassed in both breast feeding and bottle feeding.

One study of 6-month-old infants showed that 70% of the protein in their diets came from milk, 15% from meat, and 3% each from eggs, cereal, and vegetables. There is no evidence that protein deficiency in developed countries is a matter for concern among infants. In fact, a study of more than 300 infants showed protein intakes from 1½ to 2½ times recommended amounts.

Water-soluble vitamins. Breast milk usually provides the recommended dietary allowance of water-soluble vitamins if the mother's diet is adequate.

Attempts to show that thiamin is beneficial as an appetite stimulant have failed; furthermore, it has not been demonstrated that height, weight, manual dexterity, or memory retention is enhanced. Infants whose diets were adequate in thiamin were receiving enriched infant cereals, whereas those with inadequate thiamin were not.

The recommendation that infants receive 0.5 mg of riboflavin per 1000 kcal of energy intake to maintain tissue saturation means that an infant from 3 to 6 months of age needs 0.4 mg and by 6 to 12 months needs 0.6 mg. Human milk, with 0.35 mg/quart (liter) provides only 0.3 mg in the 750 ml available for the newborn, but it appears to be well utilized. The American Academy of Pediatrics recommends 0.6 mg/1000 kcal.

The recommended intake of 6 to 8 mg niacin equivalents (NE) can be met by human milk, which provides 0.15 mg of niacin and 21 mg of tryptophan (0.3 NE/dl) of milk.

The NRC recommends that a progressively increasing amount of pyridoxine be given during the first year of life. The amount in human milk reflects the amount of vitamin B_6 in the mother's diet; this increases quickly when the mother takes a supplement. Milk from mothers who used oral contraceptives for more than 30 months before pregnancy may have marginal levels of pyridoxine. Because infants have been shown to develop convulsive seizures on diets low in pyridoxine, the pyridoxine content of infant formulas is now maintained at either 0.015 mg/gram of protein or 0.04 mg/100 kcal to satisfy all the metabolic requirements of the infant.

The infant probably needs 0.005 mg of folacin/kg of body weight. However, since folacin deficiency is common among pregnant women and the reserves with which the infant enters life are minimal, intakes of up to 30 to 45 μg are recommended in the first year of life.

Although the daily intake of vitamin B_{12} from human milk is only 0.35 to 0.40 μg, the RDA during the first 5 months of life is 0.5 μg/day for formula-fed infants. Because of the reserves built up during fetal life, the possibility of vitamin B_{12} deficiency in breast-fed infants is remote, except for infants of vegan mothers. There have been many claims in advertising that vitamin B_{12} acts as a growth stimulant. The American Academy of Pediatrics found that in 13 studies of 546 "normal children," only two involving 69 children reported a significant and stimulating effect on growth with either oral or intramuscular doses of vitamin B_{12}. All the children with enhanced growth were underweight at the beginning of the study.

Intakes of ascorbic acid much below the RDA of 35 mg will protect against scurvy, thus breast-fed infants usually receive adequate amounts, and formula has added amounts to replace the heat-labile ascorbic acid destroyed during pasteurization. Infants fed cow's milk are usually given a dietary supplement during the first few months.

Fat-soluble vitamins. It is assumed that the human infant enters life with a reserve of fat-soluble vitamin A stored in the liver, depending on the vitamin A status of the mother. The RDA is set at 420 μg RE—less than the amount normally supplied in 750 ml of breast milk. Toxicity has been noted when intakes are at levels of 25,000 to 50,000 RE a day for 30 days; this results in increased intracranial pressure and hydrocephalus.

The need for vitamin D during infancy, when rapid calcification of bones and teeth occurs, is well documented. Although as little as 100 IU/day will prevent rickets and 300 IU/day will cure the condition, 400 IU (10 μg vitamin D)/day promotes good calcium absorption and skeletal growth. Intakes above this apparently have no advantage, and at levels beyond 1800 IU a decrease in calcium utilization may occur. In fact, there is evidence that sensitive infants who consistently receive from 1000 to 3000 IU may exhibit hypercalcemia, depressed appetite, and retarded growth. Although the vitamin D activity of human milk at 22 IU/liter is higher than previously recognized, it is recommended that supplement of 400 IU/day be given beginning in the first week of life. For bottle-fed babies a supplement will be necessary only if the milk or formula is not itself fortified with the vitamin.

Since little vitamin E crosses the placenta, human infants are born with low concentrations in the tissues. An intake of 3 to 4 mg TE of vitamin E is advised during the first year of life. Only when large amounts of unsaturated vegetable fats are substituted for the butterfat in formula feeding will the need for vitamin E increase. Premature infants, who have both low stores and a reduced ability to absorb vitamin E, frequently develop anemia when the membranes of the red blood cells rupture, because they are without the antioxidant protection afforded by vitamin E from late prenatal period. Diets high in PUFA make the situation worse.

Vitamin K deficiency is most likely to occur in the first few days of life among breast-fed infants. They are routinely given vitamin K **parenterally.** Those infants suffering from malabsorption or diarrhea may also be deficient.

parenterally
Given directly into the blood or intramuscularly

Minerals. Because of the rapid rate of calcification of bone to support the weight of the body by the time the baby walks, calcium is needed in early infancy. This is especially important because bones are poorly calcified at birth. Although some calcification of teeth has begun in the prenatal period, the availability and utilization of calcium in the postnatal period is a crucial factor in adequate tooth formation. Milk is capable of satisfying the infant's needs, but the efficiency with which it is used is greatly enhanced when vitamin D is available simultaneously.

Breast milk provides 280 mg of calcium/liter (210 mg/day), which is apparently adequate, because as much as two thirds of the intake is retained. The recommended allowances of 360 to 540 mg/day are intended only for the bottle-fed infant, who retains only a third to a half of its intake.

The calcium/phosphorus ratio of 1.2:1 in cow's milk compared to 2:1 in human milk is too low for the newborn infant. The baby who has difficulty excreting the relatively high amounts of phosphorus in unmodified cow's milk often develops hypocalcemic neonatal tetany.

Trace elements

Iron. Infants' needs for iron are determined to a large extent by their gestational age. Normally, a full-term infant will have received a significant amount of iron from the mother during the fetal period, but a premature infant will have received less. If reserves from fetal life are present, the infant will need virtually no dietary iron for at least 3 months. However, many pediatric nutritionists now recommend that bottle-fed infants be given formula fortified with ferrous sulfate at 10 to 15 mg/liter from birth throughout the first year of life. Although only 4% of such iron is absorbed, it provides a constant and predictable source of iron sufficient to prevent anemia. Both twins and premature infants who have lower reserves need a dietary source earlier than do full-term infants.

Dietary allowances are based on an average dietary need of 1.5 mg/kg/day, although a normal full-term infant can maintain optimal hemoglobin levels on an intake of 1 mg/kg of body weight. The intake recommended from 6 to 12 months of age can be obtained only through the use of iron-fortified formulas and iron-enriched infant cereals, which are fortified at a level of 12 mg/oz.

Zinc. Recently studies showing that most infants are in negative zinc balance in the first weeks and possible months of life have focused attention on the importance of zinc in early feeding. The high levels of zinc in colostrum (4 mg/liter, declining to 1.2 mg/liter in mature milk at 6 months and 0.5 mg/liter at 1 year) may compensate for this in breast-fed infants. Both the well-documented role of zinc in promoting normal growth and its potential role in normal brain development suggest a critical function for zinc during the developmental period. If a zinc deficiency is identified in large numbers of infants, zinc supplementation may be recommended. The RDA ranges from 3 to 5 mg.

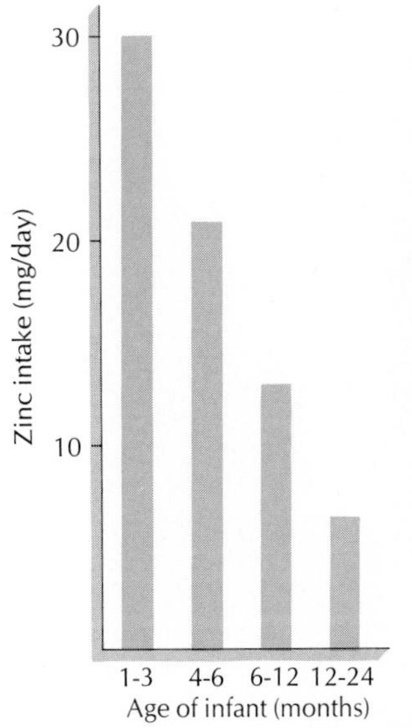

Zinc levels in human milk throughout breastfeeding period

Iodine. Past concern over inadequate iodine intake for infants has been eliminated with the increase of iodine in milk, which in turn results from the various iodine sources in the maternal food supply. However, soy-based formulas for infants must be supplemented with iodine to counteract the effect of goitrogens found in soy products. The RDA is 40 to 50 μg.

Fluorine. Fluorine, important in the development of teeth that are resistant to tooth decay, assumes particular importance in the early feeding of infants. Since relatively little fluorine crosses the placenta from the mother to the infant, it is

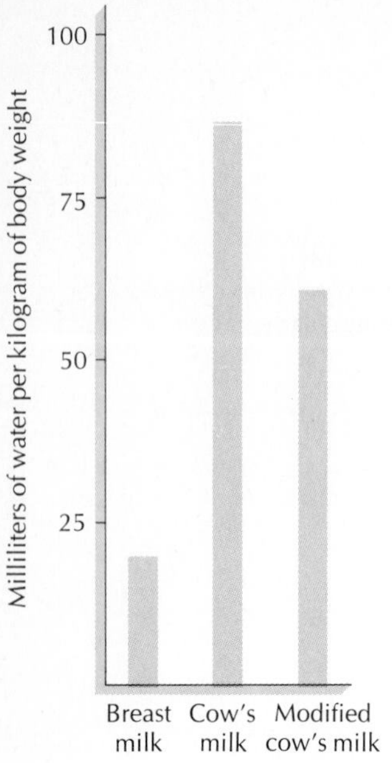

Amounts of water needed with different types of infant milks for optimal body functioning (in ml/kg of body weight)

important to provide up to 1.0 mg/day in the first year. Analysis shows that formula diluted with fluoridated water will provide as much as 0.9 mg/liter. When a variety of baby foods have been introduced, infants are ingesting 1.2 mg/day. Because the amount a bottle-fed baby receives depends on the fluorine content of the water used in the formula and food preparation, and because breast milk will have only small amounts, even if the mother is using fluoridated water, a fluorine supplement of 0.25 mg available on prescription should be provided for infants whose intake is likely to be marginal.

Other trace elements. Estimates of the requirement for other trace elements during infancy have been based largely on information on the amount present in breast milk. Because these values vary considerably among mothers, depending on the amount in their diets, and frequently vary within the same mother at different times, recommendations for daily intakes can only include a range of values. The best current estimates of need are presented in Table 16-6.

Water or fluid. Most breast-fed and formula fed infants receive enough water to meet their needs until solid foods are introduced. Although the intake of water is crucial at all stages in the life cycle, it receives a little more attention in infancy because the surface area per unit of body weight is twice that of the adult. This leads to loss of heat and water through the skin at a rate almost double that of the adult. Even more water will be required when the diet contains excessive electrolytes, such as sodium and potassium, or protein beyond needs for growth.

An infant receiving a diet of human milk requires 20 ml of water/kg of body weight to provide a sufficient amount so that the kidneys can handle waste to be excreted. If undiluted cow's milk is used, 87 ml of water is required, and if cow's milk formula, with a third of the calories coming from added carbohydrate, is used, 61 ml/kg is required. At a normal room temperature of 70° F (21° C) any one of these milk sources alone would provide enough water, but at 93° F (34° C) the cow's milk would not provide enough, since proportionately more water is lost through the skin. Thus even with a formula providing the usual 20 kcal/oz, parents should offer the child additional water when the environmental temperature is high. Formula with a calorie density greater than 30 kcal/oz should not be used.

Since a thirsty baby acts like a hungry baby, it is not uncommon to find parents giving a thirsty baby food when they should be offering water. This only increases the need for water and thus increases thirst.

Other considerations. Many nutritional requirements of infants may be influenced by the use of drugs. There is considerable evidence that anticonvulsant drugs increase the need for both vitamin D and folacin. Antibiotics influence the availability of several nutrients, such as vitamin B_{12}, carotene, and iron, and the synthesis of vitamin K.

INTRODUCTION OF SOLID FOODS

At the turn of the century, pediatricians were recommending that the milk diet of infants be supplemented with a food, such as meat or cereal, only after 1 year of age. By 1917 Dr. Emmett Holt cautiously suggested that a meat broth could safely be introduced at 8 or 9 months of age but that solid foods should be withheld until 1 year. By 1956 the pendulum had swung so far in the opposite direction that some pediatricians were recommending that an infant be put on solid foods and be expected to adhere to three meals a day by 2 or 3 weeks of age.

The American Academy of Pediatrics, recognizing a trend in infant feeding practices toward progressively earlier introduction of solid foods, in the absence of any evidence of a nutritional or physiological need, surveyed practicing pediatricians to determine the bases of their recommendations. It found that the pediatricians were indeed suggesting the use of cereal by 3 to 6 weeks of age, followed by other foods, so that by 4 or 5 months the child received a full diet of meat, eggs, fruit, vegetables, and cereal. Their reasons for this practice reflected a response to the demands of parents that they follow this "progressive" procedure rather than any belief that the infant needed the solid food.

The pendulum has now swung back: the current recommendation is that milk be the sole source of nourishment in the first 4 to 6 months of life and the primary source during the rest of the first year. This recommendation reflects a rational approach to the question of the timing and sequence of additions to the infant's diet. In spite of the almost universal acceptance of these recommendations by professionals, several surveys of infant feeding practices show that a significant number of mothers continue to introduce solid foods earlier.

Solid food added to an infant's diet is called **beikost.** If beikost is not introduced until 6 months of age, the sequencing of additions is of limited concern. However, if it is done sooner, it should be done with consideration of the nutritional needs of the infant, his physiological readiness to use foods other than milk, his physical capacity to handle them, and the relative advantages and disadvantages of adding semisolid or solid foods.

beikost
Food other than milk in the infant's diet

Introduction of Solid Food Determined By
Nutrition
Physiological readiness
Physical readiness

Nutrition. From a nutritional standpoint the nutritive needs of an infant can be readily met by a milk diet supplemented with iron, fluorine, vitamin D, and sometimes vitamin C. Since these can be added by fortification of milk or formula, or as supplements, there is no need to introduce foods other than milk before 4 to 6 months of age. The major objection to the earlier introduction of solid foods is the possibility of overfeeding, because infants have little way of communicating when they have had sufficient food.

By 6 months of age a milk diet alone cannot provide the calories necessary for the increased needs of the growing infant. At that time infant cereal is usually added to the diet. It should be mixed with milk to a consistency that can be swallowed but not sucked from the spoon. After several cereal grains, such as rice, wheat, or oats, have been introduced individually for about 1 week at a time so that it is possible to identify any cereal allergy, the child is offered a variety of strained fruits, again one at a time for several weeks. The addition of sugar to fruit is unnecessary from a nutritional standpoint, but it is used in small amounts in some commercial products to ensure consistent flavor by standardizing the natural variation in sweetness from batch to batch. Bananas that are fully ripened so that the starch is changed to sugar are a very acceptable fruit for infants. Fruits are followed by vegetables, again one at a time. These solid foods contribute an increasingly large proportion of the infant's energy requirement, with cereals providing 8% to 10% of the calories and other baby foods 30% to 40% by 9 months of age.

The protein needs of the infant at 6 months also exceed those provided for by breast milk alone, and the diet must be supplemented by a source of protein. Egg yolk with 33% protein, meat with 20%, and cottage cheese with 17% are considered suitable additions to the diet. Egg, which is **allergenic,** should be avoided by infants in families with a history of food allergy and egg whites avoided by all infants.

allergenic
Causing an allergy

As additional foods are introduced, it is desirable to maintain the distribution of calories from protein at 7% to 16%, from fat at 35% to 45%, and from carbohydrate at 29% to 58%, proportions close to those in human milk. The percentage of calories from various energy sources in selected baby foods is given in Table 16-7.

Physical development. Infants vary in the rate at which the normal rooting, sucking, and extrusion reflexes, natural at the time of birth, are replaced by the ability to swallow semisolid foods. As these changes occur, infants must learn to use them in the eating process, just as they learn to walk or talk. At birth the lower jaw is very poorly developed, and fat pads, located in the cheeks, aid in sucking by providing the needed shape to the mouth. As the infant matures, the contour of the jaw changes and the fat pads disappear, leaving the infant with the capability of chewing and swallowing rather than sucking food.

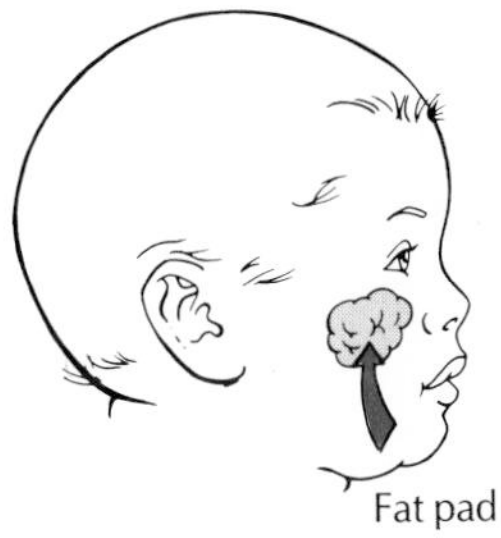

Fat pads are needed for a sucking reaction

Table 16-7 ◇ Caloric density and distribution of calories in infant foods

	Kcal/100 gram	Protein (percent)	Fat (percent)	CHO (percent)
Egg yolk	192	21	76	3
Meats	106	53	46	1
Fruits	85	2	2	96
Soups and dinners	58	16	28	56
Vegetables	45	14	6	80
Human milk	67	6	56	38
Nonfat milk	35	40	3	57
Whole milk	67	22	48	30

Physical Readiness for Solid Food Depends On
Ability to chew
Ability to swallow
Eruption of teeth

The swallowing reflex involves sufficient innervation of the tongue to enable it to form any solid food placed at the tip of the tongue into a ball and throw it to the back of the mouth, where first gravity and then the peristaltic action of the esophagus take over to convey the ball of food to the stomach. This ability usually develops at 3 to 5 months of age. Before this happens, the extrusion reflex that causes the infant to forcibly reject food or objects placed at the front of the tongue must diminish in strength. Since the ability to move food from the tip of the tongue to the throat normally develops at 3 to 5 months of age, any effort to feed solid or semisolid foods before that time means that the food is conveyed to the esophagus by some method other than swallowing. Either it must be placed sufficiently far back in the mouth that it can reach the esophagus by gravity, or the consistency of the product must be so thin that the infant is able to suck it from the spoon as a liquid, rather than using a swallowing action. Many times the infant who cannot manipulate the tongue to swallow also cannot use it to reject objects or food placed in the mouth. Thus it is not uncommon to have parents report that infants who had apparently accepted solid food at 3 to 6 weeks of age reject it at 10 to 12 weeks of age when they have the ability to push out against the spoon. Not until infants are 5 to 6 months old are they able to indicate an interest in food by moving forward or disinterest by turning away. Any effort to force them earlier may result in a frustrating and unhappy feeding experience for both the parent and the child.

Infant is Physiologically Ready for Solid Foods When
Saliva is produced
Enzymes for digestion of starch and unemulsified fat are produced
Kidneys mature to handle increased renal solute load
Gastric acidity increases

Physiological development. The ability to handle foods other than milk also depends on the physiological development of the infant. All the secretions of the digestive tract contain enzymes especially suited to the digestion of the complex nutrients of human milk, but few that are needed for other foods.

For instance, the secretion of the salivary glands is minimal at birth but increases in volume until it become sufficiently copious to cause drooling by 2 or 3 months. This is evident in the infant who has not developed the innervation of the outer part of the lips necessary to prevent it. Since salivary enzymes are involved only in the digestion of the starches, they are unnecessary as long as the child is receiving only milk, with lactose as the only carbohydrate. The appearance of salivary amylase in the saliva occurs at the time the infant is given more complex carbohydrates, such as the starch in cereals.

The proteolytic enzymes are present in adequate amounts to digest milk protein, as long as it is sufficiently dilute to produce a soft, flocculent curd on which the enzymes can act. As the child matures, the secretion of proteolytic enzymes in the intestine increases this capacity of the infant to digest nonmilk proteins. By 4 to 6 months of age, most infants are able to handle most proteins.

The kidney of the full-term infant is not completely mature. The glomeruli can satisfactorily filter the blood that passes through the kidneys, but the tubules, which are functionally less mature, are unable to reabsorb water and some solutes adequately. The tubules become efficient by 6 to 8 weeks, after which there is less concern over the use of a high-protein, high-sodium diet. Because of the poorly developed kidney function, it is important that protein, beyond that needed for growth, and extra sodium be avoided. This is especially important when the infant suffers excessive loss of fluid, such as in a hot climate, when diarrhea occurs, or when foods of high caloric density are fed.

Low gastric acidity resulting from the limited secretion of hydrochloric acid in early infancy has implications for the use of such vegetables as beets, spinach, turnips, collard greens, or broccoli, which contain nitrates. In the absence of gastric acidity, they are more readily converted to nitrites that in turn react with amines in the intestine to produce nitrosamines, which are potential carcinogens. If nitrites are absorbed, they cause the conversion of hemoglobin to methemoglobin, which has a reduced oxygen-carrying capacity. For these reasons nitrate-containing vegetables should be avoided in feeding young infants, and nitrites should be consumed only when used to control botulism in some foods.

Nitrate-Containing Vegetables
Beets
Broccoli
Carrots
Collard Greens
Spinach
Turnips

When solid foods are introduced at an extremely early age, so little is consumed and they make such an insignificant contribution to the nutrient intake that it is questionable whether the extra work, cost, and risk of contamination can be justified. If solid foods are taken in addition to milk, there is a concern about the effects of overeating; if they replace milk, the effect of the reduced calcium intake is cause for concern.

Other considerations. Many reasons have been advanced either to support or to reject the introduction of solid foods from 2 to 8 weeks of age. The belief of many parents that they can hasten the time at which the infant sleeps through the night has not been supported experimentally. One must consider that if the infant does sleep through the night at an early age, she must either reduce her total food intake or consume larger amounts at each of the remaining feedings, thus taxing the capacity of the stomach. Smaller, more frequent feedings are in keeping with the pattern of eating that an infant establishes when fed "on demand."

Some pediatricians fear that any pattern of overeating at an early age may persist throughout life and be a possible factor in obesity of children and adolescents. Such early-onset obesity is one of the most difficult types to treat.

Since the solid food consumed in the first few months is usually of minimal significance nutritionally, the major argument in favor of its use is that the child becomes accustomed early to a wider variety of flavors and textures of food and continues to accept these as he matures. Beal found that the age at which a child was offered solid foods bore little relationship to the age at which the food was accepted. As a result, she reported a period during which the child and mother experienced an unpleasant feeding relationship, with the mother trying to feed an infant who was not yet ready for the food. She believed that the feeding of semisolids before the ninth to twelfth weeks tended to increase the incidence of feeding problems and food dislikes in the infant.

Although findings are not consistent, many studies report an increased incidence of food allergy among infants who are introduced to a variety of foods at an early age. This is an especially important consideration among infants with a family history of allergy. For these, allergists suggest delaying the time of initial feeding of solid foods and choosing foods that are minimally allergenic, such as vegetables, fruits, and rice cereal. They also advise feeding each food for a relatively short time and then switching to another to avoid the sensitization that may arise from excessive use of one food.

In addition to an immature secretion of digestive enzymes, the young infant has low levels of many cellular enzymes. One that has been known for some time is phenylalanine hydroxylase, which is required for the metabolism of the essential amino acid phenylalanine. A diet high in protein in the neonatal period will tax the infant's ability to utilize the amino acid phenylalanine.

Concern over the safety of food additives in infant foods has focused on the use of salt (sodium chloride), monosodium glutamate, sugar, and modified starch.

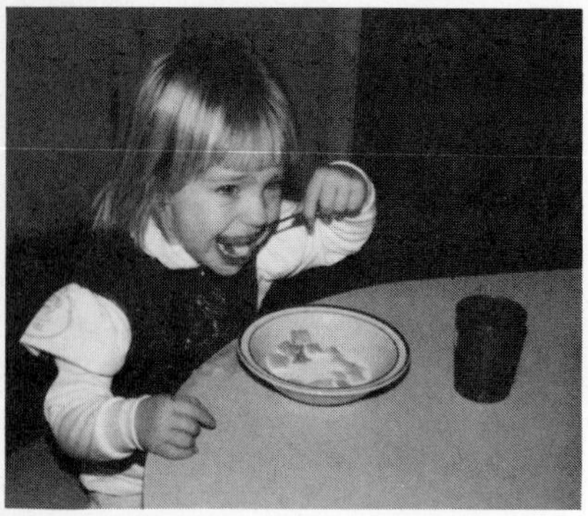

When offered at an age at which child is ready, feeding solid food can be a pleasant experience for both parent and child

All have been added to many commercially prepared infant foods, primarily to make them more palatable to the mother who was feeding them, rather than to the child who was eating them. Since no physiological or nutritional reason exists for adding them, and as long as the question of their safety remains unresolved, the FDA has ruled that the level of salt in infant foods be restricted to 0.25%, in contrast to the 1% previously found in many commercially prepared products. Since then several food processors have discontinued the addition of salt in baby foods and have issued a label statement asking the parents not to season it to their taste at feeding time. Concern about the use of salt stems from the possibility that the young infant with immature kidneys cannot excrete the increased electrolyte. If the infant retains it, there is a resultant increase in fluid volume and the potential of predisposing the infant to hypertension. The earlier children begin eating solid foods, the earlier their salt intake will increase. Studies of the preference of infants showed that they ate the same amount of food regardless of whether salt was added.

For monosodium glutamate, a flavor enhancer, the concern arises from reports that mice fed high intakes developed brain tumors. So far there is no evidence of potential danger in the amounts consumed by the young infant, but baby food manufacturers have voluntarily discontinued the use of monosodium glutamate.

The addition of sugar to infant foods has been questioned by many who fear that the child will develop a "sweet tooth." Many fruits that are labeled with sugar as an ingredient may not in reality have it added or will contain only enough to adjust the natural sweetness of the fruit to a consistent and acceptable level.

Modified starch used in baby foods are primarily starches from corn, potato, wheat, and cassava that have been treated chemically to eliminate some of their undesirable characteristics and give them the qualities needed for use in baby food. These qualities are primarily stability and the ability to thicken the product with a minimum of starch to get a desirable texture and consistency. The relatively small amount (4% of a 4.5 oz jar) provides about 20 kcal of easily digested carbohydrate. It has been determined to be readily digested and safe for use with young infants.

Order of Adding Solid Foods

- Cereal
  - Rice
  - Oats
  - Wheat
  - Mixed cereals
- Fruit
  - Bananas
- Vegetables
  - (Avoid nitrate-containing vegetables)
- Egg yolk
- Meat

Additions to the diet. The American Academy of Pediatrics, after a careful consideration of all the factors involved, has recommended that the optimal time for introducing solid foods into the infant's diet is 4 to 6 months of age. Although the Academy agrees that no nutritional or psychological benefit results from any earlier introduction, as many as 50% of mothers feed solid foods by 3 months of age.

Once the child is physically and physiologically capable of handling solid foods, the sequence and timing with which they are introduced should be determined by the nutritional needs of the child. Single-grain enriched cereals are frequently used first because of their iron content, ease of preparation and storage, and relatively low cost. Once iron-enriched cereals are given the breast-fed infant no longer needs an iron supplement. Cereal is usually followed by a variety of strained fruits and vegetables, with care being taken to avoid those that may be irritating to the gastrointestinal tract, either because of their high fiber content or their potential for inducing gas. Egg yolk, which provides vitamin A, iron, and riboflavin, is frequently used as a source of protein. Next, most infants will also receive meat. The order in which foods are introduced is not crucial, as evidenced by the number of patterns on which children thrive. Providing the nutrients needed to supplement a milk diet in a form suited to the digestive capacities of the child and the forming of a set of eating habits that will lead to good nutrition throughout childhood are much more important.

In most infants the eruption of the first teeth and thus the physical readiness to chew occur at approximately 5 to 6 months of age. It is very important that the infant be given an opportunity to develop the capacity to chew at this critical time. Dry toast is the most acceptable food to stimulate chewing. The use of hard, flintlike materials, such as crisp bacon and certain commercial biscuits, which may irritate the throat, should be avoided.

As the infant's digestive capacities develop, the strained foods of early infancy can be replaced by less finely chopped foods, with a final transition to table foods. The age at which this transition is made in a normal child varies greatly, and there is no advantage in promoting it at an early age.

EARLY FEEDING AND LATER DEVELOPMENT

Even though it is difficult to obtain adequate data, there is considerable concern about the effect of early feeding practices on later development. Interest has centered primarily on the question of whether infant feeding practices may predispose the child to later degenerative diseases. Evidence that the first year of life is one period when the number of fat cells increase in response to overfeeding led to concern that infants who form a larger number of fat cells have a greater capacity to store fat and hence have a tendency toward obesity throughout life. Studies on the relationship of infant obesity to obesity in later life have not confirmed this fear. Similarly, it is possible that high blood cholesterol levels and the deposition of lipid in the wall of the artery, risk factors in atherosclerosis, may be influenced by early feeding. Complete elimination of cholesterol from the diet of the young is, however, undesirable because cholesterol is necessary for the synthesis of many essential body compounds. Similarly, the restriction of fat in diets of children under 2 years of age is not recommended since it may result in a caloric intake incapable of supporting growth. If polyunsaturated fats are substituted for saturated fats as a way of decreasing cholesterol levels, the amount of vitamin E must be increased. The use of high levels of salt before the infant can handle excess sodium could increase the risk of hypertension (high blood pressure) in adulthood, although it would be only one of many other factors. It is also postulated that demyelinating disease, in which the material covering nerve fibers is destroyed, may be the result of a disorder of carbohydrate metabolism in early life. In all cases the effect of early diet assumes more importance for infants with a family history of any of these conditions.

Adequacy of the Diets of Infants

Relatively few studies have assessed the nutritive intake of infants. The Ten-State Nutrition Survey did obtain information on 258 infants under 6 months of age and on 340 infants between 6 and 11 months of age. These data showed clearly that intakes of iron are most likely to fall below recommended levels and that ascorbic acid intakes are frequently low in this age-group. The mean intakes for all nutrients except iron exceeded the recommended levels. Similarly, data from NHANES I and II on 892 and 672 infants, respectively, showed that for all nutrients except iron the mean intake was well above the RDAs. For iron only intakes at the 90th percentile met the standard.

The amount of calcium per kilogram of body weight and per 1000 kcal declined rapidly with age, reflecting the shift from milk to other foods with a lower content of calcium.

An analysis of the mineral content of diets of infants in the United States from 1974 to 1982 showed that intakes were above recommended levels for calcium, phosphorus, magnesium, zinc, manganese, selenium, and iodine but below these levels for iron and copper. Intakes of sodium, potassium, and iodine were much in excess of recommended levels.

The adequacy of the diets of infants is best assessed by the rate and pattern of growth and absence of illness. To help assess growth, the National Center for Health Statistics has developed growth charts representing expected patterns at varying percentiles for both boys and girls from birth to 3 years for height for age, weight for height, and head circumference for age. Some representative charts are reproduced in Figures 16-2 and 16-3.

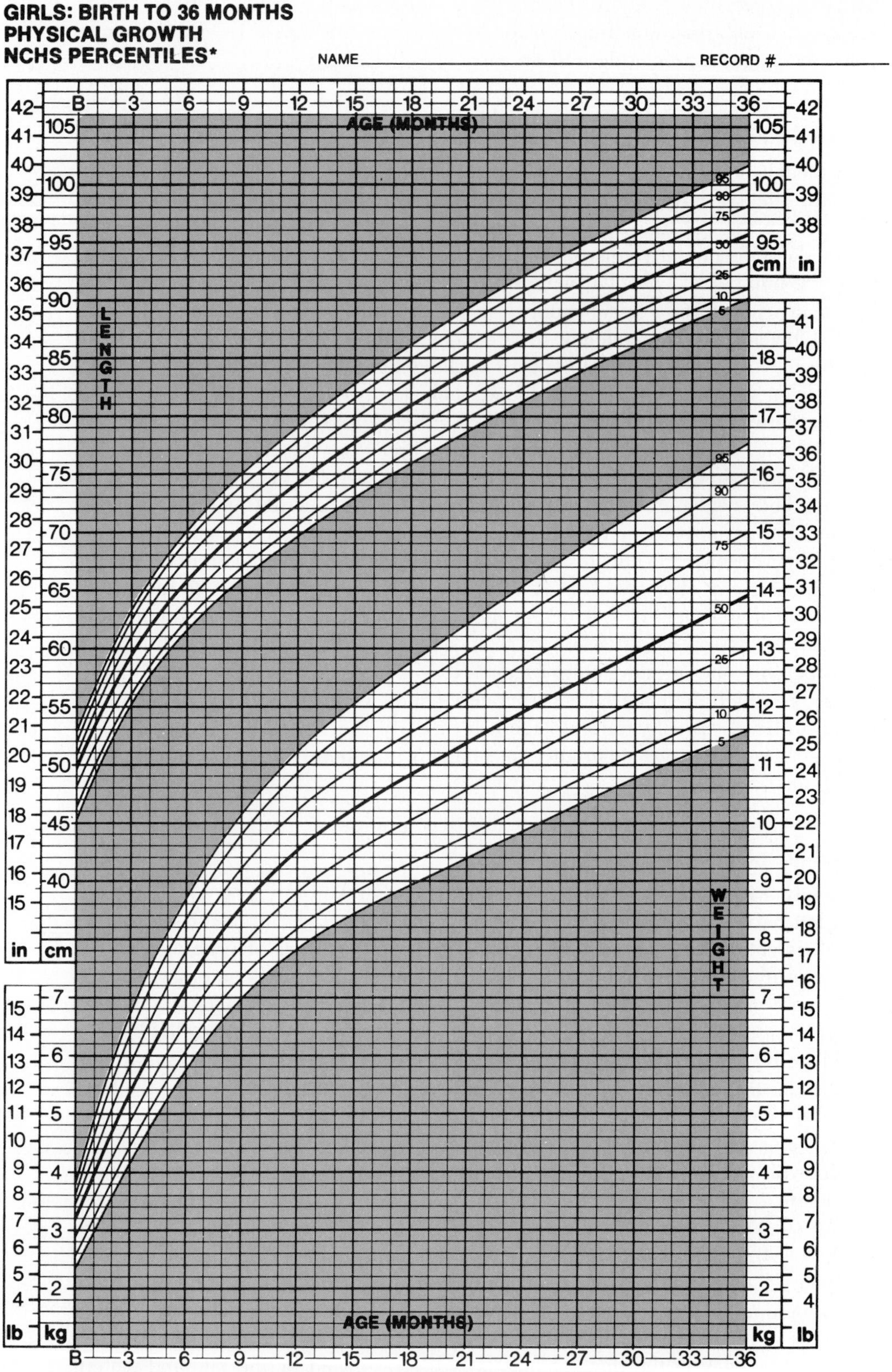

Figure 16-2 Weight and height for age for girls from birth to 36 months.

Adapted from Hamill PVV, and others: Physical growth: National Center for Health Statistics percentiles, American Journal of Clinical Nutrition 32:607, 1979. Data from the Fels Research Institute, Wright State University School of Medicine, Yellow Springs, OH © 1980 Ross Laboratories.

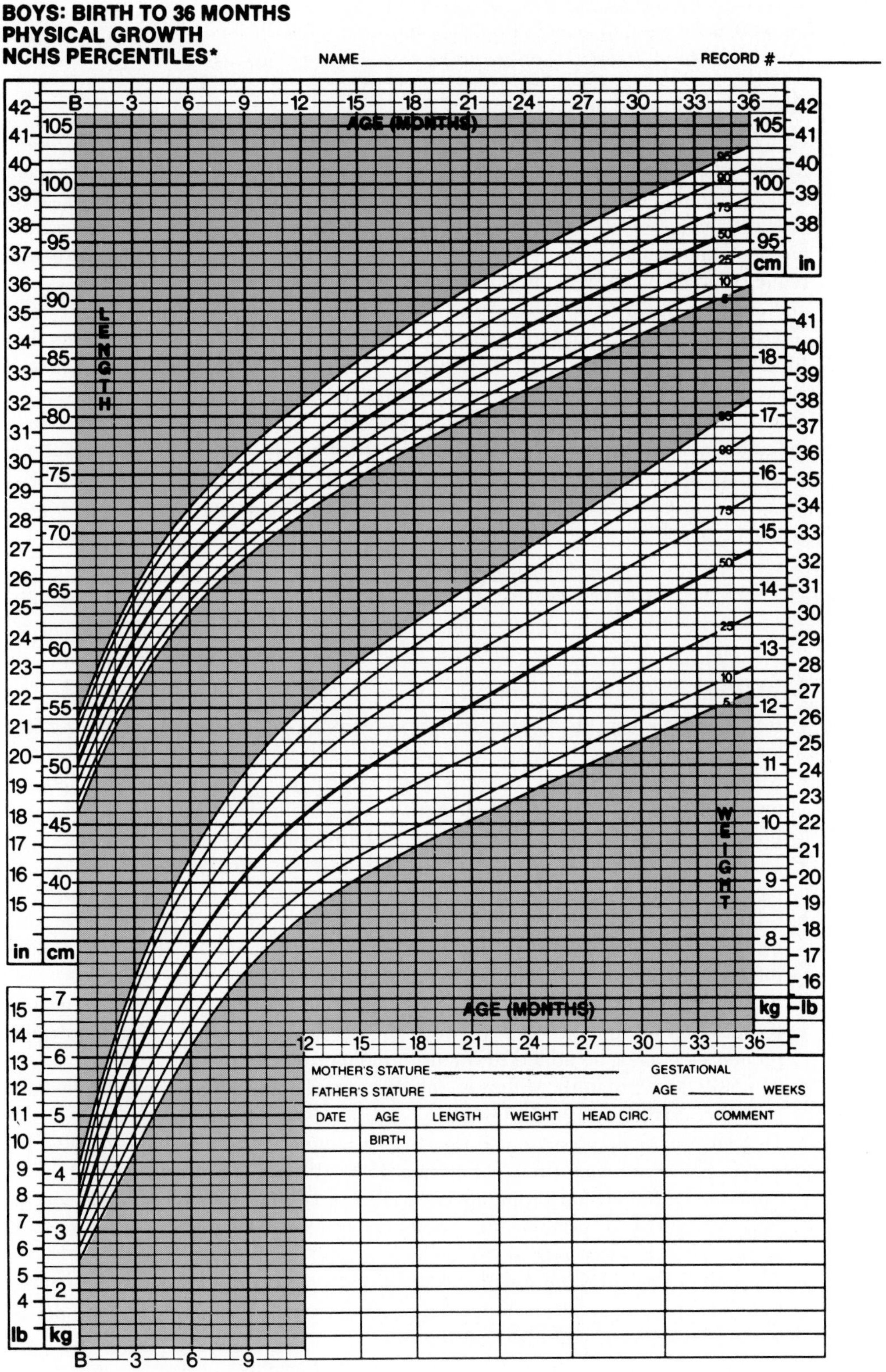

Figure 16-3 Weight and height for age for boys from birth to 36 months.

Adapted from Hamill PVV, and others: Physical growth: National Center for Health Statistics percentiles, American Journal of Clinical Nutrition 32:607, 1979. Data from the Fels Research Institute, Wright State University School of Medicine, Yellow Springs, OH © 1982 Ross Laboratories.

Failure to thrive in infants who fall below the 5th percentile in both height and weight results primarily from an inadequate food intake. This may reflect an increased need related to an illness or failure to absorb food, or it may reflect a variety of social factors, such as child abuse or vegetarianism.

Women, Infants, and Children (WIC)

Concern over the possibility that some children are disadvantaged early in life as a result of undernutrition has led to the implementation of a federally funded Special Supplemental Food Program for Women, Infants and Children, known as WIC. Since its inception in 1972, the WIC Program has provided food to help pregnant and lactating women, infants, and children age 5 and under improve their diets to reduce their chances of health problems caused by poor nutrition. To qualify, women and children at, or near, the poverty level must have some evidence of nutritional risk such as anemia, growth retardation, or previous problems during reproduction. In addition to providing food or coupons to purchase foods such as milk, cheese, eggs, cereal, peanut butter, beans, and infant formula, participants are given nutrition counseling. Evaluation of the program has found it to be cost effective in reducing fetal death rate, premature births, health care costs, and the prevalence of anemia, and it has enhanced mental performance. Its annual budget in 1988 of $1.8 billion, of which administrative costs are limited to 20%, permits the program to reach only 40% of eligible participants.

BY NOW YOU SHOULD KNOW

- Infant feeding can be divided into three chronological phases: breast or bottle feeding, transitional feeding, and modified adult diet.
- Although there are many ways in which an infant can be adequately fed, for practically all infants breast feeding is the preferable method. On the other hand, breast feeding may not be the preferable form of feeding for all mothers.
- The choice of early feeding is made on the basis of nutritional, immunological, psychological, economic, and social considerations.
- Colostrum, which is secreted from maternal breast in the first few days after birth, contains immune substances that provide protection for the infant against infection.
- Infant formulas are made from cow's milk that is modified to resemble the nutrient composition of human milk. Although the nutrients may match, immunological properties cannot be added to infant formulas.
- Foremilk and hindmilk differ in fat content and therefore effect satiety and possibly weight gain in the infant.
- The Surgeon General set a goal for 1990 of having 75% of all babies breast fed when discharged from the hospital and 35% still breast fed at 6 months.
- Breast-fed infants need supplements of vitamin D, fluorine, and, after 4 months, iron. Iron-fortified formula–fed infants require no supplements, if the formula is diluted with fluoridated water.
- The practice of allowing an infant to fall asleep with a bottle, which contains formula, milk, or juice, in the mouth results in an increased rate of tooth decay, referred to as nursing bottle syndrome.
- Solid foods should be introduced between 4 to 6 months of age.
- Solid foods should be introduced gradually and individually to monitor for allergic reactions.
- The best indication of adequacy of the diet is the growth pattern of the child.
- An infant normally doubles his weight by 4 months and triples his weight by 12 months.

STUDY QUESTIONS

1. Define the following terms: colostrum, beikost, immunoglobulin, lactalbumin, lactoferrin, foremilk, and hindmilk. What is the significance of each infant feeding?
2. What supplements should be given to an infant? When and why?
3. Enumerate the various ways in which a breast-fed infant receives additional protection against infection.
4. What are the nutritional and psychological advantages of breast feeding?
5. What are the economic factors involved in breast-feeding versus using infant formula?
6. Why is it possible to adequately feed an infant on a formula?
7. Explain how growth charts (Figures 16-2 and 16-3) are used to assess development of a child.

Applying What You've Learned

1. **Interview Two Mothers**

   Discuss with two mothers how they chose to feed their babies, the reasons, where they sought advice, and their reactions to the process.

2. **Interview Two Fathers**

   Discuss with two fathers their role in infant feeding, scheduling, preparation of formula, and their impressions of the transitional phase of infant feeding.

3. **Compare Infant Formulas**

   Go to the grocery store to read and compare labels on several infant formulas. Compare the directions for convenience of preparation versus cost of the products.

4. **Compare Baby Foods**

   While at the grocery store read and compare labels of various brands of baby food. Examine the list of ingredients for added ingredients such as sugar, salt, or modified starch.

5. **Evaluate Advice in Commercial Magazine**

   Parents Magazine has been reviewed by experts and acclaimed as being an accurate and reliable source of nutrition information. While at the grocery store or library browse through one issue. Look for articles on nutrition and the feeding of infants and or children.

6. **Review Your Feeding Habits in Infancy**

   Ask your mother about your own feeding habits, weight gain, and growth rate. Include questions about the introduction of solid foods and your food preferences.

SUGGESTED READINGS

American Dietetic Association: Position on promotion of breast feeding, Journal of the American Dietetic Association 86:1580, 1986.

Members of the American Dietetic Association are urged to play an active role in the promotion of breast feeding based on the benefits to the mother and to the infant with particular emphasis on the nutritional and immunological benefits of human milk and the physiological, social, and hygienic benefits of the breast feeding process for the mother and infant. A technical support paper elaborates on the evidence.

Brown R: Breast-feeding and family planning: a review of the relationship between breast-feeding and family planning, American Journal of Clinical Nutrition 33:162, 1982.

The author presents a very comprehensive overview of the many physiological as well as psychological and social factors that must be considered in promoting breast feeding as a factor in family planning. Of particular importance is the nutritional status of the mother and the effect of subsequent pregnancies on the health of other young children in the family. Women who breast-feed generally have longer interbirth intervals than do those who do not, but breast feeding is seldom the contraception method of choice.

Dobbing JB: Infant nutrition and later achievement, Nutrition Reviews 42:1, 1984.

Dr. Dobbing reviews the data on the relationship between early feeding and later development and concludes that growth during the last trimester of pregnancy and the first 3 years of life are major determinants of ultimate body size. He feels that fears of adult obesity as a result of early feeding should be secondary to the adverse effects on both body and brain growth of any restriction in early life.

U.S. Department of Health and Human Services: Report of the Surgeon General's Workshop on Breastfeeding and Human Lactation, Pub. No. HRS-D-MC 84-2, Washington, D.C., 1984.

This 93-page booklet covers the proceedings of a workshop that dealt with the physiology of lactation, the uniqueness of human milk, the incidence of breast feeding, and the approaches to public education being used to promote the use of human milk in the initial feeding of infants. This publication is directed toward health workers and professionals dealing with young mothers during pregnancy and their young children.

ADDITIONAL READINGS

American Academy of Pediatrics: Nutritional aspects of obesity in infancy and childhood, Pediatrics 68:880, 1981; Policy statement based on task force report—the promotion of breast-feeding, Pediatrics 69:654, 1982; Toward a prudent diet for children, Pediatrics 71:76, 1983; The transfer of drugs and other chemicals into human breast milk, Pediatrics 72:375, 1983; Soy-protein formulas: recommendations for use in infant feeding, Pediatrics 72:359, 1983; The use of whole cow's milk in infancy, Pediatrics 72:253, 1983; Imitation and substitute milks, Pediatrics 73: 876, 1984.

Anderson SA, Chinn SH, and Fisher KD: History and current status of infant formula, American Journal of Clinical Nutrition 35:381, 1982.

Brams M, and Maloney J: "Nursing bottle caries" in breast-fed children, Journal of Pediatrics 103:415, 1983.

Butte NF, and others: Human milk intake and growth in exclusively breast-fed infants, Journal of Pediatrics 104:187, 1984.

Chandra RK: Physical growth of exclusively breast-fed infants, Nutrition Research 2:275, 1982.

Chesney RW: Taurine, is it required for infant nutrition? Journal of Nutrition 118:6, 1988.

DeLuca HF: The vitamin D story: a collaborative effort of basic science and clinical medicine, FASEB 2:224, 1988.

Dobbing J: Infant nutrition and later achievement, Nutrition Reviews 42:39, 1984.

Endres J, Poon SW, Welch P, Sawicki M, and Duncan H: Dietary sodium intake of infants fed commercially prepared baby food and table food, Journal of the American Dietetic Association 87:750, 1987.

Filer LJ: Modified food starch—an update, Journal of the American Dietetic Association 88:342, 1988.

Fransson GB, and Lonnerdal B: Zinc, copper, calcium, and magnesium in human milk, Journal of Pediatrics 101:504, 1982.

Jelliffe DB: World trends in infant feeding, American Journal of Clinical Nutrition 29: 1227, 1976.

Lammi-Keef CJ, and Jensen RG: Lipids in human milk: a review 2. Composition and fat soluble vitamins, Journal of Pediatric Gastroenterology and Nutrition 3:172, 1984.

Lebenthal E, Lee FC, and Heitlinger LA: Impact of development of the gastrointestinal tract on infant feeding, Journal of Pediatrics 102:1, 1983.

Levander OA, Moser PB; and Morris VC: Dietary selenium intake and selenium concentrations of plasma, erythrocytes, and breast milk in pregnant and postpartum lactating women, American Journal of Clinical Nutrition 46:694, 1987.

Lonnerdal B: Effects of maternal dietary intake on human milk composition, Journal of Nutrition 116:499, 1986.

Marlin DW, Picciano MF, and Livant EC: Infant feeding practices, Journal of the American Dietetic Association 77:668, 1980.

Martinez GA, and Dodd DA: 1981 milk feeding patterns in the United States during the first 12 months of life, Pediatrics 71:166, 1983.

Matheny R, and Picciano MF: Feeding and growth characteristics of human milk-fed infants, Journal of the American Dietetic Association 86:327, 1986.

McCormick MC: The contribution of low birth weight to infant mortality and childhood morbidity, New England Journal of Medicine 308:612, 1982.

Metabolic and endocrine responses of infants to breast milk and formulas, Nutrition Reviews 42:10, 1984.

Nietora GG, and others: Is prolonged breast feeding associated with malnutrition? American Journal of Clinical Nutrition 39:307, 1984.

Ogra PL and Greene HL: Human milk and breastfeeding: an update on the state of the art, Pediatric Research 16:266, 1982.

Ojofeitimi ED: Effect of duration and frequency of breast-feeding on postpartum amenorrhea, Pediatrics 69:164, 1982.

Picciano MF: Nutrient needs of infants, Nutrition Today 22:8, 1987.

Sarett HP, Bain KR, and O'Leary JC: Decisions on breast-feeding or formula feeding and trends in infant-feeding practices, American Journal of Diseases of Children 137:719, 1983.

Sheard NF, and Walker WA: The role of breast milk in the development of the gastrointestinal tract, Nutrition Reviews 46:1, 1988.

Siimes MA, Salmenpera L, and Perheentupa J: Exclusive breast-feeding for 9 months: risk of iron deficiency, Journal of Pediatrics 104: 196, 1984.

Whitehead RG: Infant physiology, nutritional requirements, and lactational adequacy, American Journal of Clinical Nutrition 41: 447, 1986.

Widdowson E: Fetal and neonatal nutrition, Nutrition Today 22:16, 1987.

Yeung DL, and others: Infant fatness and feeding practices: a longitudinal assessment, Journal of the American Dietetic Association 79:531, 1981.

Yip R, Reeves JD, Lonnerdal B, Keen CL, and Dallman PR: Does iron supplementation compromise zinc nutrition in healthy infants? American Journal of Clinical Nutrition 42: 683, 1985.

Ziegler EE: Infants of low birth weight: special needs and problems, American Journal of Clinical Nutrition 41:440, 1985.

FOCUS Infant Formula—Choices and Controversies

Infant formulas have been the subject of considerable discussion in developed and developing countries for quite different reasons. In the developed and Western world an increasing number of women, particularly the more affluent and better educated, are choosing to breastfeed, and for a much longer time than did their mothers. Concern in these areas centers of how closely and successfully a formula simulates breast milk to meet the needs of the infant. In developing countries, infant formula has been the subject of intense criticism; it has been charged that its availability is influencing many mothers to abandon breast feeding. This in turn is blamed for an increase in infant mortality.

The recognition in the early 1930s that infants could be adequately and safely fed on a formula based on evaporated milk represented a significant advance from nineteenth century practices, when there was no acceptable substitute for breast feeding, and few infants who were not suckled by their mothers or by a wet nurse survived the first year of life. By the 1930s it was recognized that many of the infectious conditions of early infancy could be controlled by pasteurization or heat treatment of milk to destroy the disease-producing organisms. Careful storage under refrigeration then maintained the quality of the milk. Even though a large number of children thrived on this feeding routine, it soon became evident that there was much to be done to modify evaporated milk so that the formula more closely resembled human milk. Conditions such as rickets, scurvy, and anemia were common during infancy.

The problem of rickets was handled first by the recommendation that infants be given a supplement of cod-liver oil each day, and later by fortifying evaporated milk with vitamin D. The incidence of scurvy prompted the use of orange juice as a supplement for infants, in spite of the fact that a good many children had an allergic reaction to the oil that had been extracted from the rind. It was not until 1948 that vitamin C was added to commercial formula. The lack of vitamin C had been implicated in megaloblastic anemia. This was actually caused by a lack of folate, since vitamin C was necessary before the low levels of folacin in the diet could be converted to the active form.

Microcytic anemia, on the other hand, generally results from lack of dietary iron and is corrected by the addition of iron to infant formula. There is still considerable discussion of the relative merits of providing an iron-enriched formula to infants from birth or waiting until 4 months of age, when the reserves present in the liver and in the high hemoglobin levels at birth become depleted.

In addition to having a nutrient profile that is well suited to the needs of the infant, human milk has certain physical characteristics that make it ideal for the newborn and that we attempt to replicate in formula feeding. The stability of the mixture of emulsified fats, proteins, carbohydrates, vitamins, and minerals that make up most formulas is ensured by the addtition of a thickening or stabilizing agent to the formula. Many substances have been approved to play this role. The electrolyte composition of the formula is important, because it determines the exchange of fluids within the intestine and if levels are too high, diarrhea, dehydration, and disruption of electrolyte balance may result.

Most milk-based formulas start with fat-free cow's milk solids to which lactose is added to make the carbohydrate/protein ratio closer to that of human milk. Vegetable oils are added to provide a digestible form of fat. To better simulate the lactalbumin/casein ratio of human milk that is partially responsible for the softer curd formed during digestion, a demineralized whey is substituted for some of the milk protein. Essential vitamins and minerals are then added to bring the total amount up to the standards spelled out in the U.S. Infant Formula Act of 1980. To reduce the amount of some electrolytes, such as sodium, to appropriate levels, it may be necessary to dialyze the formula, in which case care must be taken to add back any other elements that might be withdrawn at the same time.

Soy-based formulas, which represent about 20% of the formulas produced, are used primarily for infants with allergies or a family history of allergy. They include a water-soluble soy isolate, vegetable oils, corn syrup or sucrose, and the appropriate minerals and vitamins.

Although it is added in only 40% of the formulas sold in ready-to-feed prepackaged form, water is an extremely important variable in determining the concentration of electrolytes. Instructions on the concentrated formula and the powdered product must be followed carefully.

We have made substantial progress in simulating the nutritional quality of human milk but have been less successful in trying to reproduce any of its important immunological properties. This may not be accomplished in the near future, but with the tremendous technological advances of the last 10 years, it would be unwise to predict that it could not be done. Because many of the immunological properties result from proteins and because we have already synthesized some proteins, there is little reason to say that this would not be possible once the amino acid composition and arrangement within the molecule have been determined. In the meantime, because we have made great advances in controlling disease, the lack of this immunological protection in a country with high environmental standards is not as important as in countries in which there is much greater chance of contamination.

While this question is commanding the attention of food scientists and nutritionists, the availability of infant formula in developing countries has become more of a moral and legal issue than a nutritional one. After balancing a great many persuasive arguments, the United States voted in the United Nations against a code to govern the sale of infant formula in developing countries. They maintained that they supported the consensus that breast feeding was the preferred method of feeding and that it should be maintained at a high level in all countries, developed as well as developing, and would continue to provide bilateral support to the World Health Organization to promote breast feeding wherever possible. They did not feel, however, that they could support a code that imposed a complete ban on advertising of infant formula and interfered with the flow of information between manufacturers and consumers about a product for which there is a legitimate market. Since they would not have implemented such a code in the United States, it seemed inappropriate to recommend that it be adopted by other countries.

Those who argued in favor of the code felt that the promotional activities of the companies selling infant formula in developing countries were a major factor in the decline in breast feeding and the purported increase in infant mortality associated with it. While there were indeed some inappropriate marketing practices by representatives of some companies, there was no convincing evidence that either advertising or the availability of free samples in hospitals was directly responsible for the decline in breast feeding, which had been going on for some time before advertising began. There was evidence that mothers who received samples were often not adequately informed about how to use them and thus prepared them in an unsanitary way, often using contaminated water, which may have been all that was available, or fed the formulas in excessively diluted form. In many developing countries, the vast majority of women still deliver their babies at home and make their decisions about breast feeding or bottle feeding based on what is traditional. Many live so far from a store that might sell formula that even if they had the money, they would find it almost impossible to purchase the formula. Many of the samples that were distributed to physicians found their way into the market, where they were sold at regular retail price to many of the more affluent patients who were already bottle feeding. These patients were usually better educated women who would be more likely to understand the importance of using formulas in an appropriate way.

Most of the evidence garnered against the sale of formula tended to be emotional and anecdotal. Infant deaths in developing countries were related more to low birth weight, mother's age and health, the number of previously borne offspring *(parity)*, and the type of bottle feeding (as distinguished form formula feeding). For many infants, whose mothers were not able to breast feed for a variety of physiological, social, and emotional reasons, the availability of formula made the difference between life and death.

In summary, there is almost complete agreement that we have perfected the formulation of supplemental feedings to the point that infants can thrive without breast feeding. This assumes that the formula is prepared according to directions and in a sanitary way. There is no question that breast feeding is the preferred method and that it should be used whenever possible, even if only for a short period. It is completely unacceptable to persuade a mother who is capable and willing to feed her baby at the breast to switch to bottle feeding. There are, however, many situations in which bottle feeding will be the method of choice. Under those circumstances it should be readily available, and all precautions should be used to see that it is appropriately used.

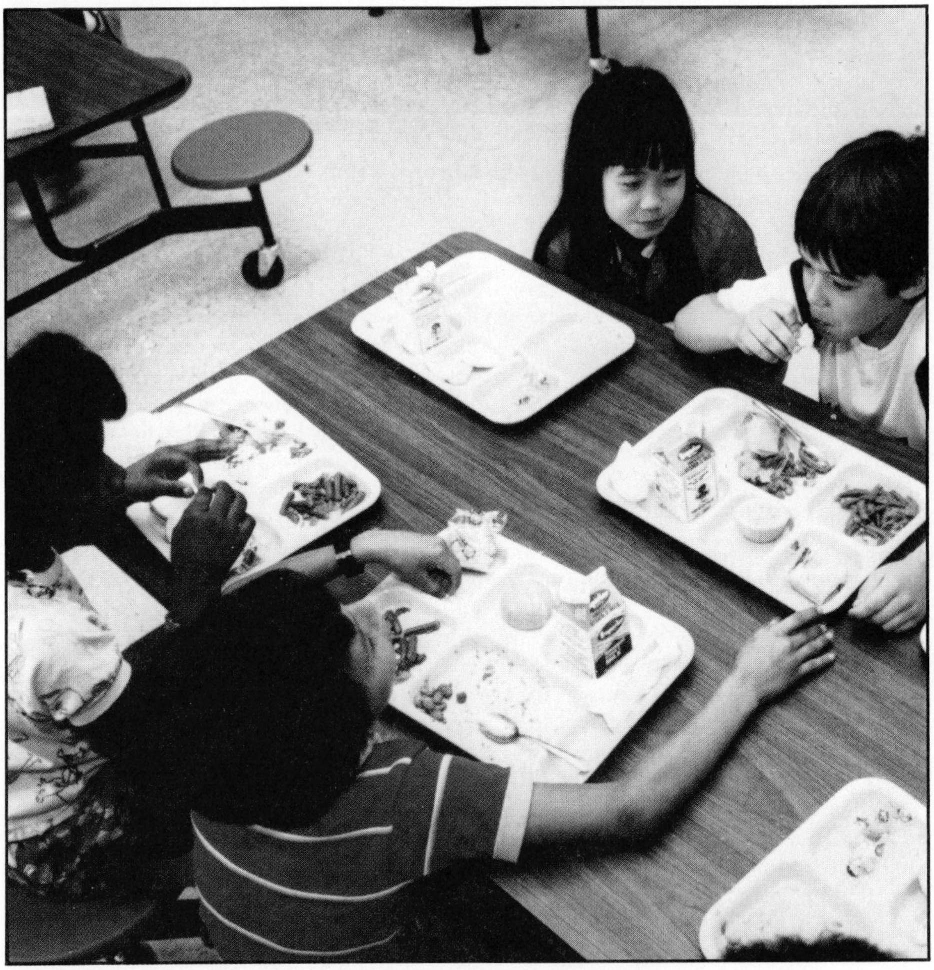

AWARENESS CHECK

Truth or Fiction?

- Snacks can be an important component of the diet of both children and adolescents.
- Teenagers who skip breakfast can perform adequately as long as they make up the nutrients later in the day.
- Milk is an important part only of the infant and childhood diet. Once a person reaches adolescence the need for calcium diminishes.
- Children have more taste buds than adults and therefore are more sensitive to the strong flavors of foods.
- Sugar causes hyperactivity in children.
- Anorexia nervosa and bulimia are two eating disorders more prevalent in young women than any other sex or age group.

Nutrition from Childhood through Adulthood

CHAPTER 17

Relatively little research has been done on the nutritional needs and problems of people from 2 to 16 years of age—largely because it represents a time when there are few severe nutritional problems. In addition, in spite of the fact that this period is critical to adult health, children and adolescents are amazingly resilient to short-term nutrient lack. We have little information on which to judge the long-term consequences of the very diverse eating patterns of this age-group. We have every reason to believe—and no reason not to believe—that nutrient adequacy, but not excess, during this time provides a form of insurance against some of the degenerative changes of aging.

In Chapter 16 we dealt with the character of the infant's diet and the gradual change in food variety and quantity as the child's nutritive needs and ability to handle a greater complexity of foods increase during the first year of life. By 1 year of age the capacity of the stomach has increased so that smaller, more frequent feedings are no longer necessary. The digestive system, the liver, and the kidneys are mature enough to handle a wide variety of foods, the products of metabolism and the waste products that need to be excreted and the *rate* of growth has slowed.

There is a great variability in the age at which an infant makes the transition from bottle feeding or breast feeding and eating pureed or chopped baby foods to drinking from a cup and eating selected items from the regular family diet. Some children make the adjustment as early as 8 months of age, whereas others may not reach this stage of maturity until 2 years of age or later. In either case, it is important to encourage children to chew when the ability to do so is established and to feed themselves when they have the manual dexterity to manipulate a spoon. Otherwise, there is no reason to encourage the change before the child is ready. The infant should probably not be denied the work of sucking from either the breast or bottle for at least the first year, because this may predispose the child to thumb-sucking or to poorly developed jaws and crowding of the teeth.

CHILDHOOD

Although growth is relatively slower in childhood than in infancy, it is extremely important that the diet provide appropriate kinds and amounts of nutrients. Children who triple their birth weight in the first year require the whole preschool period to double it again. In spite of the varying rate of growth throughout childhood, there appears to be a continuing, generally increased need for all nutrients. The pattern of increase varies for different nutrients in relation to their role in growth of specific tissues.

The dietary standards proposed by the Food and Nutrition Board represent the level of intake believed to provide optimal health benefits to practically all children in each age-group. The recognition that growth of children occurs in spurts—a period of rapid increase in skeletal height followed by a slow increase in height but a more rapid increase in weight—suggests that these values represent an excessive margin of safety at one time and a realistic goal at another. In a few instances the recommendations are based on firm experimental evidence; for some nutrients they are calculated from growth needs; for some they have been extrapolated from information on adult needs; for others they merely reflect the level of intake observed in apparently healthy children. They remain, however, our only standard for assessing dietary adequacy and are the nutritional goal used in planning food intakes. Although total nutritional need increases with age, requirements decline on the basis of body weight.

Nutrients Needed as Energy Needs Increase
Thiamin
Riboflavin
Niacin
Pantothenic acid

Nutrients Needed for Muscle Growth
Protein
Pyridoxine
Potassium
Folacin
Vitamin B_{12}
Zinc

Nutrients Needed for Blood Formation
Protein
Iron
Pyridoxine
Folacin
Vitamins B_{12}, C
Copper

Nutrients Needed for Bone Formation
Calcium
Phosphorus
Vitamins A, D, C
Protein
Manganese

Figure 17-1 represents the change in nutritive needs for boys and girls during childhood and adolescence in relation to needs in the second year of life. The suggested increment obviously varies from one nutrient to another. Fortunately for ease of diet planning, the increment for calories is frequently at least as large as the increment for other nutrients. As one would expect, the increase in energy needs represents the amount of energy needed for basal metabolism, larger increases in activity, and the amount (about 2%) stored as new muscle or adipose tissue. Requirements for basal metabolism and activity will increase proportionately with body size, whereas those for growth will vary with the rate of growth, which fluctuates from one age to another. Although the recommended energy intakes (REI) do not make a distinction between the needs for boys and girls until age 11, several studies show that boys have higher energy needs than girls and eat more as early as 6 years of age.

Since many of the water-soluble vitamins, such as thiamin, riboflavin, niacin, and pantothenic acid, are involved primarily in energy metabolism, it is not surprising to find their requirements increasing in proportion to total energy needs. Pyridoxine, involved in the utilization of dietary protein and in the synthesis of tissue protein, will be required in greater amounts during periods of rapid tissue growth. The increase in muscle mass that must accompany bone growth requires a positive nitrogen balance that is met by protein intakes of 1.5 to 2 grams/kg of body weight. The increase in total body size necessitates a larger vascular system to transport nutrients to the tissues and waste products away from the tissues, thus making demands for nutrients needed in blood formation: iron, protein, folacin, and pyridoxine. Bone growth creates a need for protein, calcium, phosphorus, fluorine, and vitamin D. The fact that vitamin A is required for maintaining epithelial cells and vitamin C is required for the synthesis of collagen provides ample reason to believe that the amount needed will increase with growth.

Growth is influenced by factors other than nutrition. Although a person's maximum size is genetically determined, nutrition is one of the most important deter-

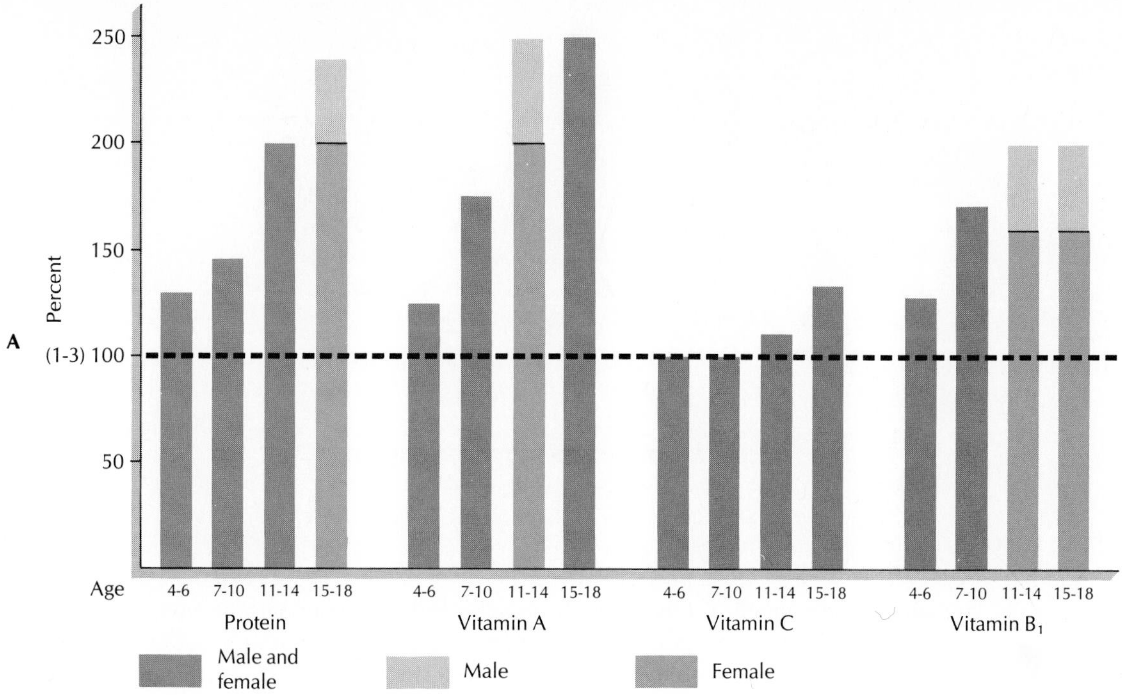

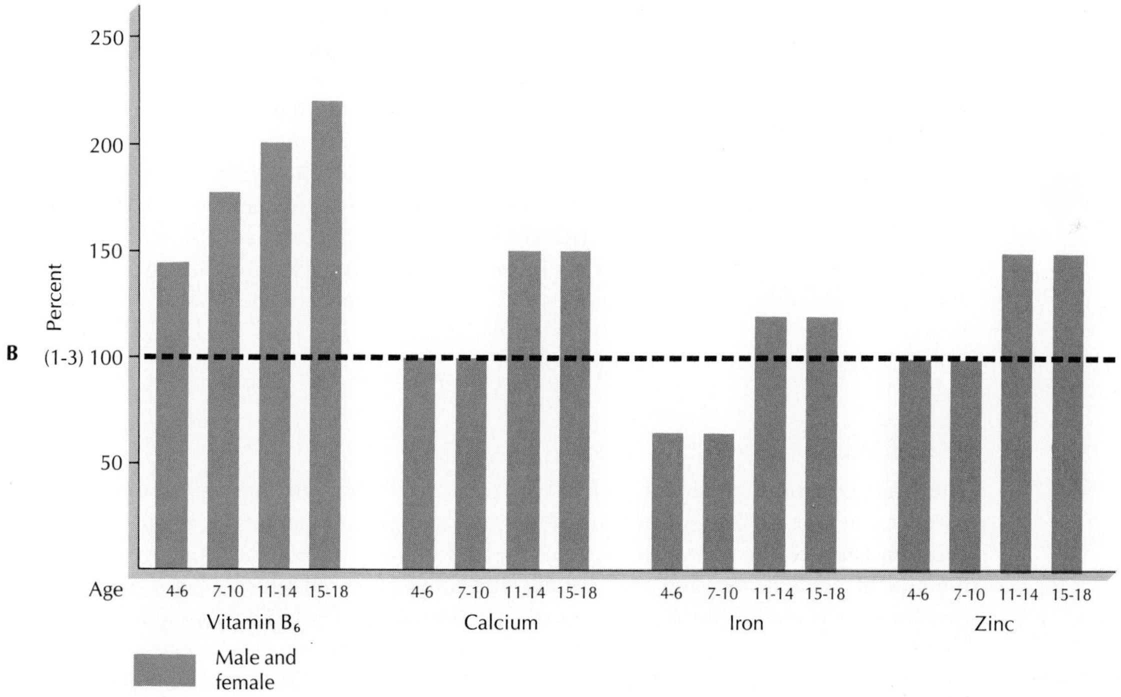

Figure 17-1 Change (by percent) in nutrient requirements from the ages of 1 to 18, in males **(A)** and females **(B)**.

Based on Recommended Dietary Allowances, ed 9, Washington, D.C., 1980, National Academy of Sciences, National Research Council, Food and Nutrition Board.

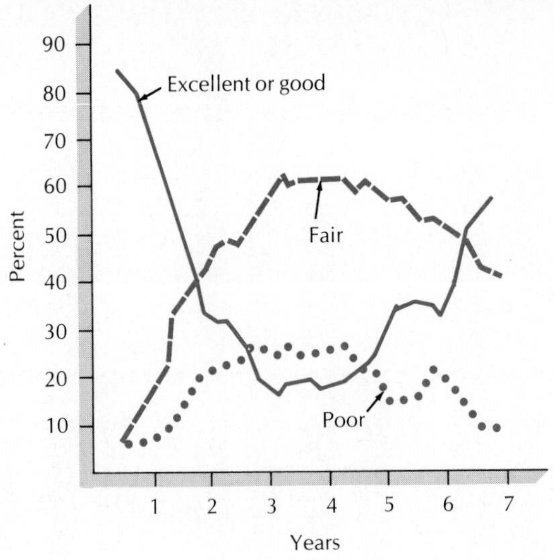

Figure 17-2 Percentage of children from 6 months old to 7 years old whose appetites were rated excellent or good, fair, or poor by their mothers.
From Beal VA: Pediatrics 20:448, 1957.

minants of how much of this potential is achieved. Other important environmental factors include medical care and sanitation to control parasites and infections. In general the overall need for nutrients increases throughout the growth period, but there will be periods when growth is slow, and the need for certain nutrients will be reduced proportionately. In their own wisdom, children reflect these changes in need by fluctuations in appetite. These changes often create a good deal of anxiety for the parents, but it is common and natural for a child who has had a hearty appetite to go through a period in which both appetite and food intake are noticeably reduced. Unless such a period is prolonged or is accompanied by signs of undernutrition, such as lethargy, fatigue, and increased susceptibility to infection, it should not cause concern. The unnecessary worry of some parents over their children's food habits is exemplified in a study showing that mothers tended to rate their children's food habits as poor, even though the children's diets met all criteria for nutritional adequacy. The fluctuations in appetite with age, as reported by mothers of Colorado children, is typical (Figure 17-2).

Although thiamin and vitamin B_{12} have been promoted as stimulants to appetite and growth in children, thiamin is of value only to correct the most severe thiamin deprivation, and B_{12} (cobalamin) has no value as an appetite stimulant. Both, of course, play essential roles in metabolism.

Transitional Foods

In planning meals for young children consider
- the food—nutrition, flavor, color, texture, and serving size
- the environment—comfort (temperature and chairs), utensils, noise level, colorful decor.
- the atmosphere—pleasant, peaceful, lacking distraction

Characteristics of Foods Children Like
Colorful
Soft
Small servings
Lukewarm
Mild flavored

The transition from an infant diet to a regular adult diet will be less traumatic if parents understand the ways children react to food. Observation suggests that children react to the color, flavor, texture, and temperature of the food, as well as the size of the servings and the attitude and atmosphere in which it is presented. Problems with any of these may lead to rejection of the food. The wise parent will try to determine the cause of the reaction; more often than not, it is something that can be easily corrected. Parents should focus on food habits that have real nutritional implications and ignore the inconsequential ones.

Children generally favor foods that are soft textured and are less accepting of foods that are dry or likely to shatter, have tough or stringy parts, or are too thick. For example, they prefer thin to thick puddings, celery with the strings removed, stewed tomatoes with the fibers cut, soft mashed potatoes to baked potatoes, moist ground meats to dry fish, and soft bread to coarse bread. This preference for moist foods may reflect the scant supply of saliva, which for older children provides a natural lubricant.

Children prefer foods that are lukewarm to extremes of hot or cold. Thus by serving the child's food first, it has usually reached the right temperature by the time others at the table are served. Milk served slightly warm is much more acceptable than ice-cold milk. The tendency of children to dawdle over ice cream until it is semisolid reflects their distaste for very cold foods.

Children are keenly sensitive to flavors, reacting to flavors that may go undetected by adults. For instance, children reject milk with a slight taint or react when food has been only slightly scorched. They will often refuse vegetables of the cabbage or onion families when these are cooked in small amounts of water to preserve nutrients and flavor, but they will accept them when the foods are cooked longer in larger amounts of water or when served with a cream sauce to modify the flavor. Once the mild flavor of the vegetable has been accepted, they can be served in a way that maximizes the nutrient content.

The quantity of food offered to children at one time is important. It is more satisfactory from a psychological point of view to offer children less than the parents anticipate they will eat and have them return for more than to present them with such a large quantity that they are defeated before they begin to eat. The use of 120- to 180-ml (4- to 6-oz) glasses that can be easily grasped in the child's chubby hands or plastic mugs with handles is preferable to a large 8- to 10-oz glass that overtaxes manual dexterity and stomach capacity. Any of these help develop good eye-hand coordination in children. Child-sized utensils are essential. Allowing children to serve themselves so that they can determine the amount of food on their plates or serving food in bite-size pieces may lead to greater acceptance of the meal. The child must also have a safe chair of appropriate size.

Appropriate Materials for Feeding Children
Small glasses or mugs with handles
Unbreakable dishes
Appropriate-sized utensils
Comfortable chair

Visually, children respond favorably to a colorful meal with color provided by the plate and setting, the combination of foods, or the judicious use of edible garnishes. It is best to avoid unnatural food shapes, inedible material, or colors not normally found in food, such as blue or purple.

Young children quite naturally like to feel both the temperature and the texture of their food. They also find that many foods are more easily manipulated with the hands than with utensils. Thus strips of meat, wedges of lettuce, or raw vegetables as finger foods allow the child to sense the feel of foods; as a result, they are often more willing to try the taste of such foods.

The age at which a child develops sufficient manual dexterity to handle a knife, fork, and spoon is again an individual matter. Success will be greater if utensils designed for the growing child are used. Until children reach the stage of motor development when they are skilled in the use of utensils, food should be served in a way that challenges them to learn but does not require so much skill that it frustrates them.

It is important to keep in mind that children are just as individual and variable in their capabilities and needs as are adults. Thus it is to be expected that many children's food preferences will not conform to the patterns suggested in these generalizations.

Meal Patterns

Data from the Nationwide Food Consumption Survey (NFCS, 1977-1978) showed that 77% of the 1- to 4-year-olds and 80% of the 4- to 6-year-olds ate at least three meals on the 3 consecutive days of record keeping, and 95% had three meals on 2 of the 3 days. The nutrient adequacy of the total days' diet was directly related to the number of days on which the child had three meals, regardless of the number of snacks.

Snacks

The role of snacks in the diet of young children remains controversial. During periods of high nutritive needs, snacks are almost essential, because small children may be unable to take in sufficient amounts of food to satisfy nutrient needs in

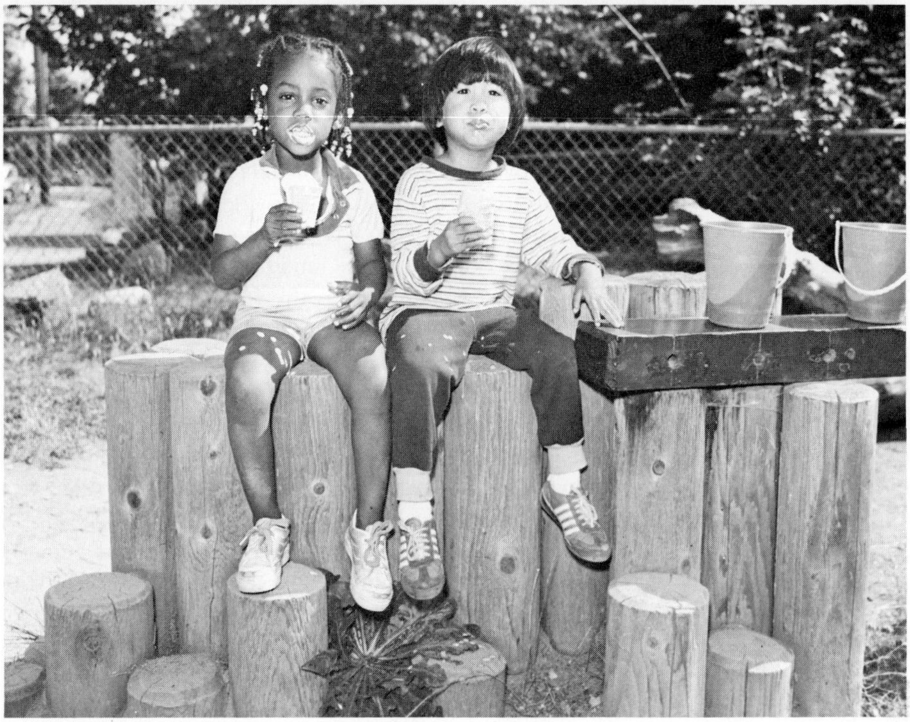

Besides being fun, snacks can play an important role in a child's nutrition.

three meals without taxing the capacity of their stomachs. On the other hand, if snacks of high satiety value are taken too near regular meal hours, they may reduce the food intake at mealtimes. One study showed that snacks given 2½ hours before lunchtime had no effect on the appetite for lunch. They did, however, reduce the caloric intake at lunch, although the combined intake from lunch and snacks was greater than from lunch alone. There is some evidence that considerable snacking takes place in front of the television. That this is a factor in sedentary life-style characteristic of a growing number of children is cause for concern.

Since adults can control the type of snacks through their control over food purchases, they have ultimate responsibility for seeing that snacks contribute to the total nutritive needs of the child. A cogent argument in favor of well-chosen snacks is provided by research showing that smaller, more frequent meals result in the formation of relatively less adipose tissue and better nutrient utilization. It is important to remember that any food, no matter how good its nutritional profile, should be used in moderation; excess use will result in the exclusion of other foods often needed to balance the nutrient intake.

An analysis of data from a USDA survey of 371 children on 4 nonconsecutive days in 1985 showed that all children had at least one snack and 47% of the 4- to 5-year-olds and 60% of the 1- to 3-year-olds had at least one a day. These provided about one fifth of the daily calories and over 15% of their intake of fiber, vitamin E, vitamin C, and riboflavin, calcium, phosphorus, magnesium, copper, and potassium. This indicates that snacks were relatively nutritious although slightly higher in calories and fat than other nutrients.

An analysis of the contribution of snacks to the total nutrient intake of these children showed that as the number of snacks increased, the adequacy of intake of both calories and other nutrients increased. This indicates that snacks tended to have an acceptable nutrient density and were not primarily sugar and refined carbohydrates. Because a pattern of snacking or smaller, more frequent meals is becoming more common, we should promote attitudes that will lead to prudent and nutritionally wise food selections.

Food Jags

Although it is desirable to educate children to accept a wide variety of foods and to be open-minded in trying new foods, it is recognized that young children go on **food jags** in which they accept a very limited number of foods and reject all others. If the accepted foods represent a nutritionally adequate but monotonous diet, as is often observed, there is little evidence that these preferences should provoke concern, unless the foods used would contribute excess amounts of additives, sugar, or salt. Jags seldom persist for prolonged periods, nor is there evidence that they lead to limited food choices in adulthood. It has been observed, however, that the quality of the diet at all ages is positively correlated with the number of different food items eaten daily. This emphasizes the importance of encouraging the use of foods from a variety of food groups during the years when food habits are forming.

food jags
Patterns of eating in which very few food items are eaten to the exclusion of all others for a long period of time (several weeks)

Adequacy of Diets of Infants and Children

The 1985 survey of children 1 to 5 years old showed that the average intake of all nutrients except iron and zinc for 1- to 3-year-olds and vitamin E and zinc for the older group exceeded the RDAs. Iron, folacin, calcium, and zinc were the nutrients for which less than 90% of the children had less than 70% of the RDA. Figure 17-3 summarizes adequacy of diets of children up to age 11 as reported in the NFCS in 1977-1978.

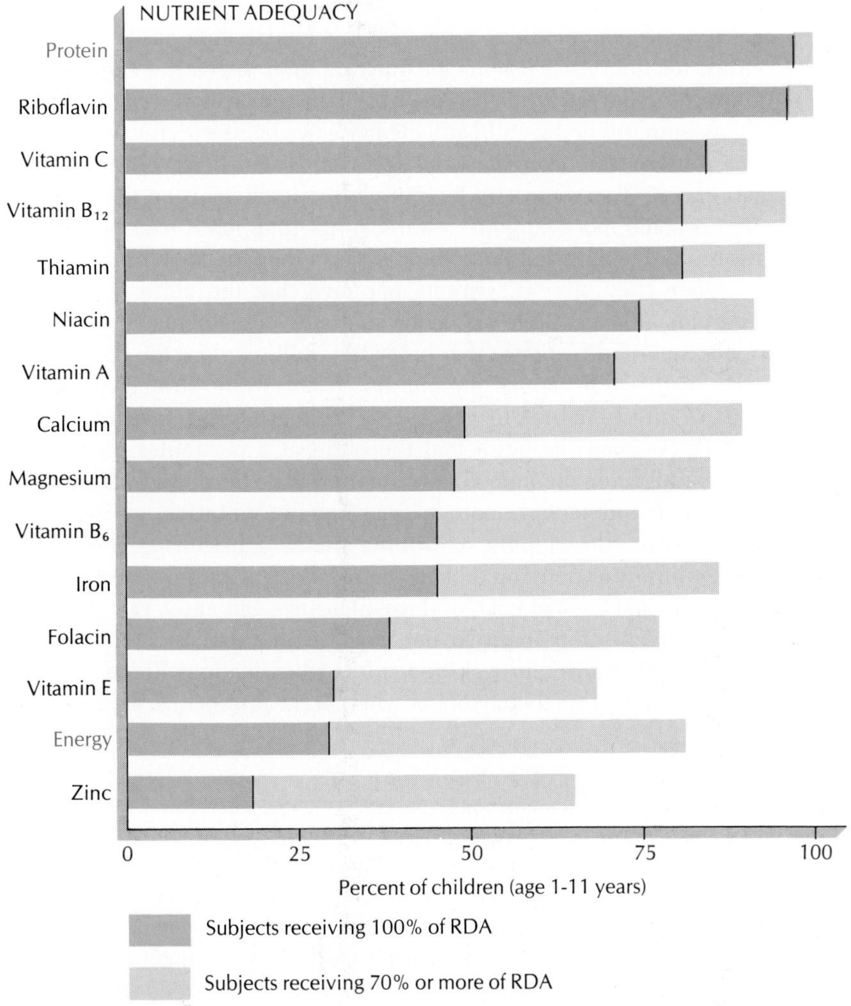

Figure 17-3 Adequacy of dietary intake of children 1 to 11 years old, as reported in the NFCS (1977-78).

Biochemical and physical assessment of the nutritional status of children in NHANES II revealed no evidence of frank deficiency conditions except that 9% of children 1 to 2 years of age and 3% to 5% of children 3 to 10 years of age had impaired iron status.

Food Preferences

Foods Liked by Children

Fruit	70%
Meat	65%
Milk	55%
Bread	48%
Vegetables	43%

Several studies to determine children's food preferences, which reflect their reactions to the appearance, taste, texture, and temperature of food, have all led to similar conclusions. Less than half the children studied liked vegetables, whereas over two thirds liked fruits. The fact that vegetables are generally unpopular may be the result of the many and possibly unsatisfactory ways in which they are prepared and the generally negative reaction of adults to the flavor of vegetables. Their attitudes may be subtly, if not overtly, communicated to children. Raw vegetables are much more popular with children than are cooked ones. Meat, milk, and bread ranked next to fruit in popularity. Food likes of youngsters are related to those of other family members, especially the father, in that food preferences influence the frequency with which specific foods are served, and even whether they are purchased. Once foods are in the home, there is little relationship between the child's food preferences and those of the parents. Children develop preferences from foods that are presented in a friendly social situation by an approving and supportive adult. The acceptance of a food by a peer or a sibling, particularly one in a leadership role, also increases the likelihood of its acceptance.

Difficulties in persuading the child to taste a new food and then to eat it frequently enough that the liking is reinforced have led to the application of the principles of behavior modification in developing food habits. This involves an immediate reward for the desired behavior (for example, vegetable eating) and the absence of any reinforcement of the undesirable behavior (refusing the food). The reward must be meaningful to the child and clearly associated with the new behavior. Once the eating pattern has been shaped, the rewards can be given intermittently and finally withdrawn. For some children praise in itself may be sufficiently rewarding; for others some more tangible reward, other than food, may be necessary.

When children fail to eat what the parent expects them to, in a form they expect it to be eaten, when they offer it, parents perceive that the child has a feeding problem. To parents unacceptable behavior includes refusing to eat, dawdling, playing with food (a normal response that helps the child explore the environment), or spitting food. In these situations parents use a variety of strategies; some are appropriate, others questionable. In general, the effectiveness varies, depending on the interactions between the adult and the child at a particular time and also whether success is judged on the immediate outcome or the long-range consequence. Most frequently used approaches include ignoring the situation, reasoning with children, coaxing them, threatening or bribing them, substituting a comparable food, punishing children, or denying them some privilege. Child psychologists have long debated the pros and cons of each of these measures but agree that the greatest problems arise when children learn to use food to manipulate their parents or caregivers. They become particularly skilled at this when food is offered as a reward for either eating or noneating behavior or when it is offered as a pacifier or a diversion.

Vegetarianism

Children raised on a strict vegetarian diet with limited intakes of available iron, protein, zinc, vitamin D, vitamin B_{12}, and calcium have an increased risk of nutritional problems such as growth retardation, rickets, anemia, and increased susceptibility to infection. Because children have a small stomach capacity they have difficulty eating enough of the high-fiber foods (fruits, vegetables, cereals, and legumes) in a vegetarian diet to meet their energy needs. Once fetal stores are depleted, vitamin B_{12} necessary for growth is very limited. As a result vegan children have heights and weights that tend to fall at the 5th to 15th percentile of growth standards more often than children on a diet that includes animal foods. Their calcium intake on a diet devoid of dairy products is alarmingly low, as is their intake of vitamin D. Both of these dietary limitations predispose them to rickets. While the intake of iron is relatively high, its bioavailability is limited because of lack of heme iron from meat products. Their increased susceptibility to infection reflects a depressed immune function which, in turn, is the result of low protein, zinc, and iron status. The lack of dietary cholesterol for myelination of nerve fibers could be a problem when caloric intake is limited. On the other hand, vitamin A, vitamin C, and magnesium are usually adequate. The distribution of calories from carbohydrate, fat, and protein of 58%, 30%, and 12% respectively approaches the recommendations of the dietary goals.

EVALUATION OF NUTRITIONAL STATUS

Children growing at the 5th percentile are shorter than 95% of children of the same age.

Because childhood is a period of active growth and a well-nourished child can be expected to have predictable increments in both height and weight, physical growth has become a readily available standard on which to assess nutritional status. Children in this generation have a more rapid rate of growth and are reaching maturity at an earlier age than children a few decades ago. This is a function not only of improved nutrition but also of favorable environmental factors and the advances in medical science that have reduced or eliminated many of the diseases that used to depress growth. As a result, it is important that any growth standard used in evaluating nutritional status be a recent one.

The National Center for Health Statistics has prepared growth curves based on cross-sectional data on the U.S. population in the last 15 years. It is recommended that these curves be used as growth standards for children. Height for age, indicating shortness or tallness, and weight for height, indicating thinness or fatness, are considered the most useful relationships. Consideration of weight for age is of limited usefulness. Curves (Figures 17-4 and 17-5) show the 5th, 10th, 25th, 50th, 75th, 90th, and 100th percentile values of weight and height for age for boys and girls, 2 to 18 years of age. Weight for height for prepubertal boys and girls is shown in Figures 17-6 and 17-7. Charts for children from birth to 3 years of age are shown in Chapter 16.

By plotting actual measurements on the appropriate chart, you can determine how a particular child is developing in comparison to other children of the same age or height. Those who fall below the 5th percentile (meaning that only 5% of the population is lighter in weight for age or height) should be screened further to determine whether nutritional or other environmental factors have caused the retarded growth or whether the child is merely genetically smaller than others. When a child is measured, that measurement should be compared to previous ones to determine whether nutritional status has improved or deteriorated. Deviations away from the median often indicate some medical or nutritional abnormality. A trend toward the upper percentiles in weight but not height is a warning to begin restriction of caloric intake and encouragement of caloric expenditure and try to determine the underlying causes of the developing obesity. Trends in the other direction may signal infection or other conditions that cause a loss of appetite and weight. Such records provide a visual record of growth trends and are therefore useful in medical evaluations in developing countries and as a diagnostic tool in many schools in Western countries.

The evaluation of weight gain in relation to expected rate of gain has been proposed as a criterion of adequacy of growth. Rate of gain is unacceptable if it is less than half the amount of gain expected. Because factors accelerating or retarding growth will affect weight earlier than stature, gain in weight that is substantially greater or less than expected from gain in stature is considered undesirable. In

Text continued on p. 532.

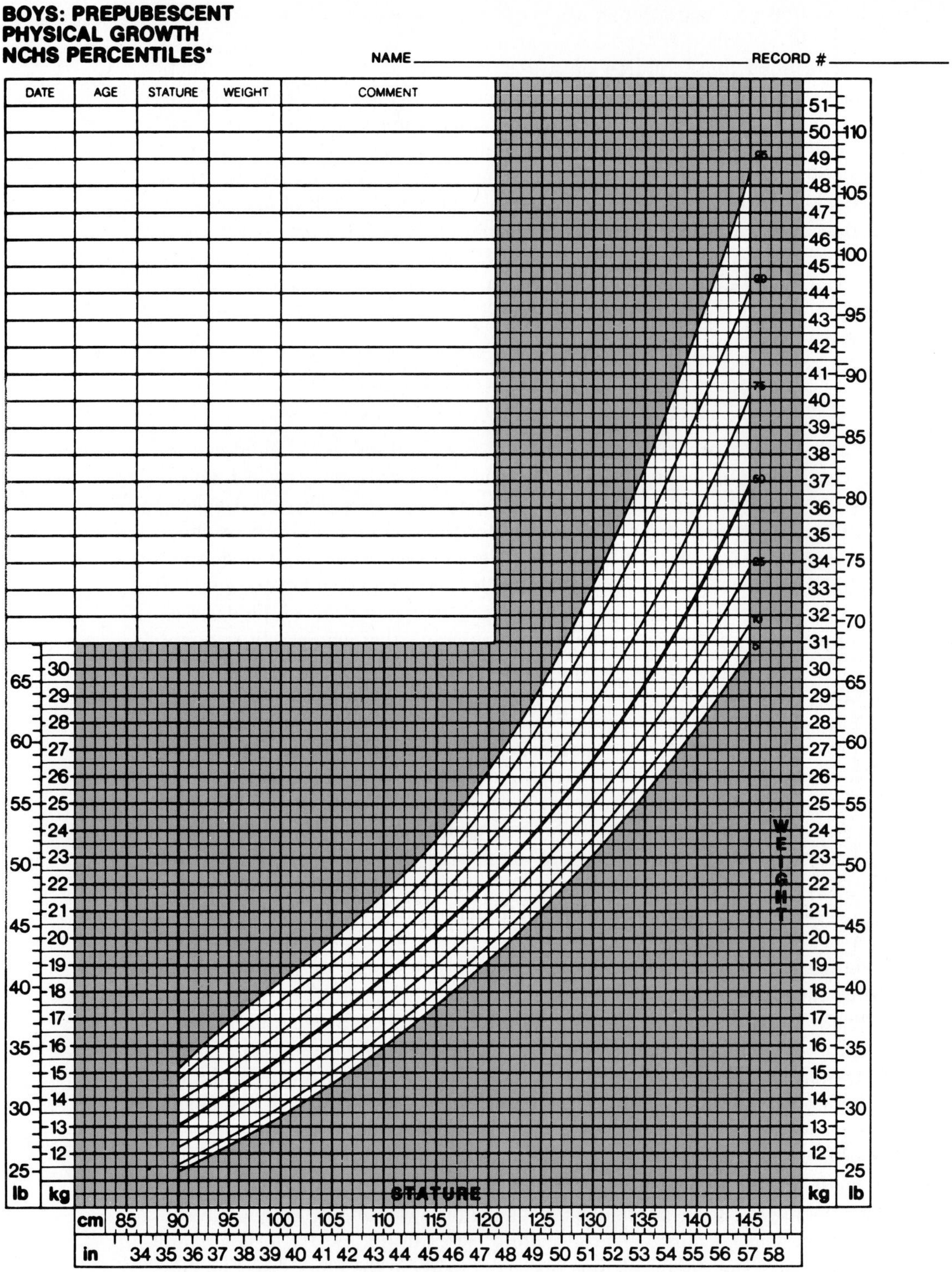

Figure 17-4 Weight for height for prepubertal boys, 2 to 11½ years of age.
Adapted from Hamill PVV, and others: Physical growth: National Center for Health Statistics percentiles, American Journal of Clinical Nutrition 32:607, 1979. Data from the National Center for Health Statistics (NCHS), Hyattsville, MD © 1982 Ross Laboratories.

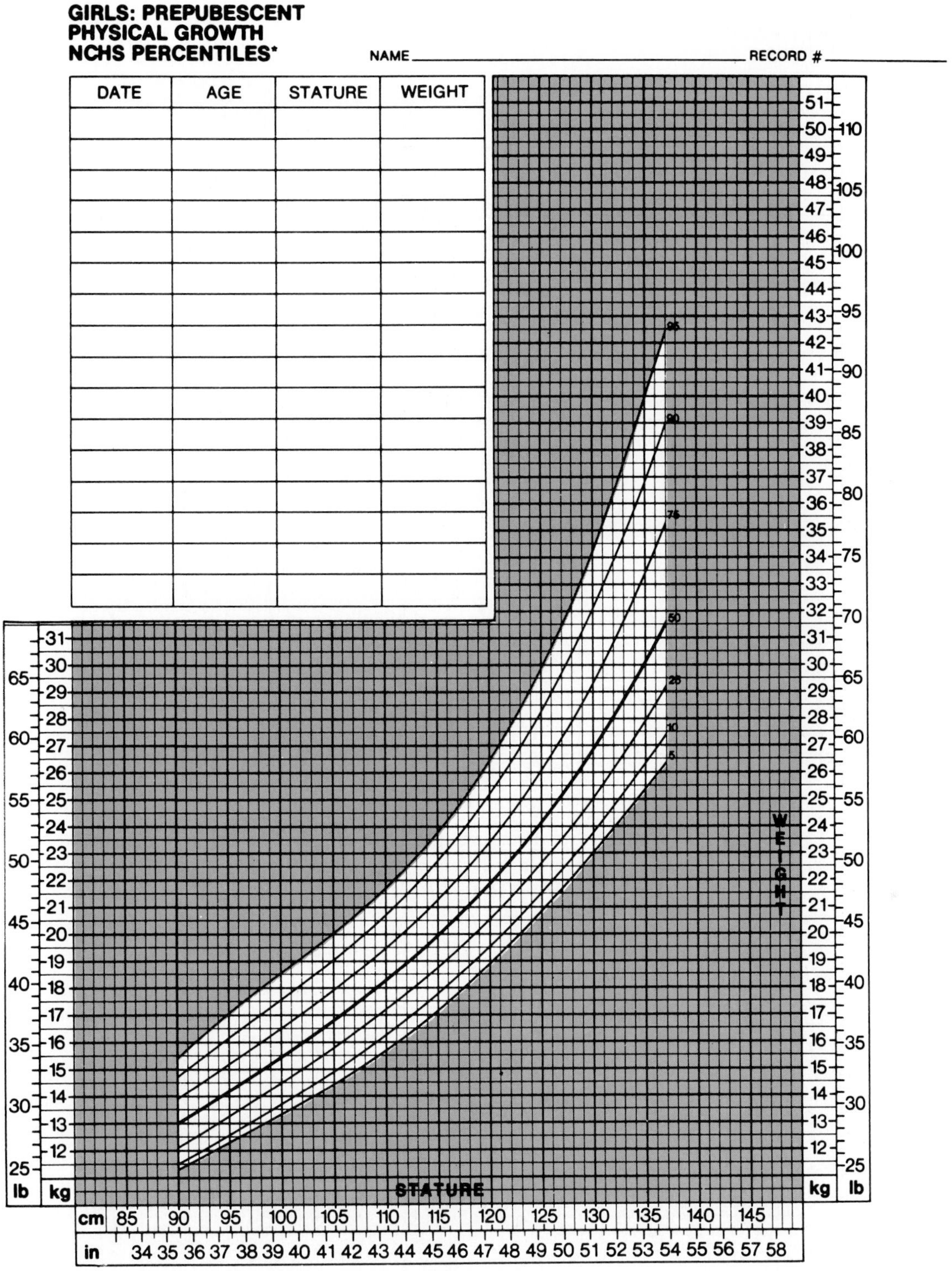

Figure 17-5 Weight for height for prepubertal girls, 2 to 10 years of age.

Adapted from Hamill PVV, and others: Physical growth: National Center for Health Statistics percentiles, American Journal of Clinical Nutrition 32:607, 1979. Data from the National Center for Health Statistics (NCHS), Hyattsville, MD © 1982 Ross Laboratories.

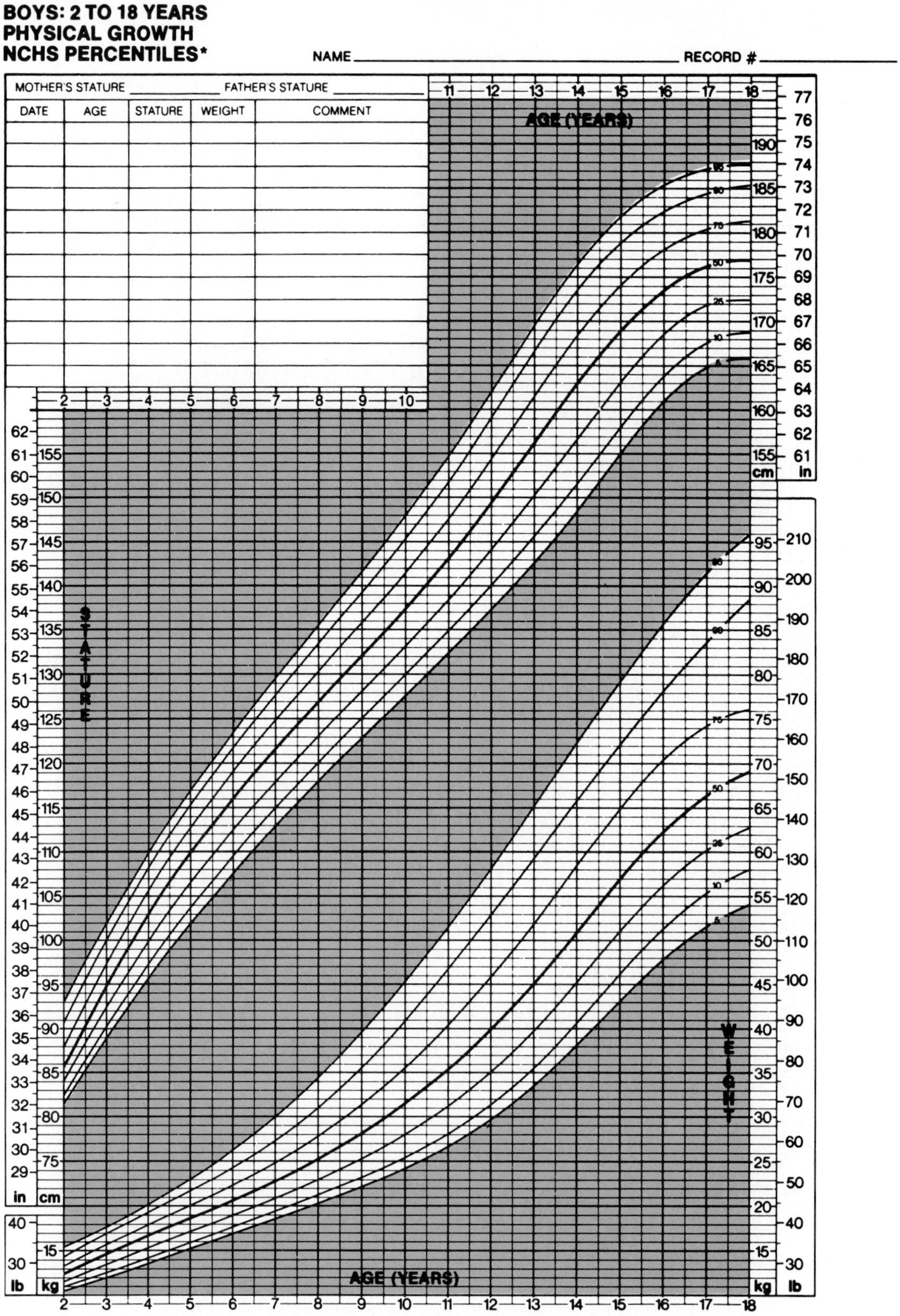

Figure 17-6 Height and weight for age for boys from 2 to 18 years of age.
Adapted from Hamill PVV, and others: Physical growth: National Center for Health Statistics percentiles, American Journal of Clinical Nutrition 32:607, 1979. Data from the National Center for Health Statistics (NCHS), Hyattsville, MD © 1982 Ross Laboratories.

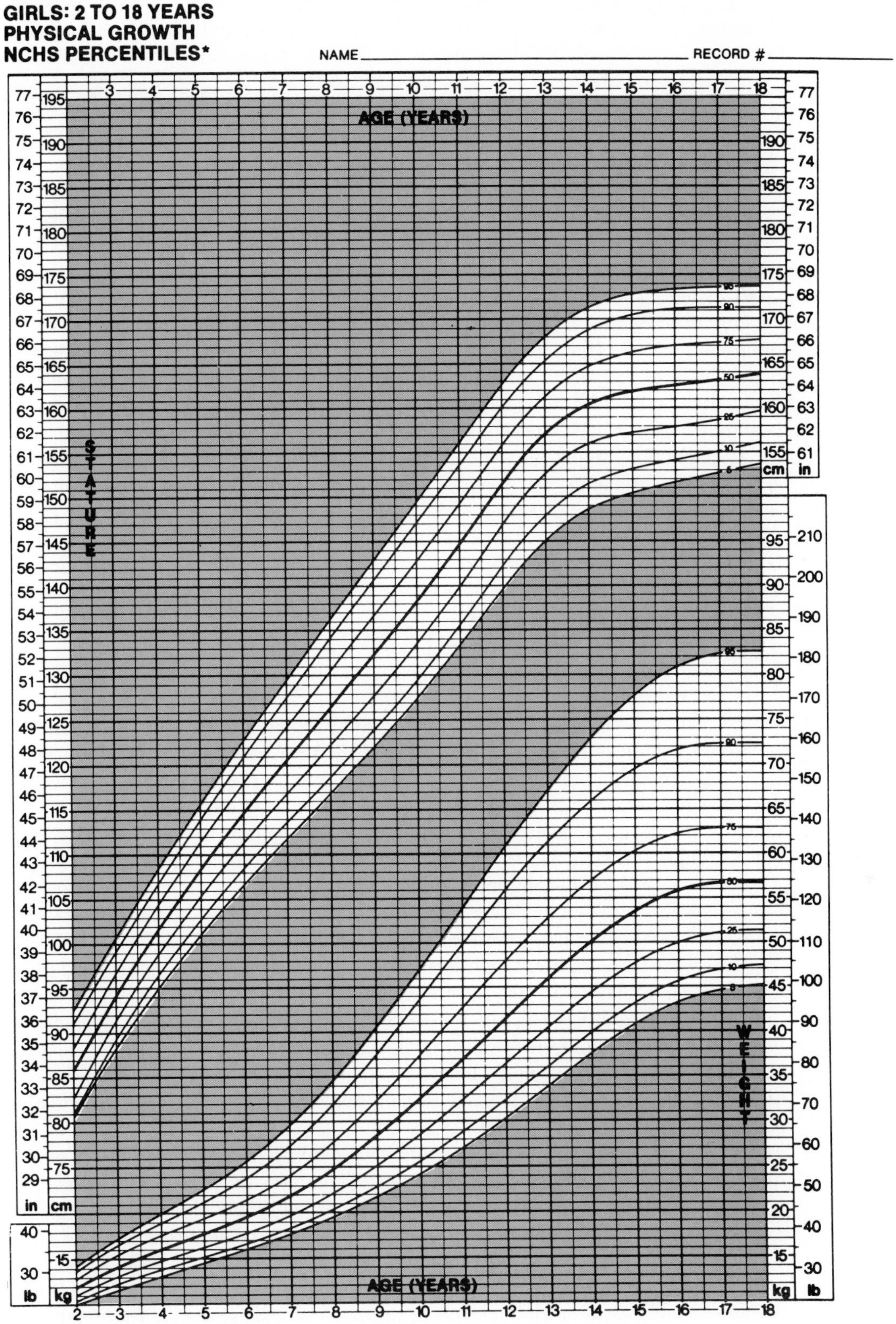

Figure 17-7 Height and weight for age for girls from 2 to 18 years of age.
Adapted from Hamill PVV, and others: Physical growth: National Center for Health Statistics percentiles, American Journal of Clinical Nutrition 32:607, 1979. Data from the National Center for Health Statistics (NCHS), Hyattsville, MD © 1982 Ross Laboratories.

general, weight for height is an excellent indicator of recent nutritional status (especially undernutrition), whereas height for age is more indicative of long-term nutritional status, which will have had an effect of stature.

Body Fatness

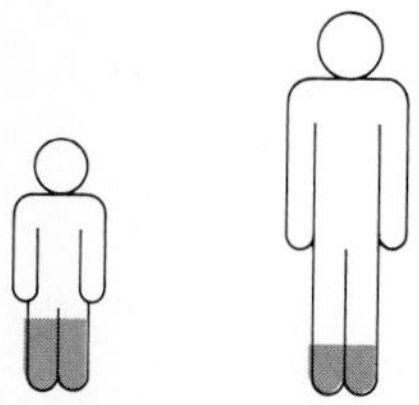

Percent of body fat at 1 year and at 7 years

With the continuing high incidence of obesity in our population and the need to recognize that people with excess body fat are distinct from those with above average body weights, attempts have been made to find a method of assessing body fatness. This assessment of body composition is also useful in evaluating growth in children. The percentage of body weight represented by fat declines from 1 to 7 years of age. Thereafter, for girls the proportion of body weight as fat increases steadily until maturity, whereas for boys it increases to puberty and then declines until maturity. Determination of body density is the most precise way of estimating body fat. It is expensive and impractical for use on large groups and may be frightening, especially for children. Calipers that exert a specific pressure have been developed to measure the thickness of a skinfold in various parts of the body as an indication of the amount of subcutaneous fat (see Figure 8-6). Although skinfold measurements are taken in many parts of the body, as an indication of body fat, measurement of a triceps skinfold is the single most accessible and useful measurement. A thickness above the 85th percentile is usually indicative of excess body fat. This is approximately 11 to 13 mm in young children, 14 to 20 mm and 19 to 25 mm in adolescent girls and boys respectively. Standards for all ages are shown in Appendix L.

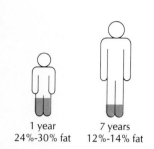

Nutrition-Related Problems in Childhood

Nutrition-Related Problems of Children
Growth retardation
Anemia
Obesity
Poor dental health

Severe malnutrition in childhood in the United States and Canada is seldom encountered now because of the availability of medical services and nutrition intervention programs and the improvement of techniques for identifying problems before they develop into a full-fledged deficiency syndrome. Pellagra and beriberi are virtually unknown, and only an occasional case of scurvy is recorded. However, the National Nutrition Survey has revealed some evidence of growth retardation. As many as 18% of the children enrolled in Head Start programs fall below the 5th percentile on height and weight standards. Similarily, 8% of Hispanic children are below this level. Such growth retardation is associated with high morbidity and some increase in mortality. Of all manifestations of malnutrition, anemia, obesity, and poor dental health are the most common.

Anemia. Resulting primarily from a lack of dietary iron, anemia is encountered most often among children in lower socioeconomic groups, in whom the reported incidence of hemoglobin levels below 10 grams/dl of blood ranges from 20% to 40%. The lack of dietary iron may result from the parents' lack of information about the importance and sources of iron; poverty, which restricts the amount and variety of foods available; or the difficulty of providing recommended levels of iron in the diet under the best of circumstances. Sometimes the situation is aggravated by intestinal parasites. A few instances are recorded of anemia resulting from the exclusive use of a milk diet, low in iron, after the first 6 months of life.

Treatment of childhood anemia usually involves the therapeutic use of iron salts at levels providing from 30 to 100 mg of iron a day, often in conjunction with vitamin C, until the hemoglobin levels have been restored to normal. This is followed by the use of a diet high in iron-rich foods, such as meat, green leafy vegetables, and enriched cereals. The child who suffers from anemia is usually lethargic, fatigues easily, is highly susceptible to infection, and may show behavioral deficits.

Obesity. A form of overnutrition, obesity represents the other end of the nutritional spectrum. Childhood or juvenile-onset obesity is a particular problem, because it is extremely refractory to treatment and tends to persist into adulthood.

This increasing problem may be attributed to several factors. Many parents, in their concern over a child's food habits, unwittingly establish a pattern of overeating when they introduce solid foods at a very early age, equate weight gain with good infant care, or use food as a reward for good behavior. Even subtle factors, such as how much a parent talks to a child at meal time both in responding to the child's behavior and in expressing approval, influence eating patterns. Thinner children and their parents may talk more and eat less at meal time. Any tendency toward obesity is further complicated by inactivity (see Chapter 7). The syndrome of the pale, flabby child who spends summers in an air-conditioned house, immobilized in front of television set, drinking beverages of low nutrient density to keep cool is observed too often and is cause for concern.

Encouraging exercise is one of the most effective strategies a parent can use to help children maintain a desirable weight. The importance of preventing obesity in childhood through an education program involving sound food selection and exercise cannot be overstressed. Encouraging children to adopt a pattern of eating and exercise that allows them to "grow into their weight" has met with more success than attempting to bring about an actual weight loss. However, this does not just happen. Every effort should be made to determine and correct the underlying cause of obesity. This is especially important to the child whose parents are obese and who probably has both a genetic and environmental predisposition to obesity. Those children with features of body build identified as endomorphic should be given special guidance.

The psychosocial effects of childhood obesity are probably as devastating as the physiological ones. Obese children are subjected to ridicule and teasing, are frequently left out of games and activities, leading them to become increasingly more sedentary and increasingly more dependent on food as an ever-available source of comfort. Obese children usually have very poor self-images and experience feelings of rejection and inferiority.

Whether or not obesity in childhood is related to obesity in later life is hotly debated. Most studies now show little relationship between weight status at birth and that at 4 years of age. Weights at 4 and 7 are closely correlated, and either may be predictive of adult status, with about 80% of obese children becoming obese adults. It is interesting to learn that children as young as 5 years of age sense the social stigma associated with obesity and are aware that it is caused by overeating. Even as early as 7 years, excess body weight in children has been found to be associated with higher blood pressure. Studies on the relationship of socioeconomic status to obesity have led to conflicting results about its impact on childhood obesity.

Dental health. During childhood, dietary factors influence dental health through their effect on both tooth formation and the character of the oral environment. Before tooth decay will occur, three conditions must be present: a caries-susceptible tooth, a fermentable carbohydrate, and microorganisms to ferment that carbohydrate. The susceptibility of the tooth to decay may be determined genetically, but few children are endowed with caries-resistant teeth. Beyond this, the integrity of the tooth structure may be a function of the nutrients that are available at a critical point in tooth formation. Vitamin A is necessary for the formation of the enamel layer, vitamin C for the dentin layer, and calcium, phosphorus, and vitamin D for the process of calcification. In addition, the availability of fluorine (fluoride) during the time the tooth is calcifying will greatly decrease the susceptibility of the tooth to decay.

Conditions Essential for Tooth Decay
Caries-susceptible tooth
Fermentable carbohydrate
Microorganisms

Nutrients Essential for Sound Tooth Development
Vitamins A, D, C
Fluorine
Calcium
Phosphorus

Once the tooth has erupted, the presence or absence of carbohydrate to adhere to the tooth surface is the major dietary factor influencing tooth decay. Thus it is not the nutrient content of the diet but rather the nature of the dietary carbohydrate and the frequency or duration of its exposure that determines the cariogenic character of the diet. The stickier the carbohydrate and the longer sugar is in the mouth, the greater the cariogenic effect. Of all dietary factors associated with control of tooth decay, fluoride has the greatest effect as a preventative, and the consumption of sucrose in a form that adheres to the tooth surface is the major detrimental factor.

Hyperactivity or hyperkinesis. In 1973 Dr. Benjamin Feingold reported success in treating children diagnosed as hyperactive by eliminating from their diets those foods containing artificial coloring and flavoring and fruits and vegetables containing naturally occurring **salicylates.** These children represented from 3% to 10% of the school-age children treated. His theory, however, was rejected by many because he had no experimental data to support it.

salicylates
Compounds similar to the active ingredient in aspirin

hyperkinesis or **hyperactivity**
A condition characterized by a high level of energy or activity
(hyper = too much; kine = energy)

Since children suffering from **hyperkinesis** are excessively restless and inattentive, have poor control of their impulses, have a consistently high level of activity, and often experience learning disabilities, they have a disruptive influence in the home and school environments. Ironically, they respond to treatment with stimulant drugs rather than tranquilizers. Sometimes they are described as "minimally brain damaged," in spite of the fact they are usually quite bright.

Because Feingold's theory implicated food as either a causative or aggravating factor in the condition, several controlled studies were undertaken to assess the behavioral effect of eliminating or including foods with artificial colors and flavors in the diet. The results are not clear-cut. There is some evidence that a *small* proportion of hyperactive children respond favorably to a diet devoid of artificial colors and flavors. Since there are no nutritional limitations associated with such a diet, in spite of the extra work involved, it is not unreasonable to recommend that it be tried. The evidence that food additives cause hyperkinesis or that sensitive children respond to very limited exposure is not strong enough to recommend a modification of our food supply or mandatory labeling of all foods containing these additives. However, parents with such children would be well advised to try the restricted diet to determine whether their child will respond to such a regimen. While the diet requires considerably more work for the family, who must avoid many processed foods and food ingredients, it is nutritionally adequate. It is recognized that there is no reason to eliminate the foods containing salicylates, including almonds, apples, grapes, tomatoes, and oranges, which Feingold originally excluded.

ADOLESCENCE

adolescence
Period from childhood to adulthood, in which physical, chemical, and emotional development is accelerated

The period of transition from childhood to adulthood, commonly called **adolescence**, is a relatively short stage in the life cycle characterized by dramatically accelerated physical, biochemical, and emotional development. The observation that the initiation of the rapid growth characteristic of adolescence is more related to weight (or possibly body composition) than to age suggests that nutritional status may be an important determinant of physiological maturity. The timing of the adolescent growth spurt signaling the onset of **puberty** depends on the child's attaining a certain critical weight, considered to be approximately 66 pounds (30 kg). This represents a critical body composition of 10% body fat. This is followed by a height growth spurt, which begins shortly after 10 years of age and peaks at 12 in girls and close to 12 and 14 years in boys. A weight growth spurt begins about 6 months later in both males and females. The period of rapid growth in both height and weight lasts from 2½ to 3 years. Thus for girls the period of greatest nutritional need relative to size is between 10 and 13 years of age and for boys between 12 and 15 years of age.

puberty
Period during growth when secondary sex characteristics appear

A growth spurt of 6 to 8 inches per year occurs in girls at 10 to 12 years of age and in boys at 12 to 14 years of age.

menarche
Time of first menstrual period

Menarche in girls occurs following the period of rapid weight gain, when weight reaches about 103 pounds (47 kg) and fat stores have doubled to 20% to 24%. The once widely held belief that menarche does not begin until body fat represents at least 17% of body weight and that ovulation ceases any time it falls below this level has been challenged. However, a body composition of 22% body fat does seem to be required to maintain regular ovulation. In males sexual development coincides with the beginning of the growth spurt; both are influenced by the adequacy of zinc status.

Both males and females attain adult stature between 18 and 20 years of age, but bone mass continues to increase until age 25. Mature women have about twice as much adipose tissue but only two thirds as much lean tissue as men.

Since growth rate and hence nutrient needs vary widely among adolescents, it has been suggested that it would be more meaningful to relate nutritional needs to a sexual maturity rating (SMR) based on the appearance of secondary sex characteristics rather than relate them to age.

The changing life-style of adolescents has a significant effect on their food habits. As they become more independent and mobile, they eat fewer meals at home and more meals outside the home, where there is little guidance on food choices; they also share more food with their peers, learn new food preferences, and discard old food habits.

Adolescence influences both nutritional needs and the absorption and utilization of nutrients. During this period, there is a rapid enlargement of organs and tissues, and sexual maturity brings about changes in physiological functions in response to hormonal changes. As reflected in the NRC recommended dietary allowances, this phase of the life cycle has some of the highest nutritive needs for males, and for females is surpassed only by needs during pregnancy and lactation.

The recommended dietary allowances for adolescents are presented in Table 17-1. These allowances represent the needs for the increase in body size and the maturation of organs. The 24 million 13- to 19-year-olds in the United States are

Table 17-1 ◇ Recommended Dietary Allowances nutrients for adolescent males, females, and pregnant adolescents (1980).

	Males		Females		Pregnant Females	
	11-14 Yr	15-18 Yr	11-14 Yr	15-18 Yr	11-14 Yr	15-18 Yr
Weight (kg)	45	66	46	55	46	55
Energy (kcal)	2700	2800	2200	2100	2500	2400
Protein (grams)	45	56	46	46	76	76
Vitamin A (μg RE)	1000	1000	800	800	1000	1000
Vitamin A (IU)	5000	5000	4000	4000	5000	5000
Vitamin D (μg)	10	10	10	10	15	15
Vitamin D (IU)	400	400	400	400	600	600
Vitamin E (mg α-TE)	8	10	8	8	10	10
Vitamin C (mg)	50	60	50	60	70	80
Folacin (μg)	400	400	400	400	800	800
Niacin (mg)	18	18	15	14	17	16
Riboflavin (mg)	1.6	1.7	1.3	1.3	1.6	1.6
Thiamin (mg)	1.4	1.4	1.1	1.1	1.5	1.5
Vitamin B_6 (mg)	1.8	2	1.8	2	2.2	2.4
Vitamin B_{12} (μg)	3	3	3	3	4	4
Calcium (mg)	1200	1200	1200	1200	1600	1600
Phosphorus (mg)	1200	1200	1200	1200	1600	1600
Iodine (μg)	150	150	150	150	175	175
Iron (mg)	18	18	18	18	18+	18+
Magnesium (mg)	350	400	300	300	450	450
Zinc (mg)	15	15	15	15	20	20
Selenium (μg)*	40	50	45	50	55	60

*As proposed, 1985.
Based on Recommended Dietary Allowances, ed 9, Washington, D.C., 1980, National Academy of Sciences, National Research Council, Food and Nutrition Board.

at a vulnerable age when their dietary patterns and food attitudes influence the health of their children and dictate the food patterns of the next generation. Teenagers, thus, are a prime and challenging target for nutrition education programs. They are also a target for marketing strategies designed to establish brand loyalties at an early age.

Specific Nutritional Needs

Recommended energy intakes (REI) approximate the average need for the age-group, while those for most other nutrients have a safety factor to include the needs of essentially all healthy adolescents. As a result, because of the very high needs for most nutrients during the period of rapid growth, requirements expressed per 1000 kcal are also higher than at almost any other time.

The requirement for energy can be judged best in relation to the amount needed to support an acceptable rate of growth and maintain a desirable weight. Data from dietary surveys show that energy intakes peak between 12 and 13 years of age for girls and at 16 for boys. For both, the peak values were higher than the average intakes suggested in the RDAs. For most adolescents, "eating to appetite" (that is, until the appetite is satisfied) offers a reasonably sensitive indicator of energy needs.

Protein tends to represent 12% to 14% of the energy intake and usually exceeds 1 gram/kg of body weight, which is considered adequate for the needs for growth and the maintenance of body tissue. Protein is a limiting factor in growth only when caloric intake is so restricted that dietary protein must be used as an energy source.

The minerals most likely to be provided in less than adequate amounts are calcium, iron, and zinc, for all of which there is a substantially increased need with rapid growth. Approximately 150 mg of calcium must be retained each day to allow for the increase in bone mass. Iron is needed for hemoglobin synthesis necessitated by the considerable expansion of blood volume and for myoglobin needed for muscle growth. The greater growth needs for boys than for girls are offset by girls' need to replace the 0.5 mg/day iron loss resulting from menstruation. Therefore the recommended iron intake is set at 18 mg daily for each. A retention of 0.4 mg of zinc, associated with muscle growth in adolescents, calls for an intake of 15 mg/day. It is not surprising that zinc intakes, especially in girls, fall below this level when one realizes that the zinc content of food parallels the protein in a ratio of 1.5 mg/10 grams of protein. Only on an intake of 100 grams of protein would the recommended level of zinc be provided.

In spite of the increase in iodine sources in the North American diet as the result of modern food processing, adolescent girls should still guard against iodine deficiency–induced goiter. At least half the salt used should be iodized to ensure an adequate intake.

Nutrient Shortfalls for Adolescents

Calcium	Vitamin A
Iron	Vitamin C
Zinc	Vitamin B_6
	Folacin

There is some concern that the tendency of some adolescents to reject milk and to respond to peer pressure and powerful marketing strategies by consuming soft drinks even in the morning, will frequently lead to a calcium/phosphorus ratio of less than 1:1. The implications of this for bone growth are not clear, but there is reason for concern. Recent studies have pointed to a problem of even greater concern. The bone mass of adolescent female gymnasts and runners suffering from amenorrhea, believed to be associated with low fat stores, is considerably reduced. Any food pattern that limits the increase in bone mass has implications for later development of osteoporosis. Thus girls, especially athletes, should be encouraged to maintain a reasonable intake of dairy products to provide adequate calcium and be discouraged from substituting carbonated beverages.

Vitamins. The need for thiamin, riboflavin, and niacin, with a major role in energy metabolism, increases directly with increased caloric intake. Folacin and vitamin B_{12}, which are essential for DNA and RNA synthesis, are needed in higher amounts when tissue synthesis is occurring rapidly. Since tissue growth involves amino acid metabolism, particularly transamination to synthesize nonessential amino acids, the requirement for vitamin B_6 is increased. Skeletal growth requires vitamin D, while the structural and functional integrity of newly formed cells depends on the availability of vitamins A, C, and E.

Of the vitamins playing a major role in the growth process, vitamins A, C, B_6, and folacin are most likely to be taken in less than adequate amounts. Biochemical assessment of nutritional status among adolescents supports this observation.

Supplements. Adolescents who meet their energy requirements from a wide selection of foods should not need supplements. About half of a group of 163 adolescents took vitamin-mineral supplements believing they would give them energy, cure colds, help their complexions, or enhance sports performance.

Adequacy of Diets

Evaluations of the nutritive adequacy of the diets of over 7000 young adults between 12 and 18 years of age in various regions in the United States (NFCS, 1977-1978) have all yielded essentially the same results, although differences in degree are found. In all instances it was observed that after boys reached age 12, their diets were more adequate and less variable than were those of girls. This can be explained in part by the fact that the quantity of food required to provide the extra 900 kcal of energy needed for boys supplies at least a minimal level of other nutrients, whereas girls, with lower caloric intakes, are forced to make more judicious choices of foods to meet the needs for all other nutrients. This is difficult at a time when they are striving for independence and are responsive to peer pressure. In general, the diets of girls provided a higher proportion of their needs for ascorbic acid and calories than did those of boys, although ascorbic acid was often low for both. Girls' diets were generally low in iron, but this was not accompanied by a higher incidence of anemia. Calcium was more frequently low in the diets of girls than of boys, and vitamin A was low in both, a reflection of a general rejection of vegetables. Protein and niacin intakes, which paralleled the use of meat, were most often adequate.

Figure 17-8 presents data on the nutrient intake of adolescent males and females in relation to the RDAs. More detailed analyses showed that the diets of girls deteriorated as the girls grew older, whereas those of boys improved throughout adolescence, and that teenagers in high-income families had more adequate intakes than those in low-income families. In general, adolescents with the poorest diets were those who skipped more meals and ate smaller amounts of food and fewer snacks. Biochemical data from NHANES II showed impaired iron status in boys 11 to 15 years old and in females 11 to 24 years old.

Concerns About Adolescents' Diets

Nutritionists express concern about the dietary habits of the 12- to 18-year-old group for many reasons. Adolescence is marked by a level of physical and emotional growth that often results in stress and anxiety. These in turn influence physiological, psychological, and social behavior. All of these factors affect nutritional behavior.

The incidence of dietary inadequacies is higher during adolescence than at any other stage of the life cycle. This is a stage at which the results of nutrient lack are far reaching, especially for girls, with a relationship often observed between abnormalities such as anemia, bone loss, and goiter and dietary practices. Emotional instability, noted especially among girls who mature early, influences the utilization of nutrients. Negative nitrogen and calcium balances have been observed among young girls under extreme emotional stress.

The possibility that many North American girls between 15 and 19 years of age will bear a child before they have fully matured is a reason to focus special attention on their nutritional status. One out of four mothers bearing her first child is less than 20 years old, and 6% of all deaths among 18- to 19-year-old girls result from complications of pregnancy. If the nutritive intake of a girl has been inadequate before she conceives, she is less able to cope with the added physical stress of pregnancy and the demands of the growing fetus and is unable to make up for her

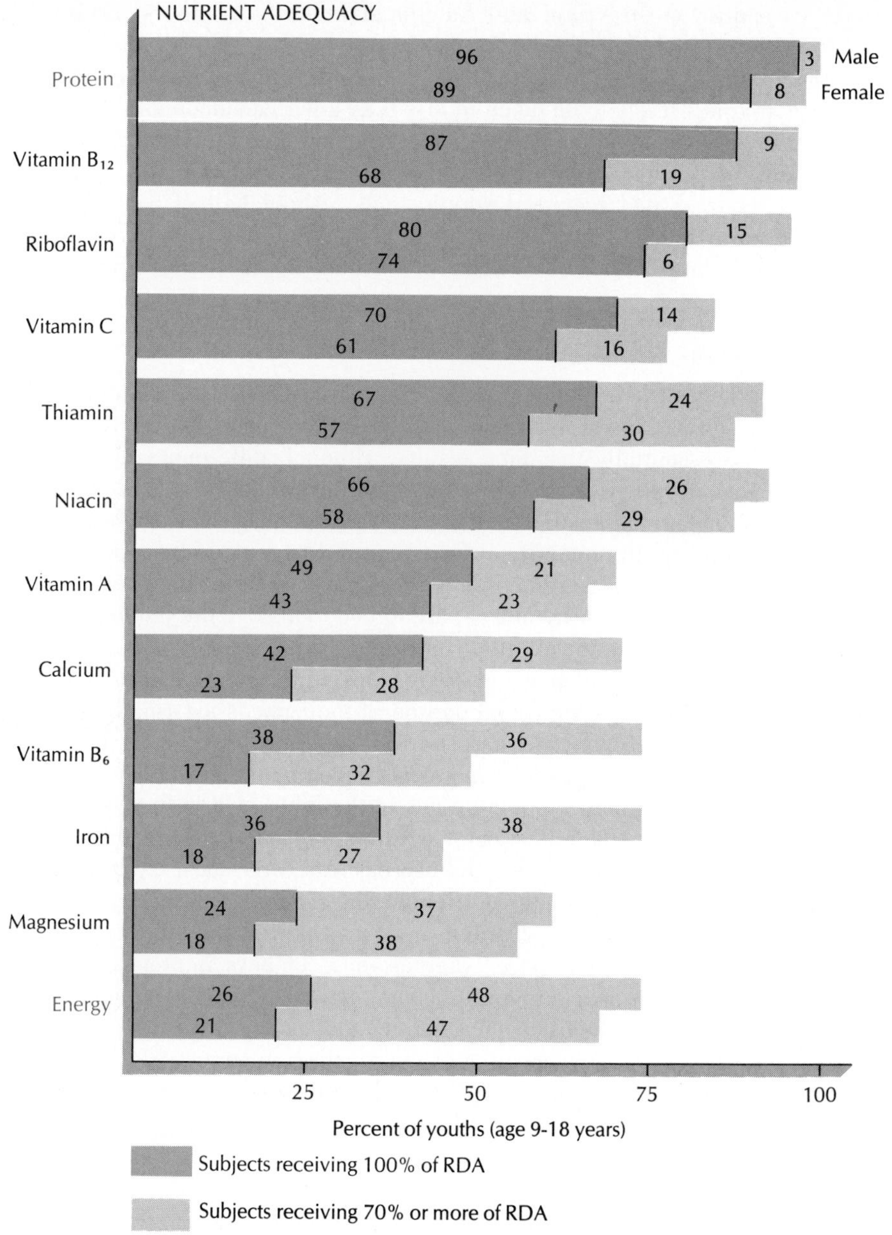

Figure 17-8 Adequacy of nutrient intake for youths 9 to 18 years of age, as reported in the NFCS (1977-1978).

own nutritive deficits. As a result, teenagers have more stillbirths and their babies are more often born prematurely, have a higher mortality rate, more congenital defects, and have inadequate nutritive stores to carry them through the initial period of extrauterine life. In all respects the malnourished mother is a poor obstetrical risk, especially when the interval between menarche and conception is short. Whether a concern over the welfare of their yet-unconceived children will provide sufficient motivation to teenage girls to modify their food habits remains to be seen. The concern of nutritionists over the diets of adolescents has prompted a concerted effort to educate and cooperate with this group.

Factors Influencing Food Habits

A few attempts have been made to determine the attitudes that influence the selection of a diet. These studies have shown that young girls who were concerned about their health, were emotionally stable, conformed to social expectations, and came from homes characterized by good family relationships made better food choices than did those motivated by considerations of group status, sociability, independence from parental control, or enjoyment of eating. Parental criticism of their eating patterns led girls to skip meals more frequently, and while skipping breakfast was found to be common, skipping lunch was more frequent. Better meals were selected in winter than in summer because their winter schedules were more regimented. The more meals an adolescent eats away from home, the less likely that individual is to consume meals of adequate nutritional content. This probably reflects conformity to the habits of peer groups. This is especially true when lunch money is used to buy lunches outside the school, a practice that may be discouraged by the trend toward short lunch periods in high schools.

Practices and beliefs that result in nutrient inadequacies are failure to eat one or more meals; inappropriate choices of snack foods; lack of supervision in the selection of meals eaten away from home; and an overriding fear of obesity, especially among girls. A concern that certain foods will aggravate adolescent acne, lack of time or companionship for regular meals, drinking no milk (perhaps a rebellion against parental influence), and the beginning of alcohol use during adolescence are additional contributors to poor nutrition.

Breakfast

The well-documented importance of breakfast for any group suggests that there is probably no nutritional substitute for a good breakfast. Having a good breakfast has two major advantages. First, the availability of a readily usable carbohydrate results in a rapid increase in blood glucose levels and the concurrent decrease in reaction time, so that performance is improved and accident rate declines. Although immediate recall is better when breakfast is omitted, problem-solving ability is poorer. Second, breakfast generally provides important nutrients, especially vitamin C, calcium, and riboflavin. Although nutritionists have maintained that these nutrients might not be provided in adequate amounts by the foods typically consumed at other meals, an analysis of NFCS data shows that adolescents and young adults do have nutritionally similar diets whether or not they eat breakfast.

Skipping breakfasts has been thought to hit a peak during adolescence, a time during which dietary habits that may persist for life are formed. Surprisingly, in NFCS 82% of the boys 11 to 18 years of age and 77% of the girls of the same age reported eating breakfast on each of 3 days. Only 3% of the boys and 4% of the girls never ate breakfast. Ninety-five percent of the breakfasts included food as well as beverages.

There are many explanations for failure to eat breakfast: lack of time, lack of appetite, preference for sleep, spending time over personal appearance, or fear of becoming fat. In one study it was observed that having someone with whom to eat breakfast, someone to prepare it, the availability of prepared foods, and the acceptance of the breakfast-eating habit in the peer group all influenced the extent to which breakfast or a preschool snack was eaten.

It should be pointed out that breakfast need not be the conventional fruit, cereal, toast, and beverage pattern. It can be any combination of foods, either liquid or solid, that provides its nutritional equivalent—at least 300 kcal—and sufficient protein and fat to provide a sense of satiety until the next meal; the breakfast should also have a nutrient density that will make a reasonable contribution of other nutrients.

Fast Foods

Many parents and health professionals express concern about the frequency with which adolescents obtain their meals from fast-food establishments. Research showing that most have only a small proportion of their meals there suggest that if there

Energy Content of Fast Foods (kcal)

Whopper	630
Sundae	570
Chocolate dipped cone	450
Fish sandwich	432
Chili dog	330

Table 17-2 ◆ Index of nutrient quality (INQ)* of menu items offered by a fast-food restaurant†

	Protein	Vitamin A	Vitamin C	Thiamin	Riboflavin	Niacin	Calcium	Iron	Nutritious?‡
Regular hamburger	2.0	0.4	0.3	1.5	1.1	2.2	0.5	1.4	Yes
Regular cheeseburger	2.0	0.5	0.2	1.2	1.3	2.0	1.1	1.1	Yes
Large hamburger	2.4	0.2	0.2	1.0	1.3	2.6	0.4	1.5	Yes
Large cheeseburger	2.4	0.6	0.2	1.0	1.5	3.2	1.1	1.0	Yes
Double patty hamburger	1.9	0.3	0.2	1.0	0.9	1.7	0.7	1.0	Yes
Fish sandwich	1.6	0.2	0.4	1.0	0.9	1.1	0.6	0.5	No
Apple pie	0.3	0.1	0.3	0.1	0.1	0.5	0.1	0.3	No
Cookies	0.6	0.1	0.2	1.4	1.0	0.3	0.1	0.6	No
Chocolate shake	1.2	0.4	0.3	0.5	3.1	0.2	2.0	0.3	Yes
Egg on English muffin	2.1	0.5	0.2	1.5	2.2	1.3	1.2	1.1	Yes
Hot cakes	0.7	0.2	0.2	1.0	1.2	0.9	0.7	0.6	No
Scrambled eggs	2.9	1.4	0.2	0.6	4.8	0.3	0.7	1.7	Yes
Pork sausage	1.9	0.1	0.1	1.8	0.9	3.5	0.2	0.6	No
English muffin, buttered	1.2	0.3	0.1	1.7	1.0	3.8	1.0	1.0	Yes
French fries	0.6	0.1	1.9	1.0	0.2	1.5	0.1	0.3	No

From Shannon BM, and Parks SC: Journal of the American Dietetic Association 76:242, 1980.

*Percent of nutrient requirement supplied by each item as purchased divided by percent of energy requirement supplied by each item, as purchased. The nutrient requirements were set as the U.S. Recommended Daily Allowance for each nutrient except protein, in which case the requirement was set as 55 grams daily. The energy requirement was set as 2200 kcal daily.

†Nutrient compositions on menu items determined by WARF Institute, Inc., Madison, WI, 1975.

‡Based on standard of 4 nutrients with INQ >1 or 2 nutrients with INQ >2. Other foods may qualify if additional nutrients are considered.

is a problem, it is overrated. The main objection is the limited selection available and the persistent belief that the foods are high in fat and salt. Criticisms that it was difficult to obtain adequate vitamins A and C and fiber from the conventional menu have led many establishments to offer a salad bar or cole slaw to improve their nutritional image. The availability of a beverage option of low-fat milk, whole milk (plain or flavored), and fruit juice in addition to coffee and soft drinks does much to further enhance the nutritional image of fast-food outlets. Data in Table 17-2 show that the majority of foods traditionally offered have considerable nutritional merit, even when assessed on a nutrient density basis. A complete analysis of foods provided in fast-food establishments is included in Appendix F. Many fast-food chains are providing nutrient information on all menu items at the point of purchase. This is a commendable trend, which might well be copied by more costly restaurants, whose customers may be nutritionally vulnerable adults.

Role of Snacks in Dietary Intake

Until recently nutritionists tended to stress the importance of three "good" meals a day and to ignore the possibility that snacks could provide anything other than foods of low-nutrient density. With the recognition that smaller, more frequent meals may have many physiological and nutritional advantages, and that snacking is a way of life with teenagers, nutritionists are focusing on improving the quality of snacks. Data on food intake patterns show that snacks are eaten by over 75% of all adolescents and provide from a fourth to a third of their caloric intake. The extent to which snacks contribute to the intake of other nutrients relates to the nature of the snacks. Contrary to general belief, there are very few foods that are used more frequently for snacks than for meals. These include ice cream and candy, but not salty snacks or soft drinks, which are used more frequently as part of a meal. About one fourth of all teenagers use milk and fruits as snacks more frequently

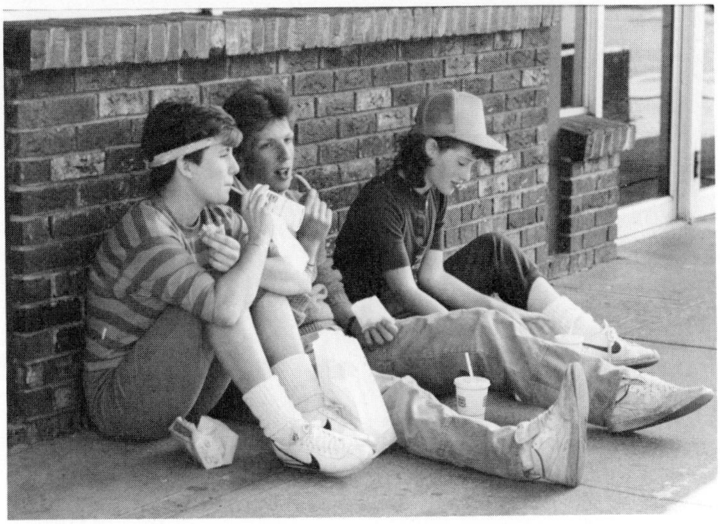

In spite of parental concerns, studies have shown that nutritional problems associated with teenagers' eating at fastfood restaurants are overrated.

than they use traditional snack foods. Cakes, cookies, milk, soft drinks, salty snack food, frozen desserts, and fruits are the snack items most often reported.

Once adults have accepted the fact that snacking is not necessarily detrimental and need not spoil the appetite for well-planned meals, they can do much to see that snacks make a significant nutrient contribution by monitoring the kinds of foods that are available. The most likely place for adults to make their influence felt are through such access points as the school lunch program, the home refrigerator, and vending machines.

Nutritious Snacks
Fresh fruit
Raw vegetables
Yogurt
Whole grain crackers
Nuts
Cheese
Fruit juice
Milk
Dried fruit

From a nutrition education standpoint, it may be better to make snacks available that have a full range of nutritional qualities, including less nutritious snacks, and give the child the information on which to base an informed decision, than to ban "nonnutritious" foods from vending machines so that the child can select only nutritious foods. In this case, he does not learn to cope in real-life situations. Studies have shown that as the number of snacks increases, the nutritional quality of the diet increases, with snacks providing about 20% of the energy and several nutrients. A Canadian study showed convincingly that given a choice, children will select wisely much of the time.

Snacking should be encouraged as an integral part of the total eating pattern but must be questioned if it constitutes overeating in disregard of the total food pattern. Snacking that is confined to the evening hours in what is described as the "night-eating syndrome" has been implicated as a contributing cause in obesity. Overeating in a short period of time results in greater production of fat, which is hard to mobilize later as an energy source.

Variety in the Diet

The widely held belief that adolescents have rather limited food experiences is not borne out by the results of the NFCS. However, as is evident from Table 17-3, some food groups, such as fish, legumes, and, surprisingly, salty snacks, were reported by only one fourth and cheese by less than one third of the respondents.

Obesity

Studies indicate that 30% to 35% of teenagers are overweight and that 80% of them will remain overweight as adults, predisposed to hypertension and diabetes. Although only 3% to 20% are actually obese, many teenagers, especially girls, are

Table 17-3 ◆ Percentage of teenagers reporting that they ate various food groups at least once in a 3-day period (NFCS, 1977-1978)

	11-15 Yr		15-19 Yr	
	M	F	M	F
Bread	98	97	99	96
Milk	96	94	93	90
Vegetables	95	96	94	96
Meat	94	91	96	94
Candy, sugar	80	78	77	73
Soft drinks	69	78	80	78
Cakes, pies, and cookies	68	75	65	63
Fruit	57	58	49	54
Eggs	50	43	54	48
Fruit juice	49	53	46	51
Poultry	40	41	43	46
Cheese	33	43	44	48
Legumes	26	23	29	23
Fish	24	23	20	22
Salty snacks	22	22	15	20

either fat, believe they are fat, or are fearful of becoming fat. Because they often try to emulate fashion models who may wear size 6 dresses, girls often aspire to an unrealistic and unhealthy body size. Thus they embark on self-directed programs of weight reduction that can easily be hazardous to health. Inadequate intakes of nutrients at a time when these young people still have high nutrient demands for growth and when they should be accumulating reserves for the reproductive period are major concerns. The problem is even greater when weight reduction is carried out intermittently, with a period of weight loss followed by one of weight gain.

For more discussion of weight control see Chapter 8.

As discussed earlier, a major cause of caloric imbalance among adolescents is a depressed level of activity rather than an excessive food intake. Whether the cause of this inactivity is more physiological, psychological, or environmental will vary with each person. Prevalence of obesity increases about 2% for every hour per day of inactivity associated with television watching. It has been observed that obese youngsters have significantly lower serum iron with normal hemoglobin levels than do nonobese youngsters. The low serum iron levels could be indicative of low levels of myoglobin and other iron-containing pigments in muscles, which may cause an unconscious reduction in activity when the oxygen available to the cells is reduced.

Adolescence, a period when energy needs for growth and maintenance are high, is a good time to initiate a life-style that helps maintain a desirable weight. Since the activity patterns developed in late adolescence often prevail throughout adulthood, adopting habits of active exercise at an early age becomes important in preventing obesity in adulthood. It is equally important that people learn early to respond to satiety signals, thus increasing their ability to adjust their food intakes to correspond to needs.

Alcohol

Although in most states the legal drinking age is 21, 80% of 12- to 17-year-olds report having at least one alcoholic drink a month and 3%, one per day. If it is true that 39% of adolescents are moderate drinkers and 28% are considered problem drinkers, alcohol consumption presents both a social and a nutritional problem. "Hard" alcohol contributes only energy, and while beer does contribute thiamin and niacin, this is hardly justification for continuing its use. Considering that people generally underreport alcohol use, the problem is undoubtedly even greater than statistics indicate. Aside from its impact on nutrient intake, alcohol has an adverse effect on the absorption of both zinc and folacin, two nutrients critical for normal growth. Its impact on the course of pregnancy has already been discussed.

Recreational Drugs

The effects of the use of "recreational drugs," such as heroin, cocaine, marijuana, and "uppers" and "downers," are not well understood. However, there is evidence that cocaine, which serves as a central nervous system stimulant similar to amphetamines, has the same effect of causing loss of appetite and consequent weight loss and possible malnutrition. Those who smoke marijuana report feelings of hunger but may or may not eat differently as a result. They usually weigh less rather than more than nonsmokers.

Smokeless Tobacco

The use of smokeless tobacco is growing among adolescents and preadolescents in the belief that it is safer than cigarette smoking. It is far from trouble-free, however, being linked to diseases of the oral cavity of which cancer is the most prevalent, high blood pressure, elevated blood glucose levels in diabetics, and low potassium levels in the blood. If oral discomfort leads to a reduction in the intake of fruit, vegetables, and meat, it has a profound effect on the intake of vitamins A and C, iron, protein, and fiber. Smokeless tobacco itself has very high sodium content (as much as 3% by weight in some products), which should be considered in assessing sodium intake. The substantial sugar content may be a contributing factor to dental caries, which may be counteracted by the copious flow of saliva to cleanse the teeth and the presence of fluoride in the tobacco.

Special Concerns of Adolescent Girls

Use of oral contraceptives. While the use of oral contraceptives is general practice among many adolescent girls to minimize the risk of unwanted pregnancies, there are undesirable nutritional consequences to their use. The most common effect is a decrease in serum and red cell folate levels associated with an increase in megaloblastic anemia. The remedy of taking a folic acid supplement poses potential problems since folic acid supplements especially in conjunction with iron supplements (frequently recommended during adolescence to prevent iron deficiency) cause a drop in serum zinc levels. This, in turn, may have adverse consequences on growth of skeletal and muscle tissues, sexual development, wound healing, and immune function. The long-term use of oral contraceptives is associated with a level of pyridoxine in mother's milk that is incapable of meeting the needs of the nursing infant.

On a positive side, the absorption of iron and a decrease in menstrual blood losses means that the iron needs of girls taking oral contraceptives may be slightly lower than those of girls not using them. Other positive nutritional effects attributed to the estrogen content of oral contraceptives are the enhanced conversion of carotene to vitamin A, elevated serum copper levels, and enhanced calcium absorption in the intestine. The biochemical changes associated with oral contraceptive use are relatively small but will vary with prior nutritional status, predisposing disease states, and concurrent use of drugs and medicines.

Premenstrual syndrome. This is a condition characterized by a group of psychological and physical symptoms that recur in some women each month between the time of ovulation and the beginning of menses. Symptoms include tension, depression, fatigue, aggression, crying spells, headaches, abdominal bloating, breast tenderness, abnormal thirst, and food cravings, in almost any combination.

It is different than the distress of menstrual cramps, headache, nausea, and diarrhea known as dysmenorrhea that is associated with the menstrual flow. In fact, the two seldom, if ever, occur in the same woman. Many nutritional therapies have been proposed but none has proved more than minimally successful. These have included supplements or megadoses of vitamin B_6, essential fatty acids, magnesium, zinc, vitamin C, and vitamin E, and the avoidance of caffeine, alcohol, and salt. The physiological theories proposed to explain the cause include hormonal imbalance, water retention, hypoglycemia, and prostaglandin deficiency. At this point there is no effective nutritional or psychological treatment for this socially debilitating condition. The adverse consequences of megadoses of some nutrients suggest that they should be used only with medical supervision.

Lactating adolescents. In spite of the fact that infants born to adolescents have an increased risk of morbidity and mortality and that breast feeding is believed to reduce this risk, there is concern about the impact of lactation on the bone mineral status of the adolescent mother. Studies have shown a significant decrease in bone mineral between 2 and 16 weeks of lactation and low dietary intakes of calcium and phosphorus. There is reason to question whether it is reasonable to expect an adolescent mother to be able to meet the nutritional demands of lactation superimposed on those of adolescent growth.

Predisposition to osteoporosis. The likelihood that postmenopausal women will develop osteoporosis is a function not only of their rate of bone loss after menopause but of their bone mass. This in turn is determined by their peak bone mass, which occurs between ages 20 and 30. It is influenced by a young woman's dietary practices during adolescence and early adulthood as well as by the regularity of her menstrual status, which is determined by her degree of physical activity and the fiber content of her diet. Excessive exercise, high fiber, and low fat intake all lead to low circulating estrogen levels, irregular menses, and decreased bone mass. Thus it appears that the prediposition to osteoporosis is in part at least the result of dietary and exercise patterns during the developmental years.

School Lunch

With 24.5 million U.S. schoolchildren participating, the National School Lunch Program can be considered an important factor in the nutrient intake of schoolchildren. The program was conceived to "safeguard the health and well-being of the nation's children and to encourage the domestic consumption of nutritious agricultural commodities and other foods." From its inception in 1946, the School Lunch Act in the United States required that a Type A lunch provide a third or more of the daily nutrient intake of the 10- to 12-year-old child, with adjustments made for younger and older children. To encourage the preparation of nutritious lunches, the USDA provided subsidies in the form of technical advice, surplus agricultural commodities, or foods purchased by the government as part of the price support programs, and a cash subsidy if the food service adhered to certain requirements. Specifically, the School Lunch Act required that each participating school operate on a nonprofit basis, serve meals at a regular meal hour, provide lunches free or at reduced cost to those unable to pay, and serve meals meeting specified nutritional standards. In addition, each state is required to match each dollar of federal money with $3 from sources within the state. In 1988 about 49%, or 11.9 million, of the children participating received free or reduced-price lunches. To qualify for reimbursement, a school must serve as a plate lunch a meal containing specific food components (as indicated in Table 17-4). The amounts required are adjusted to the age of the child.

To cope with the recognized problem of excessive plate waste, both elementary and high school students are now given the option of selecting three of the five designated items on the Type A lunch. The effect of this "offer versus serve" policy on nutrient intake has not yet been assessed. An evaluation of the adequacy of

Equivalents of Protein in 1 oz Lean Meat
- 1 oz cheese
- 1 large egg
- ½ C cooked dried peas or beans
- 2 T peanut butter

school lunches has led to concern that the lunches are failing to provide a third of the requirement for magnesium and pyridoxine. Since both these allowances are considered generous, and there is no evidence of a problem, it seems premature to make changes.

The Special Milk Program supplements the School Lunch Program and provides a subsidy for each 1 or 2 pints of milk served in a school.

Under the Child Nutrition Act of 1966, school breakfast programs have been instituted in the United States. The selected schools participating in this part of the feeding program are primarily those with many pupils from low-income families or pupils who travel great distances from their homes. About 88% of the 3.9 million children participating in 1988 received free or reduced-price breakfasts. Schools provide, at cost, one serving of fruit or juice, ½ pint of whole milk, and one serving of cereal before the regular school hour. This program has been promoted as a

Table 17-4 ◆ School lunch patterns for various age/grade groups*

	Minimum Quantities				Recommended Quantities‡
	Preschool, ages 1-2 (Group 1)	Preschool, ages 3-4 (Group II)	Grades K-3, ages 5-8 (Group III)	Grades 4-12, age 9 & over† (Group IV)	Grades 7-12, age 12 & over (Group V)
Meat or Meat Alternate					
A serving of one of the following or a combination to give an equivalent quantity:					
Lean meat, poultry, or fish (edible portion as served)	1 oz	1½ oz	1½ oz	2 oz	3 oz
Cheese	1 oz	1½ oz	1½ oz	2 oz	3 oz
Large egg(s)	½	¾	¾	1	1½
Cooked dry beans or peas	¼ cup	⅜ cup	⅜ cup	½ cup	¾ cup
Peanut butter	2 T	3 T	3 T	4 T	6 T
Vegetable and/or Fruit					
Two or more servings of vegetable or fruit or both to total	½ cup	½ cup	½ cup	¾ cup	¾ cup
Bread or Bread Alternate					
Servings of bread or bread alternate	5 per week	8 per week	8 per week	8 per week	10 per week
A serving is:					
1 slice of whole-grain or enriched bread					
A whole-grain or enriched biscuit, roll, muffin, etc.					
½ cup of cooked whole-grain or enriched rice, macaroni, noodles, whole-grain or enriched pasta products, or other cereal grains such as bulgur or corn grits					
A combination of any of the above					
Milk					
A serving of fluid milk	¾ cup (6 fl oz)	¾ cup (6 fl oz)	½ pint (8 fl oz)	½ pint (8 fl oz)	½ pint (8 fl oz)

From USDA, National School Lunch Program.

*USDA recommends, but does not require, that you adjust portions by age/grade group to better meet the food and nutritional needs of children according to their ages. If you adjust portions, Groups I-IV are minimum requirements for the age/grade groups specified. If you do *not* adjust portions, the Group IV portions are the portions to serve all children.

†Group IV is highlighted because it is the one meal pattern that will satisfy all requirements if no portion size adjustments are made.

‡Group V specifies recommended, not required, quantities for students 12 years and older. These students may request smaller portions, but not smaller than those specified in Group IV.

means of dealing with the nutritional deficits more common in the lower socioeconomic groups in the country. Although the evidence is subjective, it suggests better school performance and improved attention among children who have this breakfast before school.

In 1977 the Child Nutrition Act was amended to mandate that the federal government allocate to each state 50¢ per student for nutrition education. Following an assessment of the needs in each state, the state director of nutrition was to have responsibility for implementing a program. In most cases it was to be coordinated with the school lunch program.

A few programs demonstrated convincingly that by integrating nutrition into the academic programs in health, biology, and social science, it was possible to increase a student's understanding of nutrition. The behavioral outcomes were more difficult to measure, but there was reason for optimism that the program would help produce a generation of nutritionally informed consumers. By 1981, however, federal funding had been reduced substantially, long before the program was fully operational. Nevertheless, experience gained under the impetus of the funding moved nutrition education ahead significantly.

Other innovative intervention programs are being investigated as a possible means of improving the nutritional intake of schoolchildren, especially those from economically deprived groups.

Anorexia Nervosa and Bulimia

See *Focus* (p. 552) for more discussion of eating disorders

Anorexia nervosa is best described as a state of emaciation that has been brought on by voluntary starvation. It is seen primarily in adolescent girls from middle- and upper-class families. Unless it is recognized before it has advanced too far, it is very difficult to treat, since the victim refuses to eat. Instead of being lethargic and apathetic, as one would expect in undernutrition, anorexics have a drive to be active. Although most cases have a psychological basis, they represent a form of malnutrition far more severe than that resulting from lack of available food (for example, in famine areas).

Anorectic adolescents usually experience amenorrhea and sometimes fatal electrolyte imbalances. They deny that they are emaciated, in spite of a skeleton-like appearance, and usually continue to pursue thinness by refusing to eat and maintaining a hyperactive exercise program. Treatment consists of resolving underlying psychological problems, correcting disturbed family interactions, and restoring normal food intake and consequent weight gain. Anorexia almost always requires psychiatric as well as nutritional management.

A related phenomenon known as "gorge and purge" or *bulimia* is seen among adolescents, especially girls, from socioeconomic backgrounds similar to those who develop anorexia nervosa. These individuals consume enormous quantities of food and then immediately induce vomiting or take laxatives to purge themselves of the food (and thus the nutrients they provide). Although it has dire nutritional consequences, bulimia is primarily psychological in origin. The economic cost of maintaining such a regimen must be as high as the physiological and psychological cost.

Some of the warning signs and personal characteristics that distinguish anorexic from bulimic individuals are shown in Table 17-5. Figure 17-9 depicts some of the physical symptoms that occur with weight loss in eating disorders.

Improving Nutritional Habits

It has been well documented that nutrition knowledge is not necessarily reflected in food habits. Motivation seems to be the key to the application of sound nutritional principles to eating patterns. In adolescence the most effective motivation is the hope for vitality, good looks, and popularity. Concern over long-term effects of

Table 17-5 ◆ Warning signs and personal characteristics that distinguish anorectic from bulimic individuals

Anorexia Nervosa	Bulimia
• Turns away from food to cope	• Turns to food to cope
• Introverted	• Extroverted
• Avoids intimacy	• Seeks intimacy
• Negates feminine role	• Aspires to feminine role
• Maintains rigid control—perfectionist	• Loses control—steals, uses drugs, promiscuous
• Distorted body image	• Infrequent body distortions
• Denies illness	• Recognizes illness
• Significant and abnormal weight loss of 25% or more with no known medical illness accounting for the loss	• Within 10 to 15 pounds of normal body weight
• Intense fear of gaining weight	• Exhibit concern about their weight and make attempts to control weight by diet, vomiting or laxative and diuretic abuse.
• Reduction in food intake, denial of hunger and decrease in comsumption of fat-containing foods.	• Eating pattern may alternate between binges and fasts.
• Prolonged exercising despite fatigue and weakness.	• Most are secretive about binges and vomiting.
• Peculiar patterns of handling food.	• Food consumed during a binge has a high caloric content.
• Amenorrhea in women.	• Depressive moods may occur.
• Some exhibit bulimic episodes of binge-eating followed by vomiting or laxative abuse.	
• Symptoms of electrolyte imbalance, anemia, endocrine and immune dysfunction	
• Death resulting from starvation, hypothermia, cardiac failure.	• Death resulting from hypokalemia (low blood potassium) and suicide.

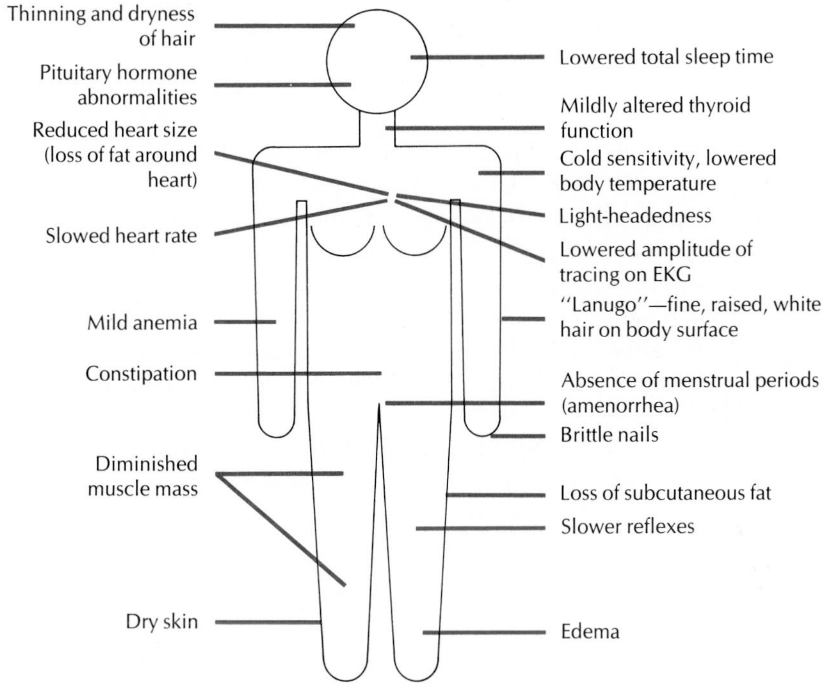

Figure 17-9 Possible signs and symptoms accompanying weight loss in eating disorders.

malnutrition or undernutrition on health has relatively little impact on the high school student or even the college student. The use of group sessions, during which the group accepts certain standards of eating and then helps provide the motivation and support to implement them, has been most effective. Sometimes it is necessary to "unlearn" sets of habits, but other times it is merely a case of modifying or improving current habits. A positive approach that builds on desirable habits rather than on correcting negative ones is preferable and more effective. It is important to start with a person's present habits, reinforce the good aspects and replace the poor with new habits, and recognize that good diets do not just happen but are planned.

BY NOW YOU SHOULD KNOW

- Needs for various nutrients are higher during the period of growth than at any other time. The rate of increase varies with time and from one nutrient to another, depending on which tissues are undergoing the most growth at any one time.
- Snacks can make a major contribution of the calories and essential nutrients needed by both children and adolescents.
- Iron, folacin, calcium, and zinc are nutrients often inadequately supplied in the diets of young children.
- Growth curves are used to determine how a child is developing in comparison to other children of the same age or height.
- During childhood the most common nutrition-related problems are growth retardation, anemia, obesity, and impaired dental health.
- During adolescence concern focuses on eating disorders and food patterns, including skipping breakfast, snacking habits, fad dieting, and the use of alcohol and drugs. Additional feminine concerns also focus on premenstrual syndrome, pregnancy, lactation, and the use of oral contraceptives.
- Food habits formed during the teen years influence health status during adulthood, and food patterns established at this time set the foundation for a lifetime of eating habits.
- The National School Lunch Program, Special Milk Program, and the Breakfast Program have all been important in contributing to adequate nutrient intake of American children while in school.

STUDY QUESTIONS

1. List the nutrients that influence normal tooth function and explain the role of each nutrient.
2. If ketchup were to be considered a vegetable in the school lunch program, explain how this is not nutritionally the same as a half a tomato.
3. You have interviewed a child on his or her food consumption patterns. You find the child skips breakfast. What are the nutritional and physical implications of skipping breakfast?
4. A child is in the 80th percentile on the growth curve. Explain what this means.
5. You are in charge of the school lunch program at a high school, and there seems to be too much wasted food. What would you do to increase the nutrient intake and decrease the amount of wasted foods?
6. You have a friend whose child is on a food jag for about 3 weeks, eating only hot dogs on buns and soda. What should your friend do?
7. How would you expect a child with iron-deficiency anemia to behave? Would you expect the child to look different?

8. Explain the differences and similarities between anorexia nervosa and bulimia.
9. What effect can recreational drugs and alcohol have on nutritional status?
10. Why are there more nutrition concerns during adolescence for girls than for boys?
11. Using Figure 17-3 found on p. 525 list the nutrients in which 25% or more of the subjects received 70% or less of the RDA. Beside each nutrient list foods that realistically could be added to the diets of children ages 1 to 11 years of age to increase nutrient consumption.

Applying What You've Learned

1. **Parental Concerns**

   Talk to parents of children from 3 to 16 years of age about the concerns they had about their children's eating habits during childhood and adolescence and how they resolved their concerns.

2. **Plot Your Growth**

   Ask your family if it has growth records from your childhood. Plot your growth on the growth curves in this chapter. How did your growth compare?

3. **Vending Machine Food Choices**

   Observe the vending machines in your local schools and assess the nutritive quality of the items available to young children and adolescents. Do they provide an opportunity to make informed choices?

4. **Assess the Lunch Program in Your School District**

   How is the school lunch program run in your school district? Does it participate in the Federal School Lunch Program? Are meals prepared on site, or are they brought to the school by a contracting organization? What proportion of schoolchildren participates?

5. **Look at the World Through the Eyes of a Child**

   Watch television on Saturday morning, making note of the foods being advertised. Go to the grocery store and look at the foods (especially breakfast cereals) that are on the eye level of children. Undoubtedly some of the foods advertised on Saturday morning were breakfast cereals. Find those cereals in the store, read the nutrition information and the list of ingredients. Can you draw any conclusions?

6. **Observe Children when Dining Out**

   Next time you are in a fast-food restaurant or a restaurant that has children or teens, observe their eating behaviors, the foods they order, how fast they eat, who they are with, and any other observations you think explain some of the eating patterns of the age-group.

7. **24-Hour Food Recall for a Child, Age 10 to 14.**

   Using Appendix F in the back of your textbook, analyze the child's nutrient intake. Compare the actual intake to the RDAs found in the text. What nutrients if any are inadequate? What foods could be added to the child's diet to improve the nutrient intake? What are the strong points about this child's diet? Remember this is just 1 day of recall, you are not in a position to prescribe dietary changes to the child or the parent.

8. **Feingold Diet**

   Write down everything you eat for 1 day. Circle the foods that you would eliminate if you were to follow the Feingold diet.

9. Plan a Meal

Plan an evening meal for a young child. What factors would you consider in meal planning and food preferences? Name the food and why you would serve those particular foods.

SUGGESTED READINGS

Committee on Nutrition, Academy of Pediatrics: Toward a prudent diet for children, Pediatrics 71:78, 1983.

The Academy of pediatrics has reviewed information on the nutritive needs of children and the relationship of diet in early life to health in adults. They recommend breast feeding for as long as is feasible, followed by formula feeding for the first year of life, addition of solid foods by 4 months of age, a varied diet after 1 year, maintenance of ideal weight, a regular exercise program, screening of children with a family history of risk factors for coronary heart disease, obesity, hypertension and diabetes, and moderation in any dietary modifications.

Foucard T: Developmental aspects of food sensitivity in childhood, Nutrition Reviews 42:98, 1984.

This article will be of interest to students who have a family history of allergy. It outlines our knowledge of food sensitivity in children, how to treat it, and the caution that there may be hazards associated with trying to manipulate the immune response.

Hertzler AA: Children's food patterns—a review: (1) Food preferences and feeding problems; (2) Family and group behavior, Journal of the American Dietetic Association 83:551, 1983.

These papers present a comprehensive review of what we do and do not know about the factors that influence the eating behavior of young children. They deal with the physical characteristics of food, such as color, flavor, and texture, as well as the very important social context in which food is offered. Questions of mealtime discipline, parent-child stimulation and interactions, and positive reinforcement are discussed.

Huse DM: Dietary treatment of anorexia nervosa, Journal of the American Dietetic Association 83:687, 1983.

The author recognizes the complex psychological and physiological bases of anorexia and describes an approach to the dietary treatment of the condition. The article deals with setting realistic goals, placing much of the responsibility on the patient, and providing sufficient but not excessive support. The importance of a weight maintenance program once the goal has been reached is stressed.

Kim WW, and others: Evaluation of long-term dietary intakes of adults consuming self-selected diets, American Journal of Clinical Nutrition 40:1327, 1984.

This report of dietary intake of 29 adults over a 1-year period showed that they selected diets that met the RDA, except for iron and calcium for females. It showed that the intake of energy and 19 other nutrients was very consistent throughout the year. Exceptions were for periods when subjects were asked to keep weighed samples of their food intake; then they reduced their intake by about 12%. This same issue contains reports of calorie, protein, calcium, phoshorus, magnesium, zinc, copper, and manganese intake and balance throughout the year of the study.

Mahan LK, and Rees JM: Nutrition in adolescence, St. Louis, 1984, Times Mirror/Mosby College Publishing.

This is an excellent book, which focuses on the second decade of life, with particular emphasis on the clinical science basis for nutrition recommendations. The authors provide practical suggestions for managing nutrition problems of adolescents and for giving advice on health promotion and disease prevention.

Rush D, editor: National evaluation of the school nutrition programs, American Journal of Clinical Nutrition 40:369, 1984.

This supplement to the journal contains 10 articles reporting findings on the effect of school programs on dietary intake, anthropometric measures, student participation, and family food expenditure. For those interested in policy decisions regarding participation in school nutrition programs, this series brings together the most current information from an evaluative study.

ADDITIONAL READINGS

Childhood

Birch LL: The relationship between children's food preferences and those of their parents, Journal of Nutrition Education 12:14, 1980.

Brownell KD, and Kaye FS: A school-based behavior modification nutrition education and physical activity program for obese children, American Journal of Clinical Nutrition 35: 277, 1982.

Conners CK, Goyette CH, and Soothwich DA: Food additives and hyperkinesis: a controlled double-bind experiment, Pediatrics 58:154, 1981.

Dwyer JT, and others: Nutritional status of vegetarian children, American Journal of Clinical Nutrition 35:204, 1982.

Edelman B: Developmental differences in conceptualization of obesity, Journal of the American Dietetic Association 80:122, 1982.

Growth of vegetarian children, Nutrition Reviews 37:108, 1979.

Newbrun E: Sugar and dental caries: a review of human studies, Science 217:418, 1982.

Patterson R, Typpo JT, Typpo MH, and Krause GF: Factors related to obesity in preschool children, Journal of the American Dietetic Association 86:1376, 1986.

Politt E, Leibel RL, and Greenfield D: Brief fasting, stress, and cognition in children, American Journal of Clinical Nutrition 34: 1526, 1981.

Weil WB: Current controversies in childhood obesity, Journal of Pediatrics 91:175, 1977.

Weiss G, and Hechtman L: The hyperactive child syndrome, Science 205:1348, 1979.

Casper RC, and others: An evaluation of trace metals, vitamins, and taste functions in anorexia nervosa, American Journal of Clinical Nutrition 33:1801, 1980.

Chan GM, Ronald N, Slater P, Hollis J, and Thomas MR: Decreased bone mineral status in lactating adolescent mothers, Journal of Pediatrics 101:767, 1982.

Clark AJ, Mossholder S, and Gates R: Folacin status in adolescent females, American Journal of Clinical Nutrition 46:302, 1987.

Dietz WH: Implications and treatment of adolescent obesity, Clinical Nutrition 4:103, 1985.

Halmi K: Anorexia and bulimia, Annual Review of Medicine 38:311, 1987.

Hertzler AA, and Schulman RS: Employed women, dieting, and support groups, Journal of the American Dietetic Association 82:153, 1983.

Huenneman RL, and others: Teenage nutrition and physique, Springfield, Ill., 1974, Charles C Thomas, Publisher.

Kirkley B: Bulimia: Clinical characteristics, development and etiology, Journal of the American Dietetic Association 86:468, 1986.

Richardson BD, and Pieters L: Menarche and growth, American Journal of Clinical Nutrition 30:2088, 1977.

Roe DA, and others: Nutritional status of women attending family planning clinics, Journal of the American Dietetic Association 81:682, 1982.

Schafer RB, and Keeth P: Influence on food decisions across the family life cycle, Journal of the American Dietetic Association 78:144, 1981.

Story M, and Resnick MD: Adolescents' views on food and nutrition, Journal of Nutrition Education 18:188, 1986.

Storz NS, and Greene WH: Body weight, body image, and perception of fad diets in adolescent girls, Journal of Nutrition Education 15:15, 1983.

Wack JT, and Rodin J: Smoking and its effects on body weight and the systems of caloric regulation, American Journal of Clinical Nutrition 35:135, 1982.

FOCUS Eating Disorders—An Adolescent Problem

Over the past 10 to 15 years it has become apparent that eating disorders have reached epidemic proportions among adolescents. There are two distinct disorders, *anorexia nervosa* and *bulimia*, which affect adolescents and college-age women more frequently than any other group. Surprisingly, they involve people with a wide range of body weights, from the emaciated to the obese, and usually result from a complex interaction of biochemical, psychological, and social factors.

"Cure" rates for persons with eating disorders are discouraging. Only 50% of recovered clients remain symptom free, 25% live with reduced symptoms, and 25% experience no meaningful remission following therapy. Thus early intervention and prevention of these insidious disorders is the only feasible approach to dealing with the problem.

The term *anorexia nervosa* was first used in 1873 by English physician William Gull to describe severely emaciated young women who refused to eat. Anorexia, meaning loss of appetite, is, in a sense, a misnomer, since only about 50% of those afflicted have loss of appetite, and then only in the latter stages. The term, however, remains in clinical and popular use.

Anorexia nervosa is found predominantly among adolescent females, affecting one in 250 girls between 12 and 18 years of age. These young women most often come from middle- to upper-class families and are described as intelligent, obedient, even "model" children until the eating disorder emerges. At that point, the constant battle over eating disrupts almost every aspect of life for the girl and her family.

The disorder is characterized by a relentless pursuit of thinness, coupled with an intense preoccupation with food, eating, and body weight. Anorexics are expert calorie counters; they eventually eliminate all "fattening" foods (most carbohydrates and all fats) and are frequently vegetarians. They often spend considerable time and effort preparing food for others and insist that others eat while they refrain from eating. Anorexics also display peculiar food-handling behaviors, such as food hoarding, cutting food into minute pieces, toying with food, and dawdling for hours over a very small meal. Transient food fads and rituals are also common.

Symptoms of anorexia nervosa include a weight loss of 20% to 25%, amenorrhea for at least 3 months, and distorted body image, with no evidence of organic disease. The disturbance of body image is so extreme that many anorexics continue to view their skeleton-like figures as grossly overweight and complain that they are "too fat" even though significant weight loss is obvious.

Other symptoms of anorexia include a sense of ineffectiveness and depression, discomfort after eating, constipation, bingeing, self-induced vomiting, laxative abuse, and hyperactivity. Despite their emaciated state, anorexics will exercise for hours, denying fatigue as they use exercise as yet another strategy to burn calories and further decrease weight.

Finally, the classic symptoms of starvation appear, including anemia, electrolyte imbalances, and endocrine and immune dysfunction. If left untreated, the deterioration of brain tissue results in apathy, coma, and death in about 1 in 20 anorexics.

The only effective treatment is hospitalization, with treatment by an interdisciplinary team giving the best results. Weight gain and restoration of adequate nutritional status are imperative. Because of the elaborate measures taken by some anorexics to refuse food, refeeding must often be by a nasogastric tube or intravenous feeding (TPN or total parenteral nutrition). Drug therapy is used to reduce hyperactivity and anxiety during mealtime, as well as to stimulate appetite. Psychotherapy, however, remains the cornerstone of treatment. Programs that incorporate behavior modification, family therapy, and nutritional counseling are most successful in the long-term rehabilitation of persons with anorexia nervosa.

Bulimia is an even more recent eating disorder, having been first publicized in 1980. The word *bulimia* means "ox hunger," an appropriate description of the voracious appetite displayed by bulimics, who constantly engage in food binges.

Bulimia usually begins as an effort to control weight. It involves alternating patterns of bingeing on large quantities of food (from 3000 to 20,000 calories is common), and then 'purging' by self-induced vomiting or by taking laxatives. Fasting and continuous strict dieting may be used separately or in conjunction with purging.

Although bulimia may be a complication of anorexia nervosa, it also affects women of normal weight. They tend to be white women of the upper and middle classes and somewhat older than those with anorexia, with 17 years being the average age of onset. Alcoholism, obesity, and depression are found among the family members of bulimics. Bulimics themselves have a tendency toward abuse of alcohol and drugs, shoplifting, and sexual promiscuity, suggesting problems in controlling their impulsive behaviors. Bulimia is further associated with feelings of low self-esteem, guilt, helplessness, and some distortion of body image.

Bulimics have recurrent episodes of binge eating, consuming high-calorie, easily ingested foods such as candy, cookies, cake, and ice cream during a binge. They tend to terminate a binge with sleep or self-induced vomiting, eat surreptitiously during a binge, make repeated attempts to lose weight, experience frequent weight fluctuations, and have fear of not being able to stop eating voluntarily. They are frequently depressed after bingeing.

The complex nature of the bulimic syndrome has critical effects on physical and emotional health. Bingeing and purging begin in an effort to control weight but gradually become a method for dealing with stress and frustration; the pattern is covert and may go on undetected for surprisingly long periods, until it eventually becomes a chronic problem. In addition to the very detrimental effects of rapid weight fluctuation, prolonged bouts of bulimia may result in electrolyte imbalances, ulceration of the gastrointestinal tract, erosion of dental enamel, loss of hair, and irregularities in the menstrual cycle; encephalograms may reveal irregular patterns.

Bulimics may go as long as 6 to 7 years before seeking help. While many bulimics respond favorably to antidepressant drug therapy, this treatment is most effective when combined with psychotherapy and behavior therapy. Nutritional counseling, aimed at regulating eating behavior and weight, further improves the treatment outcomes of bulimic clients but in itself is inadequate.

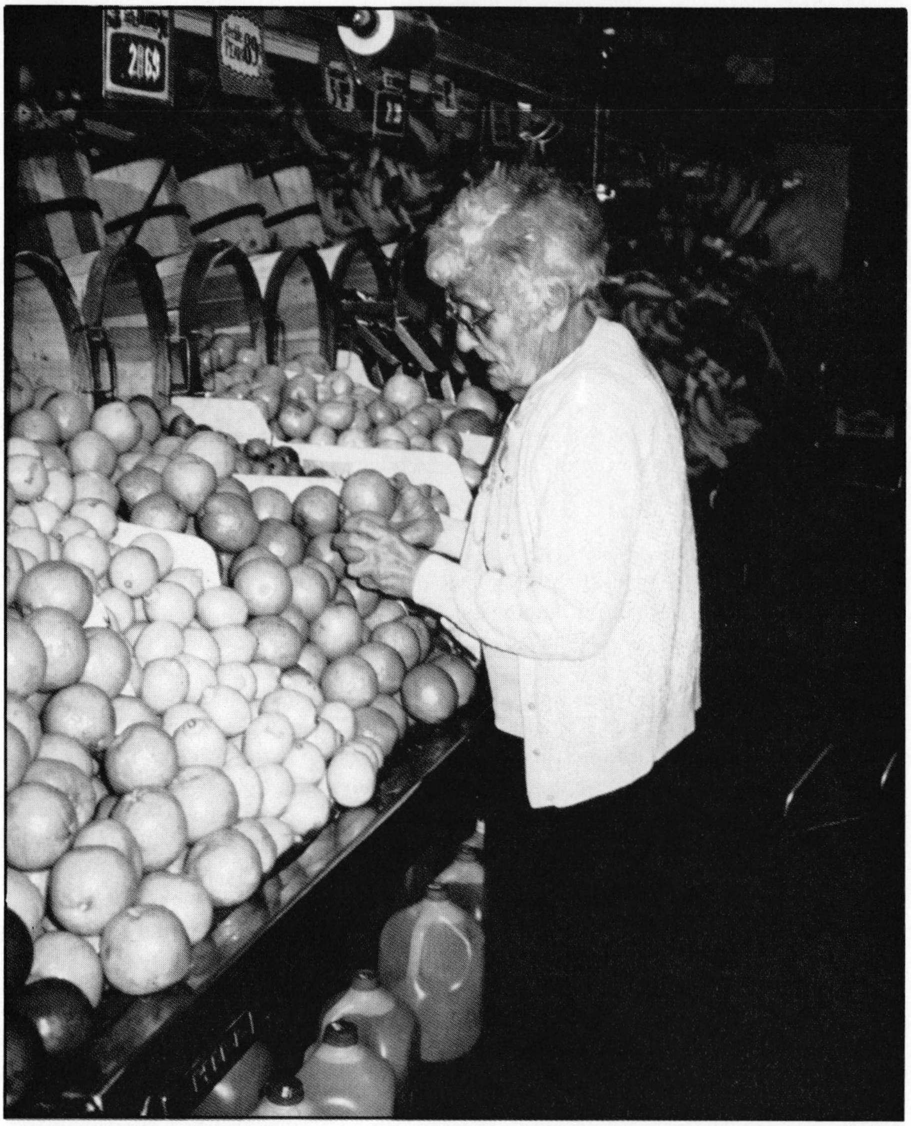

AWARENESS CHECK

Truth or Fiction?

- The elderly need less of all nutrients in comparison to active, healthy adults.
- The elderly have fewer energy needs because they cannot be as physically active as they once were.
- As we age, we experience a decreased ability to taste and smell food.
- As we age our amount of lean body mass declines, and we naturally tend to store more fat.
- More men have complications from osteoporosis than do women.
- A balanced diet will slow the aging process.

Nutrition in the Later Years

CHAPTER 18

With a growing number of people surviving to enjoy their "renaissance years," interest in learning more about nutritional needs for these mature years has increased markedly. Nutritional needs are influenced not only by the present physical state and activity of an individual but also by long-standing food habits and the many social, environmental, emotional, and physiological stresses to which a person has been subjected throughout growth and maturity. Many social programs have been developed to help senior citizens maintain nutritional adequacy to maximize their health potential. The role of nutrition in reducing causes of impaired function and ill health associated with aging is an area of research that currently has high priority, and the role of diet therapy in correcting nutrition-related problems has been long recognized.

Sooner or later, all of us will develop a very personal interest in aging. Although it is an unavoidable event, most of us would like to delay the onset and slow the process. As a result scientists, citizens, and charlatans, like modern-day Ponce de Leons, search for the "Fountain of Youth," longevity, and eternal life (or at least better quality of life, for as long as it lasts). Although eternal life remains elusive and probably unattainable, more and more people are living longer and healthier lives for many reasons, not the least of which is improved diet/nutrition. Even if all causes of premature death were eliminated, we would have a life span of about 100 years and then would succumb as the result of normal losses in physiological functioning.

Geriatrics—the branch of medicine dedicated to the care of the aging, as well as the aged—is concerned with expanding the length of the prime period of life, delaying the onset of severely degenerative aspects of aging, and treating the diseases of the aged. **Gerontology** is a broader branch of science dealing with the psychological, sociological, economic, physiological, and medical aspects of aging, with the last two often referred to as biogerontology. There has been a surge of activity in both of these fields of study in the last 3 decades.

geriatrics
The branch of medicine concerned with health problems of the elderly

gerontology
The broad area of science concerned with all social, economic, and medical problems of the elderly

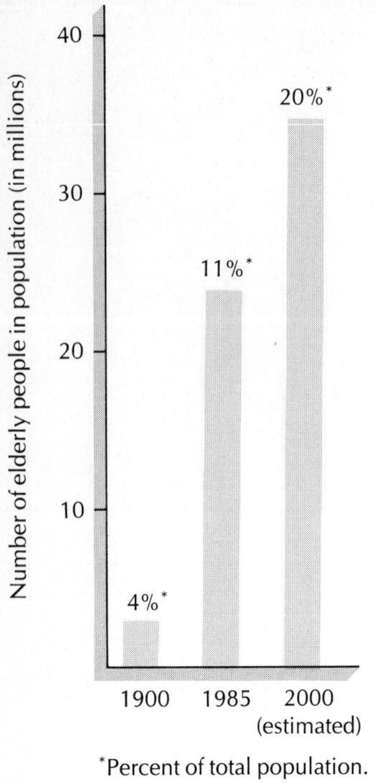

Increase in the proportion of elderly people in the United States since 1900

The creation of the National Institute on Aging, with a budget of over $200 million/year to support research on both biological and social questions of aging, represents the government's commitment to dealing with the concerns and needs of the elderly. The Institute's goal is to increase our knowledge of the changes that occur with aging as a basis for developing strategies to prevent premature aging and to enhance the quality of life for the elderly.

The establishment of a USDA Center on Aging at Tufts University in 1981, staffed by over 250 scientists, is further evidence of increased commitment to the study of nutrition and aging. The goals of this center are to explore

1. How nutrition influences various body functions during the aging process
2. The role of nutrition in retarding chronic disabilities and disorders
3. Optimal nutritional needs for older people

Growing concern over the problems of the aging population has resulted from the increase in both the total numbers and proportion of the population who are living beyond retirement age. Advances in medical technology, environmental hygiene, and nutrition have meant that more people live longer with greater freedom from disease and therefore better health. The extension of life has also made the complications of aging, both physiological and psychological, more apparent.

Recognition of the importance of good nutrition in later years is already evident from the number of intervention programs with an emphasis on nutrition that have been developed as part of government efforts to enhance the quality of life for the elderly.

In 1900, 3 million people (4% of the population in the United States) were over 65 years of age. Today, the populations of 33 million people over 60 years of age and 24 million over 65 years of age represent 15% and 11% of the total U.S. population, respectively. It is predicted that both the number and proportion of elderly people in the United States will continue to increase to 35 million and 20% of the population by the year 2000. In addition, there will be an even greater increase in the proportion of elderly people over 70 years of age, with those over 85 years the most rapidly growing segment of the population. As indicated in Table 18-1, life expectancy at birth is still increasing slowly; it continues to be greater for women than for men. At age 20, there is little increase in an individual's life expectancy from that at birth. This suggests that environmental factors over which there is some control—air and water quality, the use of drugs, alcohol, and tobacco, and proper nutrition—are only some among the many factors that determine health and longevity. Genetics continues to play a significant role and is thought to determine the upper age to which an individual will survive. The major causes of death have changed; infectious diseases have virtually disappeared and degenerative diseases have risen to the top of the list. The affluence of our life-style is a contributing factor (Table 18-2).

NUTRITION AND AGING

Cross-sectional studies include many people at one point in time; longitudinal studies follow up a group of the same people over a long period of time. For example, a cross-sectional study of aging may include one group of 40-year-olds, one of 50-year-olds, and one of 60-year-olds, all studied at the same time. In a longitudinal study of aging, a group is studied when they are 40 years old, again when they are 50, and then again when they are 60

The study of the nutritional needs of aging people is complicated by the fact that the older the people, the more complex their nutritional needs from both a social and physiological point of view. The elderly constitute a heterogeneous group in which the normal range of genetic differences is compounded by all the varying stresses, injuries, emotional and physical traumas, and nutritional imbalances to which they have been subjected throughout growth and maturity. Individual differences can be very large, and the range of values for most functions increases with age. Therefore the wide variations in the abilities of the elderly to ingest, digest, absorb, and utilize nutrients make it difficult to generalize about nutritional needs. Research in this area is further complicated by the difficulty (if not the impossibility) of studying one person throughout 50 or 60 years of life. So far, scientists have relied on data from cross-sectional studies on many different people at different ages; however, at least one longitudinal study has been completed, and another has been designed to assess the biochemical and physiological changes that occur in a group of men to be studied for 20 years. Such an investigation ought to shed considerable light on the biochemistry and physiology of the aging process to help us understand why chronological age is not a predictor of physiological age.

Studies that have been done on a few individuals, however, make it possible to provide guidelines for the nutrition of the elderly. In considering the role of nutrition in aging we are concerned not only with how nutrition influences the aging process but also how physiological changes occurring with age affect nutrient needs and use. It has been shown that diet affects longevity through (1) the development and pattern of diseases associated with old age, (2) alteration in the neuroendocrine system, (3) changes in organ and tissue protein turnover, and (4) modification of immune processes. Further knowledge of the mechanisms of the aging process will perhaps lead to either the prevention or the detection and treatment of nutritional problems of aging.

Gerontologists suggest that the best preparation for a healthy old age begins in the office of the pediatrician.

It is obvious that genetics is a major determinant of the nature of aging. Thus for almost any biological process, aging occurs at different rates in different people even under similar environmental conditions. The rate of aging also varies in different tissues within the same individual. A person with a chronological age of 80 may have a biological age of 50, and vice versa. Some elderly people are active, healthy, ambulatory, and still involved in their world. Others may be acutely ill, chronically diseased, relatively sedentary, withdrawn from society, or even immobilized.

Energy. The stresses that affect aging seem subtle and insidious. However, they accumulate over a period of years to have adverse effects on body functions. This can be vividly illustrated by the stress of a caloric imbalance of as little as 10 kcal/day, which at the end of a year results in a gain or loss of 1 pound (0.45 kg) of weight. When accumulated over a 40-year period, this imbalance represents an appreciable change in body size: 40 pounds, or 18 kg. Similarly, rather small stresses in individual cells or organs that accumulate over the years may become great enough to cause impaired cellular functioning.

Animal studies show that calorie restriction in early life results in an increase in the life span, whereas overeating after maturity increases the incidence of degenerative disease. There is no evidence from human studies to indicate how we react to a similar feeding pattern. Seemingly contradictory evidence from life insurance data suggests that there is some advantage, as far as morbidity or mortality is concerned, in weighing 10% to 15% above those weights previously considered desirable. Obesity, however, must be avoided.

Cell structure. In later years, as at any other time, the body's state of nutrition is determined by the state of nutrition of individual cells. Cells will be less than adequately nourished under conditions of dietary deficiencies or excesses, impaired digestion, incomplete absorption, inefficient distribution and utilization of nutrients, and accumulation of waste products. Many of these changes occur as the body ages. Additionally, regardless of nutrition, cells function differently as they grow older. They are less able to respond appropriately and quickly to hormones such as insulin; they are less able to synthesize needed enzymes; and they are slower to break down proteins that are normally degraded within the cell. In addition to changes in DNA and the impaired ability of RNA to direct protein synthesis, cells in older people may produce slightly defective enzymes; cellular ability to use energy is reduced when the number of mitochondria decline; and cells lining the intestine and liver cells that normally regenerate very frequently have a reduced capacity to multiply.

The changes associated with aging also result from a decrease in the number of functioning cells. The brain, for example, is unable to regenerate cells after a child reaches the ages of 2 to 4. Muscles lose their capacity after middle age, whereas the liver is able to replace cells throughout most of life. Red blood cells

Table 18-1 ◇ Life expectancy, determined at year of birth

Year of Birth	Life Expectancy (years)
1850	40
1900	47
1940	63
1950	68
1960	70
1970	70
1980	73 (men, 69; women, 77)

Table 18-2 ◇ Leading causes of death in the United States

Cause	% of Deaths
1900	
Pneumonia	12
Tuberculosis	11
Diarrhea	8
Heart disease*	8
Stroke*	6
1983	
Heart disease*	41
Cancer*	22
Stroke*	8
Accidents	8
Pneumonia	6

*NCHS-Monthly Vital Statistics Report 37(1) April 1, 1988.

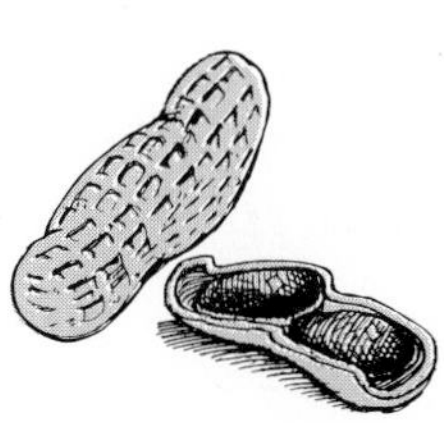

2 peanuts per day =
10 kcal per day =
1 lb body fat per year

Example of the effect of small caloric imbalance over time

cannot reproduce once they have matured, but the bone marrow is able to continue production of more red blood cells.

Collagen. Structural changes associated with collagen, the noncellular protein substance that binds the cells together, also occur with aging. Collagen, in which the rate of protein turnover is slow, becomes less elastic and more fibrous as the cells age. Connective tissue may replace some of the more active cells lost from an organ, so that the decline in functional capacity of an organ may be greater than that represented by the decrease in organ weight. In muscle, muscle fibers may be replaced by connective tissue. The accumulation of collagen is believed to contribute to the appearance of aging skin, usually the first objective evidence of advancing years, and most obvious on the face and hands.

In any case, when either the number, size, or functional capability of cells is reduced, it is reflected in the functional capability of the tissue or organ of which the cells are a part.

Growth. In recent years, physiologists have been trying to identify the nature of degenerative changes that occur with aging. In theory, aging begins with conception. However, during the period of growth, the anabolic (or building-up) processes exceed the catabolic (or degenerative) changes; therefore the net result is one of growth and increased functional capabilities of the organs and tissues of the body. Once the body has reached physiological maturity at about age 25, the process is reversed, slowly at first, until the rate of degenerative changes outweighs the rate of growth changes. Along with this process comes impaired functioning of most organs.

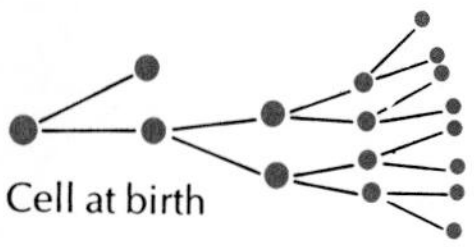

Body cells are capable of only a limited number of divisions in their lifetime—usually 50 to 55.

Studies of individual cells show that each type of cell is capable of a limited number of cell divisions during its lifetime. For most tissues, the number of divisions of a cell is somewhere between 50 and 55. After that, the cell type is incapable of any further division and therefore is unable to repair or replace itself. The age at which a cell reaches this stage is determined by a great many factors, including nutrition.

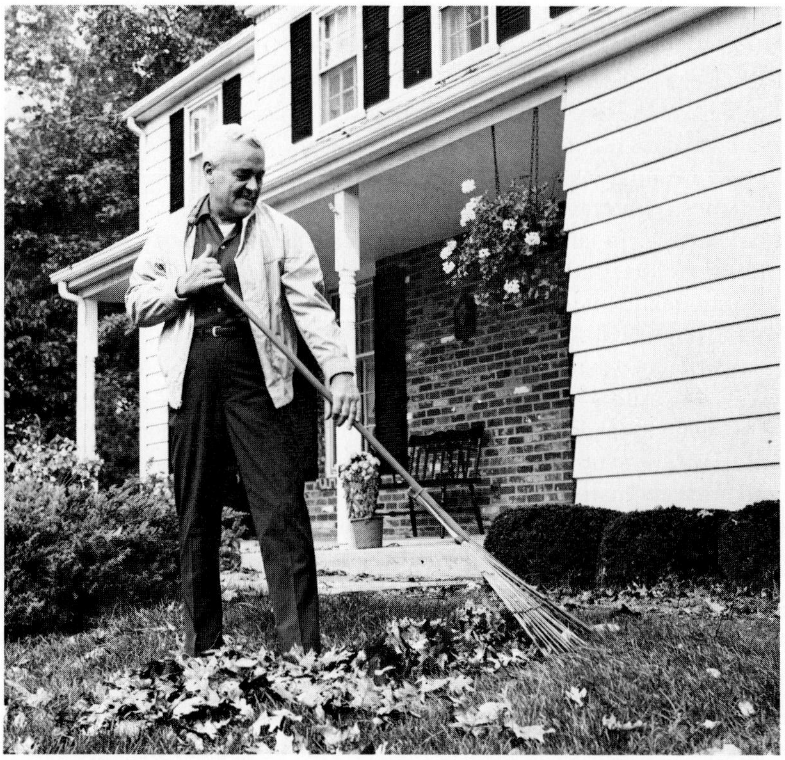

A nutritious diet throughout life combined with regular exercise contribute to good health in later years.

Table 18-3 ◇ Percentage of tissues remaining in a 75-year-old man compared to a 30-year-old man

Tissue	Percent Remaining in 75-year-old Man
Kidney weight	91
Brain weight	56
Number liver cells	92
Number of glomeruli in kidneys	69
Number of nerve trunk fibers	63
Number of taste buds	36
Body water content	75

Modified from Shock NW: Scientific American 206:100, 1962.

Exercise and activity. Maintaining an active life-style and a program of activity throughout life has many positive consequences on health. It can delay (1) the normal decrease in work capacity, (2) the decline in heart rate, (3) the loss of bone mass and muscle mass, (4) the increase in blood cholesterol and low-density lipoprotein levels, (5) the drop in high-density lipoprotein levels, and (6) the increase in glucose intolerance, all of which characterize advancing age.

Human Studies

Shock (1962) studied and measured the changes in various physiological functions in 50-year-old men and 75-year-old men, compared to 30-year-old men. Table 18-3 presents changes in tissue size from this study. Other changes such as the reduced capacities of the heart to pump blood and of the kidneys to filter the blood, the reduced reaction time for nerves, and other physiological changes in the utilization of nutrients are effects that will be discussed later.

Theories on Aging

Many theories have been advanced to explain the biochemical and physiological basis of the aging process; the following are included among them:

1. The "clinker" theory, which attributes loss of cell function with aging to the accumulation of waste or defective parts in the cells.
2. The wear-and-tear theory, which attributes aging to the chemical and mechanical exhaustion of the cells.
3. The somatic mutation theory, which suggests that somatic (growing or dividing) cells are inactivated or defective as a result of errors in DNA replication.
4. The genetic theory, which suggests that errors in DNA or RNA replication result in the death of the cell or the production of foreign proteins that limit cell function.
5. The autoimmune theory, which suggests that antibodies that usually attack only bacteria and foreign cells start to attack and destroy normal body cells.
6. The cross-linkage theory, which maintains that collagen molecules are immobilized through cross-linking by **free radicals** (the free radicals having been produced by many biochemical reactions and by the effect of ozone from the atmosphere).
7. The lipid peroxidation theory, which suggests that the oxidation of lipid in the cell membrane destroys its integrity and leads either to destruction of the cell or to the accumulation of lipofuscin granules (oxidized lipoproteins) in the cell.

Theories of Aging
"Clinker"
Wear-and-tear
Somatic mutation
Genetic
Autoimmune
Collagen cross-linkage
Lipid peroxidation

free radicals
Very reactive molecules that are released as the result of certain biochemical changes; because they cannot remain alone, they seek some other molecule with which to react

Although there is no complete agreement on the cause of aging, it is agreed that almost all changes are irreversible. Moreover, cells are interdependent; therefore if one cell dies, other cells in the same or different organs may also lose their ability to function and subsequently die.

FACTORS AFFECTING THE INTAKE OF FOOD

As with any age-group, the nutritional adequacy of the diet of the elderly is the result of a variety of factors that determine dietary intake, the utilization of nutrients, and finally the nutrient requirements. All of these factors include environmental, as well as biological, considerations. Because elderly people are so heterogeneous in terms of their past health and nutritional status during developmental and adult periods, assessing nutrient needs and adequacy is much more complex than for younger age-groups. The major influences on nutrient intake, use, and need are summarized in Table 18-4.

Table 18-4 ◊ Factors affecting food intake, nutrient utilization, and nutrient needs

	Food Intake	Nutrient Utilization	Nutrient Needs
Physical	Loss of teeth Lack of neuromuscular co-ordination Impaired hearing and vision Physical weakness and disability Immobility Discomfort on ingestion of certain foods	Immobility	Body composition Decreased activity
Physiological	Loss of sense of taste and smell Anorexia (lack of appetite)	Decreased salivation Decreased enzyme activity Decreased gastric acidity Depressed gastric motility Depressed kidney function Chronic disease Malabsorption Decreased hormonal secretion	Use of drugs Decreased metabolic efficiency
Social	Long-standing food habits Food preferences Beliefs about effects of foods Economic considerations Susceptibility to food misinformation Failure to adapt to new environment	Meal patterns	
Psychological	Living alone Depression Anxiety	Anxiety	

Physical Factors

Loss of teeth. The longer people live, the more likely they are to lose their teeth. Moreover, the lower their socioeconomic status, the less likely they will be to replace missing teeth with satisfactory dentures. The American Dental Association estimates that 50% of 65-year-olds and 66% of 75-year-olds have lost all their teeth; 80% of these groups either fail to replace them or replace them with ill-fitting dentures. Some dental problems are attributed to the loss of the supporting jawbone in **periodontal disease** (disease in tissue surrounding the teeth). Causes of periodontal disease include a low calcium/phosphorus ratio in the diet and low vitamin D intakes associated with osteoporosis in women over 50. Regardless of cause, the absence of a satisfactory method of chewing food leads a person without teeth to many modifications in eating patterns.

periodontal disease
Disease of the tissues in the mouth surrounding the teeth

Food that is inadequately chewed is difficult to swallow. Therefore people with unsatisfactory teeth tend to substitute foods requiring little chewing for those requiring more (such as raw fruits and vegetables and meat). When foods high in fiber such as the fruits and vegetables are eliminated from the diet, dietary bulk is reduced, with a resulting decrease in gastrointestinal motility and more problems of elimination. A reduced intake of meat—one of the best sources of available iron and zinc—will possibly result in impaired iron status, which in turn may influence behavior, particularly activity.

If fluoridation of the water supply, by reducing tooth decay, decreases the number of **edentulous** senior citizens, its benefits may be as great in later years as in childhood.

edentulous
Without teeth

Loss of neuromuscular coordination. The ability to maintain fine neuromuscular coordination declines with age, frequently showing up in the loss of ability to manipulate eating utensils. Rather than risk the embarrassment that would come with spilled food or inability to cut meat or eat soup, elderly people may avoid such foods. This may lead to significant dietary changes and frequent nutritional inadequacies.

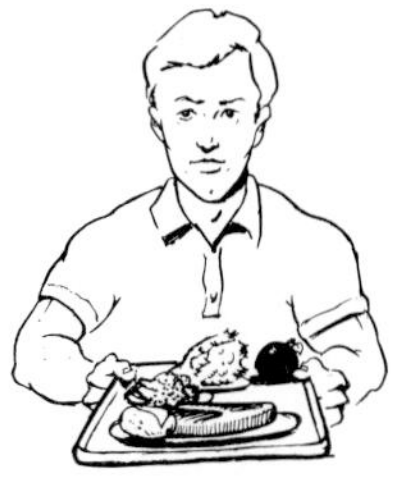
Crisp foods, regular meat

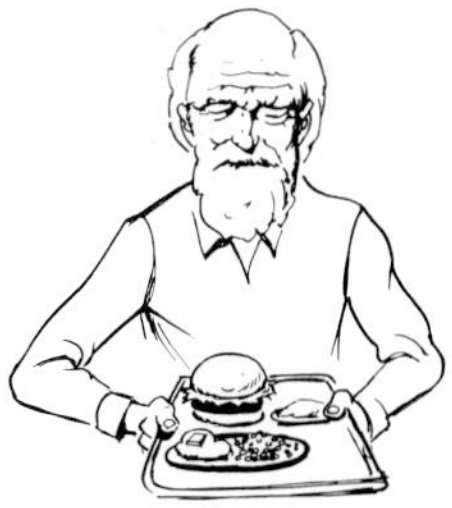
Soft foods, ground meat

People with teeth prefer crisp foods and regular meat; people without teeth or with poorly fitted dentures prefer soft food and ground meat.

People with a deteriorating ability to coordinate their movements recognize the hazards of working with boiling water or gas ranges. To avoid the danger associated with cooking food for themselves, they may choose foods that do not need cooking. These same people may also find it difficult to shop, carry food, or seek transportation to and from stores, and so rely more and more on sources of food that minimize any of these tasks. As a result, the variety of foods available for elderly people decreases as they shop near home, buy in small quantities, and do not choose food from upper shelves.

Impaired hearing and vision. The loss of visual and auditory acuity has many implications in food selection. Someone who is unable to read labels or advertisements or identify foods that are not at eye level will have trouble selecting foods in a store or taking advantage of advertised specials. Inability to read label directions decreases interest in trying new products, and poor hearing may lead to an older person's not asking for information for fear of being embarrassed.

Physical discomfort. Older people report more discomfort associated with eating certain foods. Some foods may cause heartburn, others may cause gastric distention. Still others, many elderly believe, are incompletely digested. Efforts to avoid the offending foods may lead to the exclusion of nutritious foods from the diet.

Physiological Factors

Diminished sense of taste and smell. The decline in the number of taste buds at age 70 to 36% of those at age 30 may help to explain a decreased interest in food. With fewer and less sensitive taste buds, it is understandable that the pleasure of eating is diminished. The ability to recognize odors and flavors is affected, and the ability to discriminate among varying concentrations is reduced.

dysgeusia
Condition in which taste sensations are unpleasant

The ability to taste salt declines, whereas sensitivity to sweet tastes is not diminished. A severe zinc deficiency may be involved; it too is a cause of hypogeusia (decreased taste sensitivity) and hyposmia (a loss of the sense of smell). Many older people complain of an unpleasant taste in their mouths, **dysgeusia,** that reduces their enjoyment of food by making it difficult to identify mild taste sensations. This is possibly caused by the excretion of a fluid from around the teeth during chewing and is especially a problem with cancer patients. In addition, many drugs, such as anti-hypertensive and anti-hypoglycemic agents and diuretics, used in treating health problems in the elderly, also cause a decreased taste sensitivity, compounding the problem of acceptance of food.

Anorexia. The basis for loss of appetite, or anorexia, may be either physiological or psychological. On a physiological level, depressed appetite may reflect an absolute or relative thiamin or zinc deficiency. Psychologically, it may be a manifestation of loneliness, anxiety, or unhappiness. Sometimes the use of appetizers such as light soups, tasty nibbles, or light wine will stimulate eating. An improvement in the physical or social environment, as well as frequent and smaller meals, may also improve appetite. It is extremely important that elderly people keep up not only the quality but the quantity of their food intake to maintain their nutritional status.

Social Factors

Long-standing food habits. The food patterns and preferences of the elderly are largely the result of long-standing food habits. These in turn reflect not only individual ethnic, social, and economic backgrounds but also the availability of food at the time food habits were established. People of 70 or 80 years of age have eating patterns that were established 50 or 60 years ago, in an era when the food distribution system of the United States was much simpler than it is now; these people may fail to adjust to current complex marketing strategies that give them a confusing array of foods from which to choose. For example, they may still regard fruits and vegetables as seasonal items that can be bought only at certain times. In fact, in addition to relatively high cost, this may be one of the causes of the inadequacy of vitamins A and C noted in food surveys of the elderly.

Preferences for foods associated with pleasant experiences in early life are especially strong during periods of illness, stress, or loneliness. Because the psychological and social meanings of these foods assume much more importance under these circumstances, their use becomes an important element in adjustment or recovery. Many older people crave foods such as bread and milk, brown sugar on toast, or homemade ice cream, which they associate with happy memories. These foods convey a sense of security and well-being.

Elderly people often have long-held, firmly established beliefs about the merits and adverse effects of certain foods. Common beliefs are that fish cause worms, that some fruits and milk should not be eaten together, that cheese is constipating, or that milk is appropriate only for infants. These ideas can have profound effects on nutrient intake and must be taken into account in any nutrition education effort.

Because eating patterns are deeply ingrained and have many social and psychological implications, any dietary change should be approached with the utmost sensitivity to an individual's feelings. In some cases, major modifications may be either unwise or unnecessary. In others, gradual modifications within the framework of individual food preferences over a period of time and under nonstressful conditions may be appropriate to correct apparent dietary inadequacies. When medical or metabolic problems such as ulcers, diabetes, hypertension, or allergies are identified, dietary modifications must be initiated as an essential aspect of treatment. In these cases, help from an empathetic counselor is invaluable in making the transition.

Economic considerations. Economic pressures play an important role in determining dietary adequacy. Because many elderly people are living on fixed incomes that were set when salaries and living costs were much lower, it is not surprising that they have a very limited food budget. The necessity of living on a meager income to remain financially independent forces many older people to choose the least expensive foods that provide them with energy and satisfy their hunger. This frequently means substituting relatively inexpensive carbohydrate foods such as bread and cereal products, which are often low in vitamins, minerals, and protein, for more expensive foods such as meat, milk and fresh fruits and vegetables, which are normally dependable sources of these protective nutrients. The ease with which carbohydrate-rich foods are obtained and stored enhances their appeal.

The disappearance of corner grocery stores from the older residential and downtown areas and their replacement with large supermarkets in suburban shopping plazas has compounded the problem for older residents, who characteristically choose to live in the more familiar, central, and less expensive part of town. To take advantage of lower prices at the larger supermarkets, they must either pay for public transportation to and from the store or depend on friends with cars. Once in the store, it is easy to become overwhelmed and confused by the choices available. In the end, older people may shop rather ineffectively or may resume shopping at smaller delicatessens or service stores, where prices are higher but familiar personnel provide service and a sense of security.

Nutrition misinformation. A pervading fear that they may become ill and be unable to look after themselves or bear the cost of medical care haunts many older people. This makes them ready prey for the food faddist or promoter of natural food and food supplements, who promises them excellent health, eternal youth, and increased vitality and assures them that they will avoid the debilitating diseases so feared in old age. All too frequently they are persuaded by door-to-door salespeople to invest a significant part of their income in worthless and greatly overpriced products, which cannot give the protection they seek because there are still many conditions for which no cure in known. The new ruling that any such contract can be voided within 1 to 3 days affords a certain amount of protection to someone who may have entered into an unwise agreement under the pressure of a targeted sales approach. Of even greater concern than the waste of money is the possibility that older people may rely on the **nostrums** (panaceas) of salespeople and delay seeking medical help. Their condition may then deteriorate to a point at which legitimate therapy is much less likely to succeed and treatment will be even more expensive.

Among the Nutrient-Related Products of Unproven Effectiveness Promoted for the Elderly
SOD—Superoxide dismutase
Vitamin E
Lecithin
Tryptophan
Collagen cream

nostrum
A medicine of secret ingredients; especially a quack remedy

Psychological Factors

Living alone. Older people who preserve their independence by living alone may find that this in itself leads to modified eating patterns. One third of women aged 65 to 74 years and half of those over 75 live alone. For people of either sex who live alone, the lack of motivation to cook regular meals leads to the use of

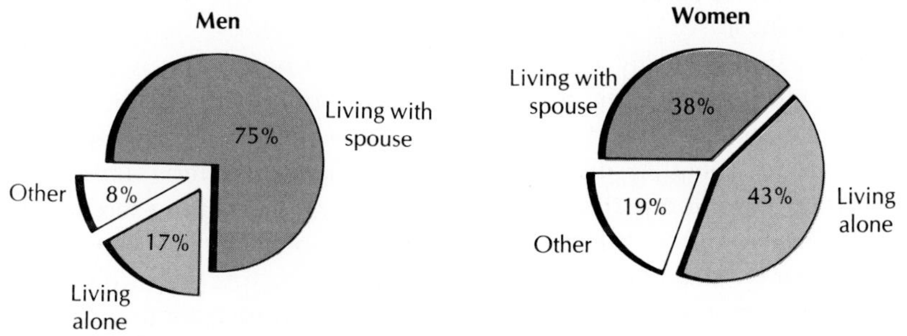

snack foods at irregular times, more often than not resulting in a poorly balanced meal. In addition, inexpensive living quarters may lack adequate cooking and refrigeration facilities. It is not unusual for an older person to have a very erratic eating pattern with days of nibbling, days of overeating, and days of very restricted intakes. Not surprisingly, it has been found that many older people eat more food with greater pleasure when they have company.

Depression. Depression, which affects other adjustments to aging, influences food intake as well. Sometimes, depression takes the form of overeating; food is seen as a pleasant and always available experience—a way of compensating for emotional poverty. Compulsive eating carries with it the problem of resulting obesity. On the other hand, depression can also lead to rejection of food. If family and friends who are concerned about the elderly person's well-being make special efforts to provide socialization, the depression may be alleviated.

Anxiety. Conditions of emotional stress or deprivation often lead to modifications both in attitudes toward food and in food habits, as well as changes in utilization of nutrients. People who are anxious or concerned frequently report a loss of appetite. In addition, the hormonal changes associated with anxiety lead to a depressed flow of digestive juices with resulting inefficiencies in the absorption of food. On the other hand, drugs used to alleviate anxiety may adversely affect appetite and utilization of nutrients.

The nutritional implications of anxiety are evident from studies showing that a diet consumed under the emotionally unhappy condition of living alone, when compared to the same diet consumed in a pleasant atmosphere with companionship results in a loss of nitrogen over a period as short as 30 days.

One of the objectives of community and federally supported congregate group feeding programs is to provide a pleasant social atmosphere at mealtime that promotes a good appetite and normal digestion.

FACTORS AFFECTING NUTRIENT USE

Decline in Physiological Functioning between 30 and 70 Years of Age

Work capacity	30%
Cardiac output	30%
Respiration	40%-50%
Basal metabolic rate	8%-10%
Hand grip	25%
Kidney function	30%-50%

Decline in physiological function. Many of the changes associated with aging occur in functions that are dependent on coordination among various organ systems, which decline at different rates. The decline in the rate at which nerve impulses are conducted is slight, but there are greater declines in the amount of blood the heart can pump and in the capacity of the lungs, which limit the amount of physical exercise an older person can tolerate. Optimal nutrition can modify some of these changes, which influence the distribution of nutrients and their utilization by various tissues.

Changes in digestive secretions. With the degeneration in the size of the salivary glands after age 60, saliva secretion decreases. The effect of this on carbohydrate digestion is minimal because other enzymes are capable of substituting for those in the saliva. However, the loss of saliva as a lubricant for food may have a very marked effect. It may lead to the use of softer and moister foods such as creamed dishes; mashed potatoes, rather than baked potatoes; and thinner, starch-thickened products, possibly as a way to compensate for the lack of natural lubricants in the saliva.

The secretion of many digestive enzymes declines, but the extent of each decrease and the age at which it occurs have not been fully established. Depending on the extent of the decrease, food may either be less completely digested or require a longer time for complete digestion. A decline in hydrochloric acid secretion is almost universal, with one third of all people over 60 failing to secrete any at all. This decline has adverse effects on the absorption of calcium, vitamin B_{12}, and iron and on the utilization of protein. Liver function remains high and there is little change in the gastric mucosa or little impairment of fat digestion.

Changes in gastric motility. The motility of the gastrointestinal tract is essential for mixing food with digestive enzymes and for the normal elimination of waste products. Decrease in gastric motility has a negative effect on digestion because the food mass may not become thoroughly mixed with digestive secretions. There are, however, benefits that may result from an increase in absorptive time. A major problem arises when decreased motility of the lower gastrointestinal tract causes constipation and in some cases leads to an increase in infections. The longer food remains in contact with the intestinal wall, the greater the possibility of adverse effects from toxicants or carcinogens. The role of thiamin in stimulating muscle tone suggests that it be used in cases where lack of motility is related to dietary deficiency. Maintaining an intake that provides 30 to 40 grams of dietary fiber will also help.

Changes in kidney function. As a person ages, the rate of blood flowing through the kidneys is decreased up to 50% of the normal adult capacity. This means that less blood reaches the kidney filtering system through which the waste products of metabolism are eliminated and the nutrients are returned to general circulation. In addition, older people have a reduced capacity to form either a more concentrated or more dilute urine. As a result, there is a decline in their ability to handle large amounts of waste products, particularly urea, sodium or water.

Kidney function influences the composition of the fluid surrounding individual cells, which is normally maintained within very narrow limits. The speed with which older people are able to cope with changes in blood and intracellular fluid composition after consuming excess acid-forming or base-forming substances may be as little as one fourth the speed of younger people. This is merely one example of changes in the rate at which the body can adjust to stress.

Alterations in the blood vessels. Alterations in the blood vessels, such as the narrowing of the lumen, thickening of the wall, and replacement of elastic muscle fibers with nonelastic material, reduce their capacity to effectively carry nutrients to body cells.

Malabsorption. Absorption of many nutrients is reduced when there is degeneration of the intestinal lining. This degeneration occurs in folacin deficiency, when new cells of the intestinal wall fail to regenerate as fast as old ones are destroyed. Chronic diseases also result in impaired absorption. Protein deficiency, which can result in a decrease in the synthesis of carrier proteins needed for absorption, reduces the uptake of nutrients such as iron and calcium.

Hormonal secretions. Changes in secretions of hormones that regulate a wide range of physiological processes have direct and indirect effects on the nutrition of the cells and therefore on the whole body. By controlling the diameter of blood vessels, the endocrine glands regulate the amount of blood and therefore the nutrients that reach the tissues. In aging people, there is a greater restriction in the size of the blood vessels leading to the kidneys than in the size of those leading to the brain, an example of ensuring a more adequate blood supply to the more vital centers. With age, body cells have fewer places to which hormones such as insulin can attach and exert their intended effect on a target cell. The adrenal gland, which normally responds to stimulation by the pituitary hormone during stress, does not respond as rapidly in older people.

Physical changes. Immobility has a negative effect on the retention of calcium in bones and the maintenance of lean body mass.

FACTORS AFFECTING NUTRIENT NEEDS

Physical Factors

Body composition. The changes in body composition that occur throughout adult life assume greater importance in later years. The decline of over 5% in lean body mass during each decade and its replacement with body fat account in part for the decline in basal metabolic rate and the decrease in body water from 70% to 50% in women and to 60% in men. Figure 18-1 depicts the change in body composition with age. An observed *slow* increase in body weight is not necessarily

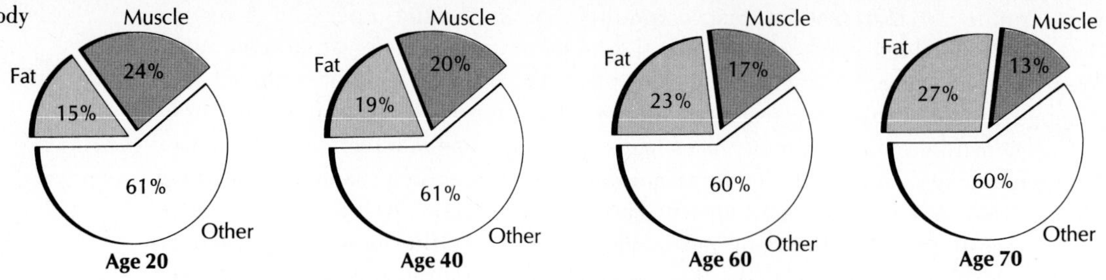

Figure 18-1 Changes in body composition with age.

bad; some studies have shown that longevity is greatest in adults with body weights slightly above ideal weight. There is more reason to be concerned about decline in body water and loss of sensitivity to thirst sensations. Dehydration has implications regarding the decreased dilution of water-soluble drugs and possible resulting toxicity.

Activity. The decline in activity associated with the decline in neuromuscular coordination and participation in sports results in a reduced need for calories and for the nutrients involved in energy metabolism.

Physiological Factors

Decrease in immune function. The loss of immunity or resistance to infection places the undernourished older person at greater risk of contracting infections or experiencing debilitating health problems. In addition, there is a decline in the response to hormones.

Decrease in metabolic efficiency. Nutrient uptake by cells may decrease by as much as 40%, leading to cellular malnutrition even when adequate nutrients are available. This helps to explain why older people do not respond as well as might be expected to nutrient supplementation.

MAJOR NUTRITION-RELATED PROBLEMS

Major Nutrition-Related Problems
- Obesity
- Osteoporosis
- Neurological dysfunction
- Anemia
- Drug-related malnutrition
- Food-induced malnutrition
- Immunity
- Impaired glucose tolerance
- Cardiovascular disease

Body mass index (a measure of the lean body mass in relation to total body size) = Body weight (kg)/height (m)^2.

Many assessments of the nutritional status of elderly people identify obesity, undernutrition, osteoporosis, diabetes, and cardiovascular disease as the most prevalent nutrition-related problems. On the basis of dietary intake studies, iron, folacin, and vitamin C appear to be the most frequent nutrient deficiencies. There is evidence of functional changes associated with lack of choline and niacin.

Obesity

Results of an assessment of 3600 people over 60 years of age in NHANES II showed that 50% of the women with a body mass index, or BMI (weight in kg/height in m^2) greater than 35 and 18% of the men with a BMI greater than 28 were obese. Among those over 80 years of age in the Ten-State Nutrition Survey, the incidence of obesity was lower. Obesity is two to three times as prevalent in women as in men. The majority of these obese elderly reported caloric intakes below recommended levels, suggesting that standards do not make adequate adjustments for a decrease in energy requirements associated with the sedentary life-style of many older citizens. The lower incidence of obesity among people over the age of 80 may reflect the high mortality rate among obese people when they are 60 to 80 years of age.

Associated with obesity is an increased incidence of diabetes. This increase reflects an impaired ability to utilize carbohydrate, possibly resulting from the decreased sensitivity of the cell to insulin. In contrast to younger adults, elderly adults who are moderately overweight have a somewhat lower mortality rate.

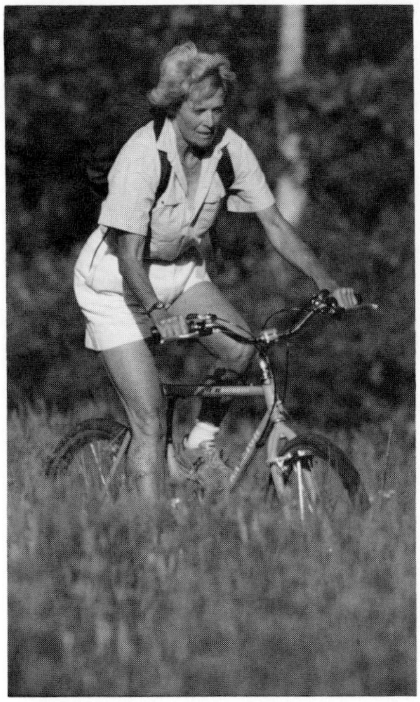

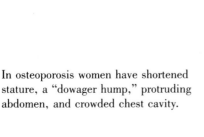

Establishing a pattern of regular exercise throughout adulthood is good preparation for continued activity in later years.

Osteoporosis

As discussed in Chapter 10, osteoporosis is characterized by a significant decrease in bone mass occurring when mineral loss proceeds at a faster rate than mineral deposition during bone remodeling. Osteoporosis is most common among postmenopausal women. Every year, approximately 200,000 people of late middle age or older break their hips, incurring hospitalization costs well in excess of $1 billion. This problem can be attributed largely to the lighter and more fragile bones of decreased mass, the result of the small but continuing loss of bone calcium that accelerates with the hormonal changes following menopause—especially loss of estrogen. Negative calcium balance, which amounts to a 25% loss of bone mass between ages 40 and 80, can be attributed to low calcium intakes, decreased intestinal absorption, decreased reabsorption in the kidneys, decreased production of the active metabolite of vitamin D normally formed in the kidneys, low protein or phosphorus intakes, high fiber intakes or low estrogen levels. Osteoporosis has many causes; however, an intake of 800 to 1200 mg of calcium throughout adulthood, kidneys that can convert vitamin D to its active form, a dietary source of fluoride to help stabilize bone mineral, and estrogen-replacement therapy for postmenopausal women all contribute to minimizing the likelihood of osteoporosis in later life. Someday, osteoporosis may indeed be a preventable consequence of aging. Currently, attempts to suppress of bone resorption appear more feasible than those to stimulate bone formation.

Vertebral fractures are also common in people with osteoporosis. The compact bone mass in the vertebrae is responsible for the height loss, low back pains, and humped backs characteristic of many elderly people. Dissolution of the jawbone is another frequent symptom of osteoporosis; it is a major contributing factor in periodontal disease, resulting in premature loss of teeth.

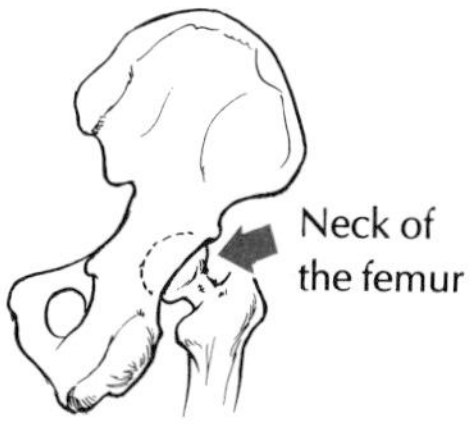

Weakness where the top of the femur is inserted in the hip joint is a cause of hip fracture in people with osteoporosis.

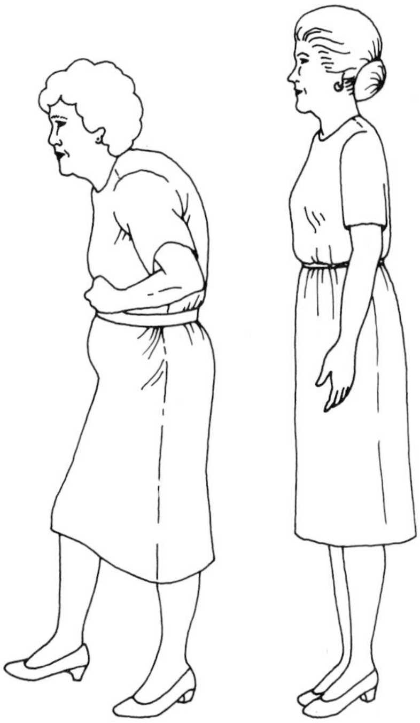

In osteoporosis women have shortened stature, a "dowager hump," protruding abdomen, and crowded chest cavity.

Neurological Dysfunction

Problems of disorientation and a slowing of neurological functioning, both seen in the elderly, have been attributed to various nutrient factors. A lack of niacin has long been associated with the dementia and depression of pellagra; a deficiency of choline hampers the synthesis of the neurotransmitter acetylcholine; deficiencies of vitamin B_6 and thiamin are associated with central nervous system problems; and folacin deficiency, the result of malabsorption, makes a significant difference in mental assessment scores.

Anemia

Anemia, characterized by feelings of fatigue, anxiety, lack of energy, and sleeplessness, is a common result of inadequate iron. Iron inadequacy can be caused by low dietary intake; impaired absorption, possibly resulting from lack of heme iron or vitamin C; or blood loss. Treatment may involve using iron supplements together with a diet providing iron sources of high bioavailability and vitamin C to enhance absorption. Megaloblastic anemia as a result of folate deficiency often occurs simultaneously with iron-deficiency anemia.

Drug-Related Malnutrition

In developed countries, people over 65 years of age understandably are often very heavy users of both over-the-counter and prescription drugs. Use of many of these influence the intake of nutrients through changes in taste, smell, or unpleasant side effects, particularly in the gastrointestinal tract, which influence appetite and food intake. They also affect absorption of nutrients by binding the nutrient in the intestinal tract or by causing changes in the intestinal mucosa that reduces its capacity to accept nutrients for absorption. Drugs may also have an effect through changes in gastrointestinal pH or motility or bacterial environment, by (1) binding or precipitating the nutrient so that it cannot be absorbed, or (2) influencing the secretion of digestive juices. Many of the commonly, and sometimes excessively, used antacids and laxatives have these effects. Metabolism of nutrients is influenced by drugs that affect the amount of an enzyme produced or inhibited in the cell. They may also increase the need for a nutrient at the cellular level or influence its excretion in the urine or bile. On the other hand, nutritional status can influence the way a drug is used. Poor nutrition or excessive intake through supplements is associated with adverse effects.

Table 18-5 lists drugs that cause an increased need for nutrients.

Fortunately not all drugs influence nutrient needs or utilization, but with the estimate of an average of 1.5 drugs prescribed per out-patient visit and 10 used in each hospitalization, the chance of some effect is great. Chances are compounded by the interactions among the drugs themselves or the nutritionally marginal diets and age-related malabsorption disorders more common with advancing age.

Because the rate of drug metabolism and detoxification in the liver is much slower in older people, drugs remain in the body longer to exert their influence on the metabolism of nutrients. Additionally, high dosages of some vitamins, such as folacin and vitamin B_6, interfere with the action of drugs such as anticonvulsants; therefore it is unwise to compensate for the adverse effects of drugs on nutrients by administering high doses of vitamins.

Food-Induced Malnutrition

The extensive use of certain foods has implications for nutritional adequacy. The use of large amounts of tea increases the need for thiamin. The high phytate content of oatmeal and the tannin in tea reduce the absorption of both iron and zinc. The

Table 18-5 ◇ Drugs that cause an increased need for various nutrients

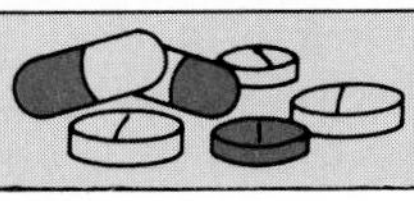

Drugs	Vitamins											Minerals		
	A	D	E	K	C	B_1	B_2	B_6	B_{12}	Niacin	Folacin	Calcium	Iron	Zinc
Alcohol						X			X		X			
Anticoagulants				X							X			
Anticonvulsants		X									X	X		
Antituberculosis drugs		X						X		X				
Antitumoral agents											X	X		
Aspirin											X			
Barbiturates					X									
Cholesterol-lowering drugs	X	X	X	X					X		X			
Laxatives	X	X	X	X								X	X	X
Mineral oil	X	X	X	X										
Neomycin	X								X					
Nicotine					X									
Penicillamine								X						
Sedatives		X												
Tetracycline					X							X		
Tranquilizers		X					X							

use of foods high in added phosphorus creates an undesirably low calcium/phosphorus ratio that leads to poor bone calcification, especially when calcium intake is low. Extensive use of alcohol not only leads to diets of reduced nutrient content and multiple deficiencies but also has adverse effects on nutrient absorption.

Immunity

While three quarters of individuals over 65 years of age have a decreased capacity to deal with illnesses such as infection, cancer, and degenerative diseases, the remainder are as responsive as young adults. This general, but not inevitable, decline in immune function is the result of a decline in the ability of the thymus gland to produce special disease-fighting cells, the failure of the red bone marrow to regenerate, a reduction of immune factors in the blood, and a delayed rate of antibody production. All of these factors respond positively to enhanced nutrition, especially among those who were seriously malnourished. Zinc, vitamin A, vitamin C, and folate are the nutrients most often identified with immune function. Although there are few cases of severe deficiencies of these nutrients, prolonged marginal intakes may be a factor in age-related depression of immune function.

Impaired Glucose Tolerance

Starting with ages in the mid to late thirties a gradual increase in blood glucose levels is characteristic in a glucose tolerance test. Between ages 60 and 70 the incidence of this increase becomes great enough to classify almost 20% of the population as non-insulin-dependent diabetics and another 13% as having impaired glucose tolerance. Both of these disorders must be treated by dietary control of the type, amount, and distribution of carbohydrate intake.

Cardiovascular Disease

Contrary to general opinion hypertension, hypercholesterolemia, glucose intolerance, and obesity continue to be factors that increase the risk of cardiovascular disease with advancing age. Also these are not inevitable consequences of aging and are influenced, modified, or delayed by appropriate diet. This usually involves adjusting caloric intake to maintain or achieve normal body weight, adjusting dietary fat, and, for hypertension-prone individuals, restricting use of discretionary or added salt.

NUTRIENT NEEDS

The information available on the nutrient needs of people over 40 years old is scarce and is based primarily on studies of the intake of healthy people rather than on experimental balance studies designed to determine needs. Some allowances are extrapolated from data on younger people; others are based on estimates of necessary losses from the body. So far we have little or no evidence that, except for calories and the nutrients involved in energy metabolism, the elderly have nutritional requirements differing significantly from those of young adults. Therefore it is suggested that the intakes proposed for most nutrients during early adulthood be maintained throughout life. Although it is reasonable to assume that there will be changes in needs of some nutrients with aging, there are few nutrients for which we can confidently propose either an increased or decreased intake. This is the result, in part, of counterbalancing influences. The decrease in lean body mass and activity should lead to a decrease in needs, but on the other hand, the decreased ability to absorb nutrients or prevent their loss suggests increased intake.

Nutrient intakes as currently proposed by the 1980 RDA committee for men and women over age 50 are presented in Table 18-6 along with the recommendations, as yet unpublished, that the 1985 RDA committee was prepared to propose. These recognized that individuals between 50 and 70 are sufficiently different than those over 70 that they should not be grouped together. However, there is very little data on which to base recommendations. From these data, it is evident that people who plan to achieve the recommended level of nutrient intake with a reduced number of calories will need to select foods of high nutrient density if they are to meet their needs through diet alone. They will have reduced opportunities to indulge in foods of low nutrient density, such as alcoholic beverages, and high-calorie foods, in which the energy is primarily from added sugar and fat.

Energy

The Food and Nutrition Board has recognized the decrease in energy needs that occurs with aging. Contributing to this decrease are the trend from active sports to spectator sports; the decline in activity with retirement; the increase in labor-saving devices; and the decline of about 3% per decade in basal metabolic needs, as the number of cells in the body decreases with the loss of tissue mass. It is suggested that energy allowances for people 50 to 69 years of age be kept at 1.6 × basal, the same as for younger mature adults, and that those for people over 70 be reduced to 1.5 × basal. With advancing age, the differences in energy expenditure among individuals become more pronounced.

FAO/WHO recommends a decrease of 5% in energy per decade from ages 39 to 59, 10% from ages 60 to 69, and an additional 10% after age 70. Regardless of recommended levels, the intake that results either in weight maintenance or a desired weight adustment is the proper energy intake.

Studies on nutritive intakes of older people have shown many low intakes, with some even less than 1400 kcal. These appear to result from efforts to reduce weight, loss of appetite, inability to buy or eat more food, failure to eat regularly, or inability to chew food or, alternatively, failure to remember or to report total food intake. In addition to not meeting needs for energy, such diets invariably are inadequate in other nutrients such as calcium, iron, and several vitamins. Even though the suggested amount of protein may be provided in these low-calorie diets, much that should go into the synthesis of body proteins is diverted to be used as a source of energy, leading to a negative nitrogen balance. Experimentally, diets of less than 1800 kcal have resulted in negative nitrogen balance.

Failure to consume adequate calories and adequate levels of other nutrients along with them may account for the fatigue, lassitude, and lack of interest in life so often experienced by elderly people. The lassitude and fatigue may depress activity to the extent that the need for calories is reduced, leading to weight gain even on a low energy intake. It is conceivable that the use of nutritionally suboptimal low-calorie meals may be responsible for the premature signs of aging.

In one study of 100 women aged 40 to 70, those whose health was rated as good consumed from 1650 to 1825 kcal daily, whereas those who health was rated

Table 18-6 ◆ Recommended dietary allowances—1980 and proposed 1985—for people over 51 years of age

	Male			Female		
	1980	1985 (proposed)		1980	1985 (proposed)	
	51+	51-69	70+	51+	51-69	70+
Protein (gram)	56	64	62	44	54	53
Calcium (mg)	800	800	800	800	1000	1000
Phosphorus (mg)	800	800	800	800	1000	1000
Magnesium (mg)	350	350	350	350		
Iron (mg)	10	10	10	10	10	10
Zinc (mg)	15	15	15	15	12	12
Iodine (μg)	150	160	160	150	160	160
Selenium (μg)	—	70	70		55	55
Vitamin A (RE)	1000	700*	700	800	600	600
Vitamin D (μg)	5	5	5	5	5	5
Vitamin E (mg)	10	10	10	8	8	8
Ascorbic Acid (mg)	60	40	40	60	30	30
Thiamin (mg)	1.2	1.3	1.1	1.0	1.1	0.9
Riboflavin (mg)	1.4	1.4	1.3	1.2	1.2	1.2
Niacin (mg)	16	16	14	13	13	13
Pyridoxine (mg)	2.2	2.0	2.0	2.0	1.7	1.7
Folacin (μg)	400	230	220	400	190	190
Vitamin B_{12} (μg)	3.0	2.0	2.0	3.0	2.0	2.0

	Provisional Recommended Dietary Intakes of Selected Minerals—1985	Estimated Safe and Adequate Daily Dietary Intake—1980
Sodium (mg)	1300	1100-3300
Potassium (mg)	2000-6000	1875-5625
Chloride (mg)	2000	1700-5100

Caloric needs vary according to physical activity and body size.
*Underlined values are lower than current 1980 RDAs

as poor consumed 1125 to 1475 kcal daily. This reinforces the recommendation that adults maintain an activity program that will allow a higher energy intake. This study also confirmed that the number of symptoms and the likelihood of other nutrient deficiencies increased when the energy value of the diet was lower. It is difficult to separate cause and effect in such a situation, however.

Protein

The total amount of protein synthesized daily declines only slightly with age, even though muscle protein turnover drops from 30% to 20% of total protein turnover and the daily synthesis of serum albumin falls. The RDAs suggests that a daily protein intake of 0.8 gram/kg of body weight be maintained throughout adulthood, although one study showed that more protein was needed to maintain nitrogen balance. In older people, protein needs will amount to 12% of energy intake. An intake greatly in excess of recommended levels is undesirable because of the added burden of excreting the urea from the deamination of protein by the less efficient kidneys.

Minerals

Calcium. There is still considerable uncertainty about whether older people, especially women, have an increased need for dietary calcium. On the one hand, their ability to absorb calcium declines, and they have increased loss of bone mass and urinary calcium excretion. On the other hand, there is evidence that without an intake of adequate vitamin D and the use of estrogens in postmenopausal women enhanced calcium intake is of limited value. It is probably more important to increase individual calcium intake to current standards than to raise the standards.

Zinc. The marginal zinc stores reported for elderly patients are attributed to intakes that generally are below the RDA, the prevalence of medical conditions, or the use of drugs that either reduce zinc absorption or increase zinc loss. Supplements to correct the problem should be used cautiously because excessive intakes may lead to gastrointestinal irritation, copper deficiency, anemia, hypercholesterolemia, and reduced immune function.

For other minerals where any deficiencies are the result of inadequate intake, impaired absorption, drug/nutrient interactions, or the effects of chronic disease, there is no indication that the recommended dietary allowance (RDA) should be increased. Each individual case should be evaluated to determine if dietary modifications or nutrient supplementation is indicated.

Vitamins

Folacin. Folacin status, which is assessed by measuring the folate level in red blood cells (as a reflection of body stores) or serum folate (as an indication of recent dietary intake), was found to be impaired in 20% of elderly people on admission to a hospital. Data on dietary intake suggest that folacin intake tends to meet recommended levels, about half of the elderly take supplements containing folic acid, and there is no evidence of a decline in the enzymes that free folacin for absorption from food. Thus it appears that the decline in gastric acidity that occurs with aging or with the use of antacids may be a factor in the poor folate status of older people, especially institutionalized patients.

Other Nutrients

For other nutrients, we have relatively little specific information about requirements. Any factor that reduces absorption calls for an increased nutrient intake. Certain drugs used in treating chronic ailments and the decline in hydrochloric acid secretion both have this effect. In general, any decline in efficiency of absorption for most nutrients counterbalances a decline in need so that the recommended intake remains essentially unchanged. In the case of fat-soluble vitamins, any factor that decreases the absorption of fat will influence the amount of fat-soluble vitamins absorbed and ultimately call for a higher intake. Even when we conduct experiments to determine needs, we find that there is such great variability among older people that it is hard to generalize from the findings.

The need for water to aid in absorption, metabolism, and the excretion of nutrients and metabolites should be one of the prime dietary considerations in nutrition for the elderly. The intake of fluid should be carefully monitored to prevent either dehydration or the retention of too much fluid. Normally an intake of 1 ml of water per kilocalorie of intake should be adequate, but for a variety of physiological and environmental reasons older people often lose their ability to adjust intake to need. Dehydration is associated with excessive losses that occur with high environmental temperature, high fever, vomiting, diarrhea, or the inability of a failing kidney to conserve water. Readily observed signs of dehydration are dryness of the lips and skin, decreased urine output, confusion, and elevated body temperature. Retention of too much fluid is usually due to physiological causes resulting in diminished ability to excrete fluid. On the other hand, since thirst becomes a less sensitive indicator of need for fluid, older people should be encouraged to continue to drink sufficient fluids to prevent dehydration.

ADEQUACY OF DIETS

The assessment of the dietary adequacy of aging people is complicated by the difficulty of obtaining subjects. In one study, only 13% of those contacted agreed to participate, which raises questions about how representative they were of the original group. In spite of these difficulties, several studies have been successfully completed to give some picture of prevailing dietary patterns.

The three major studies assessing the nutrient adequacy of the population over 60 years of age are NHANES I (1971-1974), NHANES II (1976-1980), and the Nationwide Food Consumption Survey (1977-1978). The most meaningful findings of these surveys, which are comparable to findings from smaller population surveys, are summarized in Table 18-7. From these data, it is evident that calcium, magnesium, and vitamin B_6 are the most limiting nutrients, with intakes of vitamins A

Table 18-7 ◇ Dietary intake of respondents 65 years of age and older in NHANES I (1971-74), NHANES II (1976-80), and Nationwide Food Consumption Survey (1977-78)*

	NHANES I		NHANES II		NFCS	
Nutrient	Men	Women	Men	Women	Men	Women
Protein (grams)	72	53	73	51	84	60
Calcium (mg)	602	495	597	475	729	566
Magnesium (mg)					287	227
Phosphorus (mg)			1197	880	1246	930
Iron (mg)	12.1	9.2	12.3	9.1	14.5	10.6
Thiamin (mg)	1.24	0.96	1.33	0.99	1.37	1.07
Riboflavin (mg)	1.77	1.30	1.84	1.36	1.78	1.41
Vitamin C (mg)	88	90	100	105	91	87
Vitamin B_6 (mg)					1.58	1.24
Vitamin B_{12} (μg)					5.9	4.4
Vitamin A (IU)			3929	3346	7164	6458

*Underlined values fall below recommended levels.

and C suboptimal for many people. However, adequacy of zinc and folate intakes, believed to be problem nutrients, were not assessed. A comparison of data on persons over 65 years old with younger people surveyed revealed only a slight decline in adequacy with age. NFCS and NHANES III will be held in 1989.

Findings from other studies showed a higher mortality was reported among those getting less than 40% of the recommended allowances of one or more nutrients. A large number of the subjects complained of tiredness, pains in joints, shortness of breath, constipation, and other signs of general malaise.

Of 400 Missourians over 59 years of age, 22% of the men and 59% of the women were obese, 7% had low vitamin A blood values, and 10% had deficient serum iron levels.

A Canadian study of 194 independent senior adults between the ages of 65 and 77 showed that 81% used over 50 of the 181 food items on a food frequency list. Those with more education and better health used a greater variety of foods. The most frequently used food sources in the major food groups were whole-wheat bread, breakfast cereals, eggs, cheese, chicken, potatoes, carrots, orange juice, and bananas. Fluid milk, either whole or nonfat, was used more than four times a week or not at all. Respondents tended to avoid nonfat milk, liver, nuts, and sweetened beverages, reflecting long-standing food habits, dislike of taste, digestive concerns, and health concerns, respectively. Food selection was based more on taste and perceived health benefits than on price, convenience, or status.

Several studies show a slight downward trend in intakes of all nutrients with increasing age and a sharp downward trend after age 75. Investigators also report a decrease in calories was associated with a general decrease in the amount of food consumed rather than decreases in a particular food or food group.

NUTRITIONAL STATUS

Attempts to evaluate the nutritional status of the elderly through assessment of nutrient and metabolite levels in the blood and urine have been confined almost exclusively to the Ten-State Nutrition Survey, NHANES I, and NHANES II. In the Ten-State Nutrition Survey, it was established that low biochemical levels in two or more blood and urine measures occurred in less than 8% of white people over the age of 60 but in 25% of black and Hispanic people. Over 60% of blacks and 50% of Hispanics had satisfactory levels in all measures. The NHANES studies found that 29% of blacks over the age of 60 had low hemoglobin levels, confirming the fact that this group is nutritionally vulnerable.

A similar survey in Canada revealed that low serum folate levels were the most prevalent nutritional problem in aging people. These low levels were found in 60% of the men and 61% of the women surveyed over the age of 65. Urinary thiamin values were low in about 30% of the men and 12% of the women studied.

Other, less comprehensive studies have revealed that 70% of a group of elderly people had delayed prothrombin times, indicative of vitamin K deficiency and associated with liver disease or the use of salicylates (aspirin) or antibiotics.

DIETARY SUPPLEMENTS

Older people are concerned about their health. They are usually highly motivated to take steps that they believe will help maintain a level of health sufficient for them to retain their independence. As a result, the use of dietary supplements—especially multivitamins and minerals—is widespread. One study showed that 37% of the surveyed people 55 years of age or older were using supplements. In Canada, 34% of older men and 46% of older women used supplements, and in California, 35% of the elderly did. Few of the supplements were advised by a physician, and few contained nutrients related to actual need. Some people did use supplements that provided all the nutrients lacking in their diets. Others used products that provided some but not all of the nutrients they needed or that supplemented their diets with nutrients they were already getting in adequate amounts in their regular diet. About half the respondents had nutritionally adequate diets and did not need a supplement. Few people with suboptimal intakes of calcium took supplements that included calcium. The amount of money spent on supplements may represent a large proportion of the money that older people have available for food. Therefore more guidance ought to be made available to elderly people, so that they can either choose correct supplements (if they need them) or save the money (if their diets are already adequate). Unfortunately, effective marketing strategies presently encourage unsupervised, self-prescribed supplementation among all age-groups.

A study of 500 elderly vitamin supplement users (those over 65 years of age) showed that they all had significantly lower mortality rates than did the total population of the United States. Because they also espoused life-styles that differed from the total population in other health-related ways—less smoking, limited use of alcohol, diet consciousness, and concern about the use of salt, sugar, saturated fat, and animal foods—any health benefits noted cannot be attributed solely to the use of nutrient supplements.

INTERVENTION PROGRAMS

Watkins has pointed out that, in planning programs to improve the nutritional status of the elderly, it is important to consider (1) that each person has a unique nutritional history that has been influenced by physical, emotional, and attitudinal factors; (2) that because much malnutrition is the result of disease or disability, diagnosis and treatment of the underlying cause of the disease must be made concurrent with efforts to improve the diet; and (3) that education in health, nutrition, and consumer issues can be effective in promoting improved nutritional status.

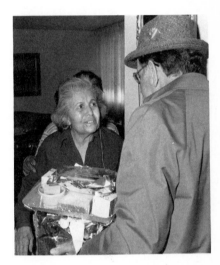

The Meals on Wheels Program provides home-delivered meals on a regular basis.

Concern about the inadequacy of food intake among the elderly, whether for social, economic, or emotional reasons, has led responsible community and government groups to develop intervention programs. Among these are the Meals-on-Wheels program and the Congregate Meals Program. In Meals-on-Wheels, a hot meal is delivered to the recipient's home 3 to 7 days a week, depending on the funding and personnel of the program. In some cases, a meal is delivered during the day along with food to be refrigerated for the evening meal and possibly also for the next day's breakfast. This program is designed for the elderly people who have inadequate cooking facilities or are unable to shop for and prepare food. The Congregate Meals Program, on the other hand, is designed to meet the social, as well as nutritional, needs of the elderly. Participants are provided with transportation to a centrally located "diners' club" where, in addition to receiving an appetizing and nutritionally adequate meal in the company of others, they are able to participate in a variety of recreational, social, and educational experiences. Both programs are designed to meet the needs of older people regardless of income. Those who can pay the full cost of the meals do so; others receive their meals at reduced or no cost and are given the opportunity to use food stamps as payment. These are the two programs receiving the most financial backing. However, other programs are also being investigated; they will try to attack the problems of hunger and social isolation that affect elderly people with stable incomes in a spiraling economy.

Nutrition Education

The Congregate Meal Program requires that participants be offered nutrition education as part of the program. A variety of approaches have been evaluated, but one of the most successful of them has involved the use of peer educators. In this approach, selected program participants are given training to qualify them to provide information. They then work with small groups of their peers in informal educational settings. The merits of this approach are that leaders are already accepted by their peer group, it is an honor for them to be selected (therefore motivation is high), and they are able to devote a significant amount of time to the effort. Most importantly, however, these peer educators are proving to be effective leaders.

Much relevant nutrition education is concerned with food purchasing and nutritive quality. Other topics of broad interest are the relationship of nutrition to health, selection and preparation of food for small families, food additives, the importance of reading labels, and inflation-related topics.

• • •

In summary, there is growing evidence that the length and quality of life are influenced by diet throughout a person's lifetime. We do not, however, have a good way to assess nutritional status in the elderly, nor do we have data on which to base estimates of nutritional requirements. Although there is little reason to think that (except for calories) older people need either more or less nutrients than they did in middle life, we do know that deficiencies exist in many older people. However, these deficiencies are more likely to be associated with socioeconomic and behavioral factors (such as low income, reduced mobility, or social isolation) or with physiological factors (such as a reduced sense of taste and smell, impaired dentition, or poor absorption) than with increased nutrient requirements alone. Nutrition is a major concern of the gerontologist, and gerontology is a growing interest of the nutritionist. Both disciplines are concerned with understanding the aging process and the ways in which it may be altered to enhance the quality of life. Some of these ways include the use of a nutritionally adequate diet throughout life and the avoidance of practices that are risk factors for diseases and health problems in later life. Because the pattern of intake of most older people differs little from what they developed at a much earlier age, dietary preparation for old age should begin in the pediatrician's office.

BY NOW YOU SHOULD KNOW

- There has been an increase in the proportion of people living beyond the age of 65 in the United States since 1900.
- Elderly people are such a heterogeneous group that it is difficult to generalize about their nutritional needs.
- Aging occurs at different rates in different people even under similar environmental conditions.
- There are at least seven theories about the biochemical and physiological bases of aging.
- Nutrient intake, nutrient utilization, and nutrient needs are determined by physical, physiological, social, and psychological factors.
- For almost all nutrients except calories, the decline in requirements because of lower activity and slower metabolism is counteracted by increased dietary need to compensate for the decline in the efficiency of absorption and metabolism. Therefore, nutrient needs change little throughout adulthood.
- The elderly are candidates for several nutrition-related problems such as obesity, osteoporosis, neurological dysfunction, anemia, drug-related malnutrition, food-induced malnutrition, loss of immunity, impaired glucose tolerance, and cardiovascular disease.
- Although the 1980 RDAs only have a category "age 51+" for older people, the 1985 RDA committee proposed RDAs for individuals 51 to 69 years of age and for individuals 70 years of age and older.
- The use of vitamin/mineral supplements is widespread among the elderly population.

- Federally funded programs such as Meals-on-Wheels and the Congregate Meals Program are designed to help the elderly maintain their independence and at the same time provide good nutrition and social stimulation.
- The Congregate Meal Program requires all participants be offered nutrition education. Peer education has proved extremely successful with this population.

STUDY QUESTIONS

1. Define the terms geriatrics and gerontology.
2. Why are recommended dietary intakes very similar for people under and over 50 years of age?
3. Why are we more concerned about the effects of drugs on nutrient needs in the elderly than in younger populations?
4. Describe the major nutrition-related problems of the elderly.
5. Explain why water remains to be an important nutrient for persons over 65 years of age.
6. Summarize the importance of oral hygiene throughout the entire life cycle.

Applying What You've Learned

1. **Interview at Least Two Senior Citizens**

   Ask questions concerning their food beliefs, food shopping, food preparation, changes in taste and smell, and the use of vitamin/mineral supplements. Also ask questions concerning the changes in food supply and methods of food preparation. Do these answers support the generalizations presented in this chapter?

2. **Analyze a 24-Hour Food Recall of a Senior Citizen in Your Family (i.e., a Grandparent or Great Aunt or Uncle)**

   Aside from tallying the total nutrient intake, analyze the food selection based on texture, method of preparation, portion sizes, and the source of dietary fiber and fluid in the diet.

3. **Research Early Studies of Nutrition of the Elderly**

   Go to the library and browse through some of the very early issues of the *Journal of the American Dietetic Association*. What were some of the studies being conducted on aging at that time?

4. **Volunteer Work**

   Volunteer to deliver or work in the kitchen for Meals-on-Wheels in your community.

5. **Plan a Diet**

   Plan a diet that is nutritionally adequate for a 75-year-old woman who requires only 1450 kcal.

6. **Evaluate Nutritional Products for the Elderly**

   Go to a health food store and look at the products marketed toward the aging population and promoted to enhance longevity and delay the process of degenerative diseases. Make some generalizations about the value, if any, of these products.

7. **Feeding Programs**

   Inquire about the feeding programs for the elderly in your community. Do they seem to be sufficient to meet the needs of those participating?

SUGGESTED READINGS

Munro HN: Nutrition and aging, British Medical Bulletin 37:83, 1981.

A scholarly review of the role of nutrition in aging, written by the Director of the USDA Center on Aging at Tufts University. This paper covers aging and body composition, tissue function, metabolism, and nutritional needs. The author emphasizes the importance of lifetime dietary habits in determining the nutritional health of the elderly.

Nutrition and Aging: Twelfth Maribou Symposium, Nutrition Reviews 46:38, 1988.

This whole issue of Nutrition Reviews is devoted to a report of papers presented by eminent scientists at the Maribou symposium on aging held in Sweden, late in 1987. Edited by Dr. Robert Olson, it covers the aging process, particularly as it affects and as it can be influenced by nutritional factors; the role of diet and exercise in the aging process; the relationship of dietary risk factors in the diseases of aging—hypertension, cardiovascular disease, osteoporosis, immune function, and obesity. It is one of the most complete and balanced discussions of the topic available. It dispels many of the myths and generalizations about practices and dietary needs of the aging population.

Roe DA: Therapeutic effects of drug-nutrient interactions in the elderly, Journal of the American Dietetic Association 85:174, 1985.

This article deals with the complexities of the interrelationships between drugs and nutrients, which are of increasing concern as the elderly are given multiple drugs to control or prevent various conditions of aging. Drugs can influence nutrient utilization through their effects on absorption, excretion, or metabolism. The nature and timing of meals can affect the utilization of drugs, creating a two-way interaction between food/nutrients and drugs. The overuse of vitamins and minerals is included in this discussion because of their pharmacological effects.

Schneider EL, Vining EM, Hadley EC, and Farnhamd SA: Recommended dietary allowances and the health of the elderly, New England Journal of Medicine 314:157, 1986.

This paper provides an excellent overview of the factors that must be considered in establishing recommended dietary allowances for the elderly, the sources of data available, and the limitations in interpreting it for the total elderly population, which is physiologically a very heterogeneous group.

ADDITIONAL READINGS

Avioli LV: Postmenopausal osteoporosis: prevention versus cure, Federation Proceedings 40: 2418, 1981.

Baylink KJ, and Ivey JI: Sodium fluoride for osteoporosis—some unanswered questions, Journal of the American Dietetic Association 243:463, 1980.

Bidlack WR, Kirsch A, and Meskin MS: Nutritional requirements of the elderly, Food Technology 40:2, 1986.

Chauhan J, and others: Age-related olfactory and taste changes and interrelationships between taste and nutrition, Journal of the American Dietetic Association 87:1543, 1987.

Chernoff R: Aging and nutrition, Nutrition Today 22(2):4, 1987.

Dawson-Hughes B, Jacques P, and Shepp C: Dietary calcium intake and bone loss from the spine in healthy postmenopausal women, American Journal of Clinical Nutrition 46:685, 1987.

Garry PJ, Goodwin JS, Hunt WC, and others: Nutritional status in a healthy elderly population: dietary and supplemental intakes, American Journal of Clinical Nutrition 36: 319, 1982.

Geissler GA, and Bates JF: The nutritional effects of tooth loss, American Journal of Clinical Nutrition 39:478, 1984.

Gersovitz M, and others: Human protein requirements: assessment of the adequacy of the current Recommended Dietary Allowances for dietary protein in elderly men and women, American Journal of Clinical Nutrition 35:6, 1982.

Guthrie, HA: Nutrient requirements of the elderly. In Chernoff R, and Lipschitz DL, editors: Nutrition and aging, New York, 1988, Raven Press.

Harper AE: Nutrition, aging and longevity, American Journal of Clinical Nutrition 36: 737, 1982.

Kannel WD: Nutrition and the occurrence and prevention of cardiovascular disease in the elderly, Nutrition Reviews 45:68, 1988.

Kohrs MB: Symposium on nutrition and aging, American Journal of Clinical Nutrition 36: 735, 1982.

Leaf A: The aging process: lessons from observations in man, Nutrition Reviews 45:40, 1988.

Lindeman RD: Mineral metabolism in the aging and aged, Journal of the American College of Nutrition 1:49, 1982.

Lynch SR, Finch CA, Monsen ER, and others: Iron status of elderly Americans, American Journal of Clinical Nutrition 36:1032, 1982.

Masaro EJ: Nutrition and aging—a current assessment, Journal of Nutrition 115:842, 1985.

Morrison SD: Nutrition and longevity, Nutrition Reviews 41:133, 1983.

Munro HN, and others: Protein nutrition of a group of free living elderly, American Journal of Clinical Nutrition 46:586, 1987.

Reggs BL, and Melton LJ: Involutional osteoporosis, New England Journal of Medicine 314:1676, 1986.

Rivlin RS, and Young EA, editors: Evidence relating selected vitamins and minerals to health and disease in the elderly population, American Journal of Clinical Nutrition 36: 977, 1982.

Shock NW: The role of nutrition in aging, Journal of the American College of Nutrition 1:3, 1982.

Sutter PM, and Russell RM: Vitamin requirements of the elderly, American Journal of Clinical Nutrition 45:50, 1987.

Walford RR, Harris SB, and Weindruck R: Dietary restriction and aging: historical phases, mechanisms, and current directions, Journal of Nutrition 117:1650, 1987.

Watkins DM: Physiology of aging, American Journal of Clinical Nutrition 36:750, 1982.

FOCUS Coronary Heart Disease—An Ever-Present Threat for the Aging

Although the mortality rate from coronary heart disaease (CHD), in which decreased blood flow causes heart attacks, has been declining steadily, it still poses the major health threat to most people past middle age. Both strokes and heart attacks reflect the effects of a general condition known as arteriosclerosis, in which the diameter of the blood vessels becomes increasingly narrow until the flow of blood is cut off. In the case of strokes, it is the flow of blood to the brain that is impeded; in the case of heart attacks, it is the muscles of the heart that are deprived. Since 1948, CHD has claimed an average of 800,000 lives every year in the United States.

After many years of research it is fairly well established that the development of arteriosclerotic plaque begins in early childhood. At that time, fatty streaks begin to form in the wall of the blood vessels. As a person ages, cholesterol from the blood and from other material tends to accumulate in the fatty streaks. Most of this cholesterol seems to come from low-density lipoproteins (LDL), which carry lipids with a higher percentage of cholesterol. As more and more cholesterol is deposited, increasingly thick plaques develop on the inside of the arterial walls. Eventually the walls become so thick that it is almost impossible for the blood to flow through the narrowed lumen, or passageway. Finally, blood trying to flow through this narrow passage clots and completely cuts off the flow. Of course this also cuts off the critical supply of oxygen to either the brain or the heart muscle, which are thus unable to function. Whether or not a stroke or heart attack is fatal depends on how much time the tissue is deprived of oxygen.

The possibility that diet is a determining factor in the development of arteriosclerosis has attracted a great deal of attention. Because plaque represents the deposition of cholesterol in the arterial wall, it seemed reasonable for researchers to look for a relationship between blood cholesterol levels and CHD. Epidemiological evidence showed clearly that elevated blood cholesterol levels along with hypertension, obesity, and stress were risk factors. The next logical question was whether or not serum cholesterol levels could be lowered through the use of drugs or by dietary manipulation.

It made sense to think that lowering the intake of dietary cholesterol might make it possible to lower blood cholesterol. We soon learned that humans have the capacity to synthesize even more cholesterol than they take in from the diet and that they synthesize more when the proportion of calories from fat rises above 35%. By substituting carbohydrate (particularly complex carbohydrate) for some of the fat calories, researchers were able to lower blood cholesterol levels. They also learned that, in addition to the total amount of fat in the diet, the *kind* of fat was important. For example, when polyunsaturated fat constituted up to one third of dietary fat, primarily from vegetable oils, less cholesterol was synthesized. From a practical standpoint, this meant using more vegetable oils and margarine and less animal fat and butter and reducing the total amount of fat.

We also know that by exercising more we can increase the proportion of cholesterol that is carried in the blood as high-density lipoproteins; this seems to protect against arteriosclerosis. Reducing calories, of course, helps us stay in energy balance and reduces the chance of gaining weight—another risk factor in CHD.

Since 1957, the American Heart Association has been issuing recommendations to the American public about guidelines for a prudent diet—one that association members feel will help keep body weight, blood pressure, and blood cholesterol levels within ranges that will minimize the possibility of CHD. Initially, they recognized only that diet could play an important role in the susceptibility to heart disease and proposed that total calories and type of fat were probably the most important considerations.

The Association's most recent recommendations are based on evidence that elevated blood cholesterol (especially if carried in low-density lipoproteins), blood pressure, smoking, diabetes, and obesity are the major risk factors in CHD. They recommend that the total fat in the diet be reduced from the current 43% to 30% to 35% of total energy intake and that saturated fats provide no more than 10% of total calories. To replace these calories, they suggest using unsaturated fats or complex carbohydrates such as cereal grains and potatoes and other vegetables. Because there is some uncertainty about how much of dietary fat should be polyunsaturated, they suggest that it not represent above 10% of the intake of calories. Although there is now evidence that monounsaturated fatty acids function in much the same beneficial way as polyunsaturated fatty acids, because many of them come from animal fats increasing them this way also increases total fat and saturated fatty acid intake. Olive oil and chocolate also contain monounsaturated fatty acids. In general, it is recommended that more complex carbohydrates from plants be used because they usually also provide more fiber than refined carbohydrates do.

A recent study of several hundred subjects with elevated blood cholesterol levels showed that those who were able to lower their blood cholesterol were less likely to suffer from CHD. However, once someone's cholesterol level was elevated, it was almost impossible to lower it by dietary intervention alone. Those who succeeded relied on the use of the drug cholestyramine, which is quite expensive and has a very unpleasant taste that discourages many subjects from continuing treatment.

Although there are now many investigators trying to unravel the complexities of CHD, we know that diet is only one of several factors involved in both prevention and treatment. However, the current consensus is that adherence to a prudent diet is the most effective method of dietary control. It is recommended that daily dietary cholesterol be kept below 300 mg, that body weight be maintained within 10% of ideal weight for height, that polyunsaturated fats provide about 10%, saturated fat no more than 10%, and monounsaturated fat the remainder of total fat to provide no more than 30% of total calories, and that complex carbohydrates rather than simple sugars replace fat calories. More recently, the recommendation to increase the use of fish is receiving much attention; fish contain a polyunsaturated fat designated EPA, believed to help reduce blood cholesterol levels. Because of the strong genetic influence in the development of CHD, there are of course many people who will not benefit from the dietary regimen and some who are unlikely to suffer from the disease no matter what they eat. An important point to remember is that a recommendation to increase polyunsaturated fats to provide 10% of calories does not suggest eating unlimited fat in this form; nor is a recommendation to reduce cholesterol a recommendation to eliminate cholesterol. In addition, following these guidelines cannot ensure freedom from CHD. It is entirely possible that many current recommendations will be modified or replaced even within the next decade as medical science acquires even more sophisticated methods of studying the problem.

Although CHD is only one of several diet-related degenerative diseases (including hypertension, diabetes, and possibly cancer) that contribute to premature death in Western societies, we have chosen to discuss it because it is the one commanding the most public attention today and has been the subject of intensive study. In reality, the diet recommended to protect against CHD does not differ appreciably from diets recommended to protect against other health problems.

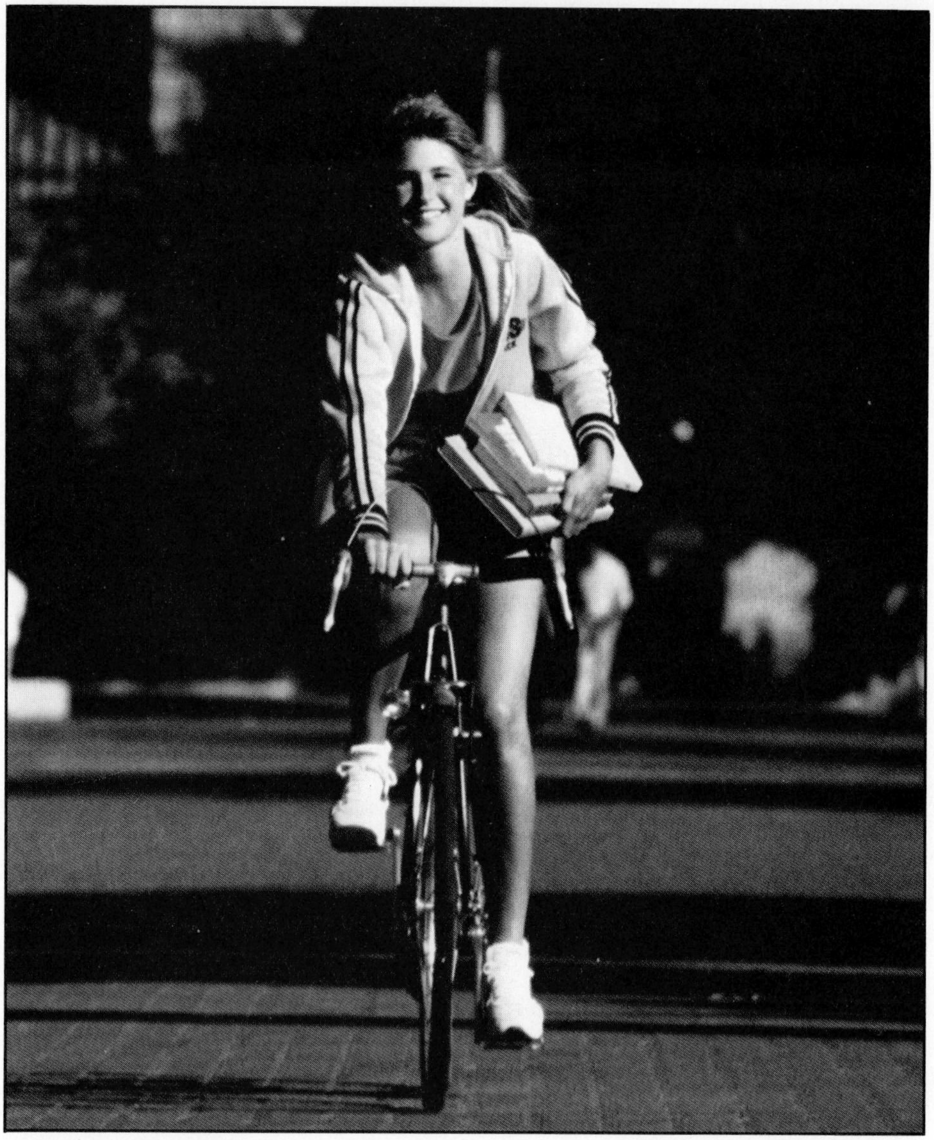

AWARENESS CHECK

Truth or Fiction?

- An athlete needs more calories because he or she has a larger calorie output than a nonathlete.
- Concentrated sweets provide quick energy and improved athletic performance.
- Athletes should never drink water before or during competition.
- Going to a sauna to sweat off extra pounds is safe weight loss for the wrestler trying to "make weight."
- To allow for proper digestion, athletes should eat about 3 to 4 hours before competing.
- Carbohydrate loading is not recommended for the average recreational athlete.

Nutrition and Physical Fitness

CHAPTER 19

It is not difficult to convince people concerned with physical fitness and most athletes that good nutrition is an important factor in fitness and athletic performance. However, it is often much more difficult to make them realize that their nutritional requirements are not much different from the requirements of less athletic people. In general, athletes need more calories and more water but a very small amount of additional protein, and little extra minerals, or vitamins. Optimal performance is influenced more by a lifetime of good food habits than by the use or avoidance of particular foods at the time of competition. There is no magic food or combination of foods that will compensate for lack of ability and training, but good nutrition may provide the competitive edge. For people concerned with general good health rather than athletic prowess, attention to both diet and exercise will provide a good basis for fitness.

For centuries, athletes have been experimenting in the hope of finding the perfect diet to ensure optimal performance during competition. Only since 1960, however, has there been much systematic research to try to identify dietary practices that might be recommended to athletes and coaches. If someone reads this chapter in the hope of finding a set of dietary rules that will definitely lead to enhanced performance, he or she will be disappointed. However, for the person interested in fitness and nutrition, the chapter should provide both guidance and reassurance. Although some nutritional practices are specific for the athlete, dietary guidelines for the most part are not appreciably different for those who exercise and those who are more sedentary. For both types of people, the first rule is to eat a variety of foods in amounts that will maintain a desired body weight. These foods should be chosen to provide protein, minerals, and vitamins in amounts suggested in the RDAs for the appropriate age group. Calories should be provided by carbohydrate, lipid, and protein in the proportions suggested in dietary guidances, 50% to 60%, 30% to 35%, and 10% to 15% of total, respectively. Among those who exercise regularly, the need will generally be higher for nutrients such as thiamin, riboflavin, and niacin, in which the requirement is directly proportionate to energy need.

Usually, intake will increase along with the increase in calorie intake. Those who exercise strenuously in warm, humid climates should be especially careful to ingest adequate amounts of water. Having laid out some general considerations, we will devote the rest of the chapter to a discussion of what we know about the ways in which activity affects nutrient requirements and the basis of many of the food beliefs of athletes.

WATER

Water is the first nutrient to be discussed because it has possibly a greater effect on athletic performance than any other nutrient. Water is the only nutrient that is lost during exercise in amounts several times greater than amounts lost from a nonexercising individual. The losses are part of water's major role in regulating body temperature through evaporation from the skin. If the fluid is not replaced, blood volume drops. This causes a decrease in the amount of the energy source, glucose, that is delivered to the cells, and in the removal of waste products of metabolism as blood is filtered through the kidney or is carried to the lungs. Although a small amount of water results from the metabolism that produces more energy, the amount of water produced is insignificant compared to the amount lost. Most people get about half their water intake (or more) from drinking fluids; they get a little less (20% to 40%) from solid foods. Athletes, on the other hand, must increase their fluid intake so that beverages account for as much as 90% of their available water.

Dehydration and Water Needs

Dehydration, or excessive water loss, can reduce the maximal oxygen consumption so essential for maximal performance. It can also interfere with the loss of body heat, resulting in an increase in body temperature and a loss of coordination. As body fluids are depleted by excessive losses, the thirst sensation normally intensifies so that most people automatically drink enough water or other beverages to replace the fluids. However, for both recreational and serious athletes, water loss can be very rapid, making dehydration a serious problem. For them, the sense of thirst does not respond fast enough to stimulate drinking a sufficient amount of water to replace fluid losses. Therefore, the athlete should make a conscious effort to consume fluids before, after, and often during exercise, and should be aware of the consequences of failure to do so.

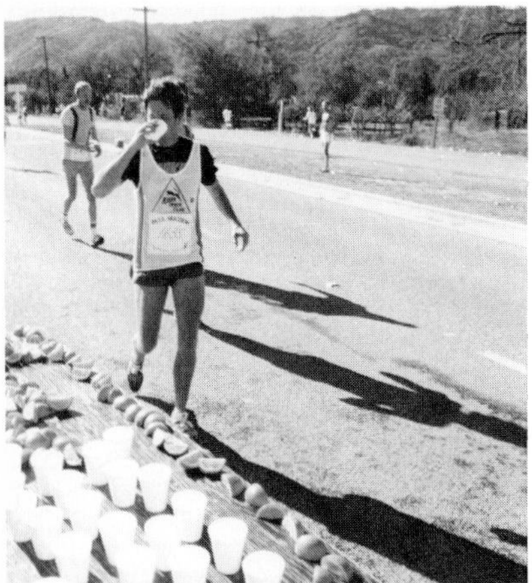

It is well known that the loss of as little as 2% of body water can cause performance to deteriorate. It is also known that in 90 minutes of exercise at 70° F, with humidity as low as 40%, a 180-pound athlete can lose 3½ to 4 pounds of water—enough to reduce the level of performance and lessen chances of appearing in the winner's circle. When the temperature is 90° F and the humidity is 80% to 100%, water losses can amount to 6 to 7 pounds—enough to cause fatigue, apathy, and both unwillingness and inability to continue strenuous exercise. Greater losses of 5% of body weight can lead to cramps and heat exhaustion, while losses as high as 7% body weight can cause hallucinations and heat stroke.

Loss of water causes a decline in blood volume, a resulting drop in blood pressure, and increases in both heart rate and body temperature. It may take several hours to restore water balance and performance. A person can soon determine how much fluid is needed during an exercise period by weighing oneself before and after the event. If the loss of weight exceeds 2% of body weight, fluid intake has been inadequate and should be increased on subsequent occasions of similar exercise (2 cups water for each pound lost). Ideally, water intake before and during a competition or exercise session should equal loss in sweat so that there is no change in body weight. In general, 2 cups of water 2 hours before, and another 2 cups 15 to 20 minutes before an event is adequate. In hot environments, additional

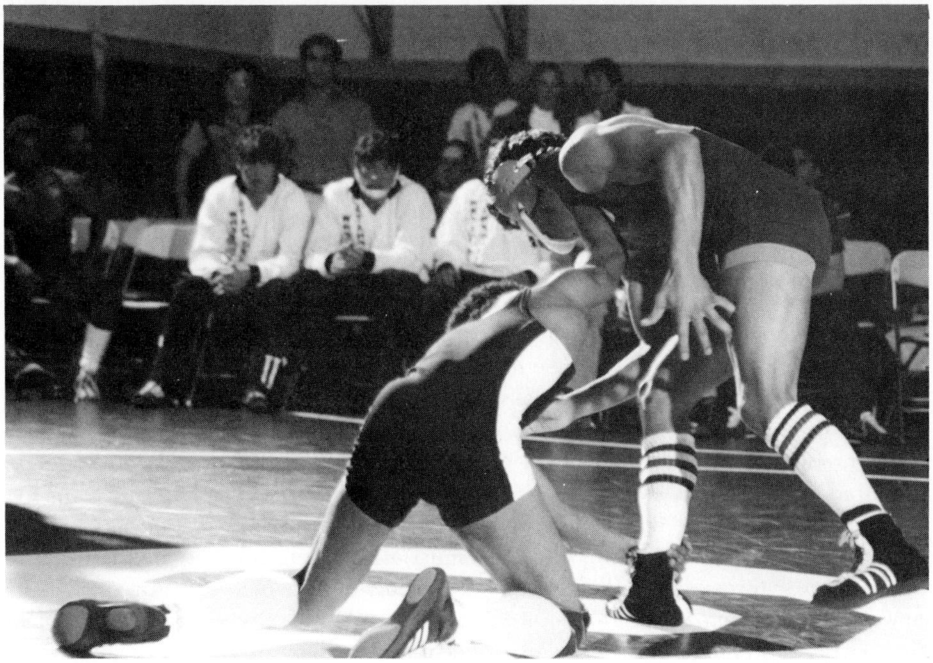

Water loss can be a serious problem for wrestlers, who sometimes go to extreme lengths, including excessive sweating, to lose weight before competition

small ½-cup drinks of cool water every 10 to 15 minutes during an event is recommended. Because there is no evidence that drinking too much water interferes with performance, there is no reason to restrict water intake before exercise. If however, there has been excessive sodium loss, large quantities of water should not be taken during exercise.

Although loss of water in sweat is accompanied by a very small loss of salt relative to the amount in the blood, there is a very persistent myth that athletes replacing water should take salt tablets at the same time. Normally, the typical diet provides enough sodium, chloride, potassium, and magnesium to replace losses. In the few cases when extra salt is needed, the best way to get it is by salting food; then there is little chance of getting too much. Some athletes experience a lot of discomfort resulting from the irritating effect of excess salt on the stomach, and sometimes they also experience additional dehydration if salt pills are taken. In response to this problem, a variety of "sports beverages" consisting of a weak-flavored solution of sodium, potassium, and glucose to replace electrolytes and energy reserves of glycogen are being promoted commercially. Except that they taste good and are popular with athletes, there is little or no reason to recommend them. If they are used, most (depending on their composition) should be diluted so that the fluid is absorbed as quickly as possible. Table 19-1 gives recommended dilutions for the various beverages that are used to replace fluid lost during exercise.

Optimal Composition of a Sports Drink (per Quart)

Sugar	2 T
Salt	1/10 tsp
Potassium chloride	1/16 tsp
Protein	0
Fat	0

Table 19-1 ◇ Recommended dilutions for replacement fluids following loss of body water

Fluid	Dilution
Fruit juices	1 part to 3-7 parts water
Soft drinks	1 part to 3 parts water
Vegetable juices	1 part to 1 part water
Sugar-free soft drinks	Drink as is
Special athletic drinks	1 part to 2 parts water

Special glucose electrolyte replacement solutions should be diluted so that they contain no more than 2.5% glucose (approximately 1 oz (2 T) sugar per quart).

The best way to prevent dehydration, an increase in body temperature, heat exhaustion, and heat stroke is to drink water before, during, and after exercise. If problems do arise, they must be treated by cooling the body as fast as possible in a cold shower or bath, by rubbing the body with ice cubes, and by drinking cold water, which is absorbed faster than warm water.

The two groups of athletes most vulnerable to water loss are marathon runners and wrestlers. Runners can lose 8 to 13 pounds of fluid during a race. This must be replaced during the event to prevent the runner from suffering very severe cardiovascluar problems as a result of the drop in blood volume. Wrestlers, on the other hand, have problems because they purposely dehydrate themselves to qualify for competition in a lower weight class. Although the use of diuretics, hot showers, whirlpools, and sweatboxes is prohibited in competition, the use of laxatives, intense sweat-producing exercise, and food and fluid restriction is not and can result in impaired performance even if partial rehydration occurs between weigh-in and competition. The large fluctuations in body weight to which a wrestler may subject himself are bound to stress the body and must almost certainly reduce his chances of performing to capacity. However, it is difficult to convince a young man eager to win that his chances are greater at the bottom end of his appropriate weight class than at the top end of the lower weight class.

ENERGY REQUIREMENTS

As discussed in Chapter 7, the energy cost of an activity is determined by the type of exercise, the duration of the exercise, and the weight of the person doing the exercise. Obviously, the more intense and longer the exercise and the heavier the individual, the higher the energy cost of almost any activity. For a 125-pound (58-kg) person, the energy cost of activity ranges from 176 kcal/hour for walking slowly, to 241 kcal for swimming the crawl, to 495 kcal for vigorous basketball, to 777 kcal for running 9 miles/hour. Comparable figures for a 205-pound person are, respectively, 266, 392, 807, and 1269 kcal/hour. It is not unusual for a swimmer with 5 hours of daily training to expend as much as 7000 kcal/day. Figure 19-1 illustrates the techniques and equipment used in determining the energy cost of an activity.

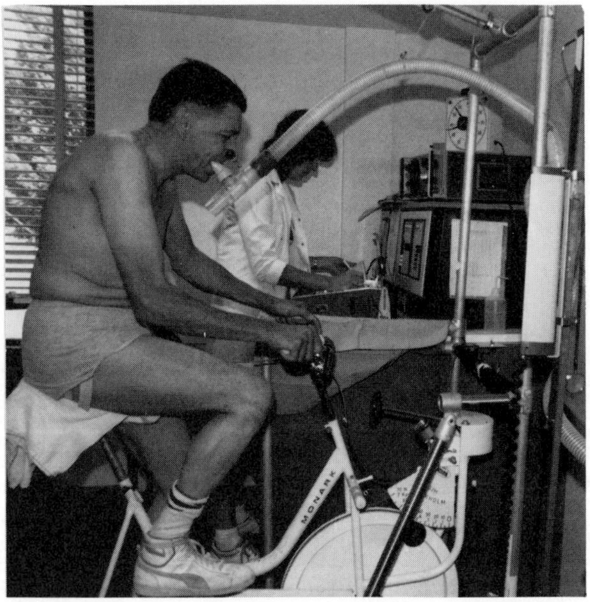

Figure 19-1 Test to determine the energy cost of bicycling.
Courtesy Jos. Loomis, Human Performance Laboratory, The Pennsylvania State University.

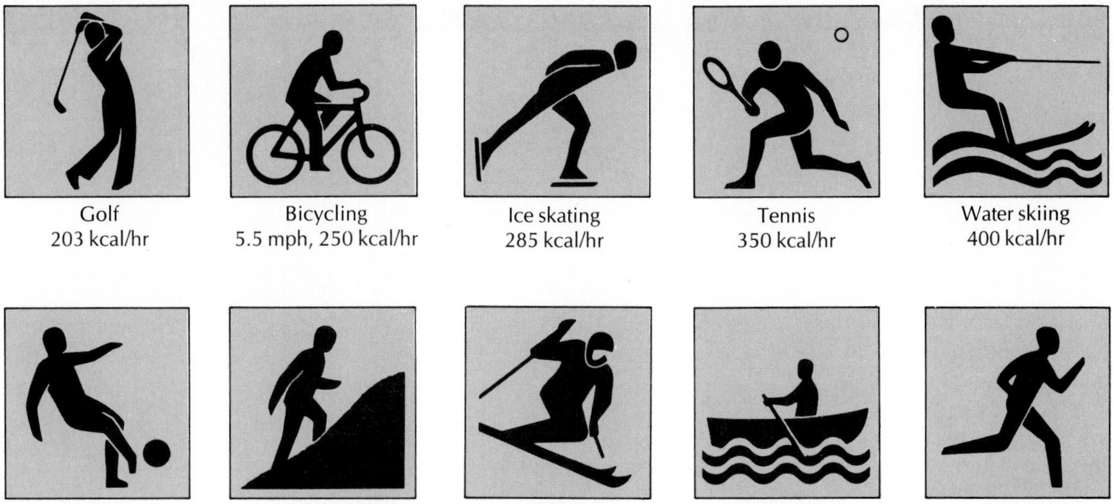
Golf
203 kcal/hr
Bicycling
5.5 mph, 250 kcal/hr
Ice skating
285 kcal/hr
Tennis
350 kcal/hr
Water skiing
400 kcal/hr
Soccer
450 kcal/hr
Mountain climbing
500 kcal/hr
Skiing
5 mph, 600 kcal/hr
Rowing
684 kcal/hr
Running
9 mph, 900 kcal/hr
7 mph, 669 kcal/hr

Energy costs of various kinds of exercise
Courtesy Rudolf Modley with the assistance of Willian R. Myers, Handbook of pictorial symbols, Dover Publications, Inc., 1976, New York, NY.

Requirements for energy among athletes vary as much as they do among more sedentary people in the population. They also vary depending on the size of each individual and the nature and intensity of the exercise under consideration. During training, daily energy requirements are usually between 3000 and 5000 kcal, but there are some reports of requirements at least twice as high. Appetite and satiety usually serve as indicators on which to base the regulation of food intake. Maintenance of desirable body weight is the best criterion of long-term adequacy or inadequacy of energy intake. Because athletes usually require considerably more sleep than other people, they must often consume their extra calories during a relatively short period of time.

Energy Sources

The energy for all body needs comes from carbohydrate, protein, and fat. For athletes and nonathletes alike, these should be provided by foods that contain enough vitamins and minerals to meet recommended intakes. Although alcohol can also provide calories, its effect on performance is such that it should be avoided by any serious athlete hoping to excel. Getting more than 10% to 15% of calories from protein is unnecessarily expensive from both a financial and a metabolic point of view. One of the most common beliefs about needs during exercise is that because exercise involves muscles and because muscles are largely protein, we need to provide large amounts of protein to meet the energy needs of exercising muscles. However, this is an erroneous conclusion. In actuality, muscles derive most of their energy from carbohydrate, provided first by blood glucose and then by the limited amount formed from muscle and liver glycogen. When that is exhausted, fat from dietary sources and body fat reserves are used. Even though body fat in most athletes, ranging from 4% to 14% of body weight, is considerably lower than that in nonathletic individuals, most athletes have fat reserves of at least 15 pounds capable of providing over 50,000 kcal, only a small portion of which would be used. Although muscle protein is not a primary source of energy, it can be broken down to amino acids, which can provide 5% to 15% of the energy used by a working muscle. There is no evidence, however, that eating more protein will increase metabolic efficiency or enhance performance or endurance. The use of protein as an energy source requires the removal and excretion of the nitrogen portion of the molecule as urea in the urine, necessitating a larger urine volume and contributing to the need for water.

Sources of Energy for Muscle
Blood glucose
Muscle glycogen
Fatty acids
Amino acids (deaminated)

Figure 19-2 Shift in the use of energy sources in the body as exercise continues.

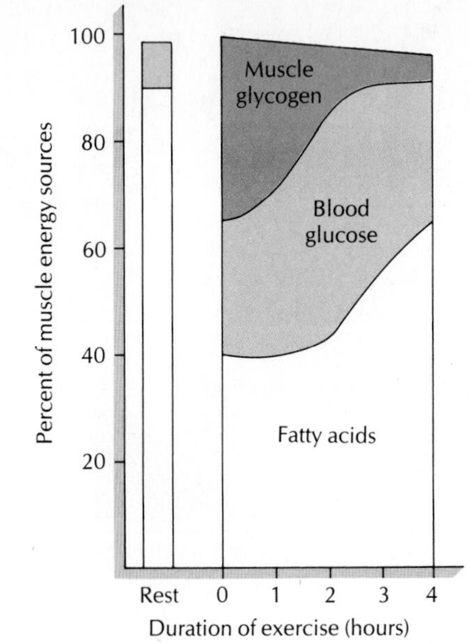

Figure 19-2 depicts the use of various energy sources with moderate exercise compared to resting.

When muscles use glucose as a source of energy, they are able to obtain only a small portion of the energy whether or not oxygen is available. If oxygen is not available, the process is called **anaerobic** metabolism (literally meaning "in the absence of air") and involves the release of a small portion of its energy as glucose is changed to pyruvic acid. Usually, most of the release of energy occurs as pyruvic acid is further oxidized in the presence of oxygen to become carbon dioxide, water, and energy; this process is described as **aerobic** (that is, "requiring air"). When sufficient oxygen is not available, the pyruvic acid is temporarily shunted to become lactic acid. When this occurs, the athlete will initially have a tingling sensation in the muscles. If the lack of oxygen continues, lactic acid will continue to accumulate; in a relatively short period of time, the muscle will feel very hard and heavy and will be unable to continue to contract in a normal fashion. As soon as the strenuous exercise is over and the body is able to provide the needed oxygen, the lactic acid changes back into pyruvic acid and the feeling in the muscle returns to normal. Athletes doing aerobic exercise can continue indefinitely, whereas those engaged in anaerobic exercise can do so for only short periods of time.

anaerobic
In the absence of air or oxygen

aerobic
In the presence of air or oxygen

Effect of Training on Energy Sources

Because there is a limited amount of stored carbohydrate available in the body and because even very lean runners (with only 5% body fat) have enough stored fat to run several marathons, the use of body fat as an energy source has the advantage of sparing the limited amount of carbohydrate. In the untrained individual, a larger proportion of energy comes from carbohydrate. However, as an athlete becomes more conditioned or trained, the ability to use fat as an energy source increases by as much as 50%. When fatty acids are more available in the blood, the muscles are more likely to use them as an energy source. The use of coffee or other caffeine-containing foods appears to increase the release of fatty acids into the blood. The efficiency with which these are used is believed to account for increases in performance and endurance that follow the use of coffee, supplying about 5 mg of caffeine per kg body weight (300 to 350 mg in 2 cups of coffee) for a 70-kg male. Higher intakes may cause anxiety, fluid loss, and increased heart rate that would counteract any benefits. The use of coffee to enhance performance is not approved.

CARBOHYDRATE LOADING

After athletes engage in strenuous exercise over a long period of time, they report an experience sometimes described as "hitting the wall"—that is, reaching a point at which it is almost impossible to keep moving. This point corresponds to the time when the reserves of the carbohydrate glycogen in the muscles are depleted. It seems reasonable to suppose that if we could find some way to increase the glycogen reserves, it would be possible for an athlete to continue to compete for a longer period of time. As a result, the dietary and exercise regimen known as "carbohydrate loading" has become quite popular. The original regimen was 3 days of a low-carbohydrate diet and strenuous exercise, followed by 4 days of a high-carbohydrate diet and minimum exercise. This program had several undesirable side effects—depression, lethargy, loss of muscle tissue, stiffness, cramps, weight gain, and early fatigue. It has been replaced by a "taper-down" regimen. With this, there is no initial depletion of glycogen. An athlete starts with a moderate amount of carbohydrate (350 grams) and by day 4 increases to 550 grams, or 60% to 65% of total calories (mainly from complex carbohydrates such as starches and cereals) during the week before the event. During this time, the level of exercise is tapered down from a normal training level to a resting level by the sixth day. This results in reserves of glycogen considerably higher than normal. These reserves are then presumably available on the seventh day, that is, the day of the competition, at which time athletes revert to their usual diet.

This program gives the athlete an advantage without the drawbacks of the original approach. It also meets the needs of some people who require more than 3 days to saturate their glycogen reserves. Perhaps the most difficult rule to follow is the requirement that there be decreasing exercise on the 3 days before the competition—the time when athletes usually do some of their most vigorous training. Carbohydrate loading will be beneficial only for events that require at least 1 to 2 hours of continuous, strenuous exercise; events that might normally deplete glycogen reserves. Carbohydrate loading is not recommended for children or teenagers. Athletes with diabetes or high blood lipid levels should do it only with medical supervision. No one should carbohydrate load more than three to four times per year.

Carbohydrate Loading Prescription

Days 1-3	Regular exercise Moderate (350g) carbohydrate diet
Days 4-5	Decreasing exercise High (550 g) complex carbohydrate diet
Day 6	Physical rest High (550g) or 60-65% calories complex carbohydrate diet
Day 7	Day of event Usual diet

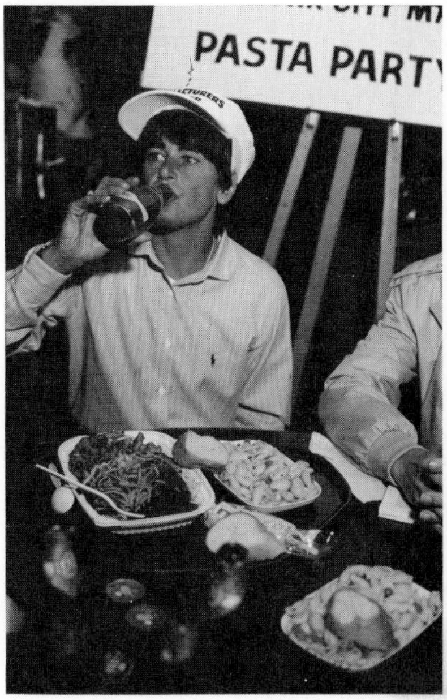

PROTEIN

One of the more common beliefs among athletes—that they have an increased need for protein—is now somewhat substantiated by recent experimental data. There is evidence that submaximal exercise may lead to some breakdown of body protein, and that an intake of 1 gram/kg body weight, and possibly as high as 1.2 to 1.6 grams/kg, is more appropriate than the 0.8 gram in which the current RDA is based. These levels, however, are still below the amount provided in the typical American diet. There is no evidence that intakes in excess of this amount will lead to increased muscle strength or protein content. Similarly, athletes following vegetarian diets are at no additional risk of protein deficiency as long as the plant protein sources are chosen based on their complimentary amino acid patterns. In general, the recommendation that 10% to 15% of calories be provided by protein assures an adequate intake.

The widely promoted practice of supplementing the diets of athletes with single amino acids or with amino acid mixtures in the form of protein hydrolysates (partially digested proteins) is of no value, and may indeed contribute to amino acid imbalances.

The term *muscle building*, along with the more colloquial term *bulking up*, is used to describe the increase in muscle mass that some athletes try to achieve. Although this increase can be gotten only through extensive conditioning and will not be influenced by diet, many people have turned to the use of dietary protein supplements in the hope that they will help to achieve the goal. Without a conditioning program, the extra protein will be converted to fat and stored, and the extra nitrogen will be excreted as urinary urea. With most diets in the United States already containing well above recommended levels of protein, there is absolutely no reason for the use of protein supplements for diets with excessive amounts of meat.

NUTRIENT SUPPLEMENTS

Nutrients Often Erroneously Promoted to Enhance Endurance and Performance
Vitamin C
Vitamin E
Zinc
Lecithin

The belief that "if a little is good, then more is better" seems to characterize beliefs and claims about the role of vitamins in athletic performance and endurance. It is true that vitamins are essential cofactors in the release of energy from food and that the higher the energy expenditure the higher the need for many of the nutrients (such as thiamin, niacin, pantothenic acid, iron, and magnesium) that are involved in energy metabolism. However, it is equally true that most diets—especially the high-calorie diets of most physically active people—will provide very adequate amounts of these nutrients if the calories are selected from a range of food items. Studies on the effects of high doses of either vitamin C or vitamin E showed that only when there had been a deficiency of the nutrient did supplements have a beneficial effect. There is absolutely no evidence of improved performance associated with megadoses of vitamins; there is, however, considerable reason to be concerned about the adverse effects of vitamins when they are taken at levels hundreds of times those needed for normal metabolism.

In the case of minerals, there is a similar lack of evidence of benefits from large intakes and considerably more evidence of toxicity from high and imbalanced intakes. Iron and calcium are the minerals most often studied. Iron supplements have some benefit when anemia is present or when tissue iron levels are low enough to reduce endurance due to lower tissue cytochromes. There seems to be no benefit from the use of supplemental calcium unless to help increase peak bone mass in amenhorreic exercising females, especially those who suffer from anorexia nervosa.

PRECOMPETITION MEAL

On this subject as on many others, there are a great many beliefs about what is nutritionally appropriate and what is not. If a person gets a psychological lift from the use of a particular food, the consequences of eliminating it from the diet can be just as devastating in terms of performance as if there were a sound physiological reason for eating the food. There may be no reason to think that performance will be better after a meal of steak and potatoes than after one of pancakes and eggs; however, if athletes have come to expect particular foods, they will undoubtedly perform less well if these foods are not provided. Similarly, if foods that they believe will interfere with top performance are included in their diet, the level of performance may suffer as much as if there were valid reasons for the effect.

In general, it is recommended that the precompetition meal be taken 3 or 4 hours before competing. It should provide anywhere from 300 to 1000 kcals and be relatively low in fat and high in complex carbohydrate such as bread, cereal, and vegetables. This will allow for almost complete digestion and absorption of the food so that the blood supply is no longer diverted to the stomach but is directed to the peripheral muscles, which are very involved in performance. Athletic performance depends on an adequate supply of blood to carry glucose and fatty acids to the exercising muscle. Liquid meals do offer advantages for athletes who have trouble digesting regular meals. These beverages are digested quickly, leave little residue, are convenient, provide substantial calories, and can be taken within an hour of competition.

Two to three cups of fluid should be taken with the meal and some fluid intake continued until competition time. The belief that consuming a candy bar causes an overshoot of insulin and reduced blood glucose level, instead of increased blood glucose, is under study.

SPECIAL ERGOGENIC FOODS

Over the years, certain beliefs have developed about the special merits of particular **ergogenic** foods or drugs in enhancing athletic performance. Investigations of many of these beliefs have failed to show any physiological basis for them. Some foods and supplements are essentially harmless in that they do not interfere with performance; they do not benefit it, either, but at least they do not interfere with normal metabolism. Other foods, however, such as wheat germ oil, kelp, vitamins C, D, and E, bee pollen, fructose, and lecithin, are often packaged especially for athletes and are exorbitantly priced—from a nutritional standpoint, they are a complete waste of money. Health food stores have been quick to recognize a lucrative market and are promoting a vast array of items that supposedly have merit in enhancing performance or stamina. Because it is likely that the list of promoted items will continue to change constantly, readers are cautioned to view all newcomers with a healthy amount of skepticism until convincing evidence of effectiveness, provided by sound scientific investigations, is presented. Testimony for products from successful athletes should be just as suspect as that provided "on the basis of unpublished scientific data." Although some of these substances have no proven physiological benefits, they may have psychological merits to the athlete.

ergogenic
Capable of producing energy

These Foods are Promoted to Enhance Endurance but Are of No Proven Benefit
Wheat germ
Wheat germ oil
Paprika
Honey
Brewer's yeast
Sunflower seeds

FOODS TO BE AVOIDED

One of the most persistent beliefs among athletes is that milk should be avoided because of a condition called "cotton mouth." This condition is characterized by a sensation of dryness in the mouth that is very distracting to athletes, who may be convinced that this interferes with their performance. At least one controlled study on swimmers regarding this problem showed no relationship between milk consumption and performance. Reports of another problem, an unpleasant and excessive secretion of mucus after drinking milk, also remain unconfirmed.

There seems to be even more controversy about the role of caffeine in performance than about almost any other food or substance. Many athletes will purposely avoid caffeine because of its diuretic effect. Others seek it out, believing that its stimulating effect on epinephrine production will improve performance. We do know that caffeine stimulates the heart rate and permits the relaxation of smooth muscles of the blood vessels so that there is less resistance to blood flow; it also stimulates the release of fatty acids into the blood, making them available as a source of energy. Because of uncertainty about the effect of caffeine on performance, it is listed among banned substances by the U.S. Olympic Committee.

CONSEQUENCES OF EXCESSIVE PHYSICAL EXERCISE

Many young women who exercise excessively and at the same time restrict their food intake to maintain a low body weight have suffered from *amenhorrea*, or cessation of menstruation, delayed menstruation (to as late as the age of 18 years), *oligomenhorrea* (infrequent or scanty menstrual periods), and decreased bone mass. The long-range consequences of these effects have not been established. In many cases, the loss of body fat is the result of either purposeful loss of weight, anorexia, or bulimia. It is to be expected that abnormal changes such as these are very likely to have long-range consequences. They are more common among gymnasts, ballet dancers, divers, and cyclists, many of whom have reduced circulating hormone levels and increased loss of bone mineral.

Some athletes, particularly (but not exclusively) young women engaged in in-

sports anemia
A condition in which there is increased destruction of red blood cells and a transient drop in hemoglobin as a result of an acute stress response to exercise

tensive exercise programs, suffer from **sports anemia.** In some individuals this is a relatively transient condition, while in others it persists throughout the period of exercise. Sports anemia is a relative iron deficiency that may be the result of a dilution of the blood, which occurs as fluid is retained and results in lower hemoglobin concentrations; alternatively, the iron deficiency may be caused by the loss of iron in sweat or urine. It is associated with training and not dietary iron deficiency. Even though the amount of iron loss is generally small, it may accumulate over time to affect hemoglobin levels. Alternatively, the friction caused by blood passing through the blood vessels in strenuous exercise may break, or *lyse,* the red blood cells, causing loss of hemoglobn. Sports anemia occurs less frequently when the diet provides 2 grams of protein/kg of body weight (as opposed to diets containing only 1 gram). It also occurs less frequently when over 50% of the protein comes from animal sources. So far, however, we have little or no information on how to correct this condition; it might not be necessary to correct it, even if we could. Because the iron is not lost and is available for synthesis of more hemoglobin, sports anemia is not considered serious. This condition is one good example of adaptation among normal, healthy people.

American Dietetic Association Guidelines to Promote Good Nutrition and Physical Fitness

Recommendations for the General Public

- Nutritionally adequate diet and exercise are major contributing factors to physical fitness and health
- Weight maintenance and weight loss should be achieved by a combination of dietary modification, change in eating behavior, and regular aerobic exercise
- Body fatness should be determined by skinfold measurements
- A diet that meets the RDA provides all nutrients needed for a physical conditioning program
- Intensity, duration, and frequency of exercise should be determined according to the age, physical condition, and health status of the individual
- Habits for a nutritionally balanced diet and physical fitness should be established during childhood and maintained throughout life

Recommendations for Athletes Involved in Training or Competition

- Increased calorie and nutrient needs should be met by increasing the number of selections from the "calories plus nutrients" foods
- A hydrated state should be maintained by consuming fluids before, during, and after exercise
- Needs for additional electrolytes should be met from foods ordinarily consumed
- Electrolyte solutions should be used only on the advice of the team physician
- A high carbohydrate intake prior to competition can be beneficial to some athletes engaging in endurance events
- No unique ergogenic value is recognized for products such as wheat germ, vitamin E, vitamin C, lecithin, honey, gelatin, phosphates, sunflower seeds, bee pollen, kelp, and brewer's yeast. Alcoholic beverages are not recommended as a source of calories, as a muscle relaxant, or as an ergogenic aid
- A light pregame meal should be eaten 3 to 4 hours prior to the competition
- Athletes not currently involved in training or competition should reduce their caloric intake to balance their energy expenditure

Adapted with permission from the American Dietetic Association, Journal of the American Dietetic Association 76:437, 1980.

Overuse injuries are another concern in athletes who perform the same movements repetitively many times a day, day after day. Examples are shoulder injuries in baseball pitchers and swimmers, and knee injuries in runners.

Benefits of Moderate Exercise and Possible Adverse Consequences of Excessive Exercise Throughout the Life Cycle

Benefits of Moderate Exercise During the Life Cycle

Childhood
- Establish lifelong exercise and health habits

Adolescence
- Prevent and treat obesity and eating disorders
- Establish lifelong exercise and health habits

Adulthood
- Weight control
- Prevent and treat many diseases
- Promote mental health and feelings of well being

Pregnancy
- Control of excessive weight gain
- More favorable nutrient profile as a result of an increased energy intake
- Possibly less constipation and varicose veins

Lactation
- Promotes return to prepregnancy weight
- Possibly improve postpartum mental status

Elderly
- Favorable effects on age-related physiological changes
- Prevent and treat osteoporosis
- Socialization

Possible Adverse Consequences of Strenuous Exercise during the Life Cycle

Childhood
- Inability to meet energy needs and compromised growth and development

Adolescence
- Inadequate energy intake
- Oxidation of dietary protein for energy
- Oligomenorrhea/Amenorrhea
- Negative calcium balance and reduced bone mass
- Sports anemia
- Anorexia athletica

Adulthood
- Possible increased need for riboflavin and vitamin B_6

Pregnancy
- Low weight gain
- Low-birth-weight infant

Lactation
- Excessive rate of weight loss, which compromises milk production and infant growth

Elderly
- Exercise-related injuries leading to disability and other complications

Adapted from Kris-Etherton PM: Nutrition and the exercising female, Nutrition Today 21(April):7, 1986.

NUTRITION KNOWLEDGE OF ATHLETES AND COACHES

Several studies of the information that athletes have about nutrition have confirmed that there are many misconceptions about the role of diet in relation to exercise and athletic performance. In many cases, especially among girls, knowledge was found to be considerably better than actual practices. Boys ate considerably better than girls, but this was thought to be the result of the large quantity of food they consumed to meet their energy requirements.

In summary, students who hope to find a definitive prescription for achieving athletic prowess in dietary recommendations will be disappointed. However, it is hoped that this chapter has provided a clearer understanding of the importance of nutrition in maintaining the health of active people. At the same time, it is good to gain an appreciation of the things that nutrition cannot do, no matter how "good" it is. Moderation and variety in choosing the daily diet remain the best advice for athletes and nonathletes alike.

The American Dietetic Association has compiled current recommendations for promoting good nutrition and physical fitness in a set of guidelines for athletes and all people concerned with maintaining a good balance between nutrition and physical fitness. These recommendations are summarized in the box on p. 592. They are reviewed/revised every 5 years. For the general public who are not involved in competitive sports, there are many benefits from *moderate* exercise but also some adverse consequences of *excessive* and *strenuous* exercise. These are outlined in the box on p. 593. As in most health-related issues, moderation in exercise seems prudent.

BY NOW YOU SHOULD KNOW

- Water has probably greater effect on athletic performance than any other nutrient.
- The Dietary Goals for all healthy Americans can also be recommended to the athlete.
- Athletes should drink water before, during, and after competition.
- Athletes have a need for increased calories, to meet the energy cost of their activities, and a proportional increase in other nutrients, especially those involved in energy metabolism.
- Although athletes may have a slightly greater protein need than nonathletes, their need is easily met in the typical American diet. There are no advantages—and even some disadvantages—to increasing protein intakes above suggested amounts.
- Many products on the market that are promoted for athletes cannot deliver the competitive edge that the advertising suggests.
- Water intake is extremely important for those who exercise, especially for those exercising in high temperatures and humidity. Thirst is not an adequate gauge of water need; the athlete should consume enough water to restore his or her weight before, during, and after exercising.
- Vitamin mineral supplements will not supply energy or provide the winning edge for the athlete. Iron supplements are of benefit only for the anemic athlete.
- The precompetition meal should be taken 3 to 4 hours before the event, and the nutrient composition should be such that the stomach is empty at the start of the event.
- Intake of additional salt to replace sodium lost during exercise is not needed and should be avoided in most cases, because it leads to dehydration and other adverse consequences.

- Sports anemia, amenorrhea, and bone loss occur among female athletes who exercise very strenuously and restrict their energy intake to the point that body fat falls below 20% of body weight.
- Ample fluid intake, moderation, and variety in food selection are the keys to dietary adequacy for athletes.
- As we have learned to use food in moderation, exercise should also be performed in moderation.

STUDY QUESTIONS

1. At the beginning of the event, a marathon runner weighs 135 pounds; at the end of the event the weight is 129 pounds. How many cups of water would that runner need to drink to make up for the fluid loss?
2. Explain why water is an essential nutrient, especially to the athlete.
3. What are several nutritional problems seen specifically in wrestlers? Explain why these are stereotypical of wrestlers.
4. What is the difference between anaerobic metabolism and aerobic metabolism?
5. Argue against protein or amino acid supplementation.
6. What are the positive and negative effects of coffee (caffeine) consumption by the athlete before competition?

Applying What You've Learned

1. **Discuss Nutrition with Athletes**

   Talk to at least two athletes involved in competitive sports. Find out what dietary adjustments they have made to increase their skills. Ask them about their food and nutrient supplement beliefs. Where do they get their nutrition information?

2. **Go to a Health Food Store and Look for Ergogenic Aids**

   What are the claims made in the literature available at the store?

3. **Leaf Through a "Fitness" Magazine in a Bookstore or Library**

   Note the number and kind of food products advertised for those interested in building physique and athletic ability.

4. **Calculate the Amount of Energy You Expend When Engaged in a Strenuous Physical Activity**

   How much more food than you normally eat would you need to provide the required number of calories?

5. **Plan an Appropriate Precompetition Meal**

   Plan a precompetition meal with approximately 800 calories. Distribute the calories so that less than 30% are from fat, less than 12% from protein, and more than 58% from carbohydrate.

6. **Analyze Your Intake**

   Using the chart, " American Dietetic Association Guidelines to Promote Good Nutrition and Physical Fitness" on p. 592, find the recommendations for the general public. Are you living by what is recommended?

SUGGESTED READINGS

American Dietetic Association: Position of the American Dietetic Association: Nutrition for physical fitness and athletic performance for adults, Journal of the American Dietetic Association 87:933, 1987.

This position paper is accompanied by a technical support paper that deals with body composition/ideal weight, energy, carbohydrate loading, protein, vitamins, minerals, hydration, ergogenic aids, alcohol, caffeine, and the precompetition meal. These discussions provide the reader with the rationale for the position that accurate and appropriate nutrition education is needed to promote optimal fitness and well-being.

National Association for Sport and Physical Education, and others: Nutrition for sport success, Washington, D.C., 1984, The Nutrition Foundation.

This publication by four organizations with interests in either sports or nutrition is a revision of the first widely available guidebook on the role of nutrition in sports. It is an attractive, practical, and sound presentation of the essence of our knowledge of good dietary practices for young athletes. It is well illustrated and should appeal to both students and their coaches.

O'Neil FT, Hynak-Hankinson MT, and Gorman J: Research and application of current topics in sports nutrition, Journal of the American Dietetic Association 86:1007, 1986.

The authors review the role of caffeine in endurance performance, iron status, and physical performance; fluid and electrolytes in relation to exercise; and calcium and exercise from physiological and biochemical perspectives. They discuss the application of these to concerns in sports nutrition.

Sherman W, and Costill D: The marathon: dietary manipulation to optimize performance, American Journal of Sports Medicine 12:44, 1984.

This paper reviews the factors that may improve marathon performance. It includes discussions of glycogen loading, premarathon meals, increasing fat oxidation to spare muscle glycogen, and carbohydrate feedings during the competition.

Williams MA: Nutrition for fitness and sport, Dubuque, Iowa, 1983, Wm. C. Brown Co.

A comprehensive and complete discussion of normal nutrition and the special needs of the athlete, presented in a style that motivates and informs. Topics include losing weight; gaining weight; the roles of carbohydrate, fat, and protein; vitamins and minerals; vegetarianism; caffeine, drugs, and alcohol; and special foods for athletes. Highly recommended for the athlete with no training in nutrition.

ADDITIONAL READINGS

American College of Sports Medicine: Weight loss in wrestlers, Sports Medicine Bulletin 11:1, 1976.

American Dietetic Association: Position paper on nutrition and physical fitness, Journal of the American Dietetic Association 76:447, 1980.

Beggood BL, and Tuck MB: Nutrition knowledge of high school athletic coaches in Texas, Journal of the American Dietetic Association 83:672, 1983.

Belko AZ: Vitamins and exercise—an update, Medicine and Science in Sports and Exercise 19:S191, 1987.

Buskirk ER: Some nutritional considerations in the conditioning of athletes, Annual Review of Nutrition 1:319, 1980.

Costill DL: Dietary potassium and heavy exercise: effects on muscle, water, and electrolytes, American Journal of Clinical Nutrition 36:266, 1982.

Costill DL: Carbohydrate nutrition before, during, and after exercise, Federal Proceedings 44:364, 1985.

Evans WJ, and Hughes VA: Dietary carbohydrates and endurance exercise, American Journal of Clinical Nutrition 41:1146, 1985.

Forbes GB: Body composition as affected by physical activity and nutrition, Federal Proceedings 44:343, 1985.

Forgac M: Carbohydrate loading—a review, Journal of the American Dietetic Association 75:42, 1979.

Haymes E: Nutritional concerns: need for iron, Medicine and Science in Sports and Exercise 19:S197, 1987.

Kris-Etherton PM: Nutrition and the exercising female, Nutrition Today 21(April): 7, 1986.

Layman D: Dietary protein needs for the athlete, Physician and Sports Medicine 15:182, 1987.

Lemon PWR: Protein and exercise: update 1987, Medicine and Science in Sports and Exercise 19:S179, 1987.

Lloyd T, and others: Interrelationships of diet, athletic activity, menstrual status, and bone density in collegiate women, American Journal of Clinical Nutrition 46:681, 1987.

National Institute of Nutrition, (Canada): Caffeine: a perspective on current concerns, Nutrition Today 22:36, 1987.

Slavin JL, Lanners G, and Engstrom MA: Amino acid supplements: Beneficial or risky? Physician and Sports Medicine 16:221, 1988.

Williams M: Ergogenic nutrition aids, Nutrition Today 23(Dec):8, 1988.

Wilmore JH, and Freund BJ: Nutritional enhancment of athletic performance, Nutrition Abstracts and Reviews 54:1, 1984.

FOCUS Are Supplements Necessary for Athletes?

When there is a suggestion in the scientific literature of a possible association between a dietary factor, drug, or form of exercise and some aspect of health, enterprising individuals or companies are often all too eager to promote an easy-to-take, conveniently packaged product for those who feel they will be helped by the use of a substance. This has been particularly true in the case of the association between diet and physical performance. Health food stores and stores catering to athletes, as well as magazines directed toward people who wish to enhance their physique or their athletic ability, are quick to cater to this market.

There are many terms that seem to have particular appeal in promoting a product. Among the ingredients that recur with predictable frequency in advertisements are electrolytes, enzymes, bee pollen, royal jelly, fructose, lecithin, soya, sterols, glandulars, herbals, wheat germ, emulsifiers, catalysts, ginseng, and spirulina. These are liberally interspersed with descriptive terms such as sustained release, dynamic, mega, ultimate, raw, all natural, pure, life essence, and ergogenic.

To illustrate the good and bad aspects of available products, this Focus section will assess the ingredients of one typical product. The product we will discuss is a powder sold in a half-pound can (227 grams) at $7.95/can (3.5¢/gram), or $15.90/pound. It is billed as a "scientifically balanced pre-athletic-event meal." As a basis for comparison, nonfat dried milk powder, a much more nutritious product, sells in the grocery store for $2.00/pound.

The ingredients are listed (in descending order, as required by law, according to the amount present in the product) as dried bananas, brewer's yeast, sesame seeds, wheat germ, bone meal, dolomite, oyster shell, bee pollen with royal jelly, almond, sunflower seed, soy protein, ginseng, lecithin, pumpkin seed, dried apricot, date, apple, peach, bromelin, and papain. In addition, the user is assured that the product contains absolutely no added sugars, salt, milk products, preservatives, artificial or synthetic ingredients, animal protein, or animal fat. The suggested serving size is one tablespoon (11 grams), with 20 servings per container. Thus cost per serving is 40¢.

What is the nutrition provided by this single-serving amount? The product itself provides 36 kcal/tablespoon. These kilocalories come from 4 grams of carbohydrate, 3 grams of protein, and 1.4 grams of fat. Obviously this amount of energy is not going to carry an athlete through many minutes of athletic competition. It does meet the basal energy needs of an 80-kg (176-pound) male for 30 minutes. If this male were engaged in a moderately strenuous activity such as tennis for 2 hours, he would require 900 kcal, which he could obtain only by consuming 25 tablespoons of this "scientifically balanced pre-athletic-event meal"—in other words, slightly over one can of the product! He could get the same number of calories and much more nutrition from a meal of one glass of milk, one slice of bread with butter, and one serving each of beef, potatoes, and tossed salad—at a cost considerably less than that of the powder.

As far as electrolytes are concerned, the "potassium-rich" dried bananas provide 100 mg, or from 2% to 5% of 1 day's need. The 10 mg of sodium in a single serving of the powder will not replace the 25 mg that even a nonexercising person will lose in 1 day. In spite of this, the label emphasizes that this product is a "convenient and efficient" way to replace important electrolytes that are lost during periods of vigorous physical exercise. The 600 mg of calcium in a single serving does come close to providing the recommended dietary allowance for calcium for men; however, the calcium/phosphorus ratio, which is 6:1, far exceeds the 1:1 or 1:2 ratio recommended. The product is a significant contributor of elements such as magnesium (550 mg/serving) and iron (5.4 mg/serving). However, the actual availability of iron is probably low because the product contains no animal protein or vitamin C, both of which increase availability of iron. As would be expected in a product that contains no ingredients of animal origin, the powder provides less than 2% of the zinc requirement.

In addition, the contributions of this "scientifically balanced" meal to our requirements for vitamins are negligible (less than 2%) for thiamin, riboflavin, niacin, vitamin B_6, folacin, pantothenic acid, vitamin A, and vitamin C. The label information reports a significant amount of vitamin B_{12}. This is hard to understand because we have previously been told that the product contains no animal products, and we know that animal products are the only sources of vitamin B_{12}. The label on the powder, which reports the amount of a vitamin such as vitamin C in micrograms (225 μg, to be exact), is typical of many that lead users to think they are getting a significant amount. Vitamin C would normally be reported in milligrams, and in this case the amount would have been 0.22 mg—a very small portion of the recommended daily amount of at least 30 mg!

What about the functions of the many "special" ingredients, other than to provide nutrients? Apparently 9% of the product is a mixture of bee pollen and royal jelly, both of which have been promoted as having special, although undefined, nutritional merit. These claims are usually substantiated by an exhaustive list detailing the amino acid composition of the product. This is impressive to some people because the names of the amino acids in themselves create a scientific aura, and even a few micrograms seems like a lot. In this case, the total amount of the bee pollen and royal jelly in the container is only 1 gram, making it impossible for the powder to provide more than 1 gram of protein—an insignificant amount, considering the average protein intake for a male is over 80 grams/day, and many people consume well over 100 grams/day. Bananas are considered a good source of potassium but seem to have no particular merit in this formulation. The emphasis on "raw" ingredients is undoubtedly to impress those who feel that by cooking or heating food ingredients we destroy some of their unique nutritional properties. If the ingredients are indeed raw and the total product has not been heat treated, there is always the possibility of microbial contamination and spoilage of the product. The fourteenth ingredient on the list is "complex carbohydrate-rich apricot, date, apple, and peach." These fruits are considered carbohydrate-rich in their natural form, but the carbohydrate in the ripe fruit is sugar, mainly sucrose and fructose, rather than the complex carbohydrate starch found in some unripe fruits. Absolutely the maximum amount of this fruit mix that could be contained in a 1-tablespoon serving is 1 gram—hardly important when we consider that almost all of us, with much lower energy requirements than athletes, will eat over 300 grams of carbohydrate a day.

The enzymes bromelin, from pineapple, and papain, from papaya, are sometimes used commercially as meat tenderizers. They are strictly proteolytic enzymes and thus digest only protein. In addition, because they themselves are proteins, they are digested in the stomach and have no effect in helping to digest the 3 grams of protein in a serving of this product. Moreover, there is little or no evidence that healthy people have any difficulty digesting protein; thus they do not have to worry about helping their bodies by buying and eating enzymes, important as enzymes may be. The inclusion of soy protein merely reflects the fact that soy provides the highest quality vegetable protein readily available; if people want protein but also want to avoid ingredients of animal origin, as is probably the case if they buy this product, then the powder may have some value for them. Almonds and sunflower and pumpkin seeds have no particular merit, although they seem to be popular items in these types of products. They do contain protein, but they also all have a relatively high fat content, making it difficult to get desired protein without the calories that come with ingesting fat.

This analysis of only one of the many products of this type on the market points to our need to consider the real nutritional significance of the ingredients and the label claims before investing in products that may not be able to deliver the value we expect. The most important questions to ask are, " What does it contain?" "What are the merits of these ingredients?" "Do I need them?" and "Could I get them in a more palatable, less expensive form?" These same questions pertain to products directed to any segment of the population for any number of reasons. The motto "Caveat emptor" ("Let the buyer beware") is never more meaningful than when we evlauate nutritional supplements.

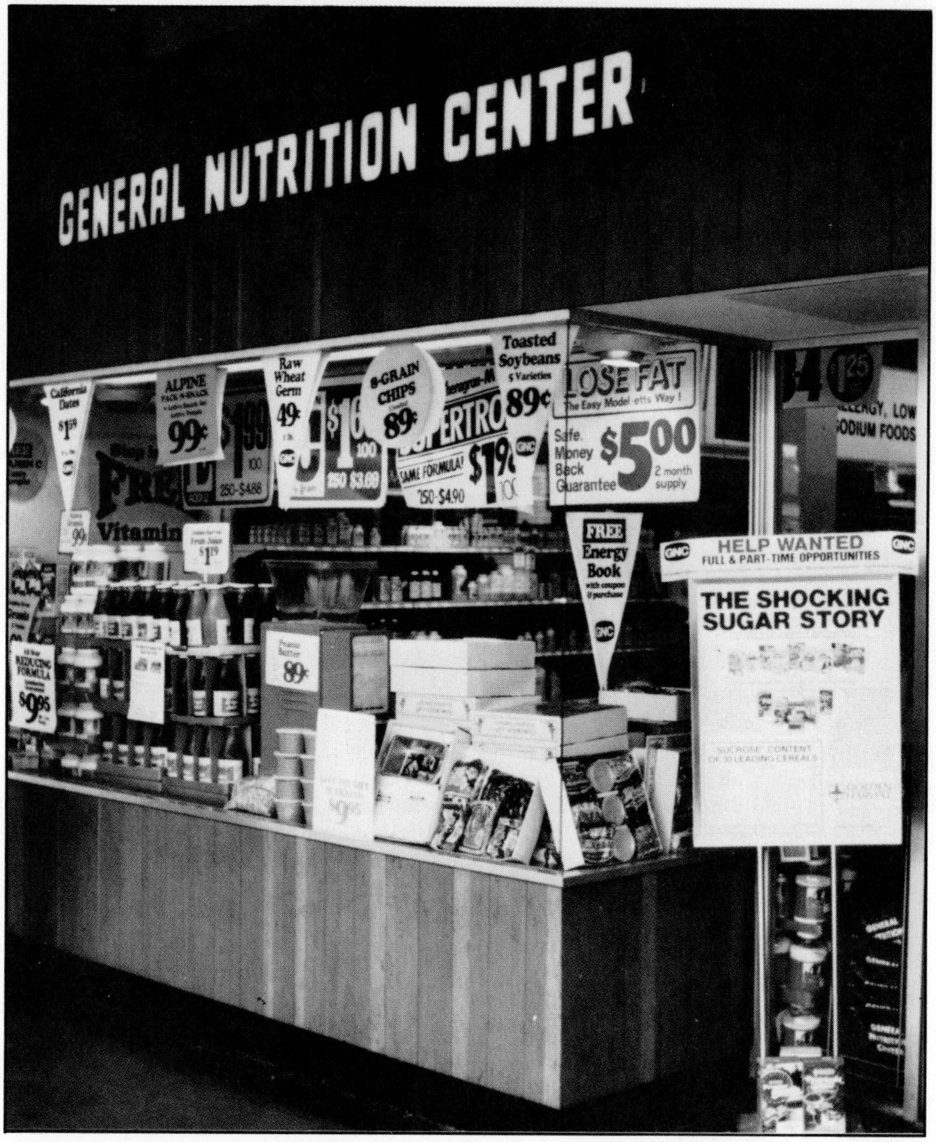

AWARENESS CHECK

Truth or Fiction?

- "Natural" on the label is well defined and regulated by the Food and Drug Administration.
- Vegans should take multiple vitamin or mineral supplements daily because they cannot get all the nutrients they need.
- Foods at health food stores may cost more than those from conventional grocery stores, but it is worth the price to know they are organically grown.
- Because so many nutrients are available in a wide variety of foods, there should be no nutritional problem from omitting one food group from an otherwise well-planned diet.

CHAPTER 20

Alternative Food Patterns

Concern over the safety of our food supply is increasing, and more and more people are questioning the ecological consequences of eating more animal foods than needed to meet nutrient needs. As a result, there is a trend toward the use of alternatives to conventional food and food patterns. Some of these alternatives are nutritionally sound and acceptable. Others, especially those that severely restrict the variety of foods used, may result in nutritionally limited diets. The booming health food industry is a questionable response to a legitimate concern. As a student of nutrition and also as a consumer, you will be called on to make judgments about many alternative food patterns. This chapter and other parts of the text are designed to give you a sufficient grasp of the principles of nutrition to help you make informed decisions.

The title "Alternative Food Patterns" has been chosen to convey the notion that there are many food patterns that lead to nutritionally adequate diets. Although some alternative food patterns represent faddism and quackery, many are good and are now finding wide acceptance by professionals and the public alike. They reflect a genuine concern about the quality of the food supply and the impact of nutrition on health. Of those that are not nutritionally sound, some are the result of attempts by unscrupulous, misdirected, or uninformed people to influence food practices for monetary gain. However, when the rationale for a food plan is founded on accepted scientific knowledge, the alternatives represent an acceptable answer to real or perceived shortcomings of conventional eating patterns. In many instances, it is hard to explain why some modifications in dietary practices are accepted with such fervor.

Reasons for Alternative Food Patterns
Distrust of food supply
Uncertainty about environment
Concern about health
Fear of additives
Antiestablishment motives

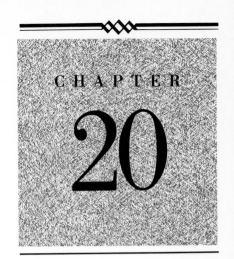

Those who choose alternatives to traditional or more conventional food patterns do so for a variety of reasons. They may be expressing antiestablishment sentiments; seeking "super health," notoriety, or truth; hoping for a miracle cure for a disease such as cancer; following fashions; expressing distrust of the food industry or the medical profession; or showing concern about uncertainties in their environment. Whatever the immediate motivation may be, any food behavior is the result of complex external influences such as friends, family, advertising, education, and availability of food and of internal influences such as attitudes, self-concepts, values, beliefs, and biological, psychological, and sociological needs. Regardless of why they are chosen, many alternative food patterns are a source of concern to nutritionists because of health, economic, and social implications.

Among the various diet patterns now enjoying popularity are vegetarian diets; ovolactovegetarian diets; macrobiotic, single-food diets; liquid diets; and natural, organic, or "health food" diets. Essentially, this is the same list we could have compiled 10 or 20 years ago, although some may have had different names then. The specifics change from year to year; however, the motivation to obtain special health-giving properties through the use of certain foods or the elimination of others remains unchanged. The resulting diets are not necessarily inadequate, but the chance of inadequacy increases as the number of foods in a diet decreases. An examination of trends in popular diets and beliefs confirms that there are few genuinely new approaches. Many "new diets" are merely revivals or slight modifications of old ones that were discarded earlier as ineffective, unpopular, unpalatable, or all three.

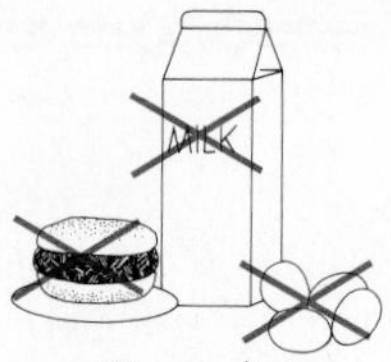

Vegan diet

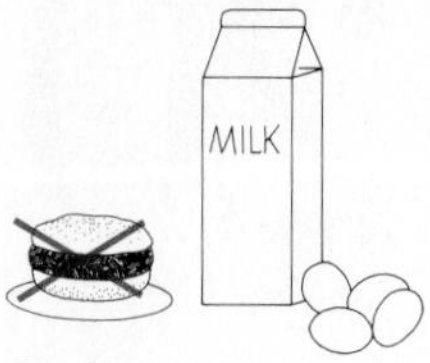

Ovolactovegetarian diet

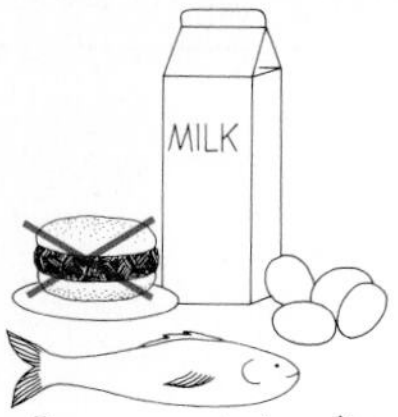

Pescovegetarian diet

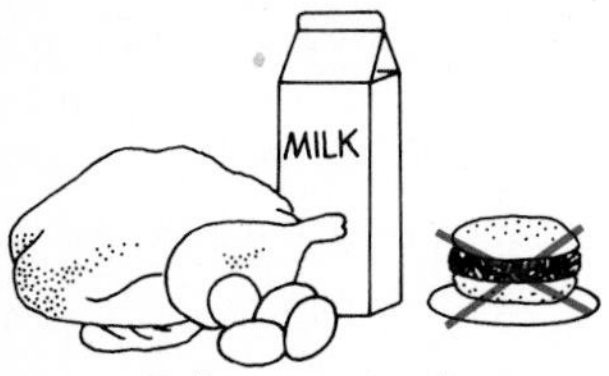

Pollovegetarian diet

Animal foods restricted or permitted on different kinds of vegetarian diets

VEGETARIANISM

The early 1970s saw a reemergence of interest in vegetarianism. Actually, vegetarianism has been practiced since biblical times as an alternative food pattern. It is estimated that about 1% of the population, most of whom are young and from middle-class and upper-class backgrounds, follow this diet to varying degrees for a variety of reasons—sometimes as individuals and sometimes in a communal setting. For some people, vegetarianism represents an aspect of religion or spiritual release and a way to purify the body. For others, it is a way to reject many aspects of affluent society, especially corporate influences. Some have a genuine concern over the wisdom, ethics, economy, esthetics, and safety of using animal products as a source of food; still others feel that a vegetarian diet can replace medicine in curing illness. For members of long-established religious groups (such as the Seventh Day Adventists), vegetarianism is an integral part of organized religion.

For more information on the aspects of vegetarian diets see *Focus,* Chapter 6.

Although vegetarianism is usually defined as the abstinence from meat, fish, and fowl, it also includes "true vegetarians," or vegans, who eat no animal products, including milk and eggs. An even more limited diet of fruit, honey, and nuts is used by a group known as fruitarians. Ovolactovegetarians, who eat eggs and milk in addition to foods of plant origin; pollovegetarians, who permit the use of poultry; and pescovegetarians, who permit the use of fish, are specific forms of vegetarianism. The 1980s has seen the rise of the "new vegetarians," who restrict their use of red meat to no more than once a week.

The nutritional adequacy or inadequacy of vegetarian diets varies with the type of diet, but for an adult only the very restricted pose any real health threat. On the positive side, vegetarian diets make it easier to achieve weight control, contain sufficient fiber to promote gastrointestinal motility, and may be associated with lower blood total and LDL cholesterol levels as a result of the intake of a plant sterol called sitosterol and limited saturated fat. Vegetarians also have a lower incidence of hypertension, diabetes, colon cancer, and possibly other problems such as osteoporosis, kidney stones, and diverticulosis. On the other hand, infants and children raised as vegans are at higher risk of anemia, rickets, and growth retardation than are those fed a more varied diet of both animal and plant foods. Lactating women and people recovering from illness can meet their needs on an ovolactovegetarian diet, but not on a vegan diet.

Macrobiotic Diets

Macrobiotic diets are vegetarian diets based on a balance of foods with "yin" (weak) and "yang" (strong) characteristics. Macrobiotic diets consist mostly of whole grains and vegetables but include the use of special teas, herbs, seaweed, and fermented soybean products. Most adherents to this diet participate in a variety of spiritual rituals and eat at least one daily meal in a communal setting. An extreme form is the Zen macrobiotic diet, which requires its followers to proceed in 7 to 10 steps to reduce the number and kinds of foods in the diet until a balance of "strong" and "weak" foods is achieved and finally only brown rice is consumed. Followers believe that any disease can be cured with this diet. Although such a diet is lacking in vitamins, calcium, and high-quality protein, the lack of vitamin C is the first deficiency to develop. Scurvy has been reported among those who adhere to the regimen, especially pregnant women and young children. The restricted fluid intake designed to "spare" the kidneys represents an additional hazard because this diet is high in sodium, which increases thirst and a need for fluid. The use of seawater (with its high salt content) to alleviate thirst only serves to make the problem worse.

Yin Foods	Yang Foods	Neutral Foods
Pork	Beef	Rice
Potatoes	Tomatoes	Noodles
Grains	Peanuts	Sugar

Single-Food Diets

Food patterns that restrict food intake to a single item or a limited number of foods lead to nutritional inadequacies. Even a food that is recognized as an important source of a nutrient should not be used as the sole source of nourishment. Spinach, with its high oxalic acid content, may prove toxic; orange juice, devoid of protein, will not support growth; and milk, low in iron, leads to anemia. All these foods, if used alone, will have severe health consequences. However, they make significant contributions as part of a balanced diet.

Many of the diets containing only one or two food items are promoted as weight-reducing aids. Such diets usually achieve that goal primarily because their monotony results in a restricted food intake. However, they are invariably deficient in several nutrients, and the longer they are used, the greater the risks. These diets also fail because they do not train people in a new, socially acceptable set of eating habits, thus providing no long-range solution to weight gain.

NATURAL (HEALTH FOOD) DIETS

The terms "health foods" and "natural foods" are used broadly and inconsistently, largely because they are undefined. Thus so-called health food diets do not fall into a set pattern. In general, people who follow them eat only food that they believe has been grown on unfertilized soil or soil fertilized with organic fertilizers and has not been subjected to any treatments with chemicals during growth, harvesting, or processing. Food that meets these criteria is expensive to produce and is usually sold either in small retail stores or mail-order outlets with a relatively small volume of business. The number of health food stores has increased sevenfold in the last two decades, to close to 7000 in the United States alone. Their annual sales are in excess of $1.5 billion.

Some foods reported to be "organically grown" are sold in stores that are part of national chains that can be found in almost any shopping mall. Many grocery stores now have a section designated "health foods," offering items such as unsweetened applesauce, yogurt, water-packed tuna, oat bran, tofu, brown rice, unsulfured raisins, and lowfat cheese also often available in conventional food stores. As can be seen in the margin, prices for conventional foods at a health food store compared to a conventional store are variable. They are sometimes the same, sometimes lower, but often higher. If items are actually made without chemical preservatives or additives, they may have very poor "keeping" qualities. Bread

Health Food Store Prices Relative to Conventional Store Prices

Brown rice	+ 77%	(that is, 77% higher)
Tofu	− 2%	
Cream cheese	+ 104%	
Bananas	+ 147%	
Tomatoes	+ 33%	
Raisins	+ 45%	
Honey	+ 24%	

From Journal of the American Dietetic Association 83:286, 1983.

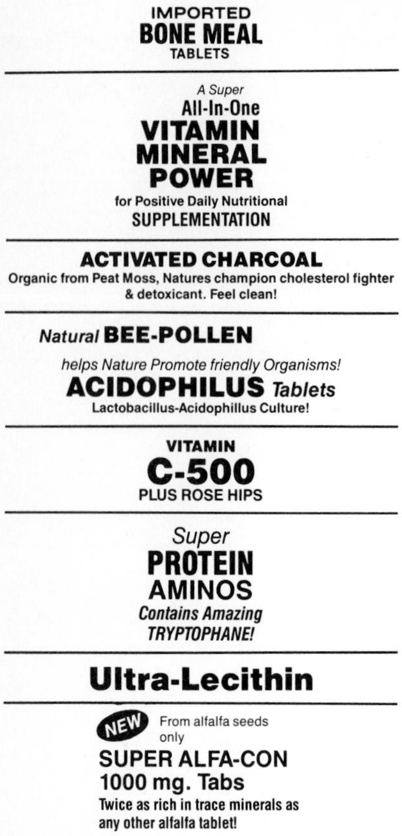

IMPORTED
BONE MEAL
TABLETS
A Super
All-In-One
VITAMIN
MINERAL
POWER
for Positive Daily Nutritional
SUPPLEMENTATION
ACTIVATED CHARCOAL
Organic from Peat Moss, Natures champion cholesterol fighter & detoxicant. Feel clean!
Natural BEE-POLLEN
helps Nature Promote friendly Organisms!
ACIDOPHILUS Tablets
Lactobacillus-Acidophillus Culture!
VITAMIN
C-500
PLUS ROSE HIPS
Super
PROTEIN
AMINOS
Contains Amazing
TRYPTOPHANE!
Ultra-Lecithin
NEW
From alfalfa seeds only
SUPER ALFA-CON
1000 mg. Tabs
Twice as rich in trace minerals as any other alfalfa tablet!

Figure 20-1 A composite of items offered for sale in a health food store.

without a mold inhibitor will become moldy in 1 or 2 days at room temperature, and almost as fast when refrigerated. Oil without either a natural or added antioxidant becomes rancid quickly if unrefrigerated, and unpreserved whole wheat may be more susceptible to insect infestation.

As illustrated in Figure 20-1, the health food store inventory also includes many other less traditional "health foods" such as carrot powder, alfalfa, alfalfa concentrates, rose hips, miracle wafers, amino acid tablets, royal jelly, millet, special formula tablets of natural vitamins and minerals, bone meal, brewer's yeast, desiccated liver, fish-liver oil, kelp, parsley, and iron. For many health food items, there is little information on nutritive content, but Table 20-1 provides some representative data.

If animal foods are to meet the usual criteria for health foods, they should come from livestock raised only on nonchemically treated feed and given no antibiotics, hormones, or other growth-stimulating chemicals. "Natural" eggs are usually fertile, and milk is unpasteurized. The safety of food that is produced and processed to meet these criteria is questionable; there is no reason to believe that such food is either more or less nutritious than other food.

In assessing the merits of natural, or organic, foods, several facts should be kept in mind. First, the elements in a fertilizer must be in an inorganic form, separated from organic material, before a plant can use them. When organic fertilizer is used, separation is usually accomplished by bacteria or microorganisms in the soil. Organic fertilizers provide only the elements excreted by the animal, which in turn got them from the food it consumed. Therefore, an animal grazing on crops grown on depleted soil recycles a manure that is also deficient in trace elements. Second, even if organically grown food were established as being superior, most Western countries are incapable of providing the quantity of organic fertilizer needed to use on the vast acreage devoted to food production. It is even questionable that the relatively small amount of food now sold as organically grown could have been produced this way. In addition, because weeds and pests are often controlled

Table 20-1 ◇ Nutritive content of 28 grams (1 oz) of foods featured in health food stores

Food	kcal	Protein (g)	Calcium (mg)	Iron (mg)	Thiamin (mg)	Riboflavin (mg)	Vitamin C (mg)	Vitamin A (IU)
Brown rice	102	2.1	3	0.2	0.04	0.01	0	0
Sunflower seeds	140	6.0	30	2.8	0.5	0.06	0	0
Dried apples	22	0.1	3	0.1	—	0.01	Trace	—
Soya beans	36	3.0	20	0.7	0.1	0.2	0	8
Wheat germ	104	7.6	20	2.6	0.42	0.2	0	0
Pumpkin seeds	180	9.8	11	3.3	0.06	0.04	0	20
Natural seaweed	104	0.4	252	2.6	0.003	0.07	0	—
Honey	90	Trace	6	0.2	Trace	Trace	1	0
Carob flour	51	1.2	99	—	—	—	—	—
Sesame seeds	163	5.0	28	0.7	0.1	0.04	0	—
Blackstrap molasses	43	—	116	2.3	0.5	0.5	—	—
Soybean sprouts	13	1.7	13	2.3	0.06	—	4	22
Desiccated liver	120	28	10	6	0.2	4.4	70	0
Wheat bran	100	4	—	—	0.19	1.0	—	—
Tofu	20	2.2	36	0.5	0.02	0.008	0	0
Brewer's yeast	78	11	78	5.0	4.0	1.2	—	—
Alfalfa sprouts	10	1.0	0	0.4	0.02	0.02	—	200
Miso	48	3.0	19	0.5	0.02	0.03	0	11.2
Bulgur wheat	47	1.7	6	0.4	0.01	Trace	0	0
Granola*	140	4	20	1.1	0.17	0.07	0	0

*Content varies greatly depending on ingredients.

manually in organic farming, labor costs are high and quality quite often low. The contention that organically grown food tastes better may be supportable, especially if it is locally produced and marketed; it may also be fresher than much food available through regular channels. As we discussed earlier, people who begin to eat this food often do feel better as a result of having changed and improved their total diets and life-styles rather than as a function of a specific "organic" or "natural" food.

Many people who adhere to "health or natural food diets" engage in intermittent fasts that can last from 1 to 30 days. They believe that fasting cleanses the digestive system, gives the organs a rest, purges the body of any toxins, and creates a heightened awareness. Fasting is dangerous and should be confined to situations where there is competent medical supervision. Drastic changes in food intake are bound to stress the body's adaptive capabilities.

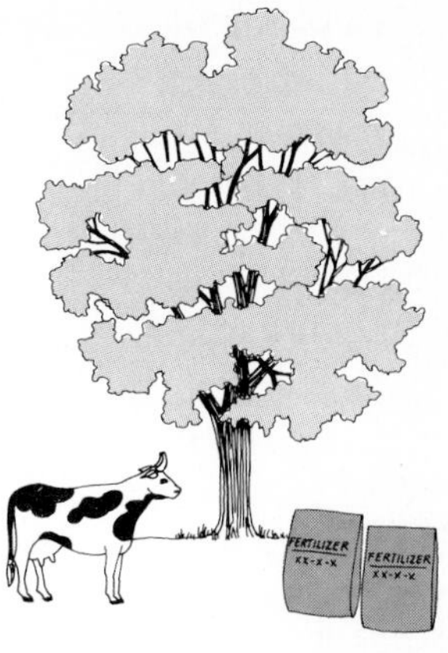

Plants are equally well nourished with either chemical or organic fertilizers

FOOD-NUTRIENT SUPPLEMENTS

Nutritionists and other health professionals are increasingly concerned about the health consequences of the trend toward using both nutrient and nonnutrient supplements. The promotion and sale of nutrient supplements is a rapidly growing and profitable business estimated at $3 billion annually with projected sales that may top $10 billion by 1990. Products are readily available to all segments of the population. They are being offered through many channels, including direct door-to-door sales; mail-order catalogs; and drug, grocery, department, and special "health food" stores.

The products are marketed or distributed either as private label brands or as well-recognized brands of reputable pharmaceutical houses. They are sold variously as multinutrient supplements, ranging from those containing rational, well-balanced, moderate-level formulas to those with high-potency and often irrational formulations; as megadoses of single nutrients; as other nonnutrient factors including RNA, rutin, and hesperidin; and as food-based products such as parsley tablets, powdered mangos, and kelp. The use and promotion of these supplements are generally based on unrealistic expectations or implied, unsubstantiated claims of their effectiveness, sometimes with endorsement from authority figures such as athletes, movie stars, or self-styled health experts. Use of these products is seldom based on an evaluation of nutrient needs or a realistic assessment of the health benefits or hazards associated with them.

The extensive popularity of food-nutrient supplements is the result of many factors. Nutrition educators have created an awareness of the role of nutrition in health promotion and in the treatment and prevention of deficiency diseases. At the same time, educators have failed to provide adequate assurance that nutritional needs can be met with a diet of foods that are available through traditional channels, chosen by informed consumers. In addition, public confidence in the nutritional quality of our food supply is being eroded by a number of vocal individuals who claim that processed foods have greatly reduced nutrient content and that depleted soils are incapable of yielding nutritious crops. Many people, hearing this, turn to supplements as a form of nutritional insurance to compensate for perceived deficiencies.

For more discussion of nutrient supplements, see Chapter 13.

For further information on hair analysis, see *Focus,* Chapter 11.

A food-nutrient supplement industry usually thrives in affluent populations, where people can afford to buy nonfood items; in "pill-oriented" societies, where people attribute almost magical properties to supplements; or in cultures where the prevailing philosophy is "if a little is good, a lot is better." Many people are attracted to the use of supplements by unscientific but authoritative-looking itemizations of needs based on analyses of hair samples, dietary profiles, or even problem-oriented questionnaires.

Concerns about the growing dependence of some people on self-directed supplementation can be categorized at three levels: low, moderate, and high. At the

Health Frauds—Not Miracles
Herbal teas
Vitamin B_{17}
Bee pollen
Protein tablets
Lecithin
Ornithine
Flavonoids
Pangamic acid
Glandular extracts
DNA
Raw milk

Some items sold as dietary supplements may be potential poisons when used in amounts greater than advised. These include:
Selenium
Zinc
Iron
Vitamin A
Dolomite
Laetrile

level of lowest concern is the economic waste involved in the use of unnecessary supplements that will be harmlessly excreted but will definitely not provide the expected benefits. Some ingredients such as rutin do not have any known nutritional function or chemical identity, while others such as dextrose or lecithin seldom if ever need to be supplied separately. Many formulas with an irrational mixture of components mislead the user into believing that all the nutrients in a long list of ingredients are present at equally effective dosages. Many people who use nutrient supplements become complacent about their nutritional status, feeling that they no longer need to have any responsibility for or concern about selecting a varied diet. Because product quality may not be monitored, a consumer has no assurance that a particular supplement is accurately labeled, either in terms of nutrient amounts or sources (natural or synthetic).

Issues of a moderate level of concern include the possibilities that people may have unrealistic and unfounded expectations of the health benefits of a product; that they may delay seeking competent medical treatment for a health problem while using a self-selected supplement; that products may be contaminated (for example, the lead content of dolomite); that interaction among nutrients within a supplement may result in loss of biological activity of one or more ingredients (for example, the interaction between vitamin D and calcium salts) or the production of an analog with antinutrient activity (for example, vitamin B_{12} analogs reported to be produced in the presence of vitamin C or iron); and that people will combine single supplements in such a way that undesirable nutrient interactions or imbalances will be created.

High-level concerns are directed toward the unknown or dangerous consequences of using inappropriately high levels of nutrients (for example, the oxalate excretion that results from high intakes of vitamin C). Of additional concern are the development of a nutrient dependency, with a rebound deficiency as a result of rapid withdrawal of high intakes; the possibility of toxic reactions to high intakes of nutrients such as trace elements and fat-soluble vitamins, for which the range of individual sensitivity to high levels is wide and the spread between requirements and toxic levels is small; and the known effects of imbalances of trace elements on the absorption, metabolism, and excretion of other elements (for example, the relationship between copper and iron or zinc and calcium).

Types of Products

"Shotgun" Formulas

Products characterized as shotgun formulas may list as many as 50 different nutrients on the label; this is designed to impress the gullible consumer, who presumably is awed by the range of items included. Some of these are nutrients for which RDAs have been established; others are those that are known to be essential but for which no requirements have been established; and still others are harmless but of no recognized nutritional significance. Of those known to be required, some will be present at many times the recommended level in shotgun formulas, whereas others will be present in insignificant amounts. The formulation of two products—one a vitamin, the other a vitamin/mineral supplement—exemplifies the problem (Table 20-2). The mixtures are obviously irrational both nutritionally and physiologically, providing from 12% to 5000% of the RDA for different nutrients, but they may seem impressive from the point of view of the uninformed consumer.

"Loaded" Formulas

The term "loaded formula" is applied to the high-potency product that competes with products from rival companies by providing more of a nutrient. One company simply adds more of a nutrient for a very insignificant difference in price than does its competitor. Average consumers do not realize that they merely excrete excess amounts of water-soluble vitamins and, more importantly, that they may develop

Table 20-2 ◇ Formulation of two typical over-the-counter nutrient supplements

Product A ("Shotgun" Formulas)	Content	Percentage of Adult RDA	Product B ("Loaded" Formulas)	Content	Percentage of Adult RDA
Vitamin A	10,000 IU	250	B_1 (Thiamine mononitrate)	50 mg	5000
Vitamin D	400 IU	100	B_2 (Riboflavin)	50 mg	4000
Vitamin C	300 mg	500	B_6 (Pyridoxine hydrochloride)	50 mg	2500
Vitamin E	30 IU	350	B_{12} (Cyanocobalamin)	100 μg	3300
Vitamin B_1	15 mg	1500	Folacin	400 μg	100
Vitamin B_2	10 mg	800	Biotin	400 μg	200
Vitamin B_6	10 mg	500	Pantothenic acid (D-Calcium pantothenate)	100 mg	1400
Vitamin B_{12}	5 μg	160			
Folacin	400 μg	100	Niacinamide	300 mg	2500
Biotin	200 μg	100			
Niacinamide	100 mg	900			
Calcium pantothenate	20 mg	300			
Iron	15 mg	150			
Calcium	100 mg	12			
Iodine	0.15 mg	50			
Magnesium	75 mg	25			
Zinc	15 mg	100			
Copper	1 mg	33			
Manganese	1 mg	20			

toxic reactions from excessive levels of fat-soluble vitamins or trace mineral elements.

In 1973, the FDA introduced legislation that would limit the number of nutrients that could be used in dietary supplements to those for which need had been demonstrated. In addition, it tried to establish limits that would ensure an effective but nontoxic dose of any nutrient. Unfortunately, a powerful lobby headed by the National Health Federation succeeded in promoting the passage of a legislative amendment that prohibited the FDA from limiting the potency, number, combinations, or variety of any synthetic or natural vitamin, mineral, other nutritional substance, or ingredient of any nutritional supplement, unless the amount recommended was found to be injurious to health. The FDA has a policy of limiting amounts in nutrient supplements to include from 50% to 150% of the U.S. RDA for children under 12 and for pregnant and lactating women, and it requires that multinutrient supplements contain a certain list of nutrients. However, as a result of the amendment, the FDA has no authority to enforce these standards.

Technically, all supplements are considered "food for special dietary purposes." If a health claim is made, the supplement is classified either as an illegal food (if the claim is not approved) or as an over-the-counter drug (if it is approved). In no case does the FDA have control over the amount of a nutrient that may be included in a supplement, although the supplement must be accurately labeled. It is the responsibility of the producer to provide evidence that the product is safe and effective, rather than for the FDA to prove that it is unsafe. Any printed material displayed close to the product is considered labeling and must accurately represent the product. The only regulatory control that is available to the FDA is to establish that a certain level of supplementation is toxic. So far, they have not chosen to do this.

Protein Supplements

The use of protein supplements by the North American population, which already has adequate protein, is a questionable practice. One firm cast doubts on the adequacy of protein in the U.S. diet to create a large market for its protein pills,

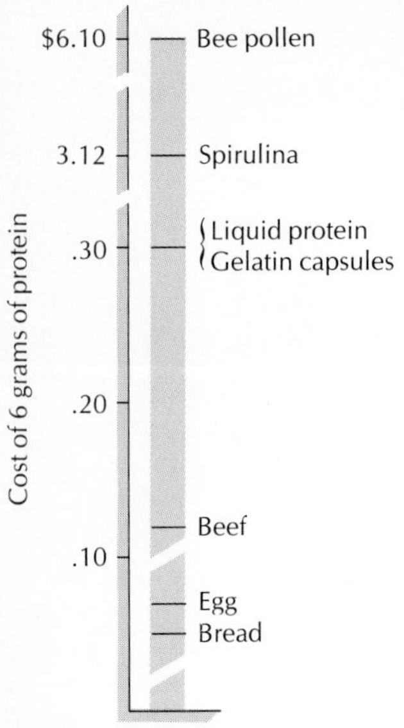

Relative cost of 6 grams of protein from traditional and nontraditional food sources

each of which contained 728 mg of protein. There are 20 grams of protein in one serving of meat; it would require 28 pills of one supplement at a cost of 25¢ per pill, or $7.00, to provide the protein of the meat serving. Liquid protein diets made from hydrolyzed collagen provide protein at a cost of 30¢/20-gram portion. This can be compared to costs of 12¢ to 69¢ from conventional food sources that are more palatable and safer and that provide other nutrients in addition to protein. Reports of deaths after the use of these products have resulted in label warnings that they can be dangerous. Powdered protein supplements, composed primarily of casein or soy protein, are not hazardous but are equally unnecessary.

More recently there has been an upsurge in the promotion of supplements of single amino acids. These are advocated for concerns ranging from the control of fever blisters, the promotion of normal sleep patterns, the improvement in body building, and the control of mood. Because a high intake of one amino acid interferes with the utilization of another, any use of single amino acids is potentially dangerous.

If the amount of money spent in the United States on dietary supplements, which are used by 75% of all households, were really an indication of the nation's nutritional need, one would conclude that we must be the most poorly nourished nation in the world. Obviously, this is not the case. However, as long as the power of the FDA to control the abuse of nutrient supplementation continues to be restricted, there is little hope that the growth of the health food and supplement business will be curbed or controlled.

Orthomolecular (Megavitamin) Therapy

Passage of the Proxmire Amendment, limiting the power of the FDA to regulate the potency of nutrient supplements, has removed any barrier to megavitamin, or **orthomolecular (megavitamin) therapy.** In orthomolecular therapy, massive doses of vitamins and excessively high intakes of minerals are administered to cure a whole host of human illnesses, ranging from the common cold to senility, from schizophrenia to sexual impotence. Because vitamins act primarily as coenzymes in the release of energy or in the synthesis or degradation of body compounds, amounts needed are determined by whether or not these reactions are taking place. Any excess must either be stored, excreted, or used for some nonvitamin function, in which case it would be considered a drug rather than a nutrient. In the case of minerals, which are needed in very small amounts, excesses may lead to serious internal imbalances and may impair rather than improve functioning.

orthomolecular (megavitamin) therapy Treatment that involves the use of vitamins at levels 10 to 1000 times the recommended amounts.

Although unfounded claims for a product cannot be made at the point of purchase, either on the label or in close proximity to the product, there are no restrictions on information that can be printed in the popular press and trade magazines or on the content of radio and television talk shows, where many claims for megadoses of nutrients are made. It should be noted, however, that in some cases, supervised megavitamin or orthomolecular therapy has been beneficial in the treatment of disease.

Because this therapy has been used only recently, we have little accumulated information from either animal or human studies on which to judge potential hazards. With the increasing number of people using supplements well in excess of recommended levels, it is reasonable to expect additional metabolic and possibly druglike problems in the future.

Naturopathy and iridology are two other treatments of medical conditions that have nutritional implications. In the former, practiced by graduates of unaccredited schools, plants and herbs alone or in combination with physical manipulation is used to "rid the body of toxins." Even though the herbs may contain only small amounts of the "active ingredient," this amount may be toxic. Additionally, herb products are poorly and inaccurately labeled. Iridology involves making nutritional diagnoses on the basis of a visual judgment relating to the color, texture, and location of various pigment flecks in the eye—a totally unacceptable method.

FOOD MISINFORMATION

It is becoming increasingly clear that promoters of food supplements, with their strongly emotional appeals, exaggerated claims, and powers of persuasion, are undermining the teaching of legitimate nutritionists. So far, the latter have had little success in competing with faddists, mostly because of their unwillingness to misrepresent or distort scientific knowledge by making unrealistic or unsubstantiated claims. It is understandable when uninformed people are easily influenced by fads; it is more difficult to fathom when others, with ready access to sound scientific information in the field, also become victims of faddism. The forces that operate to keep food faddism alive are a complex mixture of economic, sociocultural, emotional, and educational factors.

In addition to attacking the problem of food fads, the nutritionist is constantly dealing with food misinformation. The latter problem is often more difficult to fight, because it ranges from scientific half-truths, distortions, or misrepresentations of scientific information, to outright fallacies and untruths. Food quacks pretend to have information they do not possess, perpetrate their ideas or products on large groups, and are usually motivated by personal financial gain. If confronted with arguments that discredit them, quacks frequently abandon one food fad and espouse another with equal fervor.

The FDA believes that millions of Americans are being bilked by vendors of books and special devices that claim to solve the nutritional ills of the country. If a comparable amount were spent on improved food intakes, both the consumer and the food industry would benefit. Such a large expenditure of money on unnecessary supplementation is possible only in an affluent society; it reflects the health consciousness of the nation and our eternal quest for a longer and healthier life. Although food quackery was once confined to technically developed countries that enjoyed a high standard of living, it is now infiltrating some developing countries, which have no surplus resources to waste on unethical and ineffective panaceas.

Nature of Food Fads

Food fads follow several prescribed patterns, usually stressing a food concept rather than a nutrient concept. A discussion of these patterns follows.

Exaggeration of the Virtues of a Particular Food

Many fads revolve around the belief that specific foods have almost magical medicinal properties—usually in the cure of conditions for which medical science has produced no effective control or cure. Among the more common beliefs are that fruits cure cancer, carrot juice relieves leukemia, and royal jelly delays old age and leads to sexual rejuvenation. It is interesting to note that different cultures ascribe different properties to the same food. For example, the tomato is considered poisonous in some cultures, an aphrodisiac in others, and a cancer cure in still others. The folk belief that honey and vinegar cures ailments ranging from warts to hypertension to cataracts was popularized in a book by a New England physician; it is a relatively innocuous cure that has been promoted from time to time in other cultures. Of greater concern is the promotion as a cancer cure of laetrile (vitamin B_{17}), a potentially toxic cyanide compound found primarily in apricot pits.

Typical "Health Foods"
Wheat germ
Blackstrap molasses
Carob
Honey
Alfalfa sprouts
Unsulfured raisins
Bulgur wheat
Brown eggs
Seaweed

Food quacks constantly refer to the "secret formula" of a product, to which they attribute its special merits. In one example, the secret formula was alfalfa, ground bones, and the germ from cereal products; in another it was garlic, lecithin, and wheat germ; and in still another dried nonfat milk, sold at greatly inflated prices, was the special formula.

The labeling on a product may also purposely be misleading. For example, 10-mg capsules of gelatin promoted to strengthen fingernails bore a listing of the percentage of total protein, represented by 17 different amino acids; their names would give the average consumer the impression that the gelatin was highly nutritious. However, the fact that the whole capsule provided about 0.0014% of the day's protein requirement was not pointed out.

Avoidance of Foods

The omission of certain foods in the diet can be as much a food fad as the exaggerated use of other foods. The notion that any food enriched with nutrients (referred to in this context as "chemicals") is poisonous has led to the rejection of such staples in the diet as enriched white bread or milk fortified with vitamin D. The belief in a relationship between fruit and fever has led to the exclusion of fruit.

Many natural-food organizations with very impressive, "authoritative" names perpetuate the philosophy that all mental and metabolic diseases are caused by commercially processed foods. In several instances, the president of an organization or the editor of its publication has turned out to be the owner of a natural-food store that provides the kinds of foods advocated.

Avoidance of Chemicals in Food

The Delaney Clause, which is an amendment to the Food, Drug and Cosmetic Act, requires the FDA to ban the use of any substance in food for which there is any evidence, from animal or human studies, of possible carcinogenicity at any level. This clause has resulted in a ban on several coloring materials that had previously been considered safe, which in turn has led to a general distrust of any additives in foods. Some people have developed a complete disregard of the essential role of some additives in maintaining the food supply. Their fear is further compounded by the fact that many additives have awesome and mysterious names such as calcium silicate, butylated hydroxytoluene, and monostearate. These names are meaningless to most consumers but (understandably) imply something "chemical" and therefore undesirable.

The FDA is constantly seeking the help of the scientific community in assessing the safety of chemicals that appear intentionally or incidentally in the food supply. Without those chemicals that serve as preservatives (such as salt and propionate), that prevent botulism (such as nitrites), or that provide color and give foods an acceptable appearance (such as the carotene used in butter), the food supply would be costly, much less safe, and unacceptable in color, flavor, and texture.

Although there is a real need to be assured of the safety of additives, it is unrealistic to promote a total ban on their use. Instead there should be a constant monitoring of their safety, both individually and in conjunction with other additives. Many "additives," such as nitrites used in curing meats, are also formed in the body when naturally occurring nitrates found in vegetables such as beets, celery, carrots, and spinach are converted to nitrites by bacteria in the digestive tract. Nitrites from either source can react with amines in the intestinal tract to form nitrosamines, which are known carcinogens.

Antioxidants may either be naturally occurring substances such as vitamin E or added chemicals that are used to prevent rancidity and the formation of carcinogenic substances from unsaturated fats. Other additives serve to inhibit mold and bacterial growth, increase shelf life, enhance flavor, and improve color. Although they have become an integral part of our food processing system, additives must be constantly evaluated. Table 20-3 summarizes information on the functions of some additives.

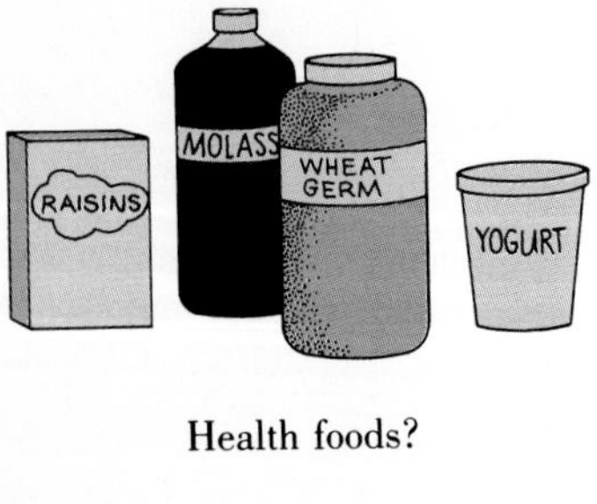

Health foods?

In apparent contradiction to the belief that chemicals in food should be avoided, the same stores selling unprocessed natural foods have shelves stacked with bottles of lecithin granules, vitamin E, selenium, protein powder, and tocopherol, often in megadose units. This gives the impression that health food advocates approve of feeding nutrients (that is, chemicals) to human beings directly but disapprove of using them as fertilizer to nourish plants that will subsequently be eaten!

Table 20-3 ◇ Role of some common additives in food

Additive	Function	Examples of Products
Agar	Stabilizer, thickener	Ice cream, whipped cream
Algin	Alginic acid stabilizer, thickener	Ice cream, cheese, yogurt
Alpha-tocopherol	Antioxidant, nutrient (vitamin E)	Cereals, oils, potato chips
Aluminum sulfate	Firming agent	
Ammonium chloride	Dough conditioner	Baked products
Autolyzed yeast	Flavor enhanced, nutrient (protein)	
Benzoate of soda	Antimicrobial agent	Margarine, fruit products
BHA, BHT	Antioxidants	Cereals, vegetable oils
Calcium lactate	Acidity controller for dough	Bread, cake filling
Carrageenan	Stabilizer, thickener	Ice cream, chocolate milk
Diglycerides	Emulsifier	Peanut butter, cereal
Disodium EDTA	Antioxidant, sequestrant	Dressings, sauces
Guar gum	Stabilizer, thickener	Beverages, salad dressing
Magnesium stearate	Anticaking agent	Candies
Modified starch	Thickener	Baby food
Pectin	Stabilizer, thickener	Fruit jellies
Polyethylene glycol	Emulsifier, stabilizer	Baked goods
Potassium sorbate	Antimicrobial agent	Cheeses, syrups
Sodium hydroxide	Acidity control	Black olives
Stearic acid	Emulsifier	Chewing gum
Sulfur dioxide	Antimicrobial agent, antioxidant	Sliced fruit, grape juice

From "Shopper's Guide to Commonly Used Food Ingredients," with the permission of Patricia Thorney and Carole Bisogni, Cornell Cooperative Extension, Cornell University, Ithaca, NY, 1983

Besides health food stores, there are health food farms, located in pastoral settings uncontaminated by herbicides, pesticides, and chemical fertilizers; some enthusiasts travel to them for the "privilege" of paying two or three times the regular grocery price for various products. (Practically all of these outlets also offer mail-order service.)

Special equipment for food preparation has been another lucrative approach for the food quack. This equipment is often demonstrated at fairs, summer resorts, arcades, department stores, or invitational parties in private homes. Promoters rely heavily on impulse buying. They attribute a wide range of merits to the equipment, such as increasing the consumption of fruits and vegetables, eliminating poisons from foods, conserving vitamins, or incorporating oxygen into food.

Mode of Operation of the Quack

Merchandising Approaches of Quacks
Public lecturers
Special equipment
Mail-order books
Pyramid sales

Food quacks create a market for their products or ideas by making a variety of highly emotional appeals. Besides capitalizing on some people's fear of being made helpless through illness, the quack provides a crutch for people with organic and psychic ailments. Quacks undermine the public's faith in the adequacy of the nation's food supply. They suggest that available foods are incapable of providing essential nutrients and claim that certain substances used in food production and processing endanger health and lead to many negative consequences. Although the indiscriminate use of some substances is unwise, there is no reason to condemn all substances at every level.

Quacks contend that all disease is caused by faulty diet, that the population suffers from widespread malnutrition, that food processing destroys the nutritive value of foods, and that soil depletion is an underlying cause of faulty diets. Because of these statements, quacks are able to create such a fear of sickness in their victims that it is very easy for them to sell their panaceas. They describe imaginary illnesses in such vague terms as "roundness of corpuscles," "tired blood," and "vitagenic," which are meaningless but have scientific overtones.

Food quacks frequently pose as members of legitimate-sounding professional organizations. It is unrealistic to expect the general public to know that the American Institute of Nutrition is an organization of recognized nutrition scientists, whereas the American Academy of Applied Nutrition and the American Nutrition Society are both nonscientific organizations. Many of these unrecognized organizations publish their own monthly journals with "scientific" articles by members. The authors naturally tend to support the use of products sold in outlets that are connected with the organizations or advertised as available by mail from their catalogs. Even reputable scientific groups have at times been temporarily misled into accepting these organizations as scientific.

Quacks promote themselves partly by using self-conferred titles such as "world-renowned nutritionist," "dietician" (as opposed to the correct "dietitian"), "international authority," and "certified metabolic technician." To further confuse the situation, those who have earned degrees that qualify them to use the title of "Doctor" have occasionally been diverted into the lucrative business of food faddism. Others have bought their degrees by mail-order houses from so-called **degree mills.** By quoting scientific data completely out of context or by inappropriately applying the findings from animal studies to humans, they are able to create an illusion of scientific expertise.

degree mills
Organizations that award degrees without requiring students to meet any educational standards; Donsbach University is one giving such degrees in nutrition

The faddist is quick to capitalize on new scientific developments, cleverly using them to market a product and turn it into a profitable venture. For example, the promoters of safflower oil, which is high in polyunsaturated fatty acids, were able for a short period of time to convince the public to buy it at the drugstore in 1100-mg capsules at 6¢ each, or approximately $25/quart, because it was found to aid in reducing blood cholesterol levels. The same product was available in the grocery store at 80¢/quart. Similarly, the ingredients in one widely distributed pill that sold for 12¢ each were found to be the same as those in half a cent's worth of dried nonfat milk solids, whereas 10 cents' worth of gelatin packaged in capsules sells for $2. Fish oil capsules often containing an inexpensive menhaden oil are a more recent promotion.

Characteristics of a Quack

If any of the following claims are made by those promoting diets or food plans, quackery can be suspected.

1. Claims that the food they are promoting has miraculous powers, usually in curing conditions that are still baffling medical science (such as arthritis, leukemia, and arteriosclerosis). Faddists usually claim to have information that is unavailable through regular medical channels.
2. Claims that they are being persecuted by medical "trusts and cartels" whose livelihood would be threatened by the success of the fad product.
3. Claims that the soil is depleted and no longer capable of supplying enough good-quality food to meet the nutritional needs of the population; solutions usually are limited to the use of food supplements or the exclusive use of "nutritious" foods grown in soil fertilized only with organic fertilizers.
4. Claims that practically everyone is suffering from some degree of malnutrition that cannot possibly be corrected by foods readily available; this is attributed to the following dietary habits:
   - Use of pasteurized rather than raw milk
   - Use of nonfertile rather than fertile eggs
   - Ingestion of "mixed meals" (that is, a variety of foods that are supposedly harmful if eaten together)
   - Use of canned fruits and vegetables

Common Misconceptions About Quackery

- Quackery is easy to spot.
- Personal experience is the best way to tell whether something works.
- Most victims of quackery are gullible.
- Quackery's victims deserve what they get.
- Quacks are frauds and crooks.
- Most quackery is promoted by quacks.
- Most quackery is dangerous.
- "Minor" forms of quackery are harmless.
- The media are reliable.
- Advertising outlets are ethical.
- Education is the answer.
- The government protects us.
- Quackery's success represents medicine's failure.
- Quackery is medicine's responsibility.
- The American Medical Association has the power to stop quackery.
- Fighting quackery is hopeless.
- Fighting quackery is risky.

Reprinted with permission from Steven Barrett, Nutrition Forum, 4:41, 1987.

Use of white flour, rather than freshly milled whole grains or sprouted grains
Use of refined sugars
Use of plant foods of all types grown on impoverished soils
Use of chemically pure or synthetic vitamins
Use of chemically contaminated foodstuff resulting from such substances as pesticides (addition to fluorine to water supplies is also opposed)

5. Claims that testimonials and anecdotal evidence are adequate support of their product.

Methods of Merchandising

Although food quacks can be found in the mainstream food-marketing business, they have often tended to rely on less conventional merchandising procedures. Common marketing strategies are high-pressure advertising in their own publications, in Sunday supplements, and in magazines, where an introductory offer (with refund privileges for dissatisfied customers) is often made. These promoters are astute enough to realize that very few disillusioned buyers will bother to seek a refund.

Door-to-door salespeople or "doorbell doctors" are often successful in convincing consumers that the only way they can protect their own and their families' health is through the use of the products they are promoting, be they special cooking pans, recipe books, food supplements, or potential cures for asthma. Usually these products are available at "special low prices" for quantity purchases on a cash basis. Victims often realize (too late) that, in supposedly "safeguarding" the health of their families, they have spent a large and unreasonable part of the family income. In some door-to-door selling situations, the parent company protects itself against responsibility for the claims of its salespeople, making it difficult to take effective legal action to stop the sales. Some states have introduced legislation that allows a victim of high-pressure sales techniques to cancel any contract within a specified time period (usually 1 to 3 days). Profits are high, with one company claiming that its successful salespeople earn in excess of $250,000 in 3 months—even a five-fold exaggeration leaves a living wage!

Books and articles on nutrition food fads have been a source of much misinformation and many half-truths for the consumer, as well as a source of tremendous income for the successful writer—especially one who can legitimately use the title "M.D." Because food quacks are not limited in their claims to established findings, they can make a much stronger and more emotional appeal than legitimate scientists, who tend to be overly cautious by comparison. Although some of the information is based on sound basic principles of nutrition, the authors, in their zeal to sell books, distort facts to achieve a strong emotional appeal. The sale of half a million copies of a book can earn an author a million dollars and the publisher, 2 million, so there is great motivation to appeal to a wide audience. By the time the fraudulent nature of a book's content is exposed, it may have earned sizable royalties for its author, who is often not upset by adverse publicity. In fact, authors often republish old books under new titles for greater profit.

The success of nutrition books is evident from the *New York Times* best-seller list. On one occasion, six out of the top 20 books on that list dealt with nutrition. Only one of these, which happened to be the most expensive, presented a rational, sound view of the topic. Authors of many of these books enhance their sales through appearances on talk shows, personal appearances in bookstores, and securing testimonials from popular public figures.

COMBATING MISINFORMATION AND FOOD FADDISM

Sources of Antiquackery Help
- Food and Drug Administration
- Federal Trade Commission
- U.S. Postal Service
- Better Business Bureaus
- National Council Against Health Fraud

Efforts to protect the public against dietary misinformation and worthless or harmful food products are the concern of several government and community agencies.

Better business bureaus in many communities attempt to police, restrict, or regulate the activities of peddlers of health foods, special cooking devices, or nutrition supplements within their regions. They describe their efforts to combat food misinformation as preventive, corrective, and educational.

The FDA is constantly concerned with protecting the consumer against mislabeling and harmful, contaminated, and worthless products. However, it is faced with an overwhelming job, considering the resources available. After the FDA believes it has sufficient evidence to press charges, court proceedings are extremely slow and costly for both parties. In some instances, by the time enforcement agencies are prepared to take action, defendants have already profited so much from a product that they do not contest the action. Regulations were enacted in 1963 that require a company to present evidence that the product it proposes to sell is safe for human consumption; these regulations have done much to lighten the load of the FDA, which previously had to prove that a product was harmful before its sale could be restricted.

For sources of reliable nutrition information, see Appendix J

Another difficulty is the reluctance of many people to initiate charges against companies that have victimized them; this hampers the operation of enforcement agencies. For people to admit that they have been "taken" is to disclose a human frailty—one they might prefer not to publicize.

Other professional groups, such as the American Public Health Association, the American Institute of Nutrition, the American Dietetic Association, the Institute of Food Technology, and the American Home Economics Association, are sources of information to help the public separate fiction from fact. The Society for Nutrition Education focuses its efforts on educating the public, from elementary schoolchildren to adult groups, on the principles of nutrition so that they can function as informed decision makers on nutrition issues, the nature of which is constantly changing.

The involvement of the Federal Trade Commission (FTC) in the fight against food quackery centers on its responsibility to protect the American public against false and misleading advertising. While cases involving charges of false advertising may take several years to try and often involve hundreds of hours of testimony, the public has a responsibility to report fraudulent practices or products.

Since 1975, the FTC has been developing regulations about nutrition information in advertising. These regulations have concerned defining terms such as "nutritious," "nourishing," "rich," and "excellent" and establishing the conditions under which foods can be compared on the basis of nutrient content.

The Lehigh Valley Committee Against Health Fraud and the American Council on Science and Health are examples of privately funded groups that have assumed responsibility for informing the public about false, misleading, and harmful health claims. The possibility of costly litigation, however, may deter some scientists from taking a firm stand in the attempt to combat fraud and quackery in nutrition.

The U.S. Postal Service performs a watchdog function, regulating the use of the mails to prevent fraud and protect the public against nutrition hoaxes.

Targets for Nutritional Quackery

- Teenagers
  - Weight loss
  - Body building
  - Growth promoters
- Elderly
  - Longevity
  - Disease prevention
  - Memory
- Athletes
  - Enhanced performance
  - Muscle building

NUTRITION EDUCATION

If an informed public is a less gullible public, nutrition education should be one of the most effective ways of combating food fads and quackery—especially with the potential of all the available media to spread accurate information. It is valid to wonder about what level of education is necessary to protect consumers from becoming victims of promoters who claim their products will cure everything from corns to sterility to leukemia. To combat nutrition faddism, we must recognize the emotional and psychological influences that perpetuate it. An educational campaign aimed at combating it must be multifaceted, attacking as many of the forces that support it as possible.

Only with a constant flow of legitimate nutrition information can progress be made in combating the high-pressure salesmanship surrounding much of food faddism. It appears that for each person involved in merchandising sound nutritional information, there are several hundred who are merchandising their own pet schemes. Several nutritionists who write regular syndicated columns for daily or weekly newspapers use the printed word to help enlighten the public. Dietitians in some larger cities operate a service known as Dial-A-Dietitian, in which people with nutrition-related questions call and are referred to the staff people most qualified to answer them. Nutrition information and resource centers are being established in various cities. The local nutrition extension specialist and the local dietetic association are sources of sound, authoritative answers regarding nutrition.

There are more difficulties in combating misinformation in the press than on labels or in advertisement for products, mainly because freedom of the press precludes monitoring the message.

The saga of food faddism is far from over. Our hope is that it can be brought under reasonable control before the health of too many people is jeopardized. On the other hand, we should not overlook the fact that the faddists have done much to dramatize the importance of nutrition and have created a nutrition consciousness in a large segment of the population. The challenge to nutritionists is to tap this interest and divert the attention of concerned people to reasonable and appropriate solutions.

BY NOW YOU SHOULD KNOW

- Many people choose alternative food patterns that differ from conventional patterns for a variety of health, emotional, and environmental reasons.
- Vegetarianism, the most popular alternative food pattern, can be nutritionally adequate if foods are chosen on the basis of a knowledge of nutrition.
- There are several different degrees of vegetarianism.
- Natural, health, or organic foods, which are seldom adequately defined, have little or no advantage over traditional foods and most often cost a great deal more.
- Nutrient supplements may be harmless, useful, or harmful; in most cases, they are unnecessary and frequently bear little relationship to a person's needs.
- The value of megavitamin therapy is unsubstantiated by scientific data; when self-prescribed, it may be potentially dangerous.
- Food fads may call for the use of certain foods or the avoidance of others for special reasons, the avoidance of chemicals in foods, or the use of special combination of foods.
- Food quacks claim that some foods have miraculous qualities; that it is impossible to be adequately nourished by conventional foods; that special products, books, or devices are necessary for good health; and that they have information that conventional medical professionals are trying to suppress.
- The FDA and the Better Business Bureau are among the groups that are constantly trying to combat food and nutrition misinformation.
- Most food additives are present for legitimate reasons to protect or maintain the quality of the food supply.

STUDY QUESTIONS

1. List several reasons for choosing an alternative food pattern.
2. Explain the harm of nutrition quackery.
3. What are the nutritional concerns of placing a child on a strict vegetarian diet?
4. List several ways to determine the reliability of nutrition information.
5. Argue as to why nutrition education should be mandatory in our school system and at all grade levels.
6. What kinds of regulatory controls exist to protect the public from health frauds?
7. Why is the "health food" business such a thriving industry in a country with an ample food supply?

Applying What You've Learned

1. **Compare Foods in Grocery Stores and Health Food Stores**

   Make a list of ten foods you eat most often. Go to a local supermarket and then to a health food store. Compare the availability of the foods and the prices. While in the health food store, look around for at least ten products you have never seen before.

2. **Read the Labels on Processed Food Products**

   Try to identify the functions of the various ingredients. Use Table 20-3 to help you with the function of some common food additives. Also note the forms in which sugars and fats are listed.

3. **Interview Several People on Their Beliefs Surrounding Natural Foods**

   Do they believe foods labeled "natural" are better? Ask them to define what natural means to them.

4. **Write Down Everything You Eat in a Day**

   How many of the items are close to their natural state? How many are convenience or processed items?

SUGGESTED READINGS

American Dietetic Association. Vegetarian diets position paper and technical support paper, Journal of the American Dietetic Association 88:351, 1988.

The Association feels that vegetarian diets are healthful and nutritionally adequate when appropriately planned. This article discusses the many types of vegetarianism practiced; the lower rates of coronary heart disease, hypertension, obesity, diabetes, colon cancer, osteoporosis, and other degenerative diseases; and the need to monitor the quality of the protein, the amount of vitamins B_{12} and D in the diet, and the effect of the diet on calcium absorption. The Association cautions about the difficulty of meeting the needs of young children and lactating women on a strict vegan diet.

Dubick MA, and Rucker RB: Dietary supplements and health aids—a critical evaluation. I. Vitamins and minerals, Journal of Nutrition Education 15:47, 1983.

Dubick MA, and Rucker RB: Dietary supplements and health aids—a critical evaluation. II. Macronutrients and fiber, Journal of Nutrition Education 15:88, 1983.

Dubick MA, and Rucker RB: Dietary supplements and health aids—a critical evaluation. III. Natural and miscellaneous products, Journal of Nutrition Education 15:123, 1983.

This series of articles spells out the range of products being sold as food supplements and health aids and describes what they are, what they can do, what they are reported to do, and what they can't do. The articles carefully identify products and warn the reader against placing undue faith in them. This series is invaluable to professionals and laypeople alike.

ADDITIONAL READINGS

Academy of Pediatrics: Nutritional aspects of vegetarianism, health foods and fad diets, Pediatrics 59:460, 1977.

American Dietetic Association: Position paper on the vegetarian approach to eating, Journal of the American Dietetic Association 77:61, 1988.

Bergan JG, and Brown PT: Nutritional status of "new" vegetarians, Journal of the American Dietetic Association 76:151, 1980.

Coon JM: Natural toxicants in foods, Journal of the American Dietetic Association 67:213, 1975.

Deutsch R: The new nuts among the berries, New York, 1977, Ballantine Books, Inc.

Dwyer JT, and others: The new vegetarians: the natural high? Journal of the American Dietetic Association 65:529, 1974.

Freeland-Graves J, Greninger SA, and Young RR: A demographic and social profile of age- and sex-matched vegetarians and non-vegetarians, Journal of the American Dietetic Association 86:907, 1986.

Grivetti LE: Cultural nutrition, Annual Review of Nutrition 1:47, 1981.

Grivetti LE: Food fact, food myth: the scientific dilemma, Food Technology, p. 14, August, 1984.

Helman AD, and Darton-Hill I: Vitamin and iron status of new vegetarians, American Journal of Clinical Nutrition 45:785, 1987.

Hogan RP: Hemorrhagic diathesis caused by drinking an herbal tea, Journal of the American Medical Association 249:2679, 1983.

Jarvis WT: Food faddism, cultism and quackery, Annual Review of Nutrition 3:35, 1983.

Kowalski R, Johnston PK, Burke KI, and Stanton H: Congress investigates vegetarian nutrition; Nutrition Today 22(4):30, 1987.

Lekon B, and Kris-Etherton P: Meal cost analysis: health food stores versus conventional food sources, Journal of the American Dietetic Association 70:456, 1981.

Looker A, and others: Vitamin/mineral supplement use: Association with dietary intake and iron status of adults, Journal of the American Dietetic Association 88:808, 1988.

Mutch PB, and Johnson PK, editors: Proceedings of First International Congress on Vegetarian Nutrition. American Journal of Clinical Nutrition 48:707, 1988.

Register UD, and Sonnenberg LM: The vegetarian diet—scientific and practical considerations, Journal of the America Dietetic Association 63:253, 1973.

Rudman D, and Williams PJ: Megadose vitamins. New England Journal of Medicine 309:488, 1983.

Rynearson EH: Americans love hogwash, Nutrition Reviews 32(suppl.1):1, 1974.

Saegert J, and Young EA: Nutrition knowledge and health food consumption, Nutrition and Behavior 1:103, 1983.

Simons FJ: Traditional use and avoidance of foods of animal origin: a cultural historical view, BioScience 28:178, 1980.

Sims LS: Communication characteristics of recommended and nonrecommended nutrition books, Home Economics Research Journal 6:2, 1977.

Young JH, and Stitt RS: Nutrition quackery—upholding the right to criticize, Food Technology 35:42, 1981.

FOCUS Health Claims—A New Look

The long established policy of the FDA, dictated by the Food, Drug, and Cosmetic Act of 1938, to prohibit implicit health claims on the label or in the advertising of food products has recently been challenged. The challenge has come in the form of explicit statements on food packages that the use of a particular food product would prevent or reduce the risk of cancer or coronary heart disease. Under 1971 laws such a statement should have led to the designation of the food in question as a drug, subject to "new drug" provisions asking for rigorous scientific scrutiny of the validity of this claim. This would have required that the processors provide evidence that the food was safe and would indeed prevent cancer or heart disease. Alternatively they would run the risk of having the foods judged to be misbranded and subject to confiscation. Instead the FDA issued a statement in 1985 of its intent to publish a revised policy. This was followed in 1987 with a proposed amendment to permit truthful and nonmisleading health claims on labels provided that the claims could be substantiated by scientific evidence.

The release of this proposed amendment gave rise to an immediate and heated debate. Proponents felt that it was possible to use this as means of providing the public with important health information to which it was entitled—clearly a significant change. Opponents on the other hand were convinced that such action would open the flood gates to irresponsible, unsubstantiated health claims for food products merely for trade advantages. They felt it would be impossible for a group of scientists to agree on appropriate health messages to be included in advertising or on the label of food products.

The difference between an implicit and an explicit health claim is the basis of the argument. The former is exemplified by statements such as "low in sodium," "contains vitamin C," "reduced calories," or "enriched with 4 vitamins and 2 minerals." Each of these implies some health benefit from the use of the food but does not make the claim. Such statements would trigger full nutrient labeling but nothing more. On the other hand explicit claims, such as "Calcium prevents osteoporosis," "Eat product X, high in calcium," or "Eating high fiber foods prevents colon cancer," "Product Y provides 2 grams for fiber per serving," the claim of an association between a specific disease and the food is considered to be articulated, not merely implied. This, by current law, makes these foods drugs and subject to all laws governing the sale of drugs—mainly that the manufacturer must provide incontroversial evidence that the food is not only safe but effective as recommended. Many look on the proposed changes as permitting "the practice of medicine on a food package, " when it is impossible to give enough detail to deliver a responsible message.

As the debate heated up most concerned professional groups voiced their opposition feeling that the proposal "flouted" the laws regarding false and misleading claims and urged that scientists collaborate to assure that claims in advertising conform to sound scientific principles. They felt it was not in the interest of public health that information regarding specific diseases appear on food labels. They emphasized that the honest claims on the relation of food to health must recognize that any benefits are a function of the total diet rather than a specific food in the diet. Many stressed the importance of providing a balanced picture, the whole truth, giving the public any information on the problems associated with the excessive use of the food as well as any benefits that might occur from more moderate uses. It was considered equally deceptive to omit any adverse facts or to make false and unsubstantiated claims of benefit. There was concern that a message to "eat more" of anything could be bad advice to someone who is already getting enough! Similarly eating "less" of something that was already used in marginal amounts could precipitate a relative deficiency.

The FDA has confirmed that it intends to move ahead with a resolution to permit advertising that foods, supplements, and nutrients would provide possible protection against certain chronic illnesses. This decision has been made in spite of a report from a legislative committee urging that they reverse their decision and back the old regulations. Thus it appears that we will no longer be protected against widespread, inadequate, inaccurate, and misleading claims to the public concerning health benefits from the use of certain food products. The FDA still backs its contention that it is important to consider ways to improve the public's understanding about reported health benefits associated with the use of certain foods, maintaining that the food label is one appropriate mechanism for public health education.

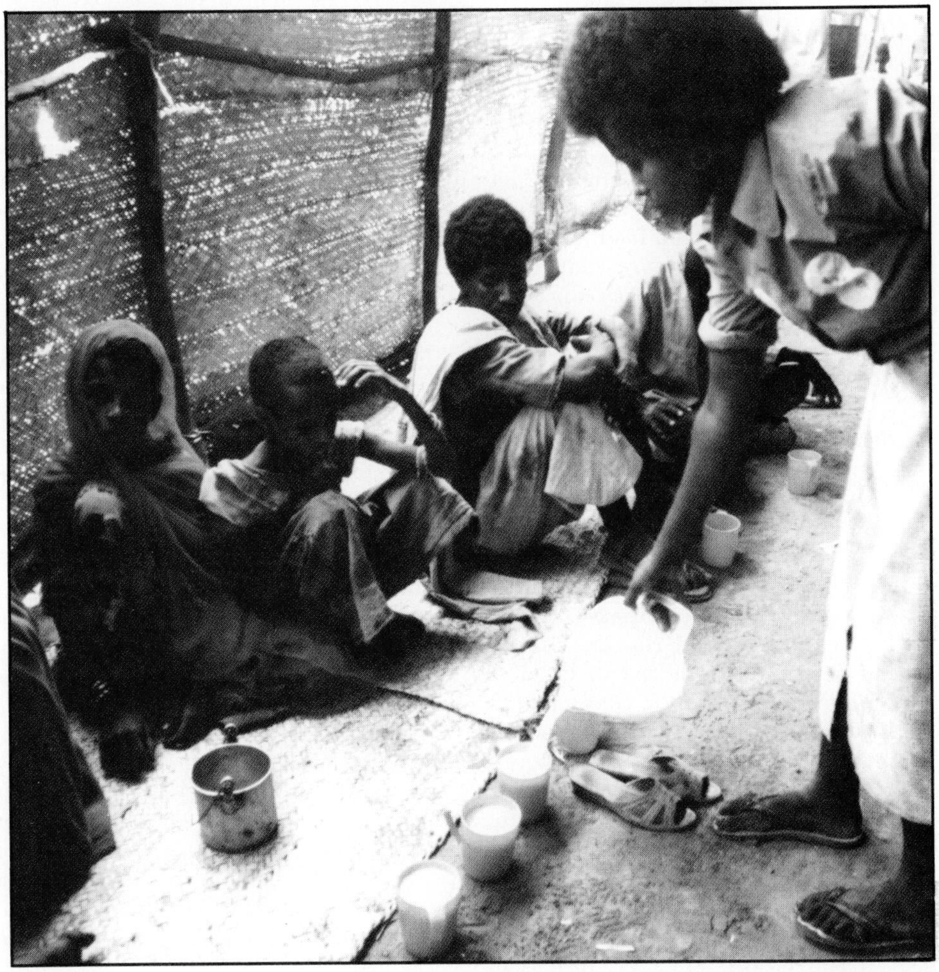

AWARENESS CHECK

Truth or Fiction?

- Protein malnutrition is now considered less critical than calorie malnutrition.
- Current nutrition intervention programs help enhance nutritional status of high-risk groups.
- Enrichment of food products is one way of improving some aspects of undernutrition.
- Not all nutrition scientists agree on how much cholesterol is recommended in the average American diet.
- The sea is a potential source of food for the world.
- Obesity is a form of malnutrition.

Nutrition: A National and International Concern

CHAPTER

21

In the early 1950s interest in nutrition focused largely on concerns about malnutrition and undernutrition in Third World countries. Western countries were providing both food and technical assistance to help alleviate the problems. By the early 1970s, North Americans began to recognize that malnutrition could exist in their own country of food surpluses. This led to the initiation and expansion of several federally funded intervention programs to reduce the incidence of poor nutrition. A rapidly growing number of North Americans are making nutrition a major concern as they strive to improve their personal health. Although research in agriculture, aquaculture, and plant and animal breeding promises to provide some solutions to problems of food quality and quantity, the skills of social scientists and communicators will be needed to help educate the public to accept and use these technological advances.

Nutrition as a national and an international concern has attracted public attention only in the latter part of this century. At the international level, concern stems from a realization that the world population is increasing at a rate that could soon exceed the capacity of the world to provide and distribute adequate amounts of food. Because two thirds of the world's children are undernourished, the problem is one of improving the level of nutrition for the current generation and also of providing this same or a more adequate level for an expanding population.

The magnitude of the problem became evident with the recognition in 1950 that the protein-deficiency disease kwashiorkor was a major cause of infant mortality in developing countries. Less dramatic effects included retarded physical growth, increased susceptibility to infection, and in very severe cases, depressed development of the central nervous system. In countries where large numbers of people must be fed from the production of a finite amount of land, it is too costly to raise animal protein unless the land is unsuitable for cultivation. Because an acre yields 25 times as much protein from soybeans and 10 times as much from rice as from beef, vegetable protein mixtures and legumes must be used whenever possible.

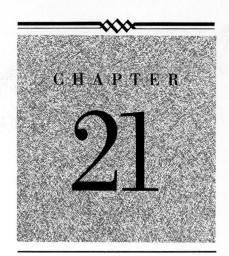

Recently those concerned with world food problems have concentrated on increasing the energy value of the food supply on the assumption that, if calories are adequate, even a limited amount of protein will be more able to meet the needs for its primary purpose of building and repairing tissues. This shift is reflected in the use of the term *energy protein deficit* to replace the term *protein calorie malnutrition* in describing the major nutritional problem facing developing countries.

Recognition of malnutrition as a national concern for developed countries is an even more recent phenomenon. In 1968 the publication *Hunger USA* and a television documentary *Hunger in America*, both charging that there was hunger in the midst of plenty, shocked the nation. These were followed by two White House Conferences on Food, Nutrition, and Health (in 1969 and 1974) and by the Senate Hearings on Nutrition and Human Needs from 1968 to 1979. All presented evidence that malnutrition is much more prevalent than previously suspected and that we had discouragingly little information on the nutritional status of the U.S. population.

The lack of any coordinated government policy on food, nutrition, and health became increasingly evident, leading to considerable lobbying activity by nutrition advocates. As a result, nutrition has become both a national and international priority, with many agencies dedicated to alleviating malnutrition and congressional leaders staking their careers on legislation on nutritional issues. Nutrition is the subject of much research not only by nutritionists, agronomists, and biochemists, but also by social scientists such as economists, sociologists, psychologists, and anthropologists. The following discussion focuses on the factors that contribute to the problem and solutions that appear promising.

A NATIONAL CONCERN

Information on the nutrient intake of the U.S. population has come primarily from data collected by the U.S. Department of Agriculture (USDA) in the Nationwide Food Consumption Survey (NFCS) and the National Centre for Health Statistics (NCHS) in their National Health and Nutrition Evaluation Study (NHANES), which are the major components of the national nutrition monitoring system. This has been supplemented by information obtained by individual investigators on much smaller and usually geographically separated groups in the population such as teenagers in Iowa, pregnant females in Alabama, or the elderly in California.

The national monitoring system has provided data on the food, and hence nutrients, available for consumption in the United States every year since 1909; the food used by households during a 7-day period every 10 years since 1955; and the food and nutrient intake of individuals in the households in the survey since 1977 to 1978. In 1985 they also began a continuing survey of females 19 to 50 years of age and their children 1 to 5 years of age for 6 nonconsecutive days a year. One-day intakes of males 19 to 50 years old were also reported.

The first attempt to assess the nutritional status as well as dietary intake of the U.S. population was the Ten-State Survey conducted by the U.S. Public Health Service in 1967 and 1968. This survey was limited to people with the lowest incomes. In 1970 and again in 1977 to 1978, the National Center for Health Statistics assessed the health and nutritional status of a representative group of the population with the use of biochemical, physical, and anthropometric as well as dietary data. Both NFCS and NHANES are underway in 1988, using more sophisticated analytical methods and obtaining data on a larger number of nutrients.

These studies permit an assessment of nutrient intake and nutritional status for various age and sex groups and some of the demographic, economic, social, and environmental factors that influence them. The nutrients for which dietary data are being analyzed are shown in Table 21-1, and the biochemical- and nutrition-related tests included in NHANES III are shown in Tables 21-2 and 21-3. The findings of many of these studies have been used throughout the text. These studies revealed that the quality of nutrition was generally related to economic status and

Nutrients Provided to Households in Average Amounts at Least Equal to the RDA

Energy	Magnesium
Protein	Calcium
Vitamin B_{12}	Vitamin C
Thiamin	Vitamin A
Niacin	Riboflavin
Iron	Vitamin B_6

Nutrients Provided at Average Levels Below the RDA

Folacin
Zinc

Nutrients Most Often Below RDA in Individual Households

Calcium	33% households
Vitamin B_6	33% households
Magnesium	25% households
Vitamin A	20% households

USDA Household Food Consumption Survey, 1978

level of education. Infants and children from families of lower socioeconomic levels tended to be below average in height and weight. Ascorbic acid, vitamin A, calcium, and iron were commonly consumed at levels below the RDAs, but biochemical evidence of vitamin deficiencies was rare.

Obesity and iron-deficiency anemia were the most common nutrition-related health problems. Impaired iron status was found in 3% to 12% of 11- to 14-year-old boys and in 2.5% to 14% of girls and females over 11 years old (percentage depends on criteria used). Low vitamin A levels were found in the serum of children (particularly Hispanics); low serum levels of vitamin C occurred in smokers; and there was some evidence of growth retardation in children, especially recent immigrants. Overweight was most common in females in the survey group. Poor dental health was associated with poor nutrition. Major surveys conducted in the United States are listed in Table 21-4.

Mean Individual Intakes

	Percent of those with intakes below RDA
>100% RDA	
Protein	12%
Vitamin B_{12}	34%
Vitamin A	50%
Riboflavin	34%
Thiamin	45%
Phosphorus	27%
Iron	57%
80 to 90% RDA	
Calcium	68%
Magnesium	75%
<75% RDA	
Vitamin B_6	80%

USDA Nationwide Food Consumption Survey, Individuals, 1978

Table 21-1 ◇ Nutrients included in dietary analysis in NFCS (1987-1988) and NHANES III

Food energy	Niacin
Protein	Vitamin B_6
Total fat	Vitamin B_{12}
Saturated fatty acids	Calcium
Monounsaturated fatty acids	Phosphorus
Polyunsaturated fatty acids	Magnesium
Cholesterol	Iron
Carbohydrate	Carotenes
Dietary fiber	Vitamin E
Vitamin A (IU)	Folate
Vitamin A (RE)	Zinc
Vitamin C	Copper
Thiamin	Sodium
Riboflavin	Potassium

Table 21-2 ◇ Hematological and biochemical assessments planned for the NHANES III nutritional component

Complete blood count (WBC, RBC, MCV, MCHC, hematocrit, hemoglobin)
Red cell distribution width
Iron and total iron binding capacity (TIBC)
Ferritin
Folate (serum and red cell)
Protoporphyrin
Retinol and retinyl ester
Carotenoids (total and individual)
Vitamin E
Vitamin C
25-Hydroxyvitamin D
Calcium (serum and ionized)
Selenium
Cholesterol (total and HDL)
Triglycerides
Apolipoproteins A_1 and B
Lead
Cadmium

Table 21-3 ◇ Nutrition-related examination components planned for NHANES III by age group

2-11 mo	1-4 yr	5-19 yr	≥20 yr
Physician examination Body measurements Dietary interview	Physician examination Body measurements Dietary interview Dental examination (2 yr+) Biochemical blood analysis	Physician examination Body measurements Dietary interview Dental examination Biochemical blood analysis Urine Allergy skin test (6 yr+)	Physician examination Body measurements Dietary interview Dental examination Biochemical blood analysis Urine Allergy skin test Bioelectrical impedance* Hand and knee x-rays (60 yr+) Oral glucose tolerance test Bone densitometry

*See Chapter 7 for explanation.

Table 21-4 ◇ Major nutrition, food, and health surveys conducted in the United States

Survey	Agency	Frequency	Data Base
National Health and Nutrition Examination Survey (NHANES II)	NCHS	10 years*	27,000 persons surveyed; 20,000 examined 6 months—74 years
NHANES III	NCHS	10 years*	Planned 1989—60,000 surveyed–45,000 examined
Hispanic HANES (HHANES)	NCHS	First survey, 1982-1984	12,000 examined; 16,000 surveyed
Nutritional Status Surveillance System	CDC	Monthly*†	In 1983, a total of 539,000 children screened and 26,000 completed pregnancies; 80% of data compiled from WIC and MCH clinics in 34 states and D.C.
Behavior Risk Factor Surveillance System	CDC	Monthly†	Telephone survey of 12,000 persons (600 persons per year in each of 20 states) in 1983
Total Diet Study (TDS)	FDA	Annually	1700 foods representative of 54 food groups found in the U.S. food supply, as determined by Neilsen Survey data
Food Label and Package Study (FLAPS)	FDA	2 years	Varies
Multi-Purpose Annual Survey of Food Shoppers	FDA	Annually	4000
Nationwide Food Consumption Survey (NFCS)	USDA	10 years	15,000 households; 30,000 individuals, 1977-1978 9600 households; 25,000 individuals, 1987-1988
Continuing Survey of Food Intake of Individuals	USDA	Annually	1985 sample: 1200 women ages 19-50 and 500 of their children ages 1-5 years (cross section of the U.S. population), and 1200 low-income women and 500 of their children ages 1-5 years
Survey of infant feeding practices	FDA	Beginning 1989	Pregnant women

*Data gathered monthly and reports issued monthly, quarterly, and annually to the states. Summary of combined state data published annually.
†Data reported to participating states quarterly, with a summary report prepared annually.

Most of the studies have identified the poor, the elderly, Hispanics, migrant workers, Eskimos, and Native Americans as the most nutritionally vulnerable groups in the country. As a result, plans for future studies include special surveys to closely monitor the nutritional status and food intake of these groups. The studies will also provide data that will permit the evaluation of the intervention programs directed to alleviate the nutritional problems of these target groups.

Groups with Nutritional Problems
Migrant workers
The elderly
Native Americans
Eskimos
The poor
Hispanics

In many respects these groups are difficult to reach with either assistance or education, because they do not tend to belong to organized groups or to seek help. In general, their nutritional status may be a function of their cultural backgrounds, inadequate knowledge of the nutritive value of foods, economic problems resulting from low and often irregular incomes, pressures of large families, and trauma from high morbidity rates. Some of the specific factors involved for each particular group will be considered briefly.

Native Americans, numbering fewer than half a million, live on 53 million acres of largely barren, dry, unproductive land and have restricted freedom to search for food and limited opportunities to earn income. The animals and fruit on which they formerly depended for food are vanishing. Meat is less available at higher prices, which leads Native Americans, whose incomes average less than $1000 per year, to consume a less expensive, high-carbohydrate diet. Infant mortality of 140 per 1000 live births, compared with a national average of 21.4 per 1000, and a tuberculosis rate eight times the national average are evidence of poor health conditions. Studies among Native Americans indicate that low intakes of ascorbic acid and vitamin A are the most prevalent nutritional inadequacies.

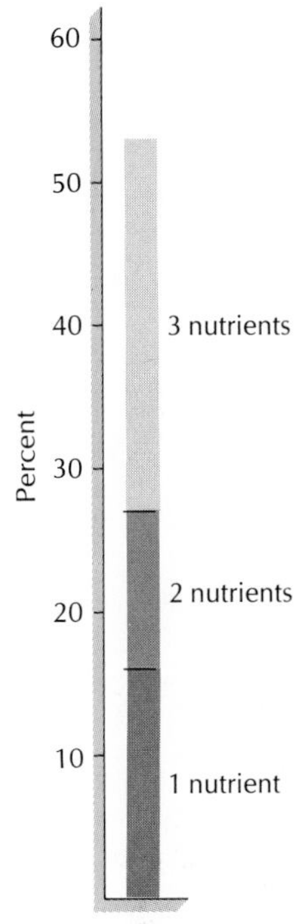

Percentage of households with intakes below 70% of the RDA

Migrant workers, dependent on agriculture for a living, have virtually no financial security. Because of the mobile nature of their existence, they have limited and irregular opportunities for education; their housing is marginal, often lacking facilities for the preparation and storage of food and for adequate sanitation. The latter factor increases the possibility of infection, to which resistance is low because of poor nutrition and possible intestinal parasitism. Frequently the mother must work in the field all day and is home to cook at most two meals a day. Older children care for younger ones and thus cannot attend school. Studies indicate that diets of migrant families are low in vitamins C and A, calcium, and riboflavin, reflecting limited use of fruit and vegetables and milk.

Eskimos traditionally obtained their food largely by hunting and fishing, and their diet was high in fat and protein and low in carbohydrates. However, they have migrated to the city in search of a steady income, and at the same time they have lost their food-gathering skills and resources. The result has been a shift to a high-carbohydrate diet, with a concurrent increase in dental cavities, reflecting an unusually high sugar intake.

The poor have been identified in many nutritional surveys as a group with generally less-than-adequate diets. This is attributed in part to their limited resources for all necessities of life, including food, and in part to the fact that low-income families generally have less education and less sound nutritional knowledge on which to base their food choices. Their problem is compounded by the fact that the cost of less expensive foods eaten by the poor, who spend 37% of their income on food, is rising faster than that of more expensive foods usually consumed by the more affluent. Interestingly, the poor get more nutrients per dollar spent on food than do those with more money.

The nutritional problems of the elderly stem from psychological and social factors such as low income, long-standing food habits, loneliness, poor housing, lack of adequate storage and preparation facilities, lack of transportation to stores, and indifference to or ignorance of adequate food habits. Physiologically they suffer from decreased ability to absorb and transport nutrients, increased excretion of nutrients, and thus relatively increased need.

For more discussion of nutrition in the elderly, see Chapter 18

Nutritional problems are by no means confined to these groups. Many others, such as adolescent girls and pregnant women, are often underfed. The overfed, another significant group, suffers from obesity and represents up to 40% of some population groups. Although the causes may be multiple, nutrition is one factor in the etiology of atherosclerosis, which is responsible for the premature death of a large number of adults.

Evaluation of Nutritional Status

Because of the multiple causes and many different ways in which deficiencies of various nutrients show up, no one method of assessing nutritional status is completely satisfactory. Some of the possible methods include:

1. Clinical observations
2. Biochemical analyses of tissues such as blood, urine, hair, or saliva
3. Physical or anthropometric measurements
4. Dietary evaluations

In addition, information from the vital statistics of a country are useful in assessing population groups.

The ways in which nutritional deficiencies develop and the techniques for detecting changes are outlined in Figure 21-1.

Clinical Observation

noninvasive
Technique that does not require "entering" the body; for example, taking a hair or saliva sample is noninvasive

clinical deficiency
A deficiency that is severe enough to cause observable changes in the body

Clinical observation is the least useful approach in identifying impending nutritional problems. However, it lends itself to use in nutritional surveys of population groups because it is **noninvasive,** involving an assessment of those parts of the body that can be readily observed in a routine physical examination. The most commonly observed tissues are the eyes, mucous membranes, skin, hair, mouth, teeth, tongue, thyroid gland, and lower extremities. As is evident in Table 21-5, many of the changes in these tissues are specific for a single nutrient. Others are nonspecific, that is, they cannot be considered as diagnostic of a specific nutrient deficiency. For example, sometimes the same condition, such as *dermatitis,* may be caused by the lack of several different nutrients. Although **clinical deficiency** signs (signs indicative of poor health) are of limited value in the early diagnosis of a deficiency or in identifying marginal intakes that prevail for short periods, the presence of

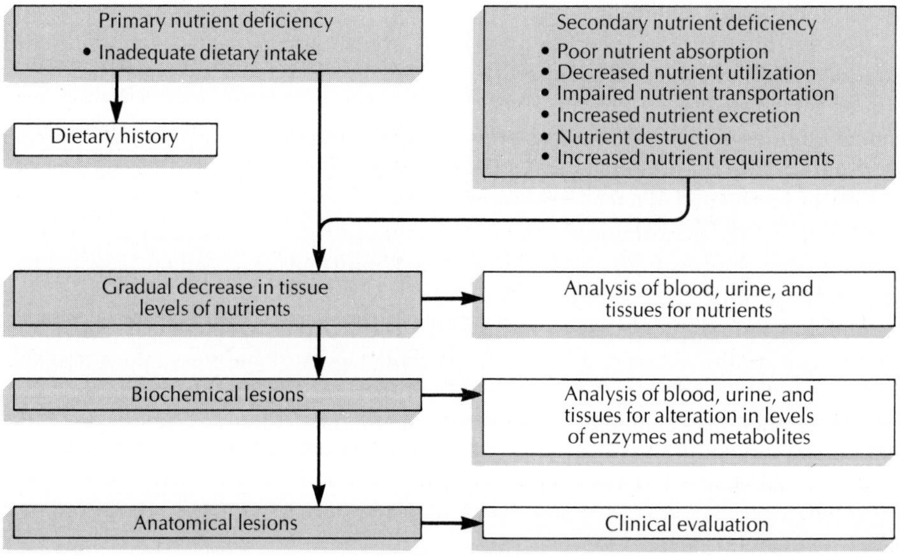

Figure 21-1 Development and assessment of nutritional deficiency symptoms. Shaded areas indicate dietary, biochemical, and physical changes; white areas indicate assessment techniques.

Table 21-5 ◇ Changes in tissues associated with loss of specific nutrients

Tissue	Nutrient	Changes
Eyes	Vitamin A	Dryness of the cornea (xerosis conjunctiva)
		Foamy spots on cornea (Bitot's spots)
		Opacity of the cornea (xerophthalmia)
	Riboflavin	Blood vessels infiltrating the cornea (corneal vascularization)
Mucous membranes	Iron	Pale membranes on the underside of the eyelid
		Pale mucous membrane
Skin	Niacin	Bilateral dermatitis on skin exposed to sunlight
	Vitamin A	Roughness at base of hair follicles (folliculosis)
	Fatty acids	Dermatitis
		Eczema in infants
	Vitamin C	Pinpoint hemorrhages
	Water	Loss of elasticity of skin
Mouth	Riboflavin	Vertical cracks in lips
	Niacin	Loss of tongue papillae
	Vitamin C	Bleeding gums

clinical deficiencies in even a few people suggests that others in the same population may be on the verge of a problem.

Because of the subjective nature of judgment in a clinical evaluation, this method is quite unreliable even when used by well-trained observers.

An examination of such tissues as hair, nails, and muscle provides information on general health but little that can be associated with a specific nutrient. Enlargement of the thyroid gland, traditionally associated with iodine deficiency or the intake of food goitrogens, is now considered to suggest an iodine excess as well (see Figure 11-10). Other clinical observations include edema, especially of the lower extremities, which suggests thiamin and protein inadequacies; depigmentation, lack of luster in the hair, and decreased hair diameter, which occur in protein deficiency; cupping of the nails, which suggests that iron is inadequate; and bowed legs and beading of the ribs, which are associated with a lack of vitamin D. Neurological abnormalities associated with thiamin and vitamin B_{12} deficiencies are identified by testing reflexes in the lower extremities.

Biochemical Analyses

The biochemical evaluation of nutritional status involves an analysis of nutrients or related metabolites in such tissues as the blood and urine. Low blood levels of a nutrient may reflect low dietary intake, defective absorption or utilization, or excessive need or excretion. Occasionally, analysis will be made with a **biopsy** sample of liver or bone, but the use of the rather hazardous and involved biopsy technique is not justified in routine nutritional evaluations.

biopsy
The removal of a small amount of tissue, such as liver or bone marrow, for analysis

The analysis of carefully sampled hair as an indicator of nutritional status, especially for micronutrient mineral elements, is being used increasingly. Readily available tissues such as saliva and the mucous membranes of the mouth and nails are being investigated to determine their usefulness in assessing nutritional status. The interpretation of biochemical data is complicated by the fact that the levels of many nutrients and metabolites in the blood and urine vary sufficiently throughout the day to make the use of values from a single determination misleading. These **diurnal variations** are also called circadian rhythms.

diurnal variation
Normal fluctuations in biochemical or physical characteristics throughout the day; for example, hemoglobin levels change merely as a function of the time of day; also called circadian rhythm (circa = about, dies = day)

Many of the analytical techniques for evaluating the constituents of the blood and urine have been adapted for use on very small samples. These microtechniques enable biochemists to make determinations for as many as 20 different nutritional factors or metabolites with a single 1-ml sample of blood. Instruments that perform several analyses simultaneously are available.

Blood Levels

Because both activity and recent food intake may influence blood biochemical data, an early morning fasting blood sample is preferred.

serum
Whole blood from which cells and clotting factors have been removed

plasma
Whole blood from which blood cells have been removed

Nutrients. The level of a nutrient in either blood **serum** or blood **plasma** may reflect either the most recent intake of a nutrient or the body's reserves. For example, levels of vitamin C in the blood reflect recent intake. Vitamin C serum levels of 0.5 mg drop to zero when reserves are only 50% depleted, whereas vitamin C levels in white blood cells drop only when tissue saturation is down to 20% of normal. This drop occurs only at the time that other symptoms of scurvy are about to appear.

On the other hand, blood levels of calcium are of little value in assessing nutritional status. The body has many mechanisms that operate to maintain normal blood levels; only when these mechanisms fail will any change occur in blood calcium levels. Amino acid analysis of blood is expensive and of little use because values are readily altered by recent intake and the breakdown of body proteins.

The large reserves of vitamin A maintained in the liver make vitamin A serum levels rather meaningless until reserves are depleted. These levels are useful, however, in detecting excessive or toxic intakes. Sometimes vitamin A blood levels may be low in spite of adequate stores in the liver if zinc or protein deficiencies prevent the vitamin's release.

Determinations of cholesterol, triglycerides, and various forms of lipoproteins are done with increasing frequency to screen people who may be at high risk of coronary heart disease.

Metabolites. Often the absence of a vitamin leads to a block in the normal series of reactions in the metabolism of carbohydrate, fat, or protein. An accumulation of one of the intermediary products in the blood often indicates a lack of the nutrient required for metabolism to proceed beyond that point. For example, an increase in pyruvic acid in the blood occurs when insufficient thiamin is available to allow carbohydrate metabolism to proceed.

Nutrients for Which Enzyme Tests Are Available
Thiamin
Riboflavin
Pyridoxine
Vitamin D

Enzymes. Because many nutrients are part of enzymes or coenzymes, it is possible to assess nutrient status by measuring an enzyme or its activity. For example, the enzyme transketolase in the red blood cells is a sensitive indicator of available thiamin; glutathione reductase of riboflavin; several transaminases of pyridoxine; and alkaline phosphatase of vitamin D status. Because all enzymes are protein, a change in all enzyme activity could be expected when protein reserves are depleted.

Carrier proteins. The determination of specific proteins that serve to transport nutrients in the blood provides some information on nutritional status. For example, the amount or saturation of transferrin or retinol-binding protein reflects the nutritional status of iron and vitamin A; ceruloplasmin reflects copper status.

Urine Analysis

Nutrients or their metabolites in the urine are useful in assessing nutritional status. Not only is the amount of a nutrient found in the urine significant, but the presence of substances not normally found in the urine is also informative.

In a saturation test, the urine is analyzed to determine the proportion of a large test dose (two to four times the requirement) of a water-soluble vitamin that is excreted. It is assumed that a person whose tissues are saturated with the nutrient will retain little and excrete most of the dose, whereas a person who has had low intakes will retain more. This test has been widely used to assess the status of vitamin C, thiamin, and riboflavin.

A variation of the saturation test is the load test, in which an abnormally large amount of a substance is fed to a subject, increasing the need for a particular nutrient. For example, in a tryptophan load test vitamin B_6, or pyridoxine, is required if the amino acid is to be metabolized and excreted in a normal manner as *N*-methyl nicotinamide. If insufficient pyridoxine is available, an abnormal urinary constituent, xanthurenic acid, appears. Histidine load tests are similarly used to evaluate folacin adequacy. In the absence of folacin, formiminoglutamic acid (FIGLU), an intermediary product of histidine metabolism, accumulates and appears in increased amounts in the urine.

Determination of hydroxyproline in the urine is a useful indicator of collagen metabolism. High levels occur during active growth and are considered desirable; low levels are undesirable.

The amount of **creatinine,** a nitrogen-containing component, in the urine is directly related to muscle mass; this information is helpful in the determination of body composition. Urinary data obtained from a **casual urine specimen** rather than a complete 24-hour specimen are more meaningful when expressed in terms of the amount of creatinine excreted at the same time.

creatinine
Nitrogen-containing component in urine, indicative of muscle mass

casual urine specimen
A urine sample collected after any one voiding of the bladder, as opposed to a complete collection of urine over a 24-hour period

Other Biochemical Tests

The rate of hemolysis, or breakdown, of red blood cell membranes is sufficiently influenced by the amount of vitamin E available to be an adequate test for vitamin E status. The prothrombin time (the length of time required for clotting) is related to vitamin K nutriture (nourishment). Plasma albumin levels are normal when adequate amounts of amino acids are available. However, serum levels usually fall only at the time other signs of protein deficiency become evident. Iron status is assessed by measuring serum ferritin.

Standards for evaluating these and other biochemical data are available. Interpretation of much of the data is difficult because of the need for more sensitive measures. Analysis of nutritional status data shows that the 30 to 40 biochemical measurements routinely used in screening population groups could be reduced to 10 tests with no loss of screening potential.

ANTHROPOMETRIC DATA

For years we have tried to establish criteria for nutritional adequacy using **anthropometric data,** that is, data from simple body measurements such as height, weight, chest circumference, and skinfold thickness. So far, we have had only limited success. Height and weight measurements can be obtained fairly easily, but the others involve considerable skill. One problem is that techniques employing calipers, which can be used to measure skinfold thickness, are difficult to master. Another problem is the interpretation of measurements once they are obtained. Standards based on recent growth data, which replace those that have been in use since the early 1930s, have provided much more valid criteria for evaluating anthropometric data.

anthropometric data
Data that include measurements of height, weight, circumference, diameter, or length of various parts of the body

Although height and weight tables, long used as growth standards, have many limitations, they still remain useful. Two general types of tables have been used for adults. The first merely records the *average* weight for height and age based on insurance statistics. The second group of tables, which is more useful in evaluating nutritional status, gives *weights for height associated with the greatest longevity and the lowest mortality*.

For more information on height and weight tables see *Focus*, Chapter 7

The anthropometric measurements used in NHANES II to provide a basis for the evaluation of nutritional status are listed in the margin. These data are useful only after being correlated with other measures of nutritional status. It is unlikely that they will provide much information beyond that provided by height, weight, and triceps skinfold measurements.

Anthropometric Measurements Used in NHANES II

Height	**Circumference**
Standing	Head
Sitting	Mid-thigh
Knee	Calf
Length	Waist
Upper leg	Buttocks
Upper arm	Mid-upper arm
Breadth	**Skinfold**
Bi-iliac	Subscapular
Elbow	Supra-iliac
Wrist	Mid-thigh
Biacromial	Triceps

The difficulties in making accurate anthropometric measurements of body structure in extremely obese people impose limitations on the usefulness of some formulas or indexes. As a result, several alternative methods have been proposed. X-ray films have made it possible to measure body fat in such areas as the hips, where caliper measurements of skinfold thickness are of little value. In addition to learning about body composition for the purpose of identifying obese people, physicians use estimates of fat-free weight to determine drug dosages.

EVALUATION OF THE DIET

Analysis of the nutrient content of food intake as part of an assessment of nutritional status provides information that is suggestive of adequacy. Unless low intakes are accompanied by some biochemical or physical evidence of a deficiency state, they are unlikely to indicate a true nutritional deficiency. Low intakes can, however, be used as a rationale for nutrition education programs or for formulating health and agricultural policies because the lower the intake, the greater the risk of inadequacies.

People with an apparently adequate diet may exhibit deficiency symptoms; conversely, people with apparently suboptimal intakes may show no evidence of deficiency. These discrepancies can be explained by wide individual variations in nutritive needs resulting from differences among people in ability to absorb a nutrient or in efficiency of utilization, as well as differences between the actual nutrient content of a food and the values used in calculating the diet. In addition, a dietary evaluation usually reflects only immediate past intake, whereas much biochemical and clinical evidence reflects long-term nutritive intake. Moreover, deficiency symptoms may persist for some time after the diet is improved. Failure to find biochemical or clinical evidence of a deficiency in conjunction with low intakes may be a reflection of the time required to deplete nutrient reserves as the quality of the diet declines. However, when a low dietary intake of a specific nutrient is found along with biochemical and clinical signs of a deficiency, the dietary data provide a basis on which to build dietary treatment.

Evaluations of nutrient intake are carried out in a number of ways, each with its own merits and limitations. Generally, however, they fall into two categories: *indirect* and *direct*.

Indirect Methods

Vital Statistics

The vital statistics of a country provide an indirect method of assessing dietary adequacy. If we have useful records that include age and causes of illness and death, we can learn something about possible nutrition-related health problems. When the incidence of conditions such as beriberi or kwashiorkor is high, malnutrition is undoubtedly present. When the recorded incidence is low, it may mean that there is a truly adequate nutrient intake; however, it is equally possible that records of mortality and morbidity statistics have not been kept precisely enough to reflect these causes of death and sickness that are less well known. For example, many times only the ultimate cause of death (such as heart failure or tuberculosis) is recorded. In any case, it is difficult to distinguish the role played by nutrition from that of environmental hygiene and medical practices. When used with a recognition of their limitations, vital statistics or public health indexes are useful tools in evaluating trends in the dietary status of a population.

Food Balance Sheet or Food Disappearance Data

The most common of the indirect methods for evaluating nutrient intake is the national food balance sheet. This includes records of agricultural productivity, the export and import of food products, and estimates of food wastage to obtain a measure of the kinds and amounts of food and therefore nutrients available to a country. Adjustments must be made for food used in animal diets and for nonfood purposes. Because no information is provided on the distribution of food within a country, it is impossible to relate the variation of intake to socioeconomic status, cultural background, age, occupation, or sex. However, food balance sheets are useful in detecting year-to-year trends on the availability of nutrients, in planning agricultural production, and in pinpointing possible nutritional shortages.

The increasing availability of computerized records of the movement of food through the distribution system (from producer to consumer) opens the possibility of alternative methods of assessing food intake patterns. Universal product codes on most packaged foods provide a precise and accurate method of identifying foods; when used in conjunction with automated checkout systems in food stores, these codes can provide information on the way in which food dollars are spent and a description of food purchases.

A menu/census approach has been used by trade groups collecting data for food companies. With this approach, representative families provide information on food purchases and their use in the home.

Direct Methods

Direct methods involve an evaluation of the dietary intake of a much smaller population unit such as an institution, a family, or one person. Some direct methods are discussed here, in increasing order of specificity of data obtained.

Food Inventory

The food inventory method is used with residents in an institution or members of a family who are fed from a common kitchen. A record is made of all the foods available at the beginning of the study; all foods purchased, contributed, or grown for consumption during the period of the study (which is usually 2 to 4 weeks long); the food remaining in the inventory at the end; and an estimate of the waste of food and the food used in feeding animals. From this information, an approximation of the nutritive value of the food available to those eating in the group during this period is calculated. Adjustments are usually made for food eaten away from home.

If a list/recall procedure is used, homemakers are given a list of food items to assist them in recalling the kinds and amounts of foods purchased or acquired during the study period.

Food inventory methods have several limitations. First, because there is no indication of who consumes the food, it is quite possible that some members of the group are adequately nourished or even overnourished, whereas others may have nutrient lacks. Second, studies on small family units have shown that homemakers modify their habits of purchasing food during a time when they are made more conscious of their buying habits. The mere presence of a person recording the food inventory creates a situation in which food habits vary from normal and may also increase the reluctance of families, especially in higher income groups, to participate. Weighed records of family food consumption may also be obtained, but these require a high level of cooperation from participating family members and still yield no data on the distribution of food among family members.

Individual Food Intake

No matter what standard is used to evaluate a person's dietary habits, it is necessary to have as complete a record as possible of the food intake for a specified period of time. This record is obtained in several ways, with the choice depending on the purpose of the study, the funds and personnel available, the target population (such as children, the elderly, or pregnant females), and the literacy level of the group.

24-Hour Recall

In the 24-hour recall method, subjects are interviewed by a trained professional who asks them to describe the kinds and amounts of food consumed during the previous 24 hours. Those interviewed are often given food models, measuring cups, or a ruler to help them describe amounts of food. This method has two major advantages. First, it is a retrospective account taken at an unannounced time; there is little possibility that subjects will modify their food habits during the time they are being assessed. The likelihood of obtaining a more complete record is high because of the short memory period. Second, it is suitable for use in illiterate populations. The trained interviewer is able to probe to elicit information on the use of such overlooked foods as condiments; beverages; snacks; and food adjuncts including catsup, mayonnaise, butter, cream, and relishes. Research has shown that data from females and younger people are more valid than data from males and older people. Probing by the interviewer increases the extent to which actual food intake is recalled by as much as 25%.

Validation studies have confirmed that large intakes are often underestimated and that small intakes are overestimated. Within the usual ranges of intake these discrepancies have limited significance, but at either very high or very low intakes, they assume greater importance.

Individual interviews are a rather expensive method of obtaining dietary information. If data are desired on a group of subjects such as schoolchildren, written 24-hour diet records are sometimes preferred. However, portable tape recorders for on-the-spot recording of food intake and telephone interviews help to overcome the problems of some people's resistance to written records and their tendency to delay recording intake.

The 24-hour recall is considered a feasible method of obtaining data that can be used to compare nutritive intakes of groups of individuals. However, the high variability in diet from day to day in Western societies precludes its use in evaluating intake for individuals or in relating daily intake to biochemical data.

Data from a 1-day period fail to provide information on variations in intake associated with season, day of the week, emotional state, or work schedule, all of which may account for variability in intake. Attempts to use longer recall periods (ranging up to 28 days) have shown that, although 4 days is a maximum for many, memory is greatly enhanced if the respondent can relate food intake to activities. In many cases, a 7-day recall is possible.

Dietary History

A dietary history is used to obtain qualitative rather than quantitative information on long-standing food habits. Used in conjunction with the 24-hour recall of food intake and a 3-day food record, it is considered an effective method of assessing nutritive adequacy. Subjects are asked for information on their past dietary habits—the number and type of meals they normally eat, the frequency and extent to which they use the various food groups (such as green and yellow vegetables, milk or milk substitutes, meat, eggs, and cereals), their food likes and dislikes, food allergies, and seasonal variations in intake. From these data it is possible to establish whether the pattern observed in the 24-hour record represents a typical or atypical food intake. Much of the success of this method depends on the cooperation of the subject and the effectiveness of the interviewer. Because a typical interview requires at least 45 minutes, it is relatively costly, both in terms of time and money. Estimates of dietary intake from a dietary history tend to be higher than those from weighed records.

Food Intake Records

When evaluating the diets of large groups of literate subjects, the use of written food intake records has proven to be an inexpensive and relatively satisfactory method of obtaining data. We still do not know how many or which days should be used and are concerned about the ability of subjects to describe food amounts accurately. In most Western countries with varied food supplies and traditions of consuming varied diets, a 1-day food record is less representative of usual dietary patterns than it is in a country where the diet seldom varies. For many people, dietary patterns on weekends differ from those on weekdays. People asked to keep a 7-day food record lose interest in the task as the time progresses and keep less satisfactory records or stop entirely, often after the fourth day. Unless there is some way to ensure that records are kept each day, there is always the possibility that the task will be put off until the end of the period, leading to errors from incomplete or inaccurate recall. The 3-day written food record gives sufficiently useful information within a short enough period of time to maintain the cooperation of subjects. Whether food intake is assessed on the basis of a food inventory, a 24-hour recall, or a written food record, the accuracy of the estimate of serving size and the investigator's interpretation of records are important.

There is a concern that, when people are asked for information on their food intake, they will change their eating habits or will record what they think they *should* have eaten rather than their actual diet. This concern has led us to look for unobtrusive measurements that involve observing subjects and not asking for information. So far, such methods have proven expensive and, in some cases, a violation of the individual's right to privacy.

Weighed Food Records

When more precise dietary analysis is required, the weighed food record is the most accurate method. With this method, all food taken by the subject must be accurately weighed and then adjusted for any plate waste. This involves training the subject to keep accurate records or assigning an investigator to be present at all times to help. However, the work involved in record keeping or the presence of an unfamiliar person often leads to a modified eating pattern. In addition, weighed food records are expensive, are appropriate only with highly motivated people or those who can be paid to participate, and cannot be used with people who eat away from home. All these factors limit their usefulness.

EVALUATION OF DIETARY RECORDS

Dietary Score

A simple scoring system for the rapid evaluation of dietary adequacy by nonprofessionals is essential. Two such approaches that do not require the extensive computations involved in using food composition tables and dietary standards have been developed. The one shown in Table 21-6, with a maximum score of 100, places slightly more emphasis on the milk and fruit/vegetable groups than on the cereal and protein groups. The use of this approach requires a judgment of the serving size of the food. Average serving sizes required to earn points are 8 oz of milk or its equivalent; ½ cup (or 4 oz) of fruits or vegetables or 6 oz of fruit juice; 1 oz of cereal (or one slice of bread) or its equivalent; and 3 oz of meat, fish, or poultry or its equivalent. To keep the scoring simple, points are seldom given for partial servings. This scoring system is typical of several with the same intent, developed by groups ranging from the USDA to commodity-oriented associations such as the National Dairy Council and the National Livestock Board. In all of these, a score of 100 is earned when all four food groups are represented.

An even simpler system, placing equal emphasis (4 points) on each of the major food groups, assigns points whenever a food item appears in the diet, regardless of the amount. This system assigns 2 points for each of two servings of milk, 2 points for each of two servings of protein food, 1 point for each of four fruits or vegetables, and 1 point for each of four cereal or bread items. It has been used in evaluating the effectiveness of nutritional intervention programs and is shown in Table 21-7. Conclusions about the adequacy of the diet using this system compare well to those obtained using much more complex systems.

Each evaluation system is based on the assumption that diets with foods from each of the four major food groups will probably (but not necessarily) provide the foundation for an adequate dietary intake. Adopting these systems to evaluate a diet that may be nutritionally adequate but that follows a less conventional pattern requires considerable knowledge of the nutritional equivalents of different foods. The agreement between the results of these simple scoring systems and more involved dietary analyses shows that they can be used with confidence as a basis for counseling.

Table 21-6 ◇ Food selection check sheet

Food		Maximum Score	Daily Score					
Milk		30						
One cup of milk or equivalent	10							
Second cup of milk	10							
Third cup of milk or more	10							
Fruits and Vegetables		30						
One serving of green or yellow vegetables	10							
One serving of citrus fruit, tomato, or cabbage	10							
Two or more servings of other fruits and vegetables, including potato	5 each							
Breads and Cereals		15						
Three servings of whole-grain or enriched cereals or breads	5 each							
Protein-rich Foods		25						
One serving of egg, meat, fish, poultry or cheese (or dried beans or peas)	15							
One or more additional servings of egg, meat, fish, poultry or cheese	10							
TOTAL		100						

Table 21-7 ◇ Dietary score*

	Score Each Time Food is Mentioned	Maximum Score
Milk and milk products	2	4
Protein foods—meat, fish, poultry, eggs	2	4
Fruits and vegetables	1	4
Cereals	1	4
TOTAL		16

*An alternative system gives an additional point for one serving of legumes, for a total score of 17.

IMPROVEMENT OF NUTRITIVE INTAKE

Targeted Intervention Programs

National programs to improve nutrient intake and to alleviate malnutrition in the United States have been directed to infants, schoolchildren, pregnant women, and the elderly. Federal policies introduced in 1981 have altered the benefits and outreach of many of these programs. All of them are subject to ongoing evaluation.

In addition to subsidizing the cost of all lunches, the National School Lunch Program (mandated by the National School Lunch Act) makes lunches available free or at reduced prices for participating children whose family incomes fall below certain levels. Participation is declining because of more stringent criteria for the extended benefits and a reduction in the subsidy available to those who are unable to pay the full price. In 1977, the Child Nutrition Act was amended to make available 50¢ per child per year, to be allocated in each state for nutrition education under the National Education Training Program. This was reduced to less than 15 cents per child in 1981 before the program had been sufficiently established to determine whether it would be cost effective. In 1985, a mere $5 million was approved for the entire program. The National School Lunch Act also provided support for the Special Milk Program for schools and child care institutions not participating in the School Lunch Program. Up to 1 pint of milk per day is provided free.

U.S. Nutrition Intervention Programs
School Lunch Program
Food Stamps
Congregate Meals
Expanded Food and Nutrition Education Program (EFNEP)
Women, Infants, and Children (WIC)
Nutrition Education and Training Program (NET)
Commodity Distribution
School Breakfast Program
Special Milk Program
Child Care Food Program

The Child Nutrition Act passed in 1966 provided funds for the purchase of equipment for schools and for a School Breakfast Program. In 1972 the Child Nutrition Act of 1966 was amended to provide a supplemental food program known as Women, Infants and Children (WIC) for pregnant and lactating women and infants and children up to 4 years of age, who are considered to be nutritional risks. This includes mothers from populations with known inadequate nutritional patterns, unacceptably high incidence of anemia, high prematurity rates, and inadequate patterns of growth; children from low-income populations known to have inadequate diets and deficient patterns of growth are also included. The program, administered by the USDA through state and local agencies, is designed to provide foods or vouchers for foods with high-quality protein, calcium, iron, vitamin A, and ascorbic acid.

Foods Distributed in WIC Program
For infants
- Iron-fortified formula
- Iron-fortified infant cereal
- Fruit juice

For children
- Vitamin D-fortified milk

For pregnant women
- Iron-enriched cereal (10 mg/serving)
- Vitamin C-rich juice
- Cheese
- Eggs

For more discussion of the WIC program, see Chapter 15

In 1969, funds for the Expanded Food and Nutrition Education Program were allocated by the USDA. In this program the Agricultural Extension Service of the USDA in each state supervises the training of nutrition aides to work one to one with low-income homemakers to help them with homemaking skills and to provide nutrition education. Most of the aides are recruited from the same socioeconomic group as those with whom they will be working. In 1970 the funds were increased, with a provision that 25% of available resources must be allocated for work by youth professionals in inner cities to integrate nutrition education in other programs for the young.

The Congregate Meals Program, designed to meet both the social and nutritional needs of the elderly, is providing meals for groups up to 5 days a week in centrally located "diners's clubs."

The Food Stamp Program, begun as a pilot program in 1961 and initiated under the Food Stamp Act of 1964, has almost totally replaced the **Commodity Distribution Program.** This latter program was started when the government had large food surpluses; it is mostly locally supported and not a government program. The Food Stamp Program, most recently amended as part of the 1985 Farm Bill, is designed to improve the diets of low-income families and at the same time to expand the market for domestically produced food. Basically the program increases the purchasing power of the eligible family by allocating sufficient food stamps to provide an adequate diet based on the cost of the Thrifty Food Plan prepared by the USDA. The value of the stamps varies with income and represents a reasonable amount to

Commodity Distribution Program
A program initiated to distribute surplus food commodities such as dried milk powder, flour, sugar, and corn meal to individuals and federally supported organizations

spend for food. As an example, in 1985 a family of five with a net income of $120 per month was allotted $265 worth of food stamps, whereas a similar family with an income of $300 received $211 in stamps. The value of the coupons decreases with income until it reaches zero. Stamps can be obtained at the bank or post office or by mail and are used as cash at participating and approved grocery stores. This program is constantly being evaluated and redesigned to provide for more equitable use of funds. It is directed by the state agency responsible for administering other federally aided assistance programs.

Enrichment

enrichment
Addition of nutrients to cereals

Terms related to "enrichment" include *restoration,* or the addition of nutrients lost in food processing; and *nutritionally enhanced,* referring to foods modified to enhance their nutrition value

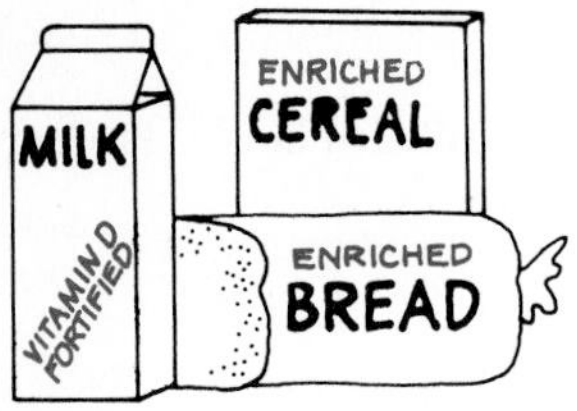

iodization
The addition of iodine to a food, usually salt

fortification
The addition of nutrients to foods other than cereals

Enrichment of food products (sometimes referred to as restoration or nutritional enhancement) has been a long-standing, effective way of correcting some aspects of undernutrition, especially since many synthetic nutrients have become available at a low cost. Compulsory enrichment of bread and flour introduced in 1940 was replaced after World War II by a voluntary program under the jurisdiction of the individual states. Currently 34 states require the enrichment of bread and flour, with thiamin, riboflavin, niacin, and iron mandatory and calcium optional within prescribed limits. Ninety percent of the bread and cereal sold in the United States is enriched. Some states require the addition of these same nutrients to cornmeal, corn grits, farina, macaroni, and noodles and the addition of thiamin, niacin, and iron to rice. In an effort to enhance effectiveness in preventing iron-deficiency anemia, the standards for iron enrichment were raised up to 25% in 1983, to 20 mg/pound of flour.

Iodization of salt contributed to a reduction in the incidence of goiter in the United States but now appears less essential because other sources of iodine are entering the food supply. **Fortification** of fresh whole and evaporated milk with vitamin D, nonfat milk with both vitamins A and D, and margarine with vitamin A is a general practice. Iron enrichment of infant cereals is not governed by any state or federal regulation other than that it be adequately labeled, but this practice has contributed to the control of iron-deficiency anemia in infants. Although many other forms of enrichment are used by the food industry, they have not received the endorsement of nutritionists for several reasons: nutrients may be used in foods that are not effective carriers; demonstrable deficiency of the nutrient may not have been found in the population consuming the product; or the nutrient may be unstable under normal conditions of preparation. With the possibility of toxicity from the excessive intake of fat-soluble vitamin D, there is concern about the indiscriminate practice of food enrichment and fortification.

In an effort to discourage ineffective and unnecessary enrichment of food products, the Food and Nutrition Board endorses the addition of nutrients to foods (fortification) when all the following conditions are met:

- **The nutrient under consideration for addition to food is judged to be significantly below the RDA in the diets of a substantial segment of the population.**
- **The food that is to carry the nutrient is consumed by most individuals in the segment of the population in need.**
- **The amount of nutrient added makes an important contribution to the total diet.**
- **The addition of the specific nutrient does not create a nutrient imbalance.**
- **The nutrient added is physiologically available and sufficiently stable so that its value will be retained during the normal shelf life of the product. Reasonable excess would be permitted to compensate for storage losses.**

- **There is reasonable assurance that excessive intake (to a level that may be harmful) will not occur.**
- **Any additional cost is affordable for the intended population.**

Specifically, the following practices in the United States continue to be endorsed: the enrichment with thiamin, riboflavin, niacin, and iron of flour, bread, degerminated cornmeal, corn grits, whole-grain cornmeal, white rice, and certain other cereal grain products; the addition of vitamin D to milk, fluid skim milk, and nonfat dry milk; the addition of vitamin A to margarine, fluid skim milk, and nonfat dry milk; and the addition of iodine to table salt. The protective action of fluoride against dental cavities is recognized, and the standardized addition of fluoride to water in areas in which the water supply has a low fluorine content is endorsed.

Dietary Guidance

The Dietary Goals developed by the Senate Select Committee on Nutrition and Human Needs marked the first attempt to provide dietary guidance for the American public to combat chronic degenerative diseases such as hypertension, coronary heart disease, and diabetes. Since then the USDA, DHHS, Food and Nutrition Board of the National Academy of Sciences, American Heart Association, American Medical Association (AMA), and Surgeon General have all issued dietary guidelines for the public. These are summarized in Table 21-8.

In general, these guidelines represent the best judgment at the time, but are considered tentative and subject to modification as more evidence is accumulated. Although there are many issues on which dietary guidelines agree, even minor points of disagreements have led to confusion. Among the most confusing points are the recommendation that dietary cholesterol be reduced; that the ratio of polyunsaturated-to-saturated fatty acids be increased to 1:1; that dietary sodium be reduced; and that dietary fat be reduced to provide 30% or less of dietary calories.

In general, at a national level in developed countries attention is focused on helping people select diets associated with maximal health benefits and minimal health risks. Programs directed at the needs of those most vulnerable to undernutrition—pregnant females, infants, children, the elderly, and the poor—are designed to provide food assistance and nutrition education. For the general public, intervention strategies such as enrichment of cereals, fluoridation of water, and iodization of salt are credited with increasing the nutritional adequacy of the diet.

To determine how much fat equals 30% of your dietary calories:

1. Estimate daily caloric intake
2. Drop the last zero
3. Divide by 3

This number equals grams of fat that would make your diet contain 30% of its calories from fat.

EXAMPLE

1. Daily calories equal 1800
2. Dropping the last zero gives you 180
3. Divide 180 by 3 and this allows you 60 grams of fat

Now you can compare that number to values on food labels and savings derived by substituting foods of lower fat content.

AN INTERNATIONAL CONCERN

At the global level efforts toward improving the nutritional health of the world's population have centered on balancing the increase in population with a comparable increase in food production. At its present rate of increase of 2% per year, world population will double in 36 years. Unfortunately this increase is not occurring evenly in all areas of the world. The largest population growth is in the poor, ill-fed areas with the most limited potential for food production. Table 21-9 graphically presents the variation in calories and protein available in different countries and areas.

The immediacy of the problem was recognized in 1974 when the United Nations (UN) convened the World Food Conference in Rome. The participants focused on ways to save the 500 million people threatened with starvation the next year because of the deficit of grain as the result of flood, drought, and fertilizer shortage. Although the conference made plans for establishing an international grain reserve and a World Food Council dedicated to minimizing the chances of such catastrophic conditions arising again, so far none have been implemented. The need for such a strategy has been reinforced by the devastation from famines in areas such as Bangladesh.

Table 21-8 ◇ Comparison of dietary advice to the public from various government and health groups

	Weight Control	Carbohydrate	Fiber	Saturated Lipid
Dietary Goals, USDA, 1978	To avoid overweight, decrease energy intake, and increase energy expenditure	Increase complex carbohydrate to 48% of energy intake; reduce refined sugar to 10% of calorie intake		Reduce to 10% of calories
Healthy People, Surgeon General, 1979		Reduce simple carbohydrate; increase complex carbohydrate		Reduce intake
National Cancer Institute, Dietary Guidelines: Rationale 1988	Avoid obesity		Increase fiber intake to 20 to 30 g/day, not >35 g	
American Heart Association, *Dietary Guidelines for Healthy Adult Americans,* 1986	Maintain desirable weight	Increase carbohydrate intake to 50% to 55% of calories, mostly complex		Reduce to <10% of calories
Dietary Guidelines, USDA, HHS, 1985	Maintain desirable weight	Avoid too much sugar	Increase fiber intake	Avoid too much
Nutritional Guidelines for Health Education in Britain, 1983	Adjust food intake and exercise to maintain optimal weight for height	Reduce sucrose to 10 kg/yr	Increase from 20 to 30 g/day	
Nutrition Recommendations for Canadians, 1979	Reduce excess consumption of calories and increase physical activity			Include source of linoleic acid
Dietary Guidelines for Americans, 1985	Maintain desirable weight	Eat adequate starch	Eat adequate fiber	Avoid too much
American Dietetic Association, 1987 *Nutrition Recommendations for Women*	Maintain desirable weight	Eat at least 50% of daily calories from carbohydrates	Include a variety of foods rich in fiber	
Nutrition and Health, Surgeon General, 1988	Achieve and maintain a desirable body weight	Increase consumption of whole-grain foods and cereal products, vegetables, and fruit	Increase fiber intake	Reduce intake

Polyunsaturated Lipid	Total Lipid	Cholesterol	Sodium	Other Advice
Increase to 10% of calories	Reduce to 30% of calories	Reduce to 300 mg/day	Decrease use of salt and foods high in salt	
	Reduce total fat intake	Reduce intake	Reduce intake	Exercise and eat a variety of foods
	Reduce to ≤30% of calories			Increase a variety of fruits, vegetables, and whole-grain cereals; avoid smoked and salt-cured food; if alcohol is used, drink in moderation
<10% of calories	Reduce to <30% of calories	<100 mg/1000 kcal, not more than 300 mg/day	Reduce to 1 g/1000 kcal, not >3 g/day	Protein should comprise 15% of caloric intake; alcohol, not >15% kcal or >50 ml ethanol
	Avoid too much	Decrease intake	Decrease intake	Eat a variety of foods
	30% of total energy intake	None	Decrease salt intake	Decrease alcohol to 4% of total energy intake; increase proportion of vegetable protein to other nutrients
	Reduce to 35% of calories			Emphasize whole-grain products, fruits, and vegetables in the diet; minimize alcohol, salt, and refined sugar
	Avoid too much	Avoid too much	Avoid too much	Moderation in alcohol use
	<33% of kilocalories		Limit salt and sodium-containing food	
	Reduce intake	Reduce intake	Reduce intake	Consume alcohol only in moderation; adolescent girls and adult women; increase foods high in calcium; community water should have optional fluoride, limit consumption and frequency of sugars if vulnerable to dental caries; children, adolescents, and women of child-bearing age, consume foods rich in iron

Table 21-9 ◆ Calorie and protein supply throughout the world (per person per day)

Area	Calories	Animal Protein (g)	Other Protein (g)
North America	3100	62	24
Western Europe	2900	40	42
South America	2700	24	40
Central America	2500	18	44
Japan	2300	19	45
China (People's Republic)	2200	4	58
Africa—south of the Sahara (excluding South Africa)	2200	6	52
North Africa	2100	8	40
India	900	4	46
Pakistan, Bangladesh	1900	8	34

From Cloud W: Science 13(8):6, 1973.

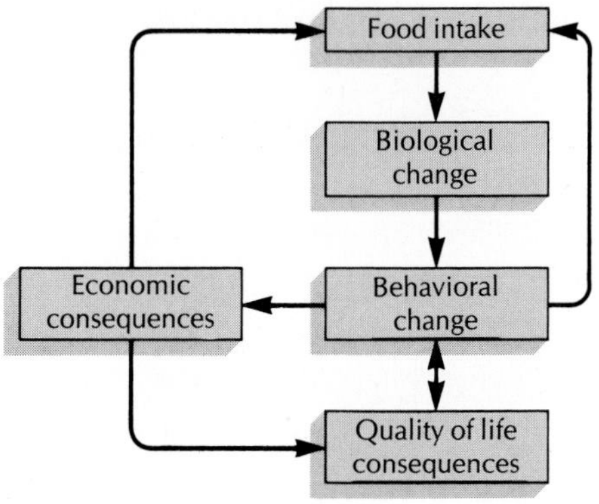

Figure 21-2 Chain of effects of either a nutrient deficiency or a nutrition intervention.

This was followed in 1977 with a report from the National Academy of Sciences entitled "World Food and Nutrition Study: the Potential Contribution of Research." Experts worked over a 2-year period to recommend research strategies to alleviate the chronic shortages of food and the debilitating effects of malnutrition. The report dealt with crop and animal productivity, aquatic food resources, food and health interventions, and nutrition education. It depicted the complex interrelationships of nutritional intervention, as shown in Figure 21-2.

At present the food-deficient areas of Asia, Africa, and Latin America have 50% of the world's population, 25% of the world's food supply, 12.5% of the income, and 50% of the arable land. On the other hand, Europe, Oceania (lands of the South Pacific Ocean), and North America have 20% of the population, 59% of the food, and 80% of the income. If the predicted population trends materialize, and if we are to maintain present nutrient intake, food supplies must increase 3.9% annually, compared with the current rate of 2.7%. If nutritional intake is to improve, the Food and Agricultural Organization (FAO) estimates food supplies would need to increase about threefold for the world and almost fourfold for the less-developed countries.

Because even the most optimistic view of the potential for increased food production does not foresee an increase of this magnitude, simultaneous efforts must be made to reverse or slow down the population growth. Should these attempts fail, the possibility of the correctives of famine, pestilence, and war is ever present.

Efforts to increase world food production must include:

1. Increasing the yield of land currently under cultivation
2. Increasing the amount of land under cultivation
3. Making maximal use of land not suitable for agriculture for the grazing of animals
4. Exploiting the sea as a potential source of food
5. Capitalizing on the capability of advancing food technology to provide unconventional food sources

The success of these efforts will depend to a certain extent on the application of agricultural technology in the form of improved plant and animal breeding; the use of herbicides, pesticides, fertilizers, and irrigation; reduction in losses after harvest; and social changes such as an available market, credit, and efficient transportation and distribution systems. Each must be evaluated in relation to its energy cost. Influences such as traditional value systems, social organization, land ownership and tenure relationships, and political climate are as important as technology in the success of innovations in agricultural production and marketing. For a more complete understanding of the complexity of the problem, a consideration of the ecology of nutritional disease is in order.

Ecology of Nutritional Disease

Epidemiologists have traditionally considered disease to be the result of a complex interaction between *host*, *environmental factors*, and *agent*. This model helps explain the varying incidence of nutritional disease under seemingly similar patterns of food consumption.

Host

The extent to which the available nutrients are utilized vary from one person to another. The factors affecting needs include age, sex, prior nutritional status, health, rate of growth, stage of development, emotional and physical stress, and genetic background. In general, the needs for nutrients are relatively high during periods of rapid growth and decline gradually after maturity. Differences attributed to sex result not only from variations in body composition, rate of growth, and the effect of different hormonal secretions, but also from different patterns of activity. The effect of genetics on the needs and utilization of nutrients has been well established. The wide range of normal requirements of specific nutrients is considered in formulating dietary allowances for healthy people.

host
An animal, plant, or human being whose health and development is influenced by an infectious agent and the environment

Whether a certain dietary intake is nutritionally inadequate is influenced by the extent to which the person can adapt to, or compensate for, suboptimal intakes. For instance, persons accustomed to low-calcium diets can use the calcium more effectively than those accustomed to higher calcium intakes. Similarly, when sodium intake is restricted or sodium needs are increased, a series of hormonal changes leads to increased retention and decreased excretion of the nutrient. The lethargy so common in the undernourished is one of several ways that the body compensates for the energy deficit.

The physiological state of the person—such as pregnancy, lactation, or growth—accounts for varying nutritional needs. Such stress factors normally result in an increased need for nutrients, but at the same time physiological adjustments increase the efficiency with which a nutrient can be utilized. Similarly, the stress of infections, such as tonsillitis, measles, tuberculosis, or pneumonia, and of parasitic infestations increases the nutrient need and in instances of marginal intake is often responsible for precipitating a nutrient inadequacy.

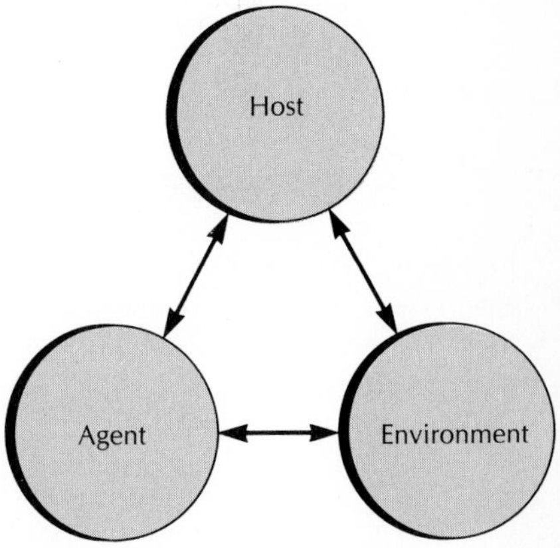

Epidemiological triad depicting relationship among agent, host, and environment as factors in nutritional disease

Environmental Factors

environmental factors
Anything in the environment that influences the health of an individual

The roles of **environmental factors** in nutritional disease are the result of their effect on the availability of nutrients, the nutritional requirements of the host, and the intake of nutrients. The environment includes both the important physical and biological environment and the social or cultural environment.

The availability of nutrients for both a population and an individual varies with the season. The phenomenon of seasonal hunger, in which food intakes hit a low point just before harvest season and a peak after harvest, is well known in developing countries. For persons dependent on sunshine as a source of vitamin D, the rainy season leads to a significant reduction in the amount of the nutrient available. Similarly, the practice in many cultures of protecting infants from exposure to sunlight deprives them of a supply of vitamin D at a time of maximal need. Seasonal fluctuations in employment such as those experienced by migrant workers, with concomitant fluctuations in income, also account for variations in availability of nutrients.

Agricultural productivity, especially in economically underdeveloped areas with poor transportation and storage facilities, obviously determines food availability. Productivity in turn depends on the nature and fertility of the soil, the climate, the topography of the land, and natural disasters such as floods, droughts, and storms. These determine the type of plant or animal that can be raised in the area and the nutritive value of food produced. For instance, cassava and soybeans can be grown on marginal land, whereas rice and wheat require more productive soil. The trace mineral content of the soil determines the mineral content of the plants produced, which influences the growth of animals feeding on the crops or the nutrient intake of persons eating the plants.

Even where the physical and biological environment would be conducive to high agricultural productivity, social factors are often the ultimate determinants. Education of the farmer in effective agricultural practices and the provision of adequate incentives to increase production are important. These may depend on the effectiveness of mass communication or the availability of a resource person who can inspire the confidence of the farmers. Adequate irrigation systems, terracing of hillsides, land tenure policies, availability of credit for seed at planting time and for herbicides and pesticides during cultivation, adequate food storage and distribution systems, and price-support policies are all socially and often politically determined factors that influence agricultural practices.

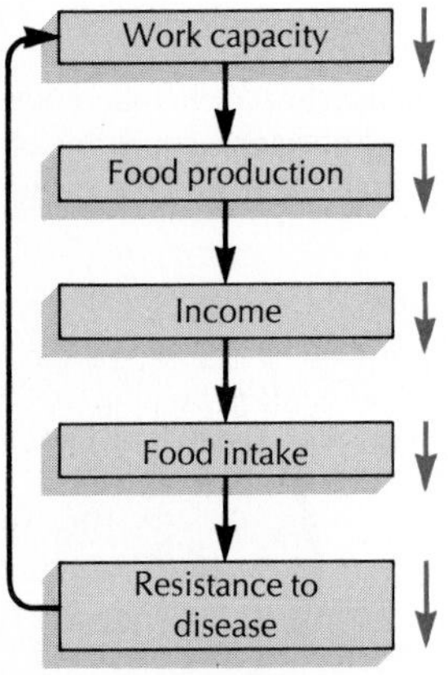

Interaction between people and their environment influencing productivity

The capacity of farmers to produce food is influenced by their health. Malaria or tuberculosis victims have reduced work capacity. Farmers with intestinal parasites experience a blood loss, anemia, and increased apathy. Reduced work capacity decreases the farmers' food production and incomes, which in turn diminishes their food intake and ability to resist intestinal parasites and infectious agents. Thus they find themselves caught in a vicious circle that must be broken if the situation is to improve.

Nutrient requirements also fall under the influence of environmental variables. Climate, as it affects heat and water and hence electrolyte losses, accounts for variations in nutrient requirements. Loss of nutrients through perspiration in a hot climate may be a precipitating factor in nutritional deficiency diseases. In developed countries the easy access to labor-saving devices reduces the requirements for calories and for nutrients involved in energy metabolism. Dietary practices, themselves an element in the environment, can influence nutrient requirements. For example, a high-carbohydrate diet calls for an increase in thiamin; a diet high in polyunsaturates, more vitamin E; a diet high in naturally occurring goitrogens, more iodine; and vegetarian diet, a supplementary source of vitamin B_{12}.

The intake of nutrients is determined to a large extent by both the physical and social environment. In the cold arctic climate only 20% of dietary calories is derived from carbohydrate, whereas in tropical regions about 80% is from the carbohydrate sources, which grow well with a high yield per acre.

Long-standing food habits are a function of the availability of food and cultural factors. Food taboos, such as the Hindus' avoidance of meat and the Jews' and Muslims' avoidance of pork, are long-standing religious restrictions. Superstitions, such as fish causing worms, eggplant causing the skin to turn dark, eggs causing sterility, and a combination of cherries and milk causing illness, have their origins in folk beliefs.

Inadequate income is an obvious factor in undernutrition. It has led older persons to adopt a high-carbohydrate diet, parents to feed diluted milk to their children, the poor to exist on a monotonous diet of rice and beans (inadequate in many nutrients), and persons in developing countries to use insignificant amounts of relatively expensive animal protein of high biological value. Although money is no guarantee of an adequate diet, when income falls below a certain point, the chances of obtaining enough nutrients decrease.

Food intake is influenced by physiological factors. The inability to chew, the loss of neuromuscular coordination, or the inability to tolerate certain foods because of allergy, gastric distress, or heartburn lead to notable changes in the character of the diet. Loss of appetite may accompany emotions such as fear or anxiety, whereas overeating may be a way of combating unhappiness or loneliness.

In developed countries, particularly among the affluent, one of the major determinants of food intake may be food fads. Faddists often advocate diets completely devoid of a particular nutrient. Scurvy has occurred among adherents of a Zen macrobiotic diet, based solely on brown rice. Some vegetarians put their children on a vitamin B_{12}–deficient diet, increasing the risk of pernicious anemia. Any diet that restricts consumption to one or two food groups increases and almost guarantees the likelihood of a nutrient deficiency. Perhaps those at greatest risk are the overweight who try successive quick weight-loss methods, almost all of which are fraught with nutritional hazards.

Agent

The third member of the epidemiological triad, the **agent,** is a relative lack of a nutrient. As just discussed, the need for a nutrient varies with host and environmental variables. Diets also vary in their nutritive content. In addition, many factors, such as the method of food processing and storage, cooking procedures, the distribution of nutrients in a day's meals, and other food components affect the amount of nutrients actually available. When nutrient stores have been depleted or cannot be mobilized, and when the amount of the available nutrient is inadequate relative to the need, a nutrient deficiency develops. The nature and severity of the symptoms vary with the specific nutrient, as does the speed with which symptoms appear. Of prime importance in prevention is the detection of biochemical changes in the blood and urine so that the condition can be corrected before physical and functional changes, which could cause severe damage, occur.

agent
The condition (malnutrition, parasite, etc.) that interacts with the environment to influence the growth and development of the host

Increasing the World Food Supply

The causes of malnutrition are multiple and interrelated. Therefore an increase in availability and utilization of food for the prevention of malnutrition may call for changes in the social, physical, or biological environment, rather than a mere increase in food production.

Increased agricultural productivity has depended to a large extent on the responsible use of pesticides and herbicides. The use of these chemicals, however, is not without hazards. Indiscriminate use may result in environmental contamination that adversely affects animals—themselves an important source of food.

Increased Agricultural Productivity is Due To
Responsible use of pesticides and herbicides
Selective breeding of plants and animals
Antibiotics and urea in animal feed

Similarly, animal food production has been increased through the use of antibiotics and hormones. Again, controls are necessary to prevent misuse so that levels remaining in animal tissues used for human consumption do not exceed established safe standards.

Selective breeding of plants has resulted in high-yielding crops particularly suited to specific areas. The Maize and Wheat Improvement Center in Mexico has produced a strain of wheat especially appropriate for the climatic and soil conditions of Central and South America. The International Rice Institute in the Philippines was responsible for a so-called "miracle" rice that is high yielding, responds well to fertilizer and irrigation, and has a shorter maturation period, making it possible

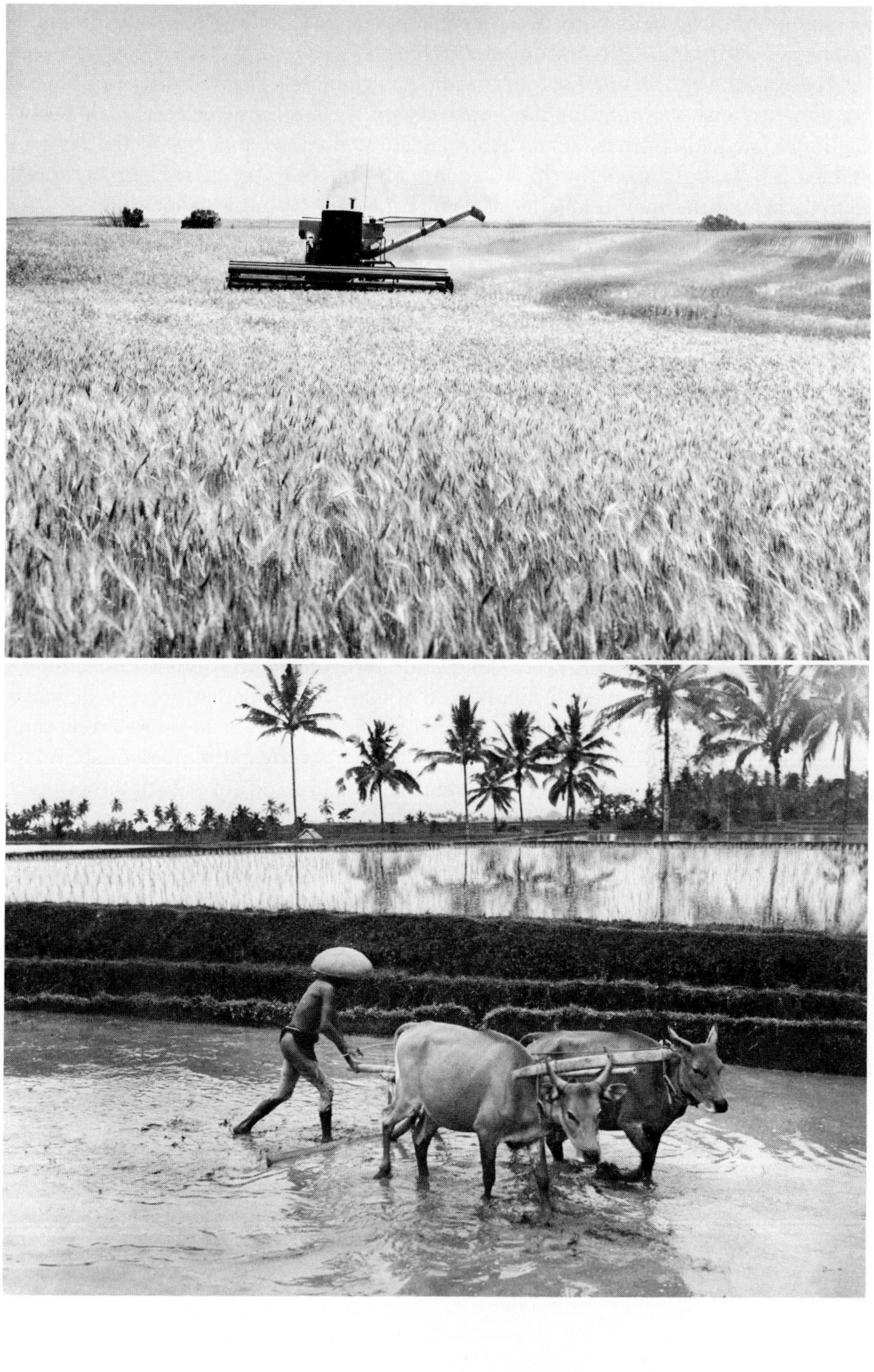

As these pictures illustrate, the difference in technology between Western (top) and Third World (bottom) agriculture is vast. Improving technology is only one key to improving agricultural productivity in developing nations

to produce more crops each year. This product has been responsible for a large increase in rice production throughout Southeast Asia—a development that has been characterized as a Green Revolution.

The Institute for Tropical Agriculture in Nigeria and one in Taiwan concentrating on vegetable production are expected to stimulate similar advances for crops such as sorghum, millet, and corn. Purdue University plant geneticists have perfected a high-yielding corn with high disease resistance. Its content of the amino acid lysine is sufficient to raise the low biological value of corn protein from a Protein Efficiency Ratio (PER) of 1.3 to 2.3, a level approaching that of casein (a high-quality milk protein). Similar advances will undoubtedly follow for other staple crops.

International Agricultural Research Centers

Mexico	Wheat
Philippines	Rice
Columbia	Cassava
	Beans
	Pasture
Nigeria	Yams
	Cowpeas
Peru	Potatoes
Liberia	Rice
India	Peanuts
	Legumes
	Sorghum
Ethiopia	Livestock
Nairobi	Animal diseases
Syria	Grains
Taiwan	Vegetables

Animal breeders are also undertaking research to improve productivity. The International Center for Tropical Agriculture in Colombia will concentrate on improving tropical livestock production. The development of a cow that thrives in the tropics, is resistant to tropical diseases, and can range on rough, marginal land has increased the potential supply of animal protein in areas where only 20% to 30% of the animal protein is now produced. Nonprotein nitrogen sources such as urea, which can be manufactured from carbon dioxide and ammonia, can be used as at least a partial source of nitrogen in feeding some animals. The development of a rapidly maturing chicken highly efficient in converting food into protein is another example of the potential of animal-breeding techniques. Governments also encourage the raising of animals such as poultry and hogs, which mature in short periods, to enhance food supplies. In addition, the "farming" of animals not now extensively used for food, such as the elephant, antelope, hippopotamus, or frog, is being investigated for countries with large game lands. The use of these animals by cultures that discourage humans from eating more conventional domestic animals, such as the cow, has great potential.

The use of fertilizer in areas of food deficiency could significantly increase the food supply from current acreage. At present only 15% of the fertilizer is used in the areas of the world that feed 50% of the world's population. To increase the use of fertilizer, it will be necessary to develop fertilizer manufacturing plants close to the areas where it is needed, to make credit readily available at the time of planting, and to provide information on its proper use. Because a cash outlay is involved, subsistence farmers who have virtually no cash reserves need to be convinced that the returns will justify the risk of borrowing. Demonstrations of its effectiveness through successful use by farmers identified as progressive community leaders have been feasible methods of increasing its acceptance.

The widespread use of chemical fertilizers to increase yield, decrease labor requirements, and lower production costs has been criticized because of the high energy cost of their production. Also, there is a possibility that nitrogen-containing fertilizers may contribute to the high nitrate content of drinking water—a potential carcinogen.

There is growing interest in natural or organic methods of pest control and of fertilizing crops. Contrary to the expectations of many, these alternative methods have been shown to be cost effective under some conditions and are applicable in large-scale agriculture. Simpler methods such as crop rotation, no-till planting, and intercropping are less expensive and accomplish much the same results.

Adequate irrigation systems have increased the productivity of land and have made it possible to use once-unproductive land. The use of either atomic or solar energy to run plants to desalinate ocean water is being explored as a means of using salt water for land irrigation. Similarly, the development of crops that thrive in brackish (slightly salty) water may make it possible to cultivate previously useless land. The importance of a water supply is evident in the inheritance patterns of many primitive societies in which the water rights to land are considered as important as the land itself.

Scientific animal-feeding techniques that include the use of cut forage crops, urea, oilseed cakes, by-products of the sugar industry, and other foods not used by humans are being promoted. Control of animal diseases such as rinderpest, hog cholera, and tuberculosis is possible, but losses from these diseases still reduce annual animal food production by 15% to 20%.

The potential of the sea as a food source has been considered; it now provides 1% of the calories and 3% of the protein in the world food supply, but opinions vary as to its potential and feasibility for future use. Some maintain that it represents an untapped resource capable of yielding over twice its current annual production and more than the projected need for 96 million metric tons in 1989. They also cite the feasibility of harvesting small fish otherwise unfit for human food that can be used in the production of fish protein concentrate, a powder containing 90% protein. This product (deodorized and defatted) has been suggested as an addition to basic cereal products, such as noodles, breads, and pasta, to enhance the biological value of the protein.

Those less optimistic about the potential of the sea as a source of protein point to the role of small fish in the food chain and suggest that by removing the small fish, we will eventually decrease the size of the schools of large fish—a more useful source of protein. Also, restrictions have already been placed on the number of big fish that can be caught to preserve the larger species. In addition, they indicate the need for considerable advances in food technology if we are to exploit the sea as a food source.

aquaculture
A science devoted to studying production of food in water

Aquaculture is now recognized as a separate discipline within the field of agriculture, concentrating on techniques to maximize the potential of the sea as a source of food. The FAO has promoted the development of fish ponds in which either brackish water or fresh water can be used for the cultivation of freshwater fish yielding as much as 4.5 metric tons/acre.

Incentives for increased food production must be great enough to counteract the old habits, customs, and traditions on which existing food production is based. Often significant changes in the social structure may be involved. In any case, increases in food production must be accompanied by comparable advances in facilities for storage and distribution. We have ample evidence that losses after harvest of food because of spoilage, insect or rodent infestation, or moisture damage reduce the food yield by as much as 25% in some parts of the world. Questions about the safety of insecticides such as ethylene dibromide necessitate a search for other methods such as irradiation or the use of carbon dioxide to reduce losses. Both of these methods kill insect larvae without leaving a harmful residue.

Improving Food Quality

soybean hydrolysates
Protein concentrates extracted from much larger amounts of soybeans and treated to make soybean use more efficient

Supplementation of food either with synthetically produced nutrients or with concentrates of natural foods holds promise. The enrichment of rice with thiamin, riboflavin, niacin, and iron; the iodization of salt; the enrichment of wheat and rice with the amino acid lysine; the addition of Fish Protein Concentrate (FPC) to cereal products; and the addition of **soybean hydrolysates** to infant foods have all had important health benefits in developing countries, although each has its inherent limitations. The effectiveness of an enrichment program depends on its use with a staple food product that is bought from major production sources, rather than from many small plants, and can be purchased by all economic segments of the population. Decentralization of rice milling and an unfavorable taxation system have hampered the success of rice enrichment in the Philippines. Similarly, in India the value of adding lysine to milled wheat has been minimal because it has been impossible to provide the machinery and control necessary in a multitude of small mills. The feasibility of using salt, which even the very poor must buy, or monosodium glutamate, a widely used flavor enhancer, as carriers for enrichment nutrients such as fluorine, vitamin A, and iron is being evaluated. Even sugar can be used as a carrier for iron or vitamin A.

USDA Research

The USDA is constantly seeking ways to improve the quality and reduce the cost of food both in the United States and throughout the world. Representative of its activities are efforts of genetic engineers and plant breeders to transfer genes from one plant to another to promote disease resistance, improved nutrient content, better storage properties, or the ability to grow under marginal conditions. New, relatively simple planting techniques allow crops to obtain and retain more water from the soil. The synthesis of plant hormones capable of stimulating growth should enhance plant yields; microbial insecticides can eliminate plant pests; and carbon dioxide or irradiation can be used to depress growth of toxic organisms.

In animal nutrition emphasis has been placed on increasing growth and fertility through the use of artificial light, temperature control, nutrient supplements, transplanting of fertilized ova into the uterus of surrogate mothers, stimulation of ovulation, and a number of forms of disease control.

Activities of International Organizations

International Agencies
Food and Agriculture Organization
World Health Organization
Aid for International Development
League for International Food Education

The World Health Organization (WHO) is primarily concerned with combating disease and other health problems and strengthening national health services. Because nutrition plays a vital role in fighting infection and reducing infant mortality and morbidity, WHO has cooperated with other agencies in seeking means of improving nutritional intake. Much of its effort has been focused on improving infant and maternal nutrition, primarily through the medical profession rather than through direct contact.

The FAO, organized under the auspices of the UN, has been charged with the responsibility of encouraging agricultural practices that will increase food production and will result in a more equitable distribution of food and improve the nutritional status of rural populations in underdeveloped areas of the world. Working in conjunction with WHO, it has formulated practical dietary standards for energy, protein, calcium, iron, vitamin A, thiamin, riboflavin, niacin, folacin, and vitamin B_{12}. FAO and WHO believe that these standards are compatible with a high level of health and that it is possible for the world to achieve this level of intake.

The United Nations Children's Emergency Fund (UNICEF) has focused its attention on the nutritional needs of children. It was responsible for the distribution of protein-rich foodstuffs in infant- and child-feeding projects throughout food-deficit areas of the world. It has also promoted school gardens through the provision of seeds and tools.

International Programs
CARE
Vista
Hope of the World
Catholic Relief Services

Many other agencies (some of which are mentioned in the margin), sponsored by both private and government groups, have contributed to the solution of the nutritional concerns of the developing nations.

In summary, today both nationally and internationally we have a vast fund of nutritional knowledge but stark evidence that much of this is not being used for the betterment of human health. Many basic questions are still unanswered, but the gap between the knowledge we have and the application of this knowledge is even more disconcerting. Correction of this situation calls for a united effort on the part of nutritionists working with anthropologists, communicators, sociologists, politicians, and agriculturists, as well as biological and physical scientists. The alleviation of human suffering is an ever-present challenge. The provision of a nutritionally adequate diet is only one—but an essential—aspect of the problem.

BY NOW YOU SHOULD KNOW

- Surveys in the United States and Canada have shown a distressing incidence of suboptimal dietary intakes of many nutrients.
- Those people most affected by suboptimal dietary intakes are the poor, the elderly, Native Americans, Eskimos, Hispanics, and migrant workers.
- Obesity affects as many as 50% of some age groups.
- Nutritional status is assessed by information on dietary intake, anthropometric measurements, physical examinations, and biochemical analyses of blood and urine.
- There is more suggestion of nutrient deficiencies from dietary research than from biochemical research. An indication of impaired iron status is the most common biochemical evidence of nutrient deficiency.
- Interpretation of data is dependent on the availability of appropriate standards.
- Although height and weight tables have many limitations, they remain useful.
- Dietary data alone are not indicative of nutritional status but provide suggestive evidence.
- Evaluation of nutrient intake can be done by both indirect and direct methods. Indirect methods are used on larger population groups and direct methods are used with smaller population units. The accuracy of direct methods depends on the honesty and accuracy of the individual reporting food intake.
- Nutrition intervention programs include the School Lunch, Food Stamp, WIC, and Congregate Feeding Programs.
- Many international research programs are directed to improving agriculture so the world can meet the food needs of a growing population.

STUDY QUESTIONS

1. What is the difference between a primary and a secondary nutritional deficiency?
2. Why are the results of clinical examinations not considered sensitive indicators of nutritional status?
3. Why can't dietary data be used alone to assess nutritional status?
4. What symptoms would you look for in deficiencies of iron, vitamin A, vitamin C, thiamin, riboflavin, iodine, and vitamin D?
5. What is the best way to detect early nutritional deficiency in children?
6. Summarize the function of each of the following: World Health Organization, Food and Agricultural Organization, Food Stamp Program, School Lunch Program, School Breakfast Program, Dietary Goals, and Food and Nutrition Board.
7. Explain the epidemiological triad.
8. What are the major differences between the Nationwide Food Consumption Survey, NHANES, and the USDA Household Food Consumption Survey?

Applying What You've Learned

1. **Undergo Biochemical Blood Screening**

   Many communities offer biochemical blood screening for a nominal fee as a yearly event at a shopping mall or in local high schools. By participating, you can have your blood levels of lipids, iron, glucose, and other components determined as well as your blood pressure. Results are sent to your physician; be sure to ask for a copy and interpretation. You owe it to yourself to at least know your blood cholesterol level.

2. **Investigate at Least One Nutritional Intervention Program Available in Your Community**

   Determine the eligibility requirements and the nature of the program benefits.

3. **Investigate Enriched or Fortified Foods**

   Identify four products in the grocery store or in your own kitchen that are enriched or fortified according to the guidelines established by the Food and Nutrition Board. Note four more that are enriched for commercial advantage.

4. **Scan Recent News Publications for Items Pertaining to Food and Nutrition**

   Identify at least one dealing with a domestic concern and one with an international concern. Apply some of the principles you have learned in interpreting the message.

5. **Getting Involved**

   Volunteer to work in a local food bank or soup kitchen.

6. **Mark October 16 on Your Calendar**

   October 16 is World Food Day; get involved! Set up a program on your campus or in your community to promote the awareness of world hunger.

7. **Evaluate Your Food Intake**

   Write down everything you have eaten today. Use Tables 21-6 and 21-7 to evaluate your nutrient intake. Do you feel your food selections have changed since the start of this course? Explain how what you have learned has influenced your food intake. Do you think these are temporary changes or permanent changes?

8. **Compare Your Food Intakes**

   Open your time capsule from the *Applying What You've Learned* section found on pp. 17 and 18 in Chapter 1. How many of these nutrition-related questions can you answer, now that you have completed this course?

SUGGESTED READINGS

Brandt EN, and McGinnis JM: Nutrition monitoring and research in the Department of Health and Human Services, Public Health Reports 99:544, 1984.

This paper describes the efforts of the federal government in monitoring the nutritional status of the U.S. population. It describes surveys planned in collaboration with USDA and those directed to low-income and Hispanic segments of the population.

Brown LR: World population growth, soil erosion, and food security, Science 214:995, 1981.

This overview of the advances that have been made in increasing the world food supply to meet the needs of an expanding population cautions about the cost in terms of soil erosion and ultimate loss of agricultural productivity. With the race between increasing population and the ability to produce enough food narrowing, the author advocates concurrent efforts to control population to avoid dire world food shortages.

Dinning JS: The role of the nutritionist in Third World agricultural policy planning, Journal of Nutrition 114:1739, 1984.

This article highlights an emerging role for nutritionists in helping to shape agricultural policy by emphasizing the nutritional impacts of various alternatives. Of special concern are polic s on imports and exports of food, agricultural subsidies, loans to farmers for agricultural inputs such as fertilizer and irrigation systems, and marketing policies. Nutritionists are uniquely qualified to provide information on the nutritional status of the population, the patterns of food intake, and distribution of food within the family and community. They must promote improved and diversified agricultural production practices that will improve the nutritional status of the population.

Sauberlich HE: Newer laboratory methods for assessing nutrition of selected B-complex vitamins, Annual Review of Nutrition 4:377, 1984.

This article deals with the merits and limitations of commonly used methods for assessing nutritional status by biochemical analyses of blood, urine, and other body tissues. It provides the reader with a basis for interpreting the data and cautions against using them in an inappropriate way.

Simko MD, Cowell C, and Gilbride JA: Nutrition assessment, Rockville, MD, 1984, Aspen Systems Corporation.

This comprehensive book presents a logical and thorough description of the techniques of nutritional assessment, provides appropriate standards for interpreting them, and discusses how they can be used in a variety of settings when nutritional assessment is desirable. It is a multiauthored book, each chapter being written by experts on a particular topic.

ADDITIONAL READINGS

Nutritional Status

Frisancho AR: New norms of upper limb fat and muscle areas for assessment of nutritional status, American Journal of Clinical Nutrition 34:2540, 1981.

Kerr GR, and others: Relationships between dietary and biochemical measures of nutritional status in HANES I data, American Journal of Clinical Nutrition 35:294, 1982.

Robinett-Weiss N, Hixson ML, Keir B, and Sieberg J: The Metropolitan Height-Weight Table: Perspective for use, Journal of the American Dietetic Association 84:1480.

Roche AF, and Himes JH: Incremental growth charts, American Journal of Clinical Nutrition 33:2041, 1980.

Shapiro LR: Streamlining and implementing nutritional assessment: the dietary approach, Journal of the American Dietetic Association 75(3):230, 1979.

Simonopoulos AD, editor: Assessment of nutritional status, American Journal of Clinical Nutrition 35(suppl):1095, 1982.

Solomons NW, and Allen LH: Functional assessment of nutritional status: principles, practice, and potential, Nutrition Reviews 41:33, 1983.

Woteki CE, Hitchcock DC, Briefel R, and Winn DN: National Health and Nutrition Examination Survey—NHANES, Nutrition Today 23:25, 1988.

Dietary Intake

Cameron M, and Von Staveren WA: Manual or methodology for food consumption studies, New York, 1988, Oxford Medical Publications, Oxford University Press.

Committee on Food Consumption Patterns, Food and Nutrition Board: Assessing changing food consumption patterns, Washington, D.C., 1981, National Academy Press.

Gersovitz M, Madden JP, and Smiciklas-Wright H: Validity of 24-hour recall and seven-day record for group comparisons, Journal of the American Dietetic Association 73:48, 1978.

Guthrie HA, and Scheer JC: Validity of Dietary Score for assessing nutrient adequacy, Journal of the American Dietetic Association 78:240, 1981.

Peterkin B, Rizek RL, and Tippett KS: Nationwide Food Consumption Survey, 1987, Nutrition Today 23:18, 1988.

Swan PB: Food consumption by individuals in the United States, Annual Review of Nutrition 3:413, 1983.

National Issues

Athrens EH Jr, and others: The evidence relating six dietary factors to the nation's health, American Journal of Clinical Nutrition 32:2621, 1979.

Brown JL: Hunger in the US, Scientific American, p. 37, Feb 1987.

Carter LJ: Organic gardening becomes legitimate, Science 209:254, July 11, 1980.

Danellson R, and Robbins L: Food consumption trends in Canada—the last 20 years, Food Market Commentary 6(4):47, 1984.

Fortmann SP, and others: Effect of health education on dietary behavior: the Stanford three-community study, American Journal of Clinical Nutrition 34:2030, 1981.

Harper AE: Dietary goals—a skeptical view, American Journal of Clinical Nutrition 31:310, 1978.

Hegsted DM: Dietary goals—a progressive view, American Journal of Clinical Nutrition 31:1504, 1978.

Hulse JH: Food science and nutrition: the gulf between the rich and the poor, Science 216:1291, 1982.

Lee SS: Health policy, a social contract: a comparison of the United States and Canada, Journal of Public Policy, p. 293, Sept., 1982.

Lockeretz W, Shearer G, and Kohl DH: Organic farming in the corn belt, Science 211:540, 1981.

McNutt, K: Dietary advice to the public: 1957 to 1980, Nutrition Reviews 38:353, 1980.

National Research Council/National Academy of Sciences: Diet and cancer, Washington, D.C., 1982, National Academy of Sciences.

Nielsen H: Nutrition in health promotion programs: a Canadian perspective, Human Nutrition: Applied Nutrition 37A:165, 1983.

The nutritive quality of processed foods: general policies for nutrient additions, Nutrition Reviews 40:93, 1982.

Ostenso GL: Nutrition policies and politics, Journal of the American Dietetic Association 88:909, 1988.

Pao E, and Mickle SJ: Problem nutrients in the United States diet, Food Technology 32:58 (Sept.), 1983.

Rose H: The microbiological production of food and drink, Scientific American 245:127, 1981.

Slater CH, and others: Ischemic heart disease: footprints through the data, American Journal of Clinical Nutrition 42:329, 1985.

International Concerns

Lunknett DL, and Smith NJH: Agricultural research and the Third World food production, Science 217:215, 1982.

National Academy of Sciences: World food and nutrition study—the potential contribution to research, Washington, D.C., 1977, National Academy of Sciences.

FOCUS Nutrition Monitoring—Why and How

Over the past few years there has been a continuing interest in promoting a systematic coordinated effort among government agencies to monitor the nutritional status of the nation. In this and other chapters we have discussed the various techniques (biochemical, dietary, anthropometric, and epidemiological) used. As the monitoring system has evolved over time, various agencies have developed, in keeping with their own objectives and priorities, their own approach to data collection. They have applied their own, often differing, standards in interpreting the findings. Thus while the United States has in place the components of a sophisticated system, the parts are sufficiently different that it is difficult, if not impossible, to compare and integrate findings from one study to another. This is an unfortunate weakness.

Efforts to facilitate coordination have given rise to the question "why nutritional surveillance?" The answer varies depending on the perspective and priorities of the agency supporting a particular aspect of the system.

The National Center for Health Statistics (NCHS) with a mandate to monitor and improve health status focuses primarily on the assessment of the nation's health. This may reflect not only the nutrient intake but also the way in which the body utilizes the nutrient to maintain health. This information is provided primarily through NHANES. For instance, while they are interested in determining the prevalence of anemia in the United States, they look at a variety of environmental and physiological factors that may be contributing to the problem. Dietary intake is only one of many possible causes and thus the assessment of dietary intake, while important, is not a shared priority.

On the other hand the USDA, which conducts surveys of food intake of householders and individuals and trends in food, and hence nutrient, availability, is involved only in assessing nutrient adequacy compared to accepted standards and does not attempt to assess health status. Their data, however, are used extensively in evaluating the relationship between dietary intake and health. The USDA directs considerable amounts of their resources into maintaining a nutrient data base, which reflects the quality of the food supply and changes in nutrient availability with changing agricultural and food processing practices. They are also concerned with developing techniques that will provide a sensitive measure of actual food intake—information that is critical to any attempt to establish the relationship between food intake and health status.

The FDA is charged with guarding the safety of our food supply and has a comparable interest in obtaining accurate information on food intake. They are interested (1) partly in judging the impact of policies such as fortification and enrichment of food products on nutrient intake and (2) partly in monitoring the level of consumption of environmental contaminants, such as pesticides and herbicides, and intentional additives, such as antioxidants, used to enhance food quality.

In addition to these three groups that invest considerable time and effort in collecting information on food practices, nutrient intake, and nutritional status, many other groups either use the techniques developed by these units to collect their own data or analyze the data collected in major national surveys to find answers to their own questions. These may range from questions about the relative health and nutritional status of participants and eligible, nonparticipants in intervention programs such as the School Lunch Program, WIC, Food Sample Program, or Congregate Meals Program. Others direct their attention to the impact of nutrition education efforts on food practices. It is very obvious that with all the questions to be answered by data collected in a national surveillance system, it is essential that monitoring efforts be not only coordinated but compatible.

In general almost all of the data on food composition come from data compiled by the USDA from analyses done in government, university, and industry laboratories, which use specified analytical techniques and reporting procedures. As a result it seems reasonable that while various tables may be more or less specific about certain classes of foods such as incorporating data in more cuts of meat or a greater variety of cereal products it should be possible to use them all interchangeably with reasonable confidence that the results are valid. In fact, the availability of different tables with minor differences in reported nutrients for the same foods is only confusing to professionals and the public alike. In most cases differences are due to minor discrepancies in serving sizes or result from rounding of data. In other instances apparent differences may be due to the specific breed of animal or species of fruit, vegetable, or cereal described calling for information that is almost impossible for the respondent to provide. Therefore such specificity is irrelevant to most dietary analysis. The assessment of nutrient intake is further complicated by uncertainty about the accuracy of estimates of food portions, which in most cases will exceed any errors that may be introduced by errors in the misuse of food composition data.

The assessment of nutritional status is a function of two factors: the sensitivity of the analytical procedures used and the availability of appropriate standards. The Centers for Disease Control devotes much of their resources toward developing the necessary techniques and standards. Once developed they should be the ones used in any attempts at surveillance. To have varying standards only introduces confusion and complicates comparison of findings from one study to the next.

Neither nutrient data base, analytical technique, nor standards of assessment should be accepted uncritically. They must be subjected to scrutiny by qualified professionals, reviewed periodically, and accepted only if judged valid and in keeping with current scientific standards. When this is achieved, the United States will have the foundation of an even more effective nutritional monitoring system with the following aims to provide:

- Data on foods, nutrient, and food additive intakes
- Data for nutrition-related risk factors and the prevalence of compromised nutritional status
- Information to study the relationships between diet, nutritional status, and health
- Data on which to revise the National Center for Health Statistics growth charts

Answers to Awareness Check: Truth or Fiction?

Chapter 1

A person hospitalized is at risk for developing malnutrition. *True*; p. 10.

The diet of a pregnant woman has little impact on the infant's physical condition at birth. *False*; p. 5.

Weightlessness changes an astronaut's nutritional status. *True*; p. 11.

Development of new foods such as low-cholesterol cheese can have only a positive effect on degenerative diseases. *False*; p. 13.

To reduce the incidence of heart disease, cancer, bone diseases, and diabetes everyone should follow dietary modifications. *True*; p. 13.

Nutrients needed in small quantities have less important functions in the body than nutrients needed in larger quantities. *False*; p. 15.

Today is described as the Naturalistic Era of nutrition. *False*; p. 6.

A dietitian is limited to working in a hospital or institutional setting, and emphasis is on diet therapy, menu planning, and food service. *False*; p. 20.

Chapter 2

The stomach is the main organ of digestion. *False*; p. 26.

External cues such as seeing or smelling food will trigger your appetite whether you are hungry or not. *True*; p. 23.

The muscular tube of the small intestine is slick like a pipe to aid in the movement of nutrients in, out, and down the gastrointestinal tract. *False*; p. 25.

The acid level of the stomach and small intestines influences digestion. *True*; p. 26.

Water passes freely across membranes by osmosis whereas solids cross by passive diffusion or active transport. *False*; p. 29.

Chapter 3

Healthy adults need at least 6 oz. of meat or meat substitute a day. *True*; p. 50.

Eggs and butter are part of the milk or dairy group. *False*; p. 48.

Eliminating all fat from the diet is the best way to reduce one's risk for heart disease. *False*; p. 45.

One half cup of cottage cheese has the same amount of calcium as one half cup of milk. *False*; p. 48.

Everyone must take in 100% of their U.S. RDA for all nutrients to maintain good health. *False*; p. 37.

Chapter 4

Carbohydrates are fattening. *False*; p. 69.

Sugar causes diabetes. *False*; p. 73.

People should avoid sugar and use sugar substitutes whenever possible. *False*; p. 97.

A person who is lactose intolerant can never eat dairy products. *False*; p. 77.

Carbohydrate loading is recommended for the weekend athlete. *False*; p. 79.

Dietary fiber may reduce one's risk of colon cancer. *True*; p. 81.

Low-carbohydrate diets are one of the most successful ways to lose weight and keep the weight off. *False*; p. 82.

Chapter 5

All fats should be eliminated from the diet. *False*; p. 101.

Butter and margarine have the same number of calories per serving. *True*; p. 127.

Prime quality meat has less fat than a less expensive cut. *False*; p. 101.

A fat is either totally saturated or totally unsaturated. *False*; p. 102.

A food product that claims to be cholesterol-free is a safe food for persons modifying their fat and cholesterol intake. *False*; p. 40.

Chapter 6

Protein is a major nutritional concern in the American diet. *False*; p. 152.

Excess dietary protein is stored as muscle or lean body tissue. *False*; p. 146.

Dietary protein eaten in amounts greater than needed for growth, maintenance of cells, or energy is converted to fat. *True*; p. 146.

Protein is necessary to produce antibodies that will fight off foreign substances such as bacteria. *True*; p. 142.

Lipoproteins will be manufactured regardless of the amount of protein in the diet. *False*; p. 142.

Amino acid supplementation is recommended to ensure nutritional well-being even in healthy individuals. *False*; p. 149.

Chapter 7

Calories have no function in the body; they only make people gain weight. *False*; p. 170.

Two people who weigh the same and are the same height will have the same basal energy requirement. *False*; p. 175.

Most people who are overweight have an underactive thyroid gland. *False*; p. 176.

Men usually have a higher calorie need than women. *True*; p. 175.

Studying very intently requires more calories than just reading for pleasure. *False*; p. 179.

Breastfeeding women have higher energy needs than pregnant women. *True*; p. 183.

Chapter 8

Weight gain occurs when energy intake exceeds energy expenditure. *True*; p. 201.

Fat weighs more than muscle. *False*; p. 202.

People who skip breakfast and lunch and overeat at night may actually store more fat than people who eat at regular intervals throughout the day. *True*; p. 211.

Except in the case of extreme obesity, it is best to lose only 1 to 1½ pounds per week. *True*; p. 214.

High-protein diets are the quickest and best way to lose excess body fat. *False*; p. 214.

Weight loss can reduce the risk for heart disease and high blood pressure. *True*; p. 206.

Chapter 9

Water is not an essential nutrient. *False*; p. 229.

Lettuce is composed almost entirely of water. *True*; p. 234.

A low-sodium product is the same as a product with no salt added. *False*; p. 245.

Pregnant women should restrict their salt intake. *False*; p. 246.

Persons living in areas with fluoridated water have protection against loss of skeletal calcium. *True*; p. 239.

Chapter 10

Calcium supplements will prevent osteoporosis. *False*; p. 276.

Most multiple vitamin supplements will provide 100% of the U.S. RDA for calcium. *False*; pp 274-276.

Osteoporosis is a disease affecting only women. *False*; p. 276.

Dolomite is a dependable and safe source of calcium. *False*; p. 275.

Long-term alcohol consumption may lead to a magnesium deficiency. *True*; p. 280.

Chapter 11

Supplements are a good way to ensure an adequate intake of trace elements. *False*; p. 321.

A cup of tea or coffee with a meal will inhibit iron absorption. *True*; p. 294.

Cooking in a cast iron skillet will increase the amount of dietary iron. *True*; p. 300.

It is simple for women to meet the RDA for iron from food alone. *False*; p. 297.

The processing of grain products reduces the zinc and selenium content of the food. *True*; p. 315.

Chapter 12

A person cannot meet all the RDAs for vitamins from food alone. *False*; p. 344.

Eating carrots will improve your eyesight. *False*; p. 348.

Vitamin A prevents cancer. *False*; p. 359.

Megadoses of vitamins can be dangerous. *True*; p. 359.

Topical vitamin A promotes smooth and youthful skin. *False*; p. 359.

Nutrient supplements are regulated and controlled by the FDA. *True*; p. 344.

Chapter 13

Vitamin C prevents and cures the common cold. *False*; p. 394.

Oranges and citrus fruits are the only dependable food sources of vitamin C. *False*; p. 391.

Megadoses of vitamin C are harmless. *False*; p. 394.

Megadoses of vitamin B_6 are harmless and should be taken to alleviate the symptoms of premenstrual syndrome. *False*; p. 409.

Cigarette smokers have an increased need for vitamin C. *True*; p. 393.

Cooking vegetables in water at a high heat and for a prolonged time will decrease their folacin content. *True*; p. 398.

Chapter 14

Thiamin, riboflavin, and niacin are nutrients used to enrich grain and cereal products. *True*; p. 417.

Body builders who eat raw egg whites may be setting themselves up for a biotin deficiency. *True*; p. 436.

Milk is one of the best food sources of riboflavin. *True*; p. 426.

It is almost impossible to meet dietary needs of pentothenic acid in our food supply. *False*; p. 433.

Milk is stored in opaque containers because it is readily destroyed by ultraviolet light. *True*; p. 425.

Chapter 15

Nutritional needs of the pregnant teen are higher than that of a woman in her 20s or 30s. *True*; p. 451.

Because the risk of degenerative diseases is greater among the obese it is recommended, as prevention, that pregnant women restrict weight gain. *False*; p. 459.

During pregnancy, a woman should restrict her intake of sodium. *False*; p. 461.

The zinc status of the pregnant woman can be adversely affected by excessive supplementation of iron and folate. *True*; p. 466.

A woman needs more calories when breast feeding than during pregnancy. *True*; p. 473.

Almost all drugs taken by a mother during lactation appear to some extent in her milk. *True*; p. 475.

Chapter 16

Breastfeeding is always the best method oi infant feeding. *False*; p. 486.

Solid foods should be introduced in the thirc month of life. *False*; p. 505.

Putting a baby to bed with a bottle of milk is a recommended pacifier that will keep the child from crying himself to sleep. *False*; p. 498.

Breastfeeding can be an expensive form of infant feeding because of the actual food dollar spent on the foods needed to meet the increased calorie and nutrient needs of the mother. *True*; p. 495.

Whole milk or cow's milk is not recommended during the first 6 months of life. *True*; p. 497.

By 6 months of age milk alone cannot provide all the calories needed by the infant. *True*; p. 505.

Chapter 17

Snacks can be an important component of the diet of both children and adolescents. *True*; p. 524.

Teenagers who skip breakfast can perform adequately as long as they make up the nutrients later in the day. *False*; p. 539.

Milk is an important part only of the infant and childhood diet. Once a person reaches adolescence the need for calcium diminishes. *False*; p. 544.

Children have more taste buds than adults and therefore are more sensitive to the strong flavors of food. *True*; p. 523.

Sugar causes hyperactivity in children. *False*; p. 534.

Anorexia nervosa and bulimia are two eating disorders more prevalent in young women than any other sex or age-group. *True*; p. 546.

Chapter 18

The elderly need less of all nutrients in comparison to active, healthy adults. *False*; p. 571.

The elderly have fewer energy needs because they cannot be as physically active as they once were. *False*; p. 571.

As we age we experience a decreased ability to taste and smell foods. *True*; p. 561.

As we age our amount of lean body mass declines and we naturally tend to store more fat. *True*; p. 565.

More men have complications from osteoporosis than do women. *False*; p. 567.

A balanced diet will slow the aging process. *False*; p. 555.

Chapter 19

An athlete needs more calories because he or she has a larger calorie output than a nonathlete. *True*; p. 586.

Concentrated sweets provide quick energy and improved athletic performance. *False*; p. 591.

Athletes should never drink water before or during competition. *False*; p. 584.

Going to a sauna to sweat off extra pounds is safe weight loss for the wrestler trying to "make weight." *False*; p. 584.

To allow for proper digestion, athletes should eat about 3 to 4 hours before competing. *True*; p. 590.

Carbohydrate loading is not recommended for the average recreational athlete. *True*; p. 589.

Chapter 20

"Natural" on the label is well defined and regulated by the Food and Drug Administration. *False*; p. 603.

Vegetarians should take multiple vitamin or mineral supplements daily because they cannot get all the nutrients they need. *False*; p. 602.

Foods at health food stores may cost more than those from conventional grocery stores, but it is worth the price to know they are organically grown. *False*; p. 603.

Because so many nutrients are available in a wide variety of foods, there should be no nutritional problems from omitting one food group from an otherwise well-planned diet. *False*; p. 603.

Chapter 21

Protein malnutrition is now considered less critical than calorie malnutrition. *True*; p. 621.

Current nutrition intervention programs are successful. *True*; p. 635.

Enrichment of food products is one way of improving some aspects of undernutrition. *True*; p. 636.

Not all nutrition scientists agree on how much cholesterol is recommended in the average American diet. *True*; p. 638.

The sea is a potential source of food for the world. *True;* p. 646.

Obesity is a form of malnutrition. *True*; p. 623.

Appendixes

APPENDIX

A Basic Principles of Chemistry and Biology

enzyme
Protein produced by a living cell to accelerate metabolic reactions; identified by the suffix "-ase" and a prefix, indicating the substrate on which it acts (for example, *amylase* = enzyme that acts on starch; *protease* = enzyme that acts on protein; *lipase* = enzyme that acts on lipid)

coenzyme
Substance that assists an enzyme in facilitating a reaction; usually has a vitamin as part of its structure

hormone
Chemical substance produced in an endocrine gland, such as the pituitary or thyroid, and transported by the blood to other tissues, where it influences function and metabolic activity

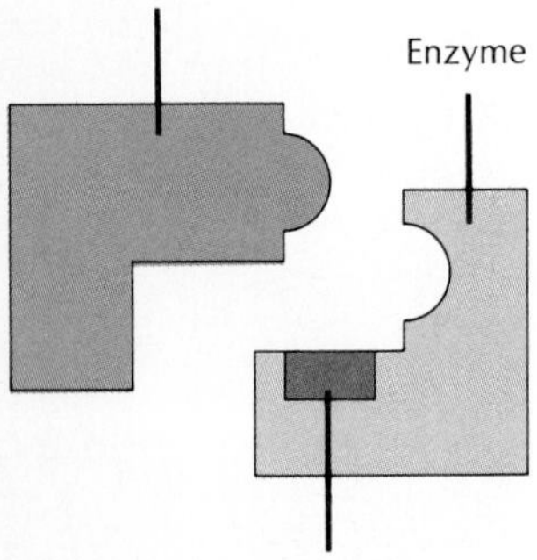

Figure A-1
Each enzyme made of protein has a unique shape that permits it to fit a specific substrate in order to bring about a specific chemical change—usually splitting off a portion of a molecule or joining two molecules to form one new one. Sometimes a vitamin-containing enzyme is necessary to allow the enzyme to fit the substrate.

An understanding of the role of both chemistry and biology involves an understanding of the roles of enzymes, coenzymes, and hormones. All of these compounds are involved in the processes by which the nutrients in food are changed into forms in which they can be utilized for growth, energy, and maintenance of the body. Some of the changes occur in the digestive tract, but the majority occur within the individual cells. **Enzymes** are proteins produced by cells. Some also have minerals as part of their structure. Each enzyme has a specific function and a unique shape that allows it to fit the substance on which it will act to bring about a specific change (Figure A-1). Sometimes an enzyme acts alone, but more often it requires the help of a **coenzyme,** or protein/vitamin complex. Enzymes, sometimes with the help of coenzymes, split a substance into two or more separate parts, remove or change some portion of the molecule, or combine two or more smaller units to synthesize or build a new substance, all of which are essential to growth.

Enzymes are easily identified because their names always end in the suffix "-ase." The first part of the name provides information about the substance on which the enzyme acts or the type of reaction that it aids. For example, a protease is an enzyme that acts on protein, and a deaminase is an enzyme that is needed for the removal of an "amino" group from a substance. Sometimes the name of the enzyme is further modified so that you can tell where or how it acts. For instance, a gastric protease is an enzyme produced by the stomach to act on protein, and a lysine deaminase is an enzyme that aids in the removal of an amino group from the amino acid, lysine. Even more specifically, the name hepatic lysine deaminase tells you that the reaction took place in the liver (*hepato* = liver). Therefore it is obvious that the name of an enzyme makes it possible to know quite a bit about what it does, where it does it, or both.

Hormones also play a very important role in many functions of the body. In contrast to enzymes, hormones are produced by specific tissues and then released into the bloodstream to be carried to other tissues on which they act. For example, the hormone *insulin,* a protein that is produced within specific cells in the pancreas, is then released into the blood to be carried to almost every cell of the body, where it assists the cells in picking up glucose from the blood. Similarly *thyroxin,* a hormone produced in the thyroid gland, is carried to other body cells where it regulates the rate of metabolism. Not all hormones are proteins; some, such as estrogens, belong to a group of nonprotein compounds called *steroids.*

CHEMISTRY

Just as it is not absolutely necessary to understand human physiology to learn about nutrition, it is not absolutely necessary to understand chemistry. However, familiarity with a few basic principles certainly does help. All nutrients are chemicals, and the way in which the body uses nutrients involves chemical changes. Therefore the reason for including this very brief discussion of chemistry should be clear.

All chemicals are made up of atoms that are held together by chemical bonds, or links. Each chemical element has a name but is usually referred to by a symbol—a sort of chemical shorthand. Thus the element carbon is referred to by the symbol C, hydrogen by H, and oxygen by O. Although we know there are at least 102 elements in our environment, there are only approximately 30 which students of nutrition need to be concerned with. These elements and the chemical shorthand by which they are identified are shown here.

Chemical Elements of Significance in Nutrition

Chemical Name	*Symbol*	*Valence*
*Hydrogen	H	1
Lithium	Li	1
*Carbon	C	4
*Nitrogen	N	3,5
*Oxygen	O	2
Fluorine	F	1
*Sodium	Na	1
Magnesium	Mg	2
Aluminum	Al	3
Silicon	SI	4
*Phosphorus	P	3
Sulfur	S	2
Chlorine	Cl	1
*Potassium	K	1
*Calcium	Ca	2
Vanadium	V	2
Manganese	Mn	2
*Iron	Fe	2
Cobalt	Co	2
Nickel	Ni	2
Copper	Cu	1
Zinc	Zn	2
Arsenic	As	3
Strontium	Sr	2
*Molybdenum	Mo	1
Tin	Sn	4
*Iodine	I	1
Lead	Pb	4

Of these, the 11 marked by an asterisk account for 99.3% of the chemical elements in living cells.

Each element has a fixed number of bonds with which it can join another element. This number is called the *valence* and is indicated after each symbol in the margin. (This number represents the number of electrons needed to fill the outer shell of an atom of the element.) Elements cannot exist with unfilled bonds and will always seek some way of satisfying this need. Therefore, if carbon (which has four unfilled electrons or bonds) joins with hydrogen (which has only one bond to be filled), it has to add four hydrogen atoms to form CH_4, or methane (in which four bonds are shared). If, however, carbon joins with oxygen, which has two unfilled bonds (or needs two electrons), it must join with only two oxygen atoms to form CO_2, or carbon dioxide. If hydrogen (with a valence of 1) joins with oxygen (with a valence of 2), the resulting compound is H_2O, which we know as water. Each of these combinations of atoms is called a *molecule*. The same rule—that each atom in a more complex molecule must have something attached to it—is followed in a compound such as glucose, with the formula $C_6H_{12}O_6$. When one hydrogen atom joins with one oxygen atom, the OH unit (called a hydroxyl group) still has one empty bond that must be attached to another bond—in the case of sugar, a C bond. When two adjacent carbon atoms have nothing else to attach to, they join each other with a second link, making a so-called double bond ($C = C$). This satisfies the carbon atoms temporarily, but as soon as they can find two free bonds to attach to, they will break apart the second bond and attach themselves to the other elements.

In discussing the basics of chemistry, we have purposely chosen to use the element *carbon* in most of our examples. Carbon is a common component in all organic matter, and all living matter is organic. When we discuss the chemistry of the body and of food, we deal almost exclusively with organic compounds in living cells, which are the subject of the branch of chemistry known as *biochemistry*.

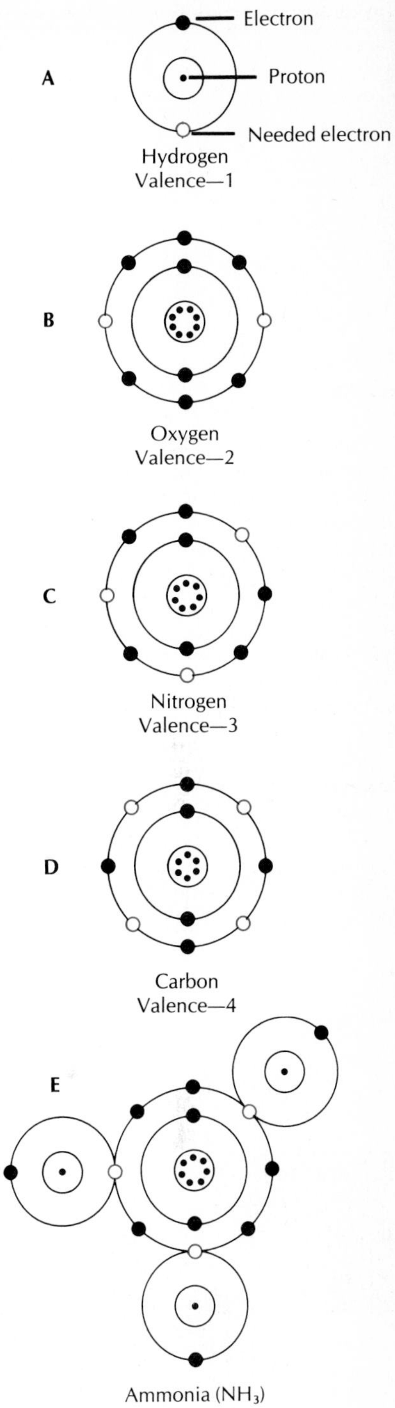

The structure of an atom of
(A) hydrogen, with one space for an electron in the outer shell,
(B) oxygen, showing two places for electrons in the outer shell,
(C) nitrogen, with three spaces for electrons, and
(D) carbon, with four spaces for electrons.
(E) Three atoms of hydrogen join one of nitrogen to make one molecule of ammonia.

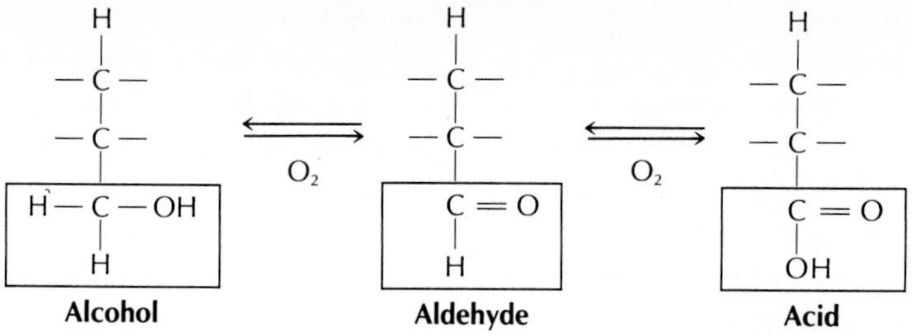

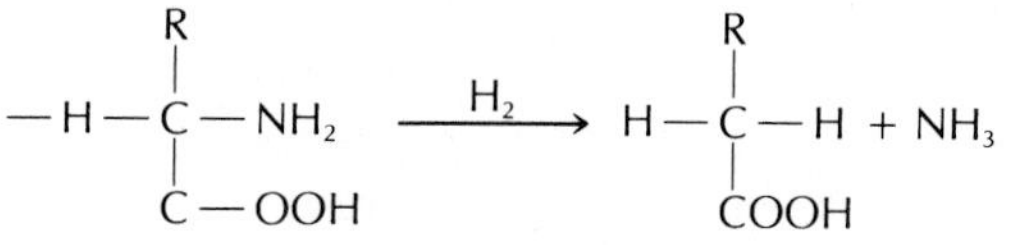

Deamination

One of the most common chemical reactions for both organic and inorganic compounds is the oxidation/reduction reaction. Oxidation includes either adding oxygen, or positive charges, to a compound, or removing hydrogen, or negative charges. Similarly, reduction of chemicals is accomplished either by adding hydrogen or taking away oxygen (a positive charge). Most of the compounds we will be concerned with exist either as an alcohol, an aldehyde, or an acid. An alcohol, which can be recognized because it has an OH group, is oxidized to an aldehyde, which is recognized by its terminal carbon atom with a hydrogen attached in one place and an oxygen occupying two bonds (CHO). An aldehyde can be further oxidized to an acid, with the end of the compound being COOH. These oxidation reactions are reversible by reduction (the addition of hydrogen or the removal of oxygen). In most cases, oxidation of one substance is paralleled by the reduction of another.

Because of the exchange of atoms that occurs, oxidation and dehydrogenation are essentially the same. Similarly, reduction and hydrogenation have much the same effect.

Other biochemical reactions that you will read about in nutrition involve the transfer of a chemical group called an amino group (NH_2), which is common in all proteins. When this amino group is removed from a compound, the process is called *deamination;* when it is transferred from one substance to another, the term is *transamination.* Similarly, many reactions involve a single carbon group (CH_3), also known as a *methyl* group. When this methyl group is transferred from one molecule to another, the process is called *transmethylation.* Actually, most biochemical reactions are named very systematically; it is usually rather easy to figure out what is described by analyzing the name of the reaction or the names of the parts of the reaction.

BIOLOGY

The cell is a basic unit of body structure. In turn, the cell is a complex structure itself with many parts analogous to the organs of the total body—such as the liver, kidneys, and heart. As illustrated in Figure A-2, cells vary considerably in size and shape, but most have the same type of internal structure and are composed of very distinctive parts called **organelles.** The general features of a typical cell are illustrated in Figure A-3. Our knowledge of the complexity of the cell structure has been made possible only with the development of the electron microscope; the complexities of the functions of the organelles were recognized only after

organelle
Structure within the cell that carries out a specific function

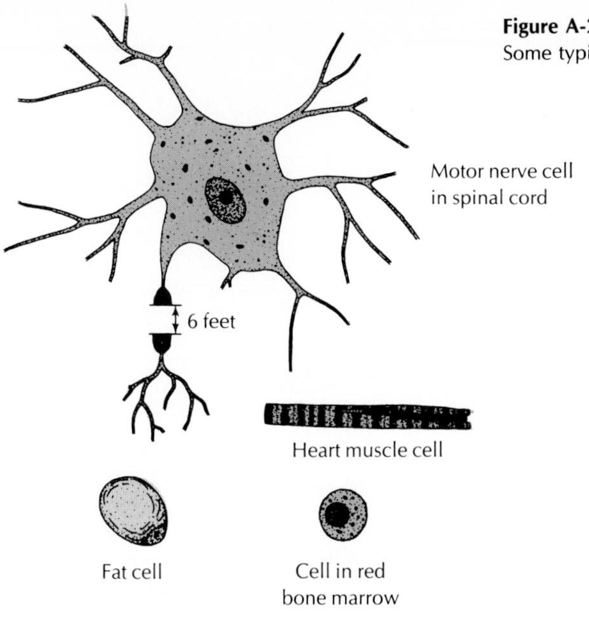

Figure A-2
Some typical mammalian cells.

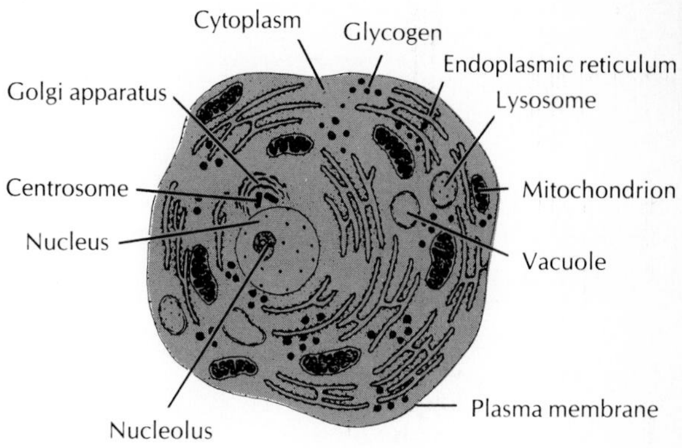

Figure A-3
Details of structure of a typical cell.

the ultracentrifuge and other sophisticated analytical techniques became available.

The *cell membrane* serves much the same function for the cell that the lining of the intestinal tract does for the body; it controls entrance of nutrients and other substances into the cell. The membrane is made up of three layers, with protein constituting the two outer layers and the third (inner) layer being a filling of lipid. The cell membrane is able to identify substances in the extracellular fluid and then determine whether they should be allowed to enter the cell or should be excluded; it also serves to keep certain substances in the cell and therefore to prevent their loss. The membrane surrounding the cell is similar to that surrounding a smaller unit within the cell, known as the **mitochondrion.** This is the cell portion responsible for the production of energy within the cell. Some cells may have only a few mitochondria, but others (such as liver cells, which are very active metabolically) may have several hundred. Each mitochondrion may contain as many as 500 different enzymes to handle the many reactions that occur within it.

The **lysosome** of the cell is similar in function to the digestive system, containing enzymes capable of breaking complex molecules into smaller, more useful ones. The lysosome is even capable of digesting the cell itself, which is essentially what happens when the cell has outlived its usefulness. It can also digest other cells that may be intruders in the human body.

Throughout the filling of the cell, known as the **cytoplasm,** is a network of canals known as *endoplasmic reticulum (ER),* which serves as a set of communication networks within and between cells. On the outside of the ER are a series of small granules known as **ribosomes,** on which new protein is synthesized. Also within the cell and separated from the cytoplasm by a membrane is the cell nucleus, which carries the genetic information needed to determine the exact nature of the protein that will be synthesized. The information is encoded in a constituent of the cell known as DNA (deoxynucleic acid); from there is is transferred to the ribosome, where the protein is synthesized by another nucleic acid known as RNA (ribonucleic acid).

lysosome
Structure within the cell that is responsible for the digestion of cell contents and for the eventual destruction of the cell itself

cytoplasm
Substance enclosed in the cell membrane exclusive of the organelles

ribosome
Protein-synthesizing organelle of the cell

mitochondrion
The specialized structure within the cell in which energy is produced

APPENDIX

B Meanings of Prefixes and Suffixes Used in Nutrition Terms

Prefix	Meaning	Example	Prefix	Meaning	Example
a-	lack of	avitaminosis	inter-	between	intercellular
ab-	away from	abnormal	interstice-	space between	interstitial
ad-	toward	addiction	intra-	within	intravascular
amyl-	starch	amylose	iso-	the same	isocaloric
an-	negative, lack of	anemia	lacto-	pertaining to milk	lactose
ana-	build-up	anabolism	lip-	fat	lipid
ante-	before, preceding	antenatal	leuko-	white	leukocyte
anti-	against	antibiotic	meta-	among	metabolic
bi-	two, double	bilateral	mono-	one	monosaccharide
calori-	heat	calorimetry	myo-	muscle	myoglobin
carcin-	cancer	carcinogen	neo-	new	neonatal
cata-	breakdown	catabolism	os-	bone	osteoblast
co-	with	coenzymes	ovo-	egg	ovulation
di-	in two parts	disaccharides	pan-	all, entire	panacea
dys-	bad	dysentery	pellis-	skin	pellagra
endo-	within	endogenous	peri-	around, on all sides	pericardium
epi-	upon, on, over, above	epithelium	poly-	many	polyneuritis
erythro-	red	erythrocyte	post-	after, behind	postnatal
ex-	out	exogenous	ren-	kidney	renal
glyce-	glucose	glycemia	syn-	with, together	synthesis
heme-	iron-containing	hemoglobin	tachy-	rapid	tachycardia
hemo-	blood	hemolysis	thio-	containing sulfur	thiamin
hepato-	pertaining to the liver	hepatitis	thrombo-	clot	thrombin
hyper-	excessive, above	hyperactive	tox-	poison	toxemia
hypo-	under, less	hypothyroidism	xero-	dry	xerophthalmia

Suffix	Meaning	Example	Suffix	Meaning	Example
-algia	suffering, pain	neuralgia	-lysis	solution, breakdown	hydrolysis
-ase	enzyme	protease	-malacia	softening	osteomalacia
-blast	cell that builds	osteoblast	-meter	instrument for measuring	calorimeter
-bole	change	metabolic	-oid	like	lipoid
-cide	causing death	pesticide	-oma	tumor, swelling	adenoma
-clast	cell that destroys	osteoclast	-ose	sugar	sucrose
-cyte	mature cell	erythrocyte	-osis	disease of, state or condition	fluorosis
-ectomy	removal	thyroidectomy	-pathy	suffering, disease	osteopathy
-emia	blood	anemia	-phagia	swallowing, eating	hyperphagia
-gen	get or produce	antigen	-phile	friend	hydrophilic
-genesis	produce	glucogenesis	-phobia	fear of, antagonism	hydrophobia
-gram	tracing or mark	cardiogram	-plasty	repair of	rhinoplasty
-graph	instrument	cardiograph	-rhea	flow, discharge	steatorrhea
-ia, iasis	disease of	cholelithiasis	-tomy	cut into	appendectomy
-itis	inflammation of	hepatitis	-trophy	growth	hypertrophy
-logy	study of	biology	-vascula	vein	intravascular

APPENDIX C

United States Recommended Daily Allowances

	Adults and children 4 or more years of age (For use in labeling conventional foods and also for "special dietary foods")	Infants	Children under 4 years of age (For use only with "special dietary foods")	Pregnant or lactating women (For use only with "special dietary foods")
Nutrients that *must* be declared on the label (in the order below)				
Protein*	45 g "high-quality protein" 65 g "proteins in general"		—	—
Vitamin A	5000 IU	1500 IU	2500 IU	8000 IU
Vitamin C (or ascorbic acid)	60 mg	35 mg	40 mg	60 mg
Thiamin (or vitamin B_1)	1.5 mg	0.5 mg	0.7 mg	1.7 mg
Riboflavin (or vitamin B_2)	1.7 mg	0.6 mg	0.8 mg	2.0 mg
Niacin	20 mg	8 mg	9 mg	20 mg
Calcium	1.0 g	0.6 g	0.8 g	1.3 g
Iron	18 mg	15 mg	10 mg	18 mg
Nutrients that *may* be declared on the label (in the order below)				
Vitamin D	400 IU	400 IU	400 IU	400 IU
Vitamin E	30 IU	5 IU	10 IU	30 IU
Vitamin B_6	2.0 mg	0.4 mg	0.7 mg	2.5 mg
Folic acid (or folacin)	0.4 mg	0.1 mg	0.2 mg	0.8 mg
Vitamin B_{12}	6 μg	2 μg	3 μg	8 μg
Phosphorus	1.0 g	0.5 g	0.8 g	1.3 g
Iodine	150 μg	45 μg	70 μg	150 μg
Magnesium	400 mg	70 mg	200 mg	450 mg
Zinc†	15 mg	5 mg	8 mg	15 mg
Copper†	2 mg	0.5 mg	1 mg	2 mg
Biotin†	0.3 mg	0.15 mg	0.15 mg	0.3 mg
Pantothenic acid†	10 mg	3 mg	5 mg	10 mg

U.S. RDA is a new term replacing "minimum daily requirement" (MDR). The U.S. RDA values chosen are derived from the highest value for each nutrient given in the NAS-NRC 1968 tables except for calcium and phosphorus. Regulations requiring declaration of sodium content of foods were introduced in July 1986.

*"High-quality protein" is defined as having a protein efficiency ratio (PER) equal to or greater than that of casein; "proteins in general" are those with a PER less than that of casein. Total protein with a PER less than 20% that of casein are considered "not a significant source of protein" and would not be expressed on the label in terms of the U.S. RDA but only as amount per serving.

†There are no NAS-NRC RDAs for biotin, pantothenic acid, zinc, and copper.

APPENDIX D

Recommended Nutrient Intakes for Canadians

Average energy requirements and summary examples of recommended nutrient intakes

Age	Sex	Average height (cm)[3]	Average weight (kg)[3]	Requirements[1,2]					
				kcal/kg[3,4]	MJ/kg[4]	kcal/day[5]	MJ/day[6]	kcal/cm[7]	MJ/cm[6]
Months									
0-2	Both	55	4.5	120-100	0.50-0.42	500	2.0	9	0.04
3-5	Both	63	7.0	100-95	0.42-0.40	700	2.8	11	0.05
6-8	Both	69	8.5	95-97	0.40-0.41	800	3.4	11.5	0.05
9-11	Both	73	9.5	97-99	0.41	950	3.8	12.5	0.05
Years									
1	Both	82	11	101	0.42	1100	4.8	13.5	0.06
2-3	Both	95	14	94	0.39	1300	5.6	13.5	0.06
4-6	Both	107	18	100	0.42	1800	7.6	17	0.07
7-9	M	126	25	88	0.37	2200	9.2	17.5	0.07
	F	125	25	76	0.32	1900	8.0	15	0.06
10-12	M	141	34	73	0.30	2500	10.4	17.5	0.07
	F	143	36	61	0.25	2200	9.2	15.5	0.06
13-15	M	159	50	57	0.24	2800	12.0	17.5	0.07
	F	157	48	46	0.19	2200	9.2	14	0.06
16-18	M	172	62	51	0.21	3200	13.2	18.5	0.08
	F	160	53	40	0.17	2100	8.8	13	0.05
19-24	M	175	71	42	0.18	3000	12.4		
	F	160	58	36	0.15	2100	8.8		
25-49	M	172	74	36	0.15	2700	11.2		
	F	160	59	32	0.13	1900	8.0		
50-74	M	170	73	31	0.13	2300	9.6		
	F	158	63	29	0.12	1800	7.6		
75+	M	168	69	29	0.12	2000	8.4		
	F	155	64	23	0.10	1500	6.0		
Pregnancy (additional)[8]									
1st Trimester									
2nd Trimester									
3rd Trimester									
Lactation (additional)[8]									

[1]Recommended nutrient intakes for Canadians, 1983—Committee for the revision of the Dietary Standard for Canada, Bureau of Nutritional Sciences, Department of National Health and Welfare. Recommended intakes of energy and of certain nutrients are not listed in this table because of the nature of the variables upon which they are based. The figures for energy are estimates of average requirements for expected patterns of activity. *For nutrients not shown, the following amounts are recommended: thiamin, 0.4 mg/100 kcal (0.48 mg/5000 kJ); riboflavin, 0.5 mg/1000 kcal (0.6 mg/5000 kJ); niacin, 6.6 NE/1000 kcal (7.9 NE/5000 kJ); vitamin B_6, 15 μg, as pyridoxine, per gram of protein intake; phosphorus, same as calcium.* Recommended intakes during periods of growth are taken as appropriate for individual representative of the midpoint in each age group. All recommended intakes are designed to cover individual variations in essentially all of a healthy population subsisting upon a variety of common foods available in Canada. It is emphasized that these are *examples* of the application of the RNI to particular classes of individuals and/or particular situations.

[2]Requirements can be expected to vary within a range of ±30%.

[3]Figures rounded to the closest whole number when ≥10 and to the closest 0.5 when <10.

[4]First and last figures are averages at the beginning and at the end of the 3-month period.

[5]Figures rounded to the nearest 50 when <1000 and to the nearest 100 when ≥1000.

[6]Figures include 2 decimal fractions if value is <1 and 1 decimal fraction if ≥1.

	Fat-soluble vitamins			Water-soluble vitamins			Minerals				
Protein (g/day)[9]	Vit A (RE/day)[10]	Vit D (μg/day)[11]	Vit E (mg/day)[12]	Vit C (mg/day)	Folacin (μg/day)[13]	Vit B_{12} (μg/day)	Ca (mg/day)	Mg (mg/day)	Fe (mg/day)	I (μg/day)	Zn (mg/day)
11[14]	400	10	3	20	50	0.3	350	30	0.4[15]	25	2[16]
14[14]	400	10	3	20	50	0.3	350	40	5	35	3
16[14]	400	10	3	20	50	0.3	400	45	7	40	3
18	400	10	3	20	55	0.3	400	50	7	45	3
18	400	10	3	20	65	0.3	500	55	6	55	4
20	400	5	4	20	80	0.4	500	65	6	65	4
25	500	5	5	25	90	0.5	600	90	6	85	5
31	700	2.5	7	35	125	0.8	700	110	7	110	6
29	700	2.5	6	30	125	0.8	700	110	7	95	7
38	800	2.5	8	40	170	1.0	900	150	10	125	6
39	800	2.5	7	40	170	1.0	1000	160	10	110	7
49	900	2.5	9	50	160	1.5	1100	220	12	160	9
43	800	2.5	7	45	160	1.5	800	190	13	160	8
54	1000	2.5	10	55	190	1.9	900	240	10	160	9
47	800	2.5	7	45	160	1.9	700	220	14	160	8
57	1000	2.5	10	60	210	2.0	800	240	8	160	9
41	800	2.5	7	45	165	2.0	700	190	14	160	8
57	1000	2.5	9	60	210	2.0	800	240	8	160	9
41	800	2.5	6	45	165	2.0	700	190	14[17]	160	8
57	1000	2.5	7	60	210	2.0	800	240	8	160	9
41	800	2.5	6	45	165	2.0	800	190	7	160	8
57	1000	2.5	6	60	210	2.0	800	240	8	160	9
41	800	2.5	5	45	165	2.0	800	190	7	160	8
15	100	2.5	2	0	305	1.0	500	15	6	25	0
20	100	2.5	2	20	305	1.0	500	20	6	25	1
25	100	2.5	2	20	305	1.0	500	25	6	25	2
20	400	2.5	3	30	120	0.5	500	80	0	50	6

[7] Figures rounded to the nearest 0.5.
[8] Pregnancy: Add 100 kcal during the first trimester and 300 for the second and third trimesters. Lactation: Add 450 kcal/day.
[9] The primary units are grams per kilogram of body weight. The figures shown here are only examples.
[10] One retinol equivalent (RE) corresponds to the biological activity of 1 μg of retinol, 6 μg of β-carotene or 12 μg of other carotenes.
[11] Expressed as cholecalciferol or ergocalciferol.
[12] Expressed as *d*-α-tocopherol equivalents, relative to which β- and γ-tocopherol and α-tocotrienol have activities of 0.5, 0.1 and 0.3 respectively.
[13] Expressed as total folate.
[14] Assumption that the protein is from breast milk or is of the same biological value as that of breast milk and that between 3 and 9 months adjustment for the quality of the protein is made.
[15] For the infant, it is assumed that breast milk is the source of iron up to 2 months of age.
[16] Based on the assumption that breast milk is the source of zinc up to 2 months of age.
[17] After the menopause the recommended intake is 7 mg/day.

APPENDIX

E Nutrient Analysis: Instructions for Keeping Food Records

To assess the nutritive adequacy of your diet, it is necessary to have a complete record of all food and beverages consumed during at least a 3-day period. To do this:

I. Record Dietary Intake

Select three 24-hour periods that you think will be representative of your normal dietary intake and activity. Most students include 2 weekdays and 1 weekend day to represent an average week's dietary intake and activity. Record everything you consume each 24-hour period starting at midnight.

Before you begin recording, look over the food composition tables in Appendix F. Become aware of the detail necessary to accurately identify a food item (for example, method of cooking and units of measurement).

List all foods and beverages consumed at or between meals for the 3 days. Record everything you put into your mouth and swallow (including vitamin/mineral supplements). Do not forget such items as gravy, jams, jellies, sauces, salad dressing, nuts, candy, margarine, butter, sugar, and milk on cereal or fruit, and social beverages. Record foods immediately after eating. Do not rely on your memory. List separately the different foods that compose one dietary item. For example, for a ham sandwich, list bun, ham, butter, mustard, and lettuce. Record time of day the food was eaten—this will help you remember all foods. Describe the food in as complete detail as possible, for example, include

Methods of preparation	Raw, broiled, fried, baked Canned, frozen
Form of food	Buttered toast Whole milk Yogurt with fruit Meat trimmed of fat Cake with frosting

Some dishes may have foods prepared differently. For example, a vegetable salad may be composed of raw spinach, cooked beans, and raw onions; potatoes may be french-fried, baked, or creamed.

Estimate the serving size.

By volume	Cups, tablespoons
By weight	Ounces, pounds
By unit	1 biscuit 1 frankfurter 1 medium apple

Express amounts of foods as specifically and accurately as possible. Indicate serving sizes of meats as ounces or measure the dimensions (for example, hamburger, 3 oz, or beef, 1 piece, 2″ × 3″ × ½″ thick). Express fruits, vegetables, and fats in terms of standard measuring cups or measuring spoons (for example, cole slaw, ½ cup; margarine, 1 teaspoon). Some items may be expressed as pieces or slices. Drinks should be recorded in fluid ounces or measuring cups.

Usual serving sizes are

Cereal	1 oz (dry weight)
Meat	3 oz
Fruit juice	6 oz
Vegetables	4 oz

II. Calculate Dietary Score

Evaluate your food intake, for each day recorded, by calculating a dietary score. Categorize the food you ate according to one of the four food groups listed. All foods will not fall into these food groups. Group others as "Miscellaneous." Each time you eat *one serving* of a food, write the specific food under the food group that includes the specific food. Do not list more than two servings for dairy or meat, or more than four servings for fruits and vegetables or breads and cereals. Thus, intake which exceeds the maximum intake is not counted. You may list combination dishes in different food groups, for example: pizza—cheese = milk and milk group, tomato sauce = fruits and vegetable group, and crust = bread and cereal group. See Canada's Food Guide (Figure 3-3 on p. 43) for examples of food categories and serving size. Table 3-6 and Table 21-6 may also be helpful.

III. Evaluate Nutrient Intake

Transfer the foods and amounts for each of the 3 days to Form E-2 and look up the amount of each nutrient in each food. Combine identical foods eaten on all 3 days (for example, if you have 1½ cups of whole milk for breakfast, 2 cups for lunch, and 3 cups for dinner, total the amount and enter on Form E-2, "whole milk, 6½ cups"). This will save space and calculations. Do this only when foods are identical. This will help you recognize the major

Form E-1 Example of food record.

Meal	Time	Food	Description	Amount	Score
Breakfast	6:30 AM	Branflakes	With raisins	3/4 Cup	
		Sugar	Brown	1 T	
		Milk	2% fat	3/4 Cup	
		Coffee	Black	1 Cup	
Snack	10:00 AM	Orange juice	Frozen, reconstituted	6 oz	
		Crackers	Graham	2	
Lunch	12:15 PM	Vegetable soup	Instant	1 Cup	
		Tomato	Raw & sliced	1/2 Medium	
		Bread	Whole-wheat	1 Thin slice	
		Milk	Chocolate	1/2 Pint	
Snack	3:30 PM	Coke	Diet/decaffeinated	8 oz	
		Corn Chips	1 Bag	1 oz	
Dinner	6:15 PM				

contributions of each food group.

Information on labels may also be used to supplement food composition data. Remember that labels list the U.S. RDA in each serving of only some nutrients. NOTE: You will need to convert % of U.S. RDA figures on the label to RDA units by calculation using Appendix C.

Example

If label says one serving has 10% U.S. RDA for iron you find that the U.S. RDA for iron is 18 mg. Thus, $.10 \times 18 = 1.8$ mg iron/serving.

IV. Compare Average Nutrient Consumption to the RDAs

Total the 3-day intake for each nutrient and then calculate the 3-day average. List the RDAs appropriate for your age and sex on Form E-2 (see inside front and back cover of the text). Compare your 3-day averages (without supplements) to the RDAs. Calculate the % RDA for each nutrient.

Example

If your average Vitamin A intake was 6,000 I.U., and the RDA is 5,000 I.U., then % RDA for Vitamin A would be:

$$\frac{\text{your intake}}{\text{RDA}} =$$

$$\frac{6000}{5000} \times 100 = 120\% \text{ RDA}$$

If the % RDA was less than 77 (without vitamin or mineral supplements), select at least two foods that would significantly improve your intake with a single serving of the food. Also choose foods you are likely to eat. If the % RDA was more than 77 (without vitamin or mineral supplements), list the foods that were the major contributors of that nutrient in *your* diet.

Form E-2 Analysis of nutrient intake.

Food and Beverages Consumed	Amount (Usual Measure)	Kcal	Protein (gm)
Milk and Milk Products			
Sub-Total			
Meat, Fish, Poultry, Eggs, Legumes			
Sub-Total			
Fruit and Vegetables			
Sub-Total			
Bread and Cereal			
Sub-Total			
Miscellaneous			
Sub-Total			
Total of All Foods			
Supplements			
Food and Supplement Total for Day			
RDA			
% RDA from Food			
% RDA from Food Plus Supplements			

Fat (gm)	CHO (gm)	Calcium (gm)	Iron (mg)	Sodium (mg)	Vit. A (IU)	Thiamin (B_1) (mg)	Ribo-flavin (B_2) (mg)	Niacin (mg)	Ascorbic Acid (Vit. C) (mg)	Choles-terol (mg)

APPENDIX

F

Nutritive Value of Edible Parts of Common Portions of Foods and Beverages

Item Number	Foods, Approximate Measures, Units, and Weight (Weight of Edible Portion Only)		Weight (grams)	Water (percent)	Food Energy (calories)	Protein (grams)	Fat (grams)	Fatty Acids		
								Saturated (grams)	Monounsaturated (grams)	Polyunsaturated (grams)
	Beverages									
	Alcoholic									
	Beer									
1	Regular	12 fl oz	360	92	150	1	0	0.0	0.0	0.0
2	Light	12 fl oz	355	95	95	1	0	0.0	0.0	0.0
	Gin, rum, vodka, whiskey									
3	80-proof	1½ fl oz	42	67	95	0	0	0.0	0.0	0.0
4	86-proof	1½ fl oz	42	64	105	0	0	0.0	0.0	0.0
5	90-proof	1½ fl oz	42	62	110	0	0	0.0	0.0	0.0
	Wines									
6	Dessert	3½ fl oz	103	77	140	Tr	0	0.0	0.0	0.0
	Table									
7	Red	3½ fl oz	102	88	75	Tr	0	0.0	0.0	0.0
8	White	3½ fl oz	102	87	80	Tr	0	0.0	0.0	0.0
	Carbonated[2]									
9	Club soda	12 fl oz	355	100	0	0	0	0.0	0.0	0.0
	Cola type									
10	Regular	12 fl oz	369	89	160	0	0	0.0	0.0	0.0
11	Diet, artificially sweetened	12 fl oz	355	100	Tr	0	0	0.0	0.0	0.0
12	Ginger ale	12 fl oz	366	91	125	0	0	0.0	0.0	0.0
13	Grape	12 fl oz	372	88	180	0	0	0.0	0.0	0.0
14	Lemon-lime	12 fl oz	372	89	155	0	0	0.0	0.0	0.0
15	Orange	12 fl oz	372	88	180	0	0	0.0	0.0	0.0
16	Pepper type	12 fl oz	369	89	160	0	0	0.0	0.0	0.0
17	Root beer	12 fl oz	370	89	165	0	0	0.0	0.0	0.0
	Cocoa and chocolate-flavored beverages. See Dairy Products (items 95-98).									
	Coffee									
18	Brewed	6 fl oz	180	100	Tr	Tr	Tr	Tr	Tr	Tr
19	Instant, prepared (2 tsp powder plus 6 fl oz water)	6 fl oz	182	99	Tr	Tr	Tr	Tr	Tr	Tr
	Fruit drinks, noncarbonated									
	Canned									
20	Fruit punch drink	6 fl oz	190	88	85	Tr	0	0.0	0.0	0.0
21	Grape drink	6 fl oz	187	86	100	Tr	0	0.0	0.0	0.0
22	Pineapple-grapefruit juice drink	6 fl oz	187	87	90	Tr	Tr	Tr	Tr	Tr
	Frozen									
	Lemonade concentrate									
23	Undiluted	6-fl-oz can	219	49	425	Tr	Tr	Tr	Tr	Tr
24	Diluted with 4⅓ parts water by volume	6 fl oz	185	89	80	Tr	Tr	Tr	Tr	Tr
	Limeade concentrate									
25	Undiluted	6-fl-oz can	218	50	410	Tr	Tr	Tr	Tr	Tr
26	Diluted with 4⅓ parts water by volume	6 fl oz	185	89	75	Tr	Tr	Tr	Tr	Tr
	Fruit juices. See type under Fruits and Fruit Juices.									
	Milk beverages. See Dairy Products (items 92-105).									

[1]Value not determined.

[2]Mineral content varies depending on water source.

							Vitamin A Value					
Cholesterol (mg)	Carbo-hydrate (grams)	Calcium (mg)	Phosphorus (mg)	Iron (mg)	Potassium (mg)	Sodium (mg)	(IU) International Units	(RE) Retinol Equivalents	Thiamin (mg)	Riboflavin (mg)	Niacin (mg)	Ascorbic Acid (mg)
0	13	14	50	0.1	115	18	0	0	0.02	0.09	1.8	0
0	5	14	43	0.1	64	11	0	0	0.03	0.11	1.4	0
0	Tr	Tr	Tr	Tr	1	Tr	0	0	Tr	Tr	Tr	0
0	Tr	Tr	Tr	Tr	1	Tr	0	0	Tr	Tr	Tr	0
0	Tr	Tr	Tr	Tr	1	Tr	0	0	Tr	Tr	Tr	0
0	8	8	9	0.2	95	9	([1])	([1])	0.01	0.02	0.2	0
0	3	8	18	0.4	113	5	([1])	([1])	0.00	0.03	0.1	0
0	3	9	14	0.3	83	5	([1])	([1])	0.00	0.01	0.1	0
0	0	18	0	Tr	0	78	0	0	0.00	0.00	0.0	0
0	41	11	52	0.2	7	18	0	0	0.00	0.00	0.0	0
0	Tr	14	39	0.2	7	32[3]	0	0	0.00	0.00	0.0	0
0	32	11	0	0.1	4	29	0	0	0.00	0.00	0.0	0
0	46	15	0	0.4	4	48	0	0	0.00	0.00	0.0	0
0	39	7	0	0.4	4	33	0	0	0.00	0.00	0.0	0
0	46	15	4	0.3	7	52	0	0	0.00	0.00	0.0	0
0	41	11	41	0.1	4	37	0	0	0.00	0.00	0.0	0
0	42	15	0	0.2	4	48	0	0	0.00	0.00	0.0	0
0	Tr	4	2	Tr	124	2	0	0	0.00	0.02	0.4	0
0	1	2	6	0.1	71	Tr	0	0	0.00	0.03	0.6	0
0	22	15	2	0.4	48	15	20	2	0.03	0.04	Tr	61[4]
0	26	2	2	0.3	9	11	Tr	Tr	0.01	0.01	Tr	64[4]
0	23	13	7	0.9	97	24	60	6	0.06	0.04	0.5	110[4]
0	112	9	13	0.4	153	4	40	4	0.04	0.07	0.7	66
0	21	2	2	0.1	30	1	10	1	0.01	0.02	0.2	13
0	108	11	13	0.2	129	Tr	Tr	Tr	0.02	0.02	0.2	26
0	20	2	2	Tr	24	Tr	Tr	Tr	Tr	Tr	Tr	4

[3]Blend of aspartame and saccharin; if only sodium saccharin is used, sodium is 75 mg; if only aspartame is used, sodium is 23 mg.
[4]With added ascorbic acid.

Continued.

Item Number	Foods, Approximate Measures, Units, and Weight (Weight of Edible Portion Only)		Weight (grams)	Water (percent)	Food Energy (calories)	Protein (grams)	Fat (grams)	Fatty Acids		
								Saturated (grams)	Monounsaturated (grams)	Polyunsaturated (grams)
	Beverages—cont'd									
	Tea									
27	Brewed	8 fl oz	240	100	Tr	Tr	Tr	Tr	Tr	Tr
	Instant, powder, prepared									
28	Unsweetened (1 tsp powder plus 8 fl oz water)	8 fl oz	241	100	Tr	Tr	Tr	Tr	Tr	Tr
29	Sweetened (3 tsp powder plus 8 fl oz water)	8 fl oz	262	91	85	Tr	Tr	Tr	Tr	Tr
	Dairy Products									
	Butter. See Fats and Oils (items 128-130).									
	Cheese									
	Natural									
30	Blue	1 oz	28	42	100	6	8	5.3	2.2	0.2
31	Camembert (3 wedges/4-oz container)	1 wedge	38	52	115	8	9	5.8	2.7	0.3
	Cheddar									
32	Cut pieces	1 oz	28	37	115	7	9	6.0	2.7	0.3
33		1 in³	17	37	70	4	6	3.6	1.6	0.2
34	Shredded	1 cup	113	37	455	28	37	23.8	10.6	1.1
	Cottage (curd not pressed down)									
	Creamed (cottage cheese, 4% fat)									
35	Large curd	1 cup	225	79	235	28	10	6.4	2.9	0.3
36	Small curd	1 cup	210	79	215	26	9	6.0	2.7	0.3
37	With fruit	1 cup	226	72	280	22	8	4.9	2.2	0.2
38	Lowfat (2%)	1 cup	226	79	205	31	4	2.8	1.2	0.1
39	Uncreamed (cottage cheese dry curd, less than ½% fat)	1 cup	145	80	125	25	1	0.4	0.2	Tr
40	Cream	1 oz	28	54	100	2	10	6.2	2.8	0.4
41	Feta	1 oz	28	55	75	4	6	4.2	1.3	0.2
	Mozzarella, made with									
	Whole milk	1 oz	28	54	80	6	6	3.7	1.9	0.2
43	Part skim milk (low moisture)	1 oz	28	49	80	8	5	3.1	1.4	0.1
44	Muenster	1 oz	28	42	105	7	9	5.4	2.5	0.2
	Parmesan, grated									
45	Cup, not pressed down	1 cup	100	18	455	42	30	19.1	8.7	0.7
46	Tablespoon	1 tbsp	5	18	25	2	2	1.0	0.4	Tr
47	Ounce	1 oz	28	18	130	12	9	5.4	2.5	0.2
48	Provolone	1 oz	28	41	100	7	8	4.8	2.1	0.2
	Ricotta, made with									
49	Whole milk	1 cup	246	72	430	28	32	20.4	8.9	0.9
50	Part skim milk	1 cup	246	74	340	28	19	12.1	5.7	0.6
51	Swiss	1 oz	28	37	105	8	8	5.0	2.1	0.3
	Pasteurized process cheese									
52	American	1 oz	28	39	105	6	9	5.6	2.5	0.3
53	Swiss	1 oz	28	42	95	7	7	4.5	2.0	0.2
54	Pasteurized process cheese food, American	1 oz	28	43	95	6	7	4.4	2.0	0.2
55	Pasteurized process cheese spread, American	1 oz	28	48	80	5	6	3.8	1.8	0.2
	Cream, sweet									
56	Half-and-half (cream and milk)	1 cup	242	81	315	7	28	17.3	8.0	1.0
57		1 tbsp	15	81	20	Tr	2	1.1	0.5	0.1
58	Light, coffee, or table	1 cup	240	74	470	6	46	28.8	13.4	1.7
59		1 tbsp	15	74	30	Tr	3	1.8	0.8	0.1
	Whipping, unwhipped (volume about double when whipped)									
60	Light	1 cup	239	64	700	5	74	46.2	21.7	2.1
61		1 tbsp	15	64	45	Tr	5	2.9	1.4	0.1
62	Heavy	1 cup	238	58	820	5	88	54.8	25.4	3.3
63		1 tbsp	15	58	50	Tr	6	3.5	1.6	0.2
64	Whipped topping, (pressurized)	1 cup	60	61	155	2	13	8.3	3.9	0.5
65		1 tbsp	3	61	10	Tr	1	0.4	0.2	Tr
66	Cream, sour	1 cup	230	71	495	7	48	30.0	13.9	1.8
67		1 tbsp	12	71	25	Tr	3	1.6	0.7	0.1

Cholesterol (mg)	Carbohydrate (grams)	Calcium (mg)	Phosphorus (mg)	Iron (mg)	Potassium (mg)	Sodium (mg)	Vitamin A Value (IU) International Units	Vitamin A Value (RE) Retinol Equivalents	Thiamin (mg)	Riboflavin (mg)	Niacin (mg)	Ascorbic Acid (mg)
0	Tr	0	2	Tr	36	1	0	0	0.00	0.03	Tr	0
0	1	1	4	Tr	61	1	0	0	0.00	0.02	0.1	0
0	22	1	3	Tr	49	Tr	0	0	0.00	0.04	0.1	0
21	1	150	110	0.1	73	396	200	65	0.01	0.11	0.3	0
27	Tr	147	132	0.1	71	320	350	96	0.01	0.19	0.2	0
30	Tr	204	145	0.2	28	176	300	86	0.01	0.11	Tr	0
18	Tr	123	87	0.1	17	105	180	52	Tr	0.06	Tr	0
119	1	815	579	0.8	111	701	1200	342	0.03	0.42	0.1	0
34	6	135	297	0.3	190	911	370	108	0.05	0.37	0.3	Tr
31	6	126	277	0.3	177	850	340	101	0.04	0.34	0.3	Tr
25	30	108	236	0.2	151	915	280	81	0.04	0.29	0.2	Tr
19	8	155	340	0.4	217	918	160	45	0.05	0.42	0.3	Tr
10	3	46	151	0.3	47	19	40	12	0.04	0.21	0.2	0
31	1	23	30	0.3	34	84	400	124	Tr	0.06	Tr	0
25	1	140	96	0.2	18	316	130	36	0.04	0.24	0.3	0
22	1	147	105	0.1	19	106	220	68	Tr	0.07	Tr	0
15	1	207	149	0.1	27	150	180	54	0.01	0.10	Tr	0
27	Tr	203	133	0.1	38	178	320	90	Tr	0.09	Tr	0
79	4	1376	807	1.0	107	1861	700	173	0.05	0.39	0.3	0
4	Tr	69	40	Tr	5	93	40	9	Tr	0.02	Tr	0
22	1	390	229	0.3	30	528	200	49	0.01	0.11	0.1	0
20	1	214	141	0.1	39	248	230	75	0.01	0.09	Tr	0
124	7	509	389	0.9	257	207	1210	330	0.03	0.48	0.3	0
76	13	669	449	1.1	307	307	1060	278	0.05	0.46	0.2	0
26	1	272	171	Tr	31	74	240	72	0.01	0.10	Tr	0
27	Tr	174	211	0.1	46	406	340	82	0.01	0.10	Tr	0
24	1	219	216	0.2	61	388	230	65	Tr	0.08	Tr	0
18	2	163	130	0.2	79	337	260	62	0.01	0.13	Tr	0
16	2	159	202	0.1	69	381	220	54	0.01	0.12	Tr	0
89	10	254	230	0.2	314	98	1050	259	0.08	0.36	0.2	2
6	1	16	14	Tr	19	6	70	16	0.01	0.02	Tr	Tr
159	9	231	192	0.1	292	95	1730	437	0.08	0.36	0.1	2
10	1	14	12	Tr	18	6	110	27	Tr	0.02	Tr	Tr
265	7	166	146	0.1	231	82	2690	705	0.06	0.30	0.1	1
17	Tr	10	9	Tr	15	5	170	44	Tr	0.02	Tr	Tr
326	7	154	149	0.1	179	89	3500	1002	0.05	0.26	0.1	1
21	Tr	10	9	Tr	11	6	220	63	Tr	0.02	Tr	Tr
46	7	61	54	Tr	88	78	550	124	0.02	0.04	Tr	0
2	Tr	3	3	Tr	4	4	30	6	Tr	Tr	Tr	0
102	10	268	195	0.1	331	123	1820	448	0.08	0.34	0.2	2
5	1	14	10	Tr	17	6	90	23	Tr	0.02	Tr	Tr

Continued.

Item Number	Foods, Approximate Measures, Units, and Weight (Weight of Edible Portion Only)		Weight (grams)	Water (percent)	Food Energy (calories)	Protein (grams)	Fat (grams)	Fatty Acids		
								Saturated (grams)	Monounsaturated (grams)	Polyunsaturated (grams)
	Dairy Products—cont'd									
	Cream products, imitation (made with vegetable fat)									
	Sweet									
	Creamers									
68	Liquid (frozen)	1 tbsp	15	77	20	Tr	1	1.4	Tr	Tr
69	Powdered	1 tsp	2	2	10	Tr	1	0.7	Tr	Tr
	Whipped topping									
70	Frozen	1 cup	75	50	240	1	19	16.3	1.2	0.4
71		1 tbsp	4	50	15	Tr	1	0.9	0.1	Tr
72	Powdered, made with whole milk	1 cup	80	67	150	3	10	8.5	0.7	0.2
73		1 tbsp	4	67	10	Tr	Tr	0.4	Tr	Tr
74	Pressurized	1 cup	70	60	185	1	16	13.2	1.3	0.2
75		1 tbsp	4	60	10	Tr	1	0.8	0.1	Tr
76	Sour dressing (filled cream type product, nonbutterfat)	1 cup	235	75	415	8	39	31.2	4.6	1.1
77		1 tbsp	12	75	20	Tr	2	1.6	0.2	0.1
	Ice cream. See Milk desserts, frozen (items 106-111).									
	Ice milk. See Milk desserts, frozen (items 112-114).									
	Milk									
	Fluid									
78	Whole (3.3% fat)	1 cup	244	88	150	8	8	5.1	2.4	0.3
	Lowfat (2%)									
79	No milk solids added	1 cup	244	89	120	8	5	2.9	1.4	0.2
80	Milk solids added, label claim less than 10 g of protein per cup	1 cup	245	89	125	9	5	2.9	1.4	0.2
	Lowfat (1%)									
81	No milk solids added	1 cup	244	90	100	8	3	1.6	0.7	0.1
82	Milk solids added, label claim less than 10 g of protein per cup	1 cup	245	90	105	9	2	1.5	0.7	0.1
	Nonfat (skim)									
83	No milk solids added	1 cup	245	91	85	8	Tr	0.3	0.1	Tr
84	Milk solids added, label claim less than 10 g of protein per cup	1 cup	245	90	90	9	1	0.4	0.2	Tr
85	Buttermilk	1 cup	245	90	100	8	2	1.3	0.6	0.1
	Canned									
86	Condensed, sweetened	1 cup	306	27	980	24	27	16.8	7.4	1.0
	Evaporated									
87	Whole milk	1 cup	252	74	340	17	19	11.6	5.9	0.6
88	Skim milk	1 cup	255	79	200	19	1	0.3	0.2	Tr
	Dried									
89	Buttermilk	1 cup	120	3	465	41	7	4.3	2.0	0.3
	Nonfat, instantized									
90	Envelope, 3.2 oz, net wt[6]	1 envelope	91	4	325	32	1	0.4	0.2	Tr
91	Cup	1 cup	68	4	245	24	Tr	0.3	0.1	Tr
	Milk beverages									
	Chocolate milk (commercial)									
92	Regular	1 cup	250	82	210	8	8	5.3	2.5	0.3
93	Lowfat (2%)	1 cup	250	84	180	8	5	3.1	1.5	0.2
94	Lowfat (1%)	1 cup	250	85	160	8	3	1.5	0.8	0.1
	Cocoa and chocolate-flavored beverages									
95	Powder containing nonfat dry milk	1 oz	28	1	100	3	1	0.6	0.3	Tr
96	Prepared (6 oz water plus 1 oz powder)	1 serving	206	86	100	3	1	0.6	0.3	Tr
97	Powder without nonfat dry milk	¾ oz	21	1	75	1	1	0.3	0.2	Tr
98	Prepared (8 oz whole milk plus ¾ oz powder)	1 serving	265	81	225	9	9	5.4	2.5	0.3
99	Eggnog (commercial)	1 cup	254	74	340	10	19	11.3	5.7	0.9
	Malted milk									
	Chocolate									
100	Powder	¾ oz	21	2	85	1	1	0.5	0.3	0.1
101	Prepared (8 oz whole milk plus ¾ oz powder)	1 serving	265	81	235	9	9	5.5	2.7	0.4

[5] Vitamin A value is largely from beta-carotene used for coloring.

[6] Yields 1 qt of fluid milk when reconstituted according to package directions.

Cholesterol (mg)	Carbo-hydrate (grams)	Calcium (mg)	Phosphorus (mg)	Iron (mg)	Potassium (mg)	Sodium (mg)	Vitamin A Value (IU) International Units	(RE) Retinol Equivalents	Thiamin (mg)	Riboflavin (mg)	Niacin (mg)	Ascorbic Acid (mg)
0	2	1	10	Tr	29	12	10[5]	1[5]	0.00	0.00	0.0	0
0	1	Tr	8	Tr	16	4	Tr	Tr	0.00	Tr	0.0	0
0	17	5	6	0.1	14	19	650[5]	65[5]	0.00	0.00	0.0	0
0	1	Tr	Tr	Tr	1	1	30[5]	3[5]	0.00	0.00	0.0	0
8	13	72	69	Tr	121	53	290[5]	39[5]	0.02	0.09	Tr	1
Tr	1	4	3	Tr	6	3	10[5]	2[5]	Tr	Tr	Tr	Tr
0	11	4	13	Tr	13	43	330[5]	33[5]	0.00	0.00	0.0	0
0	1	Tr	1	Tr	1	2	20[5]	2[5]	0.00	0.00	0.0	0
13	11	266	205	0.1	380	113	20	5	0.09	0.38	0.2	2
1	1	14	10	Tr	19	6	Tr	Tr	Tr	0.02	Tr	Tr
33	11	291	228	0.1	370	120	310	76	0.09	0.40	0.2	2
18	12	297	232	0.1	377	122	500	139	0.10	0.40	0.2	2
18	12	313	245	0.1	397	128	500	140	0.10	0.42	0.2	2
10	12	300	235	0.1	381	123	500	144	0.10	0.41	0.2	2
10	12	313	245	0.1	397	128	500	145	0.10	0.42	0.2	2
4	12	302	247	0.1	406	126	500	149	0.09	0.34	0.2	2
5	12	316	255	0.1	418	130	500	149	0.10	0.43	0.2	2
9	12	285	219	0.1	371	257	80	20	0.08	0.38	0.1	2
104	166	868	775	0.6	1136	389	1000	248	0.28	1.27	0.6	8
74	25	657	510	0.5	764	267	610	136	0.12	0.80	0.5	5
9	29	738	497	0.7	845	293	1000	298	0.11	0.79	0.4	3
83	59	1421	1119	0.4	1910	621	260	65	0.47	1.89	1.1	7
17	47	1120	896	0.3	1552	499	2160[7]	646[7]	0.38	1.59	0.8	5
12	35	837	670	0.2	1160	373	1610[7]	483[7]	0.28	1.19	0.6	4
31	26	280	251	0.6	417	149	300	73	0.09	0.41	0.3	2
17	26	284	254	0.6	422	151	500	143	0.09	0.41	0.3	2
7	26	287	256	0.6	425	152	500	148	0.10	0.42	0.3	2
1	22	90	88	0.3	223	139	Tr	Tr	0.03	0.17	0.2	Tr
1	22	90	88	0.3	223	139	Tr	Tr	0.03	0.17	0.2	Tr
0	19	7	26	0.7	136	56	Tr	Tr	Tr	0.03	0.1	Tr
33	30	298	254	0.9	508	176	310	76	0.10	0.43	0.3	3
149	34	330	378	0.5	420	138	890	203	0.09	0.48	0.3	4
1	18	13	37	0.4	130	49	20	5	0.04	0.04	0.4	0
34	29	304	265	0.5	500	168	330	80	0.14	0.43	0.7	2

[7]With added vitamin A.

Continued.

Item Number	Foods, Approximate Measures, Units, and Weight (Weight of Edible Portion Only)		Weight (grams)	Water (percent)	Food Energy (calories)	Protein (grams)	Fat (grams)	Fatty Acids: Saturated (grams)	Fatty Acids: Monounsaturated (grams)	Fatty Acids: Polyunsaturated (grams)
	Dairy Products—cont'd									
	Milk beverages—cont'd									
	Malted milk—cont'd									
	Natural									
102	Powder	¾ oz	21	3	85	3	2	0.9	0.5	0.3
103	Prepared (8 oz whole milk plus ¾ oz powder)	1 serving	265	81	235	11	10	6.0	2.9	0.6
	Shakes, thick									
104	Chocolate	10-oz container	283	72	335	9	8	4.8	2.2	0.3
105	Vanilla	10-oz container	283	74	315	11	9	5.3	2.5	0.3
	Milk desserts, frozen									
	Ice cream, vanilla									
	Regular (about 11% fat)									
106	Hardened	½ gal	1064	61	2155	38	115	71.3	33.1	4.3
107		1 cup	133	61	270	5	14	8.9	4.1	0.5
108		3 fl oz	50	61	100	2	5	3.4	1.6	0.2
109	Soft serve (frozen custard)	1 cup	173	60	375	7	23	13.5	6.7	1.0
110	Rich (about 16% fat), hardened	½ gal	1188	59	2805	33	190	118.3	54.9	7.1
111		1 cup	148	59	350	4	24	14.7	6.8	0.9
	Ice milk, vanilla									
112	Hardened (about 4% fat)	½ gal	1048	69	1470	41	45	28.1	13.0	1.7
113		1 cup	131	69	185	5	6	3.5	1.6	0.2
114	Soft serve (about 3% fat)	1 cup	175	70	225	8	5	2.9	1.3	0.2
115	Sherbet (about 2% fat)	½ gal	1542	66	2160	17	31	19.0	8.8	1.1
116		1 cup	193	66	270	2	4	2.4	1.1	0.1
	Yogurt									
	With added milk solids									
	Made with lowfat milk									
117	Fruit-flavored[8]	8-oz container	227	74	230	10	2	1.6	0.7	0.1
118	Plain	8-oz container	227	85	145	12	4	2.3	1.0	0.1
119	Made with nonfat milk	8-oz container	227	85	125	13	Tr	0.3	0.1	Tr
	Without added milk solids									
120	Made with whole milk	8-oz container	227	88	140	8	7	4.8	2.0	0.2
	Eggs									
	Eggs, large (24 oz/dozen)									
	Raw									
121	Whole, without shell	1 egg	50	75	80	6	6	1.7	2.2	0.7
122	White	1 white	33	88	15	3	Tr	0.0	0.0	0.0
123	Yolk	1 yolk	17	49	65	3	6	1.7	2.2	0.7
	Cooked									
124	Fried in butter	1 egg	46	68	95	6	7	2.7	2.7	0.8
125	Hard-cooked, shell removed	1 egg	50	75	80	6	6	1.7	2.2	0.7
126	Poached	1 egg	50	74	80	6	6	1.7	2.2	0.7
127	Scrambled (milk added) in butter; also, omelet	1 egg	64	73	110	7	8	3.2	2.9	0.8
	Fats and Oils									
	Butter (4 sticks per lb)									
128	Stick	½ cup	113	16	810	1	92	57.1	26.4	3.4
129	Tablespoon (⅛ stick)	1 tbsp	14	16	100	Tr	11	7.1	3.3	0.4
130	Pat (1-in square, ⅓ in high; 90 per lb)	1 pat	5	16	35	Tr	4	2.5	1.2	0.2
131	Fats, cooking (vegetable shortenings)	1 cup	205	0	1810	0	205	51.3	91.2	53.5
132		1 tbsp	13	0	115	0	13	3.3	5.8	3.4
133	Lard	1 cup	205	0	1850	0	205	80.4	92.5	23.0
134		1 tbsp	13	0	115	0	13	5.1	5.9	1.5
	Margarine									
135	Imitation (about 40% fat), soft	8-oz container	227	58	785	1	88	17.5	35.6	31.3
136		1 tbsp	14	58	50	Tr	5	1.1	2.2	1.9
	Regular (about 80% fat)									
	Hard (4 sticks per lb)									
137	Stick	½ cup	113	16	810	1	91	17.9	40.5	28.7
138	Tablespoon (⅛ stick)	1 tbsp	14	16	100	Tr	11	2.2	5.0	3.6
139	Pat (1-in square, ⅓ in high; 90 per lb)	1 pat	5	16	35	Tr	4	0.8	1.8	1.3

[8]Carbohydrate content varies widely because of amount of sugar added and amount and solids content of added flavoring. Consult the label if more precise values for carbohydrate and calories are needed.

[9]For salted butter; unsalted butter contains 12 mg sodium/stick, 2 mg/tbsp, or 1 mg/pat.

Cholesterol (mg)	Carbohydrate (grams)	Calcium (mg)	Phosphorus (mg)	Iron (mg)	Potassium (mg)	Sodium (mg)	Vitamin A Value (IU) International Units	Vitamin A Value (RE) Retinol Equivalents	Thiamin (mg)	Riboflavin (mg)	Niacin (mg)	Ascorbic Acid (mg)
4	15	56	79	0.2	159	96	70	17	0.11	0.14	1.1	0
37	27	347	307	0.3	529	215	380	93	0.20	0.54	1.3	2
30	60	374	357	0.9	634	314	240	59	0.13	0.63	0.4	0
33	50	413	326	0.3	517	270	320	79	0.08	0.55	0.4	0
476	254	1406	1075	1.0	2052	929	4340	1064	0.42	2.63	1.1	6
59	32	176	134	0.1	257	116	540	133	0.05	0.33	0.1	1
22	12	66	51	Tr	96	44	200	50	0.02	0.12	0.1	Tr
153	38	236	199	0.4	338	153	790	199	0.08	0.45	0.2	1
703	256	1213	927	0.8	1771	868	7200	1758	0.36	2.27	0.9	5
88	32	151	115	0.1	221	108	900	219	0.04	0.28	0.1	1
146	232	1409	1035	1.5	2117	836	1710	419	0.61	2.78	0.9	6
18	29	176	129	0.2	265	105	210	52	0.08	0.35	0.1	1
13	38	274	202	0.3	412	163	175	44	0.12	0.54	0.2	1
113	469	827	594	2.5	1585	706	1480	308	0.26	0.71	1.0	31
14	59	103	74	0.3	198	88	190	39	0.03	0.09	0.1	4
10	43	345	271	0.2	442	133	100	25	0.08	0.40	0.2	1
14	16	415	326	0.2	531	159	150	36	0.10	0.49	0.3	2
4	17	452	355	0.2	579	174	20	5	0.11	0.53	0.3	2
29	11	274	215	0.1	351	105	280	68	0.07	0.32	0.2	1
274	1	28	90	1.0	65	69	260	78	0.04	0.15	Tr	0
0	Tr	4	4	Tr	45	50	0	0	Tr	0.09	Tr	0
272	Tr	26	86	0.9	15	8	310	94	0.04	0.07	Tr	0
278	1	29	91	1.1	66	162	320	94	0.04	0.14	Tr	0
274	1	28	90	1.0	65	69	260	78	0.04	0.14	Tr	0
273	1	28	90	1.0	65	146	260	78	0.03	0.13	Tr	0
282	2	54	109	1.0	97	176	350	102	0.04	0.18	Tr	Tr
247	Tr	27	26	0.2	29	933[9]	3460[10]	852[10]	0.01	0.04	Tr	0
31	Tr	3	3	Tr	4	116[9]	430[10]	106[10]	Tr	Tr	Tr	0
11	Tr	1	1	Tr	1	41[9]	150[10]	38[10]	Tr	Tr	Tr	0
0	0	0	0	0.0	0	0	0	0	0.00	0.00	0.0	0
0	0	0	0	0.0	0	0	0	0	0.00	0.00	0.0	0
195	0	0	0	0.0	0	0	0	0	0.00	0.00	0.0	0
12	0	0	0	0.0	0	0	0	0	0.00	0.00	0.0	0
0	1	40	31	0.0	57	2178[11]	7510[12]	2254[12]	0.01	0.05	Tr	Tr
0	Tr	2	2	0.0	4	134[11]	460[12]	139[12]	Tr	Tr	Tr	Tr
0	1	34	26	0.1	48	1066[11]	3740[12]	1122[12]	0.01	0.04	Tr	Tr
0	Tr	4	3	Tr	6	132[11]	460[12]	139[12]	Tr	0.01	Tr	Tr
0	Tr	1	1	Tr	2	47[11]	170[12]	50[12]	Tr	Tr	Tr	Tr

[10]Values for vitamin A are year-round average.

[11]For salted margarine.

[12]Based on average vitamin A content of fortified margarine. Federal specifications for fortified margarine require a minimium of 15,000 IU/pound.

Continued.

Item Number	Foods, Approximate Measures, Units, and Weight (Weight of Edible Portion Only)		Weight (grams)	Water (percent)	Food Energy (calories)	Protein (grams)	Fat (grams)	Fatty Acids Saturated (grams)	Fatty Acids Monounsaturated (grams)	Fatty Acids Polyunsaturated (grams)
	Fats and Oils—cont'd									
	Margarine—cont'd									
140	Soft	8-oz container	227	16	1625	2	183	31.3	64.7	78.5
	Spread (about 60% fat)									
141	Hard (4 sticks per lb)	1 tbsp	14	16	100	Tr	11	1.9	4.0	4.8
142	Stick	½ cup	113	37	610	1	69	15.9	29.4	20.5
143	Tablespoon (⅛ stick)	1 tbsp	14	37	75	Tr	9	2.0	3.6	2.5
144	Pat (1-in square, ⅓ in high; 90 per lb)	1 pat	5	37	25	Tr	3	0.7	1.3	0.9
145	Soft	8-oz container	227	37	1225	1	138	29.1	71.5	31.3
146		1 tbsp	14	37	75	Tr	9	1.8	4.4	1.9
	Oils, salad or cooking									
147	Corn	1 cup	218	0	1925	0	218	27.7	52.8	128.0
148		1 tbsp	14	0	125	0	14	1.8	3.4	8.2
149	Olive	1 cup	216	0	1910	0	216	29.2	159.2	18.1
150		1 tbsp	14	0	125	0	14	1.9	10.3	1.2
151	Peanut	1 cup	216	0	1910	0	216	36.5	99.8	69.1
152		1 tbsp	14	0	125	0	14	2.4	6.5	4.5
153	Safflower	1 cup	218	0	1925	0	218	19.8	26.4	162.4
154		1 tbsp	14	0	125	0	14	1.3	1.7	10.4
155	Soybean oil, hydrogenated (partially hardened)	1 cup	218	0	1925	0	218	32.5	93.7	82.0
156		1 tbsp	14	0	125	0	14	2.1	6.0	5.3
157	Soybean-cottonseed oil blend, hydrogenated	1 cup	218	0	1925	0	218	39.2	64.3	104.9
158		1 tbsp	14	0	125	0	14	2.5	4.1	6.7
159	Sunflower	1 cup	218	0	1925	0	218	22.5	42.5	143.2
160		1 tbsp	14	0	125	0	14	1.4	2.7	9.2
	Salad dressings									
	Commercial									
161	Blue cheese	1 tbsp	15	32	75	1	8	1.5	1.8	4.2
	French									
162	Regular	1 tbsp	16	35	85	Tr	9	1.4	4.0	3.5
163	Low calorie	1 tbsp	16	75	25	Tr	2	0.2	0.3	1.0
	Italian									
164	Regular	1 tbsp	15	34	80	Tr	9	1.3	3.7	3.2
165	Low calorie	1 tbsp	15	86	5	Tr	Tr	Tr	Tr	Tr
	Mayonnaise									
166	Regular	1 tbsp	14	15	100	Tr	11	1.7	3.2	5.8
167	Imitation	1 tbsp	15	63	35	Tr	3	0.5	0.7	1.6
168	Mayonnaise type	1 tbsp	15	40	60	Tr	5	0.7	1.4	2.7
169	Tartar sauce	1 tbsp	14	34	75	Tr	8	1.2	2.6	3.9
	Thousand island									
170	Regular	1 tbsp	16	46	60	Tr	6	1.0	1.3	3.2
171	Low calorie	1 tbsp	15	69	25	Tr	2	0.2	0.4	0.9
	Prepared from home recipe									
172	Cooked type[13]	1 tbsp	16	69	25	1	2	0.5	0.6	0.3
173	Vinegar and oil	1 tbsp	16	47	70	0	8	1.5	2.4	3.9
	Fish and Shellfish									
	Clams									
174	Raw, meat only	3 oz	85	82	65	11	1	0.3	0.3	0.3
175	Canned, drained solids	3 oz	85	77	85	13	2	0.5	0.5	0.4
176	Crabmeat, canned	1 cup	135	77	135	23	3	0.5	0.8	1.4
177	Fish sticks, frozen, reheated (stick, 4 by 1 by ½ in)	1 fish stick	28	52	70	6	3	0.8	1.4	0.8
	Flounder or sole, baked, with lemon juice									
178	With butter	3 oz	85	73	120	16	6	3.2	1.5	0.5
179	With margarine	3 oz	85	73	120	16	6	1.2	2.3	1.9
180	Without added fat	3 oz	85	78	80	17	1	0.3	0.2	0.4
181	Haddock, breaded, fried[14]	3 oz	85	61	175	17	9	2.4	3.9	2.4
182	Halibut, broiled, with butter and lemon juice	3 oz	85	67	140	20	6	3.3	1.6	0.7
183	Herring, pickled	3 oz	85	59	190	17	13	4.3	4.6	3.1
184	Ocean perch, breaded, fried[14]	1 fillet	85	59	185	16	11	2.6	4.6	2.8

[9]For salted butter; unsalted butter contains 12 mg sodium/stick, 2 mg/tbsp, or 1 mg/pat.

[10]Values for vitamin A are year-round average.

[11]For salted margarine.

Cholesterol (mg)	Carbo-hydrate (grams)	Calcium (mg)	Phosphorus (mg)	Iron (mg)	Potassium (mg)	Sodium (mg)	Vitamin A Value (IU) International Units	Vitamin A Value (RE) Retinol Equivalents	Thiamin (mg)	Riboflavin (mg)	Niacin (mg)	Ascorbic Acid (mg)
0	1	60	46	0.0	86	2449[11]	7510[12]	2254[12]	0.02	0.07	Tr	Tr
0	Tr	4	3	0.0	5	151[11]	460[12]	139[12]	Tr	Tr	Tr	Tr
0	0	24	18	0.0	34	1123[11]	3740[12]	1122[12]	0.01	0.03	Tr	Tr
0	0	3	2	0.0	4	139[11]	460[12]	139[12]	Tr	Tr	Tr	Tr
0	0	1	1	0.0	1	50[11]	170[12]	50[12]	Tr	Tr	Tr	Tr
0	0	47	37	0.0	68	2256[11]	7510[12]	2254[12]	0.02	0.06	Tr	Tr
0	0	3	2	0.0	4	139[11]	460[12]	139[12]	Tr	Tr	Tr	Tr
0	0	0	0	0.0	0	0	0	0	0.00	0.00	0.0	0
0	0	0	0	0.0	0	0	0	0	0.00	0.00	0.0	0
0	0	0	0	0.0	0	0	0	0	0.00	0.00	0.0	0
0	0	0	0	0.0	0	0	0	0	0.00	0.00	0.0	0
0	0	0	0	0.0	0	0	0	0	0.00	0.00	0.0	0
0	0	0	0	0.0	0	0	0	0	0.00	0.00	0.0	0
0	0	0	0	0.0	0	0	0	0	0.00	0.00	0.0	0
0	0	0	0	0.0	0	0	0	0	0.00	0.00	0.0	0
0	0	0	0	0.0	0	0	0	0	0.00	0.00	0.0	0
0	0	0	0	0.0	0	0	0	0	0.00	0.00	0.0	0
0	0	0	0	0.0	0	0	0	0	0.00	0.00	0.0	0
0	0	0	0	0.0	0	0	0	0	0.00	0.00	0.0	0
0	0	0	0	0.0	0	0	0	0	0.00	0.00	0.0	0
0	0	0	0	0.0	0	0	0	0	0.00	0.00	0.0	0
3	1	12	11	Tr	6	164	30	10	Tr	0.02	Tr	Tr
0	1	2	1	Tr	2	188	Tr	Tr	Tr	Tr	Tr	Tr
0	2	6	5	Tr	3	306	Tr	Tr	Tr	Tr	Tr	Tr
0	1	1	1	Tr	5	162	30	3	Tr	Tr	Tr	Tr
0	2	1	1	Tr	4	136	Tr	Tr	Tr	Tr	Tr	Tr
8	Tr	3	4	0.1	5	80	40	12	0.00	0.00	Tr	0
4	2	Tr	Tr	0.0	2	75	0	0	0.00	0.00	0.0	0
4	4	2	4	Tr	1	107	30	13	Tr	Tr	Tr	0
4	1	3	4	0.1	11	182	30	9	Tr	Tr	0.0	Tr
4	2	2	3	0.1	18	112	50	15	Tr	Tr	Tr	0
2	2	2	3	0.1	17	150	50	14	Tr	Tr	Tr	0
9	2	13	14	0.1	19	117	70	20	0.01	0.02	Tr	Tr
0	Tr	0	0	0.0	1	Tr	0	0	0.00	0.00	0.0	0
43	2	59	138	2.6	154	102	90	26	0.09	0.15	1.1	9
54	2	47	116	3.5	119	102	90	26	0.01	0.09	0.9	3
135	1	61	246	1.1	149	1350	50	14	0.11	0.11	2.6	0
26	4	11	58	0.3	94	53	20	5	0.03	0.05	0.6	0
68	Tr	13	187	0.3	272	145	210	54	0.05	0.08	1.6	1
55	Tr	14	187	0.3	273	151	230	69	0.05	0.08	1.6	1
59	Tr	13	197	0.3	286	101	30	10	0.05	0.08	1.7	1
75	7	34	183	1.0	270	123	70	20	0.06	0.10	2.9	0
62	Tr	14	206	0.7	441	103	610	174	0.06	0.07	7.7	1
85	0	29	128	0.9	85	850	110	33	0.04	0.18	2.8	0
66	7	31	191	1.2	241	138	70	20	0.10	0.11	2.0	0

[12]Based on average vitamin A content of fortified margarine. Federal specifications for fortified margarine require a minimum of 15,000 IU/pound.

Continued.

[13]Fatty acid values apply to product made with regular margarine.

[14]Dipped in egg, milk, and breadcrumbs; fried in vegetable shortening.

Item Number	Foods, Approximate Measures, Units, and Weight (Weight of Edible Portion Only)		Weight (grams)	Water (percent)	Food Energy (calories)	Protein (grams)	Fat (grams)	Fatty Acids		
								Saturated (grams)	Monounsaturated (grams)	Polyunsaturated (grams)
	Fish and Shellfish—cont'd									
	Oysters									
185	Raw, meat only (13-19 medium selects)	1 cup	240	85	160	20	4	1.4	0.5	1.4
186	Breaded, fried[14]	1 oyster	45	65	90	5	5	1.4	2.1	1.4
	Salmon									
187	Canned (pink), solids and liquid	3 oz	85	71	120	17	5	0.9	1.5	2.1
188	Baked (red)	3 oz	85	67	140	21	5	1.2	2.4	1.4
189	Smoked	3 oz	85	59	150	18	8	2.6	3.9	0.7
190	Sardines, Atlantic, canned in oil, drained solids	3 oz	85	62	175	20	9	2.1	3.7	2.9
191	Scallops, breaded, frozen, reheated	6 scallops	90	59	195	15	10	2.5	4.1	2.5
	Shrimp									
192	Canned, drained solids	3 oz	85	70	100	21	1	0.2	0.2	0.4
193	French-fried (7 medium)[16]	3 oz	85	55	200	16	10	2.5	4.1	2.6
194	Trout, broiled, with butter and lemon juice	3 oz	85	63	175	21	9	4.1	2.9	1.6
	Tuna, canned, drained solids									
195	Oil pack, chunk light	3 oz	85	61	165	24	7	1.4	1.9	3.1
196	Water pack, solid white	3 oz	85	63	135	30	1	0.3	0.2	0.3
197	Tuna salad[17]	1 cup	205	63	375	33	19	3.3	4.9	9.2
	Fruits and Fruit Juices									
	Apples									
	Raw									
	Unpeeled, without cores									
198	2¾-in diam (about 3 per lb with cores)	1 apple	138	84	80	Tr	Tr	0.1	Tr	0.1
199	3¼-in diam (about 2 per lb with cores)	1 apple	212	84	125	Tr	1	0.1	Tr	0.2
200	Peeled, sliced	1 cup	110	84	65	Tr	Tr	0.1	Tr	0.1
201	Dried, sulfured	10 rings	64	32	155	1	Tr	Tr	Tr	0.1
202	Apple juice, bottled or canned[19]	1 cup	248	88	115	Tr	Tr	Tr	Tr	0.1
	Applesauce, canned									
203	Sweetened	1 cup	255	80	195	Tr	Tr	0.1	Tr	0.1
204	Unsweetened	1 cup	244	88	105	Tr	Tr	Tr	Tr	Tr
	Apricots									
205	Raw, without pits (about 12 per lb with pits)	3 apricots	106	86	50	1	Tr	Tr	0.2	0.1
	Canned (fruit and liquid)									
206	Heavy syrup pack	1 cup	258	78	215	1	Tr	Tr	0.1	Tr
207		3 halves	85	78	70	Tr	Tr	Tr	Tr	Tr
208	Juice pack	1 cup	248	87	120	2	Tr	Tr	Tr	Tr
209		3 halves	84	87	40	1	Tr	Tr	Tr	Tr
	Dried									
210	Uncooked (28 large or 37 medium halves per cup)	1 cup	130	31	310	5	1	Tr	0.3	0.1
211	Cooked, unsweetened, fruit and liquid	1 cup	250	76	210	3	Tr	Tr	0.2	0.1
212	Apricot nectar, canned	1 cup	251	85	140	1	Tr	Tr	0.1	Tr
	Avocados, raw, whole, without skin and seed									
213	California (about 2 per lb with skin and seed)	1 avocado	173	73	305	4	30	4.5	19.4	3.5
214	Florida (about 1 per lb with skin and seed)	1 avocado	304	80	340	5	27	5.3	14.8	4.5
	Bananas, raw, without peel									
215	Whole (about 2½ per lb with peel)	1 banana	114	74	105	1	1	0.2	Tr	0.1
216	Sliced	1 cup	150	74	140	2	1	0.3	0.1	0.1
217	Blackberries, raw	1 cup	144	86	75	1	1	0.2	0.1	0.1
	Blueberries									
218	Raw	1 cup	145	85	80	1	1	Tr	0.1	0.3
219	Frozen, sweetened	10-oz container	284	77	230	1	Tr	Tr	0.1	0.2
220		1 cup	230	77	185	1	Tr	Tr	Tr	0.1

[14] Dipped in egg, milk, and breadcrumbs; fried in vegetable shortening.
[15] If bones are discarded, value for calcium will be greatly reduced.
[16] Dipped in egg, breadcrumbs, and flour; fried in vegetable shortening.
[17] Made with drained chunk light tuna, celery, onion, pickle relish, and mayonnaise-type salad dressing.

Cholesterol (mg)	Carbohydrate (grams)	Calcium (mg)	Phosphorus (mg)	Iron (mg)	Potassium (mg)	Sodium (mg)	Vitamin A Value (IU) International Units	Vitamin A Value (RE) Retinol Equivalents	Thiamin (mg)	Riboflavin (mg)	Niacin (mg)	Ascorbic Acid (mg)
120	8	226	343	15.6	290	175	740	223	0.34	0.43	6.0	24
35	5	49	73	3.0	64	70	150	44	0.07	0.10	1.3	4
34	0	167[15]	243	0.7	307	443	60	18	0.03	0.15	6.8	0
60	0	26	269	0.5	305	55	290	87	0.18	0.14	5.5	0
51	0	12	208	0.8	327	1700	260	77	0.17	0.17	6.8	0
85	0	371[15]	424	2.6	349	425	190	56	0.03	0.17	4.6	0
70	10	39	203	2.0	369	298	70	21	0.11	0.11	1.6	0
128	1	98	224	1.4	1	1955	50	15	0.01	0.03	1.5	0
168	11	61	154	2.0	189	384	90	26	0.06	0.09	2.8	0
71	Tr	26	259	1.0	297	122	230	60	0.07	0.07	2.3	1
55	0	7	199	1.6	298	303	70	20	0.04	0.09	10.1	0
48	0	17	202	0.6	255	468	110	32	0.03	0.10	13.4	0
80	19	31	281	2.5	531	877	230	53	0.06	0.14	13.3	6
0	21	10	10	0.2	159	Tr	70	7	0.02	0.02	0.1	8
0	32	15	15	0.4	244	Tr	110	11	0.04	0.03	0.2	12
0	16	4	8	0.1	124	Tr	50	5	0.02	0.01	0.1	4
0	42	9	24	0.9	288	56[18]	0	0	0.00	0.10	0.6	2
0	29	17	17	0.9	295	7	Tr	Tr	0.05	0.04	0.2	2[20]
0	51	10	18	0.9	156	8	30	3	0.03	0.07	0.5	4[20]
0	28	7	17	0.3	183	5	70	7	0.03	0.06	0.5	3[20]
0	12	15	20	0.6	314	1	2770	277	0.03	0.04	0.6	11
0	55	23	31	0.8	361	10	3170	317	0.05	0.06	1.0	8
0	18	8	10	0.3	119	3	1050	105	0.02	0.02	0.3	3
0	31	30	50	0.7	409	10	4190	419	0.04	0.05	0.9	12
0	10	10	17	0.3	139	3	1420	142	0.02	0.02	0.3	4
0	80	59	152	6.1	1791	13	9410	941	0.01	0.20	3.9	3
0	55	40	103	4.2	1222	8	5910	591	0.02	0.08	2.4	4
0	36	18	23	1.0	286	8	3300	330	0.02	0.04	0.7	2[20]
0	12	19	73	2.0	1097	21	1060	106	0.19	0.21	3.3	14
0	27	33	119	1.6	1484	15	1860	186	0.33	0.37	5.8	24
0	27	7	23	0.4	451	1	90	9	0.05	0.11	0.6	10
0	35	9	30	0.5	594	2	120	12	0.07	0.15	0.8	14
0	18	46	30	0.8	282	Tr	240	24	0.04	0.06	0.6	30
0	20	9	15	0.2	129	9	150	15	0.07	0.07	0.5	19
0	62	17	20	1.1	170	3	120	12	0.06	0.15	0.7	3
0	50	14	16	0.9	138	2	100	10	0.05	0.12	0.6	2

[18]Sodium bisulfite used to preserve color; unsulfited product would contain less sodium.
[19]Also applies to pasteurized apple cider.
[20]Without added ascorbic acid. For value with added ascorbic acid, refer to label.

Continued.

Item Number	Foods, Approximate Measures, Units, and Weight (Weight of Edible Portion Only)		Weight (grams)	Water (percent)	Food Energy (calories)	Protein (grams)	Fat (grams)	Fatty Acids Saturated (grams)	Fatty Acids Monounsaturated (grams)	Fatty Acids Polyunsaturated (grams)
	Fruits and Fruit Juices—cont'd									
	Cantaloupe. See Melons (item 251).									
	Cherries									
221	Sour, red, pitted, canned, water pack	1 cup	244	90	90	2	Tr	0.1	0.1	0.1
222	Sweet, raw, without pits and stems	10 cherries	68	81	50	1	1	0.1	0.2	0.2
223	Cranberry juice cocktail, bottled, sweetened	1 cup	253	85	145	Tr	Tr	Tr	Tr	0.1
224	Cranberry sauce, sweetened, canned, strained	1 cup	277	61	420	1	Tr	Tr	0.1	0.2
	Dates									
225	Whole, without pits	10 dates	83	23	230	2	Tr	0.1	0.1	Tr
226	Chopped	1 cup	178	23	490	4	1	0.3	0.2	Tr
227	Figs, dried	10 figs	187	28	475	6	2	0.4	0.5	1.0
	Fruit cocktail, canned, fruit and liquid									
228	Heavy syrup pack	1 cup	255	80	185	1	Tr	Tr	Tr	0.1
229	Juice pack	1 cup	248	87	115	1	Tr	Tr	Tr	Tr
	Grapefruit									
230	Raw, without peel, membrane and seeds (3¾-in diam, 1 lb 1 oz, whole, with refuse)	½ grapefruit	120	91	40	1	Tr	Tr	Tr	Tr
231	Canned, sections with syrup	1 cup	254	84	150	1	Tr	Tr	Tr	0.1
	Grapefruit juice									
232	Raw	1 cup	247	90	95	1	Tr	Tr	Tr	0.1
	Canned									
233	Unsweetened	1 cup	247	90	95	1	Tr	Tr	Tr	0.1
234	Sweetened	1 cup	250	87	115	1	Tr	Tr	Tr	0.1
	Frozen concentrate, unsweetened									
235	Undiluted	6-fl-oz can	207	62	300	4	1	0.1	0.1	0.2
236	Diluted with 3 parts water by volume	1 cup	247	89	100	1	Tr	Tr	Tr	0.1
	Grapes, European type (adherent skin), raw									
237	Thompson seedless	10 grapes	50	81	35	Tr	Tr	0.1	Tr	0.1
238	Tokay and Emperor, seeded types	10 grapes	57	81	40	Tr	Tr	0.1	Tr	0.1
	Grape juice									
239	Canned or bottled	1 cup	253	84	155	1	Tr	0.1	Tr	0.1
	Frozen concentrate, sweetened									
240	Undiluted	6-fl-oz can	216	54	385	1	1	0.2	Tr	0.2
241	Diluted with 3 parts water by volume	1 cup	250	87	125	Tr	Tr	0.1	Tr	0.1
242	Kiwifruit, raw, without skin (about 5/lb with skin)	1 kiwifruit	76	83	45	1	Tr	Tr	0.1	0.1
243	Lemons, raw, without peel and seeds (about 4 lb with peel and seeds)	1 lemon	58	89	15	1	Tr	Tr	Tr	0.1
	Lemon juice									
244	Raw	1 cup	244	91	60	1	Tr	Tr	Tr	Tr
245	Canned or bottled, unsweetened	1 cup	244	92	50	1	1	0.1	Tr	0.2
246		1 tbsp	15	92	5	Tr	Tr	Tr	Tr	Tr
247	Frozen, single-strength, unsweetened	6-fl-oz can	244	92	55	1	1	0.1	Tr	0.2
	Lime juice									
248	Raw	1 cup	246	90	65	1	Tr	Tr	Tr	0.1
249	Canned, unsweetened	1 cup	246	93	50	1	1	0.1	0.1	0.2
250	Mangos, raw, without skin and seed (about 1½ per lb with skin and seed)	1 mango	207	82	135	1	1	0.1	0.2	0.1
	Melons, raw, without rind and cavity contents									
251	Cantaloupe, orange-fleshed (5-in diam, 2⅓ lb, whole, with rind and cavity contents)	½ melon	267	90	95	2	1	0.1	0.1	0.3
252	Honeydew (6½-in diam, 5¼ lb, whole, with rind and cavity contents)	1/10 melon	129	90	45	1	Tr	Tr	Tr	0.1
253	Nectarines, raw, without pits (about 3 per lb with pits)	1 nectarine	136	86	65	1	1	0.1	0.2	0.3
	Oranges, raw									
254	Whole, without peel and seeds (2⅝-in diam, about 2½ per lb, with peel and seeds)	1 orange	131	87	60	1	Tr	Tr	Tr	Tr
255	Sections without membranes	1 cup	180	87	85	2	Tr	Tr	Tr	Tr

[20]Without added ascorbic acid. For value with added ascorbic acid, refer to label.

[21]With added ascorbic acid.

Cholesterol (mg)	Carbohydrate (grams)	Calcium (mg)	Phosphorus (mg)	Iron (mg)	Potassium (mg)	Sodium (mg)	Vitamin A Value (IU) International Units	Vitamin A Value (RE) Retinol Equivalents	Thiamin (mg)	Riboflavin (mg)	Niacin (mg)	Ascorbic Acid (mg)
0	22	27	24	3.3	239	17	1840	184	0.04	0.10	0.4	5
0	11	10	13	0.3	152	Tr	150	15	0.03	0.04	0.3	5
0	38	8	3	0.4	61	10	10	1	0.01	0.04	0.1	108[21]
0	108	11	17	0.6	72	80	60	6	0.04	0.06	0.3	6
0	61	27	33	1.0	541	2	40	4	0.07	0.08	1.8	0
0	131	57	71	2.0	1161	5	90	9	0.16	0.18	3.9	0
0	122	269	127	4.2	1331	21	250	25	0.13	0.16	1.3	1
0	48	15	28	0.7	224	15	520	52	0.05	0.05	1.0	5
0	29	20	35	0.5	236	10	760	76	0.03	0.04	1.0	7
0	10	14	10	0.1	167	Tr	10[22]	1[22]	0.04	0.02	0.3	41
0	39	36	25	1.0	328	5	Tr	Tr	0.10	0.05	0.6	54
0	23	22	37	0.5	400	2	20	2	0.10	0.05	0.5	94
0	22	17	27	0.5	378	2	20	2	0.10	0.05	0.6	72
0	28	20	28	0.9	405	5	20	2	0.10	0.06	0.8	67
0	72	56	101	1.0	1002	6	60	6	0.30	0.16	1.6	248
0	24	20	35	0.3	336	2	20	2	0.10	0.05	0.5	83
0	9	6	7	0.1	93	1	40	4	0.05	0.03	0.2	5
0	10	6	7	0.1	105	1	40	4	0.05	0.03	0.2	6
0	38	23	28	0.6	334	8	20	2	0.07	0.09	0.7	Tr[20]
0	96	28	32	0.8	160	15	60	6	0.11	0.20	0.9	179[21]
0	32	10	10	0.3	53	5	20	2	0.04	0.07	0.3	60[21]
0	11	20	30	0.3	252	4	130	13	0.02	0.04	0.4	74
0	5	15	9	0.3	80	1	20	2	0.02	0.01	0.1	31
0	21	17	15	0.1	303	2	50	5	0.07	0.02	0.2	112
0	16	27	22	0.3	249	51[23]	40	4	0.10	0.02	0.5	61
0	1	2	1	Tr	15	3[23]	Tr	Tr	0.01	Tr	Tr	4
0	16	20	20	0.3	217	2	30	3	0.14	0.03	0.3	77
0	22	22	17	0.1	268	2	20	2	0.05	0.02	0.2	72
0	16	30	25	0.6	185	39[23]	40	4	0.08	0.01	0.4	16
0	35	21	23	0.3	323	4	8060	806	0.12	0.12	1.2	57
0	22	29	45	0.6	825	24	8610	861	0.10	0.06	1.5	113
0	12	8	13	0.1	350	13	50	5	0.10	0.02	0.8	32
0	16	7	22	0.2	288	Tr	1000	100	0.02	0.06	1.3	7
0	15	52	18	0.1	237	Tr	270	27	0.11	0.05	0.4	70
0	21	72	25	0.2	326	Tr	370	37	0.16	0.07	0.5	96

[22]For white grapefruit; pink grapefruit have about 310 IU or 31 RE.

[23]Sodium benzoate and sodium bisulfite added as preservatives.

Continued.

Item Number	Foods, Approximate Measures, Units, and Weight (Weight of Edible Portion Only)		Weight (grams)	Water (percent)	Food Energy (calories)	Protein (grams)	Fat (grams)	Fatty Acids: Saturated (grams)	Fatty Acids: Monounsaturated (grams)	Fatty Acids: Polyunsaturated (grams)
	Fruits and Fruit Juices—cont'd									
	Orange juice									
256	Raw, all varieties	1 cup	248	88	110	2	Tr	0.1	0.1	0.1
257	Canned, unsweetened	1 cup	249	89	105	1	Tr	Tr	0.1	0.1
258	Chilled	1 cup	249	88	110	2	1	0.1	0.1	0.2
	Frozen concentrate									
259	Undiluted	6-fl-oz can	213	58	340	5	Tr	0.1	0.1	0.1
260	Diluted with 3 parts water by volume	1 cup	249	88	110	2	Tr	Tr	Tr	Tr
261	Orange and grapefruit juice, canned	1 cup	247	89	105	1	Tr	Tr	Tr	Tr
262	Papayas, raw, ½-in cubes	1 cup	140	86	65	1	Tr	0.1	0.1	Tr
	Peaches									
	Raw									
263	Whole, 2½-in diam, peeled, pitted (about 4 per lb with peels and pits)	1 peach	87	88	35	1	Tr	Tr	Tr	Tr
264	Sliced	1 cup	170	88	75	1	Tr	Tr	0.1	0.1
	Canned, fruit and liquid									
265	Heavy syrup pack	1 cup	256	79	190	1	Tr	Tr	0.1	0.1
266		1 half	81	79	60	Tr	Tr	Tr	Tr	Tr
267	Juice pack	1 cup	248	87	110	2	Tr	Tr	Tr	Tr
268		1 half	77	87	35	Tr	Tr	Tr	Tr	Tr
	Dried									
269	Uncooked	1 cup	160	32	380	6	1	0.1	0.4	0.6
270	Cooked, unsweetened, fruit and liquid	1 cup	258	78	200	3	1	0.1	0.2	0.3
271	Frozen, sliced, sweetened	10-oz container	284	75	265	2	Tr	Tr	0.1	0.2
272		1 cup	250	75	235	2	Tr	Tr	0.1	0.2
	Pears									
	Raw, with skin, cored									
273	Bartlett, 2½-in diam (about 2½ per lb with cores and stems)	1 pear	166	84	100	1	1	Tr	0.1	0.2
274	Bosc, 2½-in diam (about 3 per lb with cores and stems)	1 pear	141	84	85	1	1	Tr	0.1	0.1
275	D'Anjou, 3-in diam (about 2 per lb with cores and stems)	1 pear	200	84	120	1	1	Tr	0.2	0.2
	Canned, fruit and liquid									
276	Heavy syrup pack	1 cup	255	80	190	1	Tr	Tr	0.1	0.1
277		1 half	79	80	60	Tr	Tr	Tr	Tr	Tr
278	Juice pack	1 cup	248	86	125	1	Tr	Tr	Tr	Tr
279		1 half	77	86	40	Tr	Tr	Tr	Tr	Tr
	Pineapple									
280	Raw, diced	1 cup	155	87	75	1	1	Tr	0.1	0.2
	Canned, fruit and liquid									
	Heavy syrup pack									
281	Crushed, chunks, tidbits	1 cup	255	79	200	1	Tr	Tr	Tr	0.1
282	Slices	1 slice	58	79	45	Tr	Tr	Tr	Tr	Tr
	Juice pack									
283	Chunks or tidbits	1 cup	250	84	150	1	Tr	Tr	Tr	0.1
284	Slices	1 slice	58	84	35	Tr	Tr	Tr	Tr	Tr
285	Pineapple juice, unsweetened, canned	1 cup	250	86	140	1	Tr	Tr	Tr	0.1
	Plantains, without peel									
286	Raw	1 plantain	179	65	220	2	1	0.3	0.1	0.1
287	Cooked, boiled, sliced	1 cup	154	67	180	1	Tr	0.1	Tr	0.1
	Plums, without pits									
	Raw									
288	2⅛-in diam (about 6½ per lb with pits)	1 plum	66	85	35	1	Tr	Tr	0.3	0.1
289	1½-in diam (about 15 per lb with pits)	1 plum	28	85	15	Tr	Tr	Tr	0.1	Tr
	Canned, purple, fruit and liquid									
290	Heavy syrup pack	1 cup	258	76	230	1	Tr	Tr	0.2	0.1
291		3 plums	133	76	120	Tr	Tr	Tr	0.1	Tr
292	Juice pack	1 cup	252	84	145	1	Tr	Tr	Tr	Tr
293		3 plums	95	84	55	Tr	Tr	Tr	Tr	Tr
	Prunes, dried									
294	Uncooked	4 extra large or 5 large prunes	49	32	115	1	Tr	Tr	0.2	0.1
295	Cooked, unsweetened, fruit and liquid	1 cup	212	70	225	2	Tr	Tr	0.3	0.1

[21]With added ascorbic acid.

							Vitamin A Value					
Cholesterol (mg)	Carbo-hydrate (grams)	Calcium (mg)	Phosphorus (mg)	Iron (mg)	Potassium (mg)	Sodium (mg)	(IU) International Units	(RE) Retinol Equivalents	Thiamin (mg)	Riboflavin (mg)	Niacin (mg)	Ascorbic Acid (mg)
0	26	27	42	0.5	496	2	500	50	0.22	0.07	1.0	124
0	25	20	35	1.1	436	5	440	44	0.15	0.07	0.8	86
0	25	25	27	0.4	473	2	190	19	0.28	0.05	0.7	82
0	81	68	121	0.7	1436	6	590	59	0.60	0.14	1.5	294
0	27	22	40	0.2	473	2	190	19	0.20	0.04	0.5	97
0	25	20	35	1.1	390	7	290	29	0.14	0.07	0.8	72
0	17	35	12	0.3	247	9	400	40	0.04	0.04	0.5	92
0	10	4	10	0.1	171	Tr	470	47	0.01	0.04	0.9	6
0	19	9	20	0.2	335	Tr	910	91	0.03	0.07	1.7	11
0	51	8	28	0.7	236	15	850	85	0.03	0.06	1.6	7
0	16	2	9	0.2	75	5	270	27	0.01	0.02	0.5	2
0	29	15	42	0.7	317	10	940	94	0.02	0.04	1.4	9
0	9	5	13	0.2	99	3	290	29	0.01	0.01	0.4	3
0	98	45	190	6.5	1594	11	3460	346	Tr	0.34	7.0	8
0	51	23	98	3.4	826	5	510	51	0.01	0.05	3.9	10
0	68	9	31	1.1	369	17	810	81	0.04	0.10	1.9	268[21]
0	60	8	28	0.9	325	15	710	71	0.03	0.09	1.6	236[21]
0	25	18	18	0.4	208	Tr	30	3	0.03	0.07	0.2	7
0	21	16	16	0.4	176	Tr	30	3	0.03	0.06	0.1	6
0	30	22	22	0.5	250	Tr	40	4	0.04	0.08	0.2	8
0	49	13	18	0.6	166	13	10	1	0.03	0.06	0.6	3
0	15	4	6	0.2	51	4	Tr	Tr	0.01	0.02	0.2	1
0	32	22	30	0.7	238	10	10	1	0.03	0.03	0.5	4
0	10	7	9	0.2	74	3	Tr	Tr	0.01	0.01	0.2	1
0	19	11	11	0.6	175	2	40	4	0.14	0.06	0.7	24
0	52	36	18	1.0	265	3	40	4	0.23	0.06	0.7	19
0	12	8	4	0.2	60	1	10	1	0.05	0.01	0.2	4
0	39	35	15	0.7	305	3	100	10	0.24	0.05	0.7	24
0	9	8	3	0.2	71	1	20	2	0.06	0.01	0.2	6
0	34	43	20	0.7	335	3	10	1	0.14	0.06	0.6	27
0	57	5	61	1.1	893	7	2020	202	0.09	0.10	1.2	33
0	48	3	43	0.9	716	8	1400	140	0.07	0.08	1.2	17
0	9	3	7	0.1	114	Tr	210	21	0.03	0.06	0.3	6
0	4	1	3	Tr	48	Tr	90	9	0.01	0.03	0.1	3
0	60	23	34	2.2	235	49	670	67	0.04	0.10	0.8	1
0	31	12	17	1.1	121	25	340	34	0.02	0.05	0.4	1
0	38	25	38	0.9	388	3	2540	254	0.06	0.15	1.2	7
0	14	10	14	0.3	146	1	960	96	0.02	0.06	0.4	3
0	31	25	39	1.2	365	2	970	97	0.04	0.08	1.0	2
0	60	49	74	2.4	708	4	650	65	0.05	0.21	1.5	6

Continued.

F

Item Number	Foods, Approximate Measures, Units, and Weight (Weight of Edible Portion Only)		Weight (grams)	Water (percent)	Food Energy (calories)	Protein (grams)	Fat (grams)	Fatty Acids: Saturated (grams)	Fatty Acids: Monounsaturated (grams)	Fatty Acids: Polyunsaturated (grams)
	Fruits and Fruit Juices—cont'd									
296	Prune juice, canned or bottled	1 cup	256	81	180	2	Tr	Tr	0.1	Tr
	Raisins, seedless									
297	Cup, not pressed down	1 cup	145	15	435	5	1	0.2	Tr	0.2
298	Packet, ½ oz (1½ tbsp)	1 packet	14	15	40	Tr	Tr	Tr	Tr	Tr
	Raspberries									
299	Raw	1 cup	123	87	60	1	1	Tr	0.1	0.4
300	Frozen, sweetened	10-oz container	284	73	295	2	Tr	Tr	Tr	0.3
301		1 cup	250	73	255	2	Tr	Tr	Tr	0.2
302	Rhubarb, cooked, added sugar	1 cup	240	68	280	1	Tr	Tr	Tr	0.1
	Strawberries									
303	Raw, capped, whole	1 cup	149	92	45	1	1	Tr	0.1	0.3
304	Frozen, sweetened, sliced	10-oz container	284	73	275	2	Tr	Tr	0.1	0.2
305		1 cup	255	73	245	1	Tr	Tr	Tr	0.2
	Tangerines									
306	Raw, without peel and seeds (2⅜-in diam, about 4 per lb, with peel and seeds)	1 tangerine	84	88	35	1	Tr	Tr	Tr	Tr
307	Canned, light syrup, fruit and liquid	1 cup	252	83	155	1	Tr	Tr	Tr	0.1
308	Tangerine juice, canned, sweetened	1 cup	249	87	125	1	Tr	Tr	Tr	0.1
	Watermelon, raw, without rind and seeds									
309	Piece (4 by 8 in wedge with rind and seeds; 1/16 of 32⅔-lb melon, 10 by 16 in)	1 piece	482	92	155	3	2	0.3	0.2	1.0
310	Diced	1 cup	160	92	50	1	1	0.1	0.1	0.3
	Grain Products									
311	Bagels, plain or water, enriched, 3½-in diam[24]	1 bagel	68	29	200	7	2	0.3	0.5	0.7
312	Barley, pearled, light, uncooked	1 cup	200	11	700	16	2	0.3	0.2	0.9
	Biscuits, baking powder, 2-in diam (enriched flour, vegetable shortening)									
313	From home recipe	1 biscuit	28	28	100	2	5	1.2	2.0	1.3
314	From mix	1 biscuit	28	29	95	2	3	0.8	1.4	0.9
315	From refrigerated dough	1 biscuit	20	30	65	1	2	0.6	0.9	0.6
	Breadcrumbs, enriched									
316	Dry grated	1 cup	100	7	390	13	5	1.5	1.6	1.0
	Soft. See White bread (item 351).									
	Breads									
317	Boston brown bread, canned, slice, 3¼ in by ½ in[25]	1 slice	45	45	95	2	1	0.3	0.1	0.1
	Cracked-wheat bread (¾ enriched wheat flour, ¼ cracked wheat flour)[25]									
318	Loaf, 1 lb	1 loaf	454	35	1190	42	16	3.1	4.3	5.7
319	Slice (18 per loaf)	1 slice	25	35	65	2	1	0.2	0.2	0.3
320	Toasted	1 slice	21	26	65	2	1	0.2	0.2	0.3
	French or vienna bread, enriched[25]									
321	Loaf, 1 lb	1 loaf	454	34	1270	43	18	3.8	5.7	5.9
	Slice									
322	French, 5 by 2½ by 1 in	1 slice	35	34	100	3	1	0.3	0.4	0.5
323	Vienna, 4¾ by 4 by ½ in	1 slice	25	34	70	2	1	0.2	0.3	0.3
	Italian bread, enriched									
324	Loaf, 1 lb	1 loaf	454	32	1255	41	4	0.6	0.3	1.6
325	Slice, 4½ by 3¼ by ¾ in	1 slice	30	32	85	3	Tr	Tr	Tr	0.1
	Mixed grain bread, enriched[25]									
326	Loaf, 1 lb	1 loaf	454	37	1165	45	17	3.2	4.1	6.5
327	Slice (18 per loaf)	1 slice	25	37	65	2	1	0.2	0.2	0.4
328	Toasted	1 slice	23	27	65	2	1	0.2	0.2	0.4
	Oatmeal bread, enriched[25]									
329	Loaf, 1 lb	1 loaf	454	37	1145	38	20	3.7	7.1	8.2
330	Slice (18 per loaf)	1 slice	25	37	65	2	1	0.2	0.4	0.5
331	Toasted	1 slice	23	30	65	2	1	0.2	0.4	0.5
332	Pita bread, enriched, white, 6½-in diam	1 pita	60	31	165	6	1	0.1	0.1	0.4

[24]Egg bagels have 44 mg cholesterol and 22 IU or 7 RE vitamin A per bagel.

[25]Made with vegetable shortening.

							Vitamin A Value					
Cholesterol (mg)	Carbo-hydrate (grams)	Calcium (mg)	Phosphorus (mg)	Iron (mg)	Potassium (mg)	Sodium (mg)	(IU) International Units	(RE) Retinol Equivalents	Thiamin (mg)	Riboflavin (mg)	Niacin (mg)	Ascorbic Acid (mg)
0	45	31	64	3.0	707	10	10	1	0.04	0.18	2.0	10
0	115	71	141	3.0	1089	17	10	1	0.23	0.13	1.2	5
0	11	7	14	0.3	105	2	Tr	Tr	0.02	0.01	0.1	Tr
0	14	27	15	0.7	187	Tr	160	16	0.04	0.11	1.1	31
0	74	43	48	1.8	324	3	170	17	0.05	0.13	0.7	47
0	65	38	43	1.6	285	3	150	15	0.05	0.11	0.6	41
0	75	348	19	0.5	230	2	170	17	0.04	0.06	0.5	8
0	10	21	28	0.6	247	1	40	4	0.03	0.10	0.3	84
0	74	31	37	1.7	278	9	70	7	0.05	0.14	1.1	118
0	66	28	33	1.5	250	8	60	6	0.04	0.13	1.0	106
0	9	12	8	0.1	132	1	770	77	0.09	0.02	0.1	26
0	41	18	25	0.9	197	15	2120	212	0.13	0.11	1.1	50
0	30	45	35	0.5	443	2	1050	105	0.15	0.05	0.2	55
0	35	39	43	0.8	559	10	1760	176	0.39	0.10	1.0	46
0	11	13	14	0.3	186	3	590	59	0.13	0.03	0.3	15
0	38	29	46	1.8	50	245	0	0	0.26	0.20	2.4	0
0	158	32	378	4.2	320	6	0	0	0.24	0.10	6.2	0
Tr	13	47	36	0.7	32	195	10	3	0.08	0.08	0.8	Tr
Tr	14	58	128	0.7	56	262	20	4	0.12	0.11	0.8	Tr
1	10	4	79	0.5	18	249	0	0	0.08	0.05	0.7	0
5	73	122	141	4.1	152	736	0	0	0.35	0.35	4.8	0
3	21	41	72	0.9	131	113	0[26]	0[26]	0.06	0.04	0.7	0
0	227	295	581	12.1	608	1966	Tr	Tr	1.73	1.73	15.3	Tr
0	12	16	32	0.7	34	106	Tr	Tr	0.10	0.09	0.8	Tr
0	12	16	32	0.7	34	106	Tr	Tr	0.07	0.09	0.8	Tr
0	230	499	386	14.0	409	2633	Tr	Tr	2.09	1.59	18.2	Tr
0	18	39	30	1.1	32	203	Tr	Tr	0.16	0.12	1.4	Tr
0	13	28	21	0.8	23	145	Tr	Tr	0.12	0.09	1.0	Tr
0	256	77	350	12.7	336	2656	0	0	1.80	1.10	15.0	0
0	17	5	23	0.8	22	176	0	0	0.12	0.07	1.0	0
0	212	472	962	14.8	990	1870	Tr	Tr	1.77	1.73	18.9	Tr
0	12	27	55	0.8	56	106	Tr	Tr	0.10	0.10	1.1	Tr
0	12	27	55	0.8	56	106	Tr	Tr	0.08	0.10	1.1	Tr
0	212	267	563	12.0	707	2231	0	0	2.09	1.20	15.4	0
0	12	15	31	0.7	39	124	0	0	0.12	0.07	0.9	0
0	12	15	31	0.7	39	124	0	0	0.09	0.07	0.9	0
0	33	49	60	1.4	71	339	0	0	0.27	0.12	2.2	0

[26]Made with white cornmeal. If made with yellow cornmeal, value is 32 IU or 3 RE.

Continued.

F

Item Number	Foods, Approximate Measures, Units, and Weight (Weight of Edible Portion Only)		Weight (grams)	Water (percent)	Food Energy (calories)	Protein (grams)	Fat (grams)	Fatty Acids: Saturated (grams)	Fatty Acids: Monounsaturated (grams)	Fatty Acids: Polyunsaturated (grams)
	Grain Products—cont'd									
	Breads—cont'd									
	Pumpernickel (2/3 rye flour, 1/3 enriched wheat flour)[25]									
333	Loaf, 1 lb	1 loaf	454	37	1160	42	16	2.6	3.6	6.4
334	Slice, 5 by 4 by 3/8 in	1 slice	32	37	80	3	1	0.2	0.3	0.5
335	Toasted	1 slice	29	28	80	3	1	0.2	0.3	0.5
	Raisin bread, enriched[25]									
336	Loaf, 1 lb	1 loaf	454	33	1260	37	18	4.1	6.5	6.7
337	Slice (18 per loaf)	1 slice	25	33	65	2	1	0.2	0.3	0.4
338	Toasted	1 slice	21	24	65	2	1	0.2	0.3	0.4
	Rye bread, light (2/3 enriched wheat flour, 1/3 rye flour)[25]									
339	Loaf, 1 lb	1 loaf	454	37	1190	38	17	3.3	5.2	5.5
340	Slice, 4 3/4 by 3 3/4 by 7/16 in	1 slice	25	37	65	2	1	0.2	0.3	0.3
341	Toasted	1 slice	22	28	65	2	1	0.2	0.3	0.3
	Wheat bread, enriched[25]									
342	Loaf, 1 lb	1 loaf	454	37	1160	43	19	3.9	7.3	4.5
343	Slice (18 per loaf)	1 slice	25	37	65	2	1	0.2	0.4	0.3
344	Toasted	1 slice	23	28	65	3	1	0.2	0.4	0.3
	White bread, enriched[25]									
345	Loaf, 1 lb	1 loaf	454	37	1210	38	18	5.6	6.5	4.2
346	Slice (18 per loaf)	1 slice	25	37	65	2	1	0.3	0.4	0.2
347	Toasted	1 slice	22	28	65	2	1	0.3	0.4	0.2
348	Slice (22 per loaf)	1 slice	20	37	55	2	1	0.2	0.3	0.2
349	Toasted	1 slice	17	28	55	2	1	0.2	0.3	0.2
350	Cubes	1 cup	30	37	80	2	1	0.4	0.4	0.3
351	Crumbs, soft	1 cup	45	37	120	4	2	0.6	0.6	0.4
	Whole-wheat bread[25]									
352	Loaf, 1 lb	1 loaf	454	38	1110	44	20	5.8	6.8	5.2
353	Slice (16 per loaf)	1 slice	28	38	70	3	1	0.4	0.4	0.3
354	Toasted	1 slice	25	29	70	3	1	0.4	0.4	0.3
	Bread stuffing (from enriched bread), prepared from mix									
355	Dry type	1 cup	140	33	500	9	31	6.1	13.3	9.6
356	Moist type	1 cup	203	61	420	9	26	5.3	11.3	8.0
	Breakfast cereals									
	Hot type, cooked									
	Corn (hominy) grits									
357	Regular and quick, enriched	1 cup	242	85	145	3	Tr	Tr	0.1	0.2
358	Instant, plain	1 pkt	137	85	80	2	Tr	Tr	Tr	0.1
	Cream of Wheat®									
359	Regular, quick, instant	1 cup	244	86	140	4	Tr	0.1	Tr	0.2
360	Mix'n Eat, plain	1 pkt	142	82	100	3	Tr	Tr	Tr	0.1
361	Malt-O-Meal®	1 cup	240	88	120	4	Tr	Tr	Tr	0.1
	Oatmeal or rolled oats									
362	Regular, quick, instant, nonfortified	1 cup	234	85	145	6	2	0.4	0.8	1.0
	Instant, fortified									
363	Plain	1 pkt	177	86	105	4	2	0.3	0.6	0.7
364	Flavored	1 pkt	164	76	160	5	2	0.3	0.7	0.8
	Ready to eat									
365	All-Bran® (about 1/3 cup)	1 oz	28	3	70	4	1	0.1	0.1	0.3
366	Cap'n Crunch® (about 3/4 cup)	1 oz	28	3	120	1	3	1.7	0.3	0.4
367	Cheerios® (about 1 1/4 cup)	1 oz	28	5	110	4	2	0.3	0.6	0.7
	Corn Flakes (about 1 1/4 cup)									
368	Kellogg's®	1 oz	28	3	110	2	Tr	Tr	Tr	Tr
369	Toasties®	1 oz	28	3	110	2	Tr	Tr	Tr	Tr
	40% Bran Flakes									
370	Kellogg's® (about 3/4 cup)	1 oz	28	3	90	4	1	0.1	0.1	0.3
371	Post® (about 2/3 cup)	1 oz	28	3	90	3	Tr	0.1	0.1	0.2

[25]Made with vegetable shortening.

[27]Nutrient added.

[28]Cooked without salt. If salt is added according to label recommendations, sodium content is 540 mg.

[29]For white corn grits. Cooked yellow grits contain 145 IU or 14 RE.

[30]Value based on label declaration for added nutrients.

Cholesterol (mg)	Carbohydrate (grams)	Calcium (mg)	Phosphorus (mg)	Iron (mg)	Potassium (mg)	Sodium (mg)	Vitamin A Value (IU) International Units	Vitamin A Value (RE) Retinol Equivalents	Thiamin (mg)	Riboflavin (mg)	Niacin (mg)	Ascorbic Acid (mg)
0	218	322	990	12.4	1966	2461	0	0	1.54	2.36	15.0	0
0	16	23	71	0.9	141	177	0	0	0.11	0.17	1.1	0
0	16	23	71	0.9	141	177	0	0	0.09	0.17	1.1	0
0	239	463	395	14.1	1058	1657	Tr	Tr	1.50	2.81	18.6	Tr
0	13	25	22	0.8	59	92	Tr	Tr	0.08	0.15	1.0	Tr
0	13	25	22	0.8	59	92	Tr	Tr	0.06	0.15	1.0	Tr
0	218	363	658	12.3	926	3164	0	0	1.86	1.45	15.0	0
0	12	20	36	0.7	51	175	0	0	0.10	0.08	0.8	0
0	12	20	36	0.7	51	175	0	0	0.08	0.08	0.8	0
0	213	572	835	15.8	627	2447	Tr	Tr	2.09	1.45	20.5	Tr
0	12	32	47	0.9	35	138	Tr	Tr	0.12	0.08	1.2	Tr
0	12	32	47	0.9	35	138	Tr	Tr	0.10	0.08	1.2	Tr
0	222	572	490	12.9	508	2334	Tr	Tr	2.13	1.41	17.0	Tr
0	12	32	27	0.7	28	129	Tr	Tr	0.12	0.08	0.9	Tr
0	12	32	27	0.7	28	129	Tr	Tr	0.09	0.08	0.9	Tr
0	10	25	21	0.6	22	101	Tr	Tr	0.09	0.06	0.7	Tr
0	10	25	21	0.6	22	101	Tr	Tr	0.07	0.06	0.7	Tr
0	15	38	32	0.9	34	154	Tr	Tr	0.14	0.09	1.1	Tr
0	22	57	49	1.3	50	231	Tr	Tr	0.21	0.14	1.7	Tr
0	206	327	1180	15.5	799	2887	Tr	Tr	1.59	0.95	17.4	Tr
0	13	20	74	1.0	50	180	Tr	Tr	0.10	0.06	1.1	Tr
0	13	20	74	1.0	50	180	Tr	Tr	0.08	0.06	1.1	Tr
0	50	92	136	2.2	126	1254	910	273	0.17	0.20	2.5	0
67	40	81	134	2.0	118	1023	850	256	0.10	0.18	1.6	0
0	31	0	29	1.5[27]	53	0[28]	0[29]	0[29]	0.24[27]	0.15[27]	2.0[27]	0
0	18	7	16	1.0[27]	29	343	0	0	0.18[27]	0.08[27]	1.3[27]	0
0	29	54[30]	43[31]	10.9[30]	46	5[31,32]	0	0	0.24[30]	0.07[30]	1.5[30]	0
0	21	20[30]	20[30]	8.1[30]	38	241	1250[30]	376[30]	0.43[30]	0.28[30]	5.0[30]	0
0	26	5	24[30]	9.6[30]	31	2[33]	0	0	0.48[30]	0.24[30]	5.8[30]	0
0	25	19	178	1.6	131	2[34]	40	4	0.26	0.05	0.3	0
0	18	163[27]	133	6.3[27]	99	285[27]	1510[27]	453[27]	0.53[27]	0.28[27]	5.5[27]	0
0	31	168[27]	148	6.7[27]	137	254[27]	1530[27]	460[27]	0.53[27]	0.38[27]	5.9[27]	Tr
0	21	23	264	4.5[30]	350	320	1250[30]	375[30]	0.37[30]	0.43[30]	5.0[30]	15[30]
0	23	5	36	7.5[27]	37	213	40	4	0.50[37]	0.55[27]	6.6[27]	0
0	20	48	134	4.5[30]	101	307	1250[30]	375[30]	0.37[30]	0.43[30]	5.0[30]	15[30]
0	24	1	18	1.8[30]	26	351	1250[30]	375[30]	0.37[30]	0.43[30]	5.0[30]	15[30]
0	24	1	12	0.7[37]	33	297	1250[30]	375[30]	0.37[30]	0.43[30]	5.0[30]	0
0	22	14	139	8.1[30]	180	264	1250[30]	375[30]	0.37[30]	0.43[30]	5.0[30]	0
0	22	12	179	4.5[30]	151	260	1250[30]	375[30]	0.37[30]	0.43[30]	5.0[30]	0

[31]For regular and instant cereal. For quick cereal, phosphorus is 102 mg and sodium is 142 mg.
[32]Cooked without salt. If salt is added according to label recommendations, sodium content is 390 mg.
[33]Cooked without salt. If salt is added according to label recommendations, sodium content is 324 mg.
[34]Cooked without salt. If salt is added according to label recommendations, sodium content is 374 mg.

Continued.

F

Item Number	Foods, Approximate Measures, Units, and Weight (Weight of Edible Portion Only)		Weight (grams)	Water (percent)	Food Energy (calories)	Protein (grams)	Fat (grams)	Fatty Acids: Saturated (grams)	Fatty Acids: Monounsaturated (grams)	Fatty Acids: Polyunsaturated (grams)
	Grain Products—cont'd									
	Breakfast cereals—cont'd									
	Ready to eat—cont'd									
372	Froot Loops® (about 1 cup)	1 oz	28	3	110	2	1	0.2	0.1	0.1
373	Golden Grahams® (about ¾ cup)	1 oz	28	2	110	2	1	0.7	0.1	0.2
374	Grape-Nuts® (about ¼ cup)	1 oz	28	3	100	3	Tr	Tr	Tr	0.1
375	Honey Nut Cheerios® (about ¾ cup)	1 oz	28	3	105	3	1	0.1	0.3	0.3
376	Lucky Charms® (about 1 cup)	1 oz	28	3	110	3	1	0.2	0.4	0.4
377	Nature Valley® Granola (about ⅓ cup)	1 oz	28	4	125	3	5	3.3	0.7	0.7
378	100% Natural Cereal (about ¼ cup)	1 oz	28	2	135	3	6	4.1	1.2	0.5
379	Product 19® (about ¾ cup)	1 oz	28	3	110	3	Tr	Tr	Tr	0.1
	Raisin Bran:									
380	Kellogg's® (about ¾ cup)	1 oz	28	8	90	3	1	0.1	0.1	0.3
381	Post® (about ½ cup)	1 oz	28	9	85	3	1	0.1	0.1	0.3
382	Rice Krispies® (about 1 cup)	1 oz	28	2	110	2	Tr	Tr	Tr	0.1
383	Shredded Wheat (about ⅔ cup)	1 oz	28	5	100	3	1	0.1	0.1	0.3
384	Special K® (about 1⅓ cup)	1 oz	28	2	110	6	Tr	Tr	Tr	Tr
385	Super Sugar Crisp® (about ⅞ cup)	1 oz	28	2	105	2	Tr	Tr	Tr	0.1
386	Sugar Frosted Flakes, Kellogg's® (about ¾ cup)	1 oz	28	3	110	1	Tr	Tr	Tr	Tr
387	Sugar Smacks® (about ¾ cup)	1 oz	28	3	105	2	1	0.1	0.1	0.2
388	Total® (about 1 cup)	1 oz	28	4	100	3	1	0.1	0.1	0.3
389	Trix® (about 1 cup)	1 oz	28	3	110	2	Tr	0.2	0.1	0.1
390	Wheaties® (about 1 cup)	1 oz	28	5	100	3	Tr	0.1	Tr	0.2
391	Buckwheat flour, light, sifted	1 cup	98	12	340	6	1	0.2	0.4	0.4
392	Bulgur, uncooked	1 cup	170	10	600	19	3	1.2	0.3	1.2
	Cakes prepared from cake mixes with enriched flour[35]									
	Angelfood									
393	Whole cake, 9¾-in. diam. tube cake	1 cake	635	38	1510	38	2	0.4	0.2	1.0
394	Piece, 1/12 of cake	1 piece	53	38	125	3	Tr	Tr	Tr	0.1
	Coffeecake, crumb									
395	Whole cake, 7¾ by 5⅝ by 1¼ in	1 cake	430	30	1385	27	41	11.8	16.7	9.6
396	Piece, ⅙ of cake	1 piece	72	30	230	5	7	2.0	2.8	1.6
	Devil's food with chocolate frosting									
397	Whole, 2-layer cake, 8- or 9-in diam	1 cake	1107	24	3755	49	136	55.6	51.4	19.7
398	Piece, 1/16 of cake	1 piece	69	24	235	3	8	3.5	3.2	1.2
399	Cupcake, 2½-in diam	1 cupcake	35	24	120	2	4	1.8	1.6	0.6
	Gingerbread									
400	Whole cake, 8 in square	1 cake	570	37	1575	18	39	9.6	16.4	10.5
401	Piece, 1/9 of cake	1 piece	63	37	175	2	4	1.1	1.8	1.2
	Yellow with chocolate frosting									
402	Whole, 2-layer cake, 8- or 9-in diam	1 cake	1108	26	3735	45	125	47.8	48.8	21.8
403	Piece, 1/16 of cake	1 piece	69	26	235	3	8	3.0	3.0	1.4
	Cakes prepared from home recipes using enriched flour									
	Carrot, with cream cheese frosting[36]									
404	Whole cake, 10-in diam tube cake	1 cake	1536	23	6175	63	328	66.0	135.2	107.5
405	Piece, 1/16 of cake	1 piece	96	23	385	4	21	4.1	8.4	6.7
	Fruitcake, dark[36]									
406	Whole cake, 7½-in diam, 2¼-in high tube cake	1 cake	1361	18	5185	74	228	47.6	113.0	51.7
407	Piece, 1/32 of cake, ⅔-in arc	1 piece	43	18	165	2	7	1.5	3.6	1.6
	Plain sheet cake[37]									
	Without frosting									
408	Whole cake, 9-in square	1 cake	777	25	2830	35	108	29.5	45.1	25.6
409	Piece, 1/9 of cake	1 piece	86	25	315	4	12	3.3	5.0	2.8
	With uncooked white frosting									
410	Whole cake, 9-in square	1 cake	1096	21	4020	37	129	41.6	50.4	26.3
411	Piece, 1/9 of cake	1 piece	121	21	445	4	14	4.6	5.6	2.9
	Pound[38]									
412	Loaf, 8½ by 3½ by 3¼ in	1 loaf	514	22	2025	33	94	21.1	40.9	26.7
413	Slice, 1/17 of loaf	1 slice	30	22	120	2	5	1.2	2.4	1.6

[30] Value based on label declaration for added nutrients.

[35] Excepting angelfood cake, cakes were made from mixes containing vegetable shortening and frostings were made with margarine.

Cholesterol (mg)	Carbo-hydrate (grams)	Calcium (mg)	Phosphorus (mg)	Iron (mg)	Potassium (mg)	Sodium (mg)	Vitamin A Value		Thiamin (mg)	Riboflavin (mg)	Niacin (mg)	Ascorbic Acid (mg)
							(IU) International Units	(RE) Retinol Equivalents				
0	25	3	24	4.5[30]	26	145	1250[30]	375[30]	0.37[30]	0.43[30]	5.0[30]	15[30]
Tr	24	17	41	4.5[30]	63	346	1250[30]	375[30]	0.37[30]	0.43[30]	5.0[30]	15[30]
0	23	11	71	1.2	95	197	1250[30]	375[30]	0.37[30]	0.43[30]	5.0[30]	0
0	23	20	105	4.5[30]	99	257	1250[30]	375[30]	0.37[30]	0.43[30]	5.0[30]	15[30]
0	23	32	79	4.5[30]	59	201	1250[30]	375[30]	0.37[30]	0.43[30]	5.0[30]	15[30]
0	19	18	89	0.9	98	58	20	2	0.10	0.05	0.2	0
Tr	18	49	104	0.8	140	12	20	2	0.09	0.15	0.6	0
0	24	3	40	18.0[30]	44	325	5000[30]	1501[30]	1.50[30]	1.70[30]	20.0[30]	60[30]
0	21	10	105	3.5[30]	147	207	960[30]	288[30]	0.28[30]	0.34[30]	3.9[30]	0
0	21	13	119	4.5[30]	175	185	1250[30]	375[30]	0.37[30]	0.43[30]	5.0[30]	0
0	25	4	34	1.8[30]	29	340	1250[30]	375[30]	0.37[30]	0.43[30]	5.0[30]	15[30]
0	23	11	100	1.2	102	3	0	0	0.07	0.08	1.5	0
Tr	21	8	55	4.5[30]	49	265	1250[30]	375[30]	0.37[30]	0.43[30]	5.0[30]	15[30]
0	26	6	52	1.8[30]	105	25	1250[30]	375[30]	0.37[30]	0.43[30]	5.0[30]	0
0	26	1	21	1.8[30]	18	230	1250[30]	375[30]	0.37[30]	0.43[30]	5.0[30]	15[30]
0	25	3	31	1.8[30]	42	75	1250[30]	375[30]	0.37[30]	0.43[30]	5.0[30]	15[30]
0	22	48	118	18.0[30]	106	352	5000[30]	1501[30]	1.50[30]	1.70[30]	20.0[30]	60[30]
0	25	6	19	4.5[30]	27	181	1250[30]	375[30]	0.37[30]	0.43[30]	5.0[30]	15[30]
0	23	43	98	4.5[30]	106	354	1250[30]	375[30]	0.37[30]	0.43[30]	5.0[30]	15[30]
0	78	11	86	1.0	314	2	0	0	0.08	0.04	0.4	0
0	129	49	575	9.5	389	7	0	0	0.48	0.24	7.7	0
0	342	527	1086	2.7	845	3226	0	0	0.32	1.27	1.6	0
0	29	44	91	0.2	71	269	0	0	0.03	0.11	0.1	0
279	225	262	748	7.3	469	1853	690	194	0.82	0.90	7.7	1
47	38	44	125	1.2	78	310	120	32	0.14	0.15	1.3	Tr
598	645	653	1162	22.1	1439	2900	1660	498	1.11	1.66	10.0	1
37	40	41	72	1.4	90	181	100	31	0.07	0.10	0.6	Tr
19	20	21	37	0.7	46	92	50	16	0.04	0.05	0.3	Tr
6	291	513	570	10.8	1562	1733	0	0	0.86	1.03	7.4	1
1	32	57	63	1.2	173	192	0	0	0.09	0.11	0.8	Tr
576	638	1008	2017	15.5	1208	2515	1550	465	1.22	1.66	11.1	1
36	40	63	126	1.0	75	157	100	29	0.08	0.10	0.7	Tr
1183	775	707	998	21.0	1720	4470	2240	246	1.83	1.97	14.7	23
74	48	44	62	1.3	108	279	140	15	0.11	0.12	0.9	1
640	783	1293	1592	37.6	6138	2123	1720	422	2.41	2.55	17.0	504
20	25	41	50	1.2	194	67	50	13	0.08	0.08	0.5	16
552	434	497	793	11.7	614	2331	1320	373	1.24	1.40	10.1	2
61	48	55	88	1.3	68	258	150	41	0.14	0.15	1.1	Tr
636	694	548	822	11.0	669	2488	2190	647	1.21	1.42	9.9	2
70	77	61	91	1.2	74	275	240	71	0.13	0.16	1.1	Tr
555	265	339	473	9.3	483	1645	3470	1033	0.93	1.08	7.8	1
32	15	20	28	0.5	28	96	200	60	0.05	0.06	0.5	Tr

[36]Made with vegetable oil.
[37]Cake made with vegetable shortening; frosting with margarine.

Continued.

Item Number	Foods, Approximate Measures, Units, and Weight (Weight of Edible Portion Only)		Weight (grams)	Water (percent)	Food Energy (calories)	Protein (grams)	Fat (grams)	Fatty Acids: Saturated (grams)	Fatty Acids: Monounsaturated (grams)	Fatty Acids: Polyunsaturated (grams)
	Grain Products—cont'd									
	Cakes, commercial, made with enriched flour									
	Pound									
414	Loaf, 8½ by 3½ by 3 in	1 loaf	500	24	1935	26	94	52.0	30.0	4.0
415	Slice, 1/17 of loaf	1 slice	29	24	110	2	5	3.0	1.7	0.2
	Snack cakes									
416	Devil's food with creme filling (2 small cakes per pkg)	1 small cake	28	20	105	1	4	1.7	1.5	0.6
417	Sponge with creme filling (2 small cakes per pkg)	1 small cake	42	19	155	1	5	2.3	2.1	0.5
	White with white frosting									
418	Whole, 2-layer cake, 8- or 9-in diam	1 cake	1140	24	4170	43	148	33.1	61.6	42.2
419	Piece, 1/16 of cake	1 piece	71	24	260	3	9	2.1	3.8	2.6
	Yellow with chocolate frosting									
420	Whole, 2-layer cake, 8- or 9-in diam	1 cake	1108	23	3895	40	175	92.0	58.7	10.0
421	Piece, 1/16 of cake	1 piece	69	23	245	2	11	5.7	3.7	0.6
	Cheesecake									
422	Whole cake, 9-in diam	1 cake	1110	46	3350	60	213	119.9	65.5	14.4
423	Piece, 1/12 of cake	1 piece	92	46	280	5	18	9.9	5.4	1.2
	Cookies made with enriched flour									
	Brownies with nuts									
424	Commercial, with frosting, 1½ by 1¾ by ⅞ in	1 brownie	25	13	100	1	4	1.6	2.0	0.6
425	From home recipe, 1¾ by 1¾ by ⅞ in[36]	1 brownie	20	10	95	1	6	1.4	2.8	1.2
	Chocolate chip									
426	Commercial, 2¼-in diam, ⅜ in thick	4 cookies	42	4	180	2	9	2.9	3.1	2.6
427	From home recipe, 2⅓-in diam[25]	4 cookies	40	3	185	2	11	3.9	4.3	2.0
428	From refrigerated dough, 2¼-in diam, ⅜ in thick	4 cookies	48	5	225	2	11	4.0	4.4	2.0
429	Fig bars, square, 1⅝ by 1⅝ by ⅜ in or rectangular, 1½ by 1¾ by ½ in	4 cookies	56	12	210	2	4	1.0	1.5	1.0
430	Oatmeal with raisins, 2⅝-in diam, ¼ in thick	4 cookies	52	4	245	3	10	2.5	4.5	2.8
431	Peanut butter cookie, from home recipe, 2⅝-in diam[25]	4 cookies	48	3	245	4	14	4.0	5.8	2.8
432	Sandwich type (chocolate or vanilla), 1¾-in diam, ⅜ in thick	4 cookies	40	2	195	2	8	2.0	3.6	2.2
	Shortbread									
433	Commercial	4 small cookies	32	6	155	2	8	2.9	3.0	1.1
434	From home recipe[38]	2 large cookies	28	3	145	2	8	1.3	2.7	3.4
435	Sugar cookie, from refrigerated dough, 2½-in diam, ¼ in thick	4 cookies	48	4	235	2	12	2.3	5.0	3.6
436	Vanilla wafers, 1¾-in diam, ¼ in thick	10 cookies	40	4	185	2	7	1.8	3.0	1.8
437	Corn chips	1-oz package	28	1	155	2	9	1.4	2.4	3.7
	Cornmeal									
438	Whole-ground, unbolted, dry form	1 cup	122	12	435	11	5	0.5	1.1	2.5
439	Bolted (nearly whole-grain), dry form	1 cup	122	12	440	11	4	0.5	0.9	2.2
	Degermed, enriched									
440	Dry form	1 cup	138	12	500	11	2	0.2	0.4	0.9
441	Cooked	1 cup	240	88	120	3	Tr	Tr	0.1	0.2
	Crackers[39]									
	Cheese									
442	Plain, 1 in square	10 crackers	10	4	50	1	3	0.9	1.2	0.3
443	Sandwich type (peanut butter)	1 sandwich	8	3	40	1	2	0.4	0.8	0.3
444	Graham, plain, 2½ in square	2 crackers	14	5	60	1	1	0.4	0.6	0.4
445	Melba toast, plain	1 piece	5	4	20	1	Tr	0.1	0.1	0.1
446	Rye wafers, whole-grain, 1⅞ by 3½ in	2 wafers	14	5	55	1	1	0.3	0.4	0.3
447	Saltines[40]	4 crackers	12	4	50	1	1	0.5	0.4	0.2

[25]Made with vegetable shortening.
[36]Made with vegetable oil.
[38]Made with margarine.

Cholesterol (mg)	Carbohydrate (grams)	Calcium (mg)	Phosphorus (mg)	Iron (mg)	Potassium (mg)	Sodium (mg)	Vitamin A Value: (IU) International Units	Vitamin A Value: (RE) Retinol Equivalents	Thiamin (mg)	Riboflavin (mg)	Niacin (mg)	Ascorbic Acid (mg)
1100	257	146	517	8.0	443	1857	2820	715	0.96	1.12	8.1	0
64	15	8	30	0.5	26	108	160	41	0.06	0.06	0.5	0
15	17	21	26	1.0	34	105	20	4	0.06	0.09	0.7	0
7	27	14	44	0.6	37	155	30	9	0.07	0.06	0.6	0
46	670	536	1585	15.5	832	2827	640	194	3.19	2.05	27.6	0
3	42	33	99	1.0	52	176	40	12	0.20	0.13	1.7	0
609	620	366	1884	19.9	1972	3080	1850	488	0.78	2.22	10.0	0
38	39	23	117	1.2	123	192	120	30	0.05	0.14	0.6	0
2053	317	622	977	5.3	1088	2464	2820	833	0.33	1.44	5.1	56
170	26	52	81	0.4	90	204	230	69	0.03	0.12	0.4	5
14	16	13	26	0.6	50	59	70	18	0.08	0.07	0.3	Tr
18	11	9	26	0.4	35	51	20	6	0.05	0.05	0.3	Tr
5	28	13	41	0.8	68	140	50	15	0.10	0.23	1.0	Tr
18	26	13	34	1.0	82	82	20	5	0.06	0.06	0.6	0
22	32	13	34	1.0	62	173	30	8	0.06	0.10	0.9	0
27	42	40	34	1.4	162	180	60	6	0.08	0.07	0.7	Tr
2	36	18	58	1.1	90	148	40	12	0.09	0.08	1.0	0
0	28	21	60	1.1	110	142	20	5	0.07	0.07	1.9	0
0	29	12	40	1.4	66	189	0	0	0.09	0.07	0.8	0
27	20	13	39	0.8	38	123	30	8	0.10	0.09	0.9	0
0	17	6	31	0.6	18	125	300	89	0.08	0.06	0.7	Tr
29	31	50	91	0.9	33	261	40	11	0.09	0.06	1.1	0
25	29	16	36	0.8	50	150	50	14	0.07	0.10	1.0	0
0	16	35	52	0.5	52	233	110	11	0.04	0.05	0.4	1
0	90	24	312	2.2	346	1	620	62	0.46	0.13	2.4	0
0	91	21	272	2.2	303	1	590	59	0.37	0.10	2.3	0
0	108	8	137	5.9	166	1	610	61	0.61	0.36	4.8	0
0	26	2	34	1.4	38	0	140	14	0.14	0.10	1.2	0
6	6	11	17	0.3	17	112	20	5	0.05	0.04	0.4	0
1	5	7	25	0.3	17	90	Tr	Tr	0.04	0.03	0.6	0
0	11	6	20	0.4	36	86	0	0	0.02	0.03	0.6	0
0	4	6	10	0.1	11	44	0	0	0.01	0.01	0.1	0
0	10	7	44	0.5	65	115	0	0	0.06	0.03	0.5	0
4	9	3	12	0.5	17	165	0	0	0.06	0.05	0.6	0

[39]Crackers made with enriched flour except for rye wafers and whole-wheat wafers.

[40]Made with lard.

Continued.

Item Number	Foods, Approximate Measures, Units, and Weight (Weight of Edible Portion Only)		Weight (grams)	Water (percent)	Food Energy (calories)	Protein (grams)	Fat (grams)	Fatty Acids		
								Saturated (grams)	Monounsaturated (grams)	Polyunsaturated (grams)
	Grain Products—cont'd									
	Crackers—cont'd									
448	Snack-type, standard	1 round cracker	3	3	15	Tr	1	0.2	0.4	0.1
449	Wheat, thin	4 crackers	8	3	35	1	1	0.5	0.5	0.4
450	Whole-wheat wafers	2 crackers	8	4	35	1	2	0.5	0.6	0.4
451	Croissants, made with enriched flour, 4½ by 4 by 1¾ in	1 croissant	57	22	235	5	12	3.5	6.7	1.4
	Danish pastry, made with enriched flour									
	Plain without fruit or nuts									
452	Packaged ring, 12 oz	1 ring	340	27	1305	21	71	21.8	28.6	15.6
453	Round piece, about 4¼-in diam, 1 in high	1 pastry	57	27	220	4	12	3.6	4.8	2.6
454	Ounce	1 oz	28	27	110	2	6	1.8	2.4	1.3
455	Fruit, round piece	1 pastry	65	30	235	4	13	3.9	5.2	2.9
	Doughnuts, made with enriched flour									
456	Cake type, plain, 3¼-in diam, 1 in high	1 doughnut	50	21	210	3	12	2.8	5.0	3.0
457	Yeast-leavened, glazed, 3¾-in diam, 1¼ in high	1 doughnut	60	27	235	4	13	5.2	5.5	0.9
458	English muffins, plain, enriched	1 muffin	57	42	140	5	1	0.3	0.2	0.3
459	Toasted	1 muffin	50	29	140	5	1	0.3	0.2	0.3
460	French toast, from home recipe	1 slice	65	53	155	6	7	1.6	2.0	1.6
	Macaroni, enriched, cooked (cut lengths, elbows, shells)									
461	Firm stage (hot)	1 cup	130	64	190	7	1	0.1	0.1	0.3
	Tender stage									
462	Cold	1 cup	105	72	115	4	Tr	0.1	0.1	0.2
463	Hot	1 cup	140	72	155	5	1	0.1	0.1	0.2
	Muffins made with enriched flour, 2½-in diam, 1½ in high									
	From home recipe									
464	Blueberry[25]	1 muffin	45	37	135	3	5	1.5	2.1	1.2
465	Bran[36]	1 muffin	45	35	125	3	6	1.4	1.6	2.3
466	Corn (enriched, degermed cornmeal and flour)[25]	1 muffin	45	33	145	3	5	1.5	2.2	1.4
	From commercial mix (egg and water added)									
467	Blueberry	1 muffin	45	33	140	3	5	1.4	2.0	1.2
468	Bran	1 muffin	45	28	140	3	4	1.3	1.6	1.0
469	Corn	1 muffin	45	30	145	3	6	1.7	2.3	1.4
470	Noodles (egg noodles), enriched, cooked	1 cup	160	70	200	7	2	0.5	0.6	0.6
471	Noodles, chow mein, canned	1 cup	45	11	220	6	11	2.1	7.3	0.4
	Pancakes, 4-in diam.									
472	Buckwheat, from mix (with buckwheat and enriched flours), egg and milk added	1 pancake	27	58	55	2	2	0.9	0.9	0.5
	Plain									
473	From home recipe using enriched flour	1 pancake	27	50	60	2	2	0.5	0.8	0.5
474	From mix (with enriched flour), egg, milk, and oil added	1 pancake	27	54	60	2	2	0.5	0.9	0.5
	Piecrust, made with enriched flour and vegetable shortening, baked									
475	From home recipe, 9-in diam	1 pie shell	180	15	900	11	60	14.8	25.9	15.7
476	From mix, 9-in diam	Piecrust for 2-crust pie	320	19	1485	20	93	22.7	41.0	25.0
	Pies, piecrust made with enriched flour, vegetable shortening, 9-in diam.									
	Apple									
477	Whole	1 pie	945	48	2420	21	105	27.4	44.4	26.5
478	Piece, ⅙ of pie	1 piece	158	48	405	3	18	4.6	7.4	4.4
	Blueberry									
479	Whole	1 pie	945	51	2285	23	102	25.5	44.4	27.4
480	Piece, ⅙ of pie	1 piece	158	51	380	4	17	4.3	7.4	4.6
	Cherry									
481	Whole	1 pie	945	47	2465	25	107	28.4	46.3	27.4
482	Piece, ⅙ of pie	1 piece	158	47	410	4	18	4.7	7.7	4.6

[25]Made with vegetable shortening.

[36]Made with vegetable oil.

Cholesterol (mg)	Carbo-hydrate (grams)	Calcium (mg)	Phosphorus (mg)	Iron (mg)	Potassium (mg)	Sodium (mg)	Vitamin A Value (IU) International Units	Vitamin A Value (RE) Retinol Equivalents	Thiamin (mg)	Riboflavin (mg)	Niacin (mg)	Ascorbic Acid (mg)
0	2	3	6	0.1	4	30	Tr	Tr	0.01	0.01	0.1	0
0	5	3	15	0.3	17	69	Tr	Tr	0.04	0.03	0.4	0
0	5	3	22	0.2	31	59	0	0	0.02	0.03	0.4	0
13	27	20	64	2.1	68	452	50	13	0.17	0.13	1.3	0
292	152	360	347	6.5	316	1302	360	99	0.95	1.02	8.5	Tr
49	26	60	58	1.1	53	218	60	17	0.16	0.17	1.4	Tr
24	13	30	29	0.5	26	109	30	8	0.08	0.09	0.7	Tr
56	28	17	80	1.3	57	233	40	11	0.16	0.14	1.4	Tr
20	24	22	111	1.0	58	192	20	5	0.12	0.12	1.1	Tr
21	26	17	55	1.4	64	222	Tr	Tr	0.28	0.12	1.8	0
0	27	96	67	1.7	331	378	0	0	0.26	0.19	2.2	0
0	27	96	67	1.7	331	378	0	0	0.23	0.19	2.2	0
112	17	72	85	1.3	86	257	110	32	0.12	0.16	1.0	Tr
0	39	14	85	2.1	103	1	0	0	0.23	0.13	1.8	0
0	24	8	53	1.3	64	1	0	0	0.15	0.08	1.2	0
0	32	11	70	1.7	85	1	0	0	0.20	0.11	1.5	0
19	20	54	46	0.9	47	198	40	9	0.10	0.11	0.9	1
24	19	60	125	1.4	99	189	230	30	0.11	0.13	1.3	3
23	21	66	59	0.9	57	169	80	15	0.11	0.11	0.9	Tr
45	22	15	90	0.9	54	225	50	11	0.10	0.17	1.1	Tr
28	24	27	182	1.7	50	385	100	14	0.08	0.12	1.9	0
42	22	30	128	1.3	31	291	90	16	0.09	0.09	0.8	Tr
50	37	16	94	2.6	70	3	110	34	0.22	0.13	1.9	0
5	26	14	41	0.4	33	450	0	0	0.05	0.03	0.6	0
20	6	59	91	0.4	66	125	60	17	0.04	0.05	0.2	Tr
16	9	27	38	0.5	33	115	30	10	0.06	0.07	0.5	Tr
16	8	36	71	0.7	43	160	30	7	0.09	0.12	0.8	Tr
0	79	25	90	4.5	90	1100	0	0	0.54	0.40	5.0	0
0	141	131	272	9.3	179	2602	0	0	1.06	0.80	9.9	0
0	360	76	208	9.5	756	2844	280	28	1.04	0.76	9.5	9
0	60	13	35	1.6	126	476	50	5	0.17	0.13	1.6	2
0	330	104	217	12.3	945	2533	850	85	1.04	0.85	10.4	38
0	55	17	36	2.1	158	423	140	14	0.17	0.14	1.7	6
0	363	132	236	9.5	992	2873	4160	416	1.13	0.85	9.5	0
0	61	22	40	1.6	166	480	700	70	0.19	0.14	1.6	0

Continued.

Item Number	Foods, Approximate Measures, Units, and Weight (Weight of Edible Portion Only)		Weight (grams)	Water (percent)	Food Energy (calories)	Protein (grams)	Fat (grams)	Fatty Acids		
								Saturated (grams)	Monounsaturated (grams)	Polyunsaturated (grams)
	Grain Products—cont'd									
	Pies, piecrust made with enriched flour, vegetable shortening, 9-in diam.—cont'd									
	Cream									
483	Whole	1 pie	910	43	2710	20	139	90.1	23.7	6.4
484	Piece, ⅙ of pie	1 piece	152	43	455	3	23	15.0	4.0	1.1
	Custard									
485	Whole	1 pie	910	58	1985	56	101	33.7	40.0	19.1
486	Piece, ⅙ of pie	1 piece	152	58	330	9	17	5.6	6.7	3.2
	Lemon meringue									
487	Whole	1 pie	840	47	2140	31	86	26.0	34.4	17.6
488	Piece, ⅙ of pie	1 piece	140	47	355	5	14	4.3	5.7	2.9
	Peach									
489	Whole	1 pie	945	48	2410	24	101	24.6	43.5	26.5
490	Piece, ⅙ of pie	1 piece	158	48	405	4	17	4.1	7.3	4.4
	Pecan									
491	Whole	1 pie	825	20	3450	42	189	28.1	101.5	47.0
492	Piece, ⅙ of pie	1 piece	138	20	575	7	32	4.7	17.0	7.9
	Pumpkin									
493	Whole	1 pie	910	59	1920	36	102	38.2	40.0	18.2
494	Piece, ⅙ of pie	1 piece	152	59	320	6	17	6.4	6.7	3.0
	Pies, fried									
495	Apple	1 pie	85	43	255	2	14	5.8	6.6	0.6
496	Cherry	1 pie	85	42	250	2	14	5.8	6.7	0.6
	Popcorn, popped									
497	Air-popped, unsalted	1 cup	8	4	30	1	Tr	Tr	0.1	0.2
498	Popped in vegetable oil, salted	1 cup	11	3	55	1	3	0.5	1.4	1.2
499	Coated with sugar syrup	1 cup	35	4	135	2	1	0.1	0.3	0.6
	Pretzels, made with enriched flour									
500	Stick, 2¼ in long	10 pretzels	3	3	10	Tr	Tr	Tr	Tr	Tr
501	Twisted, Dutch, 2¾ by 2⅝ in	1 pretzel	16	3	65	2	1	0.1	0.2	0.2
502	Twisted, thin, 3¼ by 2¼ by ¼ in	10 pretzels	60	3	240	6	2	0.4	0.8	0.6
	Rice									
503	Brown, cooked, served hot	1 cup	195	70	230	5	1	0.3	0.3	0.4
	White, enriched									
	Commercial varieties, all types									
504	Raw	1 cup	185	12	670	12	1	0.2	0.2	0.3
505	Cooked, served hot	1 cup	205	73	225	4	Tr	0.1	0.1	0.1
506	Instant, ready-to-serve, hot	1 cup	165	73	180	4	0	0.1	0.1	0.1
	Parboiled									
507	Raw	1 cup	185	10	685	14	1	0.1	0.1	0.2
508	Cooked, served hot	1 cup	175	73	185	4	Tr	Tr	Tr	0.1
	Rolls, enriched									
	Commerical									
509	Dinner, 2½-in diam, 2 in high	1 roll	28	32	85	2	2	0.5	0.8	0.6
510	Frankfurter and hamburger (8 per 11½-oz pkg)	1 roll	40	34	115	3	2	0.5	0.8	0.6
511	Hard, 3¾-in diam, 2 in high	1 roll	50	25	155	5	2	0.4	0.5	0.6
512	Hoagie or submarine, 11½ by 3 by 2½ in	1 roll	135	31	400	11	8	1.8	3.0	2.2
	From home recipe									
513	Dinner, 2½-in diam, 2 in high	1 roll	35	26	120	3	3	0.8	1.2	0.9
	Spaghetti, enriched, cooked									
514	Firm stage, "al dente," served hot	1 cup	130	64	190	7	1	0.1	0.1	0.3
515	Tender stage, served hot	1 cup	140	73	155	5	1	0.1	0.1	0.2
516	Toaster pastries	1 pastry	54	13	210	2	6	1.7	3.6	0.4
517	Tortillas, corn	1 tortilla	30	45	65	2	1	0.1	0.3	0.6
	Waffles, made with enriched flour, 7-in diam									
518	From home recipe	1 waffle	75	37	245	7	13	4.0	4.9	2.6
519	From mix, egg and milk added	1 waffle	75	42	205	7	8	2.7	2.9	1.5
	Wheat flours									
	All-purpose or family flour, enriched									
520	Sifted, spooned	1 cup	115	12	420	12	1	0.2	0.1	0.5
521	Unsifted, spooned	1 cup	125	12	455	13	1	0.2	0.1	0.5
522	Cake or pastry flour, enriched, sifted, spooned	1 cup	96	12	350	7	1	0.1	0.1	0.3
523	Self-rising enriched, unsifted, spooned	1 cup	125	12	440	12	1	0.2	0.1	0.5
524	Whole-wheat, from hard wheats, stirred	1 cup	120	12	400	16	2	0.3	0.3	1.1

Cholesterol (mg)	Carbohydrate (grams)	Calcium (mg)	Phosphorus (mg)	Iron (mg)	Potassium (mg)	Sodium (mg)	Vitamin A Value		Thiamin (mg)	Riboflavin (mg)	Niacin (mg)	Ascorbic Acid (mg)
							(IU) International Units	(RE) Retinol Equivalents				
46	351	273	919	6.8	796	2207	1250	391	0.36	0.89	6.4	0
8	59	46	154	1.1	133	369	210	65	0.06	0.15	1.1	0
1010	213	874	1028	9.1	1247	2612	2090	573	0.82	1.91	5.5	0
169	36	146	172	1.5	208	436	350	96	0.14	0.32	0.9	0
857	317	118	412	8.4	420	2369	1430	395	0.59	0.84	5.0	25
143	53	20	69	1.4	70	395	240	66	0.10	0.14	0.8	4
0	361	95	274	11.3	1408	2533	6900	690	1.04	0.95	14.2	28
0	60	16	46	1.9	235	423	1150	115	0.17	0.16	2.4	5
569	423	388	850	27.2	1015	1823	1320	322	1.82	0.99	6.6	0
95	71	65	142	4.6	170	305	220	54	0.30	0.17	1.1	0
655	223	464	628	8.2	1456	1947	22,480	2493	0.82	1.27	7.3	0
109	37	78	105	1.4	243	325	3750	416	0.14	0.21	1.2	0
14	31	12	34	0.9	42	326	30	3	0.09	0.06	1.0	1
13	32	11	41	0.7	61	371	190	19	0.06	0.06	0.6	1
0	6	1	22	0.2	20	Tr	10	1	0.03	0.01	0.2	0
0	6	3	31	0.3	19	86	20	2	0.01	0.02	0.1	0
0	30	2	47	0.5	90	Tr	30	3	0.13	0.02	0.4	0
0	2	1	3	0.1	3	48	0	0	0.01	0.01	0.1	0
0	13	4	15	0.3	16	258	0	0	0.05	0.04	0.7	0
0	48	16	55	1.2	61	966	0	0	0.19	0.15	2.6	0
0	50	23	142	1.0	137	0	0	0	0.18	0.04	2.7	0
0	149	44	174	5.4	170	9	0	0	0.81	0.06	6.5	0
0	50	21	57	1.8	57	0	0	0	0.23	0.02	2.1	0
0	40	5	31	1.3	0	0	0	0	0.21	0.02	1.7	0
0	150	111	370	5.4	278	17	0	0	0.81	0.07	6.5	0
0	41	33	100	1.4	75	0	0	0	0.19	0.02	2.1	0
Tr	14	33	44	0.8	36	155	Tr	Tr	0.14	0.09	1.1	Tr
Tr	20	54	44	1.2	56	241	Tr	Tr	0.20	0.13	1.6	Tr
Tr	30	24	46	1.4	49	313	0	0	0.20	0.12	1.7	0
Tr	72	100	115	3.8	128	683	0	0	0.54	0.33	4.5	0
12	20	16	36	1.1	41	98	30	8	0.12	0.12	1.2	0
0	39	14	85	2.0	103	1	0	0	0.23	0.13	1.8	0
0	32	11	70	1.7	85	1	0	0	0.20	0.11	1.5	0
0	38	104	104	2.2	91	248	520	52	0.17	0.18	2.3	4
0	13	42	55	0.6	43	1	80	8	0.05	0.03	0.4	0
102	26	154	135	1.5	129	445	140	39	0.18	0.24	1.5	Tr
59	27	179	257	1.2	146	515	170	49	0.14	0.23	0.9	Tr
0	88	18	100	5.1	109	2	0	0	0.73	0.46	6.1	0
0	95	20	109	5.5	119	3	0	0	0.80	0.50	6.6	0
0	76	16	70	4.2	91	2	0	0	0.58	0.38	5.1	0
0	93	331	583	5.5	113	1349	0	0	0.80	0.50	6.6	0
0	85	49	446	5.2	444	4	0	0	0.66	0.14	5.2	0

Continued.

Item Number	Foods, Approximate Measures, Units, and Weight (Weight of Edible Portion Only)		Weight (grams)	Water (percent)	Food Energy (calories)	Protein (grams)	Fat (grams)	Fatty Acids		
								Saturated (grams)	Monounsaturated (grams)	Polyunsaturated (grams)
	Legumes, Nuts and Seeds									
	Almonds, shelled									
525	Slivered, packed	1 cup	135	4	795	27	70	6.7	45.8	14.8
526	Whole	1 oz	28	4	165	6	15	1.4	9.6	3.1
	Beans, dry									
	Cooked, drained									
527	Black	1 cup	171	66	225	15	1	0.1	0.1	0.5
528	Great Northern	1 cup	180	69	210	14	1	0.1	0.1	0.6
529	Lima	1 cup	190	64	260	16	1	0.2	0.1	0.5
530	Pea (navy)	1 cup	190	69	225	15	1	0.1	0.1	0.7
531	Pinto	1 cup	180	65	265	15	1	0.1	0.1	0.5
	Canned, solids and liquid									
	White with									
532	Frankfurters (sliced)	1 cup	255	71	365	19	18	7.4	8.8	0.7
533	Pork and tomato sauce	1 cup	255	71	310	16	7	2.4	2.7	0.7
534	Pork and sweet sauce	1 cup	255	66	385	16	12	4.3	4.9	1.2
535	Red kidney	1 cup	255	76	230	15	1	0.1	0.1	0.6
536	Black-eyed peas, dry, cooked (with residual cooking liquid)	1 cup	250	80	190	13	1	0.2	Tr	0.3
537	Brazil nuts, shelled	1 oz	28	3	185	4	19	4.6	6.5	6.8
538	Carob flour	1 cup	140	3	255	6	Tr	Tr	0.1	0.1
	Cashew nuts, salted									
539	Dry roasted	1 cup	137	2	785	21	63	12.5	37.4	10.7
540		1 oz	28	2	165	4	13	2.6	7.7	2.2
541	Roasted in oil	1 cup	130	4	750	21	63	12.4	36.9	10.6
542		1 oz	28	4	165	5	14	2.7	8.1	2.3
543	Chestnuts, European (Italian), roasted, shelled	1 cup	143	40	350	5	3	0.6	1.1	1.2
544	Chickpeas, cooked, drained	1 cup	163	60	270	15	4	0.4	0.9	1.9
	Coconut									
	Raw									
545	Piece, about 2 by 2 by ½ in	1 piece	45	47	160	1	15	13.4	0.6	0.2
546	Shredded or grated	1 cup	80	47	285	3	27	23.8	1.1	0.3
547	Dried, sweetened, shredded	1 cup	93	13	470	3	33	29.3	1.4	0.4
548	Filberts (hazelnuts), chopped	1 cup	115	5	725	15	72	5.3	56.5	6.9
549		1 oz	28	5	180	4	18	1.3	13.9	1.7
550	Lentils, dry, cooked	1 cup	200	72	215	16	1	0.1	0.2	0.5
551	Macadamia nuts, roasted in oil, salted	1 cup	134	2	960	10	103	15.4	80.9	1.8
552		1 oz	28	2	205	2	22	3.2	17.1	0.4
	Mixed nuts, with peanuts, salted									
553	Dry roasted	1 oz	28	2	170	5	15	2.0	8.9	3.1
554	Roasted in oil	1 oz	28	2	175	5	16	2.5	9.0	3.8
555	Peanuts, roasted in oil, salted	1 cup	145	2	840	39	71	9.9	35.5	22.6
556		1 oz	28	2	165	8	14	1.9	6.9	4.4
557	Peanut butter	1 tbsp	16	1	95	5	8	1.4	4.0	2.5
558	Peas, split, dry, cooked	1 cup	200	70	230	16	1	0.1	0.1	0.3
559	Pecans, halves	1 cup	108	5	720	8	73	5.9	45.5	18.1
560		1 oz	28	5	190	2	19	1.5	12.0	4.7
561	Pine nuts (pinyons), shelled	1 oz	28	6	160	3	17	2.7	6.5	7.3
562	Pistachio nuts, dried, shelled	1 oz	28	4	165	6	14	1.7	9.3	2.1
563	Pumpkin and squash kernels, dry, hulled	1 oz	28	7	155	7	13	2.5	4.0	5.9
564	Refried beans, canned	1 cup	290	72	295	18	3	0.4	0.6	1.4
565	Sesame seeds, dry, hulled	1 tbsp	8	5	45	2	4	0.6	1.7	1.9
566	Soybeans, dry, cooked, drained	1 cup	180	71	235	20	10	1.3	1.9	5.3
	Soy products									
567	Miso	1 cup	276	53	470	29	13	1.8	2.6	7.3
568	Tofu, piece 2½ by 2¾ by 1 in	1 piece	120	85	85	9	5	0.7	1.0	2.9
569	Sunflower seeds, dry, hulled	1 oz	28	5	160	6	14	1.5	2.7	9.3
570	Tahini	1 tbsp	15	3	90	3	8	1.1	3.0	3.5
	Walnuts									
571	Black, chopped	1 cup	125	4	760	30	71	4.5	15.9	46.9
572		1 oz	28	4	170	7	16	1.0	3.6	10.6
573	English or Persian, pieces or chips	1 cup	120	4	770	17	74	6.7	17.0	47.0
574		1 oz	28	4	180	4	18	1.6	4.0	11.1

[41]Cashews without salt contain 21 mg sodium per cup, or 4 mg per oz.

[42]Cashews without salt contain 22 mg sodium per cup, or 5 mg per oz.

[43]Macadamia nuts without salt contain 9 mg sodium per cup, or 2 mg per oz.

Cholesterol (mg)	Carbo-hydrate (grams)	Calcium (mg)	Phosphorus (mg)	Iron (mg)	Potassium (mg)	Sodium (mg)	Vitamin A Value (IU) International Units	Vitamin A Value (RE) Retinol Equivalents	Thiamin (mg)	Riboflavin (mg)	Niacin (mg)	Ascorbic Acid (mg)
0	28	359	702	4.9	988	15	0	0	0.28	1.05	4.5	1
0	6	75	147	1.0	208	3	0	0	0.06	0.22	1.0	Tr
0	41	47	239	2.9	608	1	Tr	Tr	0.43	0.05	0.9	0
0	38	90	266	4.9	749	13	0	0	0.25	0.13	1.3	0
0	49	55	293	5.9	1163	4	0	0	0.25	0.11	1.3	0
0	40	95	281	5.1	790	13	0	0	0.27	0.13	1.3	0
0	49	86	296	5.4	882	3	Tr	Tr	0.33	0.16	0.7	0
30	32	94	303	4.8	668	1374	330	33	0.18	0.15	3.3	Tr
10	48	138	235	4.6	536	1181	330	33	0.20	0.08	1.5	5
10	54	161	291	5.9	536	969	330	33	0.15	0.10	1.3	5
0	42	74	278	4.6	673	968	10	1	0.13	0.10	1.5	0
0	35	43	238	3.3	573	20	30	3	0.40	0.10	1.0	0
0	4	50	170	1.0	170	1	Tr	Tr	0.28	0.03	0.5	Tr
0	126	390	102	5.7	1275	24	Tr	Tr	0.07	0.07	2.2	Tr
0	45	62	671	8.2	774	877[41]	0	0	0.27	0.27	1.9	0
0	9	13	139	1.7	160	181[41]	0	0	0.06	0.06	0.4	0
0	37	53	554	5.3	689	814[42]	0	0	0.55	0.23	2.3	0
0	8	12	121	1.2	150	177[42]	0	0	0.12	0.05	0.5	0
0	76	41	153	1.3	847	3	30	3	0.35	0.25	1.9	37
0	45	80	273	4.9	475	11	Tr	Tr	0.18	0.09	0.9	0
0	7	6	51	1.1	160	9	0	0	0.03	0.01	0.2	1
0	12	11	90	1.9	285	16	0	0	0.05	0.02	0.4	3
0	44	14	99	1.8	313	244	0	0	0.03	0.02	0.4	1
0	18	216	359	3.8	512	3	80	8	0.58	0.13	1.3	1
0	4	53	88	0.9	126	1	20	2	0.14	0.03	0.3	Tr
0	38	50	238	4.2	498	26	40	4	0.14	0.12	1.2	0
0	17	60	268	2.4	441	348[43]	10	1	0.29	0.15	2.7	0
0	4	13	57	0.5	93	74[43]	Tr	Tr	0.06	0.03	0.6	0
0	7	20	123	1.0	169	190[44]	Tr	Tr	0.06	0.06	1.3	0
0	6	31	131	0.9	165	185[44]	10	1	0.14	0.06	1.4	Tr
0	27	125	734	2.8	1019	626[45]	0	0	0.42	0.15	21.5	0
0	5	24	143	0.5	199	122[45]	0	0	0.08	0.03	4.2	0
0	3	5	60	0.3	110	75	0	0	0.02	0.02	2.2	0
0	42	22	178	3.4	592	26	80	8	0.30	0.18	1.8	0
0	20	39	314	2.3	423	1	140	14	0.92	0.14	1.0	2
0	5	10	83	0.6	111	Tr	40	4	0.24	0.04	0.3	1
0	5	2	10	0.9	178	20	10	1	0.35	0.06	1.2	1
0	7	38	143	1.9	310	2	70	7	0.23	0.05	0.3	Tr
0	5	12	333	4.2	229	5	110	11	0.06	0.09	0.5	Tr
0	51	141	245	5.1	1141	1228	0	0	0.14	0.16	1.4	17
0	1	11	62	0.6	33	3	10	1	0.06	0.01	0.4	0
0	19	131	322	4.9	972	4	50	5	0.38	0.16	1.1	0
0	65	188	853	4.7	922	8142	110	11	0.17	0.28	0.8	0
0	3	108	151	2.3	50	8	0	0	0.07	0.04	0.1	0
0	5	33	200	1.9	195	1	10	1	0.65	0.07	1.3	Tr
0	3	21	119	0.7	69	5	10	1	0.24	0.02	0.8	1
0	15	73	580	3.8	655	1	370	37	0.27	0.14	0.9	Tr
0	3	16	132	0.9	149	Tr	80	8	0.06	0.03	0.2	Tr
0	22	133	380	2.9	602	12	150	15	0.46	0.18	1.3	4
0	5	27	90	0.7	142	3	40	4	0.11	0.04	0.3	1

[44]Mixed nuts without salt contain 3 mg sodium per oz.
[45]Peanuts without salt contain 22 mg sodium per cup, or 4 mg per oz.

Continued.

Item Number	Foods, Approximate Measures, Units, and Weight (Weight of Edible Portion Only)		Weight (grams)	Water (percent)	Food Energy (calories)	Protein (grams)	Fat (grams)	Fatty Acids: Saturated (grams)	Fatty Acids: Monounsaturated (grams)	Fatty Acids: Polyunsaturated (grams)
	Meat and Meat Products									
	Beef, cooked[46]									
	Cuts braised, simmered, or pot roasted									
	Relatively fat, such as chuck blade									
575	Lean and fat, piece, 2½ by 2½ by ¾ in	3 oz	85	43	325	22	26	10.8	11.7	0.9
576	Lean only (from item 575)	2.2 oz	62	53	170	19	9	3.9	4.2	0.3
	Relatively lean, such as bottom round									
577	Lean and fat, piece, 4⅛ by 2¼ by ½ in	3 oz	85	54	220	25	13	4.8	5.7	0.5
578	Lean only (from item 577)	2.8 oz	78	57	175	25	8	2.7	3.4	0.3
	Ground beef, broiled, patty, 3 by ⅝ in									
579	Lean	3 oz	85	56	230	21	16	6.2	6.9	0.6
580	Regular	3 oz	85	54	245	20	18	6.9	7.7	0.7
581	Heart, lean, braised	3 oz	85	65	150	24	5	1.2	0.8	1.6
582	Liver, fried, one slice, 6½ by 2⅜ by ⅜ in[47]	3 oz	85	56	185	23	7	2.5	3.6	1.3
	Roast, oven cooked, no liquid added									
	Relatively fat, such as rib									
583	Lean and fat, 2 pieces, 4⅛ by 2¼ by ¼ in	3 oz	85	46	315	19	26	10.8	11.4	0.9
584	Lean only (from item 583)	2.2 oz	61	57	150	17	9	3.6	3.7	0.3
	Relatively lean, such as eye of round									
585	Lean and fat, 2 pieces, 2½ by 2½ by ⅜ in	3 oz	85	57	205	23	12	4.9	5.4	0.5
586	Lean only (from item 585)	2.6 oz	75	63	135	22	5	1.9	2.1	0.2
	Steak									
	Sirloin, broiled									
587	Lean and fat, piece, 2½ by 2½ by ¾ in	3 oz	85	53	240	23	15	6.4	6.9	0.6
588	Lean only (from item 587)	2.5 oz	72	59	150	22	6	2.6	2.8	0.3
589	Beef, canned, corned	3 oz	85	59	185	22	10	4.2	4.9	0.4
590	Beef, dried, chipped	2.5 oz	72	48	145	24	4	1.8	2.0	0.2
	Lamb, cooked									
	Chops, (3 per lb with bone)									
	Arm, braised									
591	Lean and fat	2.2 oz	63	44	220	20	15	6.9	6.0	0.9
592	Lean only (from item 591)	1.7 oz	48	49	135	17	7	2.9	2.6	0.4
	Loin, broiled									
593	Lean and fat	2.8 oz	80	54	235	22	16	7.3	6.4	1.0
594	Lean only (from item 593)	2.3 oz	64	61	140	19	6	2.6	2.4	0.4
	Leg, roasted									
595	Lean and fat, 2 pieces, 4⅛ by 2¼ by ¼ in	3 oz	85	59	205	22	13	5.6	4.9	0.8
596	Lean only (from item 595)	2.6 oz	73	64	140	20	6	2.4	2.2	0.4
	Rib, roasted									
597	Lean and fat, 3 pieces, 2½ by 2½ by ¼ in	3 oz	85	47	315	18	26	12.1	10.6	1.5
598	Lean only (from item 597)	2 oz	57	60	130	15	7	3.2	3.0	0.5
	Pork, cured, cooked									
	Bacon									
599	Regular	3 medium slices	19	13	110	6	9	3.3	4.5	1.1
600	Canadian-style	2 slices	46	62	85	11	4	1.3	1.9	0.4
	Ham, light cure, roasted									
601	Lean and fat, 2 pieces, 4⅛ by 2¼ by ¼ in	3 oz	85	58	205	18	14	5.1	6.7	1.5
602	Lean only (from item 601)	2.4 oz	68	66	105	17	4	1.3	1.7	0.4
603	Ham, canned, roasted, 2 pieces, 4⅛ by 2¼ by ¼ in	3 oz	85	67	140	18	7	2.4	3.5	0.8
	Luncheon meat									
604	Canned, spiced or unspiced, slice, 3 by 2 by ½ in	2 slices	42	52	140	5	13	4.5	6.0	1.5
605	Chopped ham (8 slices per 6-oz pkg)	2 slices	42	64	95	7	7	2.4	3.4	0.9
	Cooked ham (8 slices per 8-oz pkg)									
606	Regular	2 slices	57	65	105	10	6	1.9	2.8	0.7
607	Extra lean	2 slices	57	71	75	11	3	0.9	1.3	0.3

[46]Outer layer of fat was removed to within approximately ½ inch of the lean. Deposits of fat within the cut were not removed.

[47]Fried in vegetable shortening.

F

Cholesterol (mg)	Carbohydrate (grams)	Calcium (mg)	Phosphorus (mg)	Iron (mg)	Potassium (mg)	Sodium (mg)	Vitamin A Value (IU) International Units	Vitamin A Value (RE) Retinol Equivalents	Thiamin (mg)	Riboflavin (mg)	Niacin (mg)	Ascorbic Acid (mg)
87	0	11	163	2.5	163	53	Tr	Tr	0.06	0.19	2.0	0
66	0	8	146	2.3	163	44	Tr	Tr	0.05	0.17	1.7	0
81	0	5	217	2.8	248	43	Tr	Tr	0.06	0.21	3.3	0
75	0	4	212	2.7	240	40	Tr	Tr	0.06	0.20	3.0	0
74	0	9	134	1.8	256	65	Tr	Tr	0.04	0.18	4.4	0
76	0	9	144	2.1	248	70	Tr	Tr	0.03	0.16	4.9	0
164	0	5	213	6.4	198	54	Tr	Tr	0.12	1.31	3.4	5
410	7	9	392	5.3	309	90	30,690[48]	9120[48]	0.18	3.52	12.3	23
72	0	8	145	2.0	246	54	Tr	Tr	0.06	0.16	3.1	0
49	0	5	127	1.7	218	45	Tr	Tr	0.05	0.13	2.7	0
62	0	5	177	1.6	308	50	Tr	Tr	0.07	0.14	3.0	0
52	0	3	170	1.5	297	46	Tr	Tr	0.07	0.13	2.8	0
77	0	9	186	2.6	306	53	Tr	Tr	0.10	0.23	3.3	0
64	0	8	176	2.4	290	48	Tr	Tr	0.09	0.22	3.1	0
80	0	17	90	3.7	51	802	Tr	Tr	0.02	0.20	2.9	0
46	0	14	287	2.3	142	3053	Tr	Tr	0.05	0.23	2.7	0
77	0	16	132	1.5	195	46	Tr	Tr	0.04	0.16	4.4	0
59	0	12	111	1.3	162	36	Tr	Tr	0.03	0.13	3.0	0
78	0	16	162	1.4	272	62	Tr	Tr	0.09	0.21	5.5	0
60	0	12	145	1.3	241	54	Tr	Tr	0.08	0.18	4.4	0
78	0	8	162	1.7	273	57	Tr	Tr	0.09	0.24	5.5	0
65	0	6	150	1.5	247	50	Tr	Tr	0.08	0.20	4.6	0
77	0	19	139	1.4	224	60	Tr	Tr	0.08	0.18	5.5	0
50	0	12	111	1.0	179	46	Tr	Tr	0.05	0.13	3.5	0
16	Tr	2	64	0.3	92	303	0	0	0.13	0.05	1.4	6
27	1	5	136	0.4	179	711	0	0	0.38	0.09	3.2	10
53	0	6	182	0.7	243	1009	0	0	0.51	0.19	3.8	0
37	0	5	154	0.6	215	902	0	0	0.46	0.17	3.4	0
35	Tr	6	188	0.9	298	908	0	0	0.82	0.21	4.3	19[49]
26	1	3	34	0.3	90	541	0	0	0.15	0.08	1.3	Tr
21	0	3	65	0.3	134	576	0	0	0.27	0.09	1.6	8[49]
32	2	4	141	0.6	189	751	0	0	0.49	0.14	3.0	16[49]
27	1	4	124	0.4	200	815	0	0	0.53	0.13	2.8	15[49]

[48]Value varies widely.
[49]Contains added sodium ascorbate. If sodium ascorbate is not added, ascorbic acid content is negligible.

Continued.

Item Number	Foods, Approximate Measures, Units, and Weight (Weight of Edible Portion Only)		Weight (grams)	Water (percent)	Food Energy (calories)	Protein (grams)	Fat (grams)	Fatty Acids		
								Saturated (grams)	Monounsaturated (grams)	Polyunsaturated (grams)
	Meat and Meat Products—cont'd									
	Pork, fresh, cooked									
	Chop, loin (cut 3 per lb with bone)									
	Broiled									
608	Lean and fat	3.1 oz	87	50	275	24	19	7.0	8.8	2.2
609	Lean only (from item 608)	2.5 oz	72	57	165	23	8	2.6	3.4	0.9
	Pan-fried									
610	Lean and fat	3.1 oz	89	45	335	21	27	9.8	12.5	3.1
611	Lean only (from item 610)	2.4 oz	67	54	180	19	11	3.7	4.8	1.3
	Ham (leg), roasted									
612	Lean and fat, piece, 2½ by 2½ by ¾ in	3 oz	85	53	250	21	18	6.4	8.1	2.0
613	Lean only (from item 612)	2.5 oz	72	60	160	20	8	2.7	3.6	1.0
	Rib, roasted									
614	Lean and fat, piece, 2½ by ¾ in	3 oz	85	51	270	21	20	7.2	9.2	2.3
615	Lean only (from item 614)	2.5 oz	71	57	175	20	10	3.4	4.4	1.2
	Shoulder cut, braised									
616	Lean and fat, 3 pieces, 2½ by 2½ by ¼ in	3 oz	85	47	295	23	22	7.9	10.0	2.4
617	Lean only (from item 616)	2.4 oz	67	54	165	22	8	2.8	3.7	1.0
	Sausages (See also Luncheon meats, items 604-607)									
618	Bologna, slice (8 per 8-oz pkg)	2 slices	57	54	180	7	16	6.1	7.6	1.4
619	Braunschweiger, slice (6 per 6-oz pkg)	2 slices	57	48	205	8	18	6.2	8.5	2.1
620	Brown and serve (10-11 per 8-oz pkg), browned	1 link	13	45	50	2	5	1.7	2.2	0.5
621	Frankfurter (10 per 1-lb pkg), cooked (reheated)	1 frankfurter	45	54	145	5	13	4.8	6.2	1.2
622	Pork link (16 per 1-lb pkg), cooked[50]	1 link	13	45	50	3	4	1.4	1.8	0.5
	Salami									
623	Cooked type, slice (8 per 8-oz pkg)	2 slices	57	60	145	8	11	4.6	5.2	1.2
624	Dry type, slice (12 per 4-oz pkg)	2 slices	20	35	85	5	7	2.4	3.4	0.6
625	Sandwich spread (pork, beef)	1 tbsp	15	60	35	1	3	0.9	1.1	0.4
626	Vienna sausage (per 4-oz can)	1 sausage	16	60	45	2	4	1.5	2.0	0.3
	Veal, medium fat, cooked, bone removed									
627	Cutlet, 4⅛ by 2¼ by ½ in, braised or broiled	3 oz	85	60	185	23	9	4.1	4.1	0.6
628	Rib, 2 pieces, 4⅛ by 2¼ by ¼ in, roasted	3 oz	85	55	230	23	14	6.0	6.0	1.0
	Mixed Dishes and Fast Foods									
	Mixed dishes									
629	Beef and vegetable stew, from home recipe	1 cup	245	82	220	16	11	4.4	4.5	0.5
630	Beef pot pie, from home recipe, baked, piece, ⅓ of 9-in diam pie[51]	1 piece	210	55	515	21	30	7.9	12.9	7.4
631	Chicken a la king, cooked, from home recipe	1 cup	245	68	470	27	34	12.9	13.4	6.2
632	Chicken and noodles, cooked, from home recipe	1 cup	240	71	365	22	18	5.1	7.1	3.9
	Chicken chow mein:									
633	Canned	1 cup	250	89	95	7	Tr	0.1	0.1	0.8
634	From home recipe	1 cup	250	78	255	31	10	4.1	4.9	3.5
635	Chicken pot pie, from home recipe, baked, piece, ⅓ of 9-in diam pie[51]	1 piece	232	57	545	23	31	10.3	15.5	6.6
636	Chili con carne with beans, canned	1 cup	255	72	340	19	16	5.8	7.2	1.0
637	Chop suey with beef and pork, from home recipe	1 cup	250	75	300	26	17	4.3	7.4	4.2
	Macaroni (enriched) and cheese									
638	Canned[52]	1 cup	240	80	230	9	10	4.7	2.9	1.3
639	From home recipe[38]	1 cup	200	58	430	17	22	9.8	7.4	3.6
640	Quiche Lorraine, ⅛ of 8-in diam quiche[51]	1 slice	176	47	600	13	48	23.2	17.8	4.1

[38]Made with margarine.
[49]Contains added sodium ascorbate. If sodium ascorbate is not added, ascorbic acid content is negligible.
[50]One patty (8 per pound) of bulk sausage is equivalent to 2 links.

							Vitamin A Value					
Cholesterol (mg)	Carbo-hydrate (grams)	Calcium (mg)	Phosphorus (mg)	Iron (mg)	Potassium (mg)	Sodium (mg)	(IU) International Units	(RE) Retinol Equivalents	Thiamin (mg)	Riboflavin (mg)	Niacin (mg)	Ascorbic Acid (mg)
84	0	3	184	0.7	312	61	10	3	0.87	0.24	4.3	Tr
71	0	4	176	0.7	302	56	10	1	0.83	0.22	4.0	Tr
92	0	4	190	0.7	323	64	10	3	0.91	0.24	4.6	Tr
72	0	3	178	0.7	305	57	10	1	0.84	0.22	4.0	Tr
79	0	5	210	0.9	280	50	10	2	0.54	0.27	3.9	Tr
68	0	5	202	0.8	269	46	10	1	0.50	0.25	3.6	Tr
69	0	9	190	0.8	313	37	10	3	0.50	0.24	4.2	Tr
56	0	8	182	0.7	300	33	10	2	0.45	0.22	3.8	Tr
93	0	6	162	1.4	286	75	10	3	0.46	0.26	4.4	Tr
76	0	5	151	1.3	271	68	10	1	0.40	0.24	4.0	Tr
31	2	7	52	0.9	103	581	0	0	0.10	0.08	1.5	12[49]
89	2	5	96	5.3	113	652	8010	2405	0.14	0.87	4.8	6[49]
9	Tr	1	14	0.1	25	105	0	0	0.05	0.02	0.4	0
23	1	5	39	0.5	75	504	0	0	0.09	0.05	1.2	12[49]
11	Tr	4	24	0.2	47	168	0	0	0.10	0.03	0.6	Tr
37	1	7	66	1.5	113	607	0	0	0.14	0.21	2.0	7[49]
16	1	2	28	0.3	76	372	0	0	0.12	0.06	1.0	5[49]
6	2	2	9	0.1	17	152	10	1	0.03	0.02	0.3	0
8	Tr	2	8	0.1	16	152	0	0	0.01	0.02	0.3	0
109	0	9	196	0.8	258	56	Tr	Tr	0.06	0.21	4.6	0
109	0	10	211	0.7	259	57	Tr	Tr	0.11	0.26	6.6	0
71	15	29	184	2.9	613	292	5690	568	0.15	0.17	4.7	17
42	39	29	149	3.8	334	596	4220	517	0.29	0.29	4.8	6
221	12	127	358	2.5	404	760	1130	272	0.10	0.42	5.4	12
103	26	26	247	2.2	149	600	430	130	0.50	0.17	4.3	Tr
8	18	45	85	1.3	418	725	150	28	0.05	0.10	1.0	13
75	10	58	293	2.5	473	718	280	50	0.08	0.23	4.3	10
56	42	70	232	3.0	343	594	7220	735	0.32	0.32	4.9	5
28	31	82	321	4.3	594	1354	150	15	0.08	0.18	3.3	8
68	13	60	248	4.8	425	1053	600	60	0.28	0.38	5.0	33
24	26	199	182	1.0	139	730	260	72	0.12	0.24	1.0	Tr
44	40	362	322	1.8	240	1086	860	232	0.20	0.40	1.8	1
285	29	211	276	1.0	283	653	1640	454	0.11	0.32	Tr	Tr

[51]Crust made with vegetable shortening and enriched flour.
[52]Made with corn oil.

Continued.

Item Number	Foods, Approximate Measures, Units, and Weight (Weight of Edible Portion Only)		Weight (grams)	Water (percent)	Food Energy (calories)	Protein (grams)	Fat (grams)	Fatty Acids Saturated (grams)	Fatty Acids Monounsaturated (grams)	Fatty Acids Polyunsaturated (grams)
	Mixed Dishes and Fast Foods—cont'd									
	Mixed dishes—cont'd									
	Spaghetti (enriched) in tomato sauce with cheese									
641	Canned	1 cup	250	80	190	6	2	0.4	0.4	0.5
642	From home recipe	1 cup	250	77	260	9	9	3.0	3.6	1.2
	Spaghetti (enriched) with meatballs and tomato sauce									
643	Canned	1 cup	250	78	260	12	10	2.4	3.9	3.1
644	From home recipe	1 cup	248	70	330	19	12	3.9	4.4	2.2
	Fast food entrees									
	Cheeseburger									
645	Regular	1 sandwich	112	46	300	15	15	7.3	5.6	1.0
646	4-oz patty	1 sandwich	194	46	525	30	31	15.1	12.2	1.4
	Chicken, fried (See also Poultry and poultry products, items 656-659)									
647	Enchilada	1 enchilada	230	72	235	20	16	7.7	6.7	0.6
648	English muffin, egg, cheese, and bacon	1 sandwich	138	49	360	18	18	8.0	8.0	0.7
	Fish sandwich									
649	Regular, with cheese	1 sandwich	140	43	420	16	23	6.3	6.9	7.7
650	Large, without cheese	1 sandwich	170	48	470	18	27	6.3	8.7	9.5
	Hamburger									
651	Regular	1 sandwich	98	46	245	12	11	4.4	5.3	0.5
652	4-oz patty	1 sandwich	174	50	445	25	21	7.1	11.7	0.6
653	Pizza, cheese, 1/8 of 15-in diam pizza[51]	1 slice	120	46	290	15	9	4.1	2.6	1.3
654	Roast beef sandwich	1 sandwich	150	52	345	22	13	3.5	6.9	1.8
655	Taco	1 taco	81	55	195	9	11	4.1	5.5	0.8
	Poultry and Poultry Products									
	Chicken									
	Fried, flesh, with skin[53]									
	Batter dipped									
656	Breast, 1/2 breast (5.6 oz with bones)	4.9 oz	140	52	365	35	18	4.9	7.6	4.3
657	Drumstick (3.4 oz with bones)	2.5 oz	72	53	195	16	11	3.0	4.6	2.7
	Flour coated									
658	Breast, 1/2 breast (4.2 oz with bones)	3.5 oz	98	57	220	31	9	2.4	3.4	1.9
659	Drumstick (2.6 oz with bones)	1.7 oz	49	57	120	13	7	1.8	2.7	1.6
	Roasted, flesh only									
660	Breast, 1/2 breast (4.2 oz with bones and skin)	3.0 oz	86	65	140	27	3	0.9	1.1	0.7
661	Drumstick, (2.9 oz with bones and skin)	1.6 oz	44	67	75	12	2	0.7	0.8	0.6
662	Stewed, flesh only, light and dark meat, chopped or diced	1 cup	140	67	250	38	9	2.6	3.3	2.2
663	Chicken liver, cooked	1 liver	20	68	30	5	1	0.4	0.3	0.2
664	Duck, roasted, flesh only	1/2 duck	221	64	445	52	25	9.2	8.2	3.2
	Turkey, roasted, flesh only									
665	Dark meat, piece, 2 1/2 by 1 5/8 by 1/4 in	4 pieces	85	63	160	24	6	2.1	1.4	1.8
666	Light meat, piece, 4 by 2 by 1/4 in	2 pieces	85	66	135	25	3	0.9	0.5	0.7
	Light and dark meat									
667	Chopped or diced	1 cup	140	65	240	41	7	2.3	1.4	2.0
668	Pieces (1 slice white meat, 4 by 2 by 1/4 in and 2 slices dark meat, 2 1/2 by 1 5/8 by 1/4 in)	3 pieces	85	65	145	25	4	1.4	0.9	1.2
	Poultry food products									
	Chicken									
669	Canned, boneless	5 oz	142	69	235	31	11	3.1	4.5	2.5
670	Frankfurter (10 per 1-lb pkg)	1 frankfurter	45	58	115	6	9	2.5	3.8	1.8
671	Roll, light (6 slices per 6-oz pkg)	2 slices	57	69	90	11	4	1.1	1.7	0.9
	Turkey									
672	Gravy and turkey, frozen	5-oz package	142	85	95	8	4	1.2	1.4	0.7
673	Ham, cured turkey thigh meat (8 slices per 8-oz pkg)	2 slices	57	71	75	11	3	1.0	0.7	0.9
674	Loaf, breast meat (8 slices per 6-oz pkg)	2 slices	42	72	45	10	1	0.2	0.2	0.1

[51] Crust made with vegetable shortening and enriched flour.

[53] Fried in vegetable shortening.

F

Cholesterol (mg)	Carbo-hydrate (grams)	Calcium (mg)	Phosphorus (mg)	Iron (mg)	Potassium (mg)	Sodium (mg)	Vitamin A Value (IU) International Units	(RE) Retinol Equivalents	Thiamin (mg)	Riboflavin (mg)	Niacin (mg)	Ascorbic Acid (mg)
3	39	40	88	2.8	303	955	930	120	0.35	0.28	4.5	10
8	37	80	135	2.3	408	955	1080	140	0.25	0.18	2.3	13
23	29	53	113	3.3	245	1220	1000	100	0.15	0.18	2.3	5
89	39	124	236	3.7	665	1009	1590	159	0.25	0.30	4.0	22
44	28	135	174	2.3	219	672	340	65	0.26	0.24	3.7	1
104	40	236	320	4.5	407	1224	670	128	0.33	0.48	7.4	3
19	24	322	662	11.0	2180	4451	2720	352	0.18	0.26	Tr	Tr
213	31	197	290	3.1	201	832	650	160	0.46	0.50	3.7	1
56	39	132	223	1.8	274	667	160	25	0.32	0.26	3.3	2
91	41	61	246	2.2	375	621	110	15	0.35	0.23	3.5	1
32	28	56	107	2.2	202	463	80	14	0.23	0.24	3.8	1
71	38	75	225	4.8	404	763	160	28	0.38	0.38	7.8	1
56	39	220	216	1.6	230	699	750	106	0.34	0.29	4.2	2
55	34	60	222	4.0	338	757	240	32	0.40	0.33	6.0	2
21	15	109	134	1.2	263	456	420	57	0.09	0.07	1.4	1
119	13	28	259	1.8	281	385	90	28	0.16	0.20	14.7	0
62	6	12	106	1.0	134	194	60	19	0.08	0.15	3.7	0
87	2	16	228	1.2	254	74	50	15	0.08	0.13	13.5	0
44	1	6	86	0.7	112	44	40	12	0.04	0.11	3.0	0
73	0	13	196	0.9	220	64	20	5	0.06	0.10	11.8	0
41	0	5	81	0.6	108	42	30	8	0.03	0.10	2.7	0
116	0	20	210	1.6	252	98	70	21	0.07	0.23	8.6	0
126	Tr	3	62	1.7	28	10	3270	983	0.03	0.35	0.9	3
197	0	27	449	6.0	557	144	170	51	0.57	1.04	11.3	0
72	0	27	173	2.0	246	67	0	0	0.05	0.21	3.1	0
59	0	16	186	1.1	259	54	0	0	0.05	0.11	5.8	0
106	0	35	298	2.5	417	98	0	0	0.09	0.25	7.6	0
65	0	21	181	1.5	253	60	0	0	0.05	0.15	4.6	0
88	0	20	158	2.2	196	714	170	48	0.02	0.18	9.0	3
45	3	43	48	0.9	38	616	60	17	0.03	0.05	1.4	0
28	1	24	89	0.6	129	331	50	14	0.04	0.07	3.0	0
26	7	20	115	1.3	87	787	60	18	0.03	0.18	2.6	0
32	Tr	6	108	1.6	184	565	0	0	0.03	0.14	2.0	0
17	0	3	97	0.2	118	608	0	0	0.02	0.05	3.5	0[54]

[54]If sodium ascorbate is added, product contains 11 mg ascorbic acid.

Continued.

F

Item Number	Foods, Approximate Measures, Units, and Weight (Weight of Edible Portion Only)		Weight (grams)	Water (percent)	Food Energy (calories)	Protein (grams)	Fat (grams)	Fatty Acids Saturated (grams)	Fatty Acids Monounsaturated (grams)	Fatty Acids Polyunsaturated (grams)
	Poultry and Poultry Products—cont'd									
	Poultry food products—cont'd									
	Turkey—cont'd									
675	Patties, breaded, battered, fried (2.25 oz)	1 patty	64	50	180	9	12	3.0	4.8	3.0
676	Roast, boneless, frozen, seasoned, light and dark meat, cooked	3 oz	85	68	130	18	5	1.6	1.0	1.4
	Soups, Sauces, and Gravies									
	Soups									
	Canned, condensed									
	Prepared with equal volume of milk									
677	Clam chowder, New England	1 cup	248	85	165	9	7	3.0	2.3	1.1
678	Cream of chicken	1 cup	248	85	190	7	11	4.6	4.5	1.6
679	Cream of mushroom	1 cup	248	85	205	6	14	5.1	3.0	4.6
680	Tomato	1 cup	248	85	160	6	6	2.9	1.6	1.1
	Prepared with equal volume of water									
681	Bean with bacon	1 cup	253	84	170	8	6	1.5	2.2	1.8
682	Beef broth, bouillon, consomme	1 cup	240	98	15	3	1	0.3	0.2	Tr
683	Beef noodle	1 cup	244	92	85	5	3	1.1	1.2	0.5
684	Chicken noodle	1 cup	241	92	75	4	2	0.7	1.1	0.6
685	Chicken rice	1 cup	241	94	60	4	2	0.5	0.9	0.4
686	Clam chowder, Manhattan	1 cup	244	90	80	4	2	0.4	0.4	1.3
687	Cream of chicken	1 cup	244	91	115	3	7	2.1	3.3	1.5
688	Cream of mushroom	1 cup	244	90	130	2	9	2.4	1.7	4.2
689	Minestrone	1 cup	241	91	80	4	3	0.6	0.7	1.1
690	Pea, green	1 cup	250	83	165	9	3	1.4	1.0	0.4
691	Tomato	1 cup	244	90	85	2	2	0.4	0.4	1.0
692	Vegetable beef	1 cup	244	92	80	6	2	0.9	0.8	0.1
693	Vegetarian	1 cup	241	92	70	2	2	0.3	0.8	0.7
	Dehydrated									
	Unprepared									
694	Bouillon	1 pkt	6	3	15	1	1	0.3	0.2	Tr
695	Onion	1 pkt	7	4	20	1	Tr	0.1	0.2	Tr
	Prepared with water									
696	Chicken noodle	1 pkt (6 fl oz)	188	94	40	2	1	0.2	0.4	0.3
697	Onion	1 pkt (6 fl oz)	184	96	20	1	Tr	0.1	0.2	0.1
698	Tomato vegetable	1 pkt (6 fl oz)	189	94	40	1	1	0.3	0.2	0.1
	Sauces									
	From dry mix									
699	Cheese, prepared with milk	1 cup	279	77	305	16	17	9.3	5.3	1.6
700	Hollandaise, prepared with water	1 cup	259	84	240	5	20	11.6	5.9	0.9
701	White sauce, prepared with milk	1 cup	264	81	240	10	13	6.4	4.7	1.7
	From home recipe									
702	White sauce, medium[55]	1 cup	250	73	395	10	30	9.1	11.9	7.2
	Ready-to-serve									
703	Barbecue	1 tbsp	16	81	10	Tr	Tr	Tr	0.1	0.1
704	Soy	1 tbsp	18	68	10	2	0	0.0	0.0	0.0
	Gravies									
	Canned									
705	Beef	1 cup	233	87	125	9	5	2.7	2.3	0.2
706	Chicken	1 cup	238	85	190	5	14	3.4	6.1	3.6
707	Mushroom	1 cup	238	89	120	3	6	1.0	2.8	2.4
	From dry mix									
708	Brown	1 cup	261	91	80	3	2	0.9	0.8	0.1
709	Chicken	1 cup	260	91	85	3	2	0.5	0.9	0.4
	Sugars and Sweets									
	Candy									
710	Caramels, plain or chocolate	1 oz	28	8	115	1	3	2.2	0.3	0.1
	Chocolate									
711	Milk, plain	1 oz	28	1	145	2	9	5.4	3.0	0.3
712	Milk, with almonds	1 oz	28	2	150	3	10	4.8	4.1	0.7
713	Milk, with peanuts	1 oz	28	1	155	4	11	4.2	3.5	1.5
714	Milk, with rice cereal	1 oz	28	2	140	2	7	4.4	2.5	0.2
715	Semisweet, small pieces (60 per oz)	1 cup or 6 oz	170	1	860	7	61	36.2	19.9	1.9
716	Sweet (dark)	1 oz	28	1	150	1	10	5.9	3.3	0.3

[55]Made with enriched flour, margarine, and whole milk.

F

Cholesterol (mg)	Carbo-hydrate (grams)	Calcium (mg)	Phosphorus (mg)	Iron (mg)	Potassium (mg)	Sodium (mg)	Vitamin A Value (IU) International Units	Vitamin A Value (RE) Retinol Equivalents	Thiamin (mg)	Riboflavin (mg)	Niacin (mg)	Ascorbic Acid (mg)
40	10	9	173	1.4	176	512	20	7	0.06	0.12	1.5	0
45	3	4	207	1.4	253	578	0	0	0.04	0.14	5.3	0
22	17	186	156	1.5	300	992	160	40	0.07	0.24	1.0	3
27	15	181	151	0.7	273	1047	710	94	0.07	0.26	0.9	1
20	15	179	156	0.6	270	1076	150	37	0.08	0.28	0.9	2
17	22	159	149	1.8	449	932	850	109	0.13	0.25	1.5	68
3	23	81	132	2.0	402	951	890	89	0.09	0.03	0.6	2
Tr	Tr	14	31	0.4	130	782	0	0	Tr	0.05	1.9	0
5	9	15	46	1.1	100	952	630	63	0.07	0.06	1.1	Tr
7	9	17	36	0.8	55	1106	710	71	0.05	0.06	1.4	Tr
7	7	17	22	0.7	101	815	660	66	0.02	0.02	1.1	Tr
2	12	34	59	1.9	261	1808	920	92	0.06	0.05	1.3	3
10	9	34	37	0.6	88	986	560	56	0.03	0.06	0.8	Tr
2	9	46	49	0.5	100	1032	0	0	0.05	0.09	0.7	1
2	11	34	55	0.9	313	911	2340	234	0.05	0.04	0.9	1
0	27	28	125	2.0	190	988	200	20	0.11	0.07	1.2	2
0	17	12	34	1.8	264	871	690	69	0.09	0.05	1.4	66
5	10	17	41	1.1	173	956	1890	189	0.04	0.05	1.0	2
0	12	22	34	1.1	210	822	3010	301	0.05	0.05	0.9	1
1	1	4	19	0.1	27	1019	Tr	Tr	Tr	0.01	0.3	0
Tr	4	10	23	0.1	47	627	Tr	Tr	0.02	0.04	0.4	Tr
2	6	24	24	0.4	23	957	50	5	0.05	0.04	0.7	Tr
0	4	9	22	0.1	48	635	Tr	Tr	0.02	0.04	0.4	Tr
0	8	6	23	0.5	78	856	140	14	0.04	0.03	0.6	5
53	23	569	438	0.3	552	1565	390	117	0.15	0.56	0.3	2
52	14	124	127	0.9	124	1564	730	220	0.05	0.18	0.1	Tr
34	21	425	256	0.3	444	797	310	92	0.08	0.45	0.5	3
32	24	292	238	0.9	381	888	1190	340	0.15	0.43	0.8	2
0	2	3	3	0.1	28	130	140	14	Tr	Tr	0.1	1
0	2	3	38	0.5	64	1029	0	0	0.01	0.02	0.6	0
7	11	14	70	1.6	189	117	0	0	0.07	0.08	1.5	0
5	13	48	69	1.1	259	1373	880	264	0.04	0.10	1.1	0
0	13	17	36	1.6	252	1357	0	0	0.08	0.15	1.6	0
2	14	66	47	0.2	61	1147	0	0	0.04	0.09	0.9	0
3	14	39	47	0.3	62	1134	0	0	0.05	0.15	0.8	3
1	22	42	35	0.4	54	64	Tr	Tr	0.01	0.05	0.1	Tr
6	16	50	61	0.4	96	23	30	10	0.02	0.10	0.1	Tr
5	15	65	77	0.5	125	23	30	8	0.02	0.12	0.2	Tr
5	13	49	83	0.4	138	19	30	8	0.07	0.07	1.4	Tr
6	18	48	57	0.2	100	46	30	8	0.01	0.08	0.1	Tr
0	97	51	178	5.8	593	24	30	3	0.10	0.14	0.9	Tr
0	16	7	41	0.6	86	5	10	1	0.01	0.04	0.1	Tr

Continued.

Item Number	Foods, Approximate Measures, Units, and Weight (Weight of Edible Portion Only)		Weight (grams)	Water (percent)	Food Energy (calories)	Protein (grams)	Fat (grams)	Fatty Acids: Saturated (grams)	Fatty Acids: Monounsaturated (grams)	Fatty Acids: Polyunsaturated (grams)
	Sugars and Sweets—cont'd									
	Candy—cont'd									
717	Fondant, uncoated (mints, candy corn, other)	1 oz	28	3	105	Tr	0	0.0	0.0	0.0
718	Fudge, chocolate, plain	1 oz	28	8	115	1	3	2.1	1.0	0.1
719	Gum drops	1 oz	28	12	100	Tr	Tr	Tr	Tr	0.1
720	Hard candy	1 oz	28	1	110	0	0	0.0	0.0	0.0
721	Jelly beans	1 oz	28	6	105	Tr	Tr	Tr	Tr	0.1
722	Marshmallows	1 oz	28	17	90	1	0	0.0	0.0	0.0
723	Custard, baked	1 cup	265	77	305	14	15	6.8	5.4	0.7
724	Gelatin dessert prepared with gelatin dessert powder and water	½ cup	120	84	70	2	0	0.0	0.0	0.0
725	Honey, strained or extracted	1 cup	339	17	1030	1	0	0.0	0.0	0.0
726		1 tbsp	21	17	65	Tr	0	0.0	0.0	0.0
727	Jams and preserves	1 tbsp	20	29	55	Tr	Tr	0.0	Tr	Tr
728		1 pkt	14	29	40	Tr	Tr	0.0	Tr	Tr
729	Jellies	1 tbsp	18	28	50	Tr	Tr	Tr	Tr	Tr
730		1 pkt	14	28	40	Tr	Tr	Tr	Tr	Tr
731	Popsicle, 3-fl-oz size	1 popsicle	95	80	70	0	0	0.0	0.0	0.0
	Puddings									
	Canned									
732	Chocolate	5-oz can	142	68	205	3	11	9.5	0.5	0.1
733	Tapioca	5-oz can	142	74	160	3	5	4.8	Tr	Tr
734	Vanilla	5-oz can	142	69	220	2	10	9.5	0.2	0.1
	Dry mix, prepared with whole milk									
	Chocolate									
735	Instant	½ cup	130	71	155	4	4	2.3	1.1	0.2
736	Regular (cooked)	½ cup	130	73	150	4	4	2.4	1.1	0.1
737	Rice	½ cup	132	73	155	4	4	2.3	1.1	0.1
738	Tapioca	½ cup	130	75	145	4	4	2.3	1.1	0.1
	Vanilla									
739	Instant	½ cup	130	73	150	4	4	2.2	1.1	0.2
740	Regular (cooked)	½ cup	130	74	145	4	4	2.3	1.0	0.1
	Sugars									
741	Brown, pressed down	1 cup	220	2	820	0	0	0.0	0.0	0.0
	White									
742	Granulated	1 cup	200	1	770	0	0	0.0	0.0	0.0
743		1 tbsp	12	1	45	0	0	0.0	0.0	0.0
744		1 pkt	6	1	25	0	0	0.0	0.0	0.0
745	Powdered, sifted, spooned into cup	1 cup	100	1	385	0	0	0.0	0.0	0.0
	Syrups									
	Chocolate-flavored syrup or topping									
746	Thin type	2 tbsp	38	37	85	1	Tr	0.2	0.1	0.1
747	Fudge type	2 tbsp	38	25	125	2	5	3.1	1.7	0.2
748	Molasses, cane, blackstrap	2 tbsp	40	24	85	0	0	0.0	0.0	0.0
749	Table syrup (corn and maple)	2 tbsp	42	25	122	0	0	0.0	0.0	0.0
	Vegetables and Vegetable Products									
750	Alfalfa seeds, sprouted, raw	1 cup	33	91	10	1	Tr	Tr	Tr	0.1
751	Artichokes, globe or French, cooked, drained	1 artichoke	120	87	55	3	Tr	Tr	Tr	0.1
	Asparagus, green									
	Cooked, drained									
	From raw									
752	Cuts and tips	1 cup	180	92	45	5	1	0.1	Tr	0.2
753	Spears, ½-in diam at base	4 spears	60	92	15	2	Tr	Tr	Tr	0.1
	From frozen									
754	Cuts and tips	1 cup	180	91	50	5	1	0.2	Tr	0.3
755	Spears, ½-in diam at base	4 spears	60	91	15	2	Tr	0.1	Tr	0.1
756	Canned, spears, ½-in diam at base	4 spears	80	95	10	1	Tr	Tr	Tr	0.1
757	Bamboo shoots, canned, drained	1 cup	131	94	25	2	1	0.1	Tr	0.2
	Beans									
	Lima, immature seeds, frozen, cooked, drained									
758	Thick-seeded types (Ford hooks)	1 cup	170	74	170	10	1	0.1	Tr	0.3
759	Thin-seeded types (baby limas)	1 cup	180	72	190	12	1	0.1	Tr	0.3

[56]For regular pack; special dietary pack contains 3 mg sodium.

Cholesterol (mg)	Carbo-hydrate (grams)	Calcium (mg)	Phosphorus (mg)	Iron (mg)	Potassium (mg)	Sodium (mg)	Vitamin A Value (IU) International Units	Vitamin A Value (RE) Retinol Equivalents	Thiamin (mg)	Riboflavin (mg)	Niacin (mg)	Ascorbic Acid (mg)
0	27	2	Tr	0.1	1	57	0	0	Tr	Tr	Tr	0
1	21	22	24	0.3	42	54	Tr	Tr	0.01	0.03	0.1	Tr
0	25	2	Tr	0.1	1	10	0	0	0.00	Tr	Tr	0
0	28	Tr	2	0.1	1	7	0	0	0.10	0.00	0.0	0
0	26	1	1	0.3	11	7	0	0	0.00	Tr	Tr	0
0	23	1	2	0.5	2	25	0	0	0.00	Tr	Tr	0
278	29	297	310	1.1	387	209	530	146	0.11	0.50	0.3	1
0	17	2	23	Tr	Tr	55	0	0	0.00	0.00	0.0	0
0	279	17	20	1.7	173	17	0	0	0.02	0.14	1.0	3
0	17	1	1	0.1	11	1	0	0	Tr	0.01	0.1	Tr
0	14	4	2	0.2	18	2	Tr	Tr	Tr	0.01	Tr	Tr
0	10	3	1	0.1	12	2	Tr	Tr	Tr	Tr	Tr	Tr
0	13	2	Tr	0.1	16	5	Tr	Tr	Tr	0.01	Tr	1
0	10	1	Tr	Tr	13	4	Tr	Tr	Tr	Tr	Tr	1
0	18	0	0	Tr	4	11	0	0	0.00	0.00	0.0	0
1	30	74	117	1.2	254	285	100	31	0.04	0.17	0.6	Tr
Tr	28	119	113	0.3	212	252	Tr	Tr	0.03	0.14	0.4	Tr
1	33	79	94	0.2	155	305	Tr	Tr	0.03	0.12	0.6	Tr
14	27	130	329	0.3	176	440	130	33	0.04	0.18	0.1	1
15	25	146	120	0.2	190	167	140	34	0.05	0.20	0.1	1
15	27	133	110	0.5	165	140	140	33	0.10	0.18	0.6	1
15	25	131	103	0.1	167	152	140	34	0.04	0.18	0.1	1
15	27	129	273	0.1	164	375	140	33	0.04	0.17	0.1	1
15	25	132	102	0.1	166	178	140	34	0.04	0.18	0.1	1
0	212	187	56	4.8	757	97	0	0	0.02	0.07	0.2	0
0	199	3	Tr	0.1	2	5	0	0	0.00	0.00	0.0	0
0	12	Tr	Tr	Tr	Tr	Tr	0	0	0.00	0.00	0.0	0
0	6	Tr	Tr	Tr	Tr	Tr	0	0	0.00	0.00	0.0	0
0	100	1	Tr	Tr	4	2	0	0	0.00	0.00	0.0	0
0	22	6	49	0.8	85	36	Tr	Tr	0.02	0.08	0.1	0
0	21	38	66	0.5	82	42	40	13	0.04	0.08	0.1	0
0	22	274	34	10.1	1171	38	0	0	0.00	0.00	0.8	0
0	32	1	4	Tr	7	19	0	0	0	0	0	0
0	1	11	23	0.3	26	2	50	5	0.03	0.04	0.2	3
0	12	47	72	1.6	316	79	170	17	0.07	0.06	0.7	9
0	8	43	110	1.2	558	7	1490	149	0.18	0.22	1.9	49
0	3	14	37	0.4	186	2	500	50	0.06	0.07	0.6	16
0	9	41	99	1.2	392	7	1470	147	0.12	0.19	1.9	44
0	3	14	33	0.4	131	2	490	49	0.04	0.06	0.6	15
0	2	11	30	0.5	122	278[56]	380	38	0.04	0.07	0.7	13
0	4	10	33	0.4	105	9	10	1	0.03	0.03	0.2	1
0	32	37	107	2.3	694	90	320	32	0.13	0.10	1.8	22
0	35	50	202	3.5	740	52	300	30	0.13	0.10	1.4	10

Continued.

Item Number	Foods, Approximate Measures, Units, and Weight (Weight of Edible Portion Only)		Weight (grams)	Water (percent)	Food Energy (calories)	Protein (grams)	Fat (grams)	Fatty Acids: Saturated (grams)	Fatty Acids: Monounsaturated (grams)	Fatty Acids: Polyunsaturated (grams)
	Vegetables and Vegetables Products—cont'd									
	Beans—cont'd									
	Snap									
	Cooked, drained									
760	From raw (cut and French style)	1 cup	125	89	45	2	Tr	0.1	Tr	0.2
761	From frozen (cut)	1 cup	135	92	35	2	Tr	Tr	Tr	0.1
762	Canned, drained solids (cut)	1 cup	135	93	25	2	Tr	Tr	Tr	0.1
	Beans, mature (See Beans, dry, items 527-535; and Black-eyed peas, dry, item 536)									
	Bean sprouts (mung)									
763	Raw	1 cup	104	90	30	3	Tr	Tr	Tr	0.1
764	Cooked, drained	1 cup	124	93	25	3	Tr	Tr	Tr	Tr
	Beets									
	Cooked, drained									
765	Diced or sliced	1 cup	170	91	55	2	Tr	Tr	Tr	Tr
766	Whole beets, 2-in diam	2 beets	100	91	30	1	Tr	Tr	Tr	Tr
767	Canned, drained solids, diced or sliced	1 cup	170	91	55	2	Tr	Tr	Tr	0.1
768	Beet greens, leaves and stems, cooked, drained	1 cup	144	89	40	4	Tr	Tr	0.1	0.1
	Black-eyed peas, immature seeds, cooked and drained									
769	From raw	1 cup	165	72	180	13	1	0.3	0.1	0.6
770	From frozen	1 cup	170	66	225	14	1	0.3	0.1	0.5
	Broccoli									
771	Raw	1 spear	151	91	40	4	1	0.1	Tr	0.3
	Cooked, drained									
	From raw									
772	Spear, medium	1 spear	180	90	50	5	1	0.1	Tr	0.2
773	Spears, cut into ½-in pieces	1 cup	155	90	45	5	Tr	0.1	Tr	0.2
	From frozen									
774	Piece, 4½ to 5 in long	1 piece	30	91	10	1	Tr	Tr	Tr	Tr
775	Chopped	1 cup	185	91	50	6	Tr	Tr	Tr	0.1
	Brussels sprouts, cooked, drained									
776	From raw, 7 to 8 sprouts, 1¼ to 1½-in diam	1 cup	155	87	60	4	1	0.2	0.1	0.4
777	From frozen	1 cup	155	87	65	6	1	0.1	Tr	0.3
	Cabbage, common varieties									
778	Raw, coarsely shredded or sliced	1 cup	70	93	15	1	Tr	Tr	Tr	0.1
779	Cooked, drained	1 cup	150	94	30	1	Tr	Tr	Tr	0.2
	Cabbage, Chinese									
780	Pak-choi, cooked, drained	1 cup	170	96	20	3	Tr	Tr	Tr	0.1
781	Pe-tsai, raw, 1-in pieces	1 cup	76	94	10	1	Tr	Tr	Tr	0.1
782	Cabbage, red, raw, coarsely shredded or sliced	1 cup	70	92	20	1	Tr	Tr	Tr	0.1
783	Cabbage, savoy, raw, coarsely shredded or sliced	1 cup	70	91	20	1	Tr	Tr	Tr	Tr
	Carrots									
	Raw, without crowns and tips, scraped									
784	Whole, 7½ by 1⅛ in, or strips, 2½ to 3 in long	1 carrot, or 18 strips	72	88	30	1	Tr	Tr	Tr	0.1
785	Grated	1 cup	110	88	45	1	Tr	Tr	Tr	0.1
	Cooked, sliced, drained									
786	From raw	1 cup	156	87	70	2	Tr	0.1	Tr	0.1
787	From frozen	1 cup	146	90	55	2	Tr	Tr	Tr	0.1
788	Canned, sliced, drained solids	1 cup	146	93	35	1	Tr	0.1	Tr	0.1
	Cauliflower									
789	Raw, (flowerets)	1 cup	100	92	25	2	Tr	Tr	Tr	0.1
	Cooked, drained									
790	From raw (flowerets)	1 cup	125	93	30	2	Tr	Tr	Tr	0.1
791	From frozen (flowerets)	1 cup	180	94	35	3	Tr	0.1	Tr	0.2
	Celery, pascal type, raw									
792	Stalk, large outer, 8 by 1½ in (at root end)	1 stalk	40	95	5	Tr	Tr	Tr	Tr	Tr
793	Pieces, diced	1 cup	120	95	20	1	Tr	Tr	Tr	0.1

[57]For green varieties; yellow varieties contain 101 IU or 10 RE.
[58]For green varieties; yellow varieties contain 151 IU or 15 RE.
[59]For regular pack; special dietary pack contains 3 mg sodium.

Cholesterol (mg)	Carbo-hydrate (grams)	Calcium (mg)	Phosphorus (mg)	Iron (mg)	Potassium (mg)	Sodium (mg)	Vitamin A Value (IU) International Units	Vitamin A Value (RE) Retinol Equivalents	Thiamin (mg)	Riboflavin (mg)	Niacin (mg)	Ascorbic Acid (mg)
0	10	58	49	1.6	374	4	830[57]	83[57]	0.09	0.12	0.8	12
0	8	61	32	1.1	151	18	710[58]	71[58]	0.06	0.10	0.6	11
0	6	35	26	1.2	147	339[59]	470[60]	47[60]	0.02	0.08	0.3	6
0	6	14	56	0.9	155	6	20	2	0.09	0.13	0.8	14
0	5	15	35	0.8	125	12	20	2	0.06	0.13	1.0	14
0	11	19	53	1.1	530	83	20	2	0.05	0.02	0.5	9
0	7	11	31	0.6	312	49	10	1	0.03	0.01	0.3	6
0	12	26	29	3.1	252	466[61]	20	2	0.02	0.07	0.3	7
0	8	164	59	2.7	1309	347	7340	734	0.17	0.42	0.7	36
0	30	46	196	2.4	693	7	1050	105	0.11	0.18	1.8	3
0	40	39	207	3.6	638	9	130	13	0.44	0.11	1.2	4
0	8	72	100	1.3	491	41	2330	233	0.10	0.18	1.0	141
0	10	86	86	2.1	293	20	2540	254	0.15	0.37	1.4	113
0	9	177	74	1.8	253	17	2180	218	0.13	0.32	1.2	97
0	2	15	17	0.2	54	7	570	57	0.02	0.02	0.1	12
0	10	74	102	1.1	333	44	3500	350	0.10	0.15	0.8	74
0	13	56	87	1.9	491	33	1110	111	0.17	0.12	0.9	96
0	13	37	84	1.1	504	36	910	91	0.16	0.18	0.8	71
0	4	33	16	0.4	172	13	90	9	0.04	0.02	0.2	33
0	7	50	38	0.6	308	29	130	13	0.09	0.08	0.3	36
0	3	158	49	1.8	631	58	4370	437	0.05	0.11	0.7	44
0	2	59	22	0.2	181	7	910	91	0.03	0.04	0.3	21
0	4	36	29	0.3	144	8	30	3	0.04	0.02	0.2	40
0	4	25	29	0.3	161	20	700	70	0.05	0.02	0.2	22
0	7	19	32	0.4	233	25	20,250	2025	0.07	0.04	0.7	7
0	11	30	48	0.6	355	39	30,940	3094	0.11	0.06	1.0	10
0	16	48	47	1.0	354	103	38,300	3830	0.05	0.09	0.8	4
0	12	41	38	0.7	231	86	25,850	2585	0.04	0.05	0.6	4
0	8	37	35	0.9	261	352[62]	20,110	2011	0.03	0.04	0.8	4
0	5	29	46	0.6	355	15	20	2	0.08	0.06	0.6	72
0	6	34	44	0.5	404	8	20	2	0.08	0.07	0.7	69
0	7	31	43	0.7	250	32	40	4	0.07	0.10	0.6	56
0	1	14	10	0.2	114	35	50	5	0.01	0.01	0.1	3
0	4	43	31	0.6	341	106	150	15	0.04	0.04	0.4	8

[60]For green varieties; yellow varieties contain 142 IU or 14 RE.
[61]For regular pack; special dietary pack contains 78 mg sodium.
[62]For regular pack; special dietary pack contains 61 mg sodium.

Continued.

Item Number	Foods, Approximate Measures, Units, and Weight (Weight of Edible Portion Only)		Weight (grams)	Water (percent)	Food Energy (calories)	Protein (grams)	Fat (grams)	Fatty Acids: Saturated (grams)	Fatty Acids: Monounsaturated (grams)	Fatty Acids: Polyunsaturated (grams)
	Vegetables and Vegetables Products—cont'd									
	Collards, cooked, drained									
794	From raw (leaves without stems)	1 cup	190	96	25	2	Tr	0.1	Tr	0.2
795	From frozen (chopped)	1 cup	170	88	60	5	1	0.1	0.1	0.4
	Corn, sweet									
	Cooked, drained									
796	From raw, ear, 5 by 1¾ in	1 ear	77	70	85	3	1	0.2	0.3	0.5
	From frozen									
797	Ear, trimmed to about 3½ in long	1 ear	63	73	60	2	Tr	0.1	0.1	0.2
798	Kernels	1 cup	165	76	135	5	Tr	Tr	Tr	0.1
	Canned									
799	Cream style	1 cup	256	79	185	4	1	0.2	0.3	0.5
800	Whole kernel, vacuum pack	1 cup	210	77	165	5	1	0.2	0.3	0.5
	Cowpeas (See Black-eyed peas, immature, items 769, 770; and mature, item 536)									
801	Cucumber, with peel, slices, ⅛ in thick (large, 2⅛-in diam; small, 1¾-in diam)	6 large or 8 small slices	28	96	5	Tr	Tr	Tr	Tr	Tr
802	Dandelion greens, cooked, drained	1 cup	105	90	35	2	1	0.1	Tr	0.3
803	Eggplant, cooked, steamed	1 cup	96	92	25	1	Tr	Tr	Tr	0.1
804	Endive, curly (including escarole), raw, small pieces	1 cup	50	94	10	1	Tr	Tr	Tr	Tr
805	Jerusalem artichoke, raw, sliced	1 cup	150	78	115	3	Tr	0.0	Tr	Tr
	Kale, cooked, drained									
806	From raw, chopped	1 cup	130	91	40	2	1	0.1	Tr	0.3
807	From frozen, chopped	1 cup	130	91	40	4	1	0.1	Tr	0.3
808	Kohlrabi, thickened bulblike stems, cooked, drained, diced	1 cup	165	90	50	3	Tr	Tr	Tr	0.1
	Lettuce, raw									
	Butterhead, as Boston types									
809	Head, 5-in diam	1 head	163	96	20	2	Tr	Tr	Tr	0.2
810	Leaves	1 outer or 2 inner leaves	15	96	Tr	Tr	Tr	Tr	Tr	Tr
	Crisphead, as iceberg									
811	Head, 6-in diam	1 head	539	96	70	5	1	0.1	Tr	0.5
812	Wedge, ¼ of head	1 wedge	135	96	20	1	Tr	Tr	Tr	0.1
813	Pieces, chopped or shredded	1 cup	55	96	5	1	Tr	Tr	Tr	0.1
814	Looseleaf (bunching varieties including romaine or cos), chopped or shredded pieces	1 cup	56	94	10	1	Tr	Tr	Tr	0.1
	Mushrooms									
815	Raw, sliced or chopped	1 cup	70	92	20	1	Tr	Tr	Tr	0.1
816	Cooked, drained	1 cup	156	91	40	3	1	0.1	Tr	0.3
817	Canned, drained solids	1 cup	156	91	35	3	Tr	0.1	Tr	0.2
818	Mustard greens, without stems and midribs, cooked, drained	1 cup	140	94	20	3	Tr	Tr	0.2	0.1
819	Okra pods, 3 by ⅝ in, cooked	8 pods	85	90	25	2	Tr	Tr	Tr	Tr
	Onions									
	Raw									
820	Chopped	1 cup	160	91	55	2	Tr	0.1	0.1	0.2
821	Sliced	1 cup	115	91	40	1	Tr	0.1	Tr	0.1
822	Cooked (whole or sliced), drained	1 cup	210	92	60	2	Tr	0.1	Tr	0.1
823	Onions, spring, raw, bulb (⅜-in diam) and white portion of top	6 onions	30	92	10	1	Tr	Tr	Tr	Tr
824	Onion rings, breaded, parfried, frozen, prepared	2 rings	20	29	80	1	5	1.7	2.2	1.0
	Parsley									
825	Raw	10 sprigs	10	88	5	Tr	Tr	Tr	Tr	Tr
826	Freeze-dried	1 tbsp	0.4	2	Tr	Tr	Tr	Tr	Tr	Tr
827	Parsnips, cooked (diced or 2 in lengths), drained	1 cup	156	78	125	2	Tr	0.1	0.2	0.1
828	Peas, edible pod, cooked, drained	1 cup	160	89	65	5	Tr	0.1	Tr	0.2
	Peas, green									
829	Canned, drained solids	1 cup	170	82	115	8	1	0.1	0.1	0.3
830	Frozen, cooked, drained	1 cup	160	80	125	8	Tr	0.1	Tr	0.2
	Peppers									
831	Hot chili, raw	1 pepper	45	88	20	1	Tr	Tr	Tr	Tr

[63]For yellow varieties; white varieties contain only a trace of vitamin A.

[64]For regular pack; special dietary pack contains 8 mg sodium.

[65]For regular pack; special dietary pack contains 6 mg sodium.

Cholesterol (mg)	Carbo-hydrate (grams)	Calcium (mg)	Phosphorus (mg)	Iron (mg)	Potassium (mg)	Sodium (mg)	Vitamin A Value (IU) International Units	Vitamin A Value (RE) Retinol Equivalents	Thiamin (mg)	Riboflavin (mg)	Niacin (mg)	Ascorbic Acid (mg)
0	5	148	19	0.8	177	36	4220	422	0.03	0.08	0.4	19
0	12	357	46	1.9	427	85	10,170	1017	0.08	0.20	1.1	45
0	19	2	79	0.5	192	13	170[63]	17[63]	0.17	0.06	1.2	5
0	14	2	47	0.4	158	3	130[63]	13[63]	0.11	0.04	1.0	3
0	34	3	78	0.5	229	8	410[63]	41[63]	0.11	0.12	2.1	4
0	46	8	131	1.0	343	730[64]	250[63]	25[63]	0.06	0.14	2.5	12
0	41	11	134	0.9	391	571[65]	510[63]	51[63]	0.09	0.15	2.5	17
0	1	4	5	0.1	42	1	10	1	0.01	0.01	0.1	1
0	7	147	44	1.9	244	46	12,290	1229	0.14	0.18	0.5	19
0	6	6	21	0.3	238	3	60	6	0.07	0.02	0.6	1
0	2	26	14	0.4	157	11	1030	103	0.04	0.04	0.2	3
0	26	21	117	5.1	644	6	30	3	0.30	0.09	2.0	6
0	7	94	36	1.2	296	30	9620	962	0.07	0.09	0.7	53
0	7	179	36	1.2	417	20	8260	826	0.06	0.15	0.9	33
0	11	41	74	0.7	561	35	60	6	0.07	0.03	0.6	89
0	4	52	38	0.5	419	8	1580	158	0.10	0.10	0.5	13
0	Tr	5	3	Tr	39	1	150	15	0.01	0.01	Tr	1
0	11	102	108	2.7	852	49	1780	178	0.25	0.16	1.0	21
0	3	26	27	0.7	213	12	450	45	0.06	0.04	0.3	5
0	1	10	11	0.3	87	5	180	18	0.03	0.02	0.1	2
0	2	38	14	0.8	148	5	1060	106	0.03	0.04	0.2	10
0	3	4	73	0.9	259	3	0	0	0.07	0.31	2.9	2
0	8	9	136	2.7	555	3	0	0	0.11	0.47	7.0	6
0	8	17	103	1.2	201	663	0	0	0.13	0.03	2.5	0
0	3	104	57	1.0	283	22	4240	424	0.06	0.09	0.6	35
0	6	54	48	0.4	274	4	490	49	0.11	0.05	0.7	14
0	12	40	46	0.6	248	3	0	0	0.10	0.02	0.2	13
0	8	29	33	0.4	178	2	0	0	0.07	0.01	0.1	10
0	13	57	48	0.4	319	17	0	0	0.09	0.02	0.2	12
0	2	18	10	0.6	77	1	1500	150	0.02	0.04	0.1	14
0	8	6	16	0.3	26	75	50	5	0.06	0.03	0.7	Tr
0	1	13	4	0.6	54	4	520	52	0.01	0.01	0.1	9
0	Tr	1	2	0.2	25	2	250	25	Tr	0.01	Tr	1
0	30	58	108	0.9	573	16	0	0	0.13	0.08	1.1	20
0	11	67	88	3.2	384	6	210	21	0.20	0.12	0.9	77
0	21	34	114	1.6	294	372[66]	1310	131	0.21	0.13	1.2	16
0	23	38	144	2.5	269	139	1070	107	0.45	0.16	2.4	16
0	4	8	21	0.5	153	3	4840[67]	484[67]	0.04	0.04	0.4	109

[66]For regular pack; special dietary pack contains 3 mg sodium.
[67]For red peppers; green peppers contain 350 IU, or 35 RE.

Continued.

Item Numb	Foods, Approximate Measures, Units, and Weight (Weight of Edible Portion Only)		Weight (grams)	Water (percent)	Food Energy (calories)	Protein (grams)	Fat (grams)	Fatty Acids Saturated (grams)	Fatty Acids Monounsaturated (grams)	Fatty Acids Polyunsaturated (grams)
	Vegetables and Vegetables Products—cont'd									
	Peppers—cont'd									
	Sweet (about 5 per lb, whole), stem and seeds removed									
832	Raw	1 pepper	74	93	20	1	Tr	Tr	Tr	0.2
833	Cooked, drained	1 pepper	73	95	15	Tr	Tr	Tr	Tr	0.1
	Potatoes, cooked									
	Baked (about 2 per lb, raw)									
834	With skin	1 potato	202	71	220	5	Tr	0.1	Tr	0.1
835	Flesh only	1 potato	156	75	145	3	Tr	Tr	Tr	0.1
	Boiled (about 3 per lb, raw)									
836	Peeled after boiling	1 potato	136	77	120	3	Tr	Tr	Tr	0.1
837	Peeled before boiling	1 potato	135	77	115	2	Tr	Tr	Tr	0.1
	French fried, strip, 2 to 3½ in long, frozen									
838	Oven heated	10 strips	50	53	110	2	4	2.1	1.8	0.3
839	Fried in vegetable oil	10 strips	50	38	160	2	8	2.5	1.6	3.8
	Potato products, prepared									
	Au gratin									
840	From dry mix	1 cup	245	79	230	6	10	6.3	2.9	0.3
841	From home recipe	1 cup	245	74	325	12	19	11.6	5.3	0.7
842	Hash brown, from frozen	1 cup	156	56	340	5	18	7.0	8.0	2.1
	Mashed									
	From home recipe									
843	Milk added	1 cup	210	78	160	4	1	0.7	0.3	0.1
844	Milk and margarine added	1 cup	210	76	225	4	9	2.2	3.7	2.5
845	From dehydrated flakes (without milk), water, milk, butter, and salt added	1 cup	210	76	235	4	12	7.2	3.3	0.5
846	Potato salad, made with mayonnaise	1 cup	250	76	360	7	21	3.6	6.2	9.3
	Scalloped									
847	From dry mix	1 cup	245	79	230	5	11	6.5	3.0	0.5
848	From home recipe	1 cup	245	81	210	7	9	5.5	2.5	0.4
849	Potato chips	10 chips	20	3	105	1	7	1.8	1.2	3.6
	Pumpkin									
850	Cooked from raw, mashed	1 cup	245	94	50	2	Tr	0.1	Tr	Tr
851	Canned	1 cup	245	90	85	3	1	0.4	0.1	Tr
852	Radishes, raw, stem ends, rootlets cut off	4 radishes	18	95	5	Tr	Tr	Tr	Tr	Tr
853	Sauerkraut, canned, solids and liquid	1 cup	236	93	45	2	Tr	0.1	Tr	0.1
	Seaweed									
854	Kelp, raw	1 oz	28	82	10	Tr	Tr	0.1	Tr	Tr
855	Spirulina, dried	1 oz	28	5	80	16	2	0.8	0.2	0.6
	Southern peas. See Black-eyed peas, immature (items 769, 770), mature (item 536).									
	Spinach									
856	Raw, chopped	1 cup	55	92	10	2	Tr	Tr	Tr	0.1
	Cooked, drained									
857	From raw	1 cup	180	91	40	5	Tr	0.1	Tr	0.2
858	From frozen (leaf)	1 cup	190	90	55	6	Tr	0.1	Tr	0.2
859	Canned, drained solids	1 cup	214	92	50	6	1	0.2	Tr	0.4
860	Spinach souffle	1 cup	136	74	220	11	18	7.1	6.8	3.1
	Squash, cooked									
861	Summer (all varieties), sliced, drained	1 cup	180	94	35	2	1	0.1	Tr	0.2
862	Winter (all varieties), baked, cubed	1 cup	205	89	80	2	1	0.3	0.1	0.5
	Sunchoke. See Jerusalem-artichoke (item 805).									
	Sweet potatoes									
	Cooked (raw, 5 by 2 in; about 2½ per lb):									
863	Baked in skin, peeled	1 potato	114	73	115	2	Tr	Tr	Tr	0.1
864	Boiled, without skin	1 potato	151	73	160	2	Tr	0.1	Tr	0.2
865	Candied, 2½ by 2 in, one piece	1 piece	105	67	145	1	3	1.4	0.7	0.2
	Canned									
866	Solid pack (mashed)	1 cup	255	74	260	5	1	0.1	Tr	0.2
867	Vacuum pack, piece 2¾ by 1 in	1 piece	40	76	35	1	Tr	Tr	Tr	Tr

[68]For green peppers; red peppers contain 4220 IU, or 422 RE.

[69]For green peppers; red peppers contain 141 mg ascorbic acid.

[70]For green peppers; red peppers contain 2,740 IU, or 274 RE.

							Vitamin A Value					
Cholesterol (mg)	Carbohydrate (grams)	Calcium (mg)	Phosphorus (mg)	Iron (mg)	Potassium (mg)	Sodium (mg)	(IU) International Units	(RE) Retinol Equivalents	Thiamin (mg)	Riboflavin (mg)	Niacin (mg)	Ascorbic Acid (mg)
0	4	4	16	0.9	144	2	390[68]	39[68]	0.06	0.04	0.4	95[69]
0	3	3	11	0.6	94	1	280[70]	28[70]	0.04	0.03	0.3	81[71]
0	51	20	115	2.7	844	16	0	0	0.22	0.07	3.3	26
0	34	8	78	0.5	610	8	0	0	0.16	0.03	2.2	20
0	27	7	60	0.4	515	5	0	0	0.14	0.03	2.0	18
0	27	11	54	0.4	443	7	0	0	0.13	0.03	1.8	10
0	17	5	43	0.7	229	16	0	0	0.06	0.02	1.2	5
0	20	10	47	0.4	366	108	0	0	0.09	0.01	1.6	5
12	31	203	233	0.8	537	1076	520	76	0.05	0.20	2.3	8
56	28	292	277	1.6	970	1061	650	93	0.16	0.28	2.4	24
0	44	23	112	2.4	680	53	0	0	0.17	0.03	3.8	10
4	37	55	101	0.6	628	636	40	12	0.18	0.08	2.3	14
4	35	55	97	0.5	607	620	360	42	0.18	0.08	2.3	13
29	32	103	118	0.5	489	697	380	44	0.23	0.11	1.4	20
170	28	48	130	1.6	635	1323	520	83	0.19	0.15	2.2	25
27	31	88	137	0.9	497	835	360	51	0.05	0.14	2.5	8
29	26	140	154	1.4	926	821	330	47	0.17	0.23	2.6	26
0	10	5	31	0.2	260	94	0	0	0.03	Tr	0.8	8
0	12	37	74	1.4	564	2	2650	265	0.08	0.19	1.0	12
0	20	64	86	3.4	505	12	54,040	5404	0.06	0.13	0.9	10
0	1	4	3	0.1	42	4	Tr	Tr	Tr	0.01	0.1	4
0	10	71	47	3.5	401	1560	40	4	0.05	0.05	0.3	35
0	3	48	12	0.8	25	66	30	3	0.01	0.04	0.1	([1])
0	7	34	33	8.1	386	297	160	16	0.67	1.04	3.6	3
0	2	54	27	1.5	307	43	3690	369	0.04	0.10	0.4	15
0	7	245	101	6.4	839	126	14,740	1474	0.17	0.42	0.9	18
0	10	277	91	2.9	566	163	14,790	1479	0.11	0.32	0.8	23
0	7	272	94	4.9	740	683[72]	18.780	1878	0.03	0.30	0.8	31
184	3	230	231	1.3	201	763	3460	675	0.09	0.30	0.5	3
0	8	49	70	0.6	346	2	520	52	0.08	0.07	0.9	10
0	18	29	41	0.7	896	2	7290	729	0.17	0.05	1.4	20
0	28	32	63	0.5	397	11	24,880	2488	0.08	0.14	0.7	28
0	37	32	41	0.8	278	20	25,750	2575	0.08	0.21	1.0	26
8	29	27	27	1.2	198	74	4400	440	0.02	0.04	0.4	7
0	59	77	133	3.4	536	191	38,570	3857	0.07	0.23	2.4	13
0	8	9	20	0.4	125	21	3190	319	0.01	0.02	0.3	11

[71]For green peppers; red peppers contain 121 mg ascorbic acid.
[72]With added salt; if none is added, sodium content is 58 mg.

Continued.

Item Number	Foods, Approximate Measures, Units, and Weight (Weight of Edible Portion Only)		Weight (grams)	Water (percent)	Food Energy (calories)	Protein (grams)	Fat (grams)	Fatty Acids Saturated (grams)	Fatty Acids Monounsaturated (grams)	Fatty Acids Polyunsaturated (grams)
	Vegetables and Vegetables Products—cont'd									
	Tomatoes									
868	Raw, 2⅗-in diam (3 per 12-oz pkg)	1 tomato	123	94	25	1	Tr	Tr	Tr	0.1
869	Canned, solids and liquid	1 cup	240	94	50	2	1	0.1	0.1	0.2
870	Tomato juice, canned	1 cup	244	94	40	2	Tr	Tr	Tr	0.1
	Tomato products, canned									
871	Paste	1 cup	262	74	220	10	2	0.3	0.4	0.9
872	Puree	1 cup	250	87	105	4	Tr	Tr	Tr	0.1
873	Sauce	1 cup	245	89	75	3	Tr	0.1	0.1	0.2
874	Turnips, cooked, diced	1 cup	156	94	30	1	Tr	Tr	Tr	0.1
	Turnip greens, cooked, drained									
875	From raw (leaves and stems)	1 cup	144	93	30	2	Tr	0.1	Tr	0.1
876	From frozen (chopped)	1 cup	164	90	50	5	1	0.2	Tr	0.3
877	Vegetable juice cocktail, canned	1 cup	242	94	45	2	Tr	Tr	Tr	0.1
	Vegetables, mixed									
878	Canned, drained solids	1 cup	163	87	75	4	Tr	0.1	Tr	0.2
879	Frozen, cooked, drained	1 cup	182	83	105	5	Tr	0.1	Tr	0.1
880	Waterchestnuts, canned	1 cup	140	86	70	1	Tr	Tr	Tr	Tr
	Miscellaneous Items									
	Baking powders for home use									
	Sodium aluminum sulfate									
881	With monocalcium phosphate monohydrate	1 tsp	3	2	5	Tr	0	0.0	0.0	0.0
882	With monocalcium phosphate monohydrate, calcium sulfate	1 tsp	2.9	1	5	Tr	0	0.0	0.0	0.0
883	Straight phosphate	1 tsp	3.8	2	5	Tr	0	0.0	0.0	0.0
884	Low sodium	1 tsp	4.3	1	5	Tr	0	0.0	0.0	0.0
885	Catsup	1 cup	273	69	290	5	1	0.2	0.2	0.4
886		1 tbsp	15	69	15	Tr	Tr	Tr	Tr	Tr
887	Celery seed	1 tsp	2	6	10	Tr	1	Tr	0.3	0.1
888	Chili powder	1 tsp	2.6	8	10	Tr	Tr	0.1	0.1	0.2
	Chocolate									
889	Bitter or baking	1 oz	28	2	145	3	15	9.0	4.9	0.5
	Semisweet; see Candy (item 715).									
890	Cinnamon	1 tsp	2.3	10	5	Tr	Tr	Tr	Tr	Tr
891	Curry powder	1 tsp	2	10	5	Tr	Tr	([1])	([1])	([1])
892	Garlic powder	1 tsp	2.8	6	10	Tr	Tr	Tr	Tr	Tr
893	Gelatin, dry	1 envelope	7	13	25	6	Tr	Tr	Tr	Tr
894	Mustard, prepared, yellow	1 tsp or individual pkt	5	80	5	Tr	Tr	Tr	0.2	Tr
	Olives, canned									
895	Green	4 medium or 3 extra large	13	78	15	Tr	2	0.2	1.2	0.1
896	Ripe, Mission, pitted	3 small or 2 large	9	73	15	Tr	2	0.3	1.3	0.2
897	Onion powder	1 tsp	2.1	5	5	Tr	Tr	Tr	Tr	Tr
898	Oregano	1 tsp	1.5	7	5	Tr	Tr	Tr	Tr	0.1
899	Paprika	1 tsp	2.1	10	5	Tr	Tr	Tr	Tr	0.2
900	Pepper, black	1 tsp	2.1	11	5	Tr	Tr	Tr	Tr	Tr
	Pickles, cucumber									
901	Dill, medium, whole, 3¾ in long, 1¼-in diam	1 pickle	65	93	5	Tr	Tr	Tr	Tr	0.1
902	Fresh-pack, slices 1½-in diam, ¼ in thick	2 slices	15	79	10	Tr	Tr	Tr	Tr	Tr
903	Sweet, gherkin, small, whole, about 2½ in long, ¾-in diam	1 pickle	15	61	20	Tr	Tr	Tr	Tr	Tr
	Popcorn (See Grain products, items 497-499)									
904	Relish, finely chopped, sweet	1 tbsp	15	63	20	Tr	Tr	Tr	Tr	Tr
905	Salt	1 tsp	5.5	0	0	0	0	0.0	0.0	0.0
906	Vinegar, cider	1 tbsp	15	94	Tr	Tr	0	0.0	0.0	0.0
	Yeast									
907	Baker's, dry, active	1 pkg	7	5	20	3	Tr	Tr	0.1	Tr
908	Brewer's, dry	1 tbsp	8	5	25	3	Tr	Tr	Tr	0.0

[1]Value not determined.
[73]For regular pack; special dietary pack contains 31 mg sodium.
[74]With added salt; if none is added, sodium content is 24 mg.
[75]With no added salt; if salt is added, sodium content is 2070 mg.

Cholesterol (mg)	Carbo-hydrate (grams)	Calcium (mg)	Phosphorus (mg)	Iron (mg)	Potassium (mg)	Sodium (mg)	Vitamin A Value (IU) International Units	Vitamin A Value (RE) Retinol Equivalents	Thiamin (mg)	Riboflavin (mg)	Niacin (mg)	Ascorbic Acid (mg)
0	5	9	28	0.6	255	10	1390	139	0.07	0.06	0.7	22
0	10	62	46	1.5	530	391[73]	1450	145	0.11	0.07	1.8	36
0	10	22	46	1.4	537	881[74]	1360	136	0.11	0.08	1.6	45
0	49	92	207	7.8	2442	170[75]	6470	647	0.41	0.50	8.4	111
0	25	38	100	2.3	1050	50[76]	3400	340	0.18	0.14	4.3	88
0	18	34	78	1.9	909	1482[77]	2400	240	0.16	0.14	2.8	32
0	8	34	30	0.3	211	78	0	0	0.04	0.04	0.5	18
0	6	197	42	1.2	292	42	7920	792	0.06	0.10	0.6	39
0	8	249	56	3.2	367	25	13,080	1308	0.09	0.12	0.8	36
0	11	27	41	1.0	467	883	2830	283	0.10	0.07	1.8	67
0	15	44	68	1.7	474	243	18,990	1899	0.08	0.08	0.9	8
0	24	46	93	1.5	308	64	7780	778	0.13	0.22	1.5	6
0	17	6	27	1.2	165	11	10	1	0.02	0.03	0.5	2
0	1	58	87	0.0	5	329	0	0	0.00	0.00	0.0	0
0	1	183	45	0.0	4	290	0	0	0.00	0.00	0.0	0
0	1	239	359	0.0	6	312	0	0	0.00	0.00	0.0	0
0	1	207	314	0.0	891	Tr	0	0	0.00	0.00	0.0	0
0	69	60	137	2.2	991	2845	3820	382	0.25	0.19	4.4	41
0	4	3	8	0.1	54	156	210	21	0.01	0.01	0.2	2
0	1	35	11	0.9	28	3	Tr	Tr	0.01	0.01	0.1	Tr
0	1	7	8	0.4	50	26	910	91	0.01	0.02	0.2	2
0	8	22	109	1.9	235	1	10	1	0.01	0.07	0.4	0
0	2	28	1	0.9	12	1	10	1	Tr	Tr	Tr	1
0	1	10	7	0.6	31	1	20	2	0.01	0.01	0.1	Tr
0	2	2	12	0.1	31	1	0	0	0.01	Tr	Tr	Tr
0	0	1	0	0.0	2	6	0	0	0.00	0.00	0.0	0
0	Tr	4	4	0.1	7	63	0	0	Tr	0.01	Tr	Tr
0	Tr	8	2	0.2	7	312	40	4	Tr	Tr	Tr	0
0	Tr	10	2	0.2	2	68	10	1	Tr	Tr	Tr	0
0	2	8	7	0.1	20	1	Tr	Tr	0.01	Tr	Tr	Tr
0	1	24	3	0.7	25	Tr	100	10	0.01	Tr	0.1	1
0	1	4	7	0.5	49	1	1270	127	0.01	0.04	0.3	1
0	1	9	4	0.6	26	1	Tr	Tr	Tr	0.01	Tr	0
0	1	17	14	0.7	130	928	70	7	Tr	0.01	Tr	4
0	3	5	4	0.3	30	101	20	2	Tr	Tr	Tr	1
0	5	2	2	0.2	30	107	10	1	Tr	Tr	Tr	1
0	5	3	2	0.1	30	107	20	2	Tr	Tr	0.0	1
0	0	14	3	Tr	Tr	2132	0	0	0.00	0.00	0.0	0
0	1	1	1	0.1	15	Tr	0	0	0.00	0.00	0.0	0
0	3	3	90	1.1	140	4	Tr	Tr	0.16	0.38	2.6	Tr
0	3	17[78]	140	1.4	152	10	Tr	Tr	1.25	0.34	3.0	Tr

[76]With no added salt; if salt is added, sodium content is 998 mg.
[77]With salt added.
[78]Value may vary from 6 to 60 mg.

APPENDIX

G Nutritive Value of Fast Food Items

	Weight (g)	Energy (kcal)	Protein (g)	Carbohydrate (g)	Fat (g)	Cholesterol (mg)	Vitamins		
							A (IU)	B_1 (mg)	B_2 (mg)
Arby's									
Roast Beef, reg	147	350	22	32	15.0	39.0	X	0.23	0.43
Roast Beef, jr	86	218	12	22	8.0	20.0	X	0.15	0.26
Roast Beef, super	234	501	25	50	22.0	40.0	750	0.38	0.60
Roast Beef, deluxe	247	486	26	43	23.0	59.0	X	0.30	0.34
Beef 'n Cheddar®	190	490	24	51	21.0	51.0	X	0.12	0.34
Chicken Breast Sandwich	210	592	28	56	27.0	57.0	X	0.23	0.26
Potato Cakes (2)	85	201	2	22	14.0	1.3	X	0.09	X
French Fries	71	211	2	33	8.0	6.0	X	0.09	X
King Roast Beef	192	467	27	44	19.0	49.0	100	0.30	0.60
Bac'n Cheddar Deluxe	225	561	28	36	34.0	78.0	X	0.15	0.26
Hot Ham 'n Cheese	161	353	26	33	13.0	50.0	200	0.98	0.51
Turkey Deluxe	197	375	24	32	17.0	39.0	300	0.23	0.43
Baked Potato, Plain	312	290	8	66	0.5	0	X	0.30	0.14
Superstuffed Potato, Deluxe	312	648	18	59	38.0	72.0	1000	0.23	0.43
Broccoli and Cheddar	340	541	13	72	22.0	24.0	500	0.30	0.34
Mushroom and Cheese	300	506	16	61	22.0	21.0	750	0.23	0.43
Taco	425	619	23	73	27.0	145.0	3000	0.38	0.26
Vanilla Shake	250	295	8	44	10.0	30.0	400	0.12	0.60
Chocolate Shake	300	384	9	62	11.0	32.0	400	0.12	0.60
Jamocha Shake	305	424	8	76	10.0	31.0	300	0.09	0.51
Roasted Chicken Breast	150	254	43	2	7.0	200.0	—	—	—
Roasted Chicken Leg	161	319	41	1	16.0	214.0	—	—	—
Chicken Salad Sandwich	156	386	18	33	20.0	30.0	—	—	—
Chicken Salad & Croissant	150	472	22	16	36.0	12.0	—	—	—
Chicken Salad w/Tomato & Lettuce	270	515	25	24	36.0	12.0	—	—	—
Chicken Club Sandwich	210	621	26	57	32.0	108.0	—	—	—
Rice Pilaf	120	123	3	23	2.0	—	—	—	—
Scandinavian Vegetables, sauce	120	56	2	9	2.0	—	—	—	—
Tossed Salad, plain	210	44	3	7	tr	0	—	—	—
Tossed Salad w/20 Calorie Italian Drsg	240	57	3	9	1.0	0	—	—	—

Source: Arby's, Inc, Atlanta, Georgia. Nutritional analyses by Arby's Laboratory and other independent testing laboratories.

	Weight (g)	Energy (kcal)	Protein (g)	Carbohydrate (g)	Fat (g)	Cholesterol (mg)	A (IU)	B_1 (mg)	B_2 (mg)
Burger King									
Whopper Sandwich®	265	640	27	42	41	94	618	0.33	0.41
Whopper® w/Cheese	289	723	31	43	48	117	1001	0.34	0.48
Double Beef Whopper®	351	850	46	52	52	—	617	0.34	0.56
Double Beef Whopper® w/Cheese	374	950	51	54	60	—	1001	0.35	0.63
Whopper Junior®	136	370	15	31	17	41	296	0.23	0.25
Whopper Junior® w/Cheese	158	420	17	32	20	52	488	0.23	0.29
Hamburger	109	275	15	29	12	37	150	0.23	0.25

From Dietetic Currents 13:6, 1988.

Dashes indicate no data available; however, the food item usually provides some amount of the nutrients.

X indicates less than 2% U.S. RDA.

Tr = trace

Vitamins					Minerals									
Nia. (mg)	B_6 (mg)	B_{12} (μg)	C (mg)	D (IU)	Ca (mg)	Cu (mg)	Fe (mg)	K (mg)	Mg (mg)	P (mg)	Na (mg)	Zn (mg)	Moisture (g)	Crude Fiber (g)
7.6	—	—	X	—	80	—	3.6	—	—	—	590	—	—	—
4.0	—	—	X	—	40	—	1.8	—	—	—	345	—	—	—
9.0	—	—	36.0	—	100	—	4.5	—	—	—	800	—	—	—
5.0	—	—	X	—	100	—	6.3	—	—	—	1288	—	—	—
5.0	—	—	X	—	80	—	5.4	—	—	—	1520	—	—	—
10.0	—	—	X	—	100	—	3.6	—	—	—	1340	—	—	—
1.6	—	—	3.6	—	X	—	1.1	—	—	—	425	—	—	—
2.0	—	—	6.0	—	X	—	1.1	—	—	—	30	—	—	—
10.0	—	—	2.4	—	100	—	4.5	—	—	—	765	—	—	—
6.0	—	—	3.6	—	100	—	2.7	—	—	—	1385	—	—	—
6.0	—	—	24.0	—	200	—	1.8	—	—	—	1655	—	—	—
12.0	—	—	4.8	—	80	—	2.7	—	—	—	850	—	—	—
5.0	—	—	63.0	—	20	—	1.8	—	—	—	12	—	—	—
6.0	—	—	63.0	—	300	—	2.7	—	—	—	475	—	—	—
6.0	—	—	63.0	—	150	—	2.7	—	—	—	475	—	—	—
7.0	—	—	63.0	—	300	—	2.7	—	—	—	635	—	—	—
8.0	—	—	63.0	—	450	—	3.6	—	—	—	1065	—	—	—
X	—	—	2.4	—	300	—	0.7	—	—	—	245	—	—	—
0.4	—	—	2.4	—	300	—	1.1	—	—	—	300	—	—	—
3.0	—	—	X	—	300	—	1.1	—	—	—	280	—	—	—
—	—	—	—	—	—	—	—	—	—	—	930	—	—	—
—	—	—	—	—	—	—	—	—	—	—	995	—	—	—
—	—	—	—	—	—	—	—	—	—	—	630	—	—	—
—	—	—	—	—	—	—	—	—	—	—	725	—	—	—
—	—	—	—	—	—	—	—	—	—	—	745	—	—	—
—	—	—	—	—	—	—	—	—	—	—	1300	—	—	—
—	—	—	—	—	—	—	—	—	—	—	438	—	—	—
—	—	—	—	—	—	—	—	—	—	—	465	—	—	—
—	—	—	—	—	—	—	—	—	—	—	23	—	—	—
—	—	—	—	—	—	—	—	—	—	—	465	—	—	—
7.0	—	—	14	—	80	0.14	4.9	547	43	237	842	4.50	—	—
7.0	—	—	14	—	210	0.14	4.9	570	47	360	1126	5.10	—	—
10.0	—	—	14	—	91	0.18	7.3	760	60	387	1080	8.50	—	—
10.0	—	—	14	—	222	0.18	7.3	730	65	510	1535	9.10	—	—
4.0	—	—	6	—	40	0.07	2.8	275	24	127	486	2.30	—	—
4.0	—	—	6	—	105	0.07	2.8	287	27	189	628	2.60	—	—
4.0	—	—	3	—	37	0.06	2.7	235	23	124	509	2.40	—	—

Continued.

	Weight (g)	Energy (kcal)	Protein (g)	Carbohydrate (g)	Fat (g)	Cholesterol (mg)	Vitamins		
							A (IU)	B_1 (mg)	B_2 (mg)
Burger King—cont'd									
Cheeseburger	120	317	17	30	15	48	341	0.23	0.29
Bacon Double Cheeseburger	159	510	33	27	31	104	384	0.31	0.42
French Fries, reg	74	227	3	24	13	14	X	0.10	0.30
Onion Rings, reg	79	274	4	28	16	0	X	X	X
Apple Pie	125	305	3	44	12	4	X	0.27	0.16
Chocolate Shake, med	273	320	8	46	12	—	X	0.13	0.55
Vanilla Shake, med	273	321	9	49	10	—	X	0.11	0.57
Vanilla Shake, added syrup	284	334	9	51	10	—	—	—	—
Chocolate Shake, added syrup	284	374	8	60	11	—	X	0.12	0.51
Whaler® Fish Sandwich	189	488	19	45	27	84	36	0.28	0.21
Whaler® w/Cheese	201	530	21	46	30	95	227	0.27	0.24
Ham and Cheese	230	471	24	44	23	70	725	0.87	0.42
Chicken Sandwich	230	688	26	56	40	82	126	0.45	0.31
Chicken Tenders®	95	204	20	10	10	47	95	0.08	0.08
B'kfast Croissanwich®									
Bacon, Egg, Cheese	119	355	15	20	24	249	426	0.32	0.30
Sausage, Egg, Cheese	163	538	19	20	41	293	426	0.36	0.32
Ham, Egg, Cheese	145	335	18	20	20	262	426	0.49	0.32
Scrambled Egg Platter	195	468	14	33	30	370	375	0.31	0.35
Scrambled Egg Platter w/Sausage	247	702	22	33	52	420	375	0.42	0.40
w/Bacon	206	536	18	33	36	378	375	0.39	0.38
French Toast Platter w/Bacon	117	469	11	41	30	73	X	0.24	0.24
w/Sausage	158	635	16	41	46	115	X	0.29	0.27
Salad, plain	148	28	2	5	0	0	1583	0.06	0.12
w/House Dressing	176	159	3	8	13	11	1604	0.06	0.15
w/Bleu Cheese	176	184	3	7	16	22	1638	0.06	0.15
w/1000 Island	176	145	2	9	12	17	1659	0.06	0.13
w/French	176	152	2	13	11	0	1689	0.06	0.12
w/Golden Italian	176	162	2	7	14	0	1598	0.05	0.12
w/Creamy Italian	176	—	—	—	—	—	—	—	—
w/Reduced-Calorie Italian	176	42	2	7	1	0	1591	0.05	0.12
Cherry Pie	128	357	4	55	13	6	370	0.24	0.16
Pecan Pie	113	459	5	64	20	4	X	0.28	0.18

Source: Burger King Corp Inc. Nutritional analyses by Hazelton Laboratory of America (formerly Raltech Scientific Services Inc), Madison, Wisconsin, and Campbell Labor-

	Weight (g)	Energy (kcal)	Protein (g)	Carbohydrate (g)	Fat (g)	Cholesterol (mg)	A (IU)	B_1 (mg)	B_2 (mg)
Church's									
Fried Chicken									
Breast	93	278	21	9	17	—	—	—	—
Wing-Breast Cut	97	303	22	9	20	—	—	—	—
Thigh	93	306	19	9	22	—	—	—	—
Leg	56	147	13	5	9	—	—	—	—
Crispy Nuggets®									
Regular	18	55	3	4	3	—	—	—	—
Spicy	18	52	3	3	3	—	—	—	—
Southern Fried Catfish®	21	67	4	4	4	—	—	—	—
Hush Puppies	23	78	1	12	3	—	—	—	—
Dinner Roll	30	83	2	15	2	—	—	—	—
French Fries	90	256	4	31	13	—	—	—	—
Corn on the Cob (buttered)	270	165	5	29	3	—	—	—	—
Jalapeno Pepper	—	4	1	1	1	—	—	—	—
Pecan Pie	90	367	4	44	20	—	—	—	—
Cole Slaw	90	83	1	6	7	—	—	—	—

Source: Church's Fried Chicken, San Antonio, Texas. Nutrient analyses of chicken and catfish by Texas Testing Laboratories Inc, San Antonio; of hush puppies, Pioneer

Vitamins					Minerals									
Nia. (mg)	B_6 (mg)	B_{12} (μg)	C (mg)	D (IU)	Ca (mg)	Cu (mg)	Fe (mg)	K (mg)	Mg (mg)	P (mg)	Na (mg)	Zn (mg)	Moisture (g)	Crude Fiber (g)
4.0	—	—	3	—	102	0.06	3.8	247	26	186	651	2.60	—	—
6.0	—	—	X	—	168	0.09	3.8	363	37	328	728	5.10	—	—
7.5	—	—	X	—	X	0.08	0.5	360	21	114	160	X	—	—
X	—	—	X	—	124	0.09	0.8	173	18	195	665	0.40	—	—
0.6	—	—	5	—	X	X	1.2	122	X	31	412	X	—	—
X	—	—	X	—	260	0.09	1.6	567	46	262	202	1.00	—	—
X	—	—	X	—	295	X	X	505	32	284	205	1.00	—	—
—	—	—	—	—	—	—	—	524	—	—	213	—	—	—
X	—	—	X	—	248	0.16	1.6	590	56	264	225	1.05	—	—
4.0	—	—	X	—	X	0.11	2.2	366	40	249	592	0.09	—	—
4.0	—	—	X	—	112	0.11	2.2	378	43	311	734	1.10	—	—
6.0	—	—	7	—	195	0.12	3.2	419	42	384	1534	2.40	—	—
10.0	—	—	X	—	79	0.16	3.3	375	54	274	1423	1.20	—	—
7.0	—	—	X	—	18	0.07	0.7	200	24	236	636	0.60	—	—
2.0	—	—	X	—	136	X	2.0	182	20	249	762	1.50	—	—
4.0	—	—	X	—	145	X	2.9	284	19	292	1042	2.40	—	—
3.0	—	—	X	—	136	X	2.2	256	24	317	987	1.90	—	—
3.0	—	—	3	—	102	0.06	2.7	487	32	271	808	1.50	—	—
5.0	—	—	3	—	112	0.06	3.7	623	33	335	1213	2.70	—	—
4.0	—	—	3	—	103	0.06	2.8	532	35	299	975	1.90	—	—
3.0	—	—	X	—	59	0.01	2.7	151	19	118	448	1.30	—	—
6.0	—	—	X	—	70	X	3.7	242	18	164	686	2.30	—	—
1.0	—	—	42	—	37	0.12	1.2	382	27	57	23	0.42	—	—
1.0	—	—	42	—	44	0.11	1.3	402	27	74	293	0.52	—	—
1.0	—	—	42	—	66	0.12	1.3	382	29	83	333	0.59	—	—
1.0	—	—	43	—	42	0.12	1.4	405	28	66	251	0.50	—	—
1.0	—	—	43	—	40	0.12	1.4	410	28	60	330	0.45	—	—
1.0	—	—	42	—	40	0.12	1.3	389	28	60	292	0.43	—	—
—	—	—	—	—	—	—	—	—	—	—	—	—	—	—
1.0	—	—	42	—	40	0.12	1.4	390	30	59	430	0.42	—	—
0.5	—	—	8	—	X	X	1.1	166	12	37	204	X	—	—
0.6	—	—	X	—	24	0.14	1.1	204	16	84	374	X	—	—

atories, Camden, New Jersey.

—	—	—	—	—	—	—	—	—	—	—	560	—	43	0
—	—	—	—	—	—	—	—	—	—	—	583	—	45	0
—	—	—	—	—	—	—	—	—	—	—	448	—	42	0
—	—	—	—	—	—	—	—	—	—	—	286	—	29	0
—	—	—	—	—	—	—	—	—	—	—	125	—	8	0
—	—	—	—	—	—	—	—	—	—	—	91	—	8	0
—	—	—	—	—	—	—	—	—	—	—	151	—	9	0
—	—	—	—	—	—	—	—	—	—	—	55	—	7	0
—	—	—	—	—	—	—	—	—	—	—	—	—	—	—
—	—	—	—	—	—	—	—	—	—	—	—	—	—	—
—	—	—	—	—	—	—	—	—	—	—	—	—	—	—
—	—	—	—	—	—	—	—	—	—	—	—	—	—	—
—	—	—	—	—	—	—	—	—	—	—	—	—	—	—
—	—	—	—	—	—	—	—	—	—	—	—	—	—	—

Flour Mills Inc, San Antonio. Other products calculated from Pennington JA, Church HN (eds): *Food Values of Portions Commonly Used*, ed 14, Harper & Row, 1985.

Continued.

	Weight (g)	Energy (kcal)	Protein (g)	Carbohydrate (g)	Fat (g)	Cholesterol (mg)	Vitamins		
							A (IU)	B_1 (mg)	B_2 (mg)
Dairy Queen									
Cone, sm	85	140	3	22	4	10	100	0.03	0.17
Cone, reg	142	240	6	38	7	15	200	0.06	0.34
Cone, lg	213	340	9	57	10	25	400	0.12	0.51
Dipped Cone, sm	92	190	3	25	9	10	100	0.03	0.17
Dipped Cone, reg	156	340	6	42	16	20	200	0.06	0.34
Dipped Cone, lg	234	510	9	64	24	30	400	0.12	0.51
Sundae, sm	106	190	3	33	4	10	100	0.03	0.17
Sundae, reg	177	310	5	56	8	20	200	0.06	0.34
Sundae, lg	248	440	8	78	10	30	400	0.12	0.43
Shake, sm	291	490	10	82	13	35	500	0.15	0.60
Shake, reg	418	710	14	120	19	50	750	0.23	0.77
Shake, lg	588	990	19	168	26	70	1000	0.30	1.02
Malt, sm	291	520	10	91	13	35	500	0.15	0.60
Malt, reg	418	760	14	134	18	50	750	0.30	0.85
Malt, lg	588	1060	20	187	25	70	1000	0.38	1.19
Float	397	410	5	82	7	20	200	0.06	0.26
Banana Split	383	540	9	103	11	30	750	0.15	0.51
Parfait	283	430	8	76	8	30	400	0.09	0.43
Peanut Buster Parfait	305	740	16	94	34	30	300	0.15	0.43
Double Delight	255	490	9	69	20	25	300	0.15	0.34
Hot Fudge Brownie Delight	266	600	9	85	25	20	300	0.12	0.34
Strawberry Shortcake	312	540	10	100	11	25	400	0.23	0.51
Freeze	397	500	9	89	12	30	400	0.15	0.51
Mr. Misty®, sm	248	190	0	48	0	0	X	X	X
Mr. Misty®, reg	330	250	0	63	0	0	X	X	X
Mr. Misty®, lg	439	340	0	84	0	0	X	X	X
Mr. Misty® Kiss	89	70	0	17	0	0	X	X	X
Mr. Misty® Freeze	411	500	9	91	12	30	400	0.12	0.51
Mr. Misty® Float	411	390	5	74	7	20	200	0.06	0.26
Buster Bar	149	460	10	41	29	10	100	0.12	0.17
Dilly Bar	85	210	3	21	13	10	100	0.03	0.17
DQ Sandwich	60	140	3	24	4	5	X	0.03	0.07
Single Hamburger	148	360	21	33	16	45	100	0.30	0.17
Double Hamburger	210	530	36	33	28	85	100	0.45	0.34
Triple Hamburger	272	710	51	33	45	135	200	0.60	0.51
Single w/Cheese	162	410	24	33	20	50	200	0.30	0.17
Double w/Cheese	239	650	43	34	37	95	400	0.45	0.43
Triple w/Cheese	301	820	58	34	50	145	400	0.60	0.60
Hot Dog	100	280	11	21	16	45	X	0.12	0.14
Hot Dog w/Chili	128	320	13	23	20	55	X	0.15	0.26
Hot Dog w/Cheese	114	330	15	21	21	55	100	0.12	0.17
Super Hot Dog	175	520	17	44	27	80	X	0.23	0.26
Super Hot Dog w/Chili	218	570	21	47	32	100	X	0.23	0.43
Super Hot Dog w/Cheese	196	580	22	45	34	100	100	0.23	0.26
Fish Filet Sandwich	170	400	20	41	17	50	X	0.15	0.26
Fish Filet Sandwich w/Cheese	177	440	24	39	21	60	100	0.15	0.26
Chicken Sandwich	220	670	29	46	41	75	X	0.06	X
French Fries, sm	71	200	2	25	10	10	X	0.06	X
French Fries, lg	113	320	3	40	16	15	X	0.09	0.03
Onion Rings	85	280	4	31	16	15	X	0.09	X

Source: International Dairy Queen, Inc, Minneapolis, Minnesota. Nutrient analyses by Hazelton Laboratory of America (formerly Raltech Scientific Services Inc),

	Weight (g)	Energy (kcal)	Protein (g)	Carbohydrate (g)	Fat (g)	Cholesterol (mg)	A (IU)	B_1 (mg)	B_2 (mg)
Hardee's									
Hamburger	110	305	17	29	13	45	57	0.55	0.58
Cheeseburger	116	335	17	29	17	50	749	0.51	0.32
Big Deluxe®	248	546	29	48	26	77	398	0.50	0.73
¼-Pound Cheeseburger®	190	506	28	41	26	61	508	0.35	0.60
Roast Beef Sandwich	143	377	21	36	17	57	542	0.93	0.19
Big Roast Beef®	167	418	28	34	19	60	648	1.03	0.22

Vitamins					Minerals									
Nia. (mg)	B_6 (mg)	B_{12} (μg)	C (mg)	D (IU)	Ca (mg)	Cu (mg)	Fe (mg)	K (mg)	Mg (mg)	P (mg)	Na (mg)	Zn (mg)	Moisture (g)	Crude Fiber (g)
X	—	0.36	X	—	100	—	0.4	—	—	100	45	—	—	—
X	—	0.60	X	—	150	—	0.7	—	—	200	80	—	—	—
X	—	0.90	X	—	250	—	1.4	—	—	300	115	—	—	—
X	—	0.36	X	—	100	—	0.4	—	—	100	55	—	—	—
X	—	0.60	X	—	150	—	0.7	—	—	200	100	—	—	—
X	—	0.90	X	—	250	—	1.4	—	—	300	145	—	—	—
X	—	0.36	X	—	100	—	0.4	—	—	150	75	—	—	—
X	—	0.60	X	—	200	—	1.1	—	—	200	120	—	—	—
X	—	0.90	X	—	250	—	1.4	—	—	300	165	—	—	—
X	—	1.20	X	—	350	—	1.8	—	—	400	180	—	—	—
0.4	—	1.80	X	—	450	—	2.7	—	—	500	260	—	—	—
0.8	—	2.40	X	—	700	—	3.6	—	—	800	360	—	—	—
0.4	—	1.20	X	—	350	—	2.7	—	—	400	180	—	—	—
0.8	—	2.10	X	—	450	—	4.5	—	—	600	260	—	—	—
1.2	—	2.70	X	—	700	—	5.4	—	—	800	360	—	—	—
X	—	0.60	X	—	200	—	1.1	—	—	200	85	—	—	—
0.4	—	0.90	15.0	—	250	—	1.8	—	—	350	150	—	—	—
X	—	0.90	3.6	—	250	—	1.4	—	—	300	140	—	—	—
2.0	—	0.90	X	—	250	—	1.8	—	—	450	250	—	—	—
0.4	—	0.90	X	—	200	—	1.4	—	—	300	150	—	—	—
X	—	0.60	X	—	200	—	1.8	—	—	300	225	—	—	—
X	—	0.24	12.0	—	250	—	1.8	—	—	300	215	—	—	—
X	—	0.90	X	—	300	—	1.8	—	—	350	180	—	—	—
X	—	X	X	—	X	—	X	—	—	X	10	—	—	—
X	—	X	X	—	X	—	X	—	—	X	10	—	—	—
X	—	X	X	—	X	—	X	—	—	X	10	—	—	—
X	—	X	X	—	X	—	X	—	—	X	10	—	—	—
X	—	0.60	X	—	300	—	1.4	—	—	200	140	—	—	—
X	—	0.60	X	—	200	—	0.7	—	—	200	95	—	—	—
2.0	—	0.36	X	—	100	—	1.1	—	—	250	175	—	—	—
X	—	0.24	X	—	100	—	0.4	—	—	100	50	—	—	—
0.4	—	0.12	X	—	60	—	X	—	—	60	40	—	—	—
5.0	—	0.50	X	—	100	—	3.6	—	—	150	630	—	—	—
9.0	—	2.70	X	—	100	—	6.3	—	—	300	660	—	—	—
14.0	—	4.20	X	—	100	—	9.0	—	—	450	690	—	—	—
5.0	—	1.80	X	—	200	—	3.6	—	—	250	790	—	—	—
9.0	—	3.00	X	—	350	—	6.3	—	—	500	980	—	—	—
14.0	—	4.80	X	—	350	—	9.0	—	—	700	1010	—	—	—
3.0	—	0.90	X	—	80	—	1.4	—	—	80	830	—	—	—
4.0	—	1.20	X	—	80	—	1.8	—	—	150	985	—	—	—
3.0	—	1.20	X	—	150	—	1.4	—	—	200	990	—	—	—
5.0	—	1.50	X	—	150	—	2.7	—	—	150	1365	—	—	—
6.0	—	1.8	X	—	150	—	2.7	—	—	250	1595	—	—	—
5.0	—	1.8	X	—	250	—	1.4	—	—	300	1605	—	—	—
3.0	—	1.2	X	—	60	—	0.7	—	—	200	875	—	—	—
3.0	—	1.5	X	—	150	—	0.4	—	—	250	1035	—	—	—
0.8	—	X	9	—	X	—	0.4	—	—	60	870	—	—	—
0.8	—	X	9	—	X	—	0.34	—	—	60	115	—	—	—
1.2	—	X	15	—	X	—	1.08	—	—	100	185	—	—	—
0.4	—	X	2.4	—	20	—	0.72	—	—	60	140	—	—	—

Madison, Wisconsin.

6.4	—	—	2.0	—	23	—	3.6	231	—	—	682	—	—	—
5.5	—	—	2.0	—	48	—	2.7	197	—	—	789	—	—	—
10.6	—	—	42.0	—	98	—	6.7	594	—	—	1083	—	—	—
14.0	—	—	33.0	—	103	—	6.5	887	—	—	1950	—	—	—
3.7	—	—	3.0	—	55	—	6.3	205	—	—	1030	—	—	—
5.2	—	—	8.0	—	74	—	8.1	470	—	—	1770	—	—	—

Continued.

G

	Weight (g)	Energy (kcal)	Protein (g)	Carbohydrate (g)	Fat (g)	Cholesterol (mg)	Vitamins A (IU)	Vitamins B$_1$ (mg)	Vitamins B$_2$ (mg)
Hardee's—cont'd									
Hot Dog	120	346	11	26	22	42	tr	0.29	0.22
Hot Ham & Cheese	148	376	23	37	15	59	178	0.37	0.74
Fisherman's Fillet Sandwich®	196	514	20	50	26	41	1152	1.33	1.51
Chicken Fillet	192	510	27	42	26	57	1098	0.52	0.63
Bacon Cheeseburger	224	686	35	42	42	295	832	0.04	0.40
Sausage Biscuit	1123	413	10	34	26	29	45	0.36	0.22
Sausage & Egg Biscuit	162	521	16	34	35	293	755	0.41	0.37
Steak Biscuit	134	419	14	41	23	34	62	0.34	0.43
Steak & Egg Biscuit	162	527	20	41	31	298	772	0.39	0.58
Ham Biscuit	108	349	12	37	17	29	127	0.60	0.42
Ham & Egg Biscuit	184	458	19	37	26	293	837	0.65	0.57
Bacon & Egg Biscuit	114	405	13	30	26	305	145	0.10	0.17
French Fries, sm	71	239	3	28	13	4	tr	0.07	0.03
French Fries, lg	113	381	5	44	21	6	tr	0.11	0.05
Apple Turnover	87	282	3	37	14	5	tr	0.03	0.04
Milkshake	326	391	11	63	10	42	0	0.20	0

Source: Hardee's Food Systems Inc, Rocky Mount, North Carolina. Nutrient analyses by Webb Food Laboratory, Raleigh, North Carolina.

	Weight (g)	Energy (kcal)	Protein (g)	Carbohydrate (g)	Fat (g)	Cholesterol (mg)	Vitamins A (IU)	Vitamins B$_1$ (mg)	Vitamins B$_2$ (mg)
Jack in the Box									
Hamburger	98.0	276	13.0	30.0	12	29.0	50	0.36	0.24
Cheeseburger	113.0	323	16.0	32.0	15	42.0	300	0.36	0.27
Jumbo Jack®	205.0	485	26.0	38.0	26	64.0	348	0.51	0.21
Jumbo Jack® w/Cheese	—	630	32.0	45.0	35	110.0	750	0.53	0.34
Bacon Cheeseburger Supreme	231.0	724	34.0	44.0	46	70.0	600	0.56	0.51
Swiss & Bacon Burger	—	643	33.0	31.0	43	99.0	400	0.45	0.41
Ham & Swiss Burger	—	638	36.0	37.0	39	117.0	430	0.76	0.48
Mushroom Burger	178.7	477	28.0	30.0	27	87.0	375	0.43	0.28
Moby Jack®	137.0	444	16.0	39.0	25	47.0	300	0.40	0.25
Regular Taco	81.0	191	8.0	16.0	11	21.0	400	0.07	0.17
Super Taco	135.0	288	12.0	21.0	17	37.0	600	0.12	0.08
Club Pita	177.0	284	22.0	30.0	8	43.0	250	0.78	0.29
Chicken Supreme	228.0	601	31.0	39.0	36	60.0	450	0.52	0.37
Supreme Crescent	146.0	547	20.0	27.0	40	178.0	550	0.64	0.54
Sausage Crescent	156.0	584	22.0	28.0	43	187.0	550	0.60	0.51
Pancakes Breakfast	630.0	626	16.0	79.0	27	85.0	500	0.60	0.43
Scrambled Eggs Breakfast	720.0	719	26.0	55.0	44	260.0	750	0.68	0.59
Breakfast Jack®	126.0	307	18.0	30.0	13	203.0	450	0.47	0.41
Cooked Bacon, 2 slices	—	70	3.0	0	6	10.0	X	0.03	0.03
Chicken Strips Dinner	180.0	689	40.0	65.0	30	100.0	150	0.45	0.29
Shrimp Dinner	165.0	731	22.0	77.0	37	157.0	150	0.39	0.17
Sirloin Steak Dinner	—	699	38.0	75.0	27	75.0	150	0.68	0.51
Cheese Nachos	—	571	15.0	49.0	35	37.0	500	0.11	0.19
Supreme Nachos	—	718	23.0	66.0	40	65.0	1000	0.15	0.26
Canadian Crescent	134.0	472	18.6	24.6	31	226.0	523	0.50	0.40
Pasta Seafood Salad	15.0	394	15.0	32.0	22	47.5	2330	0.38	0.23
Taco Salad	358.0	377	31.0	10.0	24	102.0	1150	0.18	0.53
French Fries, reg	68.0	221	2.0	27.0	12	8.0	X	0.07	0.03
Onion Rings	108.0	382	5.0	39.0	23	27.0	X	0.21	0.12
Hash Brown Potatoes	90.0	68	2.0	15.0	0	0	X	0.03	X
Vanilla Shake	317.0	320	10.0	57.0	6	25.0	X	0.15	0.34
Strawberry Shake	328.0	320	10.0	55.0	7	25.0	—	0.15	0.43
Chocolate Shake	322.0	330	11.0	55.0	7	25.0	—	0.15	0.59
Apple Turnover	119.0	410	4.0	45.0	24	15.0	X	0.23	0.10

Source: Jack in the Box Restaurants, Foodmaker, Inc, San Diego, California. Nutrient analyses by Hazelton Laboratory of America (formerly Raltech Scientific Services Inc),

Vitamins					Minerals									
Nia. (mg)	B_6 (mg)	B_{12} (μg)	C (mg)	D (IU)	Ca (mg)	Cu (mg)	Fe (mg)	K (mg)	Mg (mg)	P (mg)	Na (mg)	Zn (mg)	Moisture (g)	Crude Fiber (g)
4.2	—	—	0	—	43	—	2.5	120	—	—	744	—	—	—
2.5	—	—	1.0	—	207	—	3.8	317	—	—	1067	—	—	—
7.2	—	—	5.0	—	88	—	5.1	574	—	—	314	—	—	—
9.5	—	—	12.0	—	83	—	4.8	334	—	—	360	—	—	—
6.4	—	—	3.0	—	152	—	6.3	339	—	—	1074	—	—	—
2.8	—	—	1.0	—	139	—	2.8	217	—	—	864	—	—	—
2.9	—	—	1.0	—	169	—	4.0	287	—	—	1033	—	—	—
3.3	—	—	1.0	—	121	—	4.6	265	—	—	804	—	—	—
3.4	—	—	1.0	—	151	—	5.8	335	—	—	973	—	—	—
1.8	—	—	1.0	—	181	—	3.2	235	—	—	1415	—	—	—
1.9	—	—	1.0	—	211	—	4.0	305	—	—	1584	—	—	—
1.8	—	—	2.1	—	144	—	3.0	12	—	—	823	—	—	—
1.0	—	—	10.0	—	14	—	1.0	433	—	—	121	—	—	—
0.6	—	—	16.0	—	22	—	1.0	689	—	—	192	—	—	—
0.4	—	—	21.67	—	19	—	1.0	17	—	—	—	—	—	—
0.2	—	—	0	—	450	—	1.0	652	—	—	—	—	—	—
3.20	—	—	1.2	—	70	—	2.7	—	—	—	521	—	—	—
3.30	—	—	1.2	—	160	—	2.7	—	—	—	749	—	—	—
7.03	—	—	5.1	—	97	—	6.9	—	—	—	905	—	—	—
12.0	—	—	4.8	—	250	—	4.5	—	—	—	1665	—	—	—
8.80	—	—	3.0	—	310	—	4.9	—	—	—	1307	—	—	—
6.8	—	—	3.0	—	230	—	4.7	—	—	—	1354	—	—	—
7.6	—	—	9.8	—	268	—	6.1	—	—	—	1330	—	121.0	0
7.7	—	—	2.8	—	220	—	5.3	—	—	—	906	—	88.3	1
2.80	—	—	X	—	160	—	2.2	—	—	—	820	—	—	—
1.00	—	—	X	—	100	—	1.1	—	—	—	406	—	—	—
1.40	—	—	1.8	—	150	—	1.6	—	—	—	765	—	—	—
5.89	—	—	4.2	—	80	—	2.5	—	—	—	953	—	—	—
10.6	—	—	4.2	—	240	—	3.0	—	—	—	1582	—	—	—
4.2	—	—	X	—	150	—	2.7	—	—	—	1053	—	—	—
4.6	—	—	X	—	170	—	2.9	—	—	—	1012	—	—	—
5.0	—	—	27.0	—	100	—	2.7	—	—	—	1670	—	—	—
5.0	—	—	12.0	80	250	—	0.24	—	635	—	1110	—	—	—
3.0	—	—	X	4	170	—	3.1	—	—	—	871	—	—	—
0.8	—	—	4.0	—	1	—	0.38	—	—	—	226	—	—	—
18.6	—	—	12.0	—	110	—	4.0	—	—	—	1213	—	—	—
7.0	—	—	12.0	—	370	—	4.9	—	—	—	1510	—	—	—
12.4	—	—	7.8	—	220	—	9.5	—	—	—	969	—	—	—
1.0	—	—	3.0	—	370	—	1.4	—	—	—	1154	—	—	—
3.2	—	—	8.4	—	410	—	3.2	—	—	—	1782	—	—	—
3.6	—	—	3.1	—	125	—	3.4	—	—	—	851	—	56.1	0.5
1.8	—	—	21.0	—	208	—	5.9	—	—	—	1570	—	338.0	2.0
6.0	—	—	6.6	—	280	—	4.3	—	—	—	1436	—	—	—
1.2	—	—	3.0	2	10	—	0.5	—	—	—	164	—	—	—
1.8	—	—	3.0	3	30	—	1.4	—	—	—	407	—	—	—
0.8	—	—	3.6	—	X	—	0.7	—	—	—	15	—	—	—
4.0	—	—	X	—	350	—	—	—	—	—	230	—	—	—
4.0	—	—	3.3	—	350	—	0.4	—	—	—	240	—	—	—
4.0	—	—	3.2	—	350	—	0.7	—	—	—	270	—	—	—
2.0	—	—	X	—	X	—	1.4	—	—	—	350	—	—	—

Madison, Wisconsin.

Continued.

G

	Weight (g)	Energy (kcal)	Protein (g)	Carbohydrate (g)	Fat (g)	Cholesterol (mg)	Vitamins A (IU)	Vitamins B$_1$ (mg)	Vitamins B$_2$ (mg)
Kentucky Fried Chicken									
Original Recipe®									
Wing*	56.0	181	11.8	5.77	12.3	67.0	56	0.03	0.06
Side Breast*	95.0	276	20.0	10.1	17.3	96.0	100	0.07	0.18
Center Breast*	107.0	257	25.5	8.0	13.7	93.0	100	0.09	0.14
Drumstick*	58.0	147	13.6	3.4	8.82	81.0	100	0.06	0.13
Thigh*	96.0	278	18.0	8.4	19.2	122.0	144	0.08	0.28
Extra Crispy									
Wing*	57.0	218	11.5	7.81	15.6	63.0	100	0.03	0.07
Side Breast*	98.0	354	17.7	17.3	23.7	66.0	100	0.08	0.13
Center Breast*	120.0	353	26.9	14.4	20.9	93.0	100	0.10	0.16
Drumstick*	60.0	173	12.7	5.9	10.9	65.0	100	0.05	0.14
Thigh*	112.0	371	19.6	13.8	26.3	121.0	102	0.09	0.27
Kentucky Nuggets (one)	16.0	46	2.82	2.2	2.88	11.9	100	0.02	0.03
Kentucky Nugget Sauce (oz)									
Barbeque	1.0**	35	0.3	7.1	0.57	1.0	370	0.01	0.014
Sweet and Sour	1.0**	58	0.1	13.0	0.56	1.0	60	0.01	0.02
Honey	0.5**	49	0	12.1	0.01	1.0	—	0.01	0.003
Mustard	1.0**	36	0.88	6.04	0.91	1.0	—	0.02	0.008
Kentucky Fries	119.0	268	4.8	33.3	12.8	1.8	—	0.17	0.057
Mashed Potatoes w/Gravy	86.0	62	2.1	10.3	1.4	1.0	100	0.01	0.036
Mashed Potatoes	80.0	59	1.9	11.6	0.6	1.0	100	0.01	0.038
Chicken Gravy	78.0	59	2.0	4.4	3.7	2.0	—	0.01	0.028
Buttermilk Biscuit	75.0	269	5.1	31.6	13.6	1.0	100	0.28	0.13
Potato Salad	90.0	141	1.8	12.6	9.27	11.0	90	0.07	0.023
Baked Beans	89.0	105	5.1	18.4	1.2	1.0	—	0.06	0.039
Corn on the Cob	143.0	176	5.1	31.9	3.1	1.0	272	0.14	0.113
Cole Slaw	79.0	103	1.3	11.5	5.7	4.0	269	0.03	0.026

*edible portion
**measured in ounces
Source: Kentucky Fried Chicken Corp. Nutrient analyses by Hazelton Laboratory of America (formerly Raltech Scientific Services Inc), Madison, Wisconsin.

	Weight (g)	Energy (kcal)	Protein (g)	Carbohydrate (g)	Fat (g)	Cholesterol (mg)	Vitamins A (IU)	Vitamins B$_1$ (mg)	Vitamins B$_2$ (mg)
Long John Silver's									
3 Pc Fish & Fryes	—	853	43	64	48	106	—	—	—
2 Pc Fish & Fryes	—	651	30	53	36	75	—	—	—
Fish & More	—	978	34	82	58	88	—	—	—
3 Pc Fish Dinner	—	1180	47	93	70	119	—	—	—
3 Pc Chicken Planks Dinner	—	885	32	72	51	25	—	—	—
4 Pc Chicken Planks Dinner	—	1037	41	82	59	25	—	—	—
6 Pc Chicken Nuggets Dinner	—	699	23	54	45	25	—	—	—
Fish & Chicken	—	935	36	73	55	56	—	—	—
Seafood Platter	—	976	29	85	58	95	—	—	—
Clam Dinner	—	955	22	100	58	27	—	—	—
Batter Fried Shrimp Dinner	—	711	17	60	45	127	—	—	—
Scallop Dinner	—	747	17	66	45	37	—	—	—
Oyster Dinner	—	789	17	78	45	55	—	—	—
3 Pc Kitchen-Breaded Fish Dinner	—	940	35	84	52	101	—	—	—
2 Pc Kitchen-Breaded Fish Dinner	—	818	26	76	46	76	—	—	—
Fish Sandwich Platter	—	835	30	84	42	75	—	—	—
Seafood Salad	—	426	19	22	30	113	—	—	—
Ocean Chef Salad	—	229	27	13	8	64	—	—	—
A La Carte Items									
Batter-Fried Fish	86	202	13	11	12	31	—	—	—
Kitchen-Breaded Fish	58	122	9	8	6	25	—	—	—
Chicken Plank	62	152	9	10	8	X	—	—	—
Batter-Fried Shrimp	17	47	2	3	3	17	—	—	—
Clam Chowder	185	128	7	15	5	17	—	—	—
Cole Slaw	98	182	1	11	15	12	—	—	—
Fryes	85	247	4	31	12	13	—	—	—
Hush Puppies	47	145	3	18	7	1	—	—	—

Source: Long John Silver's Inc, Lexington, Kentucky. Nutrient analyses by Department of Nutrition and Food Science, University of Kentucky.

Vitamins					Minerals									
Nia. (mg)	B_6 (mg)	B_{12} (µg)	C (mg)	D (IU)	Ca (mg)	Cu (mg)	Fe (mg)	K (mg)	Mg (mg)	P (mg)	Na (mg)	Zn (mg)	Moisture (g)	Crude Fiber (g)
3.2	—	—	3.0	—	37.7	—	0.45	—	—	—	387	—	—	—
6.8	—	—	3.0	—	48.4	—	0.79	—	—	—	654	—	—	—
10.0	—	—	3.0	—	39.3	—	0.63	—	—	—	532	—	—	—
2.9	—	—	2.0	—	12.8	—	0.597	—	—	—	269	—	—	—
4.6	—	—	2.0	—	27.6	—	1.05	—	—	—	517	—	—	—
2.8	—	—	2.0	—	21.4	—	0.52	—	—	—	437	—	—	—
6.5	—	—	2.0	—	31.9	—	0.86	—	—	—	797	—	—	—
10.0	—	—	2.2	—	34.9	—	0.86	—	—	—	842	—	—	—
2.8	—	—	2.0	—	15.2	—	0.606	—	—	—	346	—	—	—
5.2	—	—	2.0	—	46.1	—	1.21	—	—	—	766	—	—	—
1.0	—	—	1.5	—	2.4	—	0.13	—	—	—	140	—	—	—
0.19	—	—	0.36	—	6.05	—	0.24	—	—	—	450	—	—	—
0.04	—	—	0.31	—	4.66	—	0.16	—	—	—	148	—	—	—
0.04	—	—	2.5	—	0.581	—	0.11	—	—	—	15	—	—	—
0.16	—	—	1.0	—	10.2	—	0.26	—	—	—	346	—	—	—
2.7	—	—	2.7	—	24.3	—	0.94	—	—	—	89	—	—	—
1.0	—	—	1.0	—	19.1	—	0.35	—	—	—	297	—	—	—
0.96	—	—	1.0	—	20.6	—	0.28	—	—	—	228	—	—	—
0.47	—	—	—	—	8.58	—	0.48	—	—	—	398	—	—	—
1.8	—	—	1.0	—	77.0	—	1.22	—	—	—	521	—	—	—
0.6	—	—	2.7	—	10.4	—	0.32	—	—	—	396	—	—	—
0.5	—	—	2.1	—	53.6	—	1.43	—	—	—	387	—	—	—
1.8	—	—	2.3	—	7.19	—	0.39	—	—	—	21	—	—	—
0.2	—	—	18.7	—	28.5	—	0.19	—	—	—	171	—	—	—
—	—	—	—	—	—	—	—	—	—	—	2025.0	—	—	—
—	—	—	—	—	—	—	—	—	—	—	1352.0	—	—	—
—	—	—	—	—	—	—	—	—	—	—	2124.0	—	—	—
—	—	—	—	—	—	—	—	—	—	—	2797.0	—	—	—
—	—	—	—	—	—	—	—	—	—	—	1918.0	—	—	—
—	—	—	—	—	—	—	—	—	—	—	2433.0	—	—	—
—	—	—	—	—	—	—	—	—	—	—	853.0	—	—	—
—	—	—	—	—	—	—	—	—	—	—	2076.0	—	—	—
—	—	—	—	—	—	—	—	—	—	—	2161.0	—	—	—
—	—	—	—	—	—	—	—	—	—	—	1543.0	—	—	—
—	—	—	—	—	—	—	—	—	—	—	1297.0	—	—	—
—	—	—	—	—	—	—	—	—	—	—	1579.0	—	—	—
—	—	—	—	—	—	—	—	—	—	—	763.0	—	—	—
—	—	—	—	—	—	—	—	—	—	—	1900.0	—	—	—
—	—	—	—	—	—	—	—	—	—	—	1526.0	—	—	—
—	—	—	—	—	—	—	—	—	—	—	1402.0	—	—	—
—	—	—	—	—	—	—	—	—	—	—	1086.0	—	—	—
—	—	—	—	—	—	—	—	—	—	—	986.0	—	—	—
—	—	—	—	—	—	—	—	—	—	—	673.0	—	—	—
—	—	—	—	—	—	—	—	—	—	—	374.0	—	—	—
—	—	—	—	—	—	—	—	—	—	—	515.0	—	—	—
—	—	—	—	—	—	—	—	—	—	—	154.0	—	—	—
—	—	—	—	—	—	—	—	—	—	—	611.0	—	—	—
—	—	—	—	—	—	—	—	—	—	—	367.0	—	—	—
—	—	—	—	—	—	—	—	—	—	—	0.6	—	—	—
—	—	—	—	—	—	—	—	—	—	—	405.0	—	—	—

Continued.

G

	Weight (g)	Energy (kcal)	Protein (g)	Carbohydrate (g)	Fat (g)	Cholesterol (mg)	Vitamins A (IU)	Vitamins B_1 (mg)	Vitamins B_2 (mg)
McDonald's									
Chicken McNuggets®	109	323	19.1	13.7	21.3	72.8	109	0.16	0.14
Hamburger	100	263	12.4	28.3	11.3	29.1	100	0.31	0.22
Cheeseburger	114	328	15.0	28.5	16.0	40.6	353	0.30	0.24
Quarter Pounder®	160	427	24.6	29.3	23.5	81.0	128	0.35	0.32
Quarter Pounder® w/Cheese	186	525	29.6	30.5	31.6	107.0	614	0.37	0.41
Big Mac®	200	570	24.6	39.2	35.0	83.0	380	0.48	0.38
Filet-O-Fish®	143	435	14.7	35.9	25.7	45.2	186	0.36	0.23
Mc D.L.T.®	254	680	30.0	40.0	44.0	101.0	508	0.56	0.46
French Fries, reg	68	220	3.0	26.1	11.5	8.6	17	0.12	0.02
Biscuit w/Sausage, Egg	175	585	19.8	36.4	39.9	285.0	420	0.53	0.49
Biscuit w/Bacon, Egg, Cheese	145	483	16.5	33.2	31.6	263.0	653	0.30	0.43
Sausage McMuffin®	115	427	17.6	30.0	26.3	59.0	380	0.70	0.25
Sausage McMuffin® w/Egg	165	517	22.9	32.2	32.9	287.0	660	0.84	0.50
Egg McMuffin®	138	340	18.5	31.0	15.8	259.0	591	0.47	0.44
Hot Cakes w/Butter, Syrup	214	500	7.9	93.9	10.3	47.1	257	0.26	0.36
Scrambled Eggs	98	180	13.2	2.5	13.0	514.0	652	0.08	0.47
Sausage	53	210	9.8	0.6	18.6	38.8	31	0.27	0.11
English Muffin w/Butter	63	186	5.0	29.5	53.0	15.3	164	0.28	0.49
Hash Brown Potatoes	55	125	1.5	14.0	7.0	7.2	13	0.06	0.01
Vanilla Shake	291	352	9.3	59.6	8.4	30.6	349	0.12	0.70
Chocolate Shake	291	383	9.9	65.5	9.0	29.7	349	0.12	0.44
Strawberry Shake	290	362	9.0	62.1	8.7	32.2	377	0.12	0.44
Strawberry Sundae	164	320	6.0	54.0	8.7	24.6	230	0.07	0.30
Hot Fudge Sundae	164	357	7.0	58.0	10.8	26.6	230	0.07	0.31
Caramel Sundae	165	361	7.0	608.0	10.0	31.4	279	0.07	0.31
Apple Pie	85	253	1.9	29.3	14.3	12.4	34	0.02	0.02
Cherry Pie	88	260	2.0	32.1	13.6	13.4	114	0.03	0.02
McDonaldland® Cookies	67	308	4.0	49.0	10.8	10.2	27	0.23	0.23
Chocolate Chip Cookies	69	342	4.0	45.0	16.3	17.7	76	0.12	0.21

Source: McDonald's Corp, Oak Brook, Illinois. Nutrient analyses by Hazelton Laboratory of America (formerly Raltech Scientific Services Inc), Madison, Wisconsin.

	Weight (g)	Energy (kcal)	Protein (g)	Carbohydrate (g)	Fat (g)	Cholesterol (mg)	Vitamins A (IU)	Vitamins B_1 (mg)	Vitamins B_2 (mg)
Taco Bell									
Bean Burrito	166	343	11	48	12	—	1657	0.37	0.22
Beef Burrito	184	466	30	37	21	—	1675	0.30	0.39
Beefy Tostada	184	291	19	21	15	—	3450	0.16	0.27
Bellbeefer	123	221	15	23	7	—	2961	0.15	0.20
Bellbeefer w/Cheese	137	278	19	23	12	—	3146	0.16	0.27
Burrito Supreme	225	457	21	43	22	—	3462	0.33	0.35
Combination Burrito	175	404	21	43	16	—	1666	0.34	0.31
Enchilada	207	454	25	42	21	—	1178	0.31	0.37
Pintos 'N Cheese	158	168	11	21	5	—	3123	0.26	0.16
Taco	83	186	15	14	8	—	120	0.09	0.16
Tostada	138	179	9	25	6	—	3152	0.18	0.15

From (menu item portions) San Antonio, TX: Taco Bell Co., July 1976; Adams C.F.: Nutritive value of American foods in common units, in *Handbook No. 456*. Washing-

	Weight (g)	Energy (kcal)	Protein (g)	Carbohydrate (g)	Fat (g)	Cholesterol (mg)	Vitamins A (IU)	Vitamins B_1 (mg)	Vitamins B_2 (mg)
Wendy's									
Single Hamburger, multigrain bun	119	340	25	20	17	67	X	0.22	0.17
Single Hamburger, white bun	117	350	21	27	18	65	—	0.22	0.25
Double Hamburger, white bun	197	560	41	24	34	125	—	0.22	0.43
Bacon Cheeseburger, white bun	147	460	29	23	28	65	400	0.30	0.26
Chicken Sandwich, multigrain bun	128	320	25	31	10	59	X	0.15	0.14
Kid's Meal Hamburger, 2 oz	75	220	13	11	8	20	—	0.09	0.17
Chili, 8 oz	256	260	21	26	8	30	1000	0.15	0.17
French Fries, reg	98	280	4	35	14	15	—	0.15	0.03
Taco Salad	357	390	23	36	18	40	1750	0.15	0.03
Frosty Dairy Dessert	243	400	8	59	14	50	500	0.12	0.51

Vitamins					Minerals									
Nia. (mg)	B_6 (mg)	B_{12} (μg)	C (mg)	D (IU)	Ca (mg)	Cu (mg)	Fe (mg)	K (mg)	Mg (mg)	P (mg)	Na (mg)	Zn (mg)	Moisture (g)	Crude Fiber (g)
7.52	—	—	2.1	—	11	—	1.25	—	—	—	512	—	—	—
4.08	—	—	1.8	—	84	—	2.85	—	—	—	506	—	—	—
4.33	—	—	2.1	—	169	—	2.84	—	—	—	743	—	—	—
7.02	—	—	2.6	—	98	—	4.30	—	—	—	718	—	—	—
7.07	—	—	2.8	—	255	—	4.84	—	—	—	1220	—	—	—
7.20	—	—	3.0	—	203	—	4.90	—	—	—	979	—	—	—
3.0	—	—	2.1	—	133	—	2.47	—	—	—	799	—	—	—
8.0	—	—	8.0	—	230	—	6.60	—	—	—	1030	—	—	—
2.26	—	—	12.5	—	9	—	0.61	—	—	—	109	—	—	—
3.85	—	—	1.8	—	119	—	3.43	—	—	—	1301	—	—	—
2.32	—	—	1.6	—	2	—	2.57	—	—	—	1269	—	—	—
4.14	—	—	1.3	—	168	—	2.25	—	—	—	942	—	—	—
4.46	—	—	1.6	—	196	—	3.47	—	—	—	1044	—	—	—
3.77	—	—	1.4	—	226	—	2.93	—	—	—	885	—	—	—
2.27	—	—	4.7	—	103	—	2.23	—	—	—	1070	—	—	—
0.20	—	—	1.2	—	61	—	2.53	—	—	—	205	—	—	—
2.07	—	—	0.5	—	16	—	0.82	—	—	—	423	—	—	—
2.61	—	—	0.8	—	117	—	1.51	—	—	—	310	—	—	—
0.82	—	—	4.1	—	5	—	0.40	—	—	—	325	—	—	—
0.35	—	—	3.2	—	329	—	0.18	—	—	—	201	—	—	—
0.50	—	—	2.9	—	320	—	0.84	—	—	—	300	—	—	—
0.35	—	—	4.1	—	322	—	0.17	—	—	—	207	—	—	—
1.03	—	—	2.79	—	174	—	0.38	—	—	—	90	—	—	—
1.12	—	—	2.46	—	215	—	0.61	—	—	—	170	—	—	—
1.01	—	—	3.61	—	200	—	0.23	—	—	—	145	—	—	—
0.19	—	—	0.9	—	14	—	0.62	—	—	—	398	—	—	—
0.25	—	—	0.9	—	12	—	0.59	—	—	—	427	—	—	—
2.85	—	—	0.94	—	12	—	1.47	—	—	—	358	—	—	—
1.70	—	—	1.04	—	29	—	1.56	—	—	—	313	—	—	—
2.2	—	—	15.2	—	98	—	2.8	235	—	173	272	—	—	—
7.0	—	—	15.2	—	83	—	4.6	320	—	288	327	—	—	—
3.3	—	—	12.7	—	208	—	3.4	277	—	265	138	—	—	—
3.7	—	—	10.0	—	40	—	2.6	183	—	140	231	—	—	—
3.7	—	—	10.0	—	147	—	2.7	195	—	208	330	—	—	—
4.7	—	—	16.0	—	121	—	3.8	350	—	245	367	—	—	—
4.6	—	—	15.2	—	91	—	3.7	278	—	230	300	—	—	—
4.7	—	—	9.5	—	259	—	3.8	491	—	338	1175	—	—	—
0.9	—	—	9.3	—	150	—	2.3	307	—	210	102	—	—	—
2.9	—	—	0.2	—	120	—	2.5	143	—	175	79	—	—	—
0.8	—	—	9.7	—	191	—	2.3	172	—	186	101	—	—	—

ton J.B. Lippincott Co.; Valley Baptist Medical Center, Food Service Department: Descriptions of Mexican-American Foods, Fort Atkinson, WI, NASCO.

5	—	—	X	—	16	—	2.7	—	—	—	290	—	—	—
5	—	—	—	—	32	—	4.5	—	—	—	410	—	—	—
9	—	—	—	—	32	—	6.3	—	—	—	575	—	—	—
6	—	—	X	—	120	—	3.6	—	—	—	860	—	—	—
10	—	—	X	—	16	—	1.4	—	—	—	500	—	—	—
3	—	—	—	—	16	—	1.8	—	—	—	265	—	—	—
3	—	—	6	—	64	—	4.5	—	—	—	1070	—	—	—
3	—	—	12	—	X	—	1.1	—	—	—	95	—	—	—
3	—	—	21	—	160	—	4.5	—	—	—	1100	—	—	—
—	—	—	X	—	240	—	1.1	—	—	—	220	—	—	—

Continued.

G

	Weight (g)	Energy (kcal)	Protein (g)	Carbohydrate (g)	Fat (g)	Cholesterol (mg)	Vitamins A (IU)	B$_1$ (mg)	B$_2$ (mg)
Wendy's—cont'd									
Hot Stuffed Baked Potatoes									
Plain	250	250	6	52	2	tr	X	0.22	0.10
Sour Cream & Chives	310	460	6	53	24	15	500	0.22	0.14
Cheese	350	590	17	55	34	22	1000	0.22	0.26
Chili & Cheese	400	510	22	63	20	22	750	0.30	0.26
Bacon & Cheese	350	570	19	57	30	22	750	0.22	0.17
Broccoli & Cheese	365	500	13	54	25	22	1750	0.30	0.26
Ham & Cheese Omelet	114	250	18	6	17	450	1000	0.15	0.60
Ham, Cheese, & Mushroom Omelet	118	290	18	7	21	355	1000	0.23	0.60
Ham, Cheese, Onion, & Green Pepper Omelet	128	280	19	7	19	525	1000	0.15	0.60
Mushroom, Onion, & Green Pepper Omelet	114	210	14	7	15	460	750	0.09	0.51
Breakfast Sandwich	129	370	17	33	19	200	1000	0.45	0.43
French Toast, 2 slices	135	400	11	45	19	115	500	0.60	0.51
Home Fries	103	360	4	37	22	20	—	0.12	0.03

Source: Wendy's International Inc, Dublin, Ohio. Nutrient analyses: entree items, Hazelton Laboratory of America (formerly Raltech Scientific Services Inc), Madison, Wis-

	Weight (g)	Energy (kcal)	Protein (g)	Carbohydrate (g)	Fat (g)	Cholesterol (mg)	Vitamins A (IU)	B$_1$ (mg)	B$_2$ (mg)
Whataburger									
Whataburger®	302	580	32	58	24	70	211	0.79	0.54
Whataburger® w/Cheese	326	669	36	58	33	96	293	0.77	0.65
Whataburger Jr®	153	304	15	31	14	30	107	0.37	0.26
Whataburger Jr® w/Cheese	165	351	17	30	18	42	264	0.36	0.28
Justaburger®	117	265	12	28	12	25	35	0.33	0.21
Justaburger® w/Cheese	129	312	15	28	16	37	192	0.33	0.23
Whatacatch®	177	475	14	43	27	34	—	0.44	0.23
Whatacatch® w/Cheese	189	522	17	43	31	45	—	0.44	0.25
Whataburger® Doublemeat	385	806	51	59	41	154	211	0.81	0.84
Whataburger® Doublemeat w/Cheese	409	895	54	59	49	180	293	0.79	0.95
Whatachick'n® Sandwich	288	671	35	61	32	71	288	0.78	0.37
French Fries, reg	85	221	4	25	12	1	—	0.15	0.04
French Fries, lg	127	332	5	37	18	1	—	0.23	0.07
Onion Rings	73	226	4	23	13	1	—	0.12	0.05
Apple Pie	39	236	3	30	12	1	—	0.16	0.07
Vanilla Shake, sm	254	322	9	50	9	37	279	0.10	0.81
Vanilla Shake, med	340	433	12	68	13	49	375	0.14	1.10
Vanilla Shake, lg	508	647	18	101	19	74	560	0.20	1.63
Vanilla Shake, extra lg	678	861	24	134	25	98	745	0.27	2.17
Taquito	125	310	19	17	19	223	513	0.40	0.36
Taquito w/Cheese	137	357	22	17	23	235	670	0.40	0.38
Egg Omelet Sandwich	120	312	14	29	15	191	564	0.34	0.55
Breakfast on a Bun	175	520	23	29	34	234	564	0.53	0.71
Pancakes & Sausage, without syrup & butter	153	407	15	38	22	77	—	0.45	0.39
Pancakes, without syrup & butter	98	199	6	37	3	34	—	0.26	0.23
Sausage	55	208	9	1	19	43	—	0.19	0.16
Pecan Danish	63	270	5	28	16	12	223	0.31	0.19

Source: Whataburger Inc, Corpus Christi, Texas. Nutrient analyses by Hazelton Laboratory of America (formerly Raltech Scientific Services Inc), Madison, Wisconsin.

	Weight (g)	Energy (kcal)	Protein (g)	Carbohydrate (g)	Fat (g)	Cholesterol (mg)	Vitamins A (IU)	B$_1$ (mg)	B$_2$ (mg)
Zantigo									
Taco	84.5	198	10.4	12.8	11.7	30.5	—	—	—
Taco Burrito	198.7	415	20.7	41.1	19.0	43.9	—	—	—
Mild Chilito	115.0	330	13.8	36.0	14.7	26.2	—	—	—
Hot Chilito	115.3	329	14.3	35.2	14.5	31.5	—	—	—
Beef Enchilada	184.1	315	18.0	26.0	15.0	49.0	—	—	—
Cheese Enchilada	179.8	390	19.8	26.2	22.8	62.9	—	—	—

Source: Zantigo Mexican Restaurants, Columbus, Ohio.

G

Nia. (mg)	B_6 (mg)	B_{12} (µg)	C (mg)	D (IU)	Ca (mg)	Cu (mg)	Fe (mg)	K (mg)	Mg (mg)	P (mg)	Na (mg)	Zn (mg)	Moisture (g)	Crude Fiber (g)
	Vitamins				Minerals									
3	—	—	36	—	16	—	2.7	1360	—	—	60	—	—	—
3	—	—	36	—	32	—	2.7	1420	—	—	230	—	—	—
3	—	—	36	—	280	—	2.7	1380	—	—	450	—	—	—
4	—	—	36	—	200	—	3.6	1590	—	—	610	—	—	—
3	—	—	36	—	160	—	2.7	1380	—	—	1180	—	—	—
4	—	—	90	—	200	—	2.7	1550	—	—	430	—	—	—
0.8	—	—	—	—	80	—	2.7	180	—	—	405	—	—	—
1.2	—	—	—	—	80	—	2.7	190	—	—	570	—	—	—
0.8	—	—	6	—	120	—	2.7	200	—	—	485	—	—	—
X	—	—	6	—	48	—	2.7	190	—	—	200	—	—	—
3.0	—	—	—	—	120	—	3.6	155	—	—	770	—	—	—
4.0	—	—	—	—	64	—	1.8	175	—	—	850	—	—	—
0.8	—	—	5	—	16	—	0.7	615	—	—	745	—	—	—

consin; other items, US Department of Agriculture Handbook #8.

Nia. (mg)	B_6 (mg)	B_{12} (µg)	C (mg)	D (IU)	Ca (mg)	Cu (mg)	Fe (mg)	K (mg)	Mg (mg)	P (mg)	Na (mg)	Zn (mg)	Moisture (g)	Crude Fiber (g)
9.4	—	—	6.3	—	212	0.21	8.7	598	51	279	1092	4.6	181	1.5
9.5	—	—	5.9	—	358	0.17	8.0	629	56	377	1474	5.0	192	1.6
3.6	—	—	2.9	—	122	0.12	4.1	272	27	137	684	2.0	90	0.8
3.5	—	—	3.5	—	193	0.10	4.0	284	30	192	921	2.2	96	0.7
2.8	—	—	1.6	—	106	0.10	3.9	199	21	113	647	1.6	62	0.7
2.8	—	—	2.2	—	177	0.10	3.9	211	23	168	784	1.8	68	0.7
4.3	—	—	2.1	—	120	0.11	3.0	296	28	230	722	0.7	87	2.3
4.3	—	—	2.7	—	191	0.11	3.0	308	31	285	959	1.0	93	2.3
13.6	—	—	6.3	—	217	0.27	11.2	830	67	415	1296	8.1	227	1.7
13.6	—	—	5.9	—	363	0.23	10.5	861	72	513	1678	8.4	238	1.8
17.0	—	—	6.3	—	103	0.23	6.4	648	63	389	1460	1.5	154	1.0
2.0	—	—	3.2	—	9	0.13	0.6	464	28	102	30	0.3	43	0.8
3.1	—	—	4.9	—	14	0.19	0.9	695	41	153	45	0.5	64	0.9
0.7	—	—	2.5	—	21	0.06	0.7	92	14	67	410	0.3	32	0.3
1.2	—	—	—	—	9	0.05	1.0	56	8	55	265	0.1	38	0.4
0.3	—	—	—	—	261	0.03	1.7	429	28	233	169	0.8	183	0.3
0.4	—	—	1.0	—	351	0.04	2.3	576	38	312	227	1.0	245	0.3
0.6	—	—	—	—	524	0.06	3.4	860	57	466	338	1.5	366	0.5
0.8	—	—	—	—	698	0.08	4.5	1145	75	620	450	2.0	488	0.7
3.2	—	—	—	—	92	0.12	3.1	185	21	253	712	1.4	61	6.9
3.2	—	—	—	—	163	0.12	3.1	197	24	308	949	1.7	67	6.9
2.9	—	—	—	—	209	0.11	3.4	149	20	210	696	1.3	58	0.7
5.9	—	—	—	—	216	0.15	4.1	301	30	292	1051	2.3	83	0.8
5.1	—	—	—	—	60	0.08	2.6	262	24	401	1029	1.5	75	0.3

Nia. (mg)	B_6 (mg)	B_{12} (µg)	C (mg)	D (IU)	Ca (mg)	Cu (mg)	Fe (mg)	K (mg)	Mg (mg)	P (mg)	Na (mg)	Zn (mg)	Moisture (g)	Crude Fiber (g)
2.1	—	—	—	—	53	0.04	1.9	110	15	319	674	0.4	49	0.1
3.0	—	—	—	—	7	0.04	0.7	152	10	82	355	1.0	26	0.2
2.5	—	—	—	—	66	0.06	1.6	82	13	127	419	0.4	14	0.2

Nia. (mg)	B_6 (mg)	B_{12} (µg)	C (mg)	D (IU)	Ca (mg)	Cu (mg)	Fe (mg)	K (mg)	Mg (mg)	P (mg)	Na (mg)	Zn (mg)	Moisture (g)	Crude Fiber (g)
—	—	—	—	—	—	—	—	—	—	—	318	—	—	—
—	—	—	—	—	—	—	—	—	—	—	815	—	—	—
—	—	—	—	—	—	—	—	—	—	—	505	—	—	—
—	—	—	—	—	—	—	—	—	—	—	466	—	—	—
—	—	—	—	—	—	—	—	—	—	—	904	—	—	—
—	—	—	—	—	—	—	—	—	—	—	759	—	—	—

APPENDIX

H Food Sources of Nutrients in Relation to the U.S. RDA

Nutrient	Sources*			
	Excellent (75% U.S. RDA)	Good (50% U.S. RDA)	Significant (25% U.S. RDA)	Fair (10% U.S. RDA)
Vitamin C	Orange Strawberries Cauliflower Broccoli Brussels sprouts Green pepper Tomato Grapefruit Honeydew melon Mustard greens	Cabbage Spinach Tangerine Asparagus	Banana Blueberries Lima beans Raspberries Green peas Radishes Sauerkraut	Apple Peach Corn
Vitamin A	Liver Carrot Pumpkin Sweet potatoes Spinach Winter squash Turnip greens Mustard greens Beet greens	Apricots Watermelon Broccoli	Honeydew melon Peaches Prunes Tomato Nectarines	Asparagus Green beans Brussels sprouts Cheddar cheese Green peas Tomato juice
Thiamin	Pork	Dried peas Macaroni	Green peas Ham Peanuts	Orange Watermelon Dried beans Noodles Spaghetti Lamb liver Rice Cashew nuts
Riboflavin	Liver		Macaroni Cottage cheese Buttermilk Milk Yogurt	Avocado Tangerine Prunes Asparagus Broccoli Mushrooms Ice cream Beef Salmon Turkey

*Based on average serving size as follows: Meat—3 oz, edible portion; Fruit—3 to 4 oz; Vegetables—3 to 4 oz; Cereals—1 oz; Milk—8 oz.

Nutrient	Sources* Excellent (75% U.S. RDA)	Good (50% U.S. RDA)	Significant (25% U.S. RDA)	Fair (10% U.S. RDA)
Vitamin B_6		Soybeans Beef liver Tuna	Lima beans Pork Beef Veal Halibut Salmon Chicken Bananas Avocado	Cauliflower Green pepper Potatoes Spinach Raisins Perch
Vitamin B_{12}	Beef liver Clams Salmon Trappist cheese Lamb Eggs		Veal Cheese Scallops Swordfish	
Magnesium	Molasses Peanuts	Beet greens	Spinach Lima beans Green peas	Raisins Sweet potatoes Brussels sprouts Cod
Iron	Calf and pork liver Clams	Beef liver	Asparagus Ham Veal Beef Chicken Macaroni Prunes Raisins Spinach	Banana Beans Brussels sprouts Cod Green peas Noodles Rice Cashew nuts Peanuts
Calcium			Turnip greens Swiss cheese Buttermilk Milk Yogurt Salmon	Prunes Broccoli Beet greens Cottage cheese Ice cream Haddock Scallops

H

APPENDIX

I Diabetic Exchange Lists

Milk Exchange List

Skim Milk (12 g carbohydrate, 8 g protein, 0 fat, 90 kcal)

1 milk exchange

1 cup	skim or non-fat milk (½% and 1%)
⅓ cup	powdered (non-fat dry, before adding liquid)
½ cup	canned, evaporated skim milk
1 cup	buttermilk made from skim milk
1 cup	yogurt made from skim milk (plain, unflavored)

Low-Fat Milk (12 g carbohydrate, 8 g protein, 5 g fat, 120 kcal)

1 milk exchange
1 fat exchange

1 cup	2% fat fortified milk
1 cup	plain nonfat yogurt

Whole Milk (12 g carbohydrate, 8 g protein, 8 g fat, 150 kcal)

1 milk exchange
2 fat exchanges

1 cup	whole milk
½ cup	buttermilk made from whole milk
1 cup	custard style yogurt made from whole milk (plain, unflavored)

Vegetable Exchange List

(5 g carbohydrate, 2 g protein, 0 fat, 25 kcal)

1 exchange is
½ cup of cooked vegetables or vegetable juice;
1 cup of raw vegetables

artichoke (medium)
beans (green, wax)
beets
broccoli
brussels sprouts
cabbage
carrots
cauliflower
celery
eggplant
green pepper
greens
onions
pea pods
rhubarb
sauerkraut
squash, summer
string beans (green, yellow)
tomatoes
tomato juice
turnips
vegetable juice

Fruit Exchange List
(15 g carbohydrate, 0 protein, 0 fat, 60 kcal)

1 fruit exchange	
1	apple (2″ diameter)
4 rings	dried apple
½ cup	apple juice
½ cup	applesauce (unsweetened)
7 halves	apricots, fresh
½ cup	apricots, canned
4 medium	apricots, dried
½	banana, 9″ long
¾ cup	blackberries
¾ cup	blueberries
1 cup	raspberries
1¼ cup	strawberries
⅓ melon	cantaloupe (5″ diameter)
12 large	cherries (large, raw)
½ cup	cherries, canned
½ cup	cider
⅓ cup	cranberry juice
2½ medium	dates
2	figs, fresh (2″ diameter)
1½	figs, dried
½	grapefruit
½ cup	grapefruit juice
14	grapes
⅓ cup	grape juice
⅛	honeydew melon (7″ diameter)
1	kiwi (large)
¾ cup	mandarin oranges
½ small	mango
1 small	nectarine (1½″ diameter)
1 small	orange (2½″ diameter)
½ cup	orange juice
1 medium or ¾ cup	peach, fresh (2¾″ diameter)
½ cup or 2 halves	peach, canned
1 small or ½ large	pear, fresh
½ cup or 2 halves	pear, canned
¾ cup	pineapple, raw
⅓ cup	pineapple, canned
½ cup	pineapple juice
1 medium	plums (2″)
3	prunes, dried
⅓ cup	prune juice
2 T	raisins
1 medium	tangerine (2½″ diameter)
1¼ cups	watermelon (cubes)

Starch/Bread Exchange List

(15 g carbohydrate, 3 g protein, 0 fat, 80 kcal)

1 starch/bread exchange	
Bread	
1 slice	white (including French and Italian)
1 slice	whole wheat
1 slice	rye or pumpernickel
1 slice	raisin (untoasted)
2 (⅔ oz)	bread sticks (crisp, 4″ long, ½″ wide)
½ (1 oz)	bagel, small
½	English muffin
1	plain roll
½ (1 oz)	frankfurter roll
½ (1 oz)	hamburger bun
3 T	dried bread crumbs
1	tortilla (6″)
½	pita (6″ diameter)
Cereal/grains/pasta	
½ cup	bran flakes
¾ cup	other ready-to-eat unsweetened cereal
1½ cup	puffed cereal (unfrosted)
½ cup	cereal (cooked)
⅓ cup	rice or barley (cooked)
3 T	grapenuts
½ cup	shredded wheat
3 T	wheat germ
½ cup	pasta (cooked spaghetti, noodles, macaroni)
2½ cups	cornmeal (dry)
2½ T	flour (dry)
Crackers/snacks	
3	graham (2½″ square)
¾ oz	matzoh (4″ × 6″)
24	oyster
4	rye crisp (2″ × 3½″)
6	saltines
8	animal
5 slices	melba toast
3 cups	popcorn
¾ oz	pretzels
Dried beans/peas/lentils	
⅓ cup	dried beans, such as kidney, white, split, blackeye (cooked)
⅓ cup	lentils (cooked)
Starchy vegetables	
½ cup	corn
1 cup	corn on the cob (6″ long)
½ cup	lima beans
½ cup	peas, green
1 small	potato, white (3 oz baked)
½ cup	potato, mashed
¾ cup	winter squash, acorn or butternut
⅓ cup	yam or sweet potato

Starch Group (with fat)

1 starch/bread exchange
1 fat exchange

1	biscuit
½ cup	chow mein noodles
1 (2 oz)	corn bread (2″ cube)
6	cracker, round butter type
10 (1½ oz)	french fries (2″ to 3½″ long)
1	muffin, plain, small
2	pancake (4″ across)
¼ cup	stuffing, bread (prepared)
2	taco shell (6″ across)
1	waffle (4½″ sq.)
4-6 (1 oz)	whole wheat crackers (triscuits)

Meat Exchange List

(15 g carbohydrate, 3 g protein, 0 fat, 80 kcal)

Lean (0 carbohydrate, 7 g protein, 3 g fat, 55 kcal)

1 meat exchange

Beef	1 oz	baby beef (lean, chipped beef, chuck, flank steak, tenderloin, plate ribs, round (bottom, top), all cuts rump, spare ribs, tripe
Pork	1 oz	leg (whole rump, center shank), ham (center slices). USDA good or choice grades such as round, sirloin, flank, and tenderloin
Veal	1 oz	leg, loin, rib, shank, shoulder, chops, roasts, all cuts except cutlets (ground or cubed)
Poultry	1 oz	chicken, turkey, cornish hen
Fish	2 oz	fresh or frozen, any type canned salmon, tuna, mackerel, crab, or lobster
	1 oz	clams, oysters, scallops, shrimp
	3 oz	sardines, drained
Cheeses	1 oz	cottage, farmer's cheese or pot cheese (low-fat)
Dried beans and peas	½ cup	cooked

Medium Fat (0 carbohydrate, 7 g protein, 5 g fat, 75 kcal)

1 meat exchange
1 fat exchange

Beef	1 oz	all ground beef, roast (rib, chuck, rump), steak (cubed, porterhouse, T-bone), meat loaf
Lamb	1 oz	leg, rib, sirloin, loin (roast and chops), shank, shoulder
Pork	1 oz	loin (all cuts tenderloin), chops, roast, Boston butt, cutlets
Poultry	1 oz	capon, duck (domestic), goose, ground turkey
Veal	1 oz	cutlets
Organ meats	1 oz	all types
Cheeses	¼ cup	cottage (creamed), mozzarella (made with skim milk), ricotta, farmer's, neufchatel
	3 tbsp	parmesan
	1	egg

I

Meat Exchange List—cont'd

High Fat (0 carbohydrate, 7 g protein, 8 g fat, 100 kcal)

1 meat exchange
1½ fat exchange

Beef	1 oz	brisket, corned beef, ground beef (commercial), chuck (ground commercial), roasts (rib), steaks (club and rib). Most USDA prime cuts of beef
Lamb	1 oz	patties (ground lamb)
Pork	1 oz	spare ribs, loin (back ribs), pork (ground), country-style ham, deviled ham, pork sausage
Cheeses	1 oz	all regular cheeses (American, blue, brick, camembert, cheddar, gouda, limburger, muenster, swiss, monterey), all processed cheeses
Cold Cuts	1 oz	bologna, salami, pimento loaf
Frankfurter	1 oz	(turkey or chicken)
Peanut butter	1 oz	
Sausage	1 oz	(Polish, Italian)

Fat Exchange List

(0 carbohydrate, 0 protein, 5 g fat, 45 kcal)

1 fat exchange

⅛ medium	avocado
1 strip	bacon, crisp
1 tsp	butter, margarine
2 T	cream, light
2 T	cream, sour
1 T	cream, heavy
1 T	cream, cottage
Dressing	
1 T	all varieties
2 tsp	mayo type
1 T	reduced cal (mayo type)
1 T	gravy, meat
Nuts	
6	almonds, whole, dry roasted
2 large	pecans, whole
20 small or 10 large	peanuts, Spanish, whole
10	peanuts, Virginia, whole
2 whole	walnuts
1 T	cashews, dry roasted
1 T	seeds (pine, sunflower)
2 tsp	pumpkin seeds
1 T	other
Oil	
1 tsp	corn, cottonseed, safflower, soy, sunflower, olive, peanut
Olives	
10 small or 5 large	

APPENDIX

J

Selected Sources of Reliable Nutrition Information

AGENCIES

American Council on Science and Health
1995 Broadway
New York, NY 10023
212-362-7044

American Dental Association
211 E. Chicago Ave.
Chicago, IL 60611
312-440-2500

American Diabetes Association
505 8th Avenue
New York, NY 10018
212-947-9707

American Dietetic Association
Publications Department
216 W. Jackson
Chicago, IL 60604
312-899-0400

American Heart Association
7320 Greenville Avenue
Dallas, TX 75231
1-800-527-6941

American Home Economics Association
Division of Public Affairs
2010 Massachusetts Avenue, NW
Washington, D.C. 20036
202-862-8300

American Institute of Nutrition
9650 Rockville Pike
Bethesda, MD 20814
301-530-7050

American National Red Cross
Food and Nutrition Consultant
National Headquarters
431 18th Street, NW
Washington, D.C. 20006
202-737-8300

American Public Health Association
1015 18th Street, NW
Washington, D.C. 20036
202-467-5000

American School Food Service
5600 S. Quebec Street
Suite 300 B
Englewood, CO 80111
303-200-8484

Canadian Dietetic Association
385 Yonge Street
Toronto, Ontario M4T 125
CANADA

Food and Agricultural Organization
UNIPUB (United Nations International Publishers)
345 Park Avenue South
New York, NY 10016
212-686-4707

Food and Drug Administration (FDA)
Parklane Building
5600 Fishers Lane
Rockville, MD 20852

Food and Nutrition Board
National Academy of Sciences
2101 Constitution Avenue
Washington, D.C. 20418
202-389-6366

Human Nutrition Information Service
U.S. Department of Agriculture
Federal Center Building
Hyattsville, MD 20782
301-436-8457

Institute of Food Technologists
221 N. Lasalle Street
Chicago, IL 60601

ILSI Nutrition Foundation
1126 Sixteenth Street, Suite 111
Washington, D.C. 20036
202-659-0074

National Dairy Council
6300 N. River Road
Rosemont, IL 60018
312-696-1020

National Foundation—March of Dimes
1275 Mamaroneck Avenue
White Plains, NY 10605
914-428-7100

National Livestock and Meat Board
444 N. Michigan Avenue
Chicago, IL 60611
312-467-5520

Penn State Nutrition Center
Benedict House
Pennsylvania State University
University Park, PA 16802
814-865-6323

Society for Nutrition Education
1700 Broadway, Suite 300
Oakland, CA 94612
415-444-7133

Superintendent of Documents
U.S. Government Printing Office
Washington, D.C. 20402

U.S. Department of Agriculture (USDA)
Cooperative Extension Service
Home Economics
Washington, D.C. 20250

USDA Nutrition Program
Consumer and Food Economics Division
Agricultural Research Service
Hyattsville, MD 20782
301-436-8457

USDA Office of Communication
Washington, D.C. 20250

USDA School Lunch Program
Information Division
Food and Nutrition Service
Washington, D.C. 20250

World Health Organization
49 Sheridan Avenue
Albany, NY 12210
518-436-9686

PERIODIC NUTRITION UPDATES

ACHS News and Views
American Council on Science and Health
1995 Broadway
New York, NY 10023
$10 per year—6 issues

Diet and Nutrition Newsletter
Tufts University
322 W. 57th Street, Box 34T
New York, NY 10019
$18 per year—12 issues

Nutrition and the M.D.
P.O. Box 2160
Van Nuys, CA 91404
$36 per year—12 issues

Nutrition Clinics
George Stickley Company
210 West Washington Square
Philadelphia, PA 19106
$24 per year—6 issues

Nutrition Forum
George Stickley Company
210 West Washington Square
Philadelphia, PA 19106
$30 per year—12 issues

Nutrition Research Newsletter
P.O. Box 700
Palisades, NY 10964
$96 per year—12 issues

Nutrition Reviews
(ILSI-NF)
Springer Verlag, NY
175 Fifth Avenue
New York, NY 10010
$37—12 issues

Nutrition Today
Williams and Wilkins
428 Preston Street
Baltimore, MD 21202
$24.75—6 issues

Nutrition Week
Community Nutrition Institute
2001 S. Street, NW
Washington, D.C. 20009
$70 per year—weekly

Rapport
National Institute of Nutrition
210-1335 Carling Avenue
Ottawa, Ontario K1Z 8N8
613-725-1889
$20 for 2 years—4 issues

Contemporary Nutrition
General Mills
P.O. Box 1113
Minneapolis, MN 55440

Dairy Council Digests
National Dairy Council
6300 N. River Road
Rosemont, IL 60018

Dietetic Currents
Ross Laboratories
625 Cleveland Avenue
Columbus, OH 43216

Food and Nutrition News
National Livestock and Meat Board
444 N. Michigan Avenue
Chicago, IL 60611

APPENDIX

K

Process of Bone Calcification and Collagen Synthesis

THE CALCIFICATION PROCESS

A typical healthy bone calcifies to become rigid and strong and is capable of supporting the weight of the body before the infant begins to walk, sometimes as early as 8 months of age. Throughout the entire growth process, the bone shaft lengthens as the formation of new collagen matrix is followed by its calcification. At the ends and inside the shaft of the long bones is a porous crystalline structure known as the *trabeculae.* The trabeculae, which come in direct contact with the blood vessels in the bone marrow, provide a liberal supply of calcium that can be readily mobilized to maintain the critical blood calcium levels when dietary levels drop. Only when calcium reserves in the trabeculae have been depleted will decalcification of other parts of the bones occur. Under these conditions, the pelvis and the spine are the first to release calcium.

The epiphysis and epiphysial plate at the end of the bones are sections of bone that permit and regulate bone growth. Once the epiphysis loses these functions, the bones can no longer grow in length. For most bones, this occurs at the end of puberty. During growth and throughout adult life bones are remodeled and reshaped in response to changing stresses from the weight of the developing body. This constant deposition and resorption of bone is the result of the activity of cells on the bone surface, which act alternately as *osteoblasts* (bone-forming cells) and *osteoclasts* (bone-destroying cells). Once the osteoclasts have caused the destruction of the matrix and the resorption of the calcium phosphate crystals, these same cells act as osteoblasts to produce a new collagen mold that will be slightly different from the original. New crystals then grow in this mold to restore strength to the bone. The old collagen mold is gradually broken down. In young bone, bone formation predominates; in later life, bone resorption predominates, leading to critical loss of bone and therefore calcium.

In an adult, 20% of bone calcium is resorbed and replaced each year; thus every 5 years the calcium in the bone has been completely replaced. Approximately 600 to 700 mg of calcium is deposited each day in newly formed adult bone, replacing what has been resorbed. Knowledge of this dynamic, or changing, state of bone metabolism came only with the availability of radioactive isotopes of calcium that could be traced in their path through the body.

After age 40, an individual loses 3% of total compact bone mass each decade. In women, the rate of loss increases to 9% per decade from menopause until the age of 75. Trabecular bone, usually considered the more readily available calcium store, is lost at the rate of 6% to 8% per decade for both sexes, 25 to 30 years of age.

The amount of calcium needed to meet demands for bone growth varies with the rate of skeletal development. The increase in calcium content of the body from 0.8% of body weight at

K

birth (about 28 grams, or 1 oz) to 2% at maturity (about 1400 grams,or 3 pounds) represents an average daily increase of 165 mg with a reported range of 70 to 400 mg, depending on the stage of bone growth. Maximum needs occur between 13 and 14 years of age, when the body acquires about 90 grams of calcium a year, representing an increase of about 200 to 300 mg/day in body calcium. The need for calcium reflects growth in body height rather than weight.

In addition to calcium and phosphorus, other vitamins and minerals—including vitamin A, magnesium, manganese, silicon, copper, vitamin C, vitamin D, and protein—all play a role in bone growth.

COLLAGEN METABOLISM

Collagen fibrils (very small fibers) consisting of three amino acid chains are extruded from the cell as a soluble protein, *tropocollagen*. Before it is capable of performing the functions of collagen in binding cells or providing structure, tropocollagen must be changed chemically. This involves a rather simple conversion of the amino acids lysine and proline in the tropocollagen to hydroxylysine and hydroxyproline to make mature collagen. This change requires ascorbic acid (vitamin C). In the absence of ascorbic acid, collagen cannot be formed, and the tropocollagen is broken down into its component amino acids. The tissue is weakened because of a lack of collagen. This becomes evident primarily in tissues subjected to physical stress. Although vitamin C is not required for maintenance of collagen, parts of collagen in some tissues, such as scar tissue, do break down rapidly in an ascorbic acid deficiency.

Vitamin C also has a role in the synthesis of an essential material called *ground substance*, which is a gelatinous, mucuslike substance in which the mature collagen fibrils become embedded. Thus vitamin C plays a role in forming both the fibrils and the material in which they are embedded. Ground substance also serves to lubricate joints and to provide some protection against bacteria entering the body.

When collagen is not formed properly, the lack shows up in many ways. The need for ascorbic acid in the healing of wounds is most evident; in that case new connective tissue, which is primarily collagen, must be formed. The high concentration of ascorbic acid found in scar tissue and the decrease in the amount of the vitamin in blood that occurs during healing indicate that ascorbic acid is being used at the site of healing. Immediately following an injury, fibroblast cells migrate to the wound area, multiply, and begin to synthesize short collagen units of the amino acids glycine, proline, and lysine. If vitamin C is not present, neither proline nor lysine can be changed to their useful forms. If it is available, these short units are excreted into the extracellular spaces where they are united to form larger collagen fibers that bind the cells together, increase the strength of the scar tissue, and support the capillaries that accumulate in the wound area. Once a wound has healed, the collagen is constantly being remodeled, with synthesis and destruction taking place alternately. High levels of vitamin C are maintained after the scar tissue has been completely formed, indicating that the vitamin is needed in the maintenance of scar tissue. In a lack of vitamin C, the faster loss of collagen results in a weakening and breaking of the scar tissue.

APPENDIX

L

Standards for Triceps Skinfold Measurements

Age	Male					Female				
	5th	15th	50th	85th	95th	5th	15th	50th	85th	95th
0-5 mo	4	5	8	12	15	4	5	8	12	13
6-17 mo	5	7	9	13	15	6	7	9	12	15
1½-2½ yr	5	7	10	13	14	6	7	10	13	15
2½-3½	6	7	9	12	14	6	7	10	12	14
3½-4½	5	6	9	12	14	5	7	10	12	14
4½-5½	5	6	8	12	16	6	7	10	13	16
5½-6½	5	6	8	11	15	6	7	10	12	15
6½-7½	4	6	8	11	14	6	7	10	13	17
7½-8½	5	6	8	12	17	6	7	10	15	19
8½-9½	5	6	9	14	19	6	7	11	17	24
9½-10½	5	6	10	16	22	6	8	12	19	24
10½-11½	6	7	10	17	25	7	8	12	20	29
11½-12½	5	7	11	19	26	6	9	13	20	25
12½-13½	5	6	10	18	25	7	9	14	23	30
13½-14½	5	6	10	17	22	8	10	15	22	28
14½-15½	4	6	9	19	26	8	11	16	24	30
15½-16½	4	5	9	20	27	8	10	15	23	27
16½-17½	4	5	8	14	20	9	12	16	26	31
17½-24½	4	5	10	18	25	9	12	17	25	31
24½-34½	4	6	11	21	28	9	12	19	29	36
34½-44½	4	6	12	22	28	10	14	22	32	39

Adapted from Frisancho, A.: Triceps skin fold and upper arm muscle size norms for assessment of nutritional status, American Journal of Clinical Nutrition **27:**1052, 1974.

*These percentiles were derived from data obtained on all Caucasian subjects in the United States Ten-State Nutritional Survey of 1968-1970. In this survey, obesity in adults was defined as a fatfold greater than the 85th percentile.

Glossary

A

acidosis A condition in which the blood becomes too acid

active transport The process by which a substance is transported across a cell membrane, using energy and usually a protein carrier specific to the nutrient

adipocytes Special cells in the body in which fat can be stored

adipose cell /ad'ipōs/ Specialized cell in the body, capable of storing large amounts of fat

adolescence Period from childhood to adulthood, in which physical, chemical, and emotional development is accelerated

aerobic /erō'bik/ In the presence of air or oxygen

aflatoxin A mold, capable of causing cancer, that grows on nuts and legumes that are improperly stored

agent The condition (malnutrition, parasite, etc.) that interacts with the environment to influence the growth and development of the host

aldosterone /al'dōstərōn'/ A hormone secreted by the adrenal gland; it acts on the kidneys to influence the amount of sodium that is reabsorbed

aliquot A representative sample

alkalosis /al'kəlō'sis/ A condition in which the blood becomes too alkaline

allergenic Causing an allergy

alveoli Part of the ductal system of the breast into which milk is secreted and then "let down"

amenorrhea Absence of menstruation

amino acids The units from which protein is synthesized and into which it is broken down during digestion

amino acid pattern The amount of one amino acid relative to another either for requirements or in food sources

amniotic fluid /am'nē·ot'ik/ The liquid that fills the amniotic sac within the uterus, in which the baby lives during fetal development

amylase /am'ilās/ Enzyme that acts on carbohydrate

amylopectin A starch in which the glucose units are linked together in a branched arrangement

amylose /am'ilōs/ A starch in which the glucose units are linked together in one long chain (amyl = starch)

anabolism /ənab'əliz'əm/ The metabolic process that causes the synthesis or formation of a new substance

anaerobic /an'ərō'bik/ In the absence of oxygen

anion /an'ī·ən/ A negatively charged ion

anorexia /an'ōrek'sē·ə/ Loss of appetite

antagonist (antivitamin) Substance that is very similar to a vitamin but cannot take its place because of a very slight difference in chemical composition

anthropometric data Data that include measurements of height, weight, circumference, diameter, or length of various parts of the body

antibody A protein produced by the body to fight off a foreign substance such as bacteria

antidiuretic hormone (ADH) A hormone secreted by the pituitary gland that reduces the loss of fluid through the kidneys

antineuritic Substance that protects against condition affecting nerves

antioxidant Substance such as vitamin E or selenium that prevents the oxidation of another substance by taking up the oxygen itself

antirachitic Having the ability to combat rickets (anti = against or opposed; rachitic = having rickets)

apoenzyme A protein that attaches to a vitamin to form a coenzyme; facilitates specific chemical reactions

aquaculture A science devoted to studying production of food in water

ariboflavinosis /ārī'bōflā'vinō'sis/ A lack of riboflavin

aromatic amino acid An amino acid in which the carbon atoms are arranged in a ring; include phenylalanine and tyrosine

aseptic Sterile; free from contamination

ATP (adenosine triphosphate) Compound in which energy is stored when the third phosphate is added and released as it is taken away

atherogenic Causing atherosclerosis, or hardening of the arteries

B

bariatrics /ber'ē·at'riks/ The science of weight control

basal metabolism The minimum amount of energy needed to carry on the vital body processes; basal energy needs include needs for respiration, circulation, glandular activity, and muscle tonus

beikost Food other than milk in the infant's diet

beriberi /ber'ēber'ē/ A vitamin B–deficiency disease that appeared when people began eating highly milled rice and other cereal grains instead of whole-grain products

bile Substance that is made in the liver and stored in the gallbladder; it is released from the gallbladder in response to the hormone cholecystokinin; it aids in the digestion of fats

biopsy The removal of a small amount of tissue, such as liver or bone marrow, for analysis

biotechnology Using modern technology to modify living systems, including changing the structure of plant, animal, and bacteria genes

blood pressure The pressure or force exerted on the inner walls of arteries as the heart pumps blood throughout the body

blood sugar Another name for glucose, the only form in which carbohydrate can be transported in the blood

bolus A portion of food rolled into a small ball by the tongue and swallowed

bran The four outer layers of the cereal grain

buffers Substances in the body that are capable of reacting with either acid or base to neutralize them

C

calcidiol A metabolite of vitamin D, formed in the liver by adding a hydroxyl group to vitamin D, resulting in 25-hydroxycholecalciferol

calcification (or ossification) The process by which calcium and phosphorus are deposited in the flexible bone matrix to give it strength and rigidity

calcitonin /kal'sitō'nin/ Hormone produced in the thyroid gland in response to normal or elevated blood calcium levels; signals bone to stop resorption

calcitriol /kalsit'rē·ôl/ A further metabolite and active form of vitamin D, formed when the kidney further hydroxylates calcidiol to produce 1,25-dihydroxycholecalciferol

calcium rigor A condition in which the muscles are in a constant state of contraction because of high calcium levels in the blood

caliper Instrument used to measure skinfold thickness

calorie Unit of measurement; 1 calorie = 0.001 kilocalories

canola Oil extracted from rapeseed; high in polyunsaturated fatty acids; sold and first produced in Canada; allowed in the United States since 1986, where it is a major source of oil.

carbohydrate loading Process by which athletes increase their stores of glycogen in the liver; for further discussion see Chapter 21

carcinogens /kärsin'əjin/ Cancer-producing substances

cardiac sphincter The muscle between the esophagus and the stomach that controls the entrance of the digestive mass into the stomach; referred to as *cardiac* because of its proximity to the heart

cariogenic Capable of producing tooth decay (cario = tooth decay; genic = giving rise to)

carotenoids /kərot'ənoid/ Substances chemically related to beta-carotene in chemical structure

cassava A starchy root used as a dietary staple in many tropical areas

casual urine specimen A urine sample collected after any one voiding of the bladder, as opposed to a complete collection of urine over a 24-hour period

catabolism /kətab'əliz'əm/ The metabolic process that causes the breakdown or destruction of a substance; the breakdown of nutrients

catalyst /kat'əlist/ Substance that speeds up a chemical reaction but does not enter into the reaction itself

cation /kat'ī·on/ A positively charged element

ceruloplasmin A copper-containing protein synthesized in the liver; the major transport form of copper in the blood

cheilosis /kīlō'sis/ A condition characterized by cracking at the corners of the lips

chelate /kē'lāt/ Substance, usually an organic acid such as one of the amino acids, that binds to a mineral element and influences the ease with which it is absorbed, utilized, or excreted

chloride shift Transfer of choline in and out of red blood cells to maintain acid-balance in the blood

chlorophyll /klôr'əfil/ The green, magnesium-containing pigment in leaves

cholecystokinin /kol'isis'təkī'nin/ Hormone secreted in the wall of the intestine in response to the presence of fat in the small intestine

cholesterol /kəles'tərôl/ A sterol that is found in animal fats and in the blood and is part of many essential body compounds

chylomicron /kī'lōmī'kron/ A very small fat particle surrounded by a thin layer of protein to make it more soluble in the blood

chyme /kīm/ Homogenous mixture of saliva and food that enters the stomach from the esophagus

clinical deficiency A deficiency that is severe enough to cause observable changes in the body

cilia /sil'ē·ə/ Hairlike projections on the cells lining the surface of the body

coefficient of digestibility Percentage of a nutrient that is ultimately available for absorption and use by the body cells

coenzyme /kō·en'zīm/ Substance that assists an enzyme in facilitating a reaction; usually has a vitamin as part of its structure

cofactor A substance that is essential for a given reaction to occur

collagen /kol'əjən/ The protein that forms the structural material of tissues; protein forms the "mold" (matrix) for the bone

colostrum /kəlos'trəm/ The first thin, yellow, watery secretion of the human breast following birth; earliest breast milk

complex carbohydrate Carbohydrate made up of many simple monosaccharide units, such as starch and cellulose; found in cereals, potatoes, and legumes

copra Coconut meat from which oil is extracted; often exported from developing to developed countries as a cash crop

creatinine /krē'ətēn,-tin/ A nitrogen-containing substance excreted in the urine; the amount excreted is directly proportional to lean body mass

cretinism /krē'təniz'əm/ The result of an iodine deficiency over several generations; victims are physically dwarfed and mentally retarded

critical period The time in cell differentiation during which a particular issue is especially sensitive to the presence or lack of a particular nutrient

cruciferous vegetable Any member of the cabbage family; includes cabbage, broccoli, and cauliflower

crude fiber Portion of a plant that resists digestion

curd The solid portion that forms when proteins in milk are precipitated

cystic fibrosis A genetic disease in which the absorption of fat and fat-soluble nutrients is inhibited

cyanosis /sī'ənō'sis/ Too much carbon dioxide in the blood

cylomicrons Very small fat particles

cytoplasm /sī'təplaz'əm/ Substance enclosed in the cell membrane exclusive of the organelles

D

dark adaptation The ability of the eye to adapt to vision in dim light after being exposed to bright light

deamination /dē'aminā'shən/ The removal of the amino group from an amino acid

deciduous teeth /disij'o͞o·əs/ The first set of teeth, which are usually lost by age 5 to 10

deciliter (dl) 100 ml; measure in which most blood values are reported; most adults have 5 liters, or 50 deciliters, of blood

dehydration Excessive loss of body water

dehydroascorbic acid An oxidized form of vitamin C that has lost two hydrogen atoms but still can function as the vitamin

denatured Changed; a denatured protein is one in which the arrangement of the amino acids has been altered

dentin /den'tin/ The middle layer of the tooth; it is less calcified than the outer enamel layer

deoxyribonucleic acid (DNA) /dē·ok'sirī'bōno͞oklē'ic/ The genetic material in the nucleus of the cell

dermatitis /dur'mətī'tis/ A condition characterized by inflammation of the skin

desquamated /des'kwəmā'ted/ Lost or removed from the surface

detoxify To remove or destroy the toxic properties of a substance; usually occurs in the liver

dextrans /dek'strən/ Polysaccharides that adhere to the tooth surface as the result of changes in dietary carbohydrate by microorganisms in the mouth; also referred to as *dental plaque*

dibasic amino acids Amino acids that contain a second nitrogen atom; include lysine, arginine, histidine, and tryptophan

dietary fiber Any material that remains undigested in the intestines

diffusion Process by which a substance crosses a membrane from an area of high concentration to one of lower concentration; diffusion does not require energy or a carrier

digestion (hydrolysis) Process by which foods are broken down into smaller units until their size allows them to be absorbed through the intestinal wall

digestive tract The tube that passes from the mouth to the anus and includes the esophagus, the stomach, the small intestine, and the large intestine

diglyceride (diacylglycerol) Lipids with glycerol and two fatty acids

dihydroxycholecalciferol (DHCC) The active form of vitamin D after hydroxylation (addition of OH) of dietary vitamin D in the liver and then in the kidneys

dipeptide /dīpep'tīd/ Two amino acids linked together

direct calorimetry /kal'ərim'ətrē/ The direct measurement of heat by recording the change in temperature of a known volume of water

disaccharide /dīsak'ərīd/ Combination of two monosaccharides (di = two)

diuretics /dī'yo͞oret'ik/ Substances that stimulate the kidneys to excrete more fluid

diurnal variation Normal fluctuations in biochemical or physical characteristics throughout the day; for example, hemoglobin levels change merely as a function of the time of day

diverticulitis /dī'vurtik'yo͞olī'tis/ An inflammation in the wall of the intestine; usually the result of an irritation following diverticulosis

diverticulosis /dī'vurtik'yo͞olō'sis/ A condition in which there is a weakening in the wall of the intestine; usually the result of pressure from hard stools

DMF index Index that shows the number of decayed, missing, and filled teeth

double-blind study A research design in which neither the investigator nor the participants know until all data are collected whether a person was in the control or experimental groups

duodenum /do͞oədē'nəm, do͞o·od'inəm/ The first segment of the small intestine

dysgeusia A condition in which taste sensations are unpleasant

E

eclampsia /iklamp'sē·ə/ The final and more severe stage of toxemia; it usually occurs toward the end of pregnancy, is characterized by convulsive seizures, and calls for induced delivery to reduce the risk to both mother and baby

edema /idē'mə/ Condition caused by protein deficiency in which fluid collects in body tissues

edentulous Without teeth

eicosonoids Hormone-like prostacyclins with a 20-carbon structure

electrolyte /ilek'trōlīt/ Any substance that splits into charged ions when dissolved in water

embryo /em'brē·ō/ The term used to describe the developing fetus from the second to eighth week of gestation, when most of the cell differentiation takes place

emulsified Finely divided; refers to fat particles that are broken up into many small units and coated with protein film to prevent them from forming one large molecule (coalescing) again

enamel The very dense and highly calcified outer portion of the tooth; it is quite resistant to decay

endemic /endem'ik/ Restricted to a certain geographic locale—often used to refer to a nutrient deficiency

endogenous /əndoj'ənəs, ən'dojənəs/ Originating inside the body, for example, serum proteins and muscles

endosperm The center of the cereal grain bran

engineered food A food made by modifying food ingredients and combining them into a product resembling a natural food; examples are Tang and Surimi

enrichment Addition of nutrients to cereals

environmental factors Anything in the environment that influences the health of an individual

enzyme Protein produced by a living cell to accelerate metabolic reactions; identified by the suffix "ase" and a prefix, indicating the substrate on which it acts (for example *amylase* = enzyme that acts on starch; *protease* = enzyme that acts on protein; *lipase* = enzyme that acts on lipid)

epithelial cells The cells on the outer surface of the body or lining all the internal passages in the body, including the gastrointestinal tract and respiratory tract

epithelium The surface cells lining the outside of the body and all the external passages within the body

ergogenic Capable of producing energy

erythrobic acid Another name for the D form of vitamin C; it is used in meat processing to preserve the color of meat but cannot function as a vitamin in the same way as the D form found in most foods

erythroblast (*blast* = precursor cell) Earliest form of a red blood cell

erythrocyte /erith'rəsīt'/ (Gr. *erythro* = red; cyte = cell) A mature red blood cell

erythropoiesis /erith'rōpō·ē'sis/ (Gr. *poiesus* = formation) Formation of red blood cells

erythropoietin /erith'rōpō·ē'tin/ Hormone produced in the kidneys that stimulates the production of red blood cells in the bone marrow

essential amino acids (EAA) Amino acids that cannot be manufactured within the body and must be provided in the diet

essential fatty acid (EFA) A fatty acid that must be provided in the diet; the three EFAs are linoleic, arachidonic, and linolenic acids

essential nutrient A nutrient that must be provided by food because it cannot be synthesized by the body at a rate sufficient to meet bodily needs

esterfied cholesterol Cholesterol bound to another substance rather than existing free in the blood

estrogen /es'trojən/ Sex hormone that is produced in lower amounts after menopause; may inhibit bone remodelling

exogenous /igzoj'ənəs/ Originating outside the body, for example, dietary protein

exogenous fecal calcium Calcium excreted in the feces that had its origin in the diet rather than being excreted into the intestine

exophthalmic goiter /ek'softhal'mik/ Hyperthyroidism; high basal metabolic rate because of excess secretion of thyroxin (in contrast to simple goiter, which is the enlargement of the thyroid gland because of lack of iodine to produce thyroxin)

extracellular Outside the cells—includes extravascular (intravascular and intercellular)

extravascular Outside the bloodstream

extrinsic From outside the body

F

facilitated diffusion (or active transport) Process by which a substance is transported across a cell membrane using energy and usually a carrier protein specific to the nutrient

fasting glucose level One mg, or 0.001 gram, of glucose per deciliter of blood; the usual glucose level that the body tried to maintain

fatty acid A compound made up of a chain of even-numbered carbon atoms, with a methyl group at one end and a carboxyl group at the other

feces /fē'sēz/ The material, largely made up of dietary fiber and water, that is excreted through the anus from the large intestine

ferritin /fur'itin/ (L. *fer* = iron) The form in which iron is stored in the liver and spleen; a small amount of ferritin that parallels the amount of storage iron also circulates in the blood

fetus /fē'təs/ A developing human form, usually 3 months after conception to birth

fibrinogen /fībrin'əjən/ A protein that is a precursor of fibrin, which is essentially the clot in the blood

fixing, or trapping In chemistry, the conversion of a gas into solid or liquid form by chemical reactions either with or without the help of living tissue

flatulence Gas produced in the colon

fluoridation /flôr'idā'shən/ The addition of fluoride to a community water supply to bring total fluoride content to 1 ppm

fluorosis /flo͞orō'sis/ Chalky discoloration on the teeth; caused by excessive fluoride

folacin or folic acid Designates the biologically active form of the vitamin Folacin with one glutamic acid molecule; also known as pteroylmonoglutamate

folate Substances from which the vitamin folacin can be formed;

folliculosis A condition in which there is accumulation of hard material at the base of the hair follicle

fontanel /fon'tənel'/ The point at which two hemispheres of the skull merge

food jags Patterns of eating in which very few food items are eaten to the exclusion of all others for a long period of time (several weeks)

foremilk Milk secreted at the beginning of one nursing period

fortification The addition of nutrients to foods other than cereals

free radicals Very reactive molecules that are released as the result of certain biochemical changes; because they cannot remain alone, they seek some other molecule with which to react

fructose /fruk'tōs/ Monosaccharide sweeter than sucrose and found in honey and fruits

G

galactologue Medicine, food, or treatment used to stimulate the flow of milk in lactation

galactose /gəlak'tōs/ A monosaccharide found in milk

gastrin A hormone secreted from the wall of the stomach in response to the presence of food in the stomach

geophagia The practice of eating dirt

germ The small fat-containing portion of cereal grain needed for its germination

geriatrics The branch of medicine concerned with health problems of the elderly

gerontology The broad area of science concerned with all social, economic, and medical problems of the elderly

gestation The period from conception to delivery; pregnancy

globulin /glob'yo͞olin/ A protein found in the blood

glossitis /glosī'tis/ Condition characterized by a purplish tongue with a very smooth surface

glucogenic /glo͞o'kōjən'ik/ Capable of producing glucose

gluconeogenesis The formation of glucose from substances other than carbohydrate

glucose /glo͞o'kōs/ Monosaccharide found in certain foods, especially fruit, and a major source of energy

glycemic index The relative rate at which glucose appears in the blood following the ingestion of various carbohydrate-rich foods; standard for comparison is the response of glucose fed alone

glycerol /glis'ərôl/ A three-carbon compound that occurs as part of all fats

glycogen /glī'kəjən/ A polysaccharide; a carbohydrate that is stored in the muscle or liver; sometimes known as animal starch

glycolysis /glīkol'isis/ The breakdown of carbohydrate in metabolism (glyco = sugar; lysis = to break)

goitrogen A substance that interferes with the absorption or utilization of iodine and therefore may cause iodine-deficient goiter

H

heat of combustion The maximum amount of heat that can be produced by burning a substance

heme iron /hēm/ Iron provided in animal tissues as hemoglobin; about 50% of the iron in meat is heme iron

hemochromatosis /he'mōkrō'mətō'sis/ A condition in which an individual absorbs unusually high amounts of iron

hemodilution The dilution of the concentration of components in the blood, caused by an increase in blood volume during pregnancy

hemoglobin /hē'məglō'bən/ The iron-containing protein in the red blood cell that is responsible for its ability to carry oxygen to the cells and carbon dioxide away from the cells

hemolysis Breaking of red blood cells

hemosiderin /hē'mōsid'ərin/ An insoluble iron complex in which iron is stored in the liver

hexose A six-carbon sugar (hex = six; ose = sugar)

highly unsaturated fatty acids (HUFA) Long-chain fatty acids in which double bonds occur in five or six places

hindmilk Milk secreted at the end of one nursing period

holoenzyme An active enzyme made up of a protein part (apoenzyme) and either a cofactor (a mineral) or a coenzyme (a vitamin)

homeostatic mechanism Any one change or a series of changes that help prevent alterations in body biochemistry

hormone Chemical substance produced in an endocrine gland and transported by the blood to other tissues, where it influences function and metabolic activity

host An animal, plant, or human being whose health and development is influenced by an infection agent and the environment

hydrogenation The process by which hydrogen is added to an unsaturated fatty acid to make it more solid at room temperature

hydrolysis /hīdrol'isis/ The process in which a complex substance is broken down into two or more component parts, with the addition of H and OH (from water) to the parts (hydro = water; -lyze = to break)

hydrostatic pressure Pressure on fluid in blood vessels (arteries and capillaries) from pumping action of the heart

hydroxyapatite A compound made up of calcium and phosphate that is deposited into the bone matrix to give it strength and rigidity

hydroxylation A chemical process in which the OH group is added to a substance; in the formation of collagen, this must take place to make mature collagen fiber, which in turn makes strong connective tissue

hyperbilirubinemia Presence of bile pigments in the blood

hypercalcemia /hī'pərkalsē'mē·ə/ Condition in which the calcium content of the blood is above normal levels

hypercholesterolemia A blood cholesterol level greater than 240 mg/dl

hyperemesis /hī'pərem'isis/ Severe and continuing nausea

hyperglycemia /hī'pərglīsē'mē·ə/ A condition in which the level of sugar in the blood is elevated above normal

hyperkalemia /hī'pərkəlē'mē·ə/ Too much potassium in the blood

hyperkinesis or hyperactivity A condition characterized by a high level of energy or activity

hyperlipidemia High amounts of lipid in the blood

hypermagnesemia /hī'pərmag'nisē'mē·ə/ Too much magnesium in the blood

hypernatremia /hī'pərnatrē'mē·ə/ Too much sodium in the blood

hyperplasia /hī'pərplā'zhə/ Increase in cell number

hyperplastic Producing too many cells

hypertension A condition in which blood pressure is at an abnormally high level

hyperthyroidism Oversecretion of thyroxin

hypertrophy /hīpur'trəfē/ Increase in cell size

hypochromic microcytic anemia /hī'pōkrō'mik mī'krōsit'ik/ An anemia characterized by small cells with too little hemoglobin, causing a lack of color (*hypo* = too little; *-chrome* = color; *micro* = small; *-cyte* = cell)

hypogeusia Loss of sense of taste

hypoglycemia /hī'pōglīsē'mē·ə/ A condition in which the level of glucose in the blood is below normal

hyponatremia /hī'pōnatrē'mē·ə/ Too little sodium in the blood

hyposmia Loss of sense of smell

hypothalamus /hī'pōthal'əməs/ Area at the base of the brain that controls hunger, appetite, and satiety

hypothyroidism Undersecretion of thyroxin

hypovitaminosis A condition in which the level of a vitamin in the blood is too low

hypoxia /hī'poksē·ə/ A condition in which there is too little oxygen reaching body cells, particularly brain cells

I

iatrogenic /ī'atrōjen'ik/ Arising from the practice of medicine

ileocecal valve The muscle separating the small intestine from the large intestine; it controls the passage of the digestive mass into the large intestine

ileum /il'ē·əm/ The third and last section of the small intestine; between the jejunum and the large intestine

immunity Ability to resist or combat infection

immunoglobulins Antibodies that are not absorbed but are effective against viruses and bacteria in the gastrointestinal tract

implantation The process in which the fertilized ovum embeds itself in the wall of the uterus and begins to grow, receiving its nutrients from the uterine milk

in utero *Latin*, "in the womb"

indigenous /indij'ənəs/ Occurring naturally in a particular area

indirect calorimetry The measurement of energy need by calculating the energy equivalent of the amount of oxygen used

indispensable nitrogen The nitrogen needed by the body to synthesize amino acids not provided in the diet

inorganic Related to nonliving material, usually mineral in origin

insensible perspiration Loss of water through the skin that is so slow that it goes unnoticed

insulin A hormone secreted by the pancreas that regulates the rate at which cells take up glucose from the blood

intercellular Between the cells

interstitial /in'tərstish'əl/ Between the cells

intracellular Within the cells

intrauterine growth retardation (IUGR) Depressed growth of the fetus caused by poor nutrition during fetal growth; caused by congenital malformation, intrauterine infection, small or inefficient placenta, maternal smoking, alcoholism, drug addiction, or severe malnutrition

intrauterine nutrition /in'trayo͞o'tərin/ Provision of nutrients to fetus before birth

intravascular Within the bloodstream (arteries, veins, and capillaries)

intrinsic From within the body

intrinsic factor A heat-labile mucoprotein secreted from specific cells in the wall of the stomach as a normal part of gastric juice

ion Electrically charged particles

iodization The addition of iodine to a food, usually salt

irradiation Process of treating with ultraviolet light (short wavelengths)

isocaloric With the same number of calories

J

jejunum /jijo͞o'nəm/ The second segment of the small intestine, beyond the duodenum

K

keratin /ker'ətin/ A protein found in the skin and nails

kernicterus /kərnik'tərəs/ A condition characterized by mental retardation, jaundice, hemorrhaging, and neurological symptoms

ketogenic /kē'tōjen'ik/ Capable of producing ketones

ketosis /kētō'sis/ A condition in which ketones, or abnormal products of fat metabolism, accumulate in the blood

kilocalorie (kcal) Amount of heat required to raise the temperature of 1 kg of water 1° C (from 15° to 16° C); a measure used to express the energy value of food

kilojoule Unit representing the amount of energy needed to move 1 kg of weight 1 meter, by a force of 1 Newton

kwashiorkor /kwä'shē·ôr'kôr/ A protein-deficiency disease affecting young children when they are abruptly weaned from breast milk and lose their only source of protein

L

labile /lā'bil/ Easily broken down or destroyed

lactase insufficiency/lactose intolerance A lack of the enzyme lactase, which is needed to convert lactose to glucose and galactose

lactation period Period in a woman's life when her mammary glands produce milk to feed her young infant

lactoferrin Iron-containing protein found in human milk

lactose Disaccharide found in the milk of all mammals

lecithin /les'ithin/ A phospholipid, found in food (such as eggs) and in the body, in which choline is attached to the phosphate group

legumes Vegetables such as peas and beans

lesions Defects or abnormal conditions suggestive of nutritional problems

leukotrienes A special group of hormone-like substances produced in white blood cells from HUFA

limiting amino acid The amino acid in a protein that is present in the lowest amount relative to the amount needed for growth

lingual lipase A fat-splitting enzyme secreted at the base of the tongue

lipase /lī'pās, lip'ās/ Enzyme that splits fat, or lipid

lipofuscin A colored substance formed from the breakdown of the cell wall during aging

lipogenesis Formation of fat from carbohydrate or protein

lipoprotein lipase /lip'ōprō'tēn lī'pās/ The enzyme that cells use to take up lipid carried to them in the blood

lipoproteins /lip'ōprō'tēn/ Combinations of lipid and protein that are more readily transported in the blood than lipid alone

lipostat A body's regulator of appetite that responds to fat; it is located in the hypothalamus of the brain

low-birth-weight (LBW) babies Infants weighing less than 5.5 pounds (2500 grams)

lumen /loo'mən/ The inside of the digestive tube

luxus consumption The metabolism of energy-yielding nutrients for no obvious purpose; apparently an automatic adjustment that helps prevent the accumulation of fat when extra food is eaten

lymph The fluid in the circulatory system of the body that collects extra fluids

lysosome /lī'səsōm/ Structure within the cell that is responsible for the digestion of cell contents and for the eventual destruction of the cell itself

M

macrocytic anemia /mak'rōsit'ik/ An anemia characterized by very large red blood cells, which form when folate is lacking

macronutrient An element present in the body at more than 5 ppm

maltose Disaccharide; found only in germinating cereals

marasmus /məraz'məs/ A condition resulting from a lack of kilocalories and (usually) also protein

matrix The form, or "mold," for the bone made up of collagen and a carbohydrate-related material

megadose An amount of a vitamin at least 10 times the recommended intake

megaloblastic anemia /meg'əlōblas'tik/ A form of anemia characterized by large *(mega)* cells *(blast)*, in which the cells continue to grow because they fail to mature and lose their nuclei

menarche /menär'kē/ Time of physiological maturity in girls; characterized by onset of menstruation

metabolism All the chemical changes that occur in a nutrient once it is absorbed

metabolite /mitab'əlīt/ A form of a nutrient that is created during the metabolism of the nutrient

metalloenzyme An enzyme with a mineral element as an essential part of its structure

metallothionein Copper-containing protein

micelles A very small particle of lipid and bile salts

microcytic hypochromic anemia Anemia characterized by small cells and too little hemoglobin

micronutrient or **trace element** An element present in the body at less than 50 ppm

microvilli Small fingerlike projections on the surface of the villi

mitochondrion /mī'tōkon'drē·on/ The specialized structure within the cell in which energy is produced

monoglyceride (monoacylglycerol) Lipids with glycerol plus one fatty acid

monosaccharide /monō sak'ərīd/ A simple sugar unit (mono = one; sacchar = sugar)

monounsaturated fatty acids Fatty acids in which one hydrogen atom is missing from each of two adjacent carbons, resulting in a double bond between the two carbons

mucosa /myookō'sə/ The inner lining of the digestive tract

multipara /multip'ərə/ A woman who has had more than one child

myelin Protective sheath that surrounds nerve fibers and protects their ability to transmit nerve messages

myoglobin /mī'ōglō'bən/ The iron-containing compound in muscle that is responsible for providing oxygen to the cells

myxedema A condition caused by lack of thyroxin throughout the developmental period

N

National Health and Nutrition Examination Survey (NHANES) A survey of nutritional status and food intake of a representative sample of the total population, conducted on a continuing basis by the Department of Health and Human Services

Nationwide Food Consumption Survey (NFCS) A study of the food intake of individuals representative of the total population; conducted by the U.S. Department of Agriculture

neonatal (*neo* = new; *natal* = birth) First 28 days of life

neonatal hemorrhaging Bleeding soon after the time of birth

neuromotor coordination /noorō-/ The integration of the stimulus from the nerve with the contraction of the muscles

neurotransmitter A chemical substance that is able to carry a message from one nerve fiber to the next

night blindness An inability to adjust to vision in dim light

nitrogen balance The relationship between the amount of nitrogen taken into the body and the amount excreted

nonessential amino acid An amino acid that can be synthesized by body cells as long as enough nitrogen is available

nonheme iron Iron provided from plant foods and from the iron-containing parts of animal tissues other than heme

noninvasive Technique that does not require "entering" the body; for example, taking a blood or saliva sample is noninvasive

nostrum A medicine of secret ingredients; especially a quack remedy

novel food A food made by modifying food ingredients and recombining them into a product resembling a natural food; examples are Tang and Surimi

nucleic acids /nooklē'ik/ The chemicals within the nucleus of the cell that provide the code for the synthesis of thousands of body proteins

nucleus /noo'klē·əs/ A body within the cell that contains relatively large quantities of DNA

nursing-bottle syndrome The high incidence of tooth decay in infants who are allowed to fall asleep with a bottle in their mouth, which causes the fluid to be held close to the surface of the teeth; either milk or fruit juice contains enough fermentable carbohydrate to feed the bacteria in the mouth until they are capable of causing decay

nutritional adequacy Comparison of actual or estimated nutrient intake to a dietary standard

nutritional status Physical, biochemical, and anthropometric evidence of nutrition-related health

O

obligatory loss The amount of water that must be lost from the body to get rid of wastes and to regulate body temperature

oncotic pressure The force exerted by protein within the blood to pull fluid back to the bloodstream from the tissues

organelle /ôrgənel'/ Structure within the cell that carries out a specific function

organic Having its origins in living material, either plant or animal

organogenesis The process in which the fertilized cell divides and differentiates into the beginnings of the human organs and tissues

orthomolecular therapy Treatment of disease with very large doses of vitamins; at levels 10 to 1000 times the recommended amounts

osmosis /ozmō'sis/ Process in which water enters or leaves a cell to establish equilibrium between the contents of the cell and its environment

osmotic effect The tendency to attract water, usually to dilute some constituent of a fluid

osmotic pressure The pressure exerted by electrolytes in a fluid to draw liquid back across a semipermeable membrane

osteoblasts Cells that rebuild bones

osteocalcin A protein found in bone that is dependent on vitamin K for synthesis

osteoclasts Cells that destroy bones

osteomalacia /os'tē·ōməlā'shə/ A condition in which the quality but not the quantity of bone is reduced

osteoporosis A bone disease in which the amount of bone is decreased but the composition remains normal; most often affects women after menopause

ovolactovegetarian A person who will eat only milk and eggs from animals

ovo-lacto-pollovegetarian Vegetarians who include the use of milk, eggs, and poultry in their diet

oxalic acid Organic acid in spinach that binds calcium

oxidation Reaction between oxygen and unsaturated fatty acids that produces peroxides, which result in rancidity of some fats

oxidative phosphorylation The addition of a phosphate molecule to ADP to form ATP, using the energy from the release of hydrogen from NAD, which is attached to NAD and FAD in the Krebs cycle

oxytocin /ok'sitō'sin/ A hormone produced in the posterior pituitary gland; it stimulates the release of milk from the breast in response to sucking by the infant

P

parathormone Hormone secreted by the parathyroid gland in response to low blood calcium; signals kidney to resorb calcium

parathyroidectomy Removal of part of the thyroid gland

parenterally Given directly into the blood or intramuscularly

passive diffusion Process by which a substance crosses a membrane from an area of high concentration to one of lower concentration; diffusion does not require energy or a carrier

pellagra /pəlā'grə, pəlag'rə/ A condition characterized by a rough skin and caused by a lack of the vitamin niacin or the nutrients needed to convert tryptophan to niacin (pellagragenic = causing pellagra)

pentose A five-carbon sugar (pento = five; ose = sugar)

pepsin /pep'sin/ Proteolytic enzyme formed when pepsin is activated

pepsinogen /pepsin'əjən/ Inactive form of protein-splitting enzymes in the stomach

peptide bond A chemical link that joins two amino acids together, such as CO—NH, with CO from one amino acid and NH from another; water is split off

periodontal disease Disease of the tissues in the mouth surrounding the teeth

peristalsis /per'istôl'sis/ Successive wavelike contraction and relaxation of the walls of the intestinal track to mix and move ingested food

pernicious anemia /pərnish'əs/ Blood disease characterized by very large, immature red blood cells with normal amounts of hemoglobin; it is caused by a genetic defect and is manifest in the inability to absorb vitamin B_{12}

pescovegetarian A person who will eat fish but no other food of animal origin

petechiae /pētē'kē·ē/ Small patches of bleeding just under the skin; they appear as intercellular substance weakens in a vitamin C deficiency

pH (hydrogen ion concentration) A measure of the relative acidity or alkalinity of a solution; ranges from 1 to 14, with high pH levels indicating alkalinity and low pH levels indicating acidity

phenylketonuria (PKU) /fen'əlkē'tōnyo͝or'ē·ə/ Disorder in which there is a lack of the enzyme needed to handle extra amounts of the amino acid phenylalanine; results in mental retardation

phosphatase /fos'fətāz/ An enzyme that catalyzes the release of a phosphate molecule from a compound

phospholipid /fos'fōlip'id/ A lipid-related compound composed of glycerol, a phosphate molecule, and other chemical groups; helps to emulsify many fats

phosphorylation The addition of phosphate (PO_4) to a substance, usually to aid in its transfer in and out of a cell

photosynthesis /fōtōsin'thəsis/ The process by which plants, using the green pigment chlorophyll in their leaves, are able to trap energy from the sun and store it in the form of carbohydrate

physiological fuel value The maximum amount of heat that the body can receive from oxidizing the energy components in food: carbohydrate, lipid, and protein

phytic acid Substance in outer husk of grain that binds calcium and other mineral elements

phytosterol A sterol found in plant foods; sometimes causes decreased absorption of cholesterol

pica /pī'kə/ Practice of eating nonfood items such as clay or coal; sometimes used to refer to unusual cravings for food such as often occurs during pregnancy

placenta Tissue embedded in the wall of the uterus; in the placenta, maternal and fetal circulations come in close enough contact with one another that nutrients from the mother and waste from the fetus can be exchanged

plasma Whole blood from which blood cells have been removed

polychloride biphenyl (PCB) A toxic industrial chemical that can accumulate in food (fish) through contaminated water

polyneuritis Inflammation of the nerves (*poly-* = many; *neuro* = nerves; -itis = inflammation)

polysaccharide /pol'ēsak'ərīd/ Combination of many monosaccharides (*poly* = many)

polyunsaturated fatty acid (PUFA) Fatty acid in which double bonds between carbon atoms appear in two or more places

portal vein The vein that carries blood and absorbed nutrients from the intestinal wall to the liver

potassium 40 Naturally occurring stable isotope of potassium

prealbumin A protein, which is produced in the liver and is present in the blood, that serves as a carrier for vitamin A

precursor (provitamin) Substance that is chemically related to a vitamin but must be changed by the body into the active form of the vitamin

preformed The active form of a vitamin provided in foods of animal origin

pregnancy-induced hypertension A condition that occurs late in pregnancy; symptoms include high blood pressure, proteinuria, and edema

premature babies Infants who are born after less than 37 weeks of gestation

primipara /primip'ərə/ (*primus* = first; *parita* = child bearing) A woman having her first child

privo conservation The maintenance of body weight on fewer calories; apparently an automatic adjustment that keeps some people from progressive weight loss

prolactin /prōlák'tin/ A hormone produced in the anterior pituitary gland; it stimulates the production of milk in response to emptying of the breast at a feeding

prostaglandins /pros'təglan'din/ Hormone-like substances produced in the body from fatty acids, particularly arachidonic acid

protease /prō'tē·ās/ An enzyme that acts on protein, usually in the digestive system

protective foods Those foods that provide some vitamins and minerals in significant amounts in relation to needs

proteolytic enzyme /prō'tē·əlit'ik/ Protein splitting enzymes of the small intestine

proteoses and **peptones** Proteoses are protein fragments with fewer amino acids than the proteins from which they were derived; peptones are protein fragments that are even shorter than proteoses

prothrombin /prōthrom'bin/ A protein essential for the blood-clotting mechanism; a precursor of thrombin

protoporphyrin /prō'tōpôr'firin/ A compound that is a precursor of the heme in hemoglobin; accumulates when there is inadequate iron to make heme

proximate (approximate) composition Expression used to describe the percentage of macronutrients (lipid, carbohydrate, protein, fiber, and water) in a particular food

PM/S ratio The ratio of polyunsaturated and monounsaturated to saturated fatty acids in a fat

P/S ratio The ratio of polyunsaturated to saturated fatty acids in a fat

puberty Period during growth when secondary sex characteristics appear

pulses Legumes (vegetables), usually peas and beans

pylorus /pīlôr'əs/ The muscle between the stomach and the small intestine that controls the entrance of material from one to the other

R

reactive hypoglycemia A drop in blood glucose levels as a result of failure to provide the body with needed glucose

recombinant DNA /rēkom'binənt/ Genetic material that has been produced or changed in the laboratory by splicing together various parts of the DNA molecule

Recommended Dietary Allowances (RDAs) Estimates of nutrient intakes adequate to prevent deficiency in essentially all healthy Americans

Recommended Nutrient Intakes for Canadians (RNI) Estimates of nutrient needs for Canadians

remodeling Reshaping of the bones that occurs as the bones adapt to bearing the increased weight of the body

respiratory quotient (RQ) The ratio of CO_2 exhaled to O_2 inhaled

resting energy expenditure (REE) Energy needed for vital body processes plus the small amount of energy needed for sedentary activities (sedentary = "sitting")

reticulocyte /ritik'yələsīt/ An immature red blood cell

retina /ret'inə/ Inner layer of the wall at the back of the eye that contains the visual receptors

retinoids All compounds, either natural or synthetic, that are similar to retinol in chemical structure

retinol-binding protein (RBP) /ret'inôl/ A protein that serves as a carrier for vitamin A

retinol equivalent (RE) A measure of vitamin A, used for requirements and amounts in the food supply; the sum of preformed vitamin A and the amount obtained by converting the precursor to the active form

retinyl palmitate An ester formed by the combination of retinol and the fatty acid palmitic acid

rhodopsin /rōdop'sin/ A combination of the protein opsin and vitamin A in the retina of the eye; it is responsible for the ability of the eye to see in dim light

ribonuclease /rī'bōnoo͞klē'ās/ An enzyme that splits ribonucleic acid; one of the first proteins for which the amino acid composition was known

ribosome /rī'bəsōm/ Protein-synthesizing organelle of the cell

rickets A disease in which there are weaknesses and abnormalities in bone formation as the result of a vitamin D deficiency; infantile rickets is most common

ruminants Animals that chew their cud and have two stomachs

S

salicylates /səlis'əlāt/ Compounds similar to the active ingredient in aspirin

salivary amylase Starch-splitting enzyme secreted in the saliva

saturated fatty acids Fatty acids that have two hydrogen atoms (the maximum number possible) attached to each carbon in the chain

secretin /sikrē'tin/ Hormone secreted from the intestinal wall in response to food in the intestine

serotonin /ser'ətō'nin/ A neurotransmitter, produced by the brain; some research findings suggest that it triggers the desire to consume more carbohydrate

serum /sir'əm/ Whole blood from which cells and clotting factors have been removed

sickle cell anemia A genetically transmitted disease in which one amino acid in a long chain of 300 is displaced

siderosis (hemosiderosis) /sid'ərō'sis/ Condition in which there is an excessive amount of iron stored in the liver, usually because an individual does not have the ability to regulate the amount that was absorbed; this occurs in about 0.25% of the population

simple carbohydrate A carbohydrate composed of one or two monosaccharides

small for gestational age (SGA) Full-term infants who weigh less than 5.5 pounds

sodium-dependent active transport One mechanism by which nutrients are transported across a cell membrane; it requires energy and depends on an exchange of sodium from within the cell

soft tissues Organs and tissues of the body that are not normally calcified—for example, the liver, kidneys, and muscle

solute load /sō'lo͞ot, sol'yo͞ot/ The combined amount of electrolytes and waste products of metabolism that needs to be excreted by the kidneys

sorbitol A reduced form of glucose that has one additional hydrogen atom

sour krout Cabbage soup similar to sauerkraut

soybean hydrolysate A protein concentrate extracted from large amounts of soybeans

spontaneous hypoglycemia Chronically low blood glucose levels that occur because the pancreas constantly secretes too much insulin

sports anemia A condition in which there is increased destruction of red blood cells and a transient drop in hemoglobin; as a result of an acute stress response to exercise

stable isotope /ī'sətōp/ A radioactive form of an element that does not deteriorate and can be used safely in the body to measure changes during metabolism

standard of identity Precise description of the ingredients or characteristics of a specific food

steatorrhea /stē'ətərē'ə/ Condition in which the feces contains an abnormally high amount of fat; usually the result of incomplete digestion or absorption of fat

sterol A lipid-related compound in which the carbon, hydrogen, and oxygen atoms are arranged in rings

Streptococcus mutans /strep'təkok'əs/ A microorganism that acts on sucrose to produce acid; this causes tooth enamel to dissolve and leads to tooth decay

subcutaneous fat /sub'kyo͞otā'ne·əs/ Fat located just beneath the surface of the skin

substrate A substance on which an enzyme acts to change it in some way; for example, sucrose is a substrate for the enzyme sucrase because sucrase changes it to glucose and fructose

sucrose Disaccharide derived from sugar cane, sugar beets, and sorgum

superoxide dismutase (SOD) A copper-containing enzyme found in red blood cells; also known as erythrocuprein, hepatocuprein, cytocuprein, or cerebrocuprein

synergistic Helpful in a reciprocal way

T

tachycardia /tak'ikär'dē·ə/ Very rapid heartbeat (*bradycardia* is a very slow heart rate)

tannin A type of polyphenol; an astringent substance, found in tea and coffee, that binds iron

tetany /tet'ənē/ A condition in which the muscles are alternately relaxed and contracted because of low blood levels of calcium

thermic effect Changes in body temperature that reflect the composition of the diet; temperatures are higher when protein is eaten and lower when carbohydrate and fat are eaten; also called the heat-producing effect

thermic effect of food Stimulation in metabolism resulting from the availability of food for digestion, absorption, and metabolism within the cell; also known as the specific dynamic effect of food

thermogenesis /thur'mōjen'əsis/ The process by which the body produces extra heat, usually by speeding up metabolism or shivering

thiamin /thī'əmin/ A sulfur-containing vitamin (*thio* = sulfur; *amine* = nitrogen-containing)

thiaminase An enzyme that splits or destroys thiamin

thromboplastin A protein released from the blood platelets at the time of injury to a blood vessel

thyroglobulin Storage form of iodine in the thyroid gland

thyroidectomy /thī'roidek'təmē/ Removal of the thyroid gland

tocopherol One of the compounds in food having vitamin E activity

tocopherol equivalents (TE) Units of measure for vitamin E in foods and for vitamin E requirements

tocotrienol Another compound in food with vitamin E activity

tonus /tō'nəs/ The normal state of balanced tension in the tissues of the body, especially the muscles; tone is essential for many normal body functions, as holding the spine erect, the eyes open, and the jaw closed

total iron binding capacity (TIBC) The ability of the blood to remove iron from cells lining the intestine; high TIBC indicates a need for iron

total parenteral nutrition (TPN) Feeding a person totally by infusing nutrients directly into the blood

toxemia of pregnancy /toksē'mē·ə/ Severe complication late in pregnancy that threatens the life of both the mother and child; toxemia literally means blood poisoning, but this is neither a cause nor a symptom of toxemia; symptoms include high blood pressure, proteinuria, and edema

toxicity /toksis'itē/ Quality of being poisonous, or toxic

trabeculae /trəbek'yələ/ Portions of the ends of long bones that are porous to permit contact with the blood supply, so that calcium can be withdrawn to meet needs when the dietary intake is inadequate

transamination The transfer of the NH^2 group of amino acid to another substance, usually to make a different amino acid

transferrin /transfer'in/ The protein in the blood that is capable of transporting and picking up absorbed iron

transthyretin A protein which is produced in the liver and is present in the blood, that serves as a carrier for vitamin A

triacylglycerol More commonly known as triglycerides

triglycerides /trīglis'ərīd/ Class of lipids with two major components: glycerol and fatty acids

trimester /trīmes'tər/ Term applied to each of the successive 3-month periods during the 9 months of gestation

tripeptide /trīpep'tīd/ Three amino acids linked together

U

ultratrace elements Elements needed in smaller amounts than a trace element

umbilical cord /umbil'ikəl/ Narrow tube through which blood flows from the placenta to the uterus

United States Recommended Daily Allowance (U.S. RDA) Standards for nutrient intakes, used as the basis for nutrient labeling of foods and drugs; based on 1974 RDA

unphysiological levels Intake that far exceeds needed or reasonable level; such an intake could not be obtained from an unsupplemented diet

unsaturated fatty acids Fatty acids that have fewer than the maximum number of hydrogen atoms attached to the carbon chain

urea /yo͞orē'ə/ A nontoxic compound made from two molecules of toxic ammonia; produced when amino acids are deaminated

uterine milk A substance obtained from the walls of the uterus that nourishes the growing fetus before the placenta is fully developed

uterus /yo͞o'tərəs/ The female organ in which the fertilized ovum becomes embedded and in which it continues to grow throughout gestation

V

vasodilation /vā'zōdil'ətā'shən/ An increase in the size of blood vessels, usually evident in a flushing of the surface of the skin

vegan A person who will eat no food of animal origin

villi Small fingerlike projections on the internal surface of the intestine

vitamins Organic substances, needed in very small amounts, that are essential for health; they must by provided in the diet because they cannot be synthesized in the body

volatilize Change from a solid to a gas

W

waste products End products of metabolism that need to be excreted from the body either in the feces, through the kidneys in the urine, or through the lungs

water intoxication The condition that results when the water content of a cell gets so high that the cell cannot function

water-miscible Able to be mixed in water; substances that are water-miscible can be dispersed in water but not dissolved

water of metabolism The water that results from the metabolism of carbohydrate, lipid, and protein

whey The fluid portion remaining when proteins in milk precipitate out

WIC (Women, Infants, and Children) A federally funded program to provide nutrition counseling and supplemental food to pregnant women and to children who are considered at nutritional risk

whole-grain cereals Wheat, oats, corn, and other cereals from which a minimum portion of the outer husk has been removed

X

xerophthalmia A condition resulting from a deficiency of vitamin A affecting the eye

Z

zweibach Dextrinized, easily digested bread, often fed to babies; its texture is hard, crisp, and more similar to crackers than the texture of many other breads

Index

B

C

D

N

O

T

U

Photo Credits

p. **2,** Yamashita/Stock Shop
p. **11,** (bottom), NASA Lyndon B. Johnson Space Center
p. **12,** Porges/Peter Arnold
p. **22,** Brent Jones Photojournalism
p. **79,** Don Mason/West Stock
p. **162,** Frank Oberle/Photographic Resources
p. **179,** Mauritius/Stock Shop
p. **198,** Dick Luria/Stock Shop
p. **221,** H. Armstrong Roberts
p. **228,** Migdale/Photo Researchers
p. **233,** Meltzer/West Stock
p. **253,** Doug Menuez/Picture Group
p. **254,** Photo Researchers
p. **270,** Jeffrey Reed/Stock Shop
p. **288,** Photographic Resources
p. **338,** Stroheim/Stock Shop
p. **380,** Tom Tracy/Stock Shop
p. **416,** Ken Lax/Stock Shop
p. **448,** Jeffrey Reed/Medichrome
p. **470,** David Madison Photography
p. **484,** Jeffrey Reed/Stock Shop
p. **486,** Stockton/Photographic Resources
p. **497,** Bob Taylor/Stock Shop
p. **518,** Bob Daemmrich/The Image Works
p. **541,** Jeffrey Reed/Stock Shop
p. **554,** Frederic Lewis
p. **567,** Stoecklein/West Stock
p. **575,** Susanne Sucher/The Pepsis Studio
p. **582,** David Madison Photography
p. **584,** David Madison Photography
p. **585,** David Madison Photography
p. **589,** Kathryn Dudek/Photo News Photography
p. **600,** L.L.T. Rhodes/Taurus Photos
p. **620,** Doug Menuez/Picture Group

Recommended Dietary Allowances—cont'd

Mean heights and weights and recommended energy intake

Category	Age (Years)	Weight kg	Weight lb	Height cm	Height in	Energy Needs (with Range) kcal		MJ
Infants	0.0-0.5	6	13	60	24	kg × 115	(95-145)	kg × 0.48
	0.5-1.0	9	20	71	28	kg × 105	(80-135)	kg × 0.44
Children	1-3	13	29	90	35	1300	(900-1800)	5.5
	4-6	20	44	112	44	1700	(1300-2300)	7.1
	7-10	28	62	132	52	2400	(1650-3300)	10.1
Males	11-14	45	99	157	62	2700	(2000-3700)	11.3
	15-18	66	145	176	69	2800	(2100-3900)	11.8
	19-22	70	154	177	70	2900	(2500-3300)	12.2
	23-50	70	154	178	70	2700	(2300-3100)	11.3
	51-75	70	154	178	70	2400	(2000-2800)	10.1
	76+	70	154	178	70	2050	(1650-2450)	8.6
Females	11-14	46	101	157	62	2200	(1500-3000)	9.2
	15-18	55	120	163	64	2100	(1200-3000)	8.8
	19-22	55	120	163	64	2100	(1700-2500)	8.8
	23-50	55	120	163	64	2000	(1600-2400)	8.4
	51-75	55	120	163	64	1800	(1400-2200)	7.6
	76+	55	120	163	64	1600	(1200-2000)	6.7
Pregnancy						+300		
Lactation						+500		

From Recommended Dietary Allowances, revised 1979. Food and Nutrition Board National Academy of Sciences–National Research Council, Washington, D.C.

The energy allowances for the young adults are for men and women doing light work. The allowances for the two older age groups represent mean energy needs over these age spans, allowing for a 2% decrease in basal (resting) metabolic rate per decade and a reduction in activity of 200 kcal/day for men and women between 51 and 75 years, 500 kcal for men over 75 years, and 400 kcal for women over 75 . . . The customary range of daily energy output is shown for adults in parentheses, and is based on a variation in energy needs of ±400 kcal at any one age . . . emphasizing the wide range of energy intakes appropriate for any group of people.

Energy allowances for children through age 18 are based on median energy intakes of children these ages followed in longitudinal growth studies. The values in parentheses are 10th and 90th percentiles of energy intake, to indicate the range of energy consumption among children of these ages.